Swanson's Family Practice Review

A Problem-Oriented Approach

Fifth Edition

This interactive learning program is sponsored by Kaplan Medical CME for up to 79.5 hours of category 1 CME credits toward the AMA Physician's Recognition Award. These credits will be available from July 1, 2004 through June 30, 2007. Further detail is provided in the CME section on page xix.

Kaplan Medical CME is accredited by the Accreditation Council for Continuing Medical Education (ACCME) to provide continuing medical education for physicians.

Swanson's Family Practice Review
A Problem-Oriented Approach
Fifth Edition

Alfred F. Tallia, MD, MPH, FAAFP

Editor-in-Chief
Associate Professor and Vice Chair
Department of Family Medicine
Robert Wood Johnson Medical School
New Brunswick, New Jersey

Dennis A. Cardone, DO, CAQSM

Co-Editor
Associate Professor and Director of the Sports Medicine Center
Department of Family Medicine
Robert Wood Johnson Medical School
New Brunswick, New Jersey

David F. Howarth, MD, MPH

Co-Editor
Associate Professor and Director of Fellowship Programs
Department of Family Medicine
Robert Wood Johnson Medical School
New Brunswick, New Jersey

Kenneth H. Ibsen, PhD

Co-Editor
Professor Emeritus
College of Medicine
University of California
Irvine, California
Director, Kaplan Medical CME
Los Angeles, California

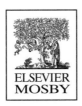

ELSEVIER
MOSBY

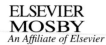

ELSEVIER
MOSBY
An Affiliate of Elsevier

The Curtis Center
170 S Independence Mall W 300E
Philadelphia, Pennsylvania 19106

Swanson's Family Practice Review
A Problem-Oriented Approach
Fifth Edition

ISBN: 0-323-03000-9

NOTICE

Medicine is an ever-changing field. Standard safety precautions must be followed, but as new research and clinical experience broaden our knowledge, changes in treatment and drug therapy may become necessary or appropriate. Readers are advised to check the most current product information provided by the manufacturer of each drug to be administered to verify the recommended dose, the method and duration of administration, and contraindications. It is the responsibility of the licensed prescriber, relying on experience and knowledge of the patient, to determine dosages and the best treatment for each individual patient. Neither the publisher nor the author assumes any liability for any injury and/or damage to persons or property arising from this publication.

Previous editions copyrighted 2001, 1996, 1991.

Library of Congress Cataloging-in-Publication Data

Swanson's family practice review : a problem-oriented approach.— 5th ed. / Alfred F.
    Tallia, editor-in-chief ... [et al.].
        p. ; cm.
    Includes bibliographical references and index.
    ISBN 0-323-03000-9
    1. Family medicine—Examinations, questions, etc. I. Title: Family practice review. II.
Tallia, Alfred F. III. Swanson, Richard W. Family practice review.
    [DNLM: 1. Family Practice—Examination Questions. WB 18.2 S972 2005]
RC58.S93 2005
616'.0076—dc22

                                                                    2004049883

Acquisitions Editor: *Thom Moore*
Developmental Editor: *Cathy Carroll*
Production Services Manager: *Joan Sinclair*
Project Manager: *Cecelia Bayruns*
Designer: *Karen O'Keefe Owens*

Printed in the United States of America

Last digit is the print number: 9 8 7 6 5 4 3 2 1

To the lasting memory of

Dr. Richard Swanson:

An extraordinary physician and educator.

CONTRIBUTORS

Dennis A. Cardone, DO, CAQSM
Associate Professor and Director
    of the Sports Medicine Center
Department of Family Medicine
Robert Wood Johnson Medical School
New Brunswick, New Jersey
*Chapters 15, 17, 24, 29, 33, 41, 42, 45, 95, 109, 115, 118,
146–155, 157–159, and 161–163*

Maria Ciminelli, MD
Assistant Professor and Associate Director
    of Family Medicine Residency
Department of Family Medicine
Robert Wood Johnson Medical School
New Brunswick, New Jersey
Chapters 22, 38, 43, 96, 100, 101, 104, 106, 112, and 119

Cathryn Heath, MD
Clinical Associate Professor
Director of Maternity Services
Department of Family Medicine
Robert Wood Johnson Medical School
New Brunswick, New Jersey
Section IV

David F. Howarth, MD, MPH
Associate Professor and Director
    of Fellowship Programs
Department of Family Medicine
Robert Wood Johnson Medical School
New Brunswick, New Jersey
Chapters 18–20, 36, 37, 39, 40, 49, and Section VIII

Kenneth H. Ibsen, PhD
Professor Emeritus
College of Medicine
University of California
Irvine, California
Director, Kaplan Medical CME
Los Angeles, California
Chapter 21 and Chapters 120–130 with Dr. Tallia

Jeffrey Levine, MD, MPH
Assistant Professor
Director of Women's Health
Department of Family Medicine
Robert Wood Johnson Medical School
New Brunswick, New Jersey
Section III with Dr. Wu

Barbara Jo McGarry, MD
Clinical Assistant Professor
Assistant Director of Family Medicine Residency
Department of Family Medicine
Robert Wood Johnson Medical School
New Brunswick, New Jersey
Chapters 12, 14, 26, 27, 31, 32, 34, 111, and 113

Beatrice Roemheld-Hamm, MD, PhD
Associate Professor
Departments of Family Medicine and Psychiatry
Medical Director, UMG
Family Medicine at Monument Square
Department of Family Medicine
Robert Wood Johnson Medical School
New Brunswick, New Jersey
Section V with Dr. Stuart

Melissa Rose, MD
Clinical Instructor
Department of Family Medicine
Robert Wood Johnson Medical School
New Brunswick, New Jersey
Chapters 93, 94, 108, 114, 117, 156, and 160

Marian R. Stuart, PhD
Clinical Professor
Director of Behavioral Sciences
Department of Family Medicine
Robert Wood Johnson Medical School
New Brunswick, New Jersey
Section V with Dr. Roemheld-Hamm

Alfred F. Tallia, MD, MPH, FAAFP
Associate Professor and Vice Chair
Department of Family Medicine
Robert Wood Johnson Medical School
New Brunswick, New Jersey
*Sections I and X plus Chapters 10, 11, 13, 16, 23, 25, 28, 30, 33,
35, 44, 46, 47, 92, 97–99, and 107, plus Chapters 120–130 with
Dr. Ibsen*

Justine Wu, MD
Clinical Instructor
Department of Family Medicine
Robert Wood Johnson Medical School
New Brunswick, New Jersey
Section III with Dr. Levine

Jabbar Zafar, DO
Assistant Professor
Assistant Director of Family Medicine Residency
Capital Health Systems
Department of Family Medicine
Robert Wood Johnson Medical School
New Brunswick, New Jersey
Chapters 102, 103, 105, 110, and 116

CONTENTS

PREFACE TO THE FIFTH EDITION

The fourth edition of *Swanson's Family Practice Review* was a marvelous educational tool; the product of a great deal of sweat, sparked by the founding genius of Dr. Swanson, the text's originator. Dr. Swanson passed away in 1996, and in the spring of 1997, Dr. Alfred F. Tallia, Vice Chairman of Family Medicine at Robert Wood Johnson Medical School, assumed the primary editorship of the text and began work on the fourth edition. User feedback indicates that the fourth edition was an effective tool not only for family physicians preparing for certification or recertification, but also for clinicians preparing for other examinations or simply desiring to hone their familiarity with the basic concepts pertinent to primary care.

The primary goals of the fifth edition are to update the content and retain the special essence that has made the fourth edition such a valued and popular educational instrument. Although the basic format of the fourth edition is retained, this edition is now arranged in a fashion designed to make it easier for the readers to find their way through the content. The book is divided into ten sections. Nine represent a clinical area tested for by the American Board of Family Physicians (ABFP), while the tenth section is an illustrated review. Each of the nine text sections contains a series of chapters covering a specific subject relevant to that section. Each chapter presents at least one clinical case that simulates a real clinical situation, providing the learner with a sense of reality and enhancing retention. Each clinical case problem is followed by questions concerning its diagnosis and management. In most chapters, this question section ends with a Clinical Case Management Problem that asks the reader to summarize the most pertinent therapeutic factors relevant to the chapter. Dr. Alicia Dermer was particularly helpful for her contributions to Chapter 97, Infant Feeding.

The question section is followed by an answer section, which provides a detailed discussion relevant to the case problems. Finally, each chapter has a short summation and a few selected readings and references, including electronic, web-based sites. The overall process is designed to increase retention and to expand and refine the readers' knowledge of the diagnostic methods, therapeutics, and patient management techniques presented in each case while providing a more holistic concept of the potential significance of the set of symptoms that define the chapter.

The chapters and most of the case problems have been chosen by a team of clinicians and subsequently reaffirmed and updated by the contributors on the basis of thorough needs analyses, including opinions of readers, participants, and faculty in live CME conferences, expert opinion, and morbidity and chart studies by Dr. Tallia and others. Content selection, designed to represent a core of knowledge that the family physician should have, was made under the direction of the editors from Robert Wood Johnson Medical School with input from other family practice physicians from across the country with special expertise in specific content areas.

The editors and contributors anticipate that the reader will both enjoy and profit from their study of this volume. Happy studying!

Alfred F. Tallia
Kenneth H. Ibsen

ACKNOWLEDGMENTS

As Editor-in-Chief, I am indebted to many individuals for their support and assistance in the preparation of the fifth edition of *Swanson's Family Practice Review*. To begin, I wish to thank my wife, Elizabeth; Dr. Cardone's wife, Silvana; and Dr. Howarth's wife, Allison, and our families, as well as those of the other authors, for their sacrifice of time and their understanding as we prepared this edition.

To Mr. Thomas Moore of Elsevier and to Drs. Richard Friedland and Rochelle Rothstein of Kaplan Medical, my thanks for their inspiration and support. To Dr. David E. Swee, Professor and Chair of Family Medicine at Robert Wood Johnson Medical School, my thanks for his encouragement and support for this important undertaking. Our thanks as well to our colleagues in the department for their help and understanding of the demands that preparation of this edition required.

Finally, to Dr. Kenneth Ibsen, Director, Continuing Medical Education at Kaplan Medical, a true scholar and gentleman, without whose tireless efforts of reading and formatting this manuscript, making excellent suggestions, and, in general, keeping us all coordinated and organized this book would not have been completed, my deepest thanks and appreciation.

Alfred F. Tallia, MD, MPH
Editor-in-Chief

This section briefly discusses the philosophy and techniques of passing board examinations or any other type of medical examination. Many examinations are moving or have moved to computer-based administration. Learn if this applies to your examination, and if so, read and use the demonstrations provided either on the web or elsewhere.

First, realize that you are "playing a game." It is, of course, a very important game, but it is nevertheless a game. When answering each question you must ask yourself the following: "What is it that the examiner wants from this question?" Let us turn our attention to the most common type of question, the multiple-choice question (MCQ).

What these tips provide the learner is a way to "outfox the fox." So, how do you outfox the fox? Following these rules will maximize the chances.

RULE 1: Allocate your time appropriately. At the beginning of the examination, divide the number of questions by the time allotted. Pace yourself accordingly, and check your progress every half hour.

RULE 2: If using a paper exam, work off of the answer sheet. Yes, you may mark up the question book, but do not wait until the end to transfer your answers from the question paper to the answer sheet. You may find that you have run out of time and your answer sheet is blank. If using a computer-administered examination, take the time before the examination to become familiar with the mechanics of maneuvering through the examination program. Learn whether you can return to questions you weren't sure about, or whether this is not allowed.

RULE 3: Answer every question in order. Do not leave an answer space blank. On paper-administered exams, you run the risk of missequencing your answers and having all answers out of order. On computer administered exams, you run the risk of not being able to return to an unanswered question.

RULE 4: Do not spend more than your allotted time on any one question. If you don't know the answer and you are not penalized for wrong answers, simply guess.

RULE 5: Even if you are penalized for wrong answers (most examinations no longer do this) and you can eliminate even one choice, answer the question anyway. The laws of mathematics indicate that you will still come out ahead.

RULE 6: If there is a question in which one choice is significantly longer than the others and you do not know the answer, select the long choice.

RULE 7: If you are faced with an "all of the above" choice, realize that these are right far more often than they are wrong. Choose "all of the above."

RULE 8: Become suspicious if you have more than three choices of the same letter in a row. Two of one choice in a row is common, three is less common, and four is almost unheard of. Something is probably wrong.

RULE 9: Answer choices tend to be very evenly distributed. In other words, the number of correct (a) choices is close to the number of correct (b) choices, and so on. However, there may be somewhat more choice (e)'s than any other, especially if there are a fair number of "all of the above" choices. If you have time, do a quick check to provide yourself with some reassurance.

RULE 10: Never, never change an answer once you have recorded it on the answer sheet unless you have an extraordinary reason for doing so. Many people taking MCQ examinations, especially if they have time on their hands after completing the examination, start second-guessing themselves and thinking of all kinds of unusual exceptions. Resist this temptation.

RULE 11: Before you choose an answer, always, always read each and every choice. Do not get caught by seeing what you believe is the correct answer jump out at you. Read all of the choices.

RULE 12: Scan the answers and the lead-in to the answers first, then read the clinical case/vignette. This way you will know what is being tested and will better attend to the necessary facts. Read each question carefully. Be especially careful to read words such as *not*, *except*, and so on. Some people find it helpful to carefully underline certain parts of the question containing such words.

Success cannot be guaranteed with these or any other rules. I do, however, believe that these rules will help you achieve better results on your board examinations.

It has been estimated that it will take 79.5 hours to complete this activity. Accordingly Kaplan Medical CME designates this educational activity for up to 79.5 hours in Category 1 credit toward the AMA Physician's Recognition Award. Each physician should claim only those hours of credit that he or she actually spent completing the educational activity. These credits will be available from July 1, 2004, through June 30, 2007.

TARGETED AUDIENCE

This activity is designed to meet the education needs of Family Practice Physicians preparing for certification or recertification and/or for a review of contemporary recommended practice behaviors. However experience with the fourth edition indicates that it will also meet the needs of physicians preparing for the other generalist examinations as well as physician assistants and other health care delivery professionals desiring an up-to-date review of the essentials of primary care.

LEARNING OBJECTIVES

Upon completion of all or selected parts of this activity, participants should have:

1. reinforced and/or expanded their preexisting knowledge in a way that will help improve the quality of their patient care
2. learned new information that will have updated their preexisting knowledge concerning current diagnostic methodologies, medications, and treatments
3. gained knowledge concerning state-of-the-art diagnostic strategies, treatment protocols, and clinical management strategies
4. gained further insight into sensitive and effective ways to communicate with patients
5. and last but not least if applicable, enhanced their knowledge concerning topics relevant to their certification, recertification, or licensing examinations

DISCLOSURE POLICY

In order to ensure balance, independence, objectivity, and scientific rigor, all contributing faculty are expected to disclose any real or apparent conflict(s) of interest that may have a direct bearing on the subject matter presented in this volume. This pertains to relationships with pharmaceutical companies, biomedical device manufacturers, or other corporations whose products or services are related to the subject matter. The intent of this policy is not to prevent a contributor with a potential conflict of interest from presenting his or her opinions, but rather to identify any potential conflict openly so that the readers may form their own judgments about the

impartiality of the content. It remains for the reader to determine whether any of the contributor's outside interests may provide a possible bias in either the exposition or the conclusions presented.

It is possible that non-FDA approved (off-label) uses of certain medications or devices may be presented. If so, it is the responsibility of the reader to identify such products before using them in his or her practice. The publisher, CME provider, or contributors cannot be held liable for misuse of any such product.

Alfred F. Tallia, MD, MPH, FAAFP: Has no conflict of interest regarding any product discussed in this enduring CME activity. No use of off-labeled products is anticipated.

Dennis A. Cardone, DO, CAQSM: Has no conflict of interest regarding any product discussed in this enduring CME activity. No use of off-labeled products is anticipated.

David F. Howarth, MD, MPH: Has no conflict of interest regarding any product discussed in this enduring CME activity. No use of off-labeled products is anticipated.

Kenneth H. Ibsen, PhD: Has no conflict of interest regarding any product discussed in this enduring CME activity. No use of off-labeled products is anticipated.

Maria Ciminelli, MD: Has no conflict of interest regarding any product discussed in this enduring CME activity. No use of off-labeled products is anticipated.

Cathryn Heath, MD: Has no conflict of interest regarding any product discussed in this enduring CME activity. No use of off-labeled products is anticipated.

Jeffery Levine, MD, MPH: Has no conflict of interest regarding any product discussed in this enduring CME activity. Use of off-labeled products in the discussion of the obstetric section may occur.

Barbara Jo McGarry, MD: Has no conflict of interest regarding any product discussed in this enduring CME activity. No use of off-labeled products is anticipated.

Beatrice Roemheld-Hamm, MD, PhD: Has no conflict of interest regarding any product discussed in this enduring CME activity. No use of off-labeled products is anticipated.

Melissa Rose, MD: Has no conflict of interest regarding any product discussed in this enduring CME activity. No use of off-labeled products is anticipated.

Marian R. Stuart, PhD: Has no conflict of interest regarding any product discussed in this enduring

CME activity. No use of off-labeled products is anticipated.

Justine Wu, MD: Has no conflict of interest regarding any product discussed in this enduring CME activity. Use of off-labeled products in the discussion of the obstetric section may occur.

Jabbar Zafar, DO: Has no conflict of interest regarding any product discussed in this enduring CME activity. No use of off-labeled products is anticipated.

PROCESS FOR OBTAINING CONTINUING MEDICAL EDUCATION CREDIT

In order to obtain CME credits, it is necessary to register first. After registration, you will be sent a questionnaire asking a little about you, how many and what type of CME credits you earned, the approximate percent improvement in your ability to answer the multiple choice questions, and pertinent evaluation data. After that form is filled out and returned with the appropriate fee, you will be sent a certificate for the credits earned.

REGISTRATION

For registration, we require your name, degree, address, telephone number, and a $25 fee. Although this registration fee is non-returnable, it will be applied to the overall fee.

Registration may be conducted by regular mail, e-mail, phone, or fax. Payment should be made to Kaplan Medical CME. The method of payment may be by check, money order, or credit card (Visa, MasterCard, American Express, or Discover).

The address for registration by mail is:

CME Administrative Secretary
c/o Kaplan Medical CME
700 South Flower Street
Suite 2900
Los Angeles, CA 90017
Fax: 231-892-1267

Registration may also be made by e-mail or phone:

E-mail: CME@kaplan.com;
Phone: 1-800-533-8850, ext. 5720

Questions may be directed to Dr. Kenneth Ibsen via e-mail at ken_ibsen@kaplan.com or phone at 1-800-533-8850, ext. 5706

To make registration by mail more convenient, a tear-out registration form is provided on page xxi.

CREDIT AND FEE SCHEDULE

Physicians requesting continuing medical education credit may do so upon completion of each individual chapter, or, alternatively, they may elect to request the credit after completing the full text. The maximum number of credit hours* and the associated fee for each chapter is indicated below. (The fees shown are based on a charge of $7.50 per credit hour for individual chapters or $6.75 when credit is granted for the complete activity [rounded off to the nearest whole dollar].)

Section	Maximal Credit Hours	Fee
1. Epidemiology & Public Health	5.5	$ 41
2. Adult Medicine	19.0	$142
3. Women's Health	5.0	$ 37
4. Maternity Care	6.0	$ 45
5. Behavioral Science & Communication	8.0	$ 60
6. Children & Adolescents	12.5	$ 94
7. General Surgery & Surgical Subspecialties	5.5	$ 41
8. Geriatric Medicine	7.0	$ 52
9. Emergency & Sports Medicine	9.0	$ 67
10. Illustrated Review	2.0	$ 15
The Whole Book (10% Discount)	79.5	$535

*These hours represent the average number of hours reported by five different readers of the 4th edition, adjusted by 3.3% to account for the greater length of the 5th edition.

Registration Form for CME Credits

Swanson's Family Practice Review, 5th Edition

Name _____   Degree _____

Address _____
                    Street   City   State   Zip

Day Phone _____   FAX _____

e-mail _____

A nonrefundable fee of $25 must be included with this registration form.

Method of Payment:
Credit card:
Type of card: Visa _____ MasterCard _____ Amer. Express. _____ Discover _____

Credit card Number _____   Expiration Date _____

Signature _____

Check _____ Money order _____

Either mail or FAX the completed form to:

CME Administrative Secretary
c/o Kaplan Medical CME
700 South Flower Street
Suite 2900
Los Angeles, CA 90017

Phone: 1-800-533-8850 ext. 5720   FAX: 231-892-1267
E-mail CME@kaplan.com

EPIDEMIOLOGY AND PUBLIC HEALTH

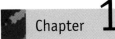
Chapter 1

The Yearly Complete Physical Examination versus the Focused Periodic Health Maintenance Examination

"Doctor, are your physical exams less thorough because you became part of an HMO?"

CLINICAL CASE PROBLEM 1:
A 51-Year-Old Male Who Presents for an "Executive" Examination

A 51-year-old male comes to your office requesting an "executive" examination. He has been in the habit of receiving a yearly "executive" examination at work but recently has switched jobs. His new employer does not offer these services. The patient had been told by a health professional at his previous job that "a complete physical—head to toe, with lots of tests—is the best method of ensuring good health." He recently heard a radio advertisement of a company that "specializes" in executive examinations but decided to see you instead.

▌ **SELECT THE BEST ANSWER TO THE FOLLOWING QUESTIONS:**

1. With regard to the relative effectiveness of a yearly complete physical examination, which of the following statements is most accurate?
   a. the effectiveness of a yearly complete physical examination has been confirmed in randomized controlled clinical trials
   b. the effectiveness of a yearly complete physical examination has been confirmed by anecdotal evidence
   c. the effectiveness of a yearly complete physical examination has been demonstrated in case–control trials
   d. the effectiveness of a yearly complete physical examination has been confirmed in population cohort studies
   e. none of the above statements is true

2. Which of the following is a criterion (or are criteria) for effective periodic health screening?
   a. the condition tested must have a significant effect on quality of life
   b. the disease must have an asymptomatic phase during which detection and treatment significantly reduce morbidity and mortality
   c. acceptable treatment methods must be available
   d. tests must be available at a reasonable cost
   e. all of the above are true

3. Good reasons to consider performing a health maintenance examination on an asymptomatic adult independent of routine screening include which of the following?
   a. to establish a good doctor–patient relationship
   b. to augment and update the patient's history
   c. to maximize your income
   d. a and b
   e. all of the above

4. Which of the following statements regarding the performance of a health maintenance examination is (are) true?
   a. the examination in itself may be therapeutic
   b. the examination may provide the patient with reassurance
   c. the examination may produce benefit to the patient through therapeutic touch
   d. the examination may play an important role in development and maintenance of the clinical skills in the physician
   e. all of the above are true

5. Which of the following statements regarding the sensitivity and specificity of a yearly complete physical examination is (are) true?
   a. the yearly complete physical examination is neither highly sensitive nor highly specific
   b. the yearly complete physical examination is both highly sensitive and highly specific
   c. the yearly complete physical examination is high in sensitivity but low in specificity
   d. the yearly complete physical examination is high in specificity but low in sensitivity
   e. none of the above statements is true

6. Which of the following is (are) valid reason(s) not to rely significantly on a yearly complete physical examination in asymptomatic adults? The yearly complete physical examination:
   a. may offer a false sense of security
   b. is an inefficient use of time

c. reinforces misperceptions about physician capabilities

d. may detract from time that could be spent on other preventive interventions

e. all of the above are true

7. Which of the following statements is (are) true regarding false-positive findings on routine complete physical examination?

a. false-positive findings create needless patient anxiety

b. false-positive findings often initiate an "intervention cascade"

c. false-positive findings place a substantial burden on the entire health care system

d. a and b

e. a, b, and c

8. Which of the following statements is true regarding patient perceptions of yearly "executive" examinations and related laboratory tests?

a. many patients believe that a routine "executive" complete examination, along with a complete laboratory profile, will diagnose the majority of illnesses

b. most patients understand the meaning of the term *periodic health maintenance examination*

c. many patients understand the importance of a focused, regional examination

d. patients are generally sensitive to the costs of routine physical examinations and routine laboratory tests

e. none of the above statements is true

CLINICAL CASE PROBLEM 2:

A 35-Year-Old Female Who Presents for a Health Maintenance Examination

A 35-year-old female has come to your office for a health maintenance examination. The physician examines the skin in an effort to identify dysplastic nevi, other unusual nevi, or other skin lesions.

9. Which of the following statements is true?

a. the examination for skin cancer in a health maintenance examination is highly sensitive and highly specific

b. the examination for skin cancer in a health maintenance examination is highly sensitive but of low specificity

c. the examination for skin cancer in a health maintenance examination is neither sensitive nor specific

d. the examination for skin cancer in a health maintenance examination is highly specific but of lower sensitivity

e. the examination for skin cancer is of variable sensitivity and specificity depending on the skill of the examiner

■ ANSWERS:

1. **e.** Although the yearly examination, including "executive" examinations, had been a primary diagnostic tool throughout much of the twentieth century, there is little, if any, evidence in the literature to support its efficacy. The yearly physical examination should not be confused with the health maintenance assessment, for which there is evidence supporting its efficacy. The health maintenance assessment is a comprehensive assessment targeted at specific age and gender causes of morbidity and mortality. Recommendations for the periodic health maintenance examination are derived from epidemiologic data that assess population risk and intervention benefit. Specific evidence-based screening and counseling interventions are part of the health maintenance examination. The United States Preventive Services Task Force is the preeminent body for the assessment and recommendation of interventions that are a part of the periodic health maintenance examination.

2. **e.** The criteria for effective periodic health screening are as follows: (1) the condition for which the physician is testing must have a significant effect on the quality of the patient's life; (2) acceptable treatment methods must be available for that particular condition; (3) the disease must have an asymptomatic phase during which detection and treatment significantly reduce morbidity and mortality; (4) treatment during the asymptomatic phase must yield a result superior to that obtained by delaying treatment until symptoms appear; (5) tests must be available at a reasonable cost; (6) tests must be acceptable to the patient; and (7) the prevalence of the condition must be sufficient to justify the cost of screening.

3. **d.** See Answer 4.

4. **e.** Reasons to perform a periodic health maintenance examination in asymptomatic adults, independent of routine screening, include the following: (1) to establish a good doctor–patient relationship; (2) to augment history taking; (3) to fulfill patient expectations; (4) to provide the therapeutic benefit of touch; (5) to maintain the physician's clinical skills; (6) to reinforce patient education, especially self-examination; (7) to realistically reassure the patient (and the physician); (8) to establish the patient's baseline health status; (9) to determine if the patient is indeed asymptomatic; and (10) to avoid giving the patient the impression that he or she must have symptoms to be examined.

5. **a.** See Answer 6.

6. **e.** The procedures entailed in the yearly complete physical examination are neither sensitive nor specific. Because of this, physicians may provide false reassurance on the basis of the findings. Consider statements such as, "Your heart sounds great" or "You've got a complete, 100% perfect bill of health." The next week you may hear from the Emergency Department doctor that your patient has just had a heart attack. Your next phone call probably will come from his lawyer. Such grandiose statements reinforce misperceptions regarding physicians' capabilities and certainly may result in legal action. Excessive concentration on physical examination detracts from time that could be spent in more productive pursuits, such as patient education and counseling about health risk behaviors and performing targeted, evidence-supported screening procedures.

7. **e.** The same excessive compulsiveness that serves as a survival skill in medical training is often dysfunctional in medical practice. False-positive findings are common in the face of low test sensitivity and specificity and low prevalence of the condition in the population tested. Even if a test has a high sensitivity and specificity, the more tests or maneuvers that are performed on the same individual, the higher the likelihood of a false-positive result. Also, the likelihood that a positive test is true positive (positive predictive value) is directly related to the prevalence of the condition in the target population. Performing examinations in populations in which the condition has a low prevalence will thus generate a high false-positive rate. False-positive test results create needless anxiety in both patients and physicians. More important, such results often lead to an "intervention cascade," initiating further testing of greater invasiveness, which increases the potential for iatrogenic harm. A good example of this is the finding of a slightly enlarged ovary (you think) on pelvic bimanual examination, a situation in which a benign cause is much more likely than a malignant cause. From that may result routine ultrasound, followed perhaps by laparoscopy to rule out a malignant tumor of very low prevalence. We all must ask ourselves before initiating any intervention, "What is the evidence that this action is likely to do the patient any good?"

8. **a.** Many patients believe that an "executive" complete examination, along with a complex laboratory profile, will diagnose the majority of illnesses. This is obviously a mistaken impression. Sadly, some health professionals have taken financial advantage of this misconception, playing off patients' needs for reassurance. Conversely, most patients are unaware of the hazards of unnecessary interventions and testing, and many physicians do not take the time to educate their patients of the hazards. As in any intervention, patients should be informed of the rationale (evidence and expected outcomes), risks, benefits, and alternatives of laboratory testing.

Despite efforts aimed at increasing public awareness and understanding, many patients do not understand the concept of the periodic health maintenance examination or of focused regional examination. In addition, patients are still not very sensitive about costs of routine examinations and routine tests. Further patient education efforts will be necessary to inform patients regarding these important issues.

9. **e.** The clinical examination of the skin has significant variability in terms of sensitivity and specificity. The major reason for the variability is the expertise of the examiner. The greater the training and expertise in skin lesion diagnosis and treatment, the higher the sensitivity and specificity of the examination. Another excellent example of this phenomenon is radiologists reading mammograms. The more training the radiologist has and the more mammograms the radiologist reads, the higher the sensitivity and specificity of mammograms.

SUMMARY OF THE YEARLY "EXECUTIVE" COMPLETE PHYSICAL EXAMINATION VERSUS THE FOCUSED PERIODIC HEALTH MAINTENANCE EXAMINATION

There is little, if any, evidence that the yearly "executive" complete physical examination is effective or addresses the issues and conditions that can be prevented or can be addressed or treated while in an asymptomatic phase.

In addition to the lack of established efficacy, there are significant risks to performing a routine complete physical examination, not the least of which is labeling someone as healthy when, in fact, he or she is not healthy.

There are reasons and situations in which it may be reasonable to perform a routine complete checkup—reasons that, when balanced against the reasons not to perform the same, come out in favor of doing a routine physical examination. These are outlined in Answer 4.

Significant misperceptions concerning the yearly physical examination exist, which often result in excess procedures and excess laboratory tests. If carried to the extreme, this is a surefire way to end up on a wild

Continued

SUMMARY OF THE YEARLY "EXECUTIVE" COMPLETE PHYSICAL EXAMINATION VERSUS THE FOCUSED PERIODIC HEALTH MAINTENANCE EXAMINATION —cont'd

goose chase. This wild goose chase, for example, may end up in a previously well person becoming ill from worry about a false-positive test result. Thus on many occasions one would not be overstating the case by saying, "Everything was fine until the patient went to the doctor."

SUGGESTED READING

These historical, classic articles challenged the established practice of yearly complete physicals:

Breslow L, Somers AR: The lifetime health-monitoring program, *New Engl J Med* 296(11):601-608, 1997.

Frame PS: A critical review of adult health maintenance. Part 1. Prevention of atherosclerotic disease, *J Fam Pract* 22(4):341-346, 1986.

Frame PS: A critical review of adult health maintenance. Part 2. Prevention of infectious diseases, *J Fam Pract* 22(5):417-422, 1986.

Frame PS: A critical review of adult health maintenance. Part 3. Prevention of cancer, *J Fam Pract* 22(6):511-520, 1986.

Frame PS: A critical review of adult health maintenance. Part 4. Prevention of metabolic, behavioral, and miscellaneous conditions, *J Fam Pract* 23(1):29-39, 1986.

Shannon KC, et al: Improving delivery of preventive health care with the comprehensive annotated reminder tool (CART). *J Fam Pract* 50(9):767-771, 2001.

Stickler GB: Are yearly physical examinations in adolescents necessary? *J Am Board Fam Pract* 13(3):172-177, 2000.

Straus SE, et al: Clinical assessment of the reliability of the examination (CARE). *ACP J Club* 133(2):A11-12, 2000.

For the American Academy of Family Physicians' policies and rationales regarding the periodic health examination, visit "clinical care and research" at their website at www.aafp.org.

Chapter **2**

Fundamental Epidemiology

"Is it sensitivity, specificity, or what?"

CLINICAL CASE PROBLEM 1:
A 25-Year-Old Medical Student Who Is Having Anxiety Attacks Regarding His Upcoming Epidemiology Examination

A 25-year-old medical student comes to your office in a state of extreme anxiety manifested by palpitations and sweating throughout the previous week. He tells you he is scheduled to have a clinical epidemiology examination in 24 hours.

On physical examination his blood pressure is 120/70 mm Hg, pulse is 90/beats per minute and regular, and respirations 24/minute. His physical examination is normal. You order a thyroid-stimulating hormone test to exclude hyperthyroidism. You explain to him that given the low prevalence of thyroid disease in his age group and the higher prevalence of anxiety in his medical school population of students, the test's negative predictive value will be helpful. He looks confused and more anxious.

In an attempt to deal with his symptoms, you decide to spend some time tutoring the student regarding basic epidemiologic concepts. You begin by explaining the basics of a 2×2 table that relates positive and negative test results to the presence or absence of disease in a specific population (Table 2-1).

Table 2-1	Relationship Between Test A and Disease B	
	Disease B Present	Disease B Absent
Test A positive	30	50
Test A negative	10	80

■ SELECT THE BEST ANSWER TO THE FOLLOWING QUESTIONS:

Use the data from Table 2-1 for Questions 1 through 6.

1. What is the sensitivity of test A for disease B?
   a. 25%
   b. 37.5%
   c. 75%
   d. 62.5%
   e. 11%

2. What is the specificity of test A for disease B?
   a. 25%
   b. 37.5%
   c. 75%
   d. 61.5%
   e. 11%

3. What is the positive predictive value (PPV) of test A in the diagnosis of disease B?
   a. 37.5%
   b. 25%
   c. 75%

d. 61.5%

e. 11%

4. What is the negative predictive value (NPV) of test A in the diagnosis of disease B?
   a. 37%
   b. 89%
   c. 25%
   d. 75%
   e. 61.5%

5. What is the likelihood ratio for test A in disease B?
   a. 0.39
   b. 1.95
   c. 3.80
   d. 0.79
   e. 1.51

6. What is the prevalence of disease A in this population?
   a. 15.5%
   b. 23.5%
   c. 40.0%
   d. 10.5%
   e. 18.4%

Consider the data in Table 2-2 illustrating the prevalence of disease X in various populations. Based on this information about disease prevalence and assuming the sensitivity of test A for disease X is 80% and the specificity of test A for disease X is 90%, answer Questions 7 through 10.

Table 2-2 Prevalence of Disease X in Certain Populations	
Setting	Prevalence (cases/100,000)
General population	50
Women, age 50 years old and older	500
Women, age 65 years old and older with a suspicious finding on clinical examination	40,000

7. What is the PPV of test A in the diagnosis of disease X in the general population?
   a. 0.4%
   b. 1.3%
   c. 5.4%
   d. 15.7%
   e. 39.6%

8. What is the PPV of test A in disease X in women age 50 and older?
   a. 0.4%
   b. 3.9%
   c. 10.7%
   d. 23.6%
   e. 52.7%

9. What is the PPV of test A in disease X in women older than 65 years of age with a suspicious finding on clinical examination?
   a. 0.4%
   b. 5.6%
   c. 34.7%
   d. 84.2%
   e. 93.0%

10. If the PPV of a test for a given disease in a given population is 4%, how many true positive test results are there in a sample of 100 positive test results?
    a. 4
    b. 10
    c. 40
    d. 96
    e. none of the above

To answer Question 11 consider the data in Table 2-3 concerning the sensitivity and specificity in the diagnosis of diabetes mellitus in the population.

Table 2-3 Sensitivity and Specificity of Blood Sugar Levels in the Diagnosis of Diabetes Mellitus		
Blood Sugar Level 2 Hours after Eating	Sensitivity	Specificity
>140 mg/100 (7.8 mmol/L)	57.1%	99.4%

11. Given that the data are correct, if the sensitivity of the test for a given blood sugar level was 38.6%, which of the following would be the most likely value for specificity?
    a. 99.2%
    b. 98.7%
    c. 92.4%
    d. 87.3%
    e. 100.0%

12. The validity of a test is best defined as which of the following?
    a. the reliability of the test
    b. the reproducibility of the test
    c. the variation in the test results

d. the degree to which the results of a measurement correspond to the true state of the phenomenon
e. the degree of biologic variation of the test

13. Which of the following terms is synonymous with the term *reliability*?
   a. reproducibility
   b. validity
   c. accuracy
   d. mean
   e. variation

14. Which of the following is not a measure of central tendency?
   a. mean
   b. median
   c. mode
   d. standard deviation
   e. none; all of the above are measures of central tendency Gaussian distribution

Consider the following experimental data: in a trial of the effect of reducing multiple risk factors on the subsequent incidence of coronary artery disease, high-risk patients were selected for study. Elevated blood pressure was one of the risk factors that caused people to be considered. People were screened for inclusion in the study on three consecutive visits. Blood pressures at those visits, before any therapeutic interventions were undertaken, were as listed in Table 2-4. Use the data in Table 2-4 to answer Question 15.

Table 2-4 Blood Pressure Readings vs. Visit Number

Visit Number	Mean Diastolic Blood Pressure (mm/Hg)
1	99.2
2	91.2
3	90.7

15. Which of the following statements regarding these data is true?
   a. these results are very strange; consider publication in any journal specializing in irreproducible results
   b. this is an example of regression to the mean
   c. this is an example of natural variation
   d. the most likely explanation is either interobserver or intraobserver variation
   e. we likely are dealing with faulty equipment in this case; the most likely reason for this would be failure to calibrate all of the blood pressure cuffs

Consider the following experimental data: a population of heavy smokers (men smoking more than 50 cigarettes per day) is divided into two groups and followed for a period of 10 years.
   Use the data from Table 2-5 to answer Question 16.

Table 2-5 10-Year Mortality Data

		Diagnosed with Lung Cancer	Average Survival Time from Diagnosis
Group 1 (experimental group)	490 individuals with annual chest x-rays	37	14 months
Group 2 (control group)	510 individuals with no annual chest x-ray	39	8 months

16. Regarding these results, which of the following statements is true?
   a. these results prove that screening chest x-rays improve survival time in lung cancer
   b. these results prove that screening chest x-rays should be considered for all smokers
   c. these results are most likely an example of lead-time bias
   d. these results are most likely an example of length-time bias
   e. these results do not make any sense; the experiment should be repeated

17. Length-time bias with respect to cancer diagnosis is defined as which of the following?
   a. bias resulting from the detection of slow-growing tumors during screening programs more often than fast-growing tumors
   b. bias resulting from the length of time a cancer was growing before any symptoms occurred
   c. bias resulting from the length of time a cancer was growing before somebody got on the ball and started to ask some questions and perform some laboratory investigations
   d. bias resulting from the length of time between the latent and more rapid growth phases of any cancer
   e. none of the above

18. Concerning population and disease measurement, *prevalence* is defined as which of the following?
   a. the fraction (proportion) of a population having a clinical condition at a given point in time

b. the fraction (proportion) of a population initially free of a disease but that develops the disease over a given period
c. equivalent to incidence
d. mathematically as $a + b/(a + b + c + d)$ in a 2×2 table relating sensitivity and specificity to PPV
e. none of the above

19. Concerning population and disease measurement, *incidence* is defined as which of the following?
a. the fraction (proportion) of a population having a clinical condition at a given point in time
b. the fraction (proportion) of a population initially free of a disease but that develops the disease over a given period
c. equivalent to prevalence
d. of little use in epidemiology
e. none of the above

20. Regarding clinical epidemiology in relation to the discipline of family practice, which of the following statements is true?
a. clinical epidemiology is higher mathematics that bears little relation to the world in general, much less the specialty of family practice
b. clinical epidemiology was invented to create anxiety and panic attacks that mimic hyperthyroidism in medical students and residents
c. clinical epidemiology is unlikely to contain any useful information for the average practicing family physician
d. clinical epidemiology is a passing fad; fortunately for all concerned, its time has passed
e. none of the above statements about clinical epidemiology is true

ANSWERS:

Table 2-6 will illustrate the answers to Questions 1 through 6.

Table 2-6 Disease X

	Disease X Present	Disease X Absent
Test A positive	30 (a) TP	50 (b) FP
Test A negative	10 (c) FN	80 (d) TN

TP, true positive; *TN*, true negative; *FP*, false positive; *FN*, false negative.

1. c. Sensitivity is defined as the proportion of people with the disease that have a positive test result. A sensitive test rarely will miss patients who have the disease. In Table 2-6, sensitivity is defined as the number of true positives (TPs) divided by the number of true positives plus the number of false negatives (FNs). That is:

$$\text{Sensitivity} = TP/(TP + FN)$$
$$\text{Sensitivity} = a/(a + c) = 30/40 = 75\%$$

A sensitive test (one that is usually positive in the presence of disease) should be selected when there is an important penalty for missing the disease. This would be so when you had reason to suspect a serious but treatable condition—for example, obtaining a chest x-ray in a patient with suspected tuberculosis or Hodgkin's disease. In addition, sensitive tests are useful in the early stages of a diagnostic workup of disease, when several possibilities are being considered, to reduce the number of possibilities. Thus, in situations like this, diagnostic tests are used to rule out diseases.

2. d. Specificity is defined as the proportion of people without the disease who have a negative test result. A specific test rarely incorrectly classifies people without the disease as having the disease. In Table 2-6, specificity is defined as the number of true negatives (TNs) divided by the number of true negatives plus the number of false positives (FPs). That is:

$$\text{Specificity} = TN/(TN + FP)$$
$$\text{Specificity} = d/(d + b) = 80/130 = 61.5\%$$

A specific test is useful to confirm, or rule in, a diagnosis that has been suggested by other tests or data. Thus a specific test is rarely positive in the absence of disease—that is, it gives very few false-positive test results. Tests with high specificity are needed when false-positive results can harm the patient physically, emotionally, or financially. Thus a specific test is most helpful when the test result is positive.

There is always a tradeoff between sensitivity and specificity. In general, if a disease has a low prevalence, choose a more specific test; if a disease has a high prevalence, choose a more sensitive test.

3. a. Positive predictive value (PPV) is defined as the probability of disease in a patient with a positive (abnormal) test result. In Table 2-6, the PPV is as follows:

$$\text{PPV} = a/(a + b) = 30/80 = 37.5\%$$

4. b. Negative predictive value (NPV) is defined as the probability of not having the disease when the test result is negative. In Table 2-6, the NPV is as follows:

$$\text{NPV} = d/(c + d) = 80/90 = 89\%$$

5. b. The likelihood ratio of a positive test result is the probability of that test result in the presence of disease divided by the probability of the test result in the absence of disease. In Table 2-6, the likelihood ratio is as follows:

Likelihood ratio (+) test results $a/(a + c)$ divided by $b/(b + d) = 30/(30 + 10)$ divided by $50/(50 + 80)$ or 1.95

6. b. The prevalence of a disease in the population at risk is the fraction or proportion of a group with a clinical condition at a given point in time. Prevalence is measured by surveying a defined population containing people with and without the condition of interest (at a given point in time). Prevalence can be equated with pretest probability. In Table 2-6 prevalence is defined as follows:

$$\text{Prevalence} = \frac{a + c}{a + b + c + d}$$

that is, $a + c$ divided by $a + b + c + d = 30 + 10/(30 + 10 + 50 + 80) = 23.5$

As prevalence decreases, PPV must decrease along with it and NPV must increase.

7. a. Answers 7 and 8 are explained in Answer 9, including Table 2-7.

Table 2-7	Calculations Involved in a General 2 x 2 Table	
	TARGET DISORDER	
	Present	Absent
Test postive	Cell a = (sensitivity)$(a + c)$	Cell b = $(b + d) - d$
Test negative	Cell c = $(a + c) - a$	Cell d = (specificity)$(b + d)$
Column sums	a + c	Total − (a + c)
Total = a + b + c + d		

8. b.

9. d. The respective PPVs for test A in the diagnosis of disease X in the general population, women older than age 50 years, and women older than 65 with a suspicious finding on clinical examination are 0.4%, 3.9%, and 84.2%.

To perform the calculations necessary to arrive at these answers the following steps are recommended:

Step 1: Identify the sensitivity and specificity of the sign, symptom, or diagnostic test that you plan to use. Many of these are published. If you are not certain, consider asking a consultant with special expertise in the area.

Step 2: Using a 2 × 2 table, set your total equal to an even number (consider, for example, 1000 as a good choice). Therefore,

$$a + b + c + d = 1000$$

Step 3: Using whatever information you have about the patient before you apply this diagnostic test, estimate his or her pretest probability (prevalence) of the disease in question. Next, put appropriate column summation numbers at the bottom of the columns $(a + c)$ and $(b + d)$. The easiest way to do this is to express your pretest probability (or prevalence) as a decimal three places to the right. This result is $(a + c)$, and 1000 minus this result is $(b + d)$.

Step 4: Start to fill in the cells of the 2 × 2 table. Multiply sensitivity (expressed as a decimal) by $(a + c)$ and put the result in cell a. You then can calculate cell c by simple subtraction.

Step 5: Similarly, multiply specificity (expressed as a decimal) by $(b + d)$ and put the result in cell d. Calculate cell b by subtraction.

Step 6: You now can calculate PPVs and NPVs for the test with the prevalence (pretest probability) used.

For example, to calculate the PPV for test A in the diagnosis of disease in women older than 65 years of age with a suspicious finding on clinical examination, use the following equation:

Prevalence = 40,000 cases/100,000 = 400/1000
Setting the total number equal to 1000,
$$(a + c)/(a + b + c + d) = 400/1000$$

Therefore $a + c = 400$ and $b + d = 600$.

Thus
$$\text{Cell a} = \text{Sensitivity} \times 400 = 0.8 \times 400 = 320$$
and
$$\text{Cell c} = 400 - 320 = 80$$

Similarly,
$$\text{Cell d} = \text{Specificity} \times 600 = 0.9 \times 600 = 540$$

Therefore
$$\text{Cell b} = 600 - 540 = 60$$
$$\text{PPV} = a/(a + b) = 320/(320 + 60) = 84.2\%$$

Similar calculations can be made for the general population (prevalence = 50/100,000) and for women older than age 50 years (prevalence = 500/100,000).

10. a. If the PPV of a test for a given disease is 4%, then only 4 of 100 positive test results will be TPs; the remainder will be FPs. Further testing (often invasive) and anxiety will be inflicted on the 96% of the population with a positive test result but without disease.

Thus careful consideration should be given to the PPV of any test for any disease in a given population before ordering it.

11. e. Remember the inverse relationship between sensitivity and specificity: if the sensitivity goes down, the specificity goes up, and if the sensitivity goes up, the specificity goes down. The only value that is greater than the previous specificity of 99.4% is 100%; therefore it is the most likely correct value of the values listed for the specificity of the test. The value in the table is actually the case at a cutoff blood sugar level of 180 mg/100 ml 2 hours after eating; if we use this value for the cutoff, there will be even more false-negative results than at 140 mg/100 ml (that is, we will incorrectly label more individuals who actually have diabetes as being normal), whereas we will not label anyone who does not have diabetes as having diabetes.

12. d. Validity is the degree to which the results of a measurement of a test actually correspond to the true state of the phenomenon being measured.

13. a. Reliability is the extent to which repeated measurements of a relatively stable phenomenon fall closely to each other. *Reproducibility* and *precision* are other words for this characteristic.

14. d. A normal, or Gaussian, distribution is characterized by the following measures of central tendency: (1) a mean: the sum of values for observations divided by the number of observations; (2) a median: the value point where the number of observations above equals the number of observations below; and (3) a mode: the most frequently occurring value.

In the same normal, or Gaussian, distribution, expressions of dispersion are the following: (1) the range: from the lowest value to the highest value in a distribution; (2) the standard deviation: the absolute value of the average difference of individual values from the mean; and (3) the percentile: the proportion of all observations falling between specified values.

The most valuable measure of dispersion in a normal, or Gaussian, distribution is the standard deviation (SD). It is defined as follows:

$$SD = \frac{\sqrt{\Sigma x - x^2}}{n - 1}$$

In a normal, or Gaussian, distribution 68.26% of the values lie within ±1 SD from the mean, 95.44% of values lie within ±2 SD from the mean, and 99.72% of values lie within ±3 SD from the mean.

15. b. As can be seen in this trial, there was a progressive and substantial decrease in mean blood pressure between the first and third visits. The explanation for this is called *regression to the mean.* The following is the best explanation of regression to the mean.

Patients who are singled out from others because they have a laboratory test that is unusually high or low can be expected, on the average, to be closer to the center of the distribution (normal, or Gaussian) if the test is repeated. Moreover, subsequent values are likely to be more accurate estimates of the true value (validity), which could be obtained if the measurement were repeated for a particular patient many times.

16. c. This is an example of lead-time bias. Lead time is the period between the detection of a medical condition by screening and when it ordinarily would have been diagnosed as a result of symptoms.

In lung cancer there is absolutely no evidence that chest x-rays have any influence on mortality. However, if, as in this case, the experimental group had chest x-rays done, their lung cancers would have been diagnosed at an earlier time and it would appear that they were longer survivors. The control group most likely would have had their lung cancers diagnosed when they developed symptoms. In fact, however, the survival time would have been exactly the same; the only difference would have been that men in the experimental group would have known that they had lung cancer for a longer period.

17. a. Length-time bias occurs because the proportion of slow-growing lesions diagnosed during a cancer screening program is greater than the proportion of those diagnosed during usual medical care. The effect of including a greater number of slow-growing cancers makes it seem that the screening and early treatment programs are more effective than they really are.

18. a. Prevalence is defined as the fraction (proportion) of a population with a clinical condition at a given point in time. Prevalence is measured by surveying a defined population in which some patients have and some patients do not have the condition of interest at a single point in time. It is not the same as incidence, and, as previously discussed in relation to sensitivity, specificity, and PPV in a 2 × 2 table, it is defined in mathematic terms as $a + c/(a + b + c + d)$.

19. b. Incidence in relation to a population is defined as the fraction (proportion) initially free of a disease or condition that go on to develop it over a given period. Commonly, it is known as the number of new cases per population in a given time, often per year.

20. e. Clinical epidemiology is a specialty that will assume increasingly more importance in the specialty of family practice. Clinical epidemiology allows us to understand disease, to understand laboratory testing, and to understand why we should do what we should do and why we should not do what we should not do. More importantly, as family physicians are called on by governments, patients, licensing bodies, and boards to justify clinical decisions and treatments, it will allow us to understand the difference between "defensive" medicine and defensible medicine (the latter being what we are trying to achieve) in the interest of optimizing the health care of patients.

SUMMARY OF FUNDAMENTAL EPIDEMIOLOGY

1. Remember the importance of sensitivity, specificity, and especially PPV; understand that the lower the prevalence (or likelihood) of a condition in the patient about to be tested, the lower the PPV of the test. In outpatient, low-prevalence situations, NPV is often more useful, if it is known.
2. Understand the importance of false-negative results and especially false-positive results in the laboratory tests that you order.
3. Be prepared to draw a 2×2 table and calculate the PPV of a test given the sensitivity, specificity, and prevalence of the condition in the population.
4. Misinterpretations that may result in survival statistics in cancer are caused by lead-time bias and length-time bias.

5. Apply the principle of regression to the mean in the diagnosis of certain conditions, hypertension being a prime example.
6. Remember the dictum *primum non nocere:* first do no harm.
7. Sensitivity and specificity are inversely related: as sensitivity of a test goes up, the specificity of the test goes down.
8. Sensitive tests should be used to rule out disease; specific tests should be used to rule in disease.
9. Although a test may be reliable, it may not have any validity.
10. Remember the definition of a normal patient: someone who has not been sufficiently investigated.

SUGGESTED READING

Jekel JF, et al: *Epidemiology, Biostatistics and Preventive Medicine,* Philadelphia, 2001, Saunders.
Oleske DM: *Epidemiology and the delivery of healthcare services: methods and applications,* New York, 2001, Kluwer Academic/Plenum Publishers.
Rothman KJ: *Epidemiology: an Introduction,* New York, 2002, Oxford University Press.

Chapter 3

Physician Intervention in Smoking Cessation

"My father lived to be 90 years old, and he smoked like a chimney. Why should I quit?"

CLINICAL CASE PROBLEM 1:
A 40-Year-Old Who Smokes Three Packs of Cigarettes a Day

A 40-year-old executive who smokes three packs of cigarettes a day comes to your office for his routine health maintenance assessment. He states that he would like to quit smoking but is having great difficulty. He has tried three times before, but he says, "Pressures at work mounted up and I just had to go back to smoking."

The patient has a history of mild hypertension. His blood cholesterol level is normal. He drinks 1 or 2 ounces of alcohol per week. His family history is significant for premature cardiovascular disease and death.

SELECT THE BEST ANSWER TO THE FOLLOWING QUESTIONS:

1. Current evidence suggests that coronary artery disease (CAD) is strongly related to cigarette smoking. What percentage of deaths from CAD is thought to be directly related to cigarette smoking?
   a. 5%
   b. 10%
   c. 20%
   d. 25%
   e. 30% to 40%

2. Which of the following diseases has not been linked to cigarette smoking?
   a. carcinoma of the larynx
   b. hypertension
   c. abruptio placenta
   d. carcinoma of the colon
   e. Alzheimer's disease

3. Which of the following statements with respect to passive smoking is false?

a. spouses of patients who smoke are not at increased risk of developing carcinoma of the lung
b. sidestream smoke contains more carbon monoxide than mainstream smoke
c. infants of mothers who smoke absorb measurable amounts of their mothers' cigarette smoke
d. children of parents who smoke have an increased prevalence of bronchitis and pneumonia
e. the most common symptom arising from passive smoking is eye irritation

4. Of the following factors listed, which is the most important factor in determining the success of a smoking cessation program in an individual?
a. the desire of the patient to quit smoking
b. a pharmacologic agent as a part of the smoking cessation program
c. the inclusion of a behavior-modification component to the program
d. physician advice to quit smoking
e. repeated office visits

5. Which of the following agents now is (are) considered first-line pharmacologic agent(s) that reliably increase long-term smoking abstinence rates?
a. bupropion SR
b. nicotine gum
c. nicotine inhalers or nasal sprays
d. nicotine patch
e. all of the above

6. Which of the following smoking cessation methods results in the highest percentage of both short-term and long-term success?
a. transdermal nicotine
b. a patient education booklet
c. physician counseling and advice
d. a contract for a "quit date"
e. a combination of all of the above

7. One of the best individual targeted smoking cessation programs is the widely recommended 5 A's approach (*Ask, Advise, Assess, Assist,* and *Arrange*) designed to help the smoker who is willing to quit. Which of the following is true about this approach?
a. the approach includes implementation of an officewide system that ensures that, for every patient at every visit, tobacco-use status is queried and documented
b. smokers should be approached intermittently and gently to avoid provoking anger
c. smokers from households with other smokers present should be advised to change domiciles

d. the approach fosters self-reliance without the support of any outside organizations or individuals
e. the use of pharmacotherapy is reserved for counseling failures

8. What is the approximate percentage of patients who relapse following successful cessation of smoking?
a. 10%
b. 50%
c. 75%
d. 85%
e. 99%

9. What is the most prevalent modifiable risk factor for increased morbidity and mortality in the United States?
a. hypertension
b. hyperlipidemia
c. cigarette smoking
d. occupational burnout
e. alcohol consumption

10. Nicotine replacement is especially important in which group of patients who smoke cigarettes?
a. those patients who smoke when work-related stressors become unmanageable
b. those patients who smoke more than 20 cigarettes a day
c. those patients who smoke within 30 minutes of awakening
d. those patients who experience withdrawal symptoms
e. all of the above
f. b, c, and d

11. Which of the following statements regarding the economic burden of smoking is (are) true?
a. the economic burden of smoking is placed not only on the individual but also on society
b. in the United States the costs related to cigarette smoking exceed $50 billion annually
c. smoking has a significant effect on work-related productivity
d. it would cost an estimated $6.3 billion annually to provide 75% of smokers ages 18 years and older with the cessation interventions of their choice
e. all of the above statements are true

■ **ANSWERS:**

1. **d.** Of deaths from CAD, 25% are directly attributable to smoking. The incidence of myocardial infarction and death from CAD is 70% higher in

cigarette smokers than in nonsmokers. In the United States 18% of all deaths are caused by cigarette smoking.

2. d. The health consequences of smoking are enormous. The major processes involved include active smoking, passive smoking, addiction, and accelerated aging. The following disease categories have been directly linked to smoking: cancer, respiratory diseases, and cardiovascular diseases. Pregnancy and infant health and other miscellaneous conditions also are affected by smoking.

The actual diseases involved include the following:
a. *Cancer*: (1) lung, (2) larynx, (3) mouth, (4) pharynx, (5) stomach, (6) liver, (7) pancreas, (8) bladder, (9) uterine cervix, (10) breast, and (11) brain
b. *Respiratory diseases*: (1) emphysema, (2) chronic bronchitis, (3) asthma, (4) bacterial pneumonia, (5) tubercular pneumonia, and (6) asbestosis
c. *Cardiovascular diseases*: (1) CAD, (2) hypertension, (3) aortic aneurysm, (4) arterial thrombosis, (5) stroke, and (6) carotid artery atherosclerosis
d. *Pregnancy and infant health*: (1) intrauterine growth restriction, (2) spontaneous abortion, (3) fetal and neonatal death, (4) abruptio placenta, (5) bleeding in pregnancy not yet discovered, (6) placenta previa, (7) premature rupture of the membranes, (8) preterm labor, (9) preeclampsia, (10) sudden infant death syndrome, (11) congenital malformations, (12) low birthweight, (13) frequent respiratory and ear infections in children, and (14) higher incidence of mental retardation
e. *Other miscellaneous conditions:* (1) peptic ulcer disease, (2) osteoporosis, (3) Alzheimer's disease, (4) wrinkling of the skin ("crow's feet" appearance on the face), and (5) impotence

The mechanisms whereby the linkage between smoking and the aforementioned diseases occur are multifactorial. What is striking, however, is the number of medical disease categories that smoking affects and the number of diseases within each category that smoking affects. Carcinoma of the colon has not been causally associated with cigarette smoking. It should be noted that research is being conducted with smoking and associated leukemia, colon cancer, and prostate cancer, and these too may prove to be associated with an increased risk.

3. a. Tobacco smoke in the environment is derived from either mainstream smoke (exhaled smoke) or sidestream smoke (smoke arising from the burning end of a cigarette). Exposure to sidestream smoking (also known as passive smoking) produces an increased prevalence of bronchiolitis, asthma, bronchitis, ear infections, and pneumonia in infants and children whose parents smoke.

The most common symptom arising from exposure to passive smoking is eye irritation. Other significant symptoms include headaches, nasal symptoms, and cough. Exposure to tobacco smoke also precipitates or aggravates allergies.

Spouses of patients who smoke are at increased risk of developing lung cancer and CAD. For lung cancer, the average relative risk is 1.34 compared to people not exposed to passive smoke. This risk, in comparison, is more than 100 times higher than the estimated effect of 20 years' exposure to asbestos while living or working in asbestos-containing buildings. It is estimated that of the 480,000 smoking-related deaths each year, 53,000 are associated with passive smoking.

4. a. The most important factor in determining the success of a smoking cessation program is the desire of the individual to quit. If the individual is not interested in quitting, the probability of success is very low. Physician advice to quit, behavior-modification aids, nicotine replacement, and repeated office visits are all important. However, without the will to quit, they will not be effective.

5. e. The first-line pharmacologic agents that may be considered for inclusion in a smoking cessation program are nicotine (delivered via inhalation, orally [via chewing gum], or transdermally) and bupropion (or bupropion SR, Zyban). The use of the antidepressant bupropion (Zyban) has proved to be effective in the treatment of cigarette smokers. The aim is to stop smoking within 1 to 2 weeks after starting the medication, with the duration of treatment between 7 and 12 weeks. This treatment modality helps address both the psychologic and physiologic aspects of smoking addiction. It acts by boosting brain levels of dopamine and norepinephrine, thus mimicking the effects of nicotine.

Second-line agents proved effective include clonidine and nortriptyline. Clonidine has proven efficacy in the relief of symptoms of opiate and alcohol withdrawal. It has been shown to be superior to placebo in helping patients remain abstinent from smoking for periods up to 1 year. Mecamylamine is a nicotine receptor antagonist that is analogous to naloxone for the treatment of opiate abuse. Mecamylamine may be useful as a method of smoking cessation in the recalcitrant smoker. It has not been studied extensively in such a population. Propranolol has been shown to relieve some of the physiologic changes associated with alcohol withdrawal–induced anxiety, but it has been shown to be ineffective in smoking cessation and has no effect on reducing subjective satisfaction and extinction of smoking behavior.

6. **e.** A meta-analysis of controlled trials of smoking cessation compared the effectiveness of smoking cessation counseling, self-help booklets, nicotine replacement, and establishing a contract and setting a quitting date. The study found that each modality was effective, but no single modality worked significantly better than the others. When treatment modalities were combined, however, the following results were obtained: two treatment modalities were more effective than one, three treatment modalities were more effective than two, and four treatment modalities were more effective than three.

7. **a.** The widely recommended 5 A's approach (*Ask, Advise, Assess, Assist,* and *Arrange*) is designed to be used with the smoker who is willing to quit. The following is taken from the helpful website "Quick Reference Guide for Clinicians Treating Tobacco Use and Dependence" at *http://www.surgeongeneral.gov/tobacco/tobaqrg.htm.*

Ask—Systematically identify all tobacco users at every visit. Implement an officewide system that ensures that, for every patient at every clinic visit, tobacco-use status is queried and documented. Expand the "vital signs" to include tobacco use, or use an alternative universal identification system such as chart stickers or an electronic medical record alert.

Advise—Strongly urge all tobacco users to quit. In a *clear, strong*, and *personalized* manner, urge every tobacco user to quit. *Clear*—"I think it is important for you to quit smoking now, and I can help you." Cutting down while you are ill is not enough." *Strong*—"As your clinician, I need you to know that quitting smoking is the most important thing you can do to protect your health now and in the future. The clinic staff and I will help you." *Personalized*—Tie tobacco use to current health/illness and/or its social and economic costs, motivation level/readiness to quit, and/or the impact of tobacco use on children and others in the household.

Assess—Determine willingness to make an attempt to quit. Ask every tobacco user if he or she is willing to make an attempt to quit at this time (e.g., within the next 30 days). Assess patient's willingness to quit. If the patient is willing to make an attempt to quit at this time, provide assistance. If the patient will participate in an intensive treatment, deliver such a treatment or refer to an intensive intervention. If the patient clearly states he or she is unwilling to make a quit attempt at this time, provide a motivational intervention. If the patient is a member of a special population (e.g., adolescent, pregnant smoker, racial/ethnic minority), consider providing additional information.

Assist—Aid the patient in quitting.

- *Help the patient with a quit plan.* A patient's preparations for quitting include the following: *Setting a quit date*—ideally, the quit date should be within 2 weeks. *Telling* family, friends, and co-workers about quitting and request understanding and support. *Anticipating* challenges to the planned quit attempt, particularly during the critical first few weeks. These include nicotine withdrawal symptoms. *Removing* tobacco products from the patient's environment. Prior to quitting, the patient should avoid smoking in places where he or she spends a lot of time (e.g., work, home, car).

- *Provide practical counseling* (problem-solving/training). Assisting patients in quitting smoking can be done as part of a brief treatment or as part of an intensive treatment program. Evidence demonstrates that the more intense and longer lasting the intervention, the more likely the patient is to stay smoke-free; even an intervention lasting fewer than 3 minutes is effective.

- *Inform them that abstinence is essential.* "Not even a single puff after the quit date." *Past quit experience (if any)*—review past quit attempts including identification of what helped during the quit attempt and what factors contributed to relapse. *Anticipate triggers or challenges in upcoming attempt*—discuss challenges/triggers and how patient will overcome them successfully. *Limit alcohol use*—because alcohol can cause relapse, the patient should consider limiting/abstaining from alcohol while quitting. *Talk to other smokers in the household*—Quitting is more difficult when there is another smoker in the household. Patients should encourage housemates to quit with them or not smoke in their presence.

- *Provide intratreatment social support.* Provide a supportive clinical environment while encouraging the patient in his or her quit attempt. "My office staff and I are available to assist you."

- *Help the patient obtain social support outside of treatment.* Help the patient develop social support for his or her quit attempt in his or her environments outside of treatment. "Ask your spouse/partner, friends, and co-workers to support you in your quit attempt."

- *Recommend the use of approved pharmacotherapy*, except in special circumstances. Recommend the use of pharmacotherapies found to be effective. Explain how these medications increase smoking cessation success and reduce withdrawal symptoms. The first-line pharmacotherapy medications include bupropion SR, nicotine gum, nicotine inhaler, nicotine nasal spray, and nicotine patch.

- *Provide supplementary materials. Sources*—federal agencies, nonprofit agencies, or local/state health departments. *Type*—culturally/racially/educationally/

age appropriate for the patient. *Location*—readily available at every clinician's workstation.

Arrange—Schedule follow-up contact. Schedule follow-up contact, either in person or via telephone. *Timing*—follow-up contact should occur soon after the quit date, preferably during the first week. A second follow-up contact is recommended within the first month. Schedule further follow-up contacts as indicated. *Actions during follow-up contact*—congratulate success. If tobacco use has occurred, review circumstances and elicit recommitment to total abstinence. Remind patient that a lapse can be used as a learning experience. Identify problems already encountered and anticipate challenges in the immediate future. Assess pharmacotherapy use and problems. Consider use or referral to more intensive treatment.

8. d. Arranging follow-up appointments for the patient is extremely important. This, in effect, prepares the patient for the support and surveillance of the physician. At the follow-up visits there is an opportunity to review concerns, review continuing plans, and discuss relapses. This last issue is extremely important because lapses occur in 85% of those who quit. The reaction and counseling of the physician following a lapse is crucial and should be framed in the context of a positive learning experience. One of the key points that needs to be reinforced by the physician is that learning to live without cigarettes is like learning any new skill—you learn from mistakes until your action becomes a new habitual behavior. Most patients take a few trials before they quit completely.

9. c. Cigarette smoking continues to be the most prevalent modifiable risk factor for increased morbidity and mortality in the United States. Not only does the smoker incur medical risks attributable to cigarette smoking, but passive smokers and society also bear the ill effects and the increased economic costs attributable to the smoker's habit.

10. f. Nicotine replacement is especially important for the following types of smokers: (1) smokers who smoke more than 20 cigarettes a day, (2) smokers who smoke within 30 minutes of waking up, and (3) smokers who experience withdrawal symptoms.

Smokers who smoke when exposed to extremely stressful work situations should be managed mainly by behavior-modification techniques, although bupropion may be a consideration for therapy.

11. e. The individual smoker and society in general incur enormous economic costs as a result of smoking. Here are some facts from the U.S. Public Health Service *Treating Tobacco Use and Dependence* Fact Sheet,

2000 (available at *www.surgeongeneral.gov/tobacco/smokfact.htm*). Surveys reveal that 25% of American adults smoke. More than 430,000 deaths in the United States each year are attributable to tobacco use, which makes tobacco the number-one cause of death and disease in the United States. Smoking prevalence among adolescents increased dramatically since 1990—more than 3000 additional children and adolescents each day become regular users of tobacco. Medical care costs attributable to smoking (or smoking-related disease) have been estimated by the Centers for Disease Control and Prevention (CDC) to be more than $50 billion annually in the United States. In addition, lost earnings and loss of productivity total at least another $47 billion a year, according to the CDC.

It would cost an estimated $6.3 billion annually to provide 75% of smokers aged 18 years and older with the intervention—counseling, nicotine patches, nicotine gum, or a combination—of their choice. This would result in 1.7 million new quitters at an average cost of $3779 per quitter—a move that would be cost-effective in relation to other medical interventions such as mammography or blood pressure screening.

Epidemiologic data suggest that more than 70% of the 50 million smokers in the United States today have made at least one prior quit attempt, and approximately 46% try to quit each year. Most smokers make several quit attempts before they successfully kick the habit. Only 21% of practicing physicians say that they have received adequate training to help their patients stop smoking, according to a recent survey of U.S. medical school deans published in the *Journal of the American Medical Association*. The majority of medical schools do not require clinical training in smoking cessation techniques. It is hoped that this guideline will serve as a call to action.

SUMMARY OF PHYSICIAN INTERVENTION IN SMOKING CESSATION

1. Identify all patients in your practice who smoke. The biggest mistake is failing to screen all patients to identify smokers. Refamiliarize yourself with the 5As approach reviewed in answer 7 above.
2. Assess the patient's readiness to change. Present all the health consequences of smoking.
3. Present the health benefits of smoking cessation.
4. Assess and develop the desire to modify smoking behavior.

5. Develop and formalize a patient-centered plan for change.
6. Establish a quitting date, and have the patient sign a contract.
7. Use transdermal nicotine or bupropion as an adjunct to counseling
8. Use behavior-modification techniques as part of counseling and advice. Have the patient keep a journal of at-risk times for smoking.
9. Consider using any and all available patient education booklets or websites from the American Lung Association (www.lungusa.org), the American Cancer Society (www.cancer.org), the American Academy of Family Physicians (www.aafp.org), the National Institutes of Health (www.nih.gov), or the Agency for Healthcare Research and Quality (www.ahrq.gov). Establish a quit date and a contract; advise and counsel the patient at regular intervals, and incorporate behavior-modification techniques; try to enlist family and workplace supports.
10. Have the patient consider times at which he or she may relapse (which will happen in 85% of patients); for example, triggers such as having a drink with friends at the end of a stressful week should be avoided for the first few months.
11. Continue surveillance for relapse prevention and plan modifications as needed. Identify alternative behaviors such as chewing gum, projects to use their hands, or a walking program.
12. Establish a reward system (i.e., take a trip with all the money you saved from no longer smoking).

SUGGESTED READING

Brosky G: Smoking cessation counseling: A practical protocol, *Can J CME* 43-60, 1994.
Healthy People 2010, chapter 27: Tobacco Use.
Jayanthi V, et al: Smoking and prevention, *Respir Med* 85:179-183, 1991.
Fiore MC, et al. *Treating Tobacco Use and Dependence.* Quick Reference Guide for Clinicians. Rockville, MD: U.S. Department of Health and Human Services. Public Health Service. October 2000.
Kottke T, et al: Attributes of successful smoking cessation interventions in medical practice, *JAMA* 259:2882, 1988.
The Agency for Health Care Policy and Research Smoking Cessation Clinical Practice Guideline, *JAMA* 275:1270-1280, 1996.
Agency for Healthcare Research and Quality at www.ahrq.gov.
National Institutes of Health at www.nih.gov.

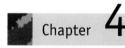 Chapter 4

Trends in Cancer Epidemiology

"Hell, Doctor! It seems like everything causes cancer so why worry?"

CLINICAL CASE PROBLEM 1:

A 74-Year-Old Farmer with Abdominal Pain

A 74-year-old grain farmer comes to your office for assessment of abdominal pain of 6 months' duration. The pain is located in the central abdomen with radiation through to the back. It is a dull, constant pain with no significant aggravating or relieving factors. It is not affected in any way by food. It is rated by the patient as a 5/10 baseline with occasional increases to 7/10. It has been getting worse for the last 2 months.

On examination, the abdomen is scaphoid. There is the suggestion of hepatomegaly, with the liver palpated 4 cm below the right costal margin. No other masses are felt.

Abdominal ultrasound reveals a solid mass lesion in the area of the head of the pancreas measuring 4 cm. There are also two or three small densities (<1 cm) in the liver.

■ SELECT THE BEST ANSWER TO THE FOLLOWING QUESTIONS:

1. What is the most likely diagnosis in this patient?
   a. benign pseudocyst of the pancreas
   b. adenocarcinoma of the pancreas
   c. squamous cell carcinoma of the pancreas
   d. pancreatitis
   e. malignant pseudocyst of the pancreas

2. With regard to the diagnosis in this patient, which of the following statements is true?
   a. the incidence of this disease has remained constant during the last 10 years in the United States
   b. the death rate from this disease has decreased significantly during the last 10 years in the United States
   c. the survival rate from this disease has increased greatly during the last 10 years in the United States
   d. there are no accurate data on death rates from this disease in the United States for the last 10 years
   e. none of the above is true

3. With regard to cancer mortality in the United States during the last 20 years, which of the following statements is true?

a. during the last 20 years, the death rate from all cancers has decreased significantly in children
b. during the last 20 years, the death rate from prostate cancer has increased by 20%
c. during the last 20 years, there has been no significant change in the death rate from lung cancers
d. during the last 20 years, the death rate from all cancers has increased by 20%
e. during the last 20 years, the death rate from breast cancer has increased by 15%

4. Which of the following statements is true regarding the leading causes of cancer mortality in the United States?
   a. the leading causes of cancer death by site in men are lung, prostate, and colon
   b. the leading causes of cancer death by site in women are breast, lung, and uterine
   c. the most prevalent cancers in women are breast, uterine, and bladder
   d. the most prevalent cancers in men are lung, bladder, and colon
   e. African Americans have a lower death rate from cancers than white Americans

5. With respect to the statistics discussed in questions 3 and 4, which of the following statements is true?
   a. the number of cancer cases can be expected to increase because of the growth and aging of the population in coming decades
   b. a major cause of the recent decline in lung cancer mortality rates in women is an increase in smoking rates
   c. high colorectal cancer screening rates continue to counterbalance the effects of diet and lack of physical activity
   d. the epidemic of obesity is unlikely to have any effect on cancer incidence and mortality trends
   e. tobacco taxes have little effect on smoking initiation in adolescents

6. With respect to secondary prevention measures for cancer, which of the following is true?
   a. the use of screening tests for breast cancer is decreasing.
   b. the use of screening tests for cervical cancer is decreasing
   c. screening rates of at-risk populations for colorectal cancer remains low
   d. physician screening rates for tobacco use in patients are satisfactory
   e. lung cancer screening tests have been shown to reduce mortality

7. What is the leading cause of cancer death in women in the United States today?

a. breast cancer
b. colon cancer
c. lung cancer
d. brain cancer
e. ovarian cancer

CLINICAL CASE PROBLEM 2:
A 50-YEAR-OLD STOCKBROKER WHO WATCHES TELEVISION

A 50-year-old stockbroker with no first-degree relatives with cancer visits you for your recommendations on colon cancer screening. She has heard about colonoscopy from a celebrity on television but wants to know what the options are and what you think. She has heard of those stool tests, but thinks the idea sounds "icky." She asks you which test you are going to have when you turn 50 years old. You spend some time providing her with information regarding screening for colorectal cancer.

8. Which of the following facts regarding colon cancer screening is correct?
   a. the United States Preventive Services Task Force (USPSTF) recommends only two screening methods: fecal occult blood testing and colonoscopy
   b. patients should be informed that the risk of perforation or serious bleeding from colonoscopy is about 1 in 1000 procedures in the community
   c. colonoscopy has been proved to reduce mortality in large-scale screening trials
   d. colon preparation for colonoscopy involves the administration of two enemas before the procedure
   e. fecal occult blood testing involves virtually no preparation on the part of the patient

CLINICAL CASE MANAGEMENT PROBLEM

Discuss the preventive measures your patients may undertake to lower their risk of cancer from all causes.

ANSWERS:

1. **b.** The most likely diagnosis in this patient is adenocarcinoma of the pancreas. With the clinical history of progressive pain, the finding of hepatomegaly (which suggests liver metastases), and the finding of a mass lesion on ultrasound, the diagnosis is almost certainly confirmed. None of the other choices are reasonable. Pseudocysts do not show solid mass lesions. Squamous cell carcinoma does not occur in the pancreas. The history, physical findings, and

ultrasound findings are not compatible with a diagnosis of pancreatitis.

2. e. During the last 10 years, the incidence of carcinoma of the pancreas has decreased by approximately 1% per year. Age-adjusted mortality from this cancer has shown a slight decrease in the past 10 years. Nevertheless, pancreatic cancer remains one of the most lethal forms of cancer, with a dismal 5-year survival rate of approximately 3%.

3. a. During the last 20 years, the overall death rate from all cancers has decreased by 40% in children in the United States. The 15- to 44-year-old age group also has experienced a decrease but not as large. Older individuals have experienced an increased mortality from cancer during the last 20 years. Leukemia is the most common cancer among children ages 0 to 14 years, and it is responsible for approximately 30% of all cancers during childhood. Acute lymphocytic cancer is the most common form of leukemia in children, whereas cancer of the brain/other nervous system is the second most common. Between 1990 and 2000, lung and prostate cancer death rates deceased in men, as did breast and colon cancer deaths in women. Nevertheless, lung cancer mortality now surpasses breast cancer mortality in woman.

4. a. In 2000 there were 553,091 cancer deaths in the United States, accounting for nearly one-fourth of deaths in the country, surpassed only by heart disease. In men, lung cancer is by far the most common fatal cancer, followed by prostate and colon and rectum cancer. In women, lung, breast, and colon and rectum cancer are the leading sites of cancer death. Overall, men experience cancer death rates that are higher than women in every racial and ethnic group. African American men and women have the highest rates of cancer mortality. Asian and Pacific Islander women have the lowest cancer death rates, at approximately half the rate for African American women. For many sites, survival rates in African Americans are 10% to 15% lower than in whites. African Americans are less likely to receive a cancer diagnosis at an early, localized stage, when treatment can improve chances of survival. Cancer prevalence rates (excluding skin cancers) by site in men are highest for prostate, lung, and colon; in women (again excluding skin cancers) it is breast, lung, and colon, respectively. (See Table 4-1.)

5. a. The huge demographic shift occurring in the North American population is likely to yield increased numbers of cancer for the foreseeable future. Age is a risk factor for the development of cancer, but it is not the only one. Because of reduced cigarette consumption, we are beginning to see a reduction in lung

Table 4-1 Cancer Death Rates (Number of deaths each year)*

The statistics are for 1992-1999, adjusted to the 2000 U.S. standard million population and represent the number of deaths per year per 100,000.

Group	Both Sexes	Males	Females
African-American	267.3	369.0	204.5
White	205.1	258.1	171.2
Asian/Pacific Islander	128.6	160.6	104.4
Hispanic/Latino	129.2	163.7	105.7
American Indian/ Alaska Native	128.6	154.5	104.4

*Table from the American Cancer Society

cancer death rates, specifically in men. Annual per capita cigarette consumption peaked in 1963 and has been decreasing ever since. In turn, after a time lag of two decades, the lung cancer death rates in men peaked in 1990, with a consistent downward trend during the rest of the decade. The lung cancer death rate among American women, who in general began regular cigarette smoking about 20 years after men, increased until 1998 but may have begun to decrease in 1999.

Obesity is a risk factor for several cancers, including female breast (among postmenopausal women), colon, and prostate. There is a definite cancer link to smoking, a possible link to dietary fat and physical inactivity, and a definite link to multiple environmental carcinogens, all of which may play a role in the changing cancer epidemiology. Despite the protestations of tobacco companies, tobacco taxes are extremely effective in curbing smoking initiation rates in children and adolescents.

6. c. Screening rates remain low in most populations despite evidence of effectiveness of many interventions. Whereas mammography and cervical cancer screening rates are increasing, colorectal cancer screening rates remain low, despite the fact that effective methodologies exist. Death rates from lung cancer, especially among women, have increased significantly over the past 20 years. Yet many clinicians fail to perform the basic screen of asking about tobacco use in their patients. Despite the proliferation of physician and health industry advertising to the contrary, currently there is no lung cancer screening methodology that has been shown to reduce mortality.

7. c. Lung cancer is now the most common cause of cancer death in American women. This primarily is associated with the significantly increased risk as a result of smoking, as previously discussed.

8. The USPSTF recommends only that screening take place, not the specific method, which should be the patient's choice after a coherent discussion of the options available with the clinician. Fecal occult blood testing, sigmoidoscopy, and colonoscopy are all acceptable screening methods. Patients should be informed of all the risks and benefits and alternatives available. That would include the risk of perforation or serious bleeding from colonoscopy, which is between 1 in 1000 to 1 in 3000 procedures, as reported in several series in the literature. As with any procedure, risks are reduced by using a colonoscopist who performs a large volume of procedures. Someday, clinician-specific outcome rates will be public knowledge, but until then, family physicians must act as information gatherers for their patients. Although colonoscopy has not yet been proved to reduce colorectal cancer mortality in large-scale screening trials, the presumption is that it will. Several trials are under way. Colon preparation for colonoscopy is extensive; it involves the administration of cathartics the night before the procedure and restricting oral intake, both of which are sometimes difficult for the elderly. Fecal occult blood testing involves careful attention to dietary intake on the part of the patient to reduce false-positive and false-negatives results.

SOLUTION TO THE CLINICAL CASE MANAGEMENT PROBLEM

The most important preventive measures that your patients may undertake to lower their risk of cancer from all causes are: (1) Discontinue cigarette, pipe, and cigar smoking, or tobacco chewing; (2) Decrease the amount of alcohol consumed; (3) Decrease the amount of dietary fat, especially saturated fat; (4) Maintain a normal weight (to be accomplished by a decrease in dietary fat, a decrease in overall caloric intake, and an exercise program); (5) Decrease exposure to environmental carcinogens whenever possible (protect yourself when applying pesticides, herbicides, and related chemicals); (6) Avoid sun exposure without a sunscreen with a sun protective factor of at least 15 or greater; (7) Follow the USPSTF recommendations concerning the Periodic Health Examination.

SUGGESTED READING

For more information, visit the following websites:

American Cancer Society: http://www.cancer.org. (This site contains a wealth of information.)

Centers for Disease Control and Prevention's Division of Cancer Prevention and Control: http://www.cdc.gov/cancer.

Centers for Disease Control and Prevention's National Center for Health Statistics mortality report: http://www.cdc.gov/nchs/about/major/dvs/mortdata.htm

National Cancer Institute: http://nci.nih.gov (This site has it all, with useful information for clinicians, patients, and researchers.)

Surveillance, Epidemiology, and End Results homepage of the National Cancer Institute: http://www.seer.cancer.gov. (This site contains all data by a variety of different variables, many of which you can graphically manipulate.)

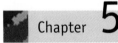

Chapter 5

Cardiovascular Epidemiology

> "Doctor, I'm an African American male. I smoke. I'm too fat. I have high cholesterol and uncontrollable hypertension. Are you going to tell me to write my will now?"

CLINICAL CASE PROBLEM 1:

A 52-YEAR-OLD MALE WITH CORONARY HEART DISEASE WHO HAS HAD BOTH A CORONARY ARTERY BYPASS GRAFTING PROCEDURE AND PERCUTANEOUS TRANSLUMINAL ANGIOPLASTY PROCEDURES DONE

A 52-year-old male with a history of coronary artery disease (CAD) treated by a coronary artery bypass grafting procedure following three percutaneous transluminal angioplasty procedures and who currently is undergoing "triple angina therapy" comes to your office for a discussion of his condition and of the implications of his condition for his children. He recently has read that family history is a strong risk factor for heart disease (HD).

■ SELECT THE BEST ANSWER TO THE FOLLOWING QUESTIONS:

1. Since 1979, cardiovascular disease mortality in women in the United States has:
   a. increased
   b. decreased by 30%
   c. stayed the same
   d. been exceeded by men
   e. decreased by more than 50%

2. Since 1979, cardiovascular disease mortality for men in the United States has:
   a. increased by 50%
   b. decreased
   c. attained parity with women
   d. increased by 20%
   e. remained unchanged

3. Which of the following regarding stroke epidemiology is correct?
   a. 50% of stroke deaths occur outside of hospitals
   b. stroke is the second leading cause of death in North America
   c. thrombotic strokes are more deadly than hemorrhagic or thromboembolic strokes
   d. age-adjusted death rates are lower in African Americans than other groupings
   e. Latinos have a higher age-adjusted death rate than other populations

4. What has been the major reason for the decline in the death rate from cardiovascular disease in the United States?
   a. new technology
   b. improved pharmacology
   c. better surgical techniques
   d. risk-factor reduction
   e. nobody really knows for sure

5. The risk of developing cardiovascular disease in patients with hypertension compared with patients who do not have hypertension is
   a. three to four times as high for HD and seven times as high for stroke
   b. twice as high for HD and five times as high for stroke
   c. six times as high for HD and eight times as high for stroke
   d. the same for HD and twice as high for stroke
   e. the same for HD and the same for stroke

6. Regarding cigarette smoking and the risk of developing HD, which of the following statements is true?
   a. cigarette smokers have a 70% greater risk of developing HD than nonsmokers
   b. cigarette smokers have a 50% greater risk of developing HD than nonsmokers
   c. cigarette smokers have a 25% greater risk of developing HD than nonsmokers
   d. cigarette smokers have a 10% greater risk of developing HD than nonsmokers
   e. there is no difference in the risk of developing HD between smokers and nonsmokers

7. Regarding cigarette smoking, which of the following statements is true?
   a. the risk of HD is increased by up to 30% for those nonsmokers exposed to workplace or at-home environmental tobacco smoke
   b. smoking costs Americans approximately $20 billion in medical care per year
   c. after quitting, smokers' HD risk drops by 50% after 10 years
   d. there is a direct correlation between smoking and education levels
   e. since 1969 prevalence of smoking has increased by 20%

8. Regarding serum cholesterol and the incidence of HD, which of the following statements is true?
   a. for each 1% reduction in serum cholesterol there is a 6% reduction in the risk of heart disease death
   b. for each 1% reduction in serum cholesterol there is a 4% reduction in the risk of heart disease death
   c. for each 1% reduction in serum cholesterol there is a 2% reduction in the risk of heart disease death
   d. for each 1% reduction in serum cholesterol there is a 1% reduction in the risk of heart disease death
   e. there is no established relationship between serum cholesterol and the risk of heart disease death

9. Regarding the risk of obesity in relation to cardiovascular disease, which of the following statements is (are) true?
   a. obesity is a risk factor for hypertension
   b. obesity is a risk factor for hypercholesterolemia
   c. obesity is a risk factor for diabetes
   d. obesity is an independent risk factor for HD
   e. all of the above statements are true

10. What is the definition of obesity?
    a. a weight 40% higher than normal weight for height
    b. a weight 30% higher than normal weight for height
    c. a weight 20% higher than normal weight for height
    d. a weight 15% higher than normal weight for height
    e. a weight 10% higher than normal weight for height

11. Body mass index (BMI) is defined as which of the following?

a. the weight in pounds divided by the square of the height in meters
b. the weight in kilograms divided by the square of the height in meters
c. the square of the height in meters divided by the weight in pounds
d. the square of the height in meters divided by the weight in kilograms
e. none of the above

12. With respect to physical inactivity (sedentary lifestyle) and the risk of cardiovascular disease, which of the following statements is (are) true?
a. sedentary lifestyle is an independent risk factor for cardiovascular disease
b. sedentary lifestyle is associated with an increased death rate from cardiovascular disease
c. sedentary lifestyle may be as strong a risk factor for cardiovascular disease as several other risk factors combined
d. sedentary lifestyle is strongly correlated with obesity
e. all of the above statements are true

13. What is the estimated percentage of Americans with hypertension whose blood pressure is under good control?
a. 50%
b. 75%
c. 25%
d. 10%
e. 5%

14. With respect to primary prevention of hypertension, all except which of the following are proven to be effective?
a. weight loss
b. reduced dietary sodium intake
c. moderation of alcohol intake
d. increased physical activity
e. calcium supplementation

15. Which of the following statements regarding the primary prevention of hypertension is true?
a. the demonstrated reductions in blood pressure using lifestyle changes can be as large as those seen in pharmacotherapy
b. lifestyle changes more effectively reduce blood pressure levels in males than in females
c. blood pressure reductions as a result of lifestyle changes are sustained for an average of 6 to 12 months
d. sodium added to processed food counts for an average of 20% of daily dietary sodium intake

e. suburbanization of living patterns in the United States has no linkage to hypertension epidemiology

ANSWERS:

1. a. Since 1979 the cardiovascular disease mortality rate for women in the United States has increased from 470,000 deaths per year to more than 500,000.

2. b. Since 1979 the cardiovascular disease mortality rate for men in the United States has decreased from 500,000 deaths per year to approximately 440,000.

3. a. Of stroke deaths, 50% occur outside of hospitals. Most patients do not make it to health care. That is why the first few hours, when thrombolytic therapy can be administered to nonhemorrhagic stroke victims, are so important. Stroke is the third leading cause of death in North America, after heart disease and cancer. Thrombotic strokes are less deadly than hemorrhagic or thromboembolic strokes, but they are more common. Age-adjusted death rates from stroke are higher in African Americans than in other groupings. In 1998 Latinos had the lowest age-adjusted death rate from stroke (19/100,000). Between 1950 and 1989 the death rate from stroke decreased by about 50%, but since 1990 there has been minimal further reduction.

4. d. The major reasons for the significant decrease in cardiovascular mortality in the United States are changes in lifestyle and risk-factor reduction. Other contributing reasons include new technology, improved pharmacology, better surgical techniques, and more effective medical managements.

5. a. Americans with hypertension have three to four times the risk of developing HD and as much as seven times the risk of stroke as do those with normal blood pressure.

6. a. Cigarette smoking is a major risk factor for cardiovascular disease. Cigarette smokers are at increased risk for fatal and nonfatal myocardial infarctions and for sudden cardiac death. Smokers have a 70% greater HD prevalence rate, a twofold to fourfold greater incidence of acquiring HD, and a twofold to fourfold greater risk for sudden death than nonsmokers.

7. a. The risk of HD is increased by up to 30% for those nonsmokers exposed to workplace or at-home environmental tobacco smoke. Smoking costs Americans more than $150 billion in medical care per year and an estimated total of $350 billion in direct and indirect (e.g., time lost from work) costs per year. With numbers like these, which don't even begin to measure the human costs, it boggles the mind how politicians in the United States still can support tobacco farming subsidies year after year. After quitting, smokers' HD risk decreases by 50% after 1 year, making the rationale for quitting all the more potent. There is a relationship between smoking and education levels. They are inversely related—the higher the education levels, the lower the smoking rate. Tobacco sellers know this and target people of lower education levels with advertising. Since 1969 prevalence of smoking in the United States has declined by 40% in people older than age 18.

8. c. Elevated serum cholesterol levels are associated with an increased risk of HD. Epidemiologic work in this area has suggested that for each 1% reduction in serum cholesterol, there is an associated 2% reduction in the risk of death from heart disease.

9. e. Being obese is a risk factor for hypertension, hypercholesterolemia, and diabetes mellitus. It is also an independent risk factor for HD. Being obese and being physically inactive increase all risks.

10. c. The definition of obesity is a weight 20% more than expected (or defined as normal) for height.

11. b. BMI is defined as the weight of a person in kilograms divided by the height of the person in meters squared. Tables are available that allow the calculation of BMI to be made easily in the office.

12. e. Physical inactivity, or a sedentary lifestyle, quickly is becoming recognized as a powerful risk factor for cardiovascular disease. It is recognized as an independent risk factor for cardiovascular disease and cardiovascular death. There is mounting evidence that a vigorous exercise program, in fact, may counteract some or all other risk factors when it comes to both the cardiovascular death rate and the cardiovascular disease prevalence rate. Physical inactivity also is associated with being obese, and these two risk factors are additive.

Weight-reduction programs are rarely successful in the absence of a reasonable exercise program. Most authorities suggest that to make a significant difference to the cardiovascular system, aerobic exercise must occur daily and last at least 30 minutes per session.

13. c. The percentage of Americans with hypertension whose blood pressure is under good control is estimated to be no more than 25%.

14. e. Weight loss, reduction of dietary sodium intake, moderation of alcohol intake, and increased physical activity are all (level of evidence A or B) effective in the prevention and control of hypertension. Calcium supplementation, although effective in some studies, has not been proved to be effective in large population studies or randomized controlled trials.

15. a. Multiple studies have demonstrated reductions in blood pressure using lifestyle changes can be as large as those seen in pharmacotherapy. Yet most physicians largely continue to ignore this fact and fail to educate their patients about this or work with them to achieve success in lifestyle changes. Imagine the cost savings to us all if clinicians were as effective in helping to change people's behaviors as they are in prescribing pharmaceuticals. Blood pressure reductions as a result of lifestyle changes are equally effective in both male and female populations and in all ethnicities, races, and socioeconomic groupings. Moreover, blood pressure reductions resulting from lifestyle changes are sustained well beyond 3 years in most studies. Sodium added to processed food counts for an astounding average of 70% of daily dietary sodium intake in North America. This is why clinicians should encourage patients to pay careful attention to food labels. Dietary sodium reduction is linked directly to primary prevention of hypertension. Suburbanization of living patterns also has been linked to obesity epidemiology in the United States. Obesity is a risk factor in hypertension. With people becoming more dependent on the automobile even for basic activities of daily living such as eating lunch, physical activity levels have declined and obesity and hypertension have increased. Think of that the next time you go to buy a house.

SUMMARY OF IMPORTANT CONCEPTS IN CARDIOVASCULAR EPIDEMIOLOGY

1. There has been a significant decrease in cardiovascular mortality rates in the United States during the last 15 years; however, the mortality rate among women is increasing.
2. The major reasons for the decrease in cardiovascular mortality rates in the United States are lifestyle modification and risk-factor reduction.
3. Lifestyle modification, particularly weight loss and physical activity, are particularly important in efforts to further reduce cardiovascular mortality.

Continued

SUMMARY OF IMPORTANT CONCEPTS IN CARDIOVASCULAR EPIDEMIOLOGY—cont'd

4. Hypertension, hypercholesterolemia, cigarette smoking, obesity, and physical inactivity are all independent risk factors for cardiovascular disease.

5. A vigorous exercise program may be enough to counteract several other cardiovascular risk factors and prevent cardiovascular morbidity and mortality.

6. Death rates from stroke are significantly higher in African Americans than in whites.

7. Cigarette smoking is estimated to account for 40% of deaths from HD in Americans younger than age 65.

8. The U.S. Department of Health and Human Services has set a number of objectives, or targets for the year 2010. Many of these targets include a further decrease in modifiable risk factors for cardiovascular disease.

9. The continuing education of the American population with respect to what they can do for themselves to decrease risk from cardiovascular disease remains our number-one priority. Aggressive intervention with risk factors through lifestyle modification, education, and counseling will remain one of the greatest and most rewarding challenges for family physicians in the next century.

10. The demonstrated reductions in blood pressure using lifestyle changes can be as large as those seen in pharmacotherapy. Clinicians need to educate their patients of this fact and learn effective means of helping to motivate patients to achieve these changes. Proven measures include restricting dietary sodium, increasing daily consumption of fruits and vegetables, increasing physical activity, losing weight, and eliminating tobacco use.

SUGGESTED READING

American Heart Association: *Heart Disease and Stroke Statistics—2003 Update*. Dallas, TX, 2003, American Heart Association. (available online at www.aha.org)

Appel LJ: Lifestyle modification as a means to prevent and treat high blood pressure. *J Am Soc Nephrol* 14(7 Suppl 2):S99-S102, 2003.

Ebrahim S: Dietary fat intake and prevention of cardiovascular disease: systematic review. *BMJ* 322(7289):757-763, 2001.

Ginsberg HN, Stalenhoef AF: The metabolic syndrome: targeting dyslipidaemia to reduce coronary risk. *J Cardiovasc Risk* 10(2):121-128, 2003.

Hooper L, et al: Reduced dietary salt for prevention of cardiovascular disease. *Cochrane Database Syst Rev* (1):CD003656, 2003.

Nabel EG: Cardiovascular disease. *N Engl J Med* 349(1):60-72, 2003.

Newell SA, et al: A critical review of interventions to increase compliance with medication-taking, obtaining medication refills, and appointment-keeping in the treatment of cardiovascular disease. *Prev Med* 29(6 Pt 1):535-548, 1999.

Smith SC: The challenge of risk reduction therapy for cardiovascular disease, *Am Fam Phys* 55:491-498, 1997.

Chapter 6

Use and Abuse of Laboratory Medicine for Routine Screening

"Doc, I want you to run every test in the book. It can't hurt to have too much data, can it?"

CLINICAL CASE PROBLEM 1:
A 45-Year-Old Male Who Requests a "Complete Laboratory Workup"

A 45-year-old "high-powered executive" (self-described) comes to your office for "the old once-over." He further tells you that he would like you to perform "every test known to humanity." From the history and physical examination of this man, you construct the following problem list: (1) obesity (body mass index 36); (2) nicotine addiction (two packs of cigarettes per day); (3) workaholic (married to his work); (4) essential hypertension (last blood pressure was 175/95 mm Hg); (5) sedentary lifestyle; and (6) history of gouty arthritis.

You get the feeling that one day soon you will be testing his troponin levels and cardiac enzymes in the emergency department. You recall some of the basic principles regarding routine laboratory screening procedures—their usefulness, cost–benefit ratio, and positive predictive value.

SELECT THE BEST ANSWER TO THE FOLLOWING QUESTIONS:

1. On the basis of the information provided, what would you do next?
   a. order a complete battery of investigations to get rid of the patient
   b. order selected investigations
   c. tell the patient that you do not specialize in his type of problems and give him the name of one of your physician friends down the street
   d. discuss the advantages and disadvantages of screening for various conditions with the patient
   e. none of the above

CLINICAL CASE PROBLEM 2:

A 53-Year-Old Male with a Slightly Elevated Serum Bilirubin Value

A 53-year-old male comes to your office for his annual checkup. The following tests were performed: complete blood count (CBC), electrolytes, blood urea nitrogen (BUN)/creatinine, liver enzymes, proteins and fractionation of same, cholesterol (fractionated) and triglycerides, prostate-specific antigen (PSA), blood sugar, serum calcium, serum phosphate, and serum uric acid.

The patient finds out that one of his liver function tests (unconjugated serum bilirubin) is slightly elevated, and he starts to worry about it. His physician then orders an abdominal ultrasound, a computed tomography scan of the abdomen, a repeat liver enzymes test, a test for an enzyme deficiency, a hepatitis panel, and a consultation with a gastroenterologist. As the patient is waiting for these tests to be performed and waiting to see the gastroenterologist, he becomes more and more anxious. After he finally sees the subspecialist, the consultant states, "Well, I can't really find anything wrong. It's probably a mild form of Gilbert's syndrome of no consequence, but we probably should check it every 6 months."

2. Which of the following statements is (are) true?
   a. because of the number of laboratory tests ordered, there was approximately a 40% chance that a positive test result (if found) would be a false-positive result rather than a true-positive result
   b. the patient who was previously healthy has now lost that status because of anxiety-creating psychologic distress
   c. even after the testing and consultations are complete, the patient still may be worried (that is, his health is negatively affected) because of the rather nondefinitive remarks by the consultant
   d. the testing and consultation process was very costly in terms of patient health
   e. all of the above statements are true

3. The percentage of "routine" laboratory tests performed in asymptomatic persons that result in a change in management strategy is estimated to be which of the following?
   a. 0.3%
   b. 3.0%
   c. 13.0%
   d. 33.3%
   e. 63.3%

4. The measure of the ability of a test to discriminate between normal and diseased states is known as which of the following?
   a. the sensitivity of the test
   b. the specificity of the test

   c. the likelihood ratio (LR) of the test
   d. the positive predictive value of the test
   e. the negative predictive value of the test

5. Which of the following reasons is (are) justifiable for ordering a laboratory or radiologic investigation?
   a. screening
   b. confirmation of clinical findings
   c. disease treatment and follow-up
   d. patient and doctor reassurance
   e. all of the above

6. Which of the following questions is (are) important to ask before implementing a screening program for a particular disorder?
   a. does the current burden of suffering justify a screening program?
   b. has the program's effectiveness been demonstrated in a clinical trial?
   c. can the health care system cope with the screening program?
   d. will people who screen positive accept advice and intervention for the condition?
   e. all of the above are important

7. Which of the following is (are) possible disadvantage(s) of some screening laboratory tests?
   a. the direct costs of the tests
   b. the direct costs of physician visits at the time of screening or to discuss results
   c. the danger of the costs of being labeled as having a disease as a result of a test
   d. the direct costs of any consultant's fees when a patient is referred to him or her for evaluation following a false-positive test result
   e. all of the above

8. In many situations walk-in clinics do not maintain the fundamental principles of family medicine. Which of the following best explains the popularity of treatment at a walk-in clinic?
   a. convenient care
   b. comprehensive care
   c. compassionate care
   d. continuous care
   e. coordinated care

9. Which of the following appears to reflect the major focus of care at a walk-in clinic?
   a. primary prevention
   b. secondary prevention
   c. tertiary prevention
   d. acute, episodic care
   e. comprehensive preventive care

10. Which of the following statements regarding "routine" laboratory panel testing in asymptomatic individuals and the standard measure of quality of care (namely quality of adjusted life years [QALY]) best describe(s) the contribution of diagnostic laboratory services in this situation?
    a. "routine" laboratory panel testing in asymptomatic patients improves QALY
    b. "routine" laboratory panel testing in asymptomatic patients decreases QALY
    c. in a randomized asymptomatic population where 50% receive "routine" panel testing and 50% did not, there was no difference in QALY
    d. in the same randomized asymptomatic population, a larger proportion of the "routine" laboratory screened group ended up in a hospital
    e. c and d

CLINICAL CASE PROBLEM 3:

AN ASYMPTOMATIC 55-YEAR-OLD MALE WHO PRESENTS FOR A PERIODIC HEALTH EXAMINATION

A 55-year-old man who had no symptoms was seen by a newly minted physician who wished to firmly establish the proper guidelines and protocols for practicing medicine. A thorough examination of the literature disclosed the following recommendations concerning screening of the male population older than 49 years with prostate specific antigen (PSA) for the detection of cancer of the prostate.
1. U.S. Preventive Services Task Force (USPSTF): insufficient evidence for or against routine screening (I recommendation).
2. American Cancer Society (ACS): recommended annually.
3. American Society of Preventive Medicine (ASPM) 1998 guideline: recommends against PSA for routine screening.
4. A certain American subspecialty association: annual PSA determination should be performed on all men older than age 50 years.
5. Canadian Task Force on the Periodic Health Examination (CTFPHE): D recommendation (not recommended)

11. Keeping the previously listed recommendations in mind, which of the following would you recommend for performing a PSA test for the man in Clinical Case Problem 3?
    a. follow the recommendation of the certain expert American subspecialty association; they are the experts, and they should know
    b. follow the recommendation of the ACS
    c. follow the recommendations of the USPSTF or the CTFPHE,

d. flip a coin: if heads, determine the level of PSA, and if tails, do not determine the level of PSA
e. forget the whole thing; this is far too complicated

12. *Screening* is defined as which of the following?
    a. any health service attempt to measure a variable that may be linked to primary prevention of a disorder
    b. any health service attempt to measure a variable that may be linked to secondary prevention of a disorder
    c. any health service attempt to measure a variable that may be linked to tertiary prevention of a disorder
    d. all of the above
    e. none of the above

13. *Case finding* is defined as which of the following?
    a. the presumptive identification of an unrecognized disease or defect by the application of tests, examinations, or other procedures in patients who happen to be in your clinical setting
    b. the presumptive identification of an unrecognized disease or defect by the application of tests, examinations, or other procedures in a non–health care setting
    c. the presumptive identification of an unrecognized disease or defect by use of a screening test among patients who are consulting the physician for unrelated symptoms
    d. b and c
    e. a and b

14. Which of the following laboratory tests is (are) indicated in an asymptomatic 49-year-old male who comes to your office for a periodic health examination?
    a. routine urinalysis
    b. routine CBC
    c. serum PSA
    d. nonfasting cholesterol
    e. a, b, and d

15. Which of the following laboratory tests is indicated in the periodic health examination of an asymptomatic 23-year-old female?
    a. serum urea nitrogen (BUN)
    b. serum creatinine
    c. serum glucose
    d. serum uric acid
    e. none of the above

16. For purposes of laboratory medicine and in recognition of the "zealous overtesting syndrome"

that many physicians seem to have acquired, a *normal patient* is defined as which of the following?

a. a patient who has had "the works"
b. a patient who has had all of the laboratory tests performed that he or she has specifically requested
c. a patient who has not been sufficiently investigated
d. a patient who has only had the absolute minimum number of tests performed
e. it all depends

CLINICAL CASE MANAGEMENT PROBLEM

As a primary care physician, you make extensive use of laboratory services. Discuss the difference between *defensive medicine* and *defensible medicine*.

ANSWERS:

1. Routine laboratory testing and the costs associated with same are increasing at an alarming rate. Although one individual test is not expensive, when taken together laboratory tests are responsible for an ever-increasing percentage of the total health care budget. There is no evidence that physicians' increased use of laboratory testing has improved the care of their patients. There is also no evidence to suggest an increase in QALY, a "gold standard" measurement for macro cost-effectiveness. The concepts of appropriate use of the laboratory at all levels of care is a clinician's patient-education responsibility that should be introduced and emphasized to patients.

2. e. Routine laboratory testing in asymptomatic patients rarely has anything to do with either quality of care or clinical practice guidelines. The most commonly cited reason for routine laboratory testing being performed on patients by their physicians is simply "because we have always done it."

Physicians are extremely concerned about "missing something" in their patients and thus tend to overinvestigate when there is no real reason for doing so. Many patients request or demand testing and will not be satisfied unless it is performed. What these patients seek is an absolute or objective form of reassurance that they incorrectly believe testing provides. The physician's responsibility is to educate themselves and their patients about the reliability, validity, predictive value, and proper place of testing in clinical decision making. Concepts relating to sensitivity, specificity, positive predictive value, and negative predictive value are detailed in Chapter 2.

3. a. The percentage of routine laboratory tests performed in asymptomatic patients that results in a change in management strategy is estimated to be between 0.3% and 0.5%. Thus 99.5% to 99.7% of routine laboratory tests are a complete waste of both time and money and may (as just illustrated) actually produce disease.

4. c. The LR is a measure of the ability of a test to discriminate between a normal and a diseased state. The LR ratio is the likelihood of finding a positive test result in a person with, rather than in a person without, the disease. The higher the LR, the more likely the disease is present if the test result is positive.

5. e. Screening for disease, case finding for disease, confirmation of clinical findings, and patient and doctor reassurance are all valid reasons for ordering a laboratory or radiologic investigation. However, the last reason (patient and physician reassurance) must be taken only so far. For example, if you believe that, by not ordering the test, the patient will suffer from significant anxiety and worry and the request is reasonable, you may choose to order the test. A good example of this would be a serologic test for hepatitis B in an unimmunized asymptomatic man who had unprotected intercourse with at least eight different partners in a 2-year period. However, limitations of the test must be explained regarding recent exposures, and patient education and immunization are more important than any reassurance a test may bring.

6. e. When trying to decide whether a screening program does more harm than good, you should consider asking the following questions: (1) Has the program's effectiveness been demonstrated in a clinical trial and was this trial double blind? (2) Are there effective treatments or effective preventive measures for the disorder? (3) Does the current burden of suffering warrant screening? (4) Is there a good screening test available (known sensitivity/specificity)? (5) Can the health care system cope with (afford in terms of financial and nonfinancial resources) the screening program? and, (6) will individuals who screen positive accept advice and intervention for the condition?

If you decide to perform a screening test, the following criteria also must be met: (1) the condition screened for must have a significant effect on the quality or quantity of life; (2) treatment for the condition must be available; (3) the condition should have an asymptomatic period during which detection and treatment significantly reduce morbidity and mortality; (4) treatment in the asymptomatic period should result in an outcome that is superior to delaying treatment until symptoms occur; (5) tests to detect the condition in the asymptomatic period must be readily available and affordable; (6) tests to detect the condition in the asymptomatic period must be acceptable to patients; and (7) there must be a high enough prevalence of the condition to justify screening.

7. e. There are many possible direct and indirect costs to the performance of laboratory tests for screening purposes:
   A. Direct costs of laboratory tests: (1) the direct cost of the laboratory test as determined by the laboratory charges; (2) the direct cost of the visit to the physician at the time the test is ordered or discussed; (3) the direct cost of any repeat laboratory test if an abnormal result is obtained; (4) the direct cost of additional laboratory and radiologic tests that are ordered because of the presence of one false-positive test result; (5) the direct cost of a referral to a consultant in the area of concern; (6) the direct cost of repeat and additional laboratory and radiologic tests that are ordered by the consultant; and (7) the direct cost of the repeat office visit to either the consultant or the family physician following the completion of consultant-ordered tests.
   B. Indirect costs of laboratory tests: (1) patient stress and anxiety caused by an abnormality found on routine laboratory testing; (2) patient stress and anxiety of waiting to complete the diagnostic testing and consultations; (3) patient's family stress and anxiety caused by the thought of what the diagnosis could be; (4) time lost from productive employment caused by physician appointments and waiting in physicians' offices; and (5) the possible inability to obtain life insurance or disability insurance following one abnormal and possibly erroneous result.

8. a. The walk-in clinic phenomenon has spread across North America like an epidemic. The reason that patients seem to seek treatment for health-related conditions in a walk-in clinic is, in most cases, convenience. Walk-in clinic use is geared, from a physician's perspective, to acute, episodic care rather than preventive medical care. Generally speaking, a walk-in clinic does not offer all the five "C" principles of family medicine, namely: (1) **C**ontinuous care; (2) **C**omprehensive care; (3) **C**oordinated care; (4) **C**ompassionate care, and (5) **C**ompetent care

9. d. Walk-in clinics are designed to provide acute, episodic care. Such provision of health care out of context from the patient's total health care needs often does not provide the patient with the holistic care required and in general is not cost-effective. Cost-effectiveness in the delivery of medical care services is a crucial issue for health care providers, health care consumers, and health care funders (government and private insurance plans, in particular).

10. e. Routine laboratory screening is, for all intents and purposes, completely devoid of any benefits to QALY. It, however, does result in a significantly higher percentage of people who end up in community and secondary care hospitals.

11. c. One of the reasons for significant confusion among physicians regarding "routine" and periodic laboratory test ordering is that there are many different and contradictory recommendations from different societies and organizations, as found out by this young physician. However, the most solid, evidence-based scientific sources regarding PSA screening are provided by the USPSTF and the CTFPHE. Rarely do these two important task forces disagree on any recommendation. Of course, always discuss conflicting recommendations with patients, and ascertain your patient's wishes in decision making.

12. b. See Question 13.

13. c. The distinction between screening, on the one hand, and case finding, on the other, is:
   • *Screening* is defined as the presumptive identification of tests, examinations, or other procedures that can be applied to a population. Screening tests sort out apparently well persons who have a disease from those who probably do not. A screening test is not intended to be diagnostic. Persons with positive or suspicious findings must be referred to their physician for diagnosis and treatment.
   • *Case finding* is defined as the identification by testing, following the clinician's search for disease, with screening tests among patients who are consulting them for unrelated reasons.
   The distinction between screening and case finding is subtle.

14. d. The only test that is indicated from those listed is the nonfasting cholesterol in a middle-aged male. This recommendation is made by the USPSTF and the CTFPHE.

15. e. Serum creatinine, BUN, serum glucose, or serum uric acid analyses are not indicated in the periodic health examination of an asymptomatic 23-year-old female.

16. c. Although somewhat tongue in cheek, it was suggested by the scientific editor of a prominent

North American family medicine journal that "a normal patient is defined as someone who has not been sufficiently investigated."

The point is that the zealous overtesting syndrome is a serious and costly problem. The major problem appears to be that physicians are not aware of the epidemiologic implications of overtesting. Epidemiologic principles will confirm that if 20 laboratory tests are done, there is a high probability that at least one of those will be abnormal and that most likely will be a false-positive result (99%). What happens from there, of course, really amounts to a wild goose chase. The goose is never caught, the patient (who was previously well) is now unhealthy because of worry caused by the condition, and the physician is frustrated (in not being able to diagnose something that is not there).

This could all be avoided if every time you ordered a laboratory test you asked yourself two simple questions: (1) Why am I doing this test?" and (2) "Is there a reasonable chance that the result of this test may change my patient management?" If the answer to the first question is valid and able to be substantiated by scientific evidence and the answer to the second question is yes, perform the test. If not, do not perform the test.

SOLUTION TO THE CLINICAL CASE MANAGEMENT PROBLEM

The major difference between defensive medicine and defensible medicine is:

Defensive medicine: A physician who practices defensive medicine practices in a manner in which he or she is afraid of possible litigation and thus orders every possible test (to avoid missing something, however esoteric). The problems with defensive medicine are as follows: (1) it does not offer you the protection you think it does; (2) it results in a pathway of decision making that has really nothing to do with hypothetic deductive or inductive reasoning; rather, it is really a blind shot in the dark with a tremendously big gun; (3) because of all of the false-positive test results that are generated, you end up spending most of your life chasing geese that you will never catch; and, (4) it is a tremendously expensive and wasteful process

Defensible medicine: A physician who practices defensible medicine practices medicine that is based on a sound approach to clinical reasoning and an inherent knowledge of the following concepts: (1) sensitivity; (2) specificity; (3) negative predictive value; (4) positive predictive value; and (5) prevalence

Each decision that the physician makes should be a well-thought-out, reasoned decision that could, with the help of a local epidemiologist, be defended from the point of optimal patient outcome.

The advantages of defensible medicine include the following: (1) improved quality of care; (2) improved physician and ultimately patient satisfaction (although the latter may be somewhat more difficult to attain); and (3) a sense of being in the"innovative group"of physicians who feel confident enough to believe in themselves and in their clinical diagnosis and clinical management.

SUMMARY OF USE AND ABUSE OF LABORATORY MEDICINE FOR ROUTINE SCREENING OF ASYMPTOMATIC PATIENTS

Estimate of abuse of laboratory medicine:
a. Conservative estimate of abuse: at least 50% of all laboratory tests performed in a primary care setting are unnecessary and cost-ineffective.
b. Estimates suggest that only 0.3% to 0.5% of all laboratory tests make any difference to the patient or have any chance of changing the patient's management.

Appropriate screening use of the laboratory:
a. Must follow the criteria described in answer 6.
b. Key questions: the following two questions must be answered in the affirmative or with a specific answer:
  i. "Why am I doing this test?"
  ii. "Is there reasonable chance that the result of this test will change my patient's management?"

Laboratory medicine and epidemiology:
a. Screening versus case finding:
  i. Screening: testing a non–self-identified population
  ii. Case finding: testing a self-identified population in a health care setting
b. Major epidemiologic concepts:
  i. Prevalence: the lower the prevalence in the population in question, the lower the positive predictive value and the higher the number of false-positive results

Continued

SUMMARY OF USE AND ABUSE OF LABORATORY MEDICINE FOR ROUTINE SCREENING OF ASYMPTOMATIC PATIENTS—cont'd

ii. Positive predictive value: the percentage of all positive test results that are actually true positives

Guidelines to follow (task force recommendations): the best guidelines to follow with respect to screening and case finding for all disorders are contained in the following two task force recommendations: the USPSTF and the CTFPHE.

The dangers of inadequate knowledge of the epidemiologic principles of effective laboratory testing:
a. The wild goose chase
b. The definition of a normal patient as a patient who has not been sufficiently investigated

c. The complete wasting of resources in an already difficult-to-manage (costwise) health care system
d. The creation of disease in patients who were previously well before their physician visit. In one controlled study of routine screening versus nonroutine screening, the only difference in the two populations was the excessive hospitalizations in the screened group. There was no effect on QALY.

SUGGESTED READING

Deyo RA: Cascade effects of medical technology. *Annu Rev Public Health*. 23:23-44, 2002.
Feldman W: On ordering tests, *Ann R Coll Phys Surg Can* 26(5):269-270, 1993.
Smetana GW, Macpherson DS: The Clinical Case Problem against routine preoperative laboratory testing. *Med Clin North Am* 87(1):7-40, 2003.

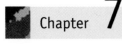

Chapter 7

Human Immunodeficiency Virus Infection

"Now with the discovery of these new drugs I can have sex with no worries, right?"

CLINICAL CASE PROBLEM 1:
A 24-YEAR-OLD MALE WITH GENERALIZED LYMPH-NODE ENLARGEMENT

A 24-year-old male comes to your office with a 2-month history of fatigue and intermittent fevers. On physical examination, his vital signs are stable, but the patient appears pale. He has significant cervical, axillary, and inguinal lymphadenopathy. The rest of the examination is normal. You ask more questions. He states that he is bisexual. He has a wife and one child but also has two other regular male partners. His human immunodeficiency virus (HIV) serology comes back positive.

■ SELECT THE BEST ANSWER TO THE FOLLOWING QUESTIONS:

1. Regarding the patient's positive test, the most appropriate next step is to:
   a. call him on the phone immediately to inform him
   b. schedule an extended visit for appropriate counseling
   c. send him a registered mail letter informing him of the results
   d. leave a message for his wife to call
   e. none of the above

2. You provide repeat confirmation of the serology and the appropriate counseling at the next visit. At this time, in addition to a CD4 count, what additional tests should be performed?
   a. a complete blood cell count (CBC) with differential
   b. serum creatinine, liver function tests, and lipid and glucose measurements
   c. hepatitis serologies and syphilis serology
   d. toxoplasma immunoglobulin G (IgG) and cytomegalovirus (CMV) IgG
   e. all of the above

3. The patient's CD4 count is normal, and serologies are normal. Assuming he has not received routine updates in more than 10 years, what immunizations are appropriate for this patient at this time?
   a. tetanus
   b. pneumococcal
   c. hepatitis A and B
   d. varicella
   e. a, b, and c

4. What prophylaxis should be considered in this patient, and at what time?

a. *Pneumocystis carinii pneumonia* (PCP) prophylaxis if the CD4 count <500 cells/mm^3
b. PCP prophylaxis if oral candidiasis develops
c. Toxoplasmosis prophylaxis if toxoplasma IgG Ab + and CD4 count <500 cells/mm^3
d. *Mycobacterium avium-intracellulare* prophylaxis if CD4 count <500 cells/mm^3
e. Tuberculosis (TB) prophylaxis if purified protein derivative (PPD) induration is >1 mm

5. Which of the following is (are) known possible routes of HIV infection?
a. sexual contact with an infected person
b. sharing needles with an infected person
c. perinatal transmission
d. transfusion with unscreened blood
e. all of the above

6. The spouse of the patient described in Clinical Case Problem 1 schedules an appointment to discuss preventive measures she should take around the house. Which of the following is (are) reasonable advice to give regarding households with an infected individual?
a. cuts, sores, or breaks on both the caregiver's and patient's exposed skin should be covered with bandages
b. practices that increase the likelihood of blood contact, such as sharing of razors and toothbrushes, should be avoided
c. gloves should be worn during contact with blood or other body fluids that could possibly contain visible blood, such as urine, feces, or vomit
d. casual contact through closed-mouth or "social" kissing of his children is not a risk for transmission of HIV
e. all of the above are reasonable recommendations

7. Which of the following is not a common life-threatening opportunistic infection in patients with acquired immune deficiency syndrome (AIDS)?
a. PCP
b. *Toxoplasma gondii* central nervous system (CNS) infection
c. *Cryptosporidium gastroenteritis*
d. *Mycobacterium avium* complex
e. none of the above

8. What is the most common malignancy associated with AIDS?
a. Kaposi's sarcoma
b. non-Hodgkin's lymphoma
c. primary lymphoma of the brain

d. acute lymphoblastic leukemia
e. Hodgkin's disease

CLINICAL CASE PROBLEM 2:
A 32-YEAR-OLD AFRICAN AMERICAN FEMALE WITH FEVER, LYMPHADENOPATHY, A RASH, AND PHARYNGITIS

A 32-year-old African American female comes to your office with a fever, lymphadenopathy, a rash, and pharyngitis. You have reasons to suspect that this patient has acute retroviral syndrome.

9. Which of the following signs and symptoms occur(s) with a frequency of greater than 50% in this syndrome?
a. diarrhea
b. myalgia or arthralgia
c. oral thrush
d. facial palsy
e. a and b

10. The rash associated with the condition described in Clinical Case Problem 2 is best described as which of the following?
a. linear streaks
b. bullae
c. confluent plaques
d. erythematous macular papular lesions
e. none of the above

CLINICAL CASE PROBLEM 3:
A 31-YEAR-OLD PATIENT WITH FULL-BLOWN AIDS

A 31-year-old patient comes to your office with a 10-day history of severe dysphagia. The dysphagia has been getting progressively worse, and the patient's oral intake is limited to liquids.

11. Based on the history, what is the most likely cause of this patient's dysphagia?
a. herpes simplex esophagitis
b. Kaposi's sarcoma of the esophagus
c. esophageal candidiasis
d. *P. carinii* esophagitis
e. none of the above

12. What is the most common cause of sight-threatening infectious disease in patients with AIDS?
a. cytomegalovirus
b. herpes simplex
c. cryptococcosis
d. toxoplasmosis
e. histoplasmosis

13. Reasons to perform plasma HIV-RNA viral load testing include all of the following except:
   a. to establish diagnosis
   b. to help decide when to begin antiviral therapy
   c. to assess drug efficacy
   d. to help decide whether to change therapy
   e. to assess a baseline viral load

CLINICAL CASE PROBLEM 4:
A 28-YEAR-OLD MALE WHO RECENTLY TESTED POSITIVE FOR HIV

A 28-year-old male comes to your office. He has recently tested positive for HIV but is asymptomatic. He wishes to discuss the pros and cons of early initiation of antiretroviral therapy with you. His CD4 T-cell count is less than 500/mm^3, and his plasma HIV-RNA is less than 10,000.

14. You tell him possible potential benefits of early initiation of therapy include all but which of the following?
   a. delayed progression to AIDS
   b. control of viral replication and mutation
   c. decreased selection of resistant virus
   d. potential maintenance of a normal immune system
   e. extended period of effectiveness of current antiviral therapies

15. You also counsel the patient in Clinical Case Problem 4 that the potential risks of early initiation of antiviral therapy include all but which of the following?
   a. quality of life reductions from adverse drug effects
   b. earlier development of drug resistance
   c. unknown long-term drug toxicities
   d. unknown duration of effectiveness of current therapies
   e. suppression of natural immune system response to infection

16. Neurologic manifestations of AIDS include which of the following?
   a. peripheral neuropathy
   b. meningitis
   c. encephalitis
   d. cognitive impairment
   e. all of the above

17. In the transmission of AIDS from mother to newborn, which of the following statements is (are) true?
   a. the baby may test negative and continue to test negative throughout his or her life
   b. only 20% to 30% of babies born to mothers who are HIV-positive seroconvert to an HIV-positive state
   c. HIV infection in infants and children has a better prognosis than HIV infection in adults
   d. all of the above statements are true
   e. none of the above statements is true

18. What is the test most frequently used to screen for HIV infection?
   a. CD4 T-cell count
   b. plasma HIV-RNA
   c. enzyme-linked immunosorbent assay (ELISA) test
   d. Western blot test
   e. none of the above

19. A 39-year-old male tests positive for HIV infection during a routine insurance medical examination. What should be your next step in testing?
   a. do nothing
   b. perform a repeat ELISA test for HIV
   c. perform an RNA viral load measurement
   d. perform a p-24 antigen level for HIV
   e. perform a CD4 T-cell count

20. Which of the following patient groups are considered at potentially higher risk for exposure to the HIV virus?
   a. men who have unprotected sex with men
   b. intravenous drug users sharing needles
   c. heterosexual females with multiple male sexual partners using nonbarrier protection
   d. a and b only
   e. all of the above

CLINICAL CASE MANAGEMENT PROBLEM

Discuss the general principles of HIV counseling and testing services in terms of the general goals and objectives and the important aspects of counseling patients before HIV testing.

ANSWERS:

1. **e.** This patient should have been counseled at the time testing was ordered, and an extended follow-up visit should have been scheduled at the time he was seen for testing. Giving information about a positive test over the telephone to the patient is inappropriate, and giving information to someone other than the patient is a violation of the patient's privacy and federal law. A wealth of information needs to be exchanged in counseling sessions. The patient's

understanding of HIV needs to be assessed, and patient education about transmission and prevention of further spread of the illness needs to take place. Information about our understanding of HIV, its prognosis, and treatment must be discussed. Referrals can be made to organizations that provide social and emotional supports. An inventory of the patient's resources should be taken, including gathering information about housing, finances (treatment is expensive), or family configurations and supports. Although the physician may not provide for all the patient's needs, he or she should be ready to make appropriate referrals. Ideally, a great deal of this exchange should have occurred during the visit when the decision was made to test for HIV.

2. **e.** Although appropriate tests are not completely agreed to by all, most would argue that there is reasonable rationale to check women who are serology positive and heterosexual men for the following: a CBC with differential, serum creatinine level, liver function tests, lipid values, glucose level, hepatitis serologies, syphilis serology, toxoplasma IgG, and cytomegalovirus (CMV) IgG. Men with positive serology results who have had multiple male sexual partners generally are positive for CMV, and a CMV IgG is not necessary in this setting. An ophthalmologist who has experience screening for retinal CMV and other opportunistic infections should evaluate patients with a CD4 count of <50 cells/mm^3. A PPD test for TB exposure should be obtained unless the patient previously has had a positive test result. A chest radiograph is reasonable, as is a Pap test in women.

3. **e.** All patients newly diagnosed with HIV infection should have their immunizations reviewed. Most patients should respond well to immunizations, if needed. Tetanus, pneumococcal, and (if serologically negative) hepatitis B vaccine are indicated. Patients who are infected with hepatitis B or C, have other underlying liver disease, or are at risk of hepatitis A because of work or travel should be immunized against hepatitis A. Although measle–mumps–rubella vaccine (MMR) has been given safely to many children with HIV, it and other live-virus vaccines, particularly varicella, generally are contraindicated. If highly active antiretroviral therapy (HAART) is to be given in the near future to a patient with a low CD4 count, consider delaying immunizations until after therapy has begun to improve the immune response. For patients who defer HAART treatment, immunization is appropriate even if severely immunosuppressed.

4. **b.** Providing prophylaxis against opportunistic infections is essential in the management of patients with HIV infection. As recommendations change, please visit the U.S. Department of Health and Human Services (USDHHS) website listed in the Suggested Reading section for the latest updates. As of this printing, the following recommendations are current. *Pneumocystis carinii pneumonia* prophylaxis is indicated for patients with any of the following: a CD4 cell count <200 cells/mm^3, oral candidiasis, or unexplained fever for >2 weeks. Prophylaxis against toxoplasmosis is indicated if the patient is toxoplasma IgG antibody positive and the CD4 cell count is <100 cells/mm^3. *Mycobacterium avium-intracellulare* prophylaxis is indicated if the CD4 cell count is <50 cells/mm^3. TB prophylaxis is given if the PPD induration is >5 mm with no history of previous treatment, if there is a history of a positive PPD without treatment, or if there is known exposure to an active case.

5. **e.** See answer 6.

6. **e.** All of these recommendations from the Centers for Disease Control and Prevention are reasonable pieces of advice to give the patient's spouse. Cuts, sores, or breaks on both a caregiver's and patient's exposed skin should be covered with bandages. Practices that increase the likelihood of blood contact, such as sharing of razors and toothbrushes, should be avoided. Gloves should be worn during contact with blood or other body fluids that could possibly contain blood, such as urine, feces, or vomit. Casual contact through closed-mouth or "social" kissing of his children is not a risk for transmission of HIV. Condoms should be used during sexual intercourse. Of course, the spouse should be offered and recommended to undergo serologic testing.

7. **e.** All the conditions listed are common life-threatening opportunistic infections in patients with AIDS. PCP is particularly common. The most characteristic symptoms of PCP are a dry cough, dyspnea, fever, and night sweats. The most characteristic signs are increased respiratory rate, acute shortness of breath at rest, rales or rhonchi heard in both lung fields, and a general look of ill health.

8. **a.** The most common malignancy associated with patients with AIDS is Kaposi's sarcoma. The characteristics of Kaposi's sarcoma are reddish/purplish skin lesions anywhere and complications including gastrointestinal obstruction causing nausea and vomiting, dyspnea from intrapulmonary lesions, or lymphatic system lesions causing lymphedema and swelling of the extremities. The second most common malignancy is lymphoma (usually non-Hodgkin's). The non-Hodgkin's lymphoma may occur as a

primary tumor in the CNS or as a primary non-CNS tumor (frequently beginning in the gut).

9. b. The most common signs and symptoms that occur with a frequency of more than 50% in acute retroviral syndrome are fever (96%), lymphadenopathy (74%), pharyngitis (70%), rash (70%), and myalgia and arthralgia (54%). Almost any other symptoms and signs are possible, but they occur at a much lower rate.

10. d. The rash usually is distributed on the face and trunk and sometimes is on the extremities including the palms and the soles. Mucocutaneous ulceration also can occur involving the mouth, esophagus, and genitals.

11. c. This patient, on the basis of the history alone, has esophageal candidiasis. This is a common opportunistic infection that often progresses from the pharynx to the esophagus. Although thrush that is limited to the pharyngeal area is well treated with a relatively simple remedy such as nystatin or clotrimazole, esophageal candidiasis should be treated aggressively. See Suggested Reading for current guidelines. Patients with esophageal candidiasis should be considered for maintenance therapy because of the significant risk of recurrence.

12. a. The major infectious disease that produces loss of sight in patients with AIDS is cytomegalovirus. Symptoms include blurring of vision or altered vision. Sight can be lost quickly with this disease.

13. a. Indications for plasma HIV-RNA testing include all of those listed except to establish a diagnosis. For this, an HIV antibody test (serology) generally is preferred. However, in the face of a syndrome consistent with acute HIV infection, the HIV-RNA viral load may be used to confirm the diagnosis if the HIV antibody test is negative or indeterminate.

14. e. Extending the period of effectiveness of current antiviral therapies is of doubtful benefit because of the possibility of resistance. Whereas all the others listed are potential benefits, many of these benefits need to be proved by further research.

15. e. Similarly, many of the potential risks need further study. However, a careful risk–benefit discussion should take place with all patients in whom early antiviral therapy is contemplated. Such discussion builds trust and keeps the patient informed of the realities of treatment.

16. e. Neurologic complications of AIDS include cognitive impairment, AIDS dementia, encephalitis, meningitis, primary lymphoma formation, and peripheral neuropathy. Peripheral neuropathy more often is associated with the treatment of AIDS (particularly nucleoside reverse transcriptase inhibitors) than the primary disease process itself.

17. d. The transmission of HIV infection from pregnant mother to infant is certainly not universal. Moreover, extremely effective prophylaxis exists and should be used. Nevertheless, it is extremely important that all health care personnel involved in delivery of the infant take meticulous precautions to avoid the transfer of blood and blood products to themselves. From the point of view of the newborn, several scenarios may occur.

- The transmission rate from a mother with HIV who has not received prophylaxis to infant is thought to be in the range of approximately 20% to 30%. Thus 70% to 80% of infants born to these mothers will not, even in the absence of prophylaxis, become infected themselves. They will continue to test negative for the rest of their lives.
- The prognosis for HIV-infection progression and the development of AIDS and AIDS-related complications is somewhat more favorable in infants than in adults, even in those whose mothers were not given prophylaxis. However, it may take up to a year for them to test positive.

18. c. HIV diagnostic testing is based on an ELISA test. This is the initial screening test. If a patient has a positive ELISA test, a confirmation test known as the Western blot routinely is carried out to confirm positivity.

19. b. A repeat ELISA screening serology should be done. If it is positive, confirm the results by performing a Western blot. See Answer 18.

20. e. High-risk behaviors include having unprotected sexual intercourse and sharing needles used for intravenous (IV) drug use. Groups historically at higher risk include men who have unprotected sex with men and IV drug users. Available data strongly suggest that the heterosexual female with many male sexual partners who uses nonbarrier methods of birth control is also at substantial risk. Such behaviorally associated risk factors are modifiable, which is why patient education is so important for the clinician to undertake.

SUMMARY AND SOLUTION TO THE CLINICAL CASE MANAGEMENT PROBLEM

Much has changed in the past two decades regarding the treatment and prognosis of individuals with HIV infection. The advent of protease inhibitors and other antiviral agents has meant that what was once a death sentence has been transformed into a problem of living with a chronic illness. Although drug resistance remains a problem, the focus has shifted to how to maintain health—in essence, secondary and tertiary prevention for those infected. Nevertheless, primary prevention should be the emphasis because in the long term it is far easier for society to prevent this illness than to deal with its consequences. Physicians have an obligation to support prevention of this illness in all its forms and to speak out for the compassionate care of those afflicted.

HIV counseling and testing are extremely important. HIV counseling and testing services are meant to achieve the following:

1. Provide an opportunity for individuals to determine their current HIV serostatus.
2. In a continued effort to avoid infection, provide behavioral counseling to prevent infection in those who are not infected. For those who are infected, provide counseling regarding prevention of transmission to others.
3. Help those who are infected to obtain appropriate services.
4. Help partners of infected individuals to receive proper preventive services.

Individuals have various degrees of understanding and knowledge about HIV transmission, testing, and risky behaviors. The physician should view all requests for HIV testing as an educational opportunity, an opportunity that cannot be missed. Among the important issues that all health care professionals associated with the counseling, testing, diagnosis, and treatment of patients with HIV face are sensitivity to sexual identity, sensitivity to culture, sensitivity to socioeconomic conditions, and an awareness of the individual's previous mental and physical conditions. The language used by the health care professional should be appropriate to the patient. An example of this last issue is the term *HIV-positive*. Frankly, patients who have the HIV virus see nothing "positive" about this at all.

Once risk factors have been identified, the decision to test for HIV seropositivity should be made by the patient. The physician has an ethical responsibility to explain the risks, benefits, and consequences of testing. Given the biologic, psychologic, and economic consequences of HIV disease, it is essential that the patient be made aware of the reasons for the test and the consequences of the test.

The following should be done before the test:

1. Ask the patient directly why he or she wants to be tested.
2. Explain the test. Explain the "window period." The body takes time to produce antibodies, usually 6 to 12 weeks. During this time the individual will continue to have negative test results.
3. Explain that positive ELISA and Western blot test results indicate that the patient has been infected. Also explain that sexual contacts need to be notified by the patient, the doctor, or the public health authorities. Requirements vary from state to state.
4. Clarify the difference between HIV infection and AIDS.
5. Discuss the benefits of testing.
6. Discuss the risks and disadvantages of testing, including insurance issues, false-positive results, false-negative results, and indeterminate test results.
7. Obtain informed consent before testing.
8. Discuss confidentiality and the circumstances under which the result must be disclosed by law or ethical obligation.

SUGGESTED READING

Estrada AL: Epidemiology of HIV/AIDS, hepatitis B, hepatitis C, and tuberculosis among minority injection drug users. *Public Health Reports* 117 Suppl 1:S126-134, 2002.

Kasten MJ: Human immunodeficiency virus: the initial physician-patient encounter. *Mayo Clin Proc* 77(9):957-62; quiz 962-963, 2002.

Watts DH: Management of human immunodeficiency virus infection in pregnancy. *N Engl J Med* 346(24):1879-1891, 2002.

NOTE: HIV management is rapidly changing. Stay up-to-date by accessing web-based information sources, including the following:

http://aidsinfo.nih.gov/guidelines (the U.S. Department of Health and Human Services/National Institutes of Health website with up-to-date treatment guidelines for adults and children)

http://www.cdc.gov/hiv/pubs/facts.htm (the CDC site with useful information regarding epidemiology and prevention)

http://sis.nlm.nih.gov/HIV/HIVMain.html (the National Library of Medicine special information services site with excellent links to everywhere and everything you might ever want to know)

http://www.hopkins-aids.edu (see the online educational resource: Medical Management of HIV Infection 2003, by Bartlett and Gallant, from the Johns Hopkins University AIDS Service)

Chapter 8

Influenza

Doctor, I was told the flu shot can cause Guillain-Barré syndrome. Why risk that in order to prevent ordinary, everyday, old-fashioned flu?"

CLINICAL CASE PROBLEM 1:
A 73-Year-Old Male with Fever, Headache, and Myalgias

You are called to see a 73-year-old boarding home resident with a 24-hour history of temperature of 103° F, headache, myalgias, cough, rhinorrhea, sore throat, and malaise. Seven other residents in the same boarding home have come down with similar symptoms. It is late winter, and there has been a significant outbreak of respiratory illness in the community. He has received no vaccinations in the previous 5 years. On examination, the patient appears acutely ill with fever, tachypnea, and tachycardia. The patient also has prominent pharyngeal erythema. There are a few expiratory rhonchi heard and intermittent bilateral rales in the lower lungs fields.

■ **SELECT THE ONE BEST ANSWER TO THE FOLLOWING QUESTIONS:**

1. What is the most likely diagnosis in this patient?
   a. influenza A
   b. bronchiolitis
   c. bacterial pneumonia
   d. septicemia secondary to an unknown focus of infection
   e. peritonsillar abscess

2. Which of the following investigations may be indicated in this patient?
   a. complete blood cell count (CBC)
   b. blood cultures
   c. chest radiograph
   d. all of the above
   e. none of the above

3. Which of the following statements regarding the influenza virus(es) is (are) true?
   a. influenza epidemics occur annually and are of major public health importance worldwide
   b. influenza viruses are subclassified as influenza A, influenza B, and influenza C
   c. excess morbidity and mortality are reported consistently during influenza epidemics
   d. all of the above
   e. none of the above

4. Concerning the use of antibiotics in influenza infection in the elderly, which of the following statements most accurately describes a high practice standard?
   a. no elderly patients with influenza should receive prophylactic antibiotics
   b. all elderly patients with influenza should receive prophylactic antibiotics
   c. in most cases of uncomplicated influenza the risk–benefit ratio favors withholding antibiotics
   d. basically, give the patient antibiotics if they ask for them; if they do not ask, do not give them
   e. nobody really knows for sure

5. What is the most common complication of the illness described in this patient?
   a. meningitis
   b. pneumonia
   c. serum sickness
   d. agranulocytosis
   e. brain abscess

6. Which of the following types of influenza is responsible for most of the world pandemics?
   a. influenza A
   b. influenza B
   c. influenza C
   d. influenza D
   e. influenza E

7. Which of the following is the drug of choice for treating the symptoms of the patient described?
   a. acetylsalicylic acid
   b. acetaminophen
   c. oseltamivir
   d. meperidine
   e. ibuprofen

8. What is the primary mode of transmission of the illness described?
   a. via blood and blood products
   b. oral–fecal contamination
   c. sneezing and coughing
   d. fomites
   e. kissing

9. What is the most reliable method for preventing influenza?
   a. gamma globulin
   b. alpha-interferon
   c. activated influenza vaccine
   d. inactivated influenza vaccine
   e. amantadine hydrochloride

10. Regarding influenza vaccine, which of the following statements is (are) true?
    a. influenza vaccine is effective only against influenza A
    b. the efficacy of influenza vaccine is approximately 95%
    c. influenza vaccine should be administered every 2 years
    d. the ideal time for administration of influenza vaccine is in the late spring
    e. none of the above is true

11. Regarding influenza vaccination, which of the following statements is (are) true?
    a. intramuscular (IM) influenza vaccination typically produces no ADRs (adverse drug reactions)
    b. the recommended dosage of the IM influenza vaccine is 0.5 mL for adults
    c. influenza vaccination reduces the severity of illness in vaccinated persons who become infected
    d. b and c
    e. a, b, and c are true

12. Which of the following statements regarding amantadine prophylaxis of influenza is (are) false?
    a. amantadine prophylaxis is effective against both influenza A and influenza B
    b. amantadine prophylaxis has been shown to reduce the duration of fever and other symptoms
    c. amantadine has been shown to reduce the duration of viral shedding
    d. amantadine prophylaxis is used in high-risk individuals in whom vaccine is contraindicated
    e. all of the above statements are false

13. Which of the following is (are) indicated for influenza prophylaxis?
    a. amantadine or rimantadine
    b. oseltamivir
    c. zanamivir
    d. a and b
    e. b and c

14. Which of the following groups should be considered for yearly vaccinations against influenza?
    a. healthy adults older than age 65 years
    b. children and adolescents receiving chronic aspirin therapy
    c. health care workers
    d. adults and children in chronic care facilities
    e. all of the above

15. Which of the following is (are) a contraindication(s) to influenza vaccine?

    a. history of asthma
    b. allergy to hens' eggs
    c. history of Ménière's disease
    d. low-risk people who developed Guillain-Barré syndrome within 6 weeks of receiving a flu shot
    e. b and d

ANSWERS:

1. **a.** This patient most likely has influenza A. Influenza A strains usually predominate in adults; influenza B strains tend to infect children. Bacterial pneumonia and a secondary septicemia may follow influenza, but at this time, with the history and physical examination reported, the most likely diagnosis is influenza. A very common symptom of influenza is a severe generalized or frontal headache, often accompanied by retro-orbital pain. Other early symptoms of influenza include diffuse myalgias, fever, and chills. Respiratory symptoms especially tend to follow the occurrence of the early symptoms. The term "flu" is used very loosely by both physicians and patients. Influenza consists of a set of symptoms that often can be used to differentiate it clinically from other viral infections. Nevertheless, because many viruses can cause symptoms like influenza, epidemiologic data are used in practice to help with diagnosis. Public health organizations gather viral cultures from sick individuals during times of high infection rates as a means to estimate influenza prevalence in the community. In children, the signs and symptoms of influenza are more subtle; they may appear simply as another upper-respiratory tract infection or "cold."

2. **d.** At this time, it would be very reasonable to perform a CBC, blood cultures, and a chest radiograph (CXR). The CXR is indicated because rales are heard in the lung fields. A CBC and blood cultures, along with the CXR, will rule out a secondary bacterial pneumonia, most often caused by *Streptococcus pneumoniae* and the bacteremia that may accompany it.

3. **d.** Influenza epidemics occur annually and are of major public health importance worldwide. The epidemics usually are associated with an antigenic drift, which may be limited, or with an antigenic shift, which is more extensive and can be more serious. The antigenic drifts (a shift in the hemagglutinin and neuraminidase antigens) in most cases provide the next year's challenge for public health practitioners. The antigenic shifts are responsible for the major "pandemics" that have occurred with influenza. They are also responsible for the major epidemics. Influenza epidemics and influenza pandemics almost always are associated with influenza A. Both

morbidity and mortality definitely are associated with influenza epidemics. This is true especially of the very old and the very young. Those with chronic disease are at even greater risk. There are three major influenza viruses, designated influenza A, influenza B, and influenza C. By far the most virulent and most significant is the influenza A virus.

4. **c.** In uncomplicated influenza viral infections, as in uncomplicated viral infections in general, there is no indication for the prescription of antibiotics. One could argue that those patients at high risk for the development of complications, such as those patients with chronic bronchitis, diabetes, renal failure, or other chronic diseases, may be treated prophylactically. However, there are no studies that support the efficacy or effectiveness of such a course.

5. **b.** The most common complication of influenza is pneumonia. This pneumonia is initially a viral pneumonia but often develops, especially in susceptible elderly patients, into a bacterial pneumonia, with *Streptococcus pneumoniae* as the most common pathogen. Other pathogens include *Staphylococcus aureus* and haemophilus. This is the reason for the recommendations of the U.S. Preventive Services Task Force on the Periodic Health Examination with respect to influenza, namely: (1) immunize all patients older than age 65 years annually with influenza vaccine, and (2) immunize all patients older than age 65 and high risk with pneumococcal vaccine.

6. **a.** All of the world's pandemics are caused by major antigenic shifts associated with influenza A. Influenza B and influenza C are associated with neither epidemics nor pandemics. There is no such thing as influenza D and E.

7. **c.** Oseltamivir is an antiviral medication effective in the treatment of all influenza variants. Thus it is a better choice than amantadine or rimantadine. It should be started within 48 hours of onset of symptoms, and its use can shorten the duration and severity of symptoms. Antivirals can be used during the influenza season as an adjunct to late vaccination, as a supplement to preseason vaccination in people who are immunodeficient, and as chemoprophylaxis in the absence of vaccination. Antivirals also can be used to reduce the spread of the virus and to minimize disruption of patient care both in the community and in the institutional setting. Influenza vaccination, however, remains the preferred method of conferring protection.

8. **c.** The influenza virus is transmitted through respiratory secretions and thus is spread easily to susceptible persons. Sneezing, coughing, and close contact while talking are thought to be the major modes of transmission.

9. **d.** The most effective method for preventing influenza A is by immunizing patients before the influenza season begins with inactivated (or killed) influenza vaccine. Influenza vaccine confers approximately 85% protection against the development of influenza and an even greater rate of protection against death from influenza.

10. **e.** Influenza vaccine is effective against both influenza A and influenza B, has an efficacy rate of approximately 85%, and should be administered yearly 1 to 2 months before the influenza season begins.

11. **d.** Influenza vaccine typically produces some minor side effects such as a sore arm, redness at the injection site, and low-grade fever. A history of anaphylactic hypersensitivity to eggs or egg products is a contraindication to receiving influenza vaccine. Details of vaccine dose are discussed in a later question, but the usual IM dose of whole virus vaccine for adults is 0.5 mL. An intranasal vaccine is now available and may supplant the injection in popularity, although it currently is a very expensive alternative. In those patients in whom immunization fails and in whom influenza does develop, influenza vaccine still reduces both the severity and the duration of symptoms.

12. **a.** Amantadine and its antiviral cousin Rimantadine are effective only against influenza A. Antivirals reduce viral shedding, and the duration and severity of influenza A symptoms (such as headache, fever, chills, myalgias, and cough) once the virus is established, and may be used as treatment in high-risk patients in whom the influenza vaccine is contraindicated.

13. **d.** Table 8-1, adapted from the Antiviral Drug Information website of the National Center for Infectious Diseases at the Centers for Disease Control and Prevention (CDC) (www.cdc.gov), summarizes comparisons among antiviral drugs for influenza.

Studies show that treatment with any of these drugs can shorten the time a person infected with influenza feels ill by approximately 1 day, if treatment is started during the first 2 days of illness.

14. **e.** Individuals who should receive yearly influenza vaccine include the following:
   1. all persons aged 50 years or older. Although some people 50 to 64 years of age who do not have chronic (long-term) medical conditions may

Table 8-1 Comparison of Antiviral Drugs for Influenza

Drug	Trade Name	Influenza Virus Type	Approved Use	Treatment Age	Prevention Age
Amantadine	Symmetrel®	A	Treatment and prevention	≥1 year	≥1 year
Rimantadine	Flumadine®	A	Treatment and prevention	Adults	≥1 year
Zanamivir	Relenza®	A and B	Treatment	≥7 years	n/a
Oseltamivir	Tamiflu®	A and B	Treatment and prevention	≥1 year	≥13 years

not be at high risk for serious complications, about 26% of people in this age group do have high-risk conditions. For this reason, beginning in 2000, yearly influenza vaccination was recommended for all people 50 to 64 years old to increase the number of high-risk individuals immunized.

2. residents of nursing homes and other long-term care facilities that house persons of any age who have long-term illnesses;

3. adults and children 6 months of age and older who have chronic heart or lung conditions, including asthma

4. adults and children 6 months of age and older who need regular medical care or had to be in a hospital because of metabolic diseases (such as diabetes), chronic kidney disease, or weakened immune system (including immune system problems caused by medicine or by infection with human immunodeficiency virus [HIV/AIDS])

5. children and teenagers (aged 6 months to 18 years) who are undergoing long-term aspirin therapy and therefore could develop Reye syndrome after the flu

6. women who will be more than 3 months pregnant during the flu season.

Other folks in whom to consider immunization include the following: young, otherwise healthy children aged 6 to 23 months who are at increased risk for influenza-related hospitalization; doctors, nurses, and other employees in hospitals and doctors' offices, including emergency response workers; employees of nursing homes and long-term care facilities who have contact with patients or residents; employees of assisted living and other residences for people in high-risk groups; people who provide home care to those in high-risk groups; and household members (including children) of people in high-risk groups. The CDC now recommends administration of the vaccine to anyone who wants to reduce their chances of getting the flu, and particularly persons who provide essential community services (such as police, firemen, etc.) and students or others in institutional settings (those who reside in dormitories).

15. People who should not get a flu shot include individuals with an allergy to hens' eggs, people with a history of a previous severe reaction to influenza vaccine, and people not at risk for complications of influenza who developed Guillain-Barré syndrome within 6 weeks after a flu shot. Asthma and other chronic illnesses are good reasons to get vaccinated.

SUMMARY OF INFLUENZA

EPIDEMIOLOGY: influenza A is responsible for all major epidemics and pandemics of influenza. It is also the most virulent of the influenza types, which include A, B, and C. Yearly outbreaks result mostly from antigenic drift in the H and N antigens. Influenza outbreaks begin in the late fall and can last until early into the new year.

SIGNS AND SYMPTOMS: headache is a common symptom. Other symptoms include fever, chills, and myalgias, followed by the symptoms of cough and congestion.

PREVENTION: influenza vaccine should be given to all high-risk groups discussed in this chapter. Ideally, immunization should take place in the fall, prior to the winter season. Vaccine efficacy averages around 85% and is effective for both influenza A and influenza B. Travelers to the tropics and winter experiencing locales also should be immunized.

ANTIVIRAL MEDICATIONS: antiviral medications may offer prophylaxis and treatment options, but they are still not a substitute for immunization. They may be used as an adjunct to vaccination in high-risk situations (especially chronic care facilities). When given early after onset of illness, they reduce the severity and duration of symptoms in persons who already have contracted the virus. As with all medications, they have potential side effects. Amantadine

Continued

SUMMARY OF INFLUENZA—cont'd

ANTIVIRAL MEDICATIONS—cont'd

and rimantadine can cause central nervous system (CNS) side effects (such as nervousness, anxiety, difficulty concentrating, and lightheadedness) and gastrointestinal side effects (such as nausea and loss of appetite). CNS side effects occur more often among persons taking amantadine than among persons taking rimantadine. Among some other persons with long-term illnesses, more serious side effects, such as delirium, hallucinations, agitation, and seizures, can occur. Side effects usually diminish and disappear after 1 week. Zanamivir is inhaled and can cause decreased respiratory function and bronchospasm, especially in those with asthma or other chronic lung disease. Therefore, zanamivir is generally not recommended for use in persons with underlying lung disease, such as asthma and chronic obstructive pulmonary disease. Other side effects reported by less than 5% of those who have used this drug are diarrhea, nausea, sinusitis, nasal infections, bronchitis, cough, headache, and dizziness. Oseltamivir can cause gastrointestinal side effects (i.e., nausea and vomiting), although these may be less severe if taken with food.

Please review answer A14 for a list of all those who should receive yearly influenza immunization.

Make sure you and your patients are immunized in a timely manner.

SUGGESTED READING

Bridges CB, et al: Prevention and control of influenza. Recommendations of the Advisory Committee on Immunization Practices (ACIP). *MMWR Morb Mortal Wkly Rep* 52(22):526, 2003.

http://www.cdc.gov (this website has up-to-date recommendations and detailed information on immunization practices for influenza)

Chapter 9

Bioterrorism

Has 9/11 defined our Brave New World?

CLINICAL CASE PROBLEM 1:
A Disturbing News Report

You are driving to your office after making hospital rounds and hear a news flash on the radio that several people in your community have come down with a mysterious respiratory illness that has caused three seemingly healthy middle-aged people to die suddenly and unexpectedly. The report says authorities have reason to suspect an act of bioterrorism. When you arrive at the office, your telephone lines are being flooded with incoming calls. Your receptionist says, "What's going on? Why is everyone panicked?"

SELECT THE BEST ANSWER TO THE FOLLOWING QUESTIONS:

1. Your best source of reliable information about the situation is?
   a. local television news reports
   b. local health department
   c. police department
   d. Centers for Disease Control and Prevention (CDC) website
   e. local newspaper

2. You receive the necessary information from the appropriate source. The next day you speak by telephone to a patient at work who gives you a plausible exposure history and relates symptoms that are of concern to you. Your most appropriate next step for this patient is?
   a. send the patient home to await instructions
   b. send the patient to the hospital emergency department
   c. bring the patient into the office for an evaluation
   d. make a home visit to the patient
   e. none of the above

3. You make the correct choice in the next step for care for this patient. Whom should you immediately notify regarding the patient and your concerns?
   a. the local health department
   b. the hospital emergency department
   c. the local police
   d. no one because it would be a violation of the patient's privacy
   e. a, b, and c

4. The agents used in bioterrorism attacks are grouped into which of the following categories?
   a. biologic and radiologic
   b. biologic, radiologic, and chemical
   c. inhaled, topical, and ingested
   d. chemical and radiologic
   e. none of the above

5. Which of the following characteristics distinguish smallpox (variola) eruptions from those of chicken-pox (varicella)?
   a. varicella eruptions are centripetal; variola are centrifugal
   b. variola eruptions break out all at once; varicella come in crops
   c. varicella eruptions are preceded by a highly febrile prodrome; variola are not
   d. variola eruptions are uncomfortable; varicella are not
   e. varicella eruptions progress slowly; variola eruptions progress to pustules in less than 12 hours

6. During which of the following times is the patient infected with variola not contagious?
   a. the incubation period
   b. the febrile prodrome
   c. during the initial rash on the tongue and in the mouth
   d. during the pustular eruptions
   e. after scab formation

7. Which of the following is true regarding smallpox?
   a. direct face-to-face contact is the most common means of smallpox spread
   b. smallpox can be spread through direct contact with infected bodily fluids or contaminated objects such as bedding or clothing
   c. smallpox can be spread through the air of enclosed buildings
   d. humans are the only natural hosts of variola
   e. all of the above

8. Which of the following is not true regarding plague?
   a. a swollen, tender lymph gland is the typical sign of the most common form of human plague
   b. signs of bubonic plague include a swollen gland with fever, chills, headache, and extreme exhaustion
   c. symptoms appear 12 to 16 days after being infected
   d. pneumonic plague causes high fever, chills, cough, difficulty breathing, and bloody sputum
   e. 14% of all plague cases in the United States are fatal

CLINICAL CASE PROBLEM 2:

Show and Tell (and Pray It Never Happens)

As part of a bioterrorism preparedness program, you are asked to lecture to a group of your colleagues at the local hospital. Here are some of the questions you get. Choose the correct response.

9. What is (are) the appropriate choice(s) of antibiotic prophylaxis for a possible inhalation anthrax exposure?
   a. ciprofloxacin
   b. doxycycline
   c. amoxicillin
   d. clarithromycin
   e. a, b, and c

10. Which of the following is (are) correct regarding inhalation anthrax?
    a. the average incubation period is 4 to 6 days
    b. the symptom complex includes fever, chills, sweats, fatigue, minimally productive cough, nausea or vomiting, and chest discomfort
    c. chest x-ray initially may show mediastinal widening, paratracheal/hilar fullness, and pleural effusions/infiltrates
    d. pleural effusions are a common complication
    e. all of the above

11. Chemical agents such as sarin typically work by causing neurotoxicity. Common routes of exposure to the agent sarin include which of the following?
    a. breathing contaminated air
    b. eating contaminated food
    c. drinking contaminated water or touching contaminated surfaces
    d. a, b, and c
    e. a and c

12. People exposed to chemical bioterrorism agents typically may experience which of the following symptoms within seconds to hours?
    a. runny nose, watery eyes, blurred vision, confusion, headache
    b. drooling and excessive sweating
    c. cough, chest tightness, rapid breathing
    d. nausea, vomiting, diarrhea
    e. all of the above

13. Which of the following is (are) an effective antidote(s) to the common neurotoxic chemical agents?
    a. atropine
    b. succinylcholine
    c. ethanol
    d. 2-PAM (pralidoxime [2-pyrididine aldoxime])
    e. a and d

14. What are the short- and long-term effects of exposure to neurotoxic chemical agents?
    a. permanent neurologic impairment at any level of exposure
    b. mild or moderately exposed people usually recover completely

c. even severely exposed people are likely to survive

d. most neurologic impairments last 1 to 2 years

e. even people who were mildly exposed are likely to die

15. Which of the following is true regarding the classic stages seen in acute radiation syndrome?

a. in the prodromal stage, classic symptoms include nausea, vomiting, and possibly diarrhea (depending on dose) and occur from minutes to days following exposure

b. the symptoms of the prodromal stage may last for up to several months

c. in the latent stage, the patient feels weak and somnolent for a few weeks

d. in the manifest illness stage, the symptoms are specific to the neurologic system and last several months

e. in the final stage, recovery or death, most patients who recover will be back to normal in a matter of days

ANSWERS:

1. b. Your local health department is your best source of information regarding any bioterrorist threats. Since the events in the United States of September and October of 2001, a massive public health effort has been made to link local health departments to the state departments of health and the federal CDC. Although notification protocols should work from local to state to federal authorities, your local health department should have the most reliable information regarding events in your area.

2. b. The local hospital emergency department is the best place for an evaluation. Most local hospitals now have protocols in place for evaluation of patients with potential exposures or symptomology suggestive of an exposure. Clinicians should familiarize themselves with the protocols in place for their area hospitals.

3. e. The family physician's responsibility for appropriate notification is an important and crucial part of the response to a potential bioterrorist agent exposure. Clinicians are on the front lines of any community event and are advised by the CDC to notify the local health department (most county health departments in the United States now have 24-hour access) and police department of any potential danger. In this case where a patient is being sent to the emergency department, the standard of care and

public health is to notify the hospital at once. Early notification is critical to an early response, and it is a critical duty of all physicians.

4. b. The agents used in bioterrorism attacks are grouped into the following categories: biologic, radiologic, and chemical. Examples of biologic agents include smallpox, plague, and anthrax. Examples of radiologic agents include traditional thermonuclear devices, so-called "dirty" bombs (small explosive devices containing radioactive materials), and radioactive waste in various delivery vehicles. Examples of chemical agents include the nerve agents sarin, VX, and mustard gases. Unfortunately, a veritable wealth of possible agents is at the disposal of determined terrorists. The clinician should become familiar with the more common agents and their effects. A good source of information is the CDC website (http://www.cdc.gov), which has multiple links to other reliable sites.

5. b. Smallpox (variola) is a serious, contagious infectious disease with an overall fatality rate of about 30% in unimmunized populations. There is no treatment for smallpox; the only prevention is vaccination. Naturally occurring smallpox was eliminated from the world in the late 1970s, after which routine vaccination was stopped. The eruptions of chickenpox (varicella) can be confused with smallpox (variola). Fortunately, there are ways to distinguish between the two. Varicella eruptions tend to be centrifugal, whereas variola are more centripetal. Variola eruptions, which typically begin on the tongue, break out all at once; varicella eruptions come in crops. Varicella eruptions are usually not proceeded by a febrile prodrome, whereas the highly febrile prodrome is characteristic of variola. Both variola and varicella eruptions are uncomfortable. Varicella eruptions progress rapidly, going from papules to vesicles sometimes in 24 hours; variola eruptions progress to pustules in several days. Pictures of each of these eruptions are available on the CDC website.

6. a. There is an incubation period of about 12 to 14 days during which time (and the only time) people are not contagious. The prodrome phase of 2-4 days consists of initial symptoms that include fever, malaise, head and body aches, and high fever to 101-104° F. Rash begins as small red spots on the tongue which develop into sores that break open. A rash will then appear on the face and spread to the arms, legs, and then to hands and feet. Within 24 hours, the rash spreads to all parts of the body. The rash then becomes raised bumps that are filled with a thick, opaque fluid and often have a depression in the center. These become pustules that crust over after two weeks.

7. **e.** Direct and prolonged face-to-face contact usually is required to spread smallpox. Smallpox also can be spread through direct contact with infected bodily fluids or contaminated objects (bedding or clothing) and rarely through the air in enclosed settings such as buildings and airplanes. Humans are the only natural hosts of variola.

8. **c.** A swollen, tender lymph gland is the typical sign of the most common form of human plague, bubonic plague. Signs of bubonic plague include a swollen gland with fever, chills, headache, and extreme exhaustion. Symptoms appear 2 to 6 days after being infected. In nonterror situations, the infection is spread most commonly by the bites of fleas from rodent carriers. Plague will spread through the bloodstream to the lungs causing pneumonic plague, which is characterized by high fever, chills, cough, difficulty breathing, and bloody sputum. Of all plague cases in the United States, 14% are fatal, but the illness is successfully treatable with antibiotics if caught early.

9. **e.** Ciprofloxacin, doxycycline, and penicillin G procaine are approved by the Food and Drug Administration (FDA) for prophylaxis of inhalational *Bacillus anthracis* infection. Amoxicillin is an option for children and pregnant or lactating women.

10. **e.** Inhalation anthrax incubation ranges from 4 to 6 days. Typical symptoms include fever, chills, sweats, fatigue, minimally productive cough, nausea or vomiting, and chest discomfort. Sounds like influenza? This is the problem during winter months. Chest x-ray initially may show mediastinal widening, paratracheal fullness, hilar fullness, and pleural effusions or infiltrates or both. Pleural effusions are common complications. Patients can survive but require aggressive supportive care and multidrug antibiotic regimens.

11. **d.** Common routes of exposure to the agent sarin include breathing contaminated air, eating contaminated food, drinking contaminated water, or touching contaminated surfaces.

12. **e.** Patients may experience any and all of the following symptoms, often within seconds or minutes of exposure: runny nose, watery eyes, blurred vision, confusion, headache, drooling and excessive sweating, cough, chest tightness, rapid breathing, nausea, vomiting, and diarrhea. Rapid treatment is essential for survival.

13. **e.** Table 9-1, adapted from the CDC (www.cdc.gov; Terrorism and Public Health), describes emergency department treatment.

14. **b.** To quote from the CDC: "Mild or moderately exposed people usually recover completely. Severely exposed people are not likely to survive. Unlike some organophosphate pesticides, nerve agents have not been associated with neurological problems lasting more than 1 to 2 weeks after the exposure."

15. **a.** The following is taken from the CDC web-based publication on acute radiation syndrome: Acute radiation syndrome (ARS) is an acute illness caused

Table 9-1 Nerve Agent Therapy in the Emergency Department

Patient Age	Mild/Moderate Symptoms[†]	Severe Symptoms[‡]	Other Treatments
Infant (0-2 y)	Atropine 0.05 mg/kg IM or 0.02 mg/kg IV; 2-PAM Cl 15 mg/kg IV slowly	Atropine 0.1 mg/kg IM or 0.02 mg/kg IV; 2-PAM Cl 15 mg/kg IV slowly	Assisted ventilation as needed. Repeat Atropine (2 mg IM or 1 mg IM for infants) at 5-10 minute intervals until secretions diminish or breathing improves. Use phentolamine for 2-PAM induced hypertension (5 mg IV adults; 1 mg IV children). Diazepam for convulsions.
Child (2-10 y)	Atropine 1 mg IM; 2-PAM Cl 15 mg/kg IV slowly	Atropine 2 mg IM; 2-PAM Cl 15 mg/kg IV slowly	
Adolescent	Atropine 2 mg IM; 2-PAM Cl 15 mg/kg IV slowly	Atropine 4 mg IM; 2-PAM Cl 15 mg/kg IV slowly	
Adult	Atropine 2-4 mg IM; 2-PAM Cl 15 mg/kg IV slowly	Atropine 6 mg IM; 2-PAM Cl 15 mg/kg IV slowly	
Frail elderly	Atropine 1 mg IM; 2-PAM Cl 5-10 mg/kg IV slowly	Atropine 2 mg IM; 2-PAM Cl 5-10 mg/kg IV slowly	

IM, intramuscularly; IV, intravenously.
[†]Mild/moderate symptoms = localized sweating, muscle fasciculations, nausea, vomiting, dyspnea.
[‡]Severe symptoms = unconsciousness, apnea, convulsions, paralysis.

by irradiation of the entire body by a high dose of ionizing radiation in a very short period (usually a matter of minutes). There are four stages of ARS:

- Prodromal stage: The classic symptoms for this stage are nausea, vomiting, and possibly diarrhea (depending on dose), which occur from minutes to days following exposure. The symptoms may last (episodically) for minutes up to several days.
- Latent stage: In this stage the patient looks and feels generally healthy for a few hours or even up to a few weeks.
- Manifest illness stage: In this stage the symptoms depend on the specific syndrome and last from hours up to several months.
- Recovery or death stage: Most patients who do not recover will die within several months of exposure. The recovery process lasts from several weeks up to 2 years.

There are three syndromes associated with the manifest illness stage: bone marrow syndrome, gastrointestinal syndrome, and cardiac syndrome (each named for the system affected). Individuals with the cardiac and gastrointestinal syndromes rarely survive. Treatment for acute radiation disease is supportive because the damage has been done; only the outcome is unknown.

SUMMARY OF BIOTERRORISM

Family physicians are likely to find themselves on the front line of response to bioterrorism. Each of us needs to familiarize ourselves with the local public health apparatus and establish lines of communication with authorities before such an event. The events of 2001 taught us that no locale is immune to the possibility of terror threats and actions. Agents used to create terror and injure the population can be biologic, chemical, and radiologic. Common agents of concern include smallpox, anthrax, plague, sarin, mustard gas, and a variety of radiologic weapons. A good source of information on this subject is the CDC. Please visit their website at http://www.cdc.gov.

SUGGESTED READING

Centers for Disease Control and Prevention: Update: investigation of bioterrorism-related anthrax and interim guidelines for exposure management and antimicrobial therapy. *MMWR Morb Mortal Wkly Rep* 50:909-919, 2001.

Dixon TC, et al: Anthrax. *N Engl J Med* 341:815-826, 1999.

ADULT MEDICINE

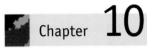

Chapter **10**

Acute ST Segment Elevation Myocardial Infarction

> "My wife had no business calling 911 just because I had a little pain in my chest. I tell you I am as healthy as a horse."

CLINICAL CASE PROBLEM 1:

A 72-Year-Old Male with Acute Chest Pain

A 72-year-old farmer is brought to the local emergency department with his wife by the county sheriff. Apparently he developed a "twinge of chest pain" while shoveling grain 3 hours ago. He insisted on staying home until "he collapsed on the floor." Even then, he wanted to stay home and rest, but his wife insisted on calling 911. The call was answered by the sheriff's department, who rushed him and his wife to the emergency room (ER) in the nearest hospital in the rural area in which he resides. At his admission he states that the pain is "almost gone"—"what a fuss about nothing." On taking a history he tells the admitting physician that he smokes two packs of cigarettes daily, that he drinks a "goodly amount of beer," and that he had been told that his serum cholesterol level is good; the doctor even told him he was one of the highest values he had ever seen for a man his age. The admitting physician also notes that the patient is obese and that he seems confused on the cholesterol issue, believing that the higher the cholesterol value, the better. On further questioning he admits to a dull, aching, viselike pain around his chest, with radiation to the left shoulder. He also discloses that when the pain was at its worst he experienced nausea and vomiting, but he adds that because he already is doing better it must have been something he ate. His wife adds that she has never seen him in so much pain, but he is a "stubborn old goat."

He still insists its just a little stomach trouble, but on physical examination, he is sweating and diaphoretic. He has vomited twice since coming to the ER. His blood pressure is 160/100 mm Hg, and his pulse is 120 and irregular. His abdomen is obese, and you believe you can detect an enlarged aorta by deep palpation.

His electrocardiogram (ECG) results reveal significant Q waves in V1 to V4 with significant ST segment eleva-

tion in the same leads. There are reciprocal ST changes (ST segment depression) in the inferior leads (II, III, avF).

■ SELECT THE BEST ANSWER TO THE FOLLOWING QUESTIONS:

1. The most likely diagnosis in this patient is:
   a. acute inferior wall myocardial infarction (MI)
   b. acute anterior wall MI
   c. acute myocardial ischemia
   d. acute pericarditis
   e. musculoskeletal chest wall pain

2. Given the history, physical examination, and ECG, your first priority is to:
   a. call the ambulance for immediate transport to another hospital that "knows how to treat this thing"
   b. admit the patient for observation
   c. administer streptokinase or tissue plasminogen activator (t-PA) intravenously (IV)
   d. administer heparin IV
   e. none of the above

3. The nearest big city hospital is a 6-hour drive. Given your attention to your first priority, you would now:
   a. call the ambulance for immediate transport to another hospital that "knows how to look after this thing"
   b. admit the patient to the coronary care unit for observation
   c. administer streptokinase or alteplase IV immediately
   d. administer heparin IV immediately
   e. none of the above

4. Which of the following criteria should be met before a patient is given thrombolytic therapy following the history, physical examination, and ECG previously described?
   a. typical chest pain suggestive of a MI
   b. ECG changes confirming MI
   c. the absence of other diseases that would explain the symptoms
   d. all of the above
   e. none of the above

5. The most correct statement regarding thrombolytic therapy in acute myocardial infarction (AMI) is:

a. patients younger than age 65 benefit more than elderly victims of MI do

b. no benefits have been realized when therapy has been instituted after 6 hours of onset of chest pain

c. thrombolytic therapy has improved the prognosis of patients with prior coronary artery bypass grafting (CABG)

d. patients with non-Q MI have benefited as well as patients who sustain Q-wave MIs with thrombolytic therapy

e. A 50% reduction in mortality has been realized when therapy is administered within 3 hours of onset of chest pain

6. Which of the following statements regarding the use of heparin in patients with AMI is (are) true?

a. heparin therapy now is used almost routinely with thrombolytic therapy during acute phase of MI treatment, providing certain criteria are met

b. heparin is recommended whenever there is echocardiographic evidence of left-ventricular thrombi

c. heparin should be administered (unless contraindicated) to all patients with acute anterior wall MI

d. heparin is contraindicated in patients with uncontrolled hypertension

e. all of the above

7. Which of the following is (are) a contraindication(s) to the use of thrombolytic therapy in patients with AMI?

a. active gastrointestinal bleeding

b. recent surgery (2 weeks postoperative)

c. history of cerebrovascular accident

d. suspected aortic dissection

e. all of the above

8. Which of the following statements regarding patients admitted to the coronary care unit following presumed MI is (are) true?

a. patients with suspected MIs should have the left-ventricular ejection fraction measured before leaving the hospital

b. patients should have an exercise tolerance test on the fourth or fifth hospital day

c. patients should have an exercise stress test performed 4 to 6 weeks after hospitalization

d. a and c

e. none of the above

9. Which of the following is (are) a significant feature(s) of the pathophysiology of MI?

a. endothelial cell wall damage

b. coronary atherosclerosis

c. thromboxane A_2 production

d. all of the above

e. a and b

10. Which of the following is (are) true concerning aspirin in the treatment of AMI?

a. aspirin may serve as a substitute for streptokinase or t-PA

b. aspirin may serve as a substitute for heparin

c. aspirin may serve as a substitute for β-blockade

d. all of the above

e. none of the above

11. Which of the following statements regarding thrombolytic therapy is false?

a. thrombolytic therapy limits myocardial necrosis

b. thrombolytic therapy preserves left-ventricular function

c. thrombolytic therapy reduces mortality

d. all of the above statements are false

e. none of the above statements is false

12. Which of the following is true regarding primary angioplasty in the treatment of acute ST segment elevated MI?

a. primary angioplasty is not a substitute for thrombolytic therapy

b. its universal adoption is likely to be limited by geography

c. it can be performed in hospitals that do not perform CABG surgery

d. stent placement worsens outcomes

e. operator variables are insignificant

13. Which of the following statements concerning dysrhythmias and dysrhythmic drugs in patients who have sustained a MI is (are) true?

a. premature ventricular contractions are common and should be treated with lidocaine

b. sustained runs of ventricular tachycardia frequently progress to ventricular fibrillation (VF)

c. prophylactic lidocaine is recommended to prevent dysrhythmias in all patients who have sustained an MI

d. none of the above

e. all of the above

14. One of the major patient concerns following an MI is the risk of a second or subsequent attack. In which of the following circumstances is the risk of reinfarction and/or mortality following MI significantly increased?

a. left-ventricular ejection fraction, 40%

b. exercise-induced ischemia

c. non Q-wave infarction (subendocardial infarction)
d. a and b
e. all of the above

15. Which of the following medications have been shown to be of benefit in some patients who have had an MI?
    a. beta blockers
    b. calcium-channel blockers
    c. aspirin
    d. a and c
    e. all of the above

16. Which of the following statements concerning rehabilitation of the patient after a MI is (are) true?
    a. sexual intercourse should not resume for at least 3 months
    b. patients who have sustained an MI should stay off work for at least 4 months
    c. patients who have sustained an MI gradually may increase activity over 6 to 8 weeks
    d. no significant psychologic distress regarding the MI has been shown to occur in the patient's spouse or significant other
    e. all of the above

17. The best single confirmatory investigation for acute myocardial infarction is:
    a. the ECG
    b. the height of ST segment elevation in the affected area (in mm) plus the depth of ST segment depression in the reciprocally affected leads (in mm)
    c. the creatine kinase isoenzyme MB fraction
    d. the presence of dysfunctional heart muscle as demonstrated by echocardiography
    e. cardiac troponin levels

18. Sudden death as a result of MI is almost always the result of:
    a. third-degree heart block resulting from infarction of the atrioventricular node
    b. ventricular tachycardia
    c. ventricular fibrillation
    d. ventricular standstill
    e. none of the above

19. Which of the following statements regarding shock and its treatment in acute MI is (are) true?
    a. the patient with AMI may develop shock secondary to hypovolemic hypotension
    b. the patient with AMI may develop shock secondary to persistent hypotension and a poor cardiac index
    c. both forms of shock respond well to treatment

with intravenous fluids (Ringer's lactate or normal saline solution)
d. a and b only
e. all of the above

20. Coronary reperfusion with thrombolytic agents has been shown to be of benefit when the onset of the pain occurs within which of the following maximum number of hours from the onset of pain?
    a. 4
    b. 6
    c. 12
    d. 24
    e. 48

21. In the Clinical Case Problem described there is a key finding on physical examination of the patient's abdomen that should be further assessed by:
    a. an abdominal ultrasound
    b. an intravenous pyelogram (IVP)
    c. a digital subtraction angiogram
    d. a computed tomography (CT) scan
    e. a magnetic resonance imaging (MRI) scan

■ ANSWERS:

1. **b.** This patient most likely has suffered an anterior wall MI. The history suggests that he is at high risk for an infarct, and the Q waves and ST segment elevations in V1 to V4 and ST segment elevation in the anterior chest leads plus reciprocal changes in the inferior wall confirm the diagnosis. An acute inferior wall MI would have ST segment elevation and possibly Q waves in the inferior leads. Acute pericarditis would have ST segment elevation in all leads. Musculoskeletal chest wall pain does not produce the abnormalities in the ECG that is seen in this patient.

2. **e.** The history, physical examination, and ECG point clearly to acute anterior wall MI. First, ascertain that the patient's airway is patent (without obstruction, vomit, or any blockage) and administer 100% oxygen.

3. **c.** Administer fibrinolytic agents such as streptokinase or alteplase (t-PA). The recombinant t-PA alteplase, a fibrin-specific agent, and streptokinase, a nonspecific agent, have been used most extensively. The recommended dose of streptokinase in AMI is 1.5 million U IV over 30 to 60 minutes. The regimen for the administration of alteplase is 15 mg IV bolus, then 0.75 mg/kg over 30 minutes (maximum 50 mg), then 0.5 mg/kg for a 60-minute period (maximum 35 mg).

Newer recombinant DNA fibrinolytic-specific agents are reteplase and tenecteplase. Reteplase is given via a 10+10 MU double bolus administered 30 minutes apart. For tenecteplase, the dose is 0.5 mg/kg single bolus (maximum 50 mg). The advantages of the recombinant DNA sources, alteplase, reteplase, and tenecteplase, are high clot selectivity and few allergic reactions. Because of ease of administration, tenecteplase often is favored as an agent.

4. d. Thrombolytic therapy should be administered only when the following criteria are met: (1) typical chest pain suggestive of an MI, (2) ECG changes confirming MI, and (3) the "absence" of other diseases that would explain the symptoms.

An age older than 70 years was formerly a criterion for exclusion of patients for thrombolytic therapy; this is no longer the case. Contraindications to thrombolytic therapy include the following: (1) active internal bleeding, (2) suspected aortic dissection, (3) prolonged or traumatic cardiopulmonary resuscitation, (4) recent head trauma or known intracranial neoplasm, (5) hemorrhagic retinopathy, (6) pregnancy, (7) history of recent (6 months or less) stroke or cerebral neoplasm, and (8) trauma or surgery within the last 2 weeks.

5. e. Although the benefits of thrombolytic therapy are greatest within the first 1 to 3 hours, a 10% mortality benefit can be achieved up to 12 hours after the onset of pain. Older patients, who have a higher complication rate, actually benefit more from thrombolytic therapy because they have a higher pretreatment hospital mortality rate. Treatment should be considered for patients as old as 80 years—or even older if the benefit-to-risk ratio seems favorable.

Patients with non–Q-wave infarcts have not benefited from thrombolytic therapy, nor have patients with prior CABG.

6. e. The role of concomitant heparin in the initial treatment of AMI has become increasingly clear over time. The HAART (highly active antiretroviral therapy) study has shown that early, effective anticoagulation with heparin maintains t-PA–induced coronary artery patency more effectively than aspirin alone. Subgroup analyses have shown that patients receiving therapeutic heparin, as measured by the activated partial thromboplastin time (APTT), have an extremely high patency approaching 95% following t-PA administration.

Heparin therapy, however, has not been found to outweigh the harms in patients receiving streptokinase, except in cases of anterior wall MI, or in patients with complications prone to thromboembolism such as atrial fibrillation or congestive heart failure.

The two most important indications for concomitant use of heparin are acute anterior wall MI and echocardiographic evidence of left-ventricular thrombi.

7. e. The major contraindications to adjunctive heparin therapy in MI are history of major surgery with time from discharge of less than 14 days, history of cardiovascular accidents, suspected aortic dissection, and acute gastrointestinal hemorrhage.

8. d. Before leaving the hospital, the patient should have his left-ventricular ejection fraction measured, and an exercise stress tolerance test should be performed after 4 to 6 weeks.

9. d. The pathophysiology of AMI centers around the formation and rupture of a vulnerable atherosclerotic plaque. The progression of atherosclerosis is as follows: (1) superficial atherosclerotic fatty streaks form in the coronary arteries even in children; (2) the fatty streaks progress to elevated fibrous plaques by the third and fourth decades of life; and (3) these fibrous plaques progress to complex, eccentric, ulcerated, and hemorrhagic plaques by the fifth and sixth decades, culminating in plaque rupture or intraplaque hemorrhage and formation of a clot leading to coronary artery occlusion.

The fragile endothelium is damaged by hypertension, elevated low-density lipoprotein (LDL) cholesterol, diabetes, smoking, and other factors. Simple denudation exposes the vascular collagen, which triggers circulating platelet adhesion and aggregation and a cascade of growth-factor release including thromboxane A_2, prostacyclin, and platelet-derived growth factor (PDGF). Smooth-muscle cell and monocyte proliferation, along with lipid accumulation under the influence of growth factors, leads to severe atherosclerosis. For reasons that are still not entirely clear, some atherosclerotic lesions, particularly those near vessel branch points and possibly triggered by viral infection or other causes of inflammation, become vulnerable and rupture, leading to the AMI syndrome.

10. e. Acetylsalicylic acid (aspirin) is the only adjunctive agent that has been shown unequivocally to reduce mortality alone or in conjunction with thrombolytic agents in patients with AMI. The ISIS-II study showed that acetylsalicylic acid (ASA) reduced mortality by 25%. However, when ASA was added to streptokinase the effect was synergistic, and mortality from MI was reduced by 42%.

Thus aspirin has been shown to reduce rethrombosis and recurrent MI. It is not, however, a substitute for anything; it should be used along with other acute agents in the treatment of MI.

11. e. Thrombolytic therapy and interventional angioplasty are the cornerstones of treatment of acute ST segment elevated MI. Thrombolytic therapy is an established, effective therapy that limits myocardial necrosis, preserves left-ventricular function, and reduces mortality.

12. b. Primary angioplasty with stenting is becoming the intervention of choice for acute ST segment elevated MI in many hospitals. Primary angioplasty with stenting is safe and confers advantages over balloon angioplasty alone. The addition of glycoprotein IIb/IIIa inhibitor abciximab treatment improves flow characteristics, prevents distal thromboembolization, and reduces the need for repeat angioplasty. A strategy of primary stenting in association with abciximab is the current gold standard of care for patients with acute MI. The use of medication-eluding stents is promising and may surpass results of primary angioplasty with stenting plus glycoprotein inhibitors. However, primary angioplasty has these limitations: outcomes vary according to skills of interventionist, and the procedure is effective only for patients presenting early (less than 12 hours after acute MI). Complications are more common than with elective angioplasty, as are ventricular arrhythmias, although the latter are generally treatable. Right coronary artery procedures have high complication rates of sinus arrest, atrioventricular block, idioventricular rhythm, and severe hypotension. Surgical backup is required because up to 5% of patients require bypass surgery. Primary angioplasty, although an effective procedural intervention, requires facilities and experienced staff, and many adults with AMI in the United States and Canada are out of timely reach of such facilities and personnel.

13. d. Premature ventricular contractions (PVCs) occur frequently following AMI but do not require treatment. Couplets, triplets, multifocal PVCs, and short runs of nonsustained ventricular tachycardia are treated effectively with intravenous lidocaine. However, although they are treated with intravenous lidocaine, no survival advantage has been shown with lidocaine in this setting.

Most clinicians do not treat these nonmalignant ventricular dysrhythmias because they rarely progress to life-threatening situations, and if they do they can be treated effectively with cardioversion or defibrillation.

Lidocaine is not recommended in the routine prophylaxis of AMI. In addition, long-term prophylaxis with oral antiarrhythmics, such as flecainide and encainide, following AMI has been shown to increase mortality drastically.

14. e. The risk of subsequent infarction and/or mortality following discharge from the hospital following an MI is increased in patients with: (1) postinfarction angina pectoris; (2) non–Q-wave infarction; (3) congestive cardiac failure; (4) left-ventricular ejection fraction less than 40%; (5) exercise-induced ischemia diagnosed by ECG or by scintigraphy; and (6) ventricular ectopy (frequency >10 PVCs/min).

15. e. Beta blockers, aspirin, and coumadin have improved the prognosis in some patients following an MI. Beta blockers appear to reduce the risk of sudden death in patients who are at increased risk. Antiplatelet agents, particularly aspirin, have been shown to be of benefit in patients who have had an MI. Aspirin reduces both rethrombosis and recurrent MI. Coumadin has been shown to decrease the risk of thromboembolic events in high-risk patients after infarction. Other antiarrhythmics have not been shown to be as effective as beta blockers as prophylactic agents.

16. c. Patients who have suffered an MI should increase activity levels gradually over a period of 6 to 8 weeks. Patients can return to work by approximately 8 weeks. Patients who have suffered an uncomplicated MI may be safely started in an activity program by 3 to 4 weeks postinfarct. Sexual intercourse can resume within 4 to 6 weeks of the infarction. There does not seem to be any logical reason for the patient to wait 3 months to resume intercourse. A good rule to follow in this case is as follows: "If the patient can climb the stairs to the bedroom, the rest is probably okay too."

In many patients the psychologic impact of an MI outweighs the physical impact. Also, in a significant percentage of families, the spouse is affected as much as, if not more than, the patient. One of the most common errors in cardiac rehabilitation is not to involve the spouse or significant other at every stage of the program.

17. e. The single best confirmatory test of the choices offered for the diagnosis of AMI is cardiac troponins. Cardiac troponins I and T are the preferred markers because they are more specific and reliable than creatine kinase or its isoenzyme creatine kinase MB. Elevation of the ST segment can result from either injury or infarction. It is neither sensitive nor specific enough for the diagnosis of infarction in the absence of Q waves. For the diagnosis of AMI, the ECG is sensitive (70% to 90% with more than 1 mm of elevation in two contiguous leads); unfortunately it is less specific. The presence of dysfunctional heart muscle on echocardiography means that there is likely to be a lowering of both the ejection fraction and the cardiac index; it says nothing about whether an MI has occurred or anything regarding the age of same.

18. c. Sudden death as a result of AMI is almost always the result of VF induced by the electrical instability of the ischemic/infarction zone. VF is most common either at the immediate onset of coronary occlusion or at the time of coronary reperfusion (reperfusion arrhythmia).

19. d. Shock in the presence of an AMI can be of two pathophysiologic varieties. Either there is hypovolemia and associated hypotension (hypovolemic shock), or there is persistent hypotension and a poor cardiac index in the presence of adequate left ventricular filling pressures.

Hypovolemic shock is best treated with volume replacement using either Ringer's lactate or normal saline solution. Care must be taken to avoid "volume overloading," which may produce pulmonary edema and congestive cardiac failure.

Cardiogenic shock generally is associated with severe left-ventricular dysfunction and occurs with large infarcts that produce damage to greater than 40% of the left ventricle. Treatment is urgent, and mortality is high. The treatments of choice include the following: (1) intraaortic balloon pump placement to increase coronary flow and decrease afterload; (2) coronary reperfusion with percutaneous transluminal balloon angioplasty (PTCA) (the mainstay of treatment); and (3) pharmacologic agents including morphine, dopamine, and dobutamine.

20. c. One clinical trial has shown unequivocally that there is a significant survival advantage to patients with AMI, even when thrombolytic agents are given up to 12 hours after the onset of the chest pain.

21. a. The finding on physical examination of the abdomen of "an enlarged aorta" should be further assessed by an abdominal ultrasound study. The patient probably has an aortic aneurysm. Although this finding also could be assessed by CT or MRI, an abdominal ultrasound is considerably less expensive and just as sensitive.

SUMMARY OF ACUTE ST SEGMENT ELEVATION MYOCARDIAL INFARCTION

1. Signs and symptoms:
Acute ST segment elevation MI occurs when a thrombus forms on a ruptured atheromatous plaque and thereby occludes a coronary artery.

The pain of MI, unlike angina pectoris, usually occurs at rest. The pain is similar to angina in location and radiation but is more severe and builds up rapidly. Usually it is described as retrosternal tightness or as a squeezing sensation or sometimes as a dull ache. Radiation to the left shoulder is common. Other common symptoms include sweating, weakness, dizziness, nausea, vomiting, and abdominal discomfort. Abdominal discomfort is especially common in inferior wall MIs.

2. ECG changes:
The classical evolution of changes is from peaked (hyperacute) T waves, to ST segment elevation, to Q-wave development, to T-wave inversion. This sequence may occur over a few hours or may take several days. (Note: If ECG changes are not present, do not assume an MI has not occurred. If signs and symptoms suggest MI, it is an MI until proved otherwise.)

3. Confirmatory evidence:
Evidence of infarction is confirmed by elevation of the cardiac troponins or creatine kinase MB fraction. Cardiac troponin I and T are the preferred markers because they are more specific and reliable than creatine kinase or its isoenzyme creatine kinase MB.

4. Other diagnostic procedures:
Scintigraphic studies including technetium-99 and thallium-201 imaging and radionuclide angiography, as well as echocardiography, may help document the extent of the damage but are not performed until after treatment.

5. Treatment of acute MI:
a. Supplementary oxygen
b. Morphine sulfate for pain relief
c. Coronary reperfusion: There currently are two means of reopening a blocked coronary artery in acute MI. They are thrombolytic therapy and primary angioplasty. Both are effective in reducing mortality but have limitations.

Thrombolysis, the most common form of treatment, is contraindicated in 20% of patients primarily because of bleeding risk. The recanalization rate is up to 55% with streptokinase and up to 60% with alteplase. There is a 5% to 15% risk of early or late reocclusion, and a 1% to 2% risk of intracranial hemorrhage with an attendant 40% mortality. Nevertheless, thrombolytic therapy is readily available and widely used. Indications for thrombolysis in acute MI are as follows: clinical history and presentation strongly suggestive of MI within 6 hours, plus one or more of a 1 to 2 mm ST elevation in two or more contiguous limb leads, new left bundle branch block, or 2-mm ST depression in V1-4 suggestive of true posterior MI. Patients presenting with the previous symptoms within 7 to 12 hours of onset with persisting chest pains and ST segment elevation are also candidates. Patients aged younger than 75 years presenting within 6 hours of anterior wall MI should be considered for recombinant t-PA. Absolute contraindications to thrombolysis include the following: aortic dissection, history of cerebral hemorrhage, cerebral aneurysm, arteriovenous malformation or intracranial neoplasm, recent (within past 6 months) thromboembolic stroke, or active internal bleeding. Patients previously treated with streptokinase should receive a recombinant t-PA (e.g., reteplase).

Primary angioplasty with stenting is becoming the intervention of choice for acute ST segment elevated MI in many hospitals. Primary angioplasty with stenting is safe and confers advantages over balloon angioplasty alone. The addition of glycoprotein IIb/IIIa inhibitor abciximab treatment improves flow characteristics, prevents distal thromboembolization, and reduces the need for repeat angioplasty. A strategy of primary stenting in association with abciximab is the current gold standard of care for patients with acute MI. The use of medication-eluding stents is promising and may surpass results of primary angioplasty with stenting plus glycoprotein inhibitors. However, primary angioplasty has these limitations: outcomes vary according to skills of interventionist, and the procedure is effective only for patients presenting early (less than 12 hours after acute MI). Complications are more common than with elective angioplasty, as are ventricular arrhythmias, although the latter are generally treatable. Right coronary artery procedures have high complication rates of sinus arrest, atrioventricular block, idioventricular rhythm, and severe hypotension. Surgical backup is required because up to 5% of patients require bypass surgery. Primary angioplasty, although an effective procedural intervention, requires facilities and experienced staff, and many adults with AMI in the United States and Canada are out of timely reach of such facilities and personnel.

  d. Aspirin one stat, 160 mg/day: Concurrent use of aspirin with a thrombolytic drug reduces mortality far more than either drug alone. In the ISIS-2 trial, aspirin with streptokinase reduced mortality by 42% without any increased incidence of stroke or major bleeding.
  e. Heparin therapy for patients receiving streptokinase: Heparin is used only for those at high risk of thromboembolism, such as those with large infarctions, atrial fibrillation, or congestive heart failure. For patients receiving fibrin-specific agents (alteplase, tenecteplase) heparin should be administered to reduce the risk of late reocclusion.
  f. Beta blockade limits the extent of infarction
  g. Nitroglycerin for pain control
  h. Warfarin: again used as was heparin, for those at high risk for thromboembolism
  i. Consider magnesium sulfate as analgesic/anxiolytic
  j. Note: Lidocaine prophylaxis is not indicated for the prevention of dysrhythmias

6. Post-MI:
  a. Submaximal stress ECG test and echocardiogram
  b. Discharge medications: aspirin; beta blocker, possibly angiotensin-converting enzyme inhibitor if there was a large infarct or thrombolytic therapy was administered, consider statin or other cholesterol lowering agent unless contraindicated. If aspirin is not tolerated, clopidogrel is an as effective, although expensive, antiplatelet alternative.
  c. Exercise program within 3 to 4 weeks
  d. Return to work within 8 weeks
  e. Sexual intercourse within 4 weeks
  f. Involvement of the spouse or significant other is critical

SUGGESTED READING

Cannon CP, Turpie AG: Unstable angina and non-ST-elevation myocardial infarction: initial antithrombotic therapy and early invasive strategy. *Circulation* 107(21):2640-2645, 2003.

Grech ED, Ramsdale DR: Acute coronary syndrome: ST segment elevation myocardial infarction. *BMJ* 326(7403):1379-1381, 2003.

Natarajan MK, Yusuf S: Primary angioplasty for ST-segment elevation myocardial infarction: ready for prime time? *CMAJ.* 169(1):32-35, 2003.

Chapter 11

Acute Coronary Symptoms and Stable Angina Pectoris

"My chest pain is getting worse. Am I dying?"

CLINICAL CASE PROBLEM 1:

A 55-YEAR-OLD MALE WITH CHEST PAIN

A 55-year-old male presents for the first time to your office for assessment of left-sided shoulder pain. The pain comes on after any strenuous activity, including walking. The pain is described as follows:

1. Quality: dull, aching
2. Quantity: 8/10 when doing any activity—otherwise he is asymptomatic
3. Location: mainly retrosternal
4. Radiation: appears to be radiating to the left shoulder area
5. Chronology: began approximately 8 months ago and has been getting worse ever since
6. Continuous/intermittent: intermittent
7. Aggravating factors: exercise of any kind
8. Relieving factors: rest
9. Associated manifestations: occasional nausea
10. Pain history: no previous pain before 8 months ago; no other significant history of pain syndromes
11. Quality of life: definitely affecting quality of life by limiting activity.

The patient tells you that the pain seems somehow worse today. For the first time, it did not go away after he stopped walking. The patient's blood pressure is 130/90 mm Hg; his pulse is 72 and regular. His heart sounds are normal. There are no extra sounds and no murmurs.

SELECT THE BEST ANSWER TO THE FOLLOWING QUESTIONS:

1. Which of the following statements regarding this patient's chest pain is (are) false?
   a. the patient may have suffered a myocardial infarction
   b. the patient's chest pain may be the result of angina pectoris
   c. the patient's chest pain may be the result of esophageal motor disorder
   d. the administration of sublingual nitroglycerin is a very sensitive test to distinguish angina pectoris from esophageal causes
   e. the patient should be admitted to the coronary care unit until the origin of the pain is firmly established

2. The patient is admitted to a chest pain unit and monitored. Which of the following investigations is not indicated at this time as part of this initial inpatient evaluation?
   a. an exercise tolerance test
   b. coronary angiography
   c. a serum thyroid stimulating hormone (TSH) level
   d. a complete blood count (CBC)
   e. a fasting blood sugar

His pain remits with aspirin and intravenous nitroglycerin. His cardiac troponin levels and ECG are normal. The patient does well and has an exercise tolerance test. This test reveals a 2.5-mm ST segment depression at 5 METS (metabolic equivalents of oxygen consumption) of activity as the patient achieved 50% of his age-predicted maximum heart rate.

3. Which of the following statements regarding this test result is (are) true?
   a. results indicate probable coronary artery disease (CAD)
   b. coronary angiography is indicated
   c. his inability to achieve maximum heart rate predicts CAD
   d. a and b
   e. all of the above statements are true

4. In addition to aspirin, which of the following medications is indicated as a first-line therapy for the treatment of this patient?
   a. diltiazem
   b. atenolol
   c. isosorbide dinitrate
   d. prazosin
   e. hydrochlorthiazide

CLINICAL CASE PROBLEM 2:

A 67-YEAR-OLD MALE WITH A HISTORY OF ANGINA PECTORIS

A 67-year-old male with a history of angina pectoris is brought to the emergency room (ER) by his wife. For the past 3 days, he has been having increasing chest pain. The retrosternal chest pain has been occurring intermittently while at rest during the day, while in bed at night, and while walking (he is able to walk only very slowly because of pain). The pain has been getting progressively persistent and worse over the past 8 hours. On physical examination, his blood pressure is 120/70 mm Hg. His pulse is 96 and regular. The rest of his examination is unchanged from previous visits to the office. His electrocardiogram (ECG) shows ST segment depression of 1.5 mm in leads V5-6. There is also flattening of the T waves seen across the precordial leads.

5. Which of the following statements regarding this patient is (are) true?
   a. this patient has unstable angina
   b. intravenous nitroglycerin and morphine may be used for pain relief
   c. the patient should be started taking heparin and clopidogrel
   d. this patient should already be taking daily aspirin
   e. all of the above are true

CLINICAL CASE PROBLEM 3:

A 50-YEAR-OLD FEMALE WITH A SHARP RETROSTERNAL CHEST PAIN

A 50-year-old female presents to the ER with a sharp retrosternal chest pain that awoke her. This is the fourth episode in as many nights, but she is sure that she is not having a heart attack because she saw her physician only 3 weeks ago. At that time, he gave her a "clean bill of health." She was told that her ECG, blood pressure, and cholesterol were completely normal. She is a nonsmoker and has no family history of CAD.

On physical examination, her blood pressure is 100/70 mm Hg. Her pulse is 96 and regular, and the remainder of the cardiovascular and respiratory examination is normal.

Her ECG reveals a significant ST segment elevation in the anterior limb leads. Within 1 hour, the ST segment has returned to normal. Cardiac troponin levels are normal.

6. Which of the following statements regarding this patient is (are) true?
   a. this patient probably has Prinzmetal's angina
   b. calcium-channel blockers are the treatment of choice for this type of angina
   c. beta blockers are advised for this type of angina
   d. a, b, and c
   e. a and b

7. Which of the following statements regarding percutaneous coronary angioplasty (PTCA) and mortality from CAD is (are) true?
   a. PTCA reduces overall mortality
   b. PTCA improves morbidity from CAD
   c. PTCA usually includes intracoronary stent placement
   d. optimal lesions for angioplasty are proximal in location, noneccentric, and located at branch (bifurcation) points in the vessel
   e. b and c

8. In which of the following patients would PTCA most likely be used?
   a. a 55-year old male smoker with left main-stem disease
   b. a diabetic patient with four-vessel disease
   c. an elderly patient with a ventricular aneurysm
   d. an obese patient with distal left anterior descending artery disease
   e. any of the above are good indications for PTCA

9. Which of the following is least likely to be used as a combination therapy in patients with angina pectoris?
   a. nitroglycerin-atenolol-nifedipine
   b. nitroglycerin-enalapril-nifedipine
   c. nitroglycerin-propranolol-verapamil
   d. nitroglycerin-metoprolol-diltiazem
   e. nitroglycerin-atenolol-nifedipine

10. Which of the following complications is seen with ticlopidine?
    a. thrombocytopenia
    b. ventricular arrhythmias
    c. atrial arrhythmias
    d. syncope
    e. b and d

11. Coronary artery bypass surgery (CABG) may be indicated as the treatment of choice for angina pectoris with which of the following patients with angina?
    a. a patient with triple-vessel disease
    b. a patient with one-vessel disease
    c. a patient with two-vessel disease
    d. CABG may be first-line therapy in any of the above
    e. b or c

CASE CLINICAL CASE PROBLEM 4:

A 65-YEAR-OLD MALE WITH ANGINA AND HYPERTENSION

A 65-year-old male presents to your office with a history strongly suggestive of angina pectoris. He also has a long history of hypertension.

On physical examination, his blood pressure is 170/100 mm Hg. Exercise tolerance testing reveals a 2.5-mm Hg ST segment depression in the lateral leads. A 2D/M mode echocardiogram reveals apical akinesis and an estimated ejection fraction of 50%.

12. Which of the following medications would you consider as the agent of first choice in the treatment of this patient?
    a. hydrochlorothiazide
    b. nifedipine
    c. clonidine
    d. atenolol
    e. prazosin

13. Which of the following investigations should be performed on a patient with possible angina pectoris?
   a. CBC
   b. chest x-ray
   c. fasting lipid profile
   d. thyroid function testing
   e. all of the above

14. The pathophysiology of angina pectoris is best explained by which of the following?
   a. significantly increased peripheral vascular resistance
   b. a balance between oxygen supply and oxygen demand
   c. an imbalance of oxygen supply and oxygen demand plus or minus coronary artery spasm
   d. significant peripheral venous and arterial vasoconstriction
   e. none of the above

15. Which of the following criteria indicate a diagnosis of unstable angina pectoris?
   a. new-onset angina (2 months) that is either severe or frequent (three episodes/day) or both
   b. patients with accelerating angina
   c. patients with angina at rest
   d. b and c
   e. all of the above

CLINICAL CASE MANAGEMENT PROBLEM

Briefly describe the phenomenon of asymptomatic coronary artery ischemia.

ANSWERS:

1. **d.** Angina pectoris simply means chest pain. Acute chest pain is a very common and often difficult diagnostic problem. Angina pectoris often is the pain of myocardial ischemia associated with acute coronary syndromes and chronic stable angina. Acute coronary syndromes include ST segment elevated myocardial infarction (discussed in Chapter 10), non-ST segment elevation myocardial infarction, and unstable angina. The distinction between unstable angina and non-ST segment myocardial infarction is the presence of elevated markers of myocardial necrosis (troponins) in infarction. The distinction between unstable angina and chronic stable angina is made on the basis of history and/or progressive ECG changes. Myocardial infarction must be assumed until proved otherwise

in patients with any significant risk factors. Of course, not all angina pectoris is the result of CAD, although this is the first hypothesis to entertain and test. Noncardiac causes of ischemia such as anemia, hyperthyroidism, musculoskeletal disorders, gastroesophageal reflux disease, pulmonary lesions, and others must be considered and ruled out. Pain from esophageal motor disorder often is confused with pain from myocardial ischemia. This differential is often exceedingly difficult. Many times (1) quality of pain, (2) quantity of pain, (3) radiation of pain, and (4) some aggravating factors are the same in both conditions. Although many physicians believe that relief with nitroglycerin is specific for myocardial ischemia and myocardial infarction, this is not the case. Sublingual nitroglycerin will relieve pain from esophageal motor disorder; it also will relieve pain from myocardial ischemia and myocardial injury.

2. **b.** We are not yet far enough down the diagnostic pathway of angina pectoris to justify the invasive procedure of coronary angiography. Normal cardiac troponin levels essentially rule out myocardial infarction. However, the origin of this patient's chest pain is still unclear and must be pursued in a systematic manner. At this time the following are diagnostic considerations: myocardial ischemia secondary to CAD or other causes, esophageal motor or reflux disorder, and musculoskeletal chest wall pain. Because this patient has other significant risk factors such as age and male gender, he should be assumed to have a cardiovascular cause for his pain until proved otherwise. Thus all testable risk factors should be measured, and the presence of underlying causes of angina should be ascertained. To rule out the possibilities of diabetes, anemia, and thyroid disease as underlying causes for his angina, a fasting blood sugar, CBC, and TSH level should be performed. Chest radiograph and pulse oximetry should be performed to evaluate for intrapulmonary causes of hypoxemia. A treadmill exercise stress test should be performed because this patient has a relatively high pretest probability of having CAD (Bayes' theorem).

3. **d.** The 2.5-mm ST segment depression quite likely represents severe coronary ischemia from CAD. Although we are not told the results of blood pressure monitoring during this patient's exercise tolerance test, if he had experienced a "hypotensive response," this would be another indication of severe ischemia. Failure to achieve his targeted maximum heart rate in and of itself does not predict CAD. However, taken together with the other information provided—ST segment depression at less than 6 METS and at less

than 70% of his predicted maximal heart rate—indicates a high probability of myocardial ischemia. With this information, coronary angiography now should be performed.

4. **b.** Medications used for treating angina pectoris of CAD include several classes of drugs: (1) antiplatelets/anticoagulants; (2) beta blockers; (3) lipid-lowering agents (3-hydroxy-3-methylglutaryl coenzyme A [HMG-CoA] reductase inhibitors); (4) nitrates; and (5) calcium channel blockers.

The underlying cause of angina of myocardial origin is the mismatch between oxygen supply and demand. There may be many causes of this mismatch, many correctable by treating the underlying condition (e.g., anemia, hyperthyroidism). Certainly the major cause to rule out or diagnose and treat is CAD. Narrowing or obstruction of the coronary arteries leads to ischemia. In the acute coronary syndromes of unstable angina and non-ST segment elevation myocardial infarction, there is generally a platelet-rich, partially occlusive thrombus present. Microthrombi can embolize and obstruct flow downstream. In the acute coronary syndrome of ST segment elevation (or Q-wave) myocardial infarction discussed in Chapter 10, a fibrin-rich, more stable occlusive thrombus is the cause of symptoms. In the past decade, much progress has been made in the development and use of several categories of medications used for the treatment of angina of CAD. Drugs listed here are the standard classes of agents used and are designed in large part to target the aforementioned pathophysiology.

Antiplatelet/anticoagulant treatment: Aspirin is the most widely used antiplatelet drug and is effective at doses from 75 to 300 mg daily. This is the agent of choice in CAD angina. Other antiplatelet agents include dipyridamole and ticlopidine. Ticlopidine is effective, but associated with the side effects of neutropenia and thrombocytopenia. Clopidogrel is another effective agent, and can be used if aspirin is contraindicated or not tolerated. Newer agents include the glycoprotein IIb/IIIa antagonists which have been used primarily in conjunction with thrombolysis in acute myocardial infarction. They are expensive, and their role is imprecisely defined in different forms of angina. Anticoagulations with low molecular weight heparin (LMWH) or standard heparin followed by warfarin have been tried in various forms of angina, and are effective in reducing morbidity primarily in persons at high risk for embolization. Warfarin should be continued for two to three months, except in atrial fibrillation, when it should be maintained indefinitely. If the patient is taking warfarin, aspirin may be taken concomitantly, but there is a higher risk of bleeding.

Use of beta-blockers is a standard therapy for the prevention of second myocardial infarction, the reduction of myocardial ischemia, and mortality reduction in the perioperative period in individuals with underlying angina. These drugs are still underutilized despite multiple guidelines and studies of effectiveness.

Good evidence exists indicating that lipid lowering HMG co-enzyme reductase inhibitors (statins) stabilize plaques of CAD and may reduce myocardial events. They are also effective in reducing LDL cholesterol, a potent risk factor in CAD.

Nitrates are the old war horses of pain relief, for which they are effective, but do little for long term mortality reduction. Still, they are popular.

A calcium-channel blocker (diltiazem) is used particularly for coronary artery spasm. These agents are applied in a cascade to the spectrum of disease ranging from chronic stable angina to the acute coronary syndromes. At a minimum, all patients with chronic stable angina and no contraindications should be on aspirin, beta-blockers and statins. Long acting nitrates, calcium channel blockers, and additional antiplatelet/anticoagulant therapy also may be considered. In acute coronary syndromes, hospitalized patients at lower risk for CAD are treated with aspirin, clopidogrel, and either heparin or LMWH until the diagnosis is made clear. For acute coronary syndrome hospitalized patients with intermittent or worsening symptoms but no ST-segment changes, with positive or negative troponins, treatment includes the use of those medications for low risk patients plus glycoprotein IIb/IIIa inhibition and early invasive intervention by cardiac catheterization.

5. **e.** The history given by this patient is one of unstable angina pectoris. Unstable angina pectoris is the term used to describe accelerating or "crescendo" angina in a patient who has previously had stable angina. Unstable angina can be diagnosed when the angina is new in onset, occurs with less exertion or at rest, lasts longer, or is less responsive to medication. Aspirin is the first treatment that should be given. For pain relief, nitrates or morphine may be used. Additionally, a beta-blocker, if not already in use, plus clopidogrel, standard heparin or LMWH, and a glycoprotein IIb/IIIa inhibitor should be started until the coronary arteries' anatomy is defined via catheterization. Nitrates are often used for the initial presentation of unstable angina. Non-parental therapy with sublingual or oral nitrates or nitroglycerin ointment may be sufficient, although IV is an option. In spite of the ECG showing only 1.5 mm of ST segment depression and no acute changes indicative of myocardial infarction, the patient should be hospitalized and placed in the coronary care unit. Serial

ECGs, and serial cardiac troponins or other markers of myocardial damage should be performed.

6. **d.** Prinzmetal's angina (coronary artery vasospasm) is angina that occurs in the absence of precipitating factors. Its symptoms most commonly occur in the early morning, often awakening the patient from sleep. It is usually associated with ST segment elevation rather than ST segment depression. Coronary angiography should be performed to rule out coexisting fixed stenotic lesions. Calcium-channel blockers are probably the drugs of choice for Prinzmetal's angina. Nitrates are also effective. Beta blockers are not indicated in patients who have vasospasm without fixed, stenotic lesions.

7. **e.** While overall mortality reduction from PTCA compared with medical treatment has not yet been shown, the procedure reduces symptoms, and in some instances, medication use. The use of new medication eluting stents inserted as part of the procedure may change mortality outcomes. Primary complications are restenosis requiring repeat procedure, arrhythmias, particularly with right coronary artery procedures, and artery rupture, necessitating surgery.

8. **d.** PTCA as a treatment for dilating stenotic coronary arterial lesions was introduced in 1977. Today successful dilatation rates per stenosis exceed 90%, complication rates have fallen to 4%, and procedure-related myocardial infarction and death remain uncommon. PTCA most often involves stent placement to maintain vessel patency. In many centers, PTCA is now the most commonly used invasive therapy for CAD. Significant restenosis used to occur within the first year in up to 40% of lesions, resulting in both symptomatic recurrence and high re-intervention rates. Various strategies – from the use of intravascular medication eluting stents to concomitant treatment with glycoprotein IIb/IIIa inhibitors – have demonstrated improvement in rates of acute closure and restenosis. In retrospective studies comparing the long-term results of PTCA and coronary artery bypass grafting (CABG), angina recurrence and event-free survival rates are better in the CABG for diabetics with multivessel disease, and patients with main stem and proximal left anterior descending artery lesions. Hence, answers a and b are incorrect. While older patients benefit from PTCA because it is better tolerated than surgery, a major ventricular aneurysm would be a contradiction. In summary, at this time the success rates of PTCA are under intensive scrutiny. Older studies comparing mortality and morbidity of PTCA with medical therapy and CABG surgery may not apply to current use of PTCA with drug eluting stents. Operator skill is another unknown with potent affects on outcomes. The family physician must stay tuned to ongoing developments in this field, and seek to know the local interventionists' rates of successful outcomes to better advise and manage the patient.

9. **b.** Of the combinations listed, the least likely combination of drugs to treat angina pectoris would be nitroglycerine-enalapril-nifedipine. Enalapril is an ACE inhibitor. Unless the patient also has congestive heart failure, ACE inhibitors are generally not used as medical therapy for angina pectoris.

10. **a.** Ticlopidine is an effective antiplatelet agent. Patients must be monitored for the possibility of thrombocytopenia and neutropenia.

11. **d.** Coronary artery bypass surgery (CABG) may be the treatment of choice in any of the choices listed, although it is specifically indicated on the basis of better mortality outcomes for individuals with left main stem disease and diabetics with multiple vessel disease.

12. **d.** A patient with both angina pectoris and hypertension should be treated with a cardioselective beta-blocker. Hydrochlorthiazide, while effective in hypertension, will not reduce his mortality as effectively as a beta-blocker. The calcium-channel blocker verapamil would be a reasonable treatment option only in addition to the beta-blocker.

13. **e.** Patients suspected of having angina pectoris need: (1) a CBC; (2) a fasting lipid profile; (3) a chest x-ray; (4) an ECG; and, (5) thyroid function testing. Moreover, renal function should be evaluated, and electrolyte and blood glucose measurements should be made. Testing for hyper-homocystinemia may also be warranted. If the patient appears to have significant COPD, then pulse-oximetry and spirometry may also be helpful.

14. **c.** The basic pathophysiology in patients with angina pectoris due to myocardial ischemia is an imbalance between oxygen supply and demand due to narrowing of the coronary arteries.

15. **e.** Unstable angina pectoris is characterized by: new onset angina (>2 months) that is severe and/or frequent (>3 episodes/day); patients with accelerating angina; or patients with angina at rest.

SOLUTION TO THE CLINICAL CASE MANAGEMENT PROBLEM

Obstructive CAD, acute myocardial infarction, and transient myocardial ischemia are frequently asymptomatic. The majority of patients with typical chronic angina pectoris are found to have objective evidence of myocardial ischemia (ST-segment depression). However, many of these same patients and some other patients who are always asymptomatic are at high risk for coronary events. Longitudinal studies have demonstrated an increased incidence of coronary events including sudden death and myocardial infarction in asymptomatic patients with positive exercise tests for ischemia. As well, patients with asymptomatic ischemia following a myocardial infarction are at far greater risk for a secondary coronary event than symptomatic patients. Patients who are found to have asymptomatic ischemia should be evaluated by stress thallium ECG. The management of asymptomatic ischemia must be individualized and depends on many factors, including the patient's age, occupation, and general medical condition. However, patients with severe asymptomatic ischemia on noninvasive testing should have aggressive risk factor modification, and at a minimum, should be placed on aspirin, beta-blockers, and possibly statins. Strong consideration should be given to referral for coronary arteriography.

SUMMARY OF ACUTE CORONARY SYMPTOMS AND STABLE ANGINA PECTORIS

DEFINITION: Angina pectoris simply means chest pain. Angina pectoris often is the pain of myocardial ischemia associated with acute coronary syndromes and chronic stable angina. Acute coronary syndromes include ST segment elevated myocardial infarction (discussed in chapter 10), non-ST segment elevation myocardial infarction, and unstable angina. The distinction between unstable angina and non-ST segment myocardial infarction is the presence of elevated markers of myocardial necrosis (troponins and others) in infarction. The distinction between unstable angina and chronic stable angina is made on the basis of history and/or progressive ECG changes. In all of the above instances, angina implies an imbalance between myocardial requirements for oxygen and the amount of oxygen delivered through the coronary arteries. This can occur via a mechanism of increased demand, diminished or extinguished delivery, or both. Acute coronary syndromes of unstable angina and non-ST segment elevation myocardial infarction have a much worse prognosis than chronic stable angina, with a 30 day mortality of between 10-20% despite treatment. These patients may also have higher long term risk of death than patients with ST segment elevation myocardial infarction. Of course, not all angina pectoris is due to CAD (CAD), although this is the first hypothesis to entertain and test. Non-cardiac causes of ischemia such as anemia, hyperthyroidism, as well as non-ischemic conditions such as musculoskeletal disorders, gastrointestinal conditions (e.g., GERD), pulmonary lesions, and others must be considered. But in the end, it is myocardial ischemia from CAD that must be examined and ruled out by the clinician, for the consequences of missing this diagnosis can be fatal.

SYMPTOMS: Patients with angina pectoris from underlying CAD frequently describe the discomfort as either an anterior chest "tightness" or "pain." Other descriptions include anterior chest "burning," "pressing," "choking," "aching," "gas," and "indigestion." These symptoms are typically located in the retrosternal area or the left chest. Usually, radiation to the left shoulder, left arm, or jaw occurs. Typical angina is aggravated by exercise and relieved by rest. Although there is no universally accepted definition of unstable angina, it has three main presentations—angina at rest, new onset angina, and increasing angina.

SIGNS: Physical examination is often normal, although hypertension is sometimes present.

RISK STRATIFICATION: Patients with chronic stable angina symptoms are at lower risk than those with unstable angina and generally can be monitored and treated as outpatients. Patients with angina at rest, new onset angina, or increasing angina should be risk stratified through ECG testing and measurement of cardiac troponins, preferably in a chest pain unit or hospital emergency department. Patients should have serial ECGs performed and cardiac biomarkers drawn, and if these are negative, early stress testing to evaluate for coronary disease. Patients with persistent or worsening symptoms, or positive cardiac troponins, despite normal ECG's, should be managed in a hospital cardiac unit as below.

Continued

SUMMARY OF ACUTE CORONARY SYMPTOMS AND STABLE ANGINA PECTORIS—cont'd

INITIAL LABORATORY EVALUATION: CBC, urinalysis, electrolytes, blood glucose, blood lipids, uric acid, renal and thyroid function tests, chest radiographs, ECG, and cardiac troponins are basic. Stress ECG testing with thallium is generally indicated in non-acute coronary syndrome initial evaluations. Radionuclide scintigraphy, echocardiography, and coronary angiography may follow.

TREATMENT: Underlying, reversible non-cardiac causes of angina should be treated as appropriate. In general, three forms of treatment exist for angina of CAD: medical therapy, percutaneous revascularization, and coronary artery bypass grafting. Older clinical trials of medical therapy must be interpreted with caution as many were completed before more recent anti-platelet, anti-fibrin, and cholesterol lowering agents were available. Patients with chronic stable angina have about a 2% average annual mortality, which is only twice that of age matched controls, a key factor to bear in mind when considering revascularization interventions. Higher risk patients, however, often stand to benefit the most from revascularization procedures. Higher risk patients include those with poor exercise capacity and easily provoked ischemia, recent onset angina, previous myocardial infarction, impaired left ventricular function, underlying diabetes, more than one stenosed artery, and those with disease that affects the left main stem or proximal left anterior descending artery.

For chronic stable angina:
a. Acute attacks:
   i. Mild: sublingual nitroglycerin or nitroglycerin spray
   ii. Severe: hospitalization and evaluation
b. Long-term prophylaxis and treatment: Risk factor reduction and aspirin, HMG co-enzyme reductase inhibitors (statins), and beta blockers with or without long-acting nitroglycerin, or long-acting calcium-channel blockers. Addition of clopidogrel and low molecular weight heparin may be considered.
c. Intervention/surgery:
   i. Percutaneous transluminal angioplasty (PTCA) has not yet demonstrated reduction in overall mortality compared to medical treatment, and patients undergo more procedures and have greater complications. However, patients do experience greater symptom relief and require fewer medications. Trials with newer medication-eluting stents may change these outcomes.
   ii. Coronary artery bypass surgery (CABG) has less mortality compared with medical treatment for patients with severe left main stem coronary disease, three vessel disease, two vessel disease with a severely affected proximal left anterior descending artery, or diabetics with multivessel disease. For lower risk patients, surgery provides symptom relief and improves exercise tolerance when medical treatment fails. Comparisons of PTCA with surgery suffer from the fact that most trials predate the more recent introduction of PTCA interventions that include medication eluting stents. In older trials examining single vessel disease, mortality is similar between surgery and PTCA, but rates of infarction, persistent symptoms, and repeat revascularization are higher in PTCA. In multivessel disease, mortality is similar, but PTCA is necessarily reserved for vessels with suitable, less tortuous, anatomy, making comparisons with surgery difficult.

For acute coronary syndromes:
a. Low risk patients: treat with aspirin, clopidogrel, and either heparin or LMWH. Consider early invasive intervention.
b. For patients with intermittent or worsening symptoms but no ST-segment changes, with positive or negative troponins, treat with the medications for low risk patients in (a.) plus glycoprotein IIb/IIIa inhibition and early invasive intervention by cardiac catheterization.
c. For treatment of ST segment elevation MI see chapter 10.
d. Prinzmetal's angina is an angina variant caused by coronary artery spasm with or without fixed stenotic lesions. It is more common in women than in men. ST segment elevation is more common than ST segment depression. Calcium-channel blockers are the treatment of choice.

SUGGESTED READING

Cannon CP, Turpie AG: Unstable angina and non-ST-elevation myocardial infarction: initial antithrombotic therapy and early invasive strategy. *Circulation.* 107(21):2640-2645, 2003.

Gibbons RJ et al: American College of Cardiology. American Heart Association clinical practice guidelines: Part I: where do they come from? *Circulation.* 107(23):2979-2986, 2003

Grech ED, Ramsdale DR: Acute coronary syndrome: unstable angina and non-ST segment elevation myocardial infarction. *BMJ.* 326(7401):1259-1261, 2003.

O'Toole L, Grech ED: Chronic stable angina: treatment options. *BMJ.* 326(7400):1185-1188, 2003.

Chapter 12

Hyperlipoproteinemia

"Where can I buy some of that good cholesterol?"

CLINICAL CASE PROBLEM 1:

A 51-YEAR-OLD MALE WITH HIGH BLOOD CHOLESTEROL

A 51-year-old male comes to your office for his "yearly workup." He is a typical type A personality: hard driving and "married to my job and proud of it." He is, however, married to his wife as well, as he points out in retrospect. He has had previous problems with "high blood cholesterol" and wishes to have his cholesterol checked today.

On examination, his blood pressure is 170/100 mm Hg. His pulse is 84 and regular. His body mass index (BMI) is 31. His abdomen is obese.

His family history is significant for hypertension in both parents. His uncle sustained a myocardial infarction (MI) at the age of 51 years, and his older brother had "heart problems" at age 53. His blood cholesterol in your office (nonfasting) is 8.2 mmol/l (328 mg/dL).

You ask the patient to return in 1 week for a fasting sample. The results are as follows: total cholesterol (TC), 288 mg/dL; triglycerides, 262 mg/dL; high-density lipoprotein (HDL), 37 mg/dL; and low-density lipoprotein (LDL), 199 mg/dL

■ SELECT THE BEST ANSWER TO THE FOLLOWING QUESTIONS:

1. Regarding this patient's lipid profile, which of the following statements is (are) true?
   a. this is a normal profile given his age and family history
   b. determination of his smoking status must be made prior to any recommendations
   c. intense dietary therapy and drug therapy should be considered immediately
   d. although this is an abnormal profile, in the absence of known coronary disease, careful observation of the cholesterol is all that is required at this time
   e. treatment decisions should be based on apoprotein levels

2. Which of the following, according to the National Cholesterol Education Program, (NCEP) defines high blood cholesterol?
   a. TC, 200 mg/dL; LDL, 130 mg/dL
   b. TC, 240 mg/dL; LDL, 160 mg/dL
   c. TC, 280 mg/dL; LDL, 190 mg/dL
   d. TC, 320 mg/dL; LDL, 220 mg/dL
   e. TC, 360 mg/dL; LDL, 250 mg/dL

3. What is the single most important risk factor for coronary artery disease (CAD)?
   a. an elevated HDL level
   b. an elevated triglyceride level
   c. an elevated LDL level
   d. a depressed HDL level
   e. an elevated total blood cholesterol

4. The NCEP defines all of the following conditions as major risk factors for CAD except?
   a. smoking
   b. obesity
   c. low HDL cholesterol
   d. hypertension
   e. age older than 45 years in males

5. All of the following conditions are at high risk for CAD except?
   a. peripheral arterial disease
   b. diabetes mellitus
   c. abdominal aortic aneurysm
   d. symptomatic carotid artery disease
   e. chronic kidney disease

6. An elevated triglyceride level is associated most closely with which of the following?
   a. impaired glycemic control
   b. hyperthyroidism
   c. weight loss
   d. low serum very low-density lipoprotein (VLDL) cholesterol
   e. elevated total serum cholesterol level

7. At what level of LDL cholesterol is treatment definitely indicated?
   a. 160 mg/dL
   b. 151 mg/dL
   c. 130 mg/dL
   d. 126 mg/dL
   e. 120 mg/dL

8. Which of the following is the treatment of choice for hypercholesterolemia?
   a. gemfibrozil
   b. colestipol
   c. nicotinic acid
   d. simvastatin
   e. none of the above

9. What is the drug class of choice for the management of mild to moderate elevations of plasma LDL?
   a. the fibric acid derivatives
   b. the nicotinic acid derivatives
   c. the 3-hydroxy-3-methylglutaryl coenzyme A (HMG-CoA) reductase inhibitors

   d. the bile acid sequestrants
   e. any of the above

10. Recommendations for lifestyle modification to reduce CAD risk include:
    a. regular aerobic exercise
    b. plant stanol ester use
    c. low-dose aspirin therapy
    d. a and c
    e. all of the above

11. Which of the following nutritional supplements helps decrease the risk of CAD?
    a. vitamin E
    b. dietary fiber
    c. hormone replacement therapy
    d. aspirin
    e. a and d

12. Which of the following is (are) independent risk factors for CAD?
    a. increased LDL concentration
    b. decreased HDL concentration
    c. increased total cholesterol concentration
    d. increased triglyceride concentration
    e. all of the above

13. Which of the following antihypertensive drugs do not have an adverse effect on plasma lipids?
    a. hydrochlorothiazide
    b. fosinopril
    c. atenolol
    d. nifedipine
    e. b and d

14. The American Heart Association's (AHA) Step 1 diet allows how much total cholesterol in the daily intake?
    a. 500 mg
    b. 400 mg
    c. 350 mg
    d. 300 mg
    e. 200 mg

15. Which of the following statements is (are) true regarding fish oil supplements?
    a. fish oils have been shown to lower plasma triglyceride levels
    b. fish oils inhibit platelet aggregation
    c. fish oils have been shown to increase HDL levels
    d. fish oils may decrease blood pressure and blood viscosity
    e. all of the above are true

16. What is the drug of choice for the treatment of hypertriglyceridemia?

   a. nicotinic acid
   b. gemfibrozil
   c. lovastatin
   d. a and b
   e. all of the above

17. Secondary causes of hyperlipidemia include all of the following except:
    a. hypothyroidism
    b. cirrhosis
    c. systemic lupus erythematosus
    d. nephrotic syndrome
    e. pregnancy

18. All of the following statements regarding abnormal lipid diagnosis and management are true except:
    a. if HDL cholesterol is greater than 60 mg/dL, then one risk factor may be subtracted from the CAD risk factor total
    b. the United States Preventive Services Task Force (USPSTF) recommends that cholesterol screening begin at age 18
    c. statin medications are best given in the evenings
    d. start a statin medication in a patient with diabetes mellitus with an LDL cholesterol of 100 mg/dL
    e. LDL cholesterol can be calculated as Total Cholesterol − (Triglycerides/5 + HDL cholesterol)

CLINICAL CASE MANAGEMENT PROBLEM

List the risk factors shown to increase the risk of CAD in the population.

ANSWERS:

   1. **c.** Given this patient's age and risk factors it was appropriate to proceed directly to a full (fasting) lipid profile. Normal serum cholesterol is defined as a value less than 5.2 mmol/l (200 mg/dL); borderline serum cholesterol is 5.2 to 6.2 mmol/l (200-240 mg/dL); and high serum cholesterol is more than 6.2 mmol/l (240 mg/dL).

   The question of which patients should be screened for hypercholesterolemia continues to be debated. The third USPSTF report recommends the following: (1) All men aged 35 and older and all women aged 45 and older should be screened routinely for lipid disorders. (This extends the recommendations of the second USPSTF, which recommended that adults not be screened until age 65.); (2) younger adults— men aged 20-35 and women aged 20-45—should be screened if they have other risk factors for heart disease. (These risk factors include tobacco use, diabetes, a family history of heart disease or high cholesterol, or high blood pressure. This recommendation expands on the recommendations of the second USPSTF, which focused on screening middle-aged men and women.); and (3) clinicians should measure HDL in addition to measuring TC or LDL. They found insufficient evidence to recommend for or against measuring triglycerides. In addition the current recommendation is to screen with a non-fasting sample.

2. b. The National Cholesterol Education Program defines a high blood cholesterol as equal or greater than the following: (1) TC, 240 mg/dL (6.2 mmol/l) and (2) LDL, 160 mg/dL (4.1 mmol/l).

3. c. The single most important risk factor for CAD is an elevated LDL. The second most important risk factor is depressed HDL.

4. b. The five major risk factors for CAD are as follows: (1) having hypertension, (2) smoking, (3) having diabetes, (4) being older than age 45 years in males and older than age 55 in females, and (5) having a family history of MI in a first-degree relative (male relative younger than age 55 or a female relative younger than age 65). Obesity is not a specific risk factor but is strongly associated with the conditions that are major risk factors.

5. e. The following conditions are considered CAD risk-factor equivalents: peripheral arterial disease, diabetes mellitus, abdominal aortic aneurysm, and symptomatic carotid artery disease.

6. a. An elevated triglyceride level, defined as 250 mg/dL or greater, often is observed in people with diabetes with poor glucose control. Weight loss and a low-carbohydrate and low-fat diet are recommended for lifestyle treatment of hypertriglyceridemia. An elevated triglyceride level is associated most closely with an elevated VLDL. TC may be elevated with high triglycerides but also can be in the normal range.

7. a. An LDL level is considered definitely elevated when it is higher than 160 mg/dL. The borderline level is between 130 and 160 mg/dL.

8. e. The treatment of choice for hypercholesterolemia is diet therapy. The AHA has produced Step 1 and Step 2 diets. The Step 1 diet includes less than 30% of total calories from fat, less than 10% of calories from saturated fat, and less than 300 mg/day of cholesterol. The Step 2 diet includes less than 30% of total daily calories as fat, less than 7% of calories from saturated fat, and less than 200 mg/day of cholesterol.

Management of hypercholesterolemia with drugs is indicated only after dietary treatment over a reasonable length of time has failed to reduce the cholesterol level to a sufficiently low level, although there is a newfound sense of more aggressive treatment, even for primary prevention, as the result of studies such as the Air Force/Texas Coronary Atherosclerosis Prevention Study (AFCAP/TexCAP). The current recommendations that diet therapy be continued for 6 months before drug therapy is started often are supplanted because this study and others have shown conclusively that aggressive treatment of even low-risk middle-aged adults with statin therapy can reduce cardiac morbidity and mortality.

9. c. The drug class of choice for mild to moderate LDL elevation is one of the HMG-CoA reductase inhibitors on the market. These include lovastatin (Mevacor), pravastatin (Pravachol), simvastatin (Zocor), and atorvastatin (Lipitor). All patients who are started taking HMG-CoA inhibitors should have not only the plasma lipids but also the liver function tests at baseline and then in 12 weeks. If no further dose changes are made, then liver function tests may be evaluated every 6 months and then yearly when stable. There is a low risk of myositis; therefore creatinine kinase levels should be measured if patients report leg pain or muscle cramps. In patients with mild to moderate isolated LDL elevation (Type IIA), plasma lipids may be normalized with 10 mg to 20 mg once daily of any of these agents. Patients with higher LDL levels may require higher doses of single-agent therapy or, alternately, multidrug therapy. With such therapy, LDL cholesterol may be lowered up to 40%, and triglyceride levels may be lowered 10% to 15%. There appears to be little change in the HDL level. All the previously mentioned drugs have been known to produce hepatic and skeletal muscle toxicity, insomnia, and weight gain. These side effects, however, are relatively uncommon, are dose related, and occur much more frequently in patients who are undergoing multidrug therapy.

The drug of second choice for Type IIA hyperlipoproteinemia is niacin. The total daily dose (500-mg tablets) is up to 3 g. All patients taking niacin require monitoring of liver function tests and creatine phosphokinase monthly for 3 months, then every 3 months for 6 months, and every 4 to 6 months thereafter. Niacin may decrease plasma LDL by up to 35% and may decrease triglyceride levels by up to 75%; at the same time it may increase the HDL by up to 100%. In addition, the apolipoprotein A level is decreased by up to 50%. Unfortunately, niacin has a considerable number of significant side effects, including the following: (1) induction of gastric irritation and gastritis; (2) activation of long-dormant peptic ulcers; (3) elevation of plasma uric acid levels, precipitating an attack of gout; (4) elevation of blood glucose levels; (5) exacerbation of diabetes; and (6) most commonly, cutaneous flushing, dry and even scaly skin, and in rare instances acanthosis nigricans.

Some of these nuance side effects can be ameliorated by coadministering aspirin and/or prescribing the long-acting formulation of niacin. Fortunately, all side effects disappear when the drug is discontinued.

Resins, including cholestyramine (Questran) and colestipol (Colestid), are the drugs of third choice for patients with Type IIA hyperlipoproteinemia. The dose ranges are 4 to 8 g once or twice daily for cholestyramine and 5 to 10 g once or twice daily for colestipol.

Their advantages include an almost complete lack of absorption and potential for systemic toxicity that goes with it. Their disadvantages include an unpleasant grittiness and multiple gastrointestinal side effects, including abdominal bloating, abdominal pain, sometimes severe constipation, and gastrointestinal bleeding. Because resins may decrease the absorption of other drugs, they and other drugs should be taken 2 hours apart.

10. e. Healthy lifestyle choices that reduce the risk of coronary events include diet, aerobic exercise, weight management, smoking cessation, multivitamin supplements with folic acid, aspirin therapy, and plant stanol ester nutritional supplements. The Food and Drug Administration (FDA) permits food labels to indicate that daily use of plant stanol esters will help reduce LDL levels. These esters are produced by the esterification of the plant steroid stanol with canola oil, and they act by blocking the intestinal absorption of cholesterol. This reduces the serum LDL but not serum HDL.

11. d. Vitamin E, although popular as an antioxidant, has not been shown to favorably or unfavorably alter the course of CAD. Dietary fiber also has no beneficial effect on heart disease, but it does show favorable effect on colorectal disease. Hormone replacement therapy was shown to increase the risk of CAD by the Women's Health Initiative. However, primary and secondary prevention trials have shown aspirin decreases CAD risk.

12. e. Risk factors for CAD include the following: (1) increased LDL concentration (most important lipid risk factor); (2) decreased HDL (second most important risk factor); (3) increased TC; and (4) increased triglyceride concentration.

13. e. Nifedipine, a calcium channel blocker, and fosinopril, an angiotensin converting enzyme (ACE) inhibitor, are the only drugs listed that do not have an adverse affect on plasma lipids. (Angiotensin receptor blockers are also neutral with respect to plasma lipids,

and alpha blockers appear to have a beneficial effect on HDL levels.) The beta blocker listed, metoprolol, and hydrochlorothiazide adversely affect plasma lipids.

14. d. As mentioned previously, the treatment of first choice for hyperlipidemia is diet. The AHA's Step 1 diet and Step 2 diets are listed in the table.

AHA Step 1 and 2 Diets		
	STEP 1	STEP 2
Cholesterol	300 mg	200 mg
Total fat	30% of calories	30% of calories
Saturated fat	10% of calories	7% of calories

15. e. Fish and fish oil supplements may reduce plasma lipid levels (especially triglycerides), inhibit platelet aggregation, decrease blood pressure and viscosity, and increase HDL cholesterol. The active ingredients are the long chain omega-3 fatty acids, eicosapentaenoic acid and docosahexaenoic acid. Well-controlled long-term studies conducted by the Brigham and Women's Hospital and the Harvard Public School of Health and released in 2002 showed an 81% decrease in sudden cardiac-related death risk in men and a 34% decrease in women who consume fish on a regular basis. Female nurses who consumed fish at least once a week also were found to have a 25% decline in nonfatal heart attacks and a significant decline in deaths in general. The authors felt both fish and fish oil supplements had a positive effect. However, the beneficial use of fish oil supplements for general use remains more controversial, perhaps because it may not generally be appreciated that efficient absorption requires the presence of other nutrients, in particular additional lipid. In addition, these polyunsaturated fatty acids readily autooxidize.

The essential C-18 omega-3 fatty acid, linolenic acid (also known as alpha-linolenic acid), can be converted to the 20 carbon eicosapentaenoic acid, which in turn is converted to the 22 carbon docosahexaenoic acid and as a consequence can substitute for fish oils. The typical U.S. diet, however, tends to limit this conversion because the linoleic/linolenic acid ratio in the diet is too high. This conversion also may be inhibited by other fatty acids; trans-fatty acids in particular have been implicated. Unfortunately the distribution of alpha-linolenic acid is limited. Studies suggest the optimal linoleic/linolenic acid ratio is between 5 to 10 to 1. The oils obtained from flax seed, walnuts, rape seed (canola), safflower, soybean, and wheat germ are the only natural substances having these fatty acids in this optimal range. The best way to assure the oils are not partially oxidized is to consume them in the foods from which they are derived.

16. **b.** The drug of choice for most cases of hypertriglyceridemia is gemfibrozil or another fibric acid derivative. Hypertriglyceridemia may be associated with Type 2a, Type 2b, Type 3, or Type 4 hyperlipoproteinemia. The usual dose of gemfibrozil is 0.6 g bid. Gemfibrozil will decrease hypertriglyceridemia by 40% to 80% and will increase HDL by 10% to 40%.

Until very recently, combining a reductase inhibitor with gemfibrozil was not recommended. This combination still should be used with caution but may be tolerated if a low dose of one drug is given 12 hours apart from a low dose of the other (e.g., pravastatin 10 mg to 20 mg in the morning with gemfibrozil 600 mg in the evening).

17. **b.** Hypothyroidism, lupus, pregnancy, oral contraceptive use, and nephritic syndrome are associated with elevations of cholesterol. Cirrhosis usually is associated with a decrease in cholesterol.

18. **b.** The USPSTF recommends general screening at age 35 years for males and age 45 years for females and targeted screening in adults age 20 to 45. If HDL cholesterol is greater than 60 mg/dL, then one risk factor may be subtracted from the CAD risk factor total.

Start a statin medication in a patient with diabetes mellitus with a LDL cholesterol of 100 mg/dL or greater. The Heart Protection Study suggests that statins may even be beneficial in people with diabetes that have LDL values of less than 100 mg/dL. LDL cholesterol can be calculated as total cholesterol − (Triglycerides/5 + HDL cholesterol). (Statin medications are best given in the evenings.)

SOLUTION TO THE CLINICAL CASE MANAGEMENT PROBLEM

The risk factors for CAD in the population are as follows: (1) family history of CAD; (2) male sex; (3) hypertension; (4) hypercholesterolemia; (5) high LDL levels; (6) low HDL levels; (7) hypertriglyceridemia: (8) high VLDL levels; (9) cigarette smoking; (10) high alcohol intake (via its effect on hypertension); (11) lack of aerobic exercise; (12) obesity; (13) Type 1 diabetes; (14) Type 2 diabetes; (15) postmenopausal women; and (16) hyperhomocystinemia.

SUMMARY OF HYPERLIPOPROTEINEMIA

A. Screening:
The third USPSTF report recommends the following: (1) all men aged 35 years and older and all women aged 45 and older should be screened routinely for lipid disorders; (2) younger adults—men aged 20-35 and women aged 20-45—should be screened if they have other risk factors for heart disease (including tobacco use, diabetes, a family history of heart disease or high cholesterol, or high blood pressure); and (3) clinicians should measure HDL in addition to measuring TC or LDL. They found insufficient evidence to recommend for or against measuring triglycerides. The current recommendation is to screen with a nonfasting sample, and all patients should receive periodic counseling regarding dietary intake of fat (especially saturated fat) and cholesterol.

B. Recommended cholesterol values:
1. TC: Normal, equal to or less than 5.2 mmol/L (200 mg/dL); borderline, 5.2-6.2 mmol/L (200-240 mg/dL); elevated, equal to or greater than 6.2 mmol/L (240 mg/dL)
2. LDL cholesterol: ideal, equal to or less than 3.4 mmol/L (130 mg/dL); borderline, 3.4-4.1 mmol/L (130-159 mg/dL); elevated, equal to or greater than 4.1 mmol/L (159 mg/dL)
3. VLDL cholesterol (triglycerides): ideal, equal to or less than 1.4 mmol/L (125 mg/dL); borderline, 1.4-2.8 mmol/L (125-250 mg/dL); elevated, equal to or greater than 2.8 mmol/L (250 mg/dL)

C. Dietary treatment of hypercholesterolemia:
Treat hypercholesterolemia if LDL cholesterol is greater than 4.1 mmol/L or 3.4 mmol/L with two or more risk factors. Dietary management is the treatment of first choice.
1. Begin with the Step 1 diet of the AHA: no more than 300 mg cholesterol; no more than 30% total fat; and no more than 10% saturated fat.
2. Continue for at least 6 months. If cholesterol levels do not normalize, consider AHA Step 2 diet: no more than 200 mg cholesterol; no more than 30% total fat and, no more than 7% saturated fat.

Continued

SUMMARY OF HYPERLIPOPROTEINEMIA—cont'd

D. Drug treatments for hypercholesterolemia to be used if dietary treatment is insufficient:
   1. Drugs of first choice are HMG Co-A reductase inhibitors. The Scandinavian Simvastatin Survival Study has shown that cholesterol-lowering drugs reduce deaths from CAD and sudden cardiac death. In this study the HMG-CoA reductase inhibitor simvastatin substantially improved survival, reducing the overall risk of death by 30% and the risk of coronary death by 42%. This adds even more credibility to the recommendation that HMG-CoA reductase inhibitors be considered the drugs of first choice for the treatment of hyperlipidemia.
   2. Drug of second choice: niacin
   3. Drug of third choice: bile acid sequestrants

E. Hypertriglyceridemia:
   Hypertriglyceridemia has been established as an independent risk factor for CAD. Always look for a secondary cause of hypertriglyceridemia, such as presence of diabetes mellitus, alcohol use, or oral contraceptive use.

   Treatments for hypertriglyceridemia include the AHA Step 1 and Step 2 diets, and the drug of choice for drug treatment of hyperlipoproteinemia primarily resulting from elevated triglycerides is gemfibrozil.

SUGGESTED READING

Albert CM, et al: Blood levels of long chain ω-3 fatty acids and the risk of sudden death. *N Engl J Med* 346:1113-1118, 2002.

Gaziano JM, et al: Cholesterol reduction: Weighing the benefits and risks. *Ann Intern Med* 124:914, 1996.

Hu FB, et al: Fish and omega-3 fatty acid intake and risk of coronary heart attack in women. *JAMA*, 287:1818-1821, 2002.

Institute for Clinical Systems Improvement: Lipid management in adults. *Institute for Clinical Systems Improvement (ICSI)*, Bloomington, MN, 2002 July.

National Heart, Lung, and Blood Institute: *National Cholesterol Education Program*, 1999.

Screening Adults for Lipid Disorders. What's New from the *USPSTF. AHRQ Publication No. APPIP* 01-0011. Agency for Healthcare Research and Quality, Rockville, MD, March 2001.

U.S. Preventive Services Task Force: *Guide to clinical preventive services*: An assessment of the effectiveness of 169 interventions, Baltimore: Williams and Wilkins, 1989.

http://www.ahrq.gov/clinic/prev/lipidwh.htm.

http://www.nhlbi.nih.gov.

Chapter 13

Congestive Heart Failure

> "I get so scared. Sometimes, in the middle of the night I can't catch my breath."

CLINICAL CASE PROBLEM 1:
A 78-YEAR-OLD FEMALE WITH SHORTNESS OF BREATH

A 78-year-old female comes to the emergency department with a 6-month history of fatigue and shortness of breath, aggravated especially when performing any exertional activity including those associated with activities of daily living. She has found that occasionally she has to get up at night and open the window to get air. There has been a weight gain of 15 pounds during the 6 months, and there has been gradual swelling of her ankles and legs. Her history reveals no previous myocardial infarction, but it does reveal the presence of type 2 diabetes for 15 years, severe hypertension for 30 years, and obesity for 8 years. Although the shortness of breath has been a significant problem for only 6 months, she does mention having "some breathing problems" intermittently for at least 4 years, and she has been treated for intermittent atrial fibrillation and moderate chronic obstructive pulmonary disease. She is taking glyburide, hydrochlorthiazide, diltiazem, coumadin, ipratropium, and captopril.

On physical examination, the patient's blood pressure is 140/90 mm Hg. The respiratory rate is 28/min, and the pulse is 98/minute and regular; she is afebrile. Head, ears, eyes, nose, and throat (HEENT) are unremarkable; there is no elevated jugular venous distention (JVD). Both S1 and S2 are normal, but a fourth heart sound is present; there are no murmurs. Chest examination reveals bibasilar rales in both lung bases. Abdominal examination is benign; the hepatojugular reflex is negative. Extremities reveal bilateral 3+ pitting edema to both knees. Pulse oximetry shows an O_2 saturation of 90% on room air. Electrocardiogram (ECG) reveals normal sinus rhythm, no acute changes, and left-ventricular (LV) hypertrophy. You suspect a form of heart failure and order a chest radiograph.

■ **SELECT THE BEST ANSWER TO THE FOLLOWING QUESTIONS:**

   1. Your working hypothesis, based on the history and physical examination, is that the patient has which of the following?

a. diastolic heart failure
b. systolic heart failure
c. biventricular heart failure
d. cor pulmonale
e. heart failure secondary to pulmonary fibrosis

2. Based on the type of failure this patient has, what is most likely to be found on chest radiograph?
a. normal chest
b. congestion and cardiomegaly
c. pulmonary edema
d. congestion with or without cardiomegaly
e. cardiomegaly

3. The chest x-ray is consistent with the history and physical examination and your diagnosis of diastolic failure. The patient is admitted for therapy. You order an echocardiogram. Again, based on the type of failure this patient has, what is this likely to show?
a. normal LV cavity size
b. an ejection fraction of more than 40%
c. a dilated left ventricle
d. an ejection size of less than 40%
e. a and b

4. The targeted range of the diastolic blood pressure in this patient should be:
a. <90 mm Hg
b. <80 mm Hg
c. between 80 and 90 mm Hg
d. it does not matter
e. >90 mm Hg to maintain perfusion

CLINICAL CASE PROBLEM 2:

A 62-YEAR-OLD MALE WITH EXERTIONAL DYSPNEA, ORTHOPNEA, AND WHEEZING.

A 62-year-old male, with a long history of smoking two packs of cigarettes a day, presents to your office with a history of worsening shortness of breath with exertion for the past 3 weeks. He also relates recent onset of fatigue, two-pillow orthopnea, and scattered wheezes when climbing a flight of stairs. Five years ago he had an anterior wall myocardial infarction but had been doing well until his recent symptoms. He has no other medical problems. He takes a baby aspirin and atenolol daily.

On examination his vital signs were as follows: pulse 100/min and regular, respiration 24 breaths/minute, blood pressure 129/89, afebrile. Weight has increased by 10 pounds since the last visit 6 months ago. There is JVD at 30 degrees elevation, rales a third of the way up in both lung fields, moderate hepatic congestion, and a positive hepatojugular reflux. Heart examination reveals an S4 but no murmurs. There is also 1+ pitting edema in both legs to his mid-calves. You perform an electrocardiogram (ECG), which shows sinus rhythm and no acute changes

but poor R-wave progression in the anterior leads. Chest radiograph reveals cardiomegaly and pulmonary vascular congestion.

5. Which of the following medications is (are) appropriate for acute management?
a. furosemide
b. captopril
c. diltiazem
d. labetalol
e. a, b, and c

6. The nonpharmacologic treatments(s) of choice for this condition may include which of the following?
a. salt restriction
b. fat restriction
c. water restriction
d. none of the above
e. a, b, and c

The patient described here is treated with the appropriate medication and improves. He returns in 2 weeks with dyspnea and fatigue, although it is not as severe as before. Vital signs are normal. At this time, the JVD has resolved and the hepatojugular reflex is absent. The cardiac examination is unchanged. There is trace pitting edema in his ankles bilaterally. He has lost 10 pounds in weight. Results of an echocardiogram are pending.

7. At this time, which of the following is (are) appropriate medication(s) to consider instituting?
a. an angiotensin-converting enzyme (ACE) inhibitor or adrenogenic receptor binder (ARB)
b. a second beta blocker
c. a calcium channel blocker
d. digitalis
e. a and d

8. Which of the following pathophysiologic mechanisms may underlie heart failure in this patient and should be searched for as part of a comprehensive evaluation?
a. LV chamber remodeling
b. coronary artery disease
c. valvular heart disease
d. abnormal excitation-contraction coupling
e. all of the above

9. What is (are) the current indication(s) for the use of digitalis in this condition?
a. a dilated left ventricle
b. an S3 or S4 gallop
c. decreased ejection fraction
d. atrial fibrillation with a rapid ventricular rate
e. c and d above

10. Which of the following is (are) correct about the effects of digitalis on patients with this condition?
   a. digoxin reduces long-term mortality
   b. digoxin decreases rates of worsening of heart failure
   c. lower digoxin maintenance doses may be as effective as higher doses
   d. digoxin use reduces hospitalizations
   e. b, c, and d

11. In evaluating a patient for systolic dysfunction, the most important characteristic found on echocardiogram is:
   a. myocardial hypertrophy
   b. valvular heart disease
   c. cor pulmonale
   d. low ejection fraction
   e. wall-motion abnormalities

12. Which of the following correctly defines the American Heart Association (AHA) stages of heart failure?
   a. Stage A are asymptomatic patients at high risk but with no identifiable structural abnormalities
   b. Stage B are asymptomatic patients with identifiable structural abnormalities
   c. Stage C are symptomatic patients with structural abnormalities
   d. Stage D are end-stage patients refractory to standard therapy
   e. all of the above

13. All but which of the following has been shown to reduce hospitalizations and mortality in selective patients with congestive heart failure (CHF)?
   a. beta blockers
   b. spironolactone
   c. ACE inhibitors
   d. biventricular pacing
   e. calcium channel blockers

CLINICAL CASE MANAGEMENT PROBLEM

A major error in treating heart failure is assuming that all patients who appear to be in heart failure need furosemide. When given furosemide, some patients actually get worse. Provide an example of a practical situation in which this could occur.

ANSWERS:

1. This patient has a classic history for diastolic heart failure. An estimated 20% to 40% of patients with CHF have preserved or normal systolic function. In these patients, contraction is normal, but diastole (relaxation phase) is abnormal. During exertion, normal filling during diastole does not occur, and cardiac output is impaired. Therefore, dyspnea is particularly profound during exertion. Dyspnea is the most common sign of both systolic and diastolic CHF. Initially, the dyspnea is present only with moderate amounts of exertion, but as the severity of the heart failure increases, the shortness of breath may occur with only minimal exertion or even at rest. Other common symptoms of heart failure are fatigue and lethargy.

Patients with diastolic cardiac failure are, like the patient presented, frequently elderly and female, with a history of hypertension, diabetes, and obesity. Atrial fibrillation, if present, is usually paroxysmal, and a fourth heart sound (S4 gallop) often is present. In systolic heart failure, which can occur in all ages and more often in males, atrial fibrillation tends to be persistent, a third heart sound is present (S3 gallop), and there is often a history of previous myocardial infarction.

In both forms of failure, lying flat often is followed by increasing shortness of breath. Paroxysms of nocturnal dyspnea (PND) are suggestive of heart failure. On careful questioning the patient describes the bouts as marked breathlessness—a "suffocating feeling"—and these symptoms often are accompanied by significant anxiety. The patient has to sit upright or even stand up to breathe and may have the urge to rush to an open window to relieve the "suffocating feeling." Extra pillows are needed to reduce the number and severity of attacks. Some patients even have to resort to sleeping upright in a chair at all times.

2. **d.** Patients with diastolic failure will present with congestion with or without cardiomegaly on chest radiograph. Do not be fooled in thinking that the absence of cardiomegaly rules out failure. In systolic failure, in contrast, cardiomegaly almost always is present. Heart failure also can be distinguished by which ventricle is failing the most. Whereas LV cardiac failure is manifested by symptoms, such as shortness of breath, right-ventricular cardiac failure is manifested by signs such as enlargement of the liver, a positive hepatojugular reflex, and an elevated jugular venous pressure. In severe cases of elevated right-sided atrial pressure, splanchnic engorgement may accompany anorexia, nausea, vomiting, ascites, and eventually cachexia. In most instances of chronic failure, however, both ventricles usually are involved, making the distinction less useful.

3. **e.** The cardinal features of diastolic heart failure are the presence on echocardiogram of a normal LV

ejection fraction and a usually normal LV cavity size. Concentric LV hypertrophy usually is present as well. In systolic heart failure, LV ejection fraction is usually less than 40% and the ventricular cavity is dilated.

4. b. This patient has diabetes and, as a result, evidence-based guidelines suggest targeting diastolic blood pressure to be less than 80 mm Hg to reduce mortality and morbidity.

5. a. The most appropriate acute pharmacotherapeutic intervention is the administration of diuretics, particularly loop diuretics, preferably intravenously. Careful attention should be given to the patient's urine output and weight as a measure of successful diuresis. Reasonable investigations in acute failure would include the following: 12 lead ECG; chest radiograph; blood chemistries including blood urea nitrogen (BUN), creatinine, glucose, and electrolytes; complete blood count (CBC); thyroid stimulating hormone (TSH); liver function tests and lipids; urinalysis for protein and sugar; and echocardiography. Diuresis should be accomplished with careful attention to electrolytes, especially potassium, with adequate replenishment of depleted salts. Oxygen should be administered to correct any hypoxia.

6. e. Nonpharmacologic therapy for CHF involves the following in order of importance: (1) bed rest; (2) salt restriction (2-3 g sodium/day); (3) fluid restriction (related to sodium restriction); and (4) fat restriction (as a reasonable approach to a healthy lifestyle using the AHA Step 1 diet, which is 300 mg cholesterol, 30% total calories from fat, and 10% of calories from saturated fat).

7. a. Two drugs have been proved particularly useful in the treatment of chronic heart failure: ACE inhibitors and beta blockers, the latter of which this patient is already taking. ACE-inhibitor drugs such as captopril, enalapril, or lisinopril have been shown to reduce both morbidity and mortality in patients with severe systolic heart failure. Little outcome difference exists between those taking higher or lower doses, so the later is preferred to reduce potential side effects. For patients who cannot tolerate ACE inhibitors, ARBs are a reasonable alternative, although no studies have produced evidence that they should be used as a first-line agent in chronic CHF. This may be more of an issue of the dosages used in trials, and a recent head-to-head study of an ACE inhibitor with or without ARB suggests the ARB agent may be as effective as an ACE alone, but the two together confer no additive advantage. Whether this is true for the entire class of ARBs remains to be seen. Beta blockers,

when used with caution and introduced carefully, also have had a positive effect on mortality and morbidity in multiple studies and are thought to work primarily by countering the harmful effects of the sympathetic nervous system. Initiation often may exacerbate symptoms, so patients must be monitored carefully and titrated slowly. Because the echocardiogram results are pending, it is uncertain whether digoxin is appropriate in this patient. Calcium channel blockers have not demonstrated the effectiveness of ACE inhibitors or beta blockers.

8. e. CHF is a syndrome in which a large number of pathophysiologic mechanisms may underlie the symptoms and signs of heart failure. Some of these include structural abnormalities of the myocardium, LV chamber, and coronary arteries and functional abnormalities of the valves and electrical systems. In this patient, a comprehensive evaluation would include a search for evidence of LV chamber remodeling, coronary artery disease, valvular heart disease, abnormal excitation-contraction coupling, and arrhythmias. Coexisting noncardiac diseases also should be identified and treated. That would include search for and control of tobacco addiction, alcohol abuse, diabetes, hypertension, obesity, anemia, sleep apnea, and renal disease.

9. e. The use of digitalis (in the form of digoxin) has come full circle. This drug, isolated from the foxglove plant, used to be the mainstay of treatment for CHF. For various reasons, it then fell into disfavor, to the point where it was virtually never used. The completion of the circle has resulted in digoxin once again being used extensively. Its primary indications are in cases of CHF with a reduced ejection fraction and atrial fibrillation with a rapid ventricular rate. Physicians should be aware of drug interactions that may increase digoxin levels. These include use of digoxin with verapamil, quinidine, procainamide, nifedipine, or amiodarone. Physicians also should be aware of electrolyte abnormalities (hypokalemia and hypomagnesemia) induced by diuretics and overdosing in the elderly, who may have decreased renal clearance.

10. e. True statement about the use and effects of digoxin include the following: digoxin decreases rates of worsening of heart failure, lower digoxin maintenance doses may be as effective as higher doses, and digoxin use in appropriate patients reduces the rate of hospitalizations in CHF. Elderly patients and those with renal insufficiency are also more prone to the toxic effects of the drug. Remember the primary indications for its use are those patients with CHF and both a low ejection fraction and atrial fibrillation with rapid ventricular rate.

11. **d.** In evaluating patients for systolic dysfunction, the most important characteristic found on echocardiogram is the ejection fraction, which is usually less than 40% in systolic heart failure. Although myocardial hypertrophy, valvular heart disease, and wall-motion abnormalities may be found, it is the ejection fraction that defines systolic dysfunction.

12. **e.** The AHA has developed a classification system that defines the different stages of heart failure, thereby emphasizing the preventive, albeit usually progressive, nature of the condition. People with Stage A heart failure are asymptomatic patients at high risk but with no identifiable structural abnormalities. People with Stage B heart failure are asymptomatic patients with identifiable structural abnormalities; Stage C is symptomatic patients with structural abnormalities; Stage D is end-stage patients refractory to standard therapy. People with Stage A disease should have risk-factor reduction, such as treatment of hyper-tension, dyslipidemia, or diabetes, and patient and family education. Stage B patients should be treated with ACE inhibitors or ARBs (all patients) and beta blockers (in selected individuals). Stage C patients should all be taking ACE inhibitors and beta blockers; should be treated with dietary sodium restriction, diuretics, and digoxin (selectively, if indicated); may be candidates for cardiac resynchronization if bundle-block is present; may be revascularized or have correction of valvular heart disease (if present); and may be treated with an aldosterone antagonist. Stage D refractory disease may be treated with all of the previously mentioned methods as appropriate plus the use of inotropics, transplantation, ventricular assistive devices, or hospice.

13. **e.** Calcium channel blockers are the exception in this list of interventions that have been found to be effective in reducing hospitalizations and mortality.

SOLUTION TO THE CLINICAL CASE MANAGEMENT PROBLEM

A practical example of a patient becoming worse after being given furosemide is the following:

A 55-year-old male with uremia and a history of CHF manifests an increasing shortness of breath and increasing edema of the extremities. You naturally assume that his CHF is worsening, and you administer furosemide. He deteriorates rapidly. The cause: uremic pericarditis. What appeared to be CHF was not. The lesson to be learned is as follows: Make sure the patient has CHF before you treat the CHF.

SUMMARY OF CONGESTIVE HEART FAILURE

1. CHF is a syndrome in which a large number of pathophysiologic mechanisms may underlie the symptoms and signs of heart failure. Some of these include structural abnormalities of the myocardium, LV chamber, and coronary arteries and functional abnormalities of the valves and electrical systems. A comprehensive evaluation includes a search for evidence of diminished pump function, LV chamber remodeling, coronary artery disease, valvular heart disease, abnormal excitation-contraction coupling, and arrhythmias. Coexisting noncardiac diseases also should be identified and treated. That would include search for and control of tobacco addiction, alcohol abuse, diabetes, hypertension, obesity, anemia, sleep apnea, and renal disease.

2. The AHA has developed a classification system that defines the different stages of heart failure, thereby emphasizing the preventive, albeit usually progressive, nature of the condition. People with Stage A heart failure are asymptomatic patients at high risk but with no identifiable structural abnormalities. People with Stage B heart failure are asymptomatic patients with identifiable structural abnormalities. Patients in Stage C are symptomatic with structural abnormalities, and Stage D consists of end-stage patients refractory to standard therapy.

3. Dyspnea is the most common symptom of both systolic and diastolic CHF. Other common symptoms of heart failure are fatigue, lethargy, and PND. An estimated 20% to 40% of patients have diastolic heart failure with preserved or normal systolic function. In these patients, contraction is normal, but diastole (relaxation phase)

is abnormal. During exertion, normal filling during diastole does not occur, and cardiac output is impaired. Therefore, dyspnea is particularly profound during exertion, and as the severity of the heart failure increases, the shortness of breath may occur with only minimal exertion or even at rest. In systolic heart failure, the more common form of heart failure, systolic function is impaired and the cardiac systolic ejection fraction is diminished (<40%) as measured by echocardiogram.

4. Patients with diastolic cardiac failure are frequently elderly and female, with a history of hypertension, diabetes, and obesity. Atrial fibrillation, if present, is usually paroxysmal, and a fourth heart sound (S4 gallop) often is present. In systolic heart failure, which can occur in all ages and more often in males, atrial fibrillation tends to be persistent, a third heart sound is present (S3 gallop), and there is often a history of previous myocardial infarction. Classic signs of both types of failure include tachypnea, tachycardia, JVD, rales, hepatojugular reflux, hepatosplenomegaly, cephalization and congestion on chest radiograph with or without cardiomegaly, and diminished oxygen saturation on pulse oximetry.

5. Reasonable investigations in acute failure would include the following: 12 lead ECG; chest radiograph; blood chemistries including BUN, creatinine, glucose, and electrolytes; CBC; TSH; liver function tests and lipids; urinalysis for protein and sugar; echocardiography; and pulse oximetry.

6. Patients with Stage A disease should have risk-factor reduction, such as treatment of hypertension, dyslipidemia, or diabetes, and patient and family education. Stage B patients should be treated with ACE inhibitors or ARBs (all patients) and beta blockers (in selected individuals). Stage C patients are symptomatic, and, in addition to oxygen, the most appropriate acute pharmacotherapeutic intervention is the administration of diuretics, particularly loop diuretics, preferably intravenously. Careful attention should be given to the patient's urine output and weight as a measure of successful diuresis. Additionally, all Stage C patients should be taking ACE and beta blockers and should be treated with dietary sodium restriction. Other therapies include the use of chronic diuretics, digoxin (selectively, if indicated), aldosterone antagonists, cardiac resynchronization if bundle block is present, and revascularization and/or correction of valvular heart disease (if present). Stage D refractory disease may be treated with all of the previously mentioned methods as appropriate plus the use of inotropics, transplantation, ventricular assistive devices, or hospice.

SUGGESTED READING

Cowie MR, Zaphiriou A: Management of chronic heart failure. *BMJ* 325(7361):422-425, 2002.

Jessup M, Brozena S: Medical progress: heart failure. *N Engl J Med.* 348(20):2007-2018, 2003.

 Chapter 14

Hypertension

"I feel fine, so I stopped taking those expensive pills you prescribed."

CLINICAL CASE PROBLEM 1:

AN OBESE 47-YEAR-OLD MALE WITH HYPERTENSION

A 47-year-old male presents to your office for a yearly checkup. He is 5 foot 10 inches tall, weighs 250 pounds, smokes two packs of cigarettes a day, and "slams down" 12 ounces of whiskey a day. He is a truck driver and is on the road a lot. He frequently eats at "fast-food joints."

On physical examination you find his blood pressure to be 180/105 mm Hg. His point of maximum impulse (PMI) is detected in the sixth intercostal space in the anterior axillary line. His funduscopic examination is normal. He has no carotid bruits.

▶ SELECT THE BEST ANSWER TO THE FOLLOWING QUESTIONS:

1. Which of the following statements about this patient's blood pressure is (are) false?
   a. a single blood pressure reading of diastolic 105 mm Hg is satisfactory for a diagnosis of hypertension
   b. this patient's alcohol intake may be a significant contributing factor to his elevated blood pressure

c. the patient should have his blood pressure rechecked after a period of rest in the office

d. the patient should return for reassessment of his blood pressure in 1 week

e. the patient's cigarette smoking may be a significant contributing factor to his elevated blood pressure

2. Which of the following blood pressure values meets the definition of prehypertension in the report on *Prevention, Detection, Evaluation and Treatment of Hypertension* of the Joint National Committee on Detection, Evaluation, and Treatment of High Blood Pressure (JNC) VII?
   a. 122/82
   b. 140/90
   c. 118/78
   d. 135/85
   e. a and d

3. The minimum goal in hypertension therapy is to reduce his blood pressure to a level less than which of the following?
   a. 150/90 mm Hg
   b. 140/90 mm Hg
   c. 130/90 mm Hg
   d. 120/80 mm Hg
   e. 110/70 mm Hg

4. A week later, the patient returns to your office with blood pressure measurements taken by his company's nurse. They are as follows: 148/95, 144/92, and 150/90. At this time you would prescribe:
   a. a thiazide diuretic
   b. a beta blocker
   c. a calcium channel blocker
   d. an angiotensin-converting enzyme (ACE) inhibitor
   e. none of the above

5. What is the first-line pharmacologic therapy now recommended for most patients with hypertension?
   a. a beta blocker
   b. a thiazide diuretic
   c. a calcium channel blocker
   d. an ACE inhibitor
   e. any of the above

6. Which of the following statements is false?
   a. in chronic congestive heart failure, ACE inhibitors, beta blockers, and aldosterone inhibitors have been shown to decrease morbidity and mortality
   b. recurrent strokes are decreased by a combination of ACE inhibitors and thiazide diuretics

c. calcium channel blockers are beneficial in reducing cardiovascular disease and stroke in patients with diabetes mellitus

d. hypertension in older individuals is best treated with calcium channel blockers

e. ACE inhibitors should be avoided in women of childbearing age or pregnant women

7. Which statement(s) is (are) true regarding the use of antihypertensive drugs with other comorbidities?
   a. thiazide diuretics are useful in slowing demineralization in osteoporosis
   b. beta blockers are useful in prophylactic treatment of migraine headache
   c. beta blockers are useful in the comanagement of Raynaud's phenomenon
   d. a and b
   e. all of the above

8. The initial diagnostic workup of a patient with hypertension should include which of the following?
   a. electrolytes
   b. blood urea nitrogen (BUN), creatinine
   c. electrocardiogram (ECG)
   d. 24-hour urine for vanillylmandelic acid (VMA) and metanephrines
   e. a, b, and c
   f. all of the above

9. Based on the patient's history and physical examination, which of the following statements concerning his hypertensive complications is most likely true?
   a. the patient is unlikely to have any hypertensive complications
   b. this patient likely has hypertensive retinopathy
   c. this patient likely has cardiac hypertrophy
   d. this patient likely has hypertensive renal failure
   e. none of the above is true

10. Which of the following statements accurately applies to mild hypertension?
    a. the term is no longer considered appropriate in defining hypertension
    b. mild hypertension describes a systolic level of 140-159 mm Hg
    c. mild hypertension describes a diastolic level of 90-104 mm Hg
    d. b and c
    e. none of the above

11. Which of the following statements regarding the treatment of hypertensive emergencies and urgencies is false?

a. patients with marked blood pressure elevations and acute target organ damage require hospitalization
b. patients with marked blood pressure elevations without target organ damage should receive immediate combination oral hypertensive therapy
c. the oral medication of choice for hypertensive urgencies is sublingual nifedipine
d. all of the above
e. none of the above

CLINICAL CASE PROBLEM 2:
A 50-YEAR-OLD MALE WITH RESISTANT HYPERTENSION

A 50-year-old male is being treated for hypertension with a low-salt diet, hydrochlorothiazide 25 mg/day, and propranolol 120 mg bid. His blood pressure at present is 180/100 mm Hg.

12. Which of the following would be a reasonable third-line agent for the treatment of this patient's blood pressure?
    a. atenolol
    b. metoprolol
    c. labetalol
    d. furosemide
    e. enalapril

13. What is the most common side effect of ACE inhibitors?
    a. cough
    b. constipation
    c. headache
    d. skin rash
    e. depression

14. What is the recommended starting dose for hydrochlorothiazide (HCTZ)?
    a. 25 mg
    b. 50 mg
    c. 75 mg
    d. 100 mg
    e. none of the above

15. Which one of the following prescribing considerations concerning HCTZ is true?
    a. it can be used without concern in patients taking digoxin
    b. it is safe for use in patients with uric acid metabolism disorders
    c. it can cause hyperkalemia
    d. it can be associated with osteoporosis development
    e. its use should be avoided in patients allergic to sulfonamides

16. Based on the history and physical examination of the patient described in Clinical Case Problem 1, which of the following additional investigations should be undertaken?
    a. digital subtraction angiography
    b. intravenous pyelogram (IVP)
    c. echocardiogram
    d. retinal ultrasound
    e. renal ultrasound

17. Which medication would be the least optimal in a patient with asthma?
    a. hydrochlorothiazide
    b. propranolol
    c. lisinopril
    d. nifedipine
    e. prazosin

18. Which antihypertensive medication is best avoided in chronic kidney disease?
    a. lisinopril
    b. furosemide
    c. amlodipine
    d. triamterene
    e. atenolol

19. Which medication is contraindicated in gout?
    a. atenolol
    b. hydrochlorothiazide
    c. lisinopril
    d. nifedipine
    e. prazosin

20. The 47-year old male patient described in Clinical Case Problem 1 is admitted to the hospital a few months later for an acute myocardial infarction. He has disregarded your previously prescribed therapies. What medications would you now prescribe for his blood pressures that average 160/90?
    a. metoprolol
    b. amlodipine
    c. lisinopril
    d. a and c
    e. a, b, and c

CLINICAL CASE PROBLEM 3:
A 49-YEAR-OLD OBESE POSTMENOPAUSAL WOMAN WITH TYPE 2 DIABETES MELLITUS

The next day, the wife of the patient described in Clinical Case Problem 2, a teacher, sees you in your office. She is a 49-year-old postmenopausal obese woman with type 2 diabetes mellitus. She brings in a list of blood pressures taken by the school nurse over the past 3 months. The blood pressure readings average 136/86.

21. Your approach to this clinical case problem could include:

   a. recommend lifestyle changes and a return visit in 3 months

   b. prescribe lisinopril, when her blood pressure is unchanged in 3 months

   c. prescribe metoprolol, when her blood pressure is unchanged in 3 months

   d. a and b

   e. a and c

CLINICAL CASE MANAGEMENT PROBLEM

Specify the recommended and contraindicated antihypertensive drugs for the following patients:

Patient 1: A young patient with hyperdynamic circulation

Patient 2: An elderly patient with no particular chronic diseases other than hypertension

Patient 3: An African American patient

Patient 4: A patient with gout

Patient 5: A patient with ischemic heart disease

Patient 6: A patient with asthma

Patient 7: A patient with peripheral vascular disease

Patient 8: A patient with non–insulin-dependent diabetes

Patient 9: A patient with insulin-dependent diabetes

Patient 10: A patient with hypercholesterolemia

Patient 11: A patient with congestive heart failure

Patient 12: A patient who is pregnant

■ **ANSWERS:**

1. a. Hypertension should not be diagnosed until a sustained, repetitive elevation of blood pressure has been documented. For diagnosis, at least three readings averaging greater than 140 mm Hg systolic or 90 mm Hg diastolic must be documented, preferably by the same observer using the same technique. The classification is based on two or more properly measured seated blood pressure readings on two or more office visits. Alcohol abuse is a significant cause of hypertension. Any patient with hypertension should be questioned regarding alcohol intake. Although a low dose of alcohol has been shown to be cardioprotective, low must be carefully defined. An absolute maximum of two drinks per day may be cardioprotective; any more than that may be harmful and, indeed, an additional risk factor for coronary artery disease.

The patient described in this clinical case problem should have his blood pressure taken again after 5 minutes of controlled rest. If his arm circumference is greater than 33 cm, obtain his blood pressure reading with the obese blood pressure cuff. Also instruct this patient to abstain from caffeine and cigarette smoking for at least 2 hours before his pressure is checked on his next visit.

A patient whose blood pressure returns to normal after a period of rest is known as a "labile hypertensive." Of patients who are labile hypertensive, approximately 50% go on to develop sustained hypertension.

2. e. JNC VII describes prehypertension as a 120-139 mm Hg systolic and 80-89 mm Hg diastolic blood pressure reading. Those with blood pressures in the 130/80 to 139/89 mm Hg range are at twice the risk to develop hypertension as those with lower values. Treatment is to prescribe lifestyle modifications. It has been well established that home blood pressure readings (if done correctly and taken with a blood pressure recording device that has been calibrated against a mercury manometer) are more accurate and a more significant predictor of cardiovascular morbidity and mortality than office blood pressure readings.

The patient should not be started taking antihypertensive medication at this time. First, the diagnosis must be established. Second, before considering antihypertensive medication you must consider nonpharmacologic therapy and attempt to lower his or her blood pressure without drugs.

3. b. The minimum goal in antihypertensive therapy is to reduce the blood pressure to a level of 140 mm Hg systolic and 90 mm Hg diastolic. Ideally the blood pressure should be less than 120/80.

4. e. The first step in treating this patient's blood pressure is to use nonpharmacologic therapy. There is no doubt that nonpharmacologic therapy has a major role to play in the management of hypertension. Nonpharmacologic therapies that have been shown to make a difference and should be prescribed for this patient include: (1) weight reduction; (2) alcohol elimination (in a person such as this, who "slams down" 12 ounces of whiskey per day, your best bet would be to attempt to eliminate the "slamming" completely); (3) cigarette smoking cessation; (4) aerobic exercise 4 hours/week or 1200 kcal; however, this patient first should be given an exercise tolerance test); (5) salt intake reduction; and (6) fat intake reduction.

The fat-reduction program should follow the American Heart Association's Step 1 Diet formula (decreasing the fat content of the diet without changing the total caloric intake will automatically begin the weight-reduction process) or the National Heart, Lung, and Blood Institute's DASH diet (a combination diet rich in fruits, vegetables, and low-fat dairy foods, and low in saturated and total fat), which has been shown to lower blood pressure.

You need to decide which of these therapies to begin with; obviously attempting to alter everything at once will not work. An alcohol rehabilitation program or a smoking cessation program would be an excellent first choice.

5. b. The JNC VII recommends thiazide diuretics for most patients and specific drugs for compelling indications. For instance, in diabetes mellitus, type 1, with proteinuria, an ACE inhibitor is recommended. In heart failure, ACE inhibitors and diuretics and aldosterone antagonists are recommended. In isolated systolic hypertension of older individuals, diuretics are preferred, and long-acting dihydropyridine calcium antagonists are also acceptable. In the face of myocardial infarction, beta blockers and ACE inhibitors are recommended. In chronic kidney disease, ACE inhibitors and antitension II receptor blockers (ARBs) have shown favorable effects on the progression of diabetic and nondiabetic renal disease. Recurrent stroke rates are lowered by a combination of ACE inhibitors and thiazide diuretics.

6. d. In chronic congestive heart failure, ACE inhibitors, beta blockers, and aldosterone inhibitors have been shown to decrease morbidity and mortality. Recurrent strokes are decreased by a combination of ACE inhibitors and thiazide diuretics. Calcium channel blockers are beneficial in reducing cardiovascular disease and stroke in patients with diabetes mellitus. Hypertension in older individuals is best treated with diuretics. ACE inhibitors should be avoided in women of childbearing age or pregnant women because they are teratogenic.

7. d. Thiazides are useful in the treatment of osteoporosis because they slow the demineralization process. Beta blockers are useful in migraine headache prophylaxis but are contraindicated in Raynaud's phenomenon.

8. e. The basic (and cost-effective) hypertensive workup includes: (1) complete urinalysis; (2) hemoglobin and hematocrit; (3) BUN and creatinine; (4) serum calcium and potassium; (5) fasting lipid profile; (6) plasma glucose; and (7) ECG.

Other tests, including renal ultrasound, IVP, or 24-hour urine for VMA and metanephrines, are indicated only under special circumstances. A patient that is, for example, 55 years old and who develops hypertension for the first time should be suspected of having a secondary cause. (As a general rule, if essential hypertension is going to develop, it will develop before the age of 50). In a 50-year-old patient the most common secondary cause of hypertension is renal artery stenosis. This would call for investigation with magnetic resonance angiography of the renal arteries or Doppler flow analysis of the renal arteries. Another secondary cause includes pheochromocytoma (hypertension, sweating, and palpitations).

9. c. This patient probably has cardiac hypertrophy. This is suspected from the physical examination of the heart, when the point of maximal impulse is found in the sixth intercostal space-anterior axillary line. The normal apical impulse is located at or medial to the midclavicular line in the fourth or fifth intercostal space. The physical examination described provided no evidence concerning retinopathy or nephropathy.

10. a. The term mild hypertension is no longer considered appropriate in defining hypertension because it may very well give some a false sense of security ("I've been told I have hypertension, but I've also been told it is mild; therefore, I really don't have to worry about it"). See the following table for the newer JNC VII classification.

Classification of Blood Pressure for Adults

Classification	Systolic mm Hg	Diastolic mm Hg
Normal	<120	<80
Prehypertension	130–139	80–89
Hypertension		
Stage 1	140–159	90–99
Stage 2	= >160	= >100

11. d. Hypertensive emergencies and hypertensive urgencies are defined as follows: A hypertensive emergency is a clinical situation in which blood pressure must be lowered immediately and carefully to prevent or limit target organ damage. Examples of hypertensive emergencies are malignant hypertension, acute myocardial ischemic syndromes, acute pulmonary edema, acute renal insufficiency, acute intracranial events, postoperative bleeding, eclampsia, and pheochromocytoma. Generally a 25% reduction in the initial blood pressure values is required to prevent further complications.

A hypertensive urgency is a clinical situation in which blood pressure should be lowered within 24 to 48 hours. Examples of hypertensive urgencies are accelerated hypertension, marked hypertension associated with congestive cardiac failure, stable angina pectoris, transient cerebral ischemic attacks, and perioperative hypertension. Previously used sublingual nifedipine was found in studies to cause acute coronary events and ischemic strokes when used in hypertensive emergencies.

Hypertensive emergency/urgency drug selection must be made on a pathophysiologic basis.

A summary of current recommendations:
1. Central nervous system disorder:
   a. Drug of choice: sodium nitroprusside
   b. Alternatives: labetalol
2. Intracranial hemorrhage:
   a. Drug of choice: sodium nitroprusside
   b. Alternatives: labetalol
3. Acute left-ventricular failure:
   a. Drug of choice: enalaprilat
   b. Contraindicated: labetalol
4. Acute coronary ischemia:
   a. Drug of choice: nitroglycerin
   b. Alternatives: labetalol, sodium nitroprusside
5. Unstable angina:
   a. Drug of choice: nitroglycerin
   b. Alternatives: labetalol
6. Aortic dissection:
   a. Drug of choice: esmolol hydrochloride
   b. Alternatives: sodium nitroprusside and propranolol
   c. Contraindicated: hydralazine
7. Eclampsia:
   a. Drug of choice: $MgSO_4$ (magnesium sulfate)
   b. Alternatives: hydralazine
8. Pheochromocytoma:
   a. Drug of choice: phentolamine
   b. Contraindicated: beta-adrenoreceptor blockers

12. e. This patient is currently on a thiazide diuretic and a beta blocker. Therefore the most reasonable alternative as a third-line agent would be either an ACE inhibitor or a calcium channel blocker.

Atenolol and metoprolol are also beta blockers and thus would not be reasonable choices.

Labetalol is a combination alpha–beta blocker and thus would also be a poor choice.

Furosemide is a loop diuretic and would not be a reasonable choice for the management of this patient's hypertension.

Enalapril is an ACE inhibitor and would be an excellent choice for a third-line agent.

13. a. The most common side effect of ACE inhibitors is cough. The mechanism of the cough appears to be bradykinin induced. It does not appear to be truly allergic in nature. Approximately 15% of patients taking chronic ACE inhibitors develop a chronic cough. ARBs do not have this side effect.

14. a. The starting dose of a hydrochlorothiazide is 25 mg. A low dose (25 mg) has been shown in many studies to be just as efficacious as a higher dose (50 mg, 75 mg, or 100 mg). The only difference between the low dose and the higher doses is the greatly increased incidence of side effects with the higher doses. The same principle, with weigh dose adjusted for molecular weight difference, holds true for other thiazides.

15. e. Thiazide diuretics may produce any of six metabolic side effects: hyperglycemia, hyperuricemia, hyperlipidemia, hypomagnesemia, hyponatremia, and hypokalemia. Some patients that are allergic to sulfonamides are also allergic to HCTZ. Because HCTZ can cause hypokalemia, concurrent digoxin use must be monitored. Thiazide diuretics slow the demineralization process in bone.

16. c. The patient's point of maximum impulse is in the sixth intercostal space in the anterior axillary line. This suggests left-ventricular hypertrophy secondary to hypertension (and perhaps also as a result of the obesity). An echocardiogram is indicated to evaluate the thickness of the left ventricle.

17. b. In a patient with asthma, a nonselective beta blocker should be avoided because it may lead to bronchoconstriction and wheezing.

18. d. Triamterene possibly would lead to hyperkalemia, which is problematic in chronic kidney disease. ACE inhibitors and ARB medications provide a favorable prognosis for kidney disease until hyperkalemia develops. To manage fluid balance in kidney disease, a loop diuretic often is needed, particularly in combination with an ACE or ARB medication.

19. b. HCTZ is contraindicated in gout because it may raise uric acid levels.

20. d. Administration of beta blockers and ACE inhibitors is associated with a favorable outcome in cases of myocardial infarction.

21. d. Lifestyle changes are the cornerstone of hypertension and diabetes mellitus management. A compelling indication is to prescribe an ACE inhibitor in a patient with diabetes. Beta blockers have not shown as compelling an indication with respect to prevention of diabetic nephropathy.

SOLUTION TO THE CLINICAL CASE MANAGEMENT PROBLEM

Patient 1: A young patient with hyperdynamic circulation

Recommended drugs: beta blockers
Contraindicated drugs: none

Patient 2: An elderly patient with no particular chronic diseases other than hypertension

Such a person is liable to suffer from isolated systolic hypertension resulting from increased vascular stiffness (decreased compliance).
Recommended drugs: First-line agents: diuretics, with reduced drug dose; second-line agents: ACE inhibitors, long-acting calcium channel blockers
Contraindicated drugs: none

Patient 3: An African American patient

Recommended drugs: thiazide diuretics are preferred for initial therapy, calcium channel antagonists also are effective
Contraindicated drugs: none, but in the absence of concomitant thiazide therapy the effect of ACE inhibitors or beta blockers is blunted

Patient 4: A patient with gout

Recommended drugs: any drug but diuretics
Contraindicated drugs: diuretics

Patient 5: A patient with ischemic heart disease

Recommended drugs: beta blockers, calcium channel blockers
Contraindicated drugs: none

Patient 6: A patient with asthma

Recommended drugs: calcium channel blockers
Contraindicated drugs: beta blockers

Patient 7: A patient with peripheral vascular disease

Recommended drugs: calcium channel blockers or other vasodilators
Contraindicated drugs: beta blockers

Patient 8: A patient with non–insulin-dependent diabetes

Recommended drugs: ACE inhibitors
Contraindicated drugs: none, although diuretics may increase blood sugar levels

Patient 9: A patient with insulin-dependent diabetes

Recommended drugs: ACE inhibitors
Contraindicated drugs: beta blockers

Patient 10: A patient with hypercholesterolemia

Recommended drugs: ACE inhibitors, calcium channel blockers, alpha blockers, beta blockers with intracarotid sodium Amytal (ISA)
Contraindicated drugs: high-dose beta blockers without ISA, high-dose diuretics

Patient 11: A patient with congestive heart failure

Recommended drugs: ACE inhibitors, diuretics
Contraindicated drugs: none, although beta blockers should be used with caution

Patient 12: A pregnant patient

Recommended drugs: alpha methyldopa, hydralazine
Contraindicated drugs: diuretics, ACE inhibitors

SUMMARY OF HYPERTENSION

1. **Diagnosis:** Blood pressure measurement in three readings, separated by a time of at least 1 week. Each of the three readings should be taken after at least 5 minutes of controlled rest and after having not consumed caffeine or smoked during the last hour. Hypertension is diagnosed if the average systolic pressure is at least 140 mm Hg and/or the average diastolic pressure is at least 90 mm Hg. A single reading of a diastolic pressure of 110 mm Hg is also probably sufficient for the diagnosis of hypertension.

2. **Evaluation:** History, physical examination, and laboratory evaluation should include the evaluation of other risk factors, including family history of hypertension and other cardiovascular disease, presence of diabetes mellitus, obesity, alcohol intake, hyperlipidemia, smoking, exercise pattern, and stress.

   Look for evidence of end-organ damage: cardiac hypertrophy (may need echocardiogram), funduscope, and renal function.

   Laboratory evaluation should include complete blood count, urinalysis, electrolytes, BUN, creatinine, calcium, cholesterol, glucose, and ECG.

Continued

SUMMARY OF HYPERTENSION —cont'd

3. **Classification:** Staging system outlined in Answer 10. Stages have replaced mild, moderate, and severe hypertension.
4. **Nonpharmacologic treatment:** Treatment with medication includes weight reduction, increase in aerobic exercise, restriction of sodium, restriction of saturated fat (DASH diet), discontinued smoking, and decreased stress.
5. **Pharmacologic treatment:** The Seventh Report of the Joint National Committee on Detection, Evaluation, and Treatment of High Blood Pressure (JNC VII) recommends use of thiazide diuretics in most patients. Optimal formulation should be effective for 24 hours, requiring only a once-daily dose, if at all possible. Long-acting formulations are preferred over short-acting agents because adherence to therapy is better, control is consistent and persistent, cost may be lower, and nighttime

protection from sudden increases in blood pressure is present. Combinations of low doses of two agents from different classes are recommended and practically inevitable in Stage 2 hypertension. JNC VII also recommends specific medications when compelling indications exist.

SUGGESTED READING

Chobanian AV, et al: The Seventh Report of the Joint National Committee on Prevention, Detection, Evaluation, and Treatment of High Blood Pressure: the JNC 7 report. *JAMA* 289(19):2560-2572, 2003.

Clinical Evidence, Cardiovascular Concerns, *British Medical Journal Publishing Group*, June 2003.

Hall WD: A rational approach for the treatment of hypertension in special populations, *Am Fam Phys* 60:156-162, 1999.

Institute for Clinical Systems Improvement: *Hypertension Diagnosis and Treatment*, www.icsi.org, April 2003.

National Heart, Lung and Blood Institute, National Institutes of Health: *High Blood Pressure Information for Health Professionals*, http://www.nhlbi.nih.gov.

World Health Association and International Society of Hypertension: Clinical update, 1999 guidelines for hypertension. *Clin Rev* 9(6):123-126, 1999.

Chapter 15

Dysrhythmia

> "Sometimes my heart forgets a beat or two."

CLINICAL CASE PROBLEM 1:
A 37-YEAR-OLD MALE WITH "SKIPPING HEART BEATS"

A 37-year-old male comes to your office for assessment of "skipping heart beats." These skipped beats have been a concern for the past 8 months. The patient reports no other symptoms accompanying these skipped beats. Specifically, he reports no increased sweating, no palpitations, no weight loss, no chest pain, no pleuritic pain, and no anxiety.

On physical examination, his blood pressure is 100/70 mm Hg. On auscultation of his heart you observe that S1 and S2 are normal—there are no extra sounds or murmurs. You hear approximately 5 premature beats/min.

■ SELECT THE BEST ANSWER TO THE FOLLOWING QUESTIONS:

1. What is the most commonly encountered "premature contraction"?
   a. a ventricular premature beat
   b. an atrial premature beat
   c. atrial flutter
   d. atrial fibrillation
   e. none of the above

2. Most atrial premature beats discovered on clinical examination are:
   a. associated with chronic obstructive pulmonary disease (COPD)
   b. completely benign
   c. associated with valvular heart disease
   d. associated with an increase in cardiovascular mortality
   e. none of the above

3. Most ventricular premature beats discovered on clinical examination are:
   a. associated with COPD
   b. completely benign
   c. associated with valvular heart disease
   d. associated with an increase in cardiovascular mortality
   e. none of the above

CLINICAL CASE PROBLEM 2:
A 51-YEAR-OLD MALE WITH ACUTE CHEST PAIN

A 51-year-old male presents to the emergency room (ER) with an acute episode of chest pain. He has a history of atrial fibrillation. On examination, his blood pressure is 80/60 mm Hg and his ventricular rate is approximately 160 beats/min. He is in acute distress. His respiratory rate is 32/min. His electrocardiogram (ECG) shows atrial fibrillation with a rapid ventricular response.

4. What should your first step in management be?
   a. digitalize the patient
   b. give the patient intravenous (IV) verapamil
   c. give the patient IV adenosine
   d. start synchronized cardioversion
   e. start rapid IV hydration

CLINICAL CASE PROBLEM 3:

A 44-YEAR-OLD WHITE MALE WITH PALPITATIONS

A 44-year-old white male comes to your ER saying he has palpitations. He denies chest pain or shortness of breath. There is no history of known heart disease or cardiac risk factors except for mild obesity. He does admit to drinking heavily the night before at an office retirement party.

On physical examination, his blood pressure is 120/80 mm Hg and his ventricular rate is 160 beats/min. His ECG confirms atrial fibrillation with a rapid ventricular response.

5. What should you do at this time?
   a. digitalize the patient
   b. treat the patient with IV verapamil
   c. treat the patient with IV procainamide
   d. cardiovert the patient
   e. have him perform a Valsalva maneuver by rebreathing into a paper bag

6. What is the recommended treatment for paroxysmal supraventricular tachycardia (PSVT) with hemodynamic compromise?
   a. synchronized cardioversion
   b. direct-current countershock
   c. IV adenosine
   d. IV verapamil
   e. IV digoxin

7. Patients with chronic atrial fibrillation are at increased risk for which of the following conditions?
   a. acute myocardial infarction (MI)
   b. ventricular tachycardia
   c. sudden cardiac death
   d. cerebrovascular accident
   e. ventricular fibrillation

8. What is the drug of choice for prevention of the complication described in Question 7?
   a. prophylactic streptokinase
   b. prophylactic warfarin
   c. prophylactic heparin
   d. prophylactic lidocaine
   e. no drug is recommended

9. Which of the following statements regarding the medical treatment of atrial premature beats with antiarrhythmic drugs is true?
   a. the benefit outweighs the risk
   b. the risk outweighs the benefit
   c. the risk and the benefit are equal
   d. the risk and benefit depend on the patient
   e. nobody really knows for sure

10. Which of the following statements regarding the medical treatment of ventricular premature beats with antiarrhythmic drugs is true?
   a. the benefit outweighs the risk
   b. the risk outweighs the benefit
   c. the risk and the benefit are equal
   d. the risk and the benefit depend on the patient
   e. nobody really knows for sure

ANSWERS:

1. **b.** Atrial premature beats are the most common premature beats encountered in the adult population. They are almost always asymptomatic and often are discovered incidentally during a medical examination. Patients with atrial premature beats often complain of "palpitations" or "a feeling of skipped heart beats" during periods of emotional stress or during periods of quiet such as while resting in bed. Atrial premature beats may be associated with tachycardias that, particularly if nonsustained (less than 30 seconds), may not be perceived by the patient.

2. **b.** Atrial premature beats require no treatment except reassurance of the patient. Reassurance is particularly important because the more convinced the patient is that something is seriously wrong, the more atrial premature beats he or she will sustain.

There are obviously other causes of palpitations that must be considered, such as thyrotoxicosis, panic disorder, and pheochromocytoma. However, benign premature atrial contractions are much more common than premature atrial contractions as a result of thyrotoxicosis, panic disorder, or pheochromocytoma.

3. **b.** Most ventricular premature contractions, as with atrial premature contractions, turn out to be completely benign. As with atrial premature contractions, most patients simply need reassurance. Also as with atrial premature contractions, most ventricular premature contractions are asymptomatic and often are discovered during a medical examination. Occasionally, premature ventricular contractions (PVCs) (unlike premature atrial contractions [PACs]) may be symptoms of more serious underlying heart disease. With runs of ventricular premature beats (ventricular tachycardia), the patient may develop angina, dyspnea, dizziness, syncope, and even cardiac arrest.

If there is a serious question about the number of ventricular premature beats per minute, a 24-hour Holter monitor is an excellent way to measure. The risk of prescribing a patient a prophylactic antiarrhythmic drug for ventricular ectopy outweighs the benefit.

4. d. This patient presents with what appears to be an acute attack of atrial fibrillation with rapid ventricular response. This is an unstable tachycardia. The treatment of choice of this patient is synchronized cardioversion at 100 joules of energy. Advanced cardiac life support (ACLS) protocol recommends cardioversion energies of (1) 100 joules, (2) 200 joules, (3) 300 joules, and (4) 360 joules, in that order, and in succession if the previous energy level was not successful.

5. b. In this case, the patient has the same condition, atrial fibrillation. However, in this case he is hemodynamically stable instead of hemodynamically unstable. Therefore a less dramatic intervention than cardioversion can be attempted at this time. The scenario of atrial fibrillation following alcohol ingestion ("holiday heart syndrome") is seen frequently over holidays and weekends. Generally the acute cardiac rhythm disturbance occurs in the background of heavy chronic alcohol consumption. Occasionally the arrhythmia may be induced acutely without chronic abuse, especially after a period of prolonged sleeplessness.

ACLS protocol would suggest that for rate control in this situation, both beta blockers and calcium channel blockers are appropriate.

6. a. Unstable PSVT is treated with immediate cardioversion.

A patient who presents with stable PSVT first should be treated with vagal maneuvers and adenosine. Vagal maneuvers have therapeutic and diagnostic value. These maneuvers can help differentiate PSVT from other rhythms such as atrial flutter. Carotid sinus massage, Valsalva maneuver, and the placement of a cold ice pack on the skin are examples of vagal maneuvers. Pressing on the eyeballs is not a recommended vagal maneuver.

7. d. These patients are at increased risk for sudden stroke.

8. b. Anticoagulation therapy is underused for patients with chronic atrial fibrillation. Because these patients are at risk for embolic cerebrovascular accidents, it is recommended they start taking warfarin prophylaxis, provided there is no contraindication. All of the trials to date have shown that chronic warfarin therapy maintained with an international normalized ratio (INR) of 2.0-3.0 significantly reduces the incidence of strokes in patients with chronic atrial fibrillation (whether persistent or intermittent). In high-risk patients, warfarin is about twice as effective as aspirin in reducing risk of stroke. Younger patients (<65 years old) with no risk factors (previous stroke or transient ischemic attack, hypertension current or in the past, diabetes, or congestive heart failure) may be treated with aspirin alone.

9. b. The risk outweighs the benefit; see Answer 10.

10. b. In patients with either PACs or PVCs it is obvious that unless the circumstances are unusual and have been documented electrophysiologically, the risk of treatment with antiarrhythmic drugs outweighs the benefit. A number of trials have confirmed this.

SUMMARY OF DYSRHYTHMIA

1. **Atrial premature beats:** These are benign and extremely common; reassurance is the only treatment recommended.
2. **Ventricular premature beats:** The vast majority are benign, they are extremely common, and reassurance is the only treatment recommended after a complete cardiovascular status is determined for the patient.

   According to the Cardiac Arrhythmia Suppression Trial (CAST), with ventricular ectopy, even in patients at high risk (that is, following an MI), the risk of treating this dysrhythmia is greater than the risk of doing nothing.
3. Treatment for PSVT when the patient is stable consists of vagal maneuvers and adenosine.
4. Treatment for atrial fibrillation is:
   a. If hemodynamically unstable: synchronized cardioversion: 100J-200J-300J-360J
   b. If hemodynamically stable: calcium channel blockers or beta blockers
   c. Prophylaxis against embolic cerebrovascular accidents with warfarin is recommended. The INR should be maintained between 2.0 and 3.0. If warfarin is contraindicated, or in younger patients with no risk factors, aspirin therapy is effective.

SUGGESTED READING

Cummins RO, ed: *ACLS Provider Manual.* Dallas, 2002, American Heart Association.

Falk RH: Medical Progress: Atrial Fibrillation. *N Engl J Med* 344(14): 1067-1078, 2001.

Khairy P, Nattel S: New insights into the mechanisms and management of atrial fibrillation. *CMAJ* 167(9):1012-1020, 2002.

Trohman RG: Supraventricular tachycardia: Implications for the intensivist. *Critical Care Med* 28(10):N129-N135, 2000.

Chapter 16

Obesity

> "My doctor has me on a diet, so please leave the nuts and cherry off of my banana split."

CLINICAL CASE PROBLEM 1:

A 45-Year-Old Male Weighing 320 Pounds and Complaining of Fatigue

A 320-lb, 45-year-old male comes to your office saying he feels fatigued. He has been obese all his life. He tells you that his obesity has nothing to do with calorie intake and everything to do with his slow metabolic rate. He has been investigated extensively at many major centers specializing in "slow metabolic rates." The result of his encounters has been a conclusion that he is simply "eating too much" (with which he disagrees). He has heard from a friend that "you are different," and has come to you for "the truth."

On examination, his body mass index (BMI) is off the scale (46). He weighs 320 lb and is 5 feet 10 inches tall. Although you cannot feel his point of maximal impulse (PMI), you believe it is in the region of the anterior axillary line, sixth intercostal space. S1 and S2 are distant, as are his breath sounds. His abdomen is obese with striae covering the abdomen. His liver and spleen can not be felt.

You refer him to your local dietician and promise that you will "investigate his slow metabolic rate" if he will agree to adhere to a diet. The dietician puts him on an 1800 kcal/day diet and calculates his ideal weight to be 170 lb.

■ SELECT THE BEST ANSWER TO THE FOLLOWING QUESTIONS:

1. Assuming that his total energy expenditure is 2300 kcal/day and he does, in fact, stick to his 1800 kcal/day diet, how long will it take for him to reach his ideal weight?
   a. 125 days
   b. 225 days
   c. 325 days
   d. 525 days
   e. 1050 days

2. How is obesity generally defined?
   a. an increase in the ponderal index of 20% above normal
   b. a decrease in the ponderal index of 30% below normal
   c. an increase in the BMI of 20% above normal
   d. a BMI of 30 kg/m^2 or greater
   e. none of the above

3. Which of the following statements is (are) true regarding obesity?
   a. obesity is associated with increased death rates from cancer
   b. obesity is associated with increased death rates from coronary artery disease
   c. obesity is associated with increased death rates from diabetes mellitus
   d. a and b are both true; c has not been proved
   e. a, b, and c are all true

4. What is the overall prevalence of obesity in the United States?
   a. 5%
   b. 10%
   c. 23%
   d. 34%
   e. 50%

5. Which of the following conditions is (are) most clearly linked with obesity?
   a. alveolar hypoventilation syndrome
   b. hypertension
   c. hyperlipidemia
   d. diabetes mellitus
   e. all of the above

6. The use of severe calorie-restricted diets (800 kcal/day) has been responsible for many deaths. What is the most common cause of death in these cases?
   a. sudden cardiac death, secondary to dysrhythmia
   b. congestive cardiac failure, secondary to anemia
   c. hepatic failure
   d. renal failure
   e. septicemia

7. Which of the following theories have been postulated to explain the physiology of obesity?
   a. the fat-cell theory
   b. the lipoprotein-lipase theory
   c. the thermogenesis-brown adipose tissue theory
   d. all of the above
   e. none of the above

8. Which of the following statements is (are) true regarding the use of anorexic drugs?
   a. short-term studies demonstrate that weight loss is greater with these agents at 1 month than with placebo agents
   b. hypertension is a documented side effect of these agents
   c. renal failure is a documented side effect of these agents
   d. long-term studies suggest that these agents are not beneficial as part of a weight-loss program
   e. all of the above

9. Which of the following is (are) advocated as part of a weight-loss program?
   a. a nutritionally balanced diet
   b. decreasing the percentage of calories derived from fat
   c. an exercise program
   d. caloric restriction to approximately 500 kcal/day less than maintenance
   e. all of the above

10. The practical management of weight loss by the family physician should involve which of the following?
   a. multiple office visits for 8 to 12 weeks
   b. changes to the act of eating
   c. keeping a daily food diary
   d. all of the above
   e. none of the above

11. Which one of the following statements concerning the use of echocardiography in obese patients is true?
   a. echocardiography is not indicated in obese patients
   b. echocardiography cannot predict future risk in obese patients
   c. echocardiography is indicated in obese patients to document the size of the right ventricle; right ventricular hypertrophy is a major predicator of future risk
   d. echocardiography may disclose the formation of "obese heart clots"
   e. none of the above are true

CLINICAL CASE MANAGEMENT PROBLEM

The vast majority of patients with obesity have essential obesity (analogous to essential hypertension). There are, however, secondary causes. List the potential secondary causes of obesity.

▶ **ANSWERS:**

1. **e.** One pound of fat is equal to 3500 kcal. Therefore, if his total energy expenditure is 2300 kcal/day and the patient is taking in only 1800 kcal/day (the recommended difference in a weight-loss program between energy expenditure and energy intake is 500 kcal), his energy deficit is 500 kcal/day. His excess weight above ideal body weight is 150 lb. This 150 lb is equal to 525,000 kcal. The corresponding time to lose this number of calories is 1050 days (2.87 years).

2. **d.** The National Institutes of Health (NIH) define obesity as a BMI of 30 kg/m² or more and a BMI of between 25 and 29.9 kg/m² as overweight. BMI is calculated by multiplying the weight in pounds by 703, and dividing the product by the height in inches squared (i.e., BMI = [(weight in pounds × 703) ÷ (height in inches)²]

3. **e.** Obesity is a major public health issue. There is a certain stigmatization to the diagnosis of obesity not present in many other conditions. Some authorities suggest that we should label obesity as essential obesity in the same way that we label hypertension as essential hypertension. The comparison between hypertension and obesity does not end there. Obesity is a major risk factor for coronary artery disease and other cardiovascular conditions including hypertension, congestive heart failure, cardiomyopathy, and angina pectoris.

Obesity is associated with an increased incidence of type 2, non–insulin-dependent diabetes mellitus (NIDDM), caused by an effective increase in insulin resistance, which, of course, is linked to increased mortality.

Obesity has been established indirectly as a risk factor for some cancers. For example, it appears from some studies that the high-fat diet usually associated with obesity also is associated with an increased risk of colon cancer.

Other diseases that have been shown to be directly linked to obesity include the following: (1) thromboembolic disease; (2) endometrial carcinoma; (3) restrictive lung disease; (4) Pickwickian syndrome; (5) gout; (6) degenerative arthritis; (7) gallstone formation and gallbladder disease; (8) infertility; (9) hyperlipoproteinemias; (10) hernias and esophageal reflux; (11) psychosocial disabilities; and (12) increased risk of obstetric and surgical morbidity.

4. **c.** The overall prevalence of obesity in the North American adult population is approximately 23% (BMI ≥30), an astounding increase from roughly 13% a decade ago. In children, the increase is even more frightening, having exceeded 14% in children 6-11 years old (at or higher than the age-specific 95th percentile) and 12% in adolescents 12-17 years old. In certain groups, such as the Pima Indians, the prevalence is 50%. A higher prevalence of obesity appears in those individuals in the lowest socioeconomic groups; the prevalence does, in fact, decrease as socioeconomic status increases. Combining the categories of overweight (BMI 25-29.9) at 32% and obesity (BMI ≥30) at 23%, fully 55% of the adult population in North America is carrying excess weight.

5. **e.** Of the conditions already postulated as linked with obesity, the strongest associations are between obesity and hypertension and obesity and diabetes.

It should be noted that the other conditions listed previously also are linked to obesity. Moreover, there is strong evidence that weight loss in an obese individual reduces blood pressure; hemoglobin A1c levels; and triglyceride, low-density lipoprotein, and total cholesterol levels, and it increases high-density lipoprotein levels.

6. a. The most common cause of death reported among patients who are on severe calorie-restricted diets is sudden cardiac death as a result of ventricular arrhythmias or dysrhythmias.

7. d. Some of the theories that have been brought forward to explain essential obesity include the following: (1) the fat-cell theory; (2) the lipoprotein-lipase theory; and (3) the thermogenesis-brown fat adipose tissue theory.

Studies done on monozygotic twins have established that 70% of the variance in BMI is the result of genetic factors, with only 30% resulting from environmental factors. This puts a different light on the whole question of slow metabolizers versus fast metabolizers. This genetic information suggests that metabolism is very much a function of genetics and genetic endowment. Recent isolation of gene products that modulate the feeding patterns of adults further support this.

8. e. Although short-term weight loss is enhanced by these agents, long-term studies demonstrate that most patients suffer a rebound effect and actually may end up even heavier. In addition, hypertension and renal failures have been documented in patients using anorexic drugs. These medications can be classified as catecholaminergic or serotonergic:
1. Catecholaminergic agents include amphetamines; appetite suppressants such as phentermine, diethylpropion, and mazindol; and phenylpropanolamine, which is sold over the counter.
2. The serotonergic agents fenfluramine and dexfenfluramine were withdrawn from the market in 1997, and although fluoxetine (Prozac) and sertraline (Zoloft) are serotonergic and often used in obesity treatment, they are not approved for the treatment of obesity. Newer medications, including sibutramine (Meridia) and orlistat, may be useful adjuncts to low-calorie diets, physical activity, and behavior therapy in carefully selected patients.

Surgical intervention to treat obesity should be limited to those with a BMI higher than 40. More than 100,000 patients have undergone gastroplasty with vertical band (Mason) gastroplasty as the treatment of choice.

9. e. A structured program is essential for successful long-term weight loss. Most successful weight-loss programs are multidisciplinary, concentrating on hypocaloric diets, behavior modification to change eating behaviors, aerobic and strengthening exercise, and social support.

The weight-loss program must contain three essential components: (1) a nutritionally balanced diet, (2) aerobic exercise, and (3) a reduction in the percentage of calories derived from fat. It now has been shown that reducing the percentage of calories derived from fat (compared to carbohydrates and proteins) by itself produces weight loss. Current recommendations suggest that the energy intake should be approximately 500 calories less than energy output in a weight-loss program. Low-carbohydrate diets, although effective in rapid short-term weight loss, have not been proved more effective long term than a balanced calorie-restricted diet. Additionally, the long-term effects of carbohydrate-restricted diets are not known. Nevertheless, new attention is being turned on these diets, and results of studies should prove interesting because this and other diets are a multimillion dollar per year industry. The importance in strength training is receiving new attention. Research has shown that larger muscle mass burns fat and calories more efficiently. Many weight-loss programs now emphasize a balance between aerobic activity and muscle strength training. There is good evidence that other benefits (e.g., improved proprioception and balance in the elderly) may derive from strength training. As also noted in Answer 7, newer research strongly implicates genetic influences. Some believe that 50% to 75% of obesity may be explained by genetic causes.

10. d. The practical management of weight loss in a patient by the patient's family physician should include the following: (1) making weekly office visits over a period of 8 to 12 weeks and gradual lengthening of time between visits after that; (2) modifying eating habits; (3) keeping a food diary; and (4) increasing aerobic and strength training exercise activity.

Home weighing is not recommended because of significant fluctuations in body weight as a result of body water. If it is necessary for the patient to weigh himself or herself at home, it should be done no more than once or twice every 2 weeks.

The modification of eating habits is an important and interesting component of the overall plan. First, patients must begin to regard eating as a conscious activity rather than something that happens while thinking of other things. Second, the suggestion of drinking two glasses of water just before the meal to decrease appetite has validity. Third, instructing the patient to eat more slowly and chew food more thoroughly also appears to be valid.

11. e. Echocardiography is an important investigational modality in patients who are obese. It measures the size of the left, not the right, ventricle and is an indicator of left-ventricular hypertrophy, not right-ventricular hypertrophy. Left-ventricular hypertrophy is a major predicator of morbidity and mortality, and hypertrophy is significantly more common in patients who are obese than in patients who are not obese. It should be noted that the Centers for Disease Control and Prevention recommend an echocardiogram for any patient who took dexfenfluramine or fenfluramine and presents with a new-onset murmur or cardiac symptoms.

SOLUTION TO THE CLINICAL CASE MANAGEMENT PROBLEM

The most common causes of secondary obesity include the following:
1. Iatrogenic disease: drugs that produce either true weight gain (more fat) as a side effect or produce salt and water retention.
2. Depression: many patients gain weight
3. Cushing's syndrome
4. Hypothyroidism
Remember, however, that less than 1% of patients who are obese have an identifiable secondary cause of obesity.

SUMMARY OF OBESITY

A. **Pathophysiology:** Evidence suggests that the etiology of obesity is at least 70% genetic and only 30% environmental.

B. **Definition:** (1) BMI ≥30 kg/m^2, or alternatively, (2) 20% higher than suggested ideal body weight.

C. **Prevalence:** An epidemic of obesity exists in the United States. In the year 2000, 23% of adults in the United States were obese; when combined with overweight (BMI 25-29.9) American adults, more than 55% of adults carry excess weight and its health consequences. Children are of particular concern because obesity rates are increasing, portending increasing rates as adults with attendant morbidities. Already the rate of type 2 diabetes has increased significantly in children.

D. **Significance:** (1) Obesity now is regarded as the most important public health problem in the United States. (Unfortunately, it often is ignored because of the social stigma attached to it.) (2) Even more important is the increase in prevalence of obesity in children and adolescents. In 1995, 14% of children and 12% of adolescents in the United States were obese. More than one-fourth of the children in the United States are now overweight.

E. **Complications:** This increase in obesity translates into increased prevalence of the following: (1) coronary artery disease; (2) myocardial infarction (obese patients are 250% more likely to develop coronary artery disease than are nonobese patients); (3) cerebrovascular disease; (4) left-ventricular hypertrophy and congestive heart failure; (5) hyperlipidemia; (6) type 2 diabetes mellitus with macrovascular complications; (7) osteoarthritis; (8) cholelithiasis and cholecystitis; (9) obstructive sleep apnea and Pickwickian syndrome; (10) restrictive lung disease; (11) cancer (associated with a high-fat diet); and (12) gout.

Because obesity is a major risk factor for type 2 diabetes, the responsibility for the complications associated with this disease also can largely be considered a consequence of diabetes. These include the following: (1) diabetic nephropathy from chronic renal failure (diabetes mellitus type 2 is the most common cause of chronic renal failure in the United States because type 2 diabetes is 10 times more frequent than type 1 diabetes); (2) diabetic retinopathy; (3) diabetic neuropathy; (4) autonomic neuropathy; and (5) generalized atherosclerotic vascular disease.

F. **Treatment:** (1) Avoid all diet fads and diet "revolutions." (2) Avoid anorexic drugs. (3) Change the composition of the diet. Maintain carbohydrate and protein, and decrease fat. Avoid simple sugars. (4) Attend multiple office visits to establish a baseline and to motivate continual weight loss; (5) Decrease caloric intake to approximately 500 kcal/day less than energy expenditure. (This produces a weight loss of approximately 1 lb/wk.) (6) Increase aerobic and strength-training exercise. (This is essential to long-term weight loss and maintenance.) (7) Receive positive reinforcement from a support group, the physician, family, and friends.

SUGGESTED READING

Clinical Guidelines on the Identification, Evaluation, and Treatment of Overweight and Obesity in Adults. *NIH publication # 9804083*, September 1998.

Hill JC, et al: What are the most effective interventions to reduce childhood obesity? *J Fam Pract* 51(10):891, 2002.

National Institute of Diabetes and Digestive and Kidney Disorders: "Medical Care for obese patients." www.niddk.nih.gov/health/nutrit/pubs/medcare/medcare2.htm (an excellent website with reliable useful information from this National Institutes of Health office).

Noel PH, Pugh JA: Management of overweight and obese adults. *BMJ* 325(7367):757-761, 2002.

Reaven GM: Importance of identifying the overweight patient who will benefit the most by losing weight. *Ann Intern Med* 138(5):420-423, 2003.

Shepherd TM: Effective management of obesity. *J Fam Pract* 52(1):34-42, 2003.

Yanovski SZ, Yanovski JA: Obesity. *N Engl J Med* 346(8):591-602, 2002.

Chapter 17

Deep Venous Thrombosis and Pulmonary Thromboembolism

"A broken leg killed my wife?"

CLINICAL CASE PROBLEM 1:

A 65-Year-Old Female with Cyanosis, Shortness of Breath, and Substernal Chest Pain

A 65-year-old female is admitted to the emergency room with a 3-hour history of cyanosis, shortness of breath, and substernal chest pain. She had been discharged 5 days earlier after having a total hip replacement for severe osteoarthritis. The hip surgery was uneventful.

On physical examination the patient is in obvious acute respiratory distress. Her respiratory rate is 40/min and her breathing is labored. Her blood pressure is 100/70 mm Hg. Cyanosis is present. There appear to be decreased breath sounds in the lower lobe of the right lung and adventitious breath sounds in all lobes.

■ **SELECT THE BEST ANSWER TO THE FOLLOWING QUESTIONS:**

1. Based on the information provided, what is the most likely diagnosis in this patient?
   a. fat embolus
   b. acute myocardial infarction
   c. dissecting aortic aneurysm
   d. acute pulmonary embolism (PE)
   e. cholesterol emboli syndrome

2. Which of the following findings on the history and physical examination increases the likelihood of a patient having a pulmonary embolism?
   a. heart rate >100 beats/min
   b. hemoptysis
   c. surgery in the previous 4 weeks
   d. previous deep venous thrombosis (DVT)
   e. all of the above

3. Which of the following statements is true concerning examination of a patient with suspected DVT?
   a. clinical examination is diagnostic in every case
   b. clinical examination is, in most cases, diagnostic
   c. clinical examination is of some value but has low sensitivity and low specificity
   d. clinical examination is of no value
   e. nobody really knows for sure

4. Which of the following blood-gas combinations occur most commonly in the condition described in Clinical Case Problem 1?
   a. decreased P_{O_2} and decreased P_{CO_2}
   b. decreased P_{O_2} and increased P_{CO_2}
   c. increased P_{O_2} and increased P_{CO_2}
   d. increased P_{O_2} and decreased P_{CO_2}
   e. none of the above

5. What is the most common cause of morbidity and mortality among hospitalized immobile patients?
   a. myocardial infarction
   b. cerebrovascular accident
   c. DVT/pulmonary embolism
   d. nosocomial infection
   e. none of the above

6. Which of the following best describes D-dimer screening for suspected venous thromboembolism (VTE)?
   a. high sensitivity, low specificity
   b. low sensitivity, high specificity
   c. high sensitivity, high specificity
   d. low sensitivity, low specificity
   e. none of the above

7. Which of the following is evidence of adequate anticoagulation with heparin in patients with DVT/pulmonary embolism?
   a. partial thromboplastin time (PTT) 1.2× that of the control
   b. PTT 1.4× that of the control
   c. PTT 1.5-2.5× that of the control
   d. PTT 2.5-3.0× that of the control
   e. none of the above

8. Which of the following is (are) a risk factor for the condition described earlier?
   a. prolonged immobilization
   b. long leg fractures
   c. pregnancy
   d. malignancy
   e. all of the above

9. Which of the following statements about treatment modalities for VTE is correct?
   a. low–molecular-weight heparin (LMWH) increases the PTT to the same degree as unfractionated heparin (UFH)
   b. protamine reverses the anticoagulant activity of UFH but not LMWH
   c. in patients who are hemodynamically stable, thrombolytic therapy has been shown to reduce mortality and the risk of recurrent pulmonary embolism (PE)
   d. leafy green vegetables can potentiate the anticoagulant effect of warfarin
   e. inferior vena cava (IVC) filters are indicated in patients with VTE and who have a contraindication to anticoagulation

10. Which of the following statements regarding DVT prophylaxis is correct?
    a. patients undergoing hip replacement surgery should receive either LMWH or warfarin
    b. low-dose subcutaneous heparin has been shown to be as effective as LMWH in patients undergoing knee replacement surgery
    c. intermittent pneumatic compression of the legs should not be used in combination with LMWH or coumadin
    d. intermittent pneumatic compression of the legs decreases endogenous fibrinolytic activity
    e. all of the above

ANSWERS:

1. **d.** VTE is a disease entity comprised of PE and DVT. This patient most likely has a PE. Hip surgery is a common predisposing factor for PE. Symptoms of PE are often subtle. It is often impossible to distinguish PE from myocardial infarction on the basis of symptoms alone. Chest pain, dyspnea, anxiety, hyperventilation, and syncope are common to both conditions. Signs of PE include adventitious breath sounds, fever, and cyanosis. PE is suggested by the triad of cough, hemoptysis, and pleuritic chest pain.

PE may lead to acute cor pulmonale. This complication produces the following: (1) distended neck veins; (2) tachycardia; (3) an accentuated and split pneumonic heart sound; (4) Kussmaul's sign (distention of the jugular veins on inspiration); and (5) pulsus paradoxus (exaggerated decrease in blood pressure on inspiration). Systemic hypotension and shock suggest massive PE.

In the postoperative setting fat and cholesterol emboli syndromes always need to be considered. A hallmark of both of these disorders is the presence of purpura. Fat embolism typically occurs on the upper body 2 to 3 days after a major injury. Through the use of special fixatives, the emboli can be demonstrated in biopsy specimens of the petechiae. Cholesterol emboli usually are seen on the lower extremities of patients with atherosclerotic vascular disease. They often follow anticoagulant therapy or an invasive vascular procedure such as an arteriogram. Associated findings include livedo reticularis, gangrene, cyanosis, subcutaneous nodules, and ischemic ulcerations.

2. **e.** When evaluating a patient for a possible embolism, risk factors that increase the probability of the diagnosis include the following: (1) signs and symptoms of DVT; (2) a heart rate >100 beats/min; (3) immobilization or surgery in the past 4 weeks; (4) a history of DVT or PE; (5) hemoptysis; or (6) cancer (receiving treatment or palliative care or received treatment within the past 6 months).

3. **c.** The clinical diagnosis of DVT is difficult and unreliable. DVT frequently is present in the absence of clinical signs (such as pain, heat, or swelling) and is absent in about 75% of patients in whom clinical signs or symptoms suggest its presence.

4. **a.** Massive embolism commonly is associated with arterial hypoxemia, hypocapnia, and respiratory alkalosis. In addition, the difference between the alveolar PO_2 and the arterial PO_2 (PAO_2-PaO_2) may be widened owing to the increase in alveolar dead space. However, a normal alveolar-arterial (A-a) gradient does not exclude the diagnosis.

5. **c.** The most common cause of morbidity and mortality among hospitalized immobile patients is DVT and pulmonary embolism. This is directly related to the immobile state.

In the United States the incidence of fatal plus nonfatal pulmonary emboli exceeds 500,000 annually. This overall incidence is verified by autopsy statistics. Evidence of recent or old embolism is detected in 25% to 30% of routine autopsies.

6. **a.** D-dimer testing (a measurement of the degradation products of cross-linked fibrin circulating in plasma) is a highly sensitive but nonspecific screening test for suspected VTE. It is most useful to help rule out VTE. If the D-dimer test is negative, VTE is highly unlikely. D-dimer is elevated in

almost all patients with an embolism but also is elevated with advancing age, pregnancy, trauma, cancer, and inflammatory conditions and during the postoperative period.

7. **c.** The value of PTT in monitoring the safety and efficacy of heparin administration remains controversial. With respect to safety, the risk of hemorrhage (the principal complication of heparin therapy) is not clearly related to coagulation test alterations; rather, it appears related to factors such as the coexistence of other diseases associated with bleeding risk (gastric or duodenal ulcer, coagulopathies, or uremia) and advanced age. Likewise, achievement of the desired effect of heparin (cessation of thrombus growth *in vivo*) has not been related consistently to coagulation tests.

Current recommendations suggest keeping the PTT measured just prior to the next intermittent dose at or above 1.5 times the control and at 1.5-2.5 times the control with the continuous infusion regimen.

8. **e.** The risk of DVT and PE is increased by the following: (1) immobility (both posttraumatic and postoperative); (2) long leg fractures; (3) a prior history of DVT; (4) oral contraceptive or estrogen use; (5) cerebrovascular accident (CVA) or a history of CVA; (6) pregnancy; (7) malignancy; (8) autoimmune disease; (9) nephrotic syndrome; (10) polycythemia; (11) inflammatory bowel disease; (12) congestive heart failure; or (13) obesity.

9. **e.** IVC filters are indicated in patients with VTE and a contraindication to anticoagulation. The filters also are indicated when there is a recurrence of VTE despite anticoagulation. LMWH does not increase the PTT. Protamine reverses the anticoagulant activity of UFH and LMWH. Thrombolytic therapy has not been shown to decrease mortality or risk of recurrent PE in patients who are hemodynamically stable. If there is no contraindication, thrombolytic therapy is indicated in patients with PE and circulatory shock. Eating leafy green vegetables, along with medications such as rifampin, griseofulvin, sucralfate, and barbiturates, can reduce the anticoagulant effect of warfarin.

10. **a.** Patients undergoing hip or knee replacement surgery should receive prophylaxis with LMWH or warfarin. Low-dose subcutaneous heparin has not been shown to be as effective as LMWH for DVT prophylaxis in patients undergoing knee replacement surgery. There can be additional benefit when intermittent pneumatic compression of the legs is used in combination with other preventive strategies. In addition to improving blood flow, intermittent pneumatic compression of the legs also increases endogenous fibrinolytic activity.

SUMMARY OF DEEP VENOUS THROMBOSIS AND PULMONARY THROMBOEMBOLISM

1. **Diagnosis:**
   Most patients who develop DVT and subsequent PE have one of the previously described risk factors. Remember that DVT is often clinically silent and the clinical diagnosis is notoriously inaccurate.

   PE often is heralded by the abrupt onset of dyspnea, chest pain, apprehension, hemoptysis, or syncope. When massive PE is present, the signs of acute cor pulmonale are evident. With PE, rhonchi frequently are heard in the chest.

2. **Laboratory diagnosis:**
   Arterial blood gases: low Po_2, low Pco_2, respiratory alkalosis

3. **The current investigational modalities for DVT and PE include:**
   a. The chest x-ray: The chest x-ray may show a parenchymal infiltrate and evidence of a pleural effusion if pulmonary infarction has occurred.
   b. Arterial blood gases: The blood gas results in PE show arterial hypoxemia, hypocapnia, and respiratory alkalosis. Blood gas results are most useful when used in conjunction with other information.
   c. D-dimer testing: This is a valuable test that, if negative, helps to rule out VTE. As already discussed, D-dimer levels are elevated in many different circumstances.
   d. The ventilation/perfusion scan: This is a valuable test when the results are definitive. A normal or low probability scan is very good for ruling out a PE, and a high probability scan is strongly associated with a PE. The problem is that many patients without a PE will have abnormal findings on V/scanning and many patients with a PE will not have findings that indicate a high probability.
   e. Computed tomography (CT) scan: This imaging allows direct visualization of emboli and detection of parenchymal abnormalities. In studies, the sensitivity of helical CT scanning for diagnosis of embolism ranged from 57% to 100%, depending on a number of variables including location of emboli and differences in technology. Newer scanners are more sensitive.
   f. Ultrasonography of leg veins: This is a good initial screening tool, but results need to be interpreted with caution. Ultrasonography is negative in up to 50% of patients with proven embolism. Also, up to 20% of patients without

Continued

SUMMARY OF DEEP VENOUS THROMBOSIS AND PULMONARY THROMBOEMBOLISM—cont'd

f. Ultrasonography of leg veins—cont'd
an embolism will have positive ultrasonographic findings.
g. Pulmonary angiography: Pulmonary angiography is the "gold standard" for the diagnosis of PE in the presence of an equivocal V/scan or CT scan.
h. Venography: Ascending venography is the "gold standard" for the diagnosis of DVT.

4. Treatment:
a. Supplemental oxygen
b. Heparin: UFH or LMWH
c. Warfarin
d. IVC filter: indicated for patients with VTE who have a contraindication to anticoagulation or for patients with recurrence of PE despite anticoagulation therapy or for some patients at high risk for initial or recurrent PE.
e. Thrombolytic therapy: reserved for patients with massive PE and cardiovascular compromise.

SUGGESTED READING

Fedullo PF, Tapson VF: The Evaluation of Suspected Pulmonary Embolism. *N Engl J Med* 349(13):1247-1256, 2003.
Nazario R, et al: Treatment of Venous Thromboembolism. *Cardiol Rev* 10(4):249-259, 2002.
Wells PS, et al: Derivation of a simple clinical model to categorize patients' probability of pulmonary embolism: increasing the model's utility with the SimpliRED D-dimer. *Thromb Haemost*, 83:416-420, 2000.

 Chapter 18

Chronic Obstructive Pulmonary Disease

"I can't have emphysema.
I quit smoking 10 years ago."

CLINICAL CASE PROBLEM 1:
A 55-YEAR-OLD MALE WITH A CHRONIC COUGH

A 55-year-old male presents to your office for assessment of a chronic cough. He complains of "coughing for the last 10 years." The cough has become more bothersome lately. The cough is productive of sputum that is usually mucoid; occasionally it becomes purulent.

He has a 35-year history of smoking two packs of cigarettes a day (a history of 70 packs per year). He quit smoking approximately 2 years ago.

On physical examination his blood pressure is 160/85 mm Hg. His pulse is 96 and regular. He has a BMI (body mass index) of 34. He weighs 280 lb. He wheezes while he talks. On auscultation, adventitious breath sounds are heard in all lobes. His chest x-ray reveals significant bronchial wall thickening. There are increased markings at both lung bases.

SELECT THE BEST ANSWER TO THE FOLLOWING QUESTIONS:

1. What is the most likely diagnosis in this patient?
   a. smoker's cough
   b. subacute bronchitis
   c. emphysema
   d. chronic bronchitis
   e. allergic bronchitis

2. What is the most likely cause of this condition?
   a. right-sided heart failure
   b. cor pulmonale
   c. cigarette smoking
   d. obstructive sleep apnea
   e. hypercarbia

3. Which of the following statements regarding this condition is (are) true?
   a. the disease develops in 10% to 15% of cigarette smokers
   b. cigarette smokers in whom this disease develops usually report the onset of cough with expectoration 10 to 12 years after smoking began
   c. dyspnea is noted initially only on extreme exertion; as the condition progresses it becomes more severe and occurs with mild activity
   d. pneumonia, pulmonary hypertension, cor pulmonale, and chronic respiratory failure characterize the late stages of the disease
   e. all of the above are true

4. Which of the following regarding the patient described above is (are) true?
   a. this patient is a "pink puffer"
   b. this patient's blood gases likely will show a decreased Pco_2

c. this patient's chest x-ray will demonstrate normal to increased lung markings
d. this patient's disease is a disease of the terminal bronchi
e. all of the above are true

5. Which of the following pulmonary function results is not associated with the condition described above?
   a. reduced FEV_1 (forced expiratory volume)
   b. reduced FEV_1/FVC (forced vital capacity)
   c. reduced FEF_{25-75} (forced expiratory flow)
   d. decreased residual volume
   e. none of the above are associated with this disease state

6. Regarding the pathophysiology of chronic bronchitis, which of the following statements is (are) false?
   a. most histologic studies in patients with chronic bronchitis have shown an increase in the size of mucus-secreting glands as measured by the Reid index (a ratio of gland to bronchial wall thickness)
   b. smooth-muscle hyperplasia occurs in patients with chronic bronchitis
   c. chronic bronchitis is characterized by chronic, excessive secretion of mucus
   d. in chronic bronchitis, there is a clear relationship between smooth-muscle hyperplasia and bronchodilator responsiveness or methacholine sensitivity
   e. none of the above are false

7. Which of the following is (are) established risk factors for chronic obstructive pulmonary disease (COPD)?
   a. smoking
   b. atopy
   c. elevated levels of immunoglobulin E (IgE)
   d. bronchial hyperresponsiveness
   e. all of the above

8. Which of the following is (are) accurate regarding the role of bacteria in chronic bronchitis?
   a. the delay in mucociliary clearance allows inhaled bacteria to colonize the normally sterile airways and to multiply, leading to further infectious exacerbations
   b. *Haemophilus influenzae, Streptococcus pneumoniae,* and *Moraxella catarrhalis* account for 75% of all exacerbations of chronic bronchitis
   c. bacteria may act synergistically with tobacco smoke to impede mucociliary clearance and allow organisms to colonize the airways further

d. nicotine stimulates the growth of *Haemophilus influenzae*
e. a, b, and c
f. all of the above

9. Which of the following is (are) a consideration in the diagnosis of chronic bronchitis?
   a. asthma
   b. postnasal drip from sinusitis
   c. chronic angiotensin-converting enzyme (ACE) inhibitor therapy
   d. a and b
   e. all of the above

10. Which of the following statements regarding smoking cessation and COPD is (are) true?
    a. cessation of smoking dramatically reduces symptoms in patients with established COPD
    b. coughing stops in 80% of patients with COPD who quit smoking
    c. coughing stops in more than 50% of patients with COPD within 4 weeks
    d. all of the above
    e. none of the above

11. Which of the following drugs is (are) the most effective for long-term pharmacologic management in a patient with chronic bronchitis?
    a. an inhaled beta agonist
    b. an inhaled anticholinergic
    c. an inhaled corticosteroid
    d. oral prednisone
    e. a, b, and c are considered to be equally efficacious

12. Which of the following drugs is (are) recommended as routine symptomatic management for a patient with chronic bronchitis?
    a. an inhaled beta agonist
    b. an inhaled anticholinergic
    c. an inhaled corticosteroid
    d. a and b
    e. all of the above

13. Long-term home oxygen therapy is indicated in which of the patients with chronic bronchitis?
    a. all patients who have established chronic bronchitis and who have met the criteria of symptoms for at least 5 years
    b. all patients who have a resting arterial partial pressure of oxygen of 55 mm Hg or less
    c. all patients who have a resting arterial partial pressure of oxygen of 60 mm Hg or less with evidence of chronic tissue hypoxia as demonstrated by cor pulmonale or polycythemia

d. b and c
e. all of the above

CLINICAL CASE PROBLEM 2:
A PATIENT WHOSE SYMPTOMS ARE EXACERBATED BY SECOND–HAND SMOKE

The patient described in Clinical Case Problem 1 is stabilized with long-term therapy. Unfortunately, during the winter holiday, he travels to his son's home in a distant state and finds himself in an environment in which six packs of cigarettes a day are being smoked by his son and his son's wife (four packs for the son and two packs for his wife). There is a layer of definite haze that hangs approximately 1 ft below all the ceilings in the house. As he sits around the house 1 day (unable to go outside or walk any distance at all because of significantly increased shortness of breath since arriving) he counts the number of ashtrays; there are 21. His son, through the haze of smoke, finally notices that his dad is out of breath and his lips appear very blue. He takes him to the nearest emergency room (ER).

The ER doctor diagnoses his condition as an acute exacerbation of chronic bronchitis. His major symptoms at this time include dyspnea, increased sputum production, and purulence. The patient's PaO_2 when measured in the ER is 44 mm Hg.

14. Which of the following should be instituted as therapy for this condition?
    a. low-flow oxygen
    b. intravenous corticosteroids
    c. oral ciprofloxacin
    d. a and b only
    e. all of the above

15. Which of the following organisms that have been implicated in the pathogenesis of acute exacerbations of chronic bronchitis has (have) exhibited resistance *in vivo* to ampicillin?
    a. *Haemophilus influenzae*
    b. *Streptococcus pneumoniae*
    c. *Moraxella catarrhalis*
    d. a and b only
    e. all of the above

CLINICAL CASE PROBLEM 3:
A 23-YEAR-OLD MALE SMOKER WITH A 10-DAY COUGH

A 23-year-old male presents to your office for assessment of a 10-day cough that has "now gone into my lungs." He complains of sputum production, which was initially clear but now has turned "yellow." He said that

he called your partner last night and your partner told him to "get in here today and we will prescribe an antibiotic and clear this thing up quick." This patient has no history of other respiratory illnesses. On examination, the patient's lungs are clear. His temperature is normal (98.6° C). No other positive physical findings are present.

16. What would you do?
    a. reach for the "good old prescription pad" and scribble down the first reasonable thing that comes to mind
    b. reach for the "good old prescription pad" but think briefly about which antibiotic you wish to prescribe before you prescribe it
    c. reach for the "good old prescription pad" but think quite a bit before deciding which antibiotic you wish to prescribe
    d. auscultate the patient's lung through his shirt, sweater, and winter jacket, and then reach for the prescription pad
    e. take the Fifth Amendment on this question
    f. none of the above

CLINICAL CASE MANAGEMENT PROBLEM

Describe the difference between the two major types of COPD in terms of: (1) part of airway affected; (2) color of lips in severely affected individual; (3) definition of both types; (4) pathophysiology; and (5) the causes.

▶ ANSWERS:

1. **d.** This patient has chronic bronchitis. Chronic bronchitis is defined as cough and sputum production on most days for at least 3 months of the year for at least 2 years. Chronic bronchitis and emphysema are the two underlying conditions in COPD.

Emphysema is a destructive process involving the lung parenchyma. It is defined as abnormal permanent enlargement of air spaces distal to the terminal bronchioles accompanied by destruction of alveolar walls.

Acute bronchitis is an inflammation of the bronchi caused by an infectious agent or acute exposure to a nonspecific irritant. Acute bronchitis most often is caused by a viral infection. Acute bronchitis may occur as a complication of chronic bronchitis.

2. **c.** Chronic bronchitis most commonly is caused by cigarette smoking. Right-sided heart failure and cor pulmonale may result from chronic bronchitis and/or emphysema. Obstructive sleep apnea is often a complication of COPD. Hypercarbia (increased PCO_2

level) is a valuable prognostic sign in chronic bronchitis and allows the prediction (along with decreased PO_2) of when certain therapies, especially home oxygen, should be used.

3. e. Chronic bronchitis usually develops in cigarette smokers approximately 10 to 12 years after smoking initiation. Patients with chronic bronchitis have an increased susceptibility to recurrent respiratory tract infections. COPD develops in 10% to 15% of patients who are cigarette smokers. In these patients, airflow obstruction worsens over time if cigarette smoking is continued.

Dyspnea initially is noted only on extreme exertion, but as the COPD progresses, it becomes more severe and occurs with mild activity. In severe disease, dyspnea may occur at rest.

Complications of COPD include pneumonia, pulmonary hypertension, cor pulmonale, and chronic respiratory failure.

4. c. Patients with COPD can be classified into two basic types: Type A COPD patients, or "pink puffers," and Type B COPD patients, or "blue bloaters." The patient described in this question is a typical blue bloater who typically has the following characteristics: (1) is stocky or obese; (2) has cough and sputum production; (3) has normal or increased lung markings; (4) has a markedly reduced PO_2 and an elevated PCO_2; and (5) often develops pulmonary hypertension and/or cor pulmonale. Blue bloaters have chronic bronchitis. Type A COPD pink puffers typically have the following characteristics: (1) are thin; (2) have dyspnea; (3) have hyperinflated lungs on chest x-ray; and (4) have a slightly decreased PO_2 and a normal or slightly decreased PCO_2. Pink puffers have emphysema.

5. d. Chronic bronchitis is characterized by several abnormalities observed on pulmonary function testing. Abnormalities noted most frequently include: (1) an increased (not decreased) residual volume, (2) a decrease in FEV_1 (the forced vital capacity in 1 second), (3) a decrease in FEV_1/FVC; and (4) a decrease in FEF_{25-75}.

COPD is divided into the following stages:

Stage 0 (at risk): FEV is normal, FEV_1/FVC is normal

Stage I (mild COPD): FEV>80%, FEV_1/FVC <70% predicted

Stage II (moderate COPD): FEV_1 50% to 80%, FEV_1/FVC <70%

Stage IIa (moderate COPD): FEV_1 30% to 50%, FEV_1/FVC <70%

Stage III (severe COPD): FEV_1 <30%, FEV_1/FVC <70%

6. d. Most mucus is secreted by subepithelial glands in the large airways. It follows that chronic bronchitis, a disorder characterized by chronic, excessive secretion of mucus, is a disease of the large airways. Most histologic studies of chronic bronchitis have shown an increase in the size of the mucus-secreting glands as measured by the Reid index (a ratio of gland to bronchial wall thickness), although no clearcut relation between this index and the degree of airflow obstruction has been established. Patients with chronic bronchitis also have smooth-muscle hyperplasia; however, unlike the situation in asthma, there is no clearcut relationship between their responsiveness or methacholine sensitivity. Bronchial hyperresponsiveness, which is present in at least 50% of patients with COPD, may lead to dyspnea and hypoxemia.

7. e. It commonly is thought that cigarette smoking is the only risk factor for COPD. In fact, a number of other risk factors are implicated: (1) exposure to tobacco smoke; (2) domestic and occupational pollutants and recurrent respiratory tract infections, particularly in infancy; (3) atopy, which is characterized by eosinophilia or an increased level of serum IgE; (4) the presence of bronchial hyperresponsiveness; (5) a family history of COPD; and (6) certain protease deficiencies such as alpha$_1$-antitrypsin deficiency, which also may be responsible for a positive family history.

8. f. Cigarette smoking, as the most common cause of chronic bronchitis, leads to loss of ciliated epithelium and more viscous secretions, compromising the local defenses of the respiratory tract. The delay in mucociliary clearance allows inhaled bacteria to colonize the normally sterile airways and to multiply, leading to further infectious exacerbations. *Haemophilus influenzae* is present in the sputum of about 60% of patients with stable chronic bronchitis. *Haemophilus influenza, Streptococcus pneumonia,* and *Moraxella catarrhalis* account for 75% of all exacerbations of chronic bronchitis and 85% to 95% of bacterial exacerbations. *H. influenzae* may act synergistically with tobacco smoke to impede mucociliary clearance and allow further multiplication and colonization of the airway. Byproducts of *H. influenzae* metabolism have been shown to cause further impairment of ciliated cells *in vitro,* stimulate mucus production, and secrete IgA protease that may further impair host defenses. In addition, nicotine has been shown to stimulate the growth of this organism, and *H. influenzae* has been shown to engender an immune reaction in the airways.

9. e. The diagnosis of chronic bronchitis rests on clinical criteria that already have been described.

There are no characteristic physical findings and no specific radiographic changes or laboratory features diagnostic of this disease.

The differential diagnosis of chronic cough, however, must be considered. This includes: (1) asthma; (2) postnasal drip; (3) gastroesophageal reflux; (4) foreign body aspiration; (5) congestive heart failure; (6) bronchiectasis; and (7) chronic ACE inhibitor therapy (15% of patients taking ACE inhibitors develop a chronic cough).

10. d. The cessation of smoking produces dramatic symptomatic benefits for patients with chronic bronchitis. Coughing stops in up to 77% of quitters and improves in another 17%. When coughing stops, it does so within 4 weeks in 54% of patients. A number of effective pharmacotherapy agents are available to assist patients in quitting. These include nicotine replacement agents and antidepressants such as bupropion (Zyban) and nortriptyline (Aventyl). These agents increase long-term quit rates.

Influenza virus can worsen the epithelial damage induced by cigarette smoke and predispose the airways to subsequent bacterial proliferation, leading to excessive mucus hypersecretion and greater airflow obstruction. Annual influenza vaccination reduces morbidity and mortality caused by influenza in patients with COPD, although its role in this disease has not been assessed in large-scale clinical trials. Patients with COPD also should receive the pneumococcal vaccine.

11. b. Ipratropium bromide is the most effective long-term pharmacologic agent used in chronic bronchitis and COPD. In the treatment of COPD, a stepwise approach should be used:

Mild intermittent: beta agonist

Mild to moderate persistent: ipratropium plus beta agonist

Suboptimal response: add theophylline and/or albuterol and/or mucolytic agent

Persistent symptoms: oral prednisone

Severe exacerbation: hospitalize

12. d. See Answer 13.

13. d. Symptomatic therapy for patients with chronic bronchitis includes the use of: (1) inhaled bronchodilators; (2) oral bronchodilators; (3) inhaled corticosteroids; (4) oral corticosteroids; (5) inhaled anticholinergics; (6) home oxygen therapy; and (7) rehabilitation programs.

The use of inhaled bronchodilators by patients with airflow obstruction may increase flow rates and reduce dyspnea. Inhaled anticholinergic agents appear to produce greater bronchodilatation than inhaled beta 2 agonists in COPD, with fewer side effects. This may be related to increased cholinergic tone in the airways as the degree of obstruction progresses. Combination therapy with agents from both groups may have an additive effect in some patients. Patients who demonstrate symptomatic or physiologic improvement, or both, with these medications should be maintained on the inhaled drugs indefinitely. In patients who remain symptomatic while taking inhaled bronchodilators, a trial of an oral theophylline medication is warranted. These medications are weaker bronchodilators than inhaled anticholinergics or beta-agonist drugs but may have additional beneficial effects in chronic bronchitis by increasing respiratory muscle strength and endurance, improving mucociliary clearance, and increasing central respiratory drive, all of which may lead to a symptomatic improvement in patients with the disease.

At present, regular use of oral or inhaled corticosteroids cannot be recommended as routine therapy for all patients with chronic bronchitis. Although steroids have clear antiinflammatory effects and decrease mucus hypersecretion, a beneficial effect can be shown in only 10% to 20% of patients.

The benefits of home oxygen therapy have been clearly demonstrated in major clinical trials. To be considered candidates for treatment, patients must (1) be in a stable clinical state, (2) have a resting arterial partial pressure of oxygen PaO_2 of 55 mm Hg or less, or (3) have a PaO_2 of 60 mm Hg with evidence of chronic tissue hypoxia as demonstrated by cor pulmonale or polycythemia. In properly selected patients, the use of home oxygen for more than 18 hours a day may increase the life span of the patients with COPD by 6 or 7 years. Oxygen also is indicated in patients with signs and symptoms of cor pulmonale or pulmonary hypertension or with desaturation during sleep.

14. e. Treatment of an acute exacerbation of chronic bronchitis provides symptomatic relief and prevents any transient decline in pulmonary function. Low-flow oxygen should be instituted if hypoxemia is present (as in this case). The goal of oxygen therapy in this case is to get the PaO_2 higher than 60 mm Hg. In addition, oral or intravenous corticosteroids should be given because they have been shown to hasten the resolution of patients in the acute exacerbation phase of chronic bronchitis.

Patients with all three of the following "acute exacerbative symptoms" have been shown to benefit from antibiotic therapy: (1) increasing dyspnea; (2) increased sputum production; and (3) purulence of sputum.

In patients with two or less of the three symptoms, the situation is less clear.

15. **e.** Antibiotic choices obviously should be based on both host and pathogen factors. The latter relate to resistance problems. The three most common isolates associated with acute exacerbations of chronic bronchitis are: (1) *Haemophilus influenzae*; (2) *Streptococcus pneumoniae*; and (3) *Moraxella catarrhalis*.

All have exhibited resistance *in vivo* to ampicillin and other first-line agents. Nevertheless, most U.S. and international guidelines recommend initial treatment of acute exacerbations of chronic bronchitis with amoxicillin or tetracycline derivatives. Other potential first-line agents include trimethoprim–sulfamethoxazole and cefaclor. In the most complicated cases of acute exacerbation of chronic bronchitis, most guidelines recommend quinolones, macrolides, and a second- or third-generation cephalosporin as the initial agent.

16. **f.** This patient has acute bronchitis and is a healthy young man with no concomitant illnesses.

The cause of acute bronchitis in a patient like this is almost always a viral infection (adenovirus, influenza virus, or rhinovirus). It has only been present for 24 hours, and at this time there is no good reason for prescribing an antibiotic. What your partner says or what your patient expects are not satisfactory reasons for doing something that, on the basis of probability, is likely to do no good whatsoever.

A reasonable treatment protocol to follow for the treatment of acute bronchitis follows:

1. Healthy middle-aged adult, no other respiratory problems, cough and purulent sputum production of short duration: no culture; no antibiotic
2. Healthy middle-aged adult, no other respiratory problems, cough and purulent sputum production persists for longer than 1 week: no culture; macrolide antibiotic (to cover mycoplasma)
3. Healthy elderly adult, no other respiratory problems, cough and purulent sputum production of short duration: no culture; no antibiotic
4. Healthy elderly adult, no other respiratory problems, cough and purulent sputum production for greater than 1 week: no culture; trimethoprim–sulfamethoxazole or amoxicillin
5. Elderly adult with chronic disease, cough and sputum production: no culture initially; macrolide no matter how long symptoms have persisted.

SOLUTION TO THE CLINICAL CASE MANAGEMENT PROBLEM

1. The two forms of COPD are chronic bronchitis and emphysema.
   a. Chronic bronchitis affects the large airways of the lung.
   b. Emphysema affects the terminal bronchi.
2. The color of lips in severely affected individuals is:
   a. Blue; the "blue bloater" equals chronic bronchitis.
   b. Pink; the "pink puffer" equals emphysema.
3. Definitions:
   a. Chronic bronchitis: Excessive cough, productive of sputum on most days for at least 3 months a year during at least 2 consecutive years
   b. Emphysema: Defined histologically by abnormal permanent enlargement, without obvious fibrosis, of the airspaces distal to the terminal bronchi, accompanied by destruction of their walls.
4. Pathophysiology:

   a. Chronic bronchitis:
      i. chronic, excessive secretion of mucus
      ii. increase in the size of the mucus-secreting cells
      iii. smooth-muscle hyperplasia
      iv. bronchial airway hyperresponsiveness
   b. Emphysema:
      i. distal airspace enlargement
      ii. no significant fibrosis
      iii. loss of alveolar attachments
      iv. decrease in elastic recoil
      v. increase in lung compliance
      vi. hyperinflation
      vii. ventilation-perfusion mismatching
5. Causes: Most cases of both chronic bronchitis and emphysema are the result of cigarette smoking; alpha-1-antitrypsin deficiency is a factor in some cases of emphysema.

SUMMARY OF CHRONIC OBSTRUCTIVE PULMONARY DISEASE

1. **Definitions:**
   See the Clinical Case Management Problem box.
2. **Pathophysiology:**
   See the Clinical Case Management Problem box.
3. **Differentiation of disease entities in COPD:**
   See the Clinical Case Management Problem box.
4. **Signs and symptoms:**
   a. Symptoms: dyspnea, cough, sputum production, and sputum purulence. When cor pulmonale and right-sided heart failure are present, there is extremity swelling.
   b. Signs: increased respiratory rate, respiratory distress, cyanosis, barrel chest, distant heart sounds, increased jugular venous pressure
   c. Three most important signs/symptoms indicating deterioration are: (i) increasing dyspnea; (ii) increased sputum volume and, (iii) increased purulence.
5. **Pulmonary function test abnormalities:**
   a. Decreased FEV_1
   b. Decreased ratio of FEV_1/FVC
   c. Decreased FEF_{25-75}
   d. Increased residual volume
   e. Normal to increased functional residual capacity
   f. Decreased diffusion capacity
6. **Pathologic organisms associated with infection in COPD:**
   a. *Haemophilus influenzae*
   b. *Streptococcus pneumoniae*
   c. *Moraxella catarrhalis*
7. **Treatment:**
   a. Bronchodilators:
      i. Best single agent for long-term treatment in chronic bronchitis is an inhaled anticholinergic-ipratropium (Atrovent).
      ii. Beta agonists should be combined with (i) above.
   b. Corticosteroids: Routine use of inhaled corticosteroids cannot be recommended in chronic care. Corticosteroids (both inhaled and intra-venous/oral) are most helpful in acute exacerbations. Macrolides in atypical cases are expected.
   c. Antibiotics: Routine prophylactic use of antibiotics cannot be recommended. They are most useful in acute exacerbations if all three of the following are present: (i) increasing dyspnea; (ii) increasing sputum production; and (iii) increasing sputum purulence.

      Antibiotics of choice include ampicillin, trimethoprim–sulfamethoxazole, amoxicillin, doxycycline, and cefaclor. Floxin is effective for severe exacerbations, and macrolides should be used if atypical organisms are suspected. Note: Resistance is constantly increasing and recommendations may rapidly change.
   d. Home oxygen: Home oxygen is indicated if PaO_2 is 55 mm Hg or less at rest or if PaO_2 is 60 mm Hg with evidence of chronic tissue hypoxia as demonstrated by cor pulmonale or polycythemia.
   e. Diuretics: Use of diuretics is indicated only for treatment of cor pulmonale and right-sided heart failure.
   f. Smoking cessation: At any time in the course of COPD smoking cessation can be and is of benefit. Do not accept "I've smoked too long and I am too old to quit."
   g. Counseling/support groups: Group therapy with other patients with COPD often helps the patient come to terms with the disease.

SUGGESTED READING

Bope E: COPD. In Rakel R, ed: *Conn's Current Therapy,* 223-226, Philadelphia, 2003, WB Saunders.

Weinstein N, et al: The Resident's Guide to Ambulatory Care. 2001-2002, 5th ed. *The Patient Care of COPD,* 145-146. Anadem Press Inc, 2003, Columbus OH.

Braunwald EF, et al: *Harrison's Manual of Medicine,* 15th ed., 626-629, 2002

Man SF, et al: Contemporary management of COPD: clinical applications. *JAMA* 290:2313-2316, 2003.

Sin DD, et al: Contemporary management of COPD: scientific review. *JAMA* 290:2301-2312, 2003.

Chapter 19

Asthma

"Some wheeze, some don't, but it's still serious."

CLINICAL CASE PROBLEM 1:
A 22-YEAR-OLD MALE WITH A CHRONIC COUGH

A 22-year-old male presents to your office for assessment of a chronic cough. He has just moved to your city and will be attending the university there. He has moved into a bachelor apartment in the basement of a house.

As soon as he moved in, he began to notice a chronic, nonproductive cough associated with shortness of breath. He has never had these symptoms before, and he has no known allergies. When he leaves for school for the day, the symptoms disappear. The symptoms are definitely worse at night.

His landlady has three cats. He didn't think he was allergic to cats, but now he thinks that might be the problem.

On examination, his respiratory rate is 16 and regular. He is in no distress at the present time. There are a few expiratory rhonchi heard in all lobes. His blood pressure is 120/70, and his pulse is 72 and regular.

■ **SELECT THE BEST ANSWER TO THE FOLLOWING QUESTIONS:**

1. What is the most likely diagnosis in this patient?
   a. paroxysmal nocturnal cough syndrome
   b. hyporesponsive airways disease
   c. cough variant asthma
   d. allergic bronchitis
   e. none of the above

2. In children, which of the following statements is (are) true?
   a. it is sometimes difficult to differentiate asthma from bronchiolitis
   b. some children with an episode of bronchiolitis do not develop asthma
   c. the relationships among bronchiolitis, ongoing bronchial hyperactivity, and asthma are unclear, although many children with bronchiolitis develop asthma
   d. all of the above
   e. none of the above

3. Which of the following is (are) included in the working definition of asthma?
   a. reversible airway obstruction
   b. bronchial airway inflammation
   c. bronchial airway hyperresponsiveness to a variety of stimuli
   d. expiratory rhonchi
   e. a, b, and c
   f. all of the above

4. Which of the following statements regarding incidence and mortality regarding asthma is (are) false?
   a. the mortality from asthma is decreasing (presumably because of improved therapies)
   b. the number of cases of asthma from various causes continues to increase at a rapid rate.
   c. in the United States in 1990, the estimated health care cost associated with asthma was approximately $3.4 billion
   d. all of the above statements are false
   e. none of the above statements are false

5. Asthma, on a pathophysiologic basis, is primarily:
   a. a bronchoconstricting process
   b. an allergenic stimulus process
   c. an inflammatory process
   d. a bronchial hyperreactivity process
   e. an immunoglobulin E-mediated antigen-antibody reaction

6. Following antigenic stimulation of the bronchial airway, which cell is most responsible for the beginning of the airway's response?
   a. the basophil
   b. the mast cell
   c. the eosinophil
   d. the bronchial epithelial cell
   e. the bronchial mucus-producing goblet cells

7. What is (are) the substance(s) released by the cell that is most responsible for the beginning of the airway's response?
   a. histamine
   b. proteolytic enzymes
   c. heparin
   d. chemotactic factors
   e. all of the above

8. The parameter most useful in evaluating a patient with asthma is?
   a. peak flow
   b. peak inspiratory flow rate
   c. the forced expiratory volume in one second (FEV_1)
   d. none of the above
   e. all of the above

9. The main classification classes for asthma as provided by the American Academy of Allergy, Asthma, and Immunology include:

a. severe persistent
b. moderate persistent
c. mild persistent
d. mild intermittent
e. all of the above

10. The reversible airflow obstruction seen in asthma results from which of the following?
    a. bronchoconstriction
    b. mucus plug formation
    c. edema
    d. a and b
    e. all of the above

11. Which of the following is (are) a clinical hallmark(s) of asthma?
    a. cough
    b. nocturnal dyspnea
    c. wheezing
    d. shortness of breath
    e. a, c, and d

CLINICAL CASE PROBLEM 2:

A 24-Year-Old Wheezer

A 24-year-old woman patient develops wheezing and shortness of breath when exposed to cold air or when exercising. These symptoms are getting worse.

12. Which of the following is the prophylactic agent of choice for the treatment of asthma in these circumstances?
    a. inhaled beta$_2$ agonists
    b. oral aminophylline
    c. inhaled anticholinergics
    d. inhaled sodium cromoglycate
    e. oral corticosteroids

13. What is the mechanism of action of the agent of choice in Question 12?
    a. mast cell stabilizer
    b. inhibitor of early-phase reaction
    c. inhibitor of late-phase reaction
    d. bronchodilator
    e. none of the above

14. What is the treatment of choice for long-term stabilization?
    a. long-acting beta$_2$ agonists
    b. leukotriene modifiers
    c. an inhaled anticholinergic
    d. inhaled steroid
    e. a and b

15. Which of the following stepped care classifications used to guide pharmacotherapy in asthma requires environmental control as the necessary first step for treatment?
    a. mild intermittent asthma
    b. mild persistent asthma
    c. moderate persistent asthma
    d. severe persistent asthma
    e. all of the above

16. All the following except which are characteristics of mild persistent asthma:
    a. symptoms occurring more than twice a week but less than once a day
    b. exacerbations that affect activity
    c. peak expiratory flow (PEF) greater than 80% of personal best
    d. PEF variability of 20% to 30%
    e. nocturnal symptoms two to three times per week

17. Which of the following most accurately describes the preferred pharmacologic treatment of moderate persistent asthma in adults?
    a. inhaled sodium cromoglycate alone
    b. inhaled beta$_2$ agonists alone
    c. inhaled corticosteroids alone
    d. daily inhaled corticosteroids plus long-acting inhaled beta$_2$ agonists, if needed
    e. inhaled sodium cromoglycate continually plus intermittent inhaled beta$_2$ agonists

18. All the following are characteristics of severe persistent asthma except:
    a. continual symptoms
    b. frequent exacerbations that may last days
    c. infrequent nighttime symptoms
    d. PEF rates less than 60% of personal best
    e. PEF variability of more than 30%

19. Pharmacotherapy of severe persistent asthma includes:
    a. high-dose steroids via mask
    b. long-acting bronchodilator
    c. sustained-released theophylline
    d. quick relief with an inhaled beta$_2$ agonist as needed
    e. all of the above

20. In a patient whose PEF rate is less than 50% of personal best, suggesting a severe exacerbation, the initial home treatment includes which of the following?
    a. an inhaled short-acting beta$_2$ agonist administered three times via metered-dosed inhaler or one time via nebulizer

b. inhaled cromolyn, three times via metered-dosed inhaler or one time via nebulizer
c. an inhaled corticosteroid, administered three times via metered-dosed inhaler or one time via nebulizer
d. subcutaneous self-administered epinephrine
e. none of the above

21. Which of the following pulmonary function tests is the most useful for diagnosis of asthma?
a. decreased forced vital capacity (FVC)
b. increased residual volume
c. a ratio of FEV_1/FVC of 75%
d. increased functional residual capacity
e. increased total lung capacity

22. Which of the following pulmonary function tests is most easily carried out at home?
a. FEV_1/FVC ratio
c. FCV
c. mid-expiratory flow rate
d. PEF rate
e. residual volume

23. Which of the following is the most common abnormality observed on the chest x-ray in a patient with asthma?
a. hyperinflation
b. increased bronchial markings
c. atelectasis
d. flattening of the diaphragm
e. all of the above are equally common

24. What is the most common abnormality seen on physical examination of a patient with asthma?
a. increased respiratory rate
b. inspiratory rales
c. inspiratory rhonchi
d. expiratory rales
e. expiratory wheezes

25. Environmental control as a part of the therapeutic intervention involves a search for and elimination of which of the following agents from the patient's environment:
a. air pollution
b. pollens, molds, mites, cockroaches, and pets
c. tobacco smoke, wood stoves, and fumes
d. workplace exposures
e. sulfates, aspirin, other nonsteroidal antiinflammatory drugs, and other potential offending drugs
f. all of the above

26. Pure cough variant asthma has which of the following characteristics?
a. patients often have to go from doctor to doctor until someone makes the diagnosis
b. patients are treated in the same manner as noncough variant asthma
c. cough variant asthma is very uncommon
d. a and b
e. all of the above

27. A patient who presents to the ER in acute respiratory distress resulting from a severe attack of asthma should be treated with all of the following except:
a. warm, humidified, high-flow-rate oxygen
b. constant bedside monitoring
c. intravenous corticosteroids
d. intravenous fluids
e. intravenous antibiotics

28. Which of the following statements regarding childhood asthma is (are) false?
a. there is a very significant hereditary component to the probability of a child acquiring asthma
b. asthma in children often is associated with parental smoking
c. asthmatic children are often allergic to aspirin (acetylsalicylic acid)
d. inhaled corticosteroids, administered properly, do not pose a major risk or hazard to childhood growth
e. many children who are asthmatic go on to outgrow it

29. Which of the following viral agents has been implicated as a cause of asthma?
a. respiratory syncytial virus
b. parainfluenza virus
c. adenovirus
d. rhinovirus
e. influenza virus

CLINICAL CASE MANAGEMENT PROBLEM

A rural family physician has noticed an interesting phenomenon. This summer there have been two very severe lightning storms. In the first instance, approximately 1 hour after the storm subsided, six children displayed signs and symptoms of asthma. In the second instance, eight children displayed signs and symptoms of asthma 1 hour after the storm. (Only three children appeared on both occasions.) How do you explain this?

ANSWERS:

1. c. This patient has cough variant asthma. Physicians should be aware that cough variant asthma is particularly common in children but can occur, as in this case, in adults as well. The diagnosis often is missed because in many cases there is no wheezing.

2. d. First, it is sometimes difficult to differentiate on the basis of symptoms, signs, and laboratory findings between asthma and bronchiolitis. Second, some children with an episode of bronchiolitis do not develop asthma. Third, the relationship between bronchiolitis and asthma is unclear. There is good evidence at this time that bronchiolitis may be a risk factor for asthma and may predispose to asthma.

3. e. The current working definition of asthma is as follows: (1) a lung disease with airway obstruction that is usually reversible; (2) a lung disease that is characterized by airway inflammation; and (3) a lung disease that is characterized by increased bronchial hyperresponsiveness to various stimuli.

4. a. The morbidity and mortality from asthma are increasing, not decreasing. Asthma often is referred to as an obstructive lung disease manifested by recurring wheezing. The obstruction is secondary to inflammation, mucosal edema, mucous hypersecretion, and smooth-muscle contraction.

Asthma affects more than 17 million Americans each year. Despite efforts to provide better diagnostics, prevention, and treatment, the prevalence and mortality from asthma continues to increase.

5. c. Our understanding of the pathophysiology of asthma has undergone considerable change in the past few years. This has had a substantial impact on treatment. Asthma now is recognized as an inflammatory disorder. Although bronchoconstriction and bronchial hyperreactivity are characteristics of asthma, the basic underlying pathophysiologic process is inflammation in the bronchial wall.

6. b. For further comment see Answer 11.

7. e. For further comment see Answer 11.

8. c. The FEV_1 is the most useful parameter in evaluating patients with asthma. The rate in disciplined patients is helpful in following lung function, especially when exposed to various allergens. For further comment see Answer 11.

9. e. These characteristic classes are important to identify because they lead to a stepwise approach to the identification and treatment of asthma. For further comment see Answer 11.

10. b. For further comment see Answer 11.

11. e. The diagnosis of asthma often is made on the basis of a typical history of abrupt dyspnea, with a dry, nonproductive cough and wheezing.

Questions 6-11 describe the pathophysiology of asthma. The events are as follows:

Event 1: Beginning of the response of the bronchial wall to the particular antigenic stimulation

Event 2: Antigenic stimulation leads to mast cell degranulation

Event 3: Mast cell degranulation leads to the following:
   a. Immediate release of preformed mediators from granules
   b. Release of secondary mediators, including: (i) histamine; (ii) chemotactic factors; (iii) proteolytic enzymes; and (iv) heparin.

Event 4: The release of these mediators leads to significant smooth-muscle bronchoconstriction.

Event 5: The initial bronchial constriction leads to recruitment of other inflammatory cells, including (a) neutrophils; (b) eosinophils; and (c) mononuclear cells.

Event 6: The recruitment of these "secondary mediator cells" has demonstrated the release of (a) cytokines; (b) vasoactive factors; and (c) arachidonic acid metabolites.

Event 7: Activation of epithelial and endothelial cells occurs, enhancing inflammatory responses.

Event 8: Release of interleukins 3 to 6, tumor necrosis factor, and interferon-gamma has been demonstrated in the inflammatory response.

The importance of these series of events is as follows:

1. The early-phase reaction of asthma is mediated by the "primary mediators": neutrophils, eosinophils, and mononuclear cells.
2. The late-phase reaction of asthma is mediated by the "secondary mediators": cytokines, vasoactive factors, and arachidonic acid metabolites.

Important summary points include the following:

• Asthma is a chronic inflammatory disorder of the lower airways characterized by episodes of acute symptomatic exacerbations overlaying chronic inflammation. Inflammation results in the following:
   1. Increased bronchial hyperresponsiveness to stimuli
   2. Reversible airflow obstruction by (a) bronchoconstriction; (b) mucus plug formation; and (c) edema.

Atopy is a predisposing factor in many patients.

12. **a.** The prophylactic agent of choice for exercise-induced or cold-air–induced asthma is a short-acting beta$_2$ agonist, albuterol.

13. **d.** Albuterol works as a bronchodilator.

14. **e.** Both prophylactic daily leukotriene modifiers and long-acting beta$_2$ agonists have been used successfully for long-term stabilization of competitive athletes' exercise-induced asthma.

15. **e.** All of the above.

16. **e.** The characteristics of mild persistent asthma include symptoms twice a week, but less than once a day. Exacerbations may effect activity. Nighttime symptoms occur more than twice per month, FEV$_1$ or PEF is 80% or more, and PEF variation is 20% to 30%.

17. **d.** The pharmacotherapy for moderate persistent asthma in adults and children 5 years of age and older includes the use of a daily medium dose inhaled corticosteroid and the addition, if needed, of a long-acting inhaled beta$_2$ agonist or sustained released theophylline.

18. **c.** Infrequent nighttime symptoms is incorrect. Nighttime symptoms occur frequently.

19. **e.** The treatment for severe persistent asthma includes the following: (1) antiinflammatory treatment with an inhaled corticosteroid; (2) long-acting bronchodilators with either inhaled beta$_2$ agonists; (3) sustained released theophylline or long-acting beta$_2$-agonist tablets; and (4) corticosteroid tablets or syrup (2 mg/kg/day, with no more than 60 mg/day). Short-acting inhaled beta$_2$ agonists can be used as needed to control symptoms.

20. **a.** A PEF measuring less than 50% of personal best suggests a severe exacerbation. Initial treatment should include an inhaled short-acting beta$_2$ agonist administered three times via metered dose inhaler or one time via nebulizer. If the PEF rate remains less than 50% of personal best or wheezing and shortness of breath persist, the patient should repeat the beta$_2$ agonist and proceed to the nearest emergency room.

21. **c.** Remember, however, that the FEV$_1$ is the most sensitive in evaluating patients with asthma.

22. **d.** The PEF rate is a useful tool for clinician assessment and patient self-assessment of their asthma. It is also useful to monitor and change therapy and to diagnosis exacerbations. Patients should establish their personal best PEF rate. This is established after

therapy extinguishes symptoms. For 2 to 3 weeks the patient records daily his or her PEF rate in the early afternoon with the same meter. An average is obtained. The PEF rate should be recalculated every 6 months to account for growth in children or disease progression.

23. **b.** Increased bronchial markings is the most common abnormality observed on the chest x-ray in a patient with asthma.

24. **a.** Following is an overview of the clinical findings and their importance in asthma.

Physical examination signs and symptoms: (1) increased respiratory rate; (2) use of accessory muscles of respiration (intercostals, sternocleidomastoid, scalene muscles); (3) dyspnea and anxiety; (4) the most characteristic lung finding on auscultation is expiratory rhonchi (wheezes); rhonchi are high-pitched sounds that occur when air has to travel through a constricted or inflamed passageway; (5) nasal flaring; (6) cyanosis in severe cases (lips); and (7) paroxysmal cough.

Chest x-ray findings: (1) the most characteristic chest x-ray abnormality in asthma is the presence of increased bronchial wall markings. (This is most prominent when viewed from the end-on position. This finding results from the increase in the thickness of the bronchial wall and changes in the epithelium, which are associated with inflammation. These changes are translated into increased radio-opacity); (2) there is also flattening of the diaphragm in some cases as a result of chronic inflammation and use of the accessory muscles of respiration.

The most useful pulmonary function tests: (1) PEF rate (this is discussed earlier); (2) FEV$_1$/FVC in percentage (normal 80%). (This measures the amount of air volume that can be expressed in 1 second over the total amount of lung air volume that can be expressed. It is by far the most important test done in a spirometry laboratory for the diagnosis and management of asthma.); (3) MEF$_{25-75}$ in percentage (normal 75%). (This is the maximum expiratory flow that occurs between 25% and 75% of the vital capacity.)

25. **f.** All of the above.

26. **d.** The following features of cough variant asthma should be borne in mind: (1) Cough variant asthma is very common. At least 33% of children with asthma will have only the cough, no wheezing; (2) Adults, as with the patient described, also may develop cough variant asthma.

27. **e.** An acute, severe asthmatic attack is an emergency. The basic elements of treatment are as follows:

(1) give agonist via nebulizer, inhaled beta₂; (2) ensure the patient is sitting up; (3) immediately give the patient warm, humidified 100% oxygen via a Venturi mask; (4) start two intravenous lines; 5) begin an intravenous corticosteroid immediately; (6) obtain blood gases and electrolytes analyses; (7) monitor vital signs continuously (with an electrocardiogram hooked into the main computer at the nurses' desk); and (8) once the patient is stable, transfer him or her to an observation unit ward if this has been a severe attack and you have had trouble controlling it; do not discharge the patient.

28. **e.** First, there is a very significant heredity component to asthma. If one parent has it, the child may have up to a 25% risk. If two parents have it, the child's risk may be up to 50%. Second, there is a very strong association between parental smoking and asthma in children. Third, many children who have asthma are allergic to aspirin and other nonsteroidal antiinflammatory drugs.

Remember that asthma, nasal polyps, and aspirin allergy constitute a recognized triad.

Finally, patients do not "outgrow" asthma. Children who have asthma may experience less severe attacks as adults, or they may never experience problems. However, they have not outgrown it.

29. **a.** There appears to be a very strong association between respiratory syncytial virus (the main virus causing bronchiolitis) and asthma. Although it is difficult to say that the relationship is cause and effect, there is enough good evidence to suggest that it might be. More research in this area may help resolve this issue.

SOLUTION TO THE CLINICAL CASE MANAGEMENT PROBLEM

Indeed, this is a fascinating situation. The town in which the physician practices is, by the way, very small, having only 3,200 people.

An environmentalist she knew suggested the possibility of ozone production as a side effect of the lightning strikes. In fact, ozone has been shown to be associated with asthma, and it appears that this is the most probable explanation.

SUMMARY OF ASTHMA

1. All that wheezes is not asthma, and all asthma does not wheeze.
2. A moderately severe to severe attack of asthma is an emergency. Do not discharge the patient unless you are very sure that the asthma attack is resolved completely.
3. Asthma is an inflammatory disease.
4. The mortality from asthma is increasing.
5. There is effective prophylaxis for exercise-induced asthma.
6. Cough variant asthma is very common.
7. There is nothing wrong with a short course of oral steroids (prednisone 20 mg to 30 mg/day) for a severe case of asthma. It works, and it will keep the patient out of the hospital and out of danger.
8. Suggest peak flow meters to all of your patients with asthma for home monitoring.
9. Stepped care provides a rational rubric for pharmacotherapy.

SUGGESTED READING

Braunwald E., et al: Asthma and Hypersensitivity Pneumonitis. In *Harrison's Manual of Medicine,* 15 ed, 620-624, McGraw-Hill, 2002, New York.

Rakel R, Bope E: Asthma in Adolescents, Adults, and Children, In Rakel R, ed: *Conn's Current Therapy* 814-827, WB Saunders, 2003, Philadelphia.

Weinstein, N, et al: The Resident's Guide to Ambulatory Care, 2001-2002, 5th ed. *The Patient Care of Asthma,* 138-144, Anadem Press Inc, 2003, Columbus OH.

Chapter 20

Pneumonia

"You gave Mrs. Jones a shot. Why can't I have one too?"

CLINICAL CASE PROBLEM 1:
A 24-YEAR-OLD UNIVERSITY STUDENT WITH A DRY HACKING COUGH

A 24-year-old university student presents to the Student Health Service with a 3-day history of a dry hacking cough that was initially nonproductive but has become productive of scant, white sputum. The patient also complains of malaise, headache, fever, and muscle aches and pains. The patient did not have any other upper–respiratory tract symptoms before this illness began (no rhinorrhea, no sore throat, and no conjunctivitis).

The patient has had no episodes like this in the past; however, her roommate developed the same symptoms 2 days ago.

On examination, the patient has a temperature of 39° C (102.2° F). You hear a few scattered rales in the left lung base. No other abnormalities are found.

■ **SELECT THE BEST ANSWER TO THE FOLLOWING QUESTIONS:**

1. Which of the following is the most cost-effective strategy at the present time?
   a. order no laboratory tests or imaging investigations; assume that it is viral and will clear up on its own
   b. order no laboratory tests or imaging investigations; treat with ampicillin just to be on the safe side
   c. order the complete workup, every possible test; no matter what the patient has, you are not the one who is going to get sued
   d. on the basis of your clinical findings order a chest x-ray
   e. forget the tests; just treat her with "big gun therapy"

2. What is the most likely diagnosis in this patient?
   a. viral pneumonia
   b. *Mycoplasma pneumoniae* pneumonia
   c. *Streptococcus pneumoniae* pneumonia
   d. *Klebsiella pneumoniae* pneumonia
   e. no pneumonia of any kind; a case of simple acute bronchitis

3. If you ordered a chest x-ray, what would be the most likely finding?
   a. nothing: clear and normal
   b. left lower-lobe pneumonia
   c. left lower-lobe interstitial pneumonia
   d. bilateral lower-lobe infiltrates
   e. bilateral upper-lobe infiltrates

4. What is the treatment of choice for the patient described in Clinical Case Problem 1?
   a. symptomatic treatment only
   b. ribavirin for respiratory syncytial virus
   c. erythromycin
   d. ampicillin
   e. penicillin G

CLINICAL CASE PROBLEM 2:
A VERY SICK 55-YEAR-OLD FEMALE

A 55-year-old female, previously healthy and recovering from an episode of bronchitis, suddenly develops a "shaking chill" followed by the onset of a high fever—40° C (104° F); pleuritic chest pain; and cough productive of purulent, rust-colored sputum.

On examination, the patient appears ill. Her respiratory rate is 30 beats/min, and bronchial breath sounds are heard in the left lower lobe. Chest x-ray reveals consolidation present in the left lower lobe.

5. On the basis of the history, the physical examination, and the chest x-ray, what is the most likely organism responsible for this patient's illness?
   a. gram-negative bacillus
   b. gram-negative cocci
   c. gram-positive bacillus
   d. gram-positive cocci (lancet-shaped)
   e. no growth on aerobic growth media

6. What is the most likely organism responsible for this patient's illness?
   a. *Streptococcus pneumoniae*
   b. *Klebsiella pneumoniae*
   c. *Mycoplasma pneumoniae*
   d. influenza A
   e. *Haemophilus influenzae*

7. What is the treatment for the patient described in Clinical Case Problem 2?
   a. penicillin
   b. ciprofloxacin
   c. gentamicin
   d. macrolide antibiotic
   e. a and c

CLINICAL CASE PROBLEM 3:
A 35-YEAR-OLD RENAL TRANSPLANT PATIENT WITH FEVER, DYSPNEA AND TWO DAYS OF DIARRHEA

A 35-year-old male patient with chronic renal failure who had a renal transplant 6 months ago and is being treated with corticosteroids and cyclosporine came to your office 4 days ago with fever, dyspnea, and 2 days of diarrhea. The chest x-ray showed an area of consolidation in the right middle lobe and a diffuse interstitial infiltrate. He has not responded to ceftriaxone and has a continued fever and cough. Today he is lethargic and confused.

8. What is the most likely organism causing his pneumonia?
   a. *Pneumocystis carinii*
   b. *Legionella pneumoniae*
   c. *Mycobacterium tuberculosis*
   d. *Mycobacterium avium intracellulare*
   e. *Cytomegalovirus*

9. What is the drug of first choice for the patient described in Clinical Case Problem 3?
   a. macrolide
   b. cephalosporin
   c. quinolone
   d. tetracycline
   e. a and c

CLINICAL CASE PROBLEM 4:
A 75-Year-Old Alcoholic with Fever, Shortness of Breath, Chest Pain, and Cough Productive of Purulent Sputum and Blood

A 75-year-old patient with alcoholism and a history of congestive heart failure is admitted to hospital suffering from fever, shortness of breath, chest pain, and cough productive of purulent sputum and blood. On physical examination, the patient has a temperature of 39° C (102.2° F), a respiratory rate of 28 beats/min, and bronchial breath sounds in the right upper lobe.

A chest x-ray confirms the diagnosis of right upper-lobe pneumonia, with a small cavitary lesion.

10. What is the most likely organism responsible for this patient's illness?
    a. *Streptococcus pneumoniae*
    b. *Klebsiella pneumoniae*
    c. *Mycoplasma pneumoniae*
    d. influenza A
    e. *Haemophilus influenzae*

11. What is (are) the treatment(s) of choice for the patient described in Clinical Case Problem 4?
    a. erythromycin
    b. ceftriaxone plus azithromycin
    c. penicillin G
    d. ampicillin
    e. ampicillin plus gentamicin

CLINICAL CASE PROBLEM 5:
A 55-Year-Old Male Smoker with Chronic Obstructive Pulmonary Disease, High Fever, Chills, Cough, and Shortness of Breath

A 55-year-old male with a history of smoking 60 packs of cigarettes a year and documented chronic obstructive pulmonary disease (COPD) presents with a high fever, chills, a productive cough (yellowish-green sputum), and shortness of breath.

On examination, there are decreased breath sounds in the right middle lobe and right lower lobe. You suspect a pneumonia.

A chest x-ray confirms right middle-lobe and right lower-lobe pneumonia. A Gram stain reveals gram-negative rods in abundance.

12. Based on his 60 pack-a-year history of smoking, the Gram stain result, and his history of chronic bronchitis, what is the most likely organism in this patient?
    a. *Moraxella catarrhalis*
    b. *Mycoplasma pneumoniae*
    c. *Haemophilus influenzae*
    d. a or b
    e. a or c

13. What is(are) treatment(s) of choice for this patient?
    a. erythromycin
    b. cefuroxime plus azithromycin
    c. penicillin G
    d. ampicillin
    e. ampicillin plus gentamicin

14. An elderly patient in a long-term care facility develops influenza A pneumonia despite both vaccination and amantadine prophylaxis. What is the organism most likely to complicate influenza pneumonia?
    a. *Streptococcus pneumoniae*
    b. *Haemophilus influenzae*
    c. *Chlamydia trachomatis*
    d. *Chlamydia pneumoniae*
    e. *Mycoplasma pneumoniae*

15. What is the most common cause of community-acquired pneumonia?
    a. *Mycoplasma pneumoniae*
    b. *Haemophilus influenzae*
    c. *Streptococcus pneumoniae*
    d. *Staphylococcus aureus*
    e. a viral pneumonia

16. What is the most common cause of nosocomial pneumonia?
  a. *Mycoplasma pneumoniae*
  b. aerobic gram-negative bacteria
  c. *Streptococcus pneumoniae*
  d. *Haemophilus influenza*
  e. viral pneumonia

CLINICAL CASE MANAGEMENT PROBLEM

Discuss the characteristics of a sputum specimen satisfactory for Gram stain and for culture.

■ ANSWERS:

1. d. Certainly the most reasonable course of action following the history and physical examination is to perform a chest x-ray.

2. b. This patient most likely has a *Mycoplasma* pneumonia. *Mycoplasma pneumoniae* is a common respiratory-tract pathogen in young adults. The most common respiratory symptom is a dry, hacking, usually nonproductive cough. Systemic symptoms include malaise, headache, and fever. Rash, serous otitis media, and joint symptoms occasionally accompany the respiratory symptoms.

3. d. Physical findings are usually either minimal or unremarkable. Auscultation of the chest usually reveals only scattered rhonchi or fine, localized rales. The chest x-ray, however, often reveals fine or patchy lower-lobe or perihilar infiltrates. The white blood cell count (WBC) often is elevated (10,000 to 15,000/mm^3). Cold agglutinins are nonspecific and found in only 30% to 50% of cases. The diagnosis can be confirmed by acute and convalescent mycoplasma complement fixation or enzyme immunoassay titers.

Clinically and radiographically, pneumonia caused by adenovirus is often difficult to differentiate from mycoplasma pneumonia. The clinical picture does not fit that of *Streptococcus pneumoniae,* and the patient has no risk factors that should produce a *Klebsiella pneumoniae.*

Mycoplasma pneumonia is the favored diagnosis over viral pneumonia (adenovirus) because of age, the absence of other upper-respiratory tract symptoms, the prevalence of *Mycoplasma* pneumonia in students of colleges and universities, and the disparity of findings on auscultation relative to the findings on chest x-ray.

4. c. The treatment of choice is either erythromycin, or one of the newer macrolides such as azithromycin or clarithromycin, or tetracycline for a period of 10 days.

5. d. The most likely organism is a lancet-shaped gram-positive cocci, *Streptococcus pneumoniae.*

6. a. This patient has a classical history of pneumococcal pneumonia. *Streptococcus pneumoniae* (pneumococcus) is the most common cause of bacterial pneumonia in the adult population.

Pneumococcal pneumonia often presents with a "shaking rigor" (as in this patient), followed by fever, pleuritic chest pain, and cough with purulent or rust-colored sputum. Viral upper or lower respiratory–tract infections may precede pneumococcal pneumonia.

In patients who are elderly or debilitated, the presentation may be atypical. Fever may be low grade, behavior disturbances may seem more significant than respiratory symptoms, and cough may not be prominent. Patients appear acutely ill, frequently with dyspnea, with minimal execution and chest splinting. Signs of consolidation frequently are present.

An elevated WBC count with left shift is common. Chest x-ray usually shows disease confined to one lobe (frequently a lower lobe), but several lobes may be involved with either consolidation or bronchopneumonia. Gram stain of the sputum shows polymorphonuclear leukocytes and lancet-shaped gram-positive diplococci.

Sputum cultures should be obtained, but up to 40% of patients with bacteremic pneumococcal pneumonia will have negative sputum cultures. Therefore blood cultures should be obtained in these patients.

7. d. Empiric treatment for streptococcal pneumonia would include macrolides such as azithromycin (Zithromax), clarithromycin (Biaxin), or a tetracycline for patients with no cardiopulmonary disease or modifying factors. It should be noted, however, that erythromycin, if used, has a little coverage for *H. influenza*. For patients with drug-resistant *Streptococcus pneumoniae* or gram-negatives, a beta-lactam-macrolide combination or a quinolone as monotherapy should be used (gatifloxin [Tequinol], levofloxacin [Levaquin] or moxifloxacin [Avelor]). Because it is impossible to exclude *Legionella* given these clinical findings, a macrolide should be added to the cephalosporin, or the quinolone could be used alone. With the patient's clinical picture including a respiratory rate of 30 beats/min and chest splinting, hospitalization with intravenous therapy is indicated.

8. b. The combination of pneumonia plus failure to respond to standard antibiotics such as ceftriaxone in an immunocompromised host points to the diagnosis of legionella.

9. a. Newer macrolides and quinolones are considered the agents of choice. It should be noted that many studies have indicated that erythromycin has weak antilegionella activity. Therefore if erythromycin is selected for therapy, rifampin also should be added. From the macrolide class, azithromycin is the most active against legionella, and the best bactericidal activity for legionella are the quinolones. In severe cases, intravenous medication should be used. A response usually is seen in 3-5 days.

10. b. Although the most likely cause of pneumonia in a person who is elderly and debilitated remains *Streptococcus pneumoniae*, the gram-negative organism *Klebsiella pneumoniae* is commonly found in alcoholics; it frequently is seen in nosocomial pneumonias. The chest x-ray results described point to this latter organism.

Although the presentation in *Klebsiella* pneumonia may be similar to pneumococcal pneumonia, the upper lobes are involved more frequently than the lower lobes. Sudden onset is common. Pleuritic chest pain and hemoptysis are common features. Sputum is thick and often bloody. Because this is a necrotizing pneumonia, cavitary lesions may be found, which do not occur with *Streptococcus pneumoniae*. Other important causes of pneumonia in elderly patients include other gram-negative organisms such

as *Escherichia coli, H. influenza,* and gram-positive organisms such as *Streptococcus pneumoniae* and *Staphylococcus aureus.*

11. b. The treatment of first choice for this patient is the cephalosporin cefuroxime (or ceftriaxone) plus azithromycin. This drug combination is effective against all the pathogens listed. An alternative is to use one of the newer quinolones (such as levofloxacin) alone.

12. e. In a patient with a pneumonia complicating chronic bronchitis, likely organisms include *Haemophilus influenzae* and *Moraxella catarrhalis.*

13. b. The treatment of choice is the same as for the patient in Clinical Case Problem 4: a cephalosporin (such as cefuroxime or ceftriaxone) plus a macrolide (such as azithromycin [Zithromax] or clarithromycin [Biaxin]).

14. a. The most likely organism to complicate influenza pneumonia is *Streptococcus pneumoniae.*

15. c. The most common cause of community-acquired pneumonia is *Streptococcus pneumoniae.*

16. b. The most common cause of nosocomial pneumonia is aerobic gram-negative bacteria, although recent studies have shown that *Staphylococcus aureus* now occurs with almost equal frequency.

SOLUTION TO THE CLINICAL CASE MANAGEMENT PROBLEM

Sputum cytology is essential to make an accurate diagnosis of pneumonia. Saliva or nasopharyngeal secretions are of little value in determining the etiology of pneumonia because colonization with gram-negative bacilli and other organisms is frequent.

If more than 25 squamous epithelial cells are seen in a low power magnification (LPM) field, the specimen is considered inadequate for culture. The ideal sputum specimen contains fewer than 10 squamous epithelial cells per LPM and many polymorphonuclear leukocytes.

SUMMARY OF PNEUMONIA

1. Community-acquired pneumonia:

The most common cause in all age groups is *Streptococcus pneumoniae*. Another common cause is *Chlamydia pneumoniae*, which causes around 15% of all pneumonias. Certain risk factors (age, underlying illness) can suggest other possible causes.

2. Young adults:

Mycoplasma pneumoniae is a common causative agent, and mycoplasma pneumonia is common among young adults. Mycoplasma pneumonia often can be differentiated from other pneumonias by the signs/symptoms as elicited on history and physical examination and the findings on chest x-ray. Diagnostic clues to mycoplasma pneumoniae are a harsh, nonproductive, constant cough with little evidence of the shaking chills and high fever seen in streptococcal pneumonia. The major differential diagnosis is adenoviral pneumonia.

3. **Middle-aged adults with COPD:**
Haemophilus influenzae: Haemophilus influenzae pneumonia is a common pneumonia complicating COPD. Another common cause is *Moraxella catarrhalis*, which is seen primarily in patients with underlying cardiopulmonary disease.

4. **Immunocompromised individuals or individuals with COPD who fail to respond to conventional therapy:**
Suspect *Legionella* pneumonia. The signs and symptoms of *Legionella* pneumonia include malaise, headache, myalgia, weakness, and fever. Following these symptoms, there are intermittent rigors within 24 hours. In addition there is a nonproductive or minimally productive cough, and scant hemoptysis and pleuritic chest pain are common.

5. **Elderly patients with immune compromise secondary to alcohol:**
Suspect *Klebsiella pneumoniae*. Klebsiella pneumonia has much the same signs and symptoms as other bacterial pneumonias (see the following section).

6. **Bacterial versus viral pneumonia:**
   a. Bacterial pneumonia: fever, chills (sudden onset of shaking chills in pneumococcal pneumonia), pleuritic chest pain, productive cough, purulent sputum, tachycardia, tachypnea, bronchial breath sounds.
   b. Viral pneumonia: gradual onset, general malaise, headache, prominent cough (often nonproductive), sometimes few abnormalities on examination of the lung (auscultation). The chest x-ray findings are more prominent.
   c. Mycoplasma pneumonia: as in viral pneumonia, except cough can be almost constant, harsh, nonproductive, and irritative.

7. **Treatment:**
   a. For patients with community-acquired pneumonia who do not require hospital admission, the treatment of choice is either a macrolide (erythromycin, azithromycin, or clarithromycin) or one of the quinolones (such as levofloxacin).
   b. For patients who require hospital admission, the treatment of choice is either a cephalosporin (such as cefuroxime or ceftriaxone) plus a macrolide (erythromycin or azithromycin) or one of the quinolones (levofloxacin) alone.

8. **Prevention:**
   a. Pneumococcal vaccine: all patients at high risk.
   b. Influenza vaccine (annually): all patients and health care workers at high risk.

SUGGESTED READING

Braunwald E, et al: Pneumonia, In *Harrison's Manual of Medicine*, 15th ed. 434-436, McGraw-Hill, 2002, New York.
Rakel R, Bope E: Asthma in Adolescents, Adults, and Children, In Rakel R, ed. *Conn's Current Therapy* 814-827, Elsevier, 2003, Philadelphia.

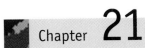
Chapter **21**

Esophageal Disorders

"Doctor, it is my heart, isn't it?"

CLINICAL CASE PROBLEM 1:
A 33-Year-Old Male with Substernal and Retrosternal Pain and Hypertension

A 33-year-old overweight male comes to the emergency room in an agitated state complaining of substernal and retrosternal pain radiating to his neck, accompanied by a congested feeling in his chest. He states that this pain started on arising that morning and he is convinced he is having a heart attack.

On physical examination, his blood pressure is 210/95 mm Hg and his pulse is 106 beats per minute (BPM) and regular. His heart sounds and electrocardiogram (ECG) pattern are normal. His lungs are clear. His abdomen is soft; no masses and no tenderness are felt. He was given nitroglycerine tablets, and his blood pressure quickly decreased.

As his blood pressure subsided and after he was told his ECG pattern was normal, he calmed down and remembered a history of intermittent upper-abdominal chest pain that was quickly relieved with antacids. A burning sensation was not predominant, but he said that on some occasions it left a feeling of pins and needles in the throat. These pains had no relationship to exercise or exertion but were exacerbated by eating and relieved by antacids. Furthermore he states he had been agitated and slept poorly the previous night because he had had been informed the day before that he will be laid off from work at the end of the month. In an attempt to console himself, before going to bed the previous night he polished off a pound of chocolates washed down with a bottle of red wine. He also smoked a pack of cigarettes in a few hours rather that at his usual rate of a pack a day.

SELECT THE BEST ANSWER TO THE FOLLOWING QUESTIONS:

1. Which of the following must be considered in the differential diagnosis of this patient's problem?
   a. acid reflux disease
   b. myocardial ischemia
   c. peptic ulcer disease
   d. panic disorder
   e. a and d only
   f. all of the above

2. Given the history and physical examination, which of the following conditions is (are) most likely responsible for the symptoms noted?
   a. acid reflux disease
   b. myocardial ischemia
   c. peptic ulcer disease
   d. panic disorder
   e. a and d

3. What is the major pathophysiologic mechanism underlying the chronic symptoms described in Clinical Case Problem 1?
   a. transient relaxation of the lower esophageal sphincter (LES)
   b. decreased resting pressure of the LES
   c. achalasia
   d. excess production of hydrogen ions (H^+) in the stomach
   e. esophageal spasm

4. Which of the following is the least acceptable treatment for gastroesophageal reflux disease (GERD)?
   a. antacids and over-the-counter histamine 2 (H_2) antagonists
   b. certain lifestyle changes
   c. prescription-strength H_2 antagonists
   d. prokinetic agents
   e. proton pump inhibitors (PPIs)

5. Which of the following is not associated with severe chronic GERD?
   a. difficulty in swallowing
   b. esophageal cancer
   c. Barrett's esophagus
   d. esophageal varices
   e. esophagitis

CLINICAL CASE PROBLEM 2:

A 68-YEAR OLD MALE WHO FINDS SWALLOWING DIFFICULT

A 68-year-old male comes to your office with a complaint about an apparent lump in his throat and difficulty swallowing. He finds that solid foods and pills tend to stick in his throat, sometimes causing him to choke. He also has some trouble swallowing liquids. He has smoked a pack or two of cigarettes since he was age 14 and admits to having a few shots of whiskey on almost a daily basis.

Vital signs are normal. No abnormalities are discerned on physical examination.

6. Which of the following is the least likely cause of his dysphagia?
   a. achalasia
   b. diffuse esophageal spasm
   c. a lower esophageal ring (Schatzki ring)
   d. pharyngeal paralysis
   e. an esophageal stricture

7. Which of the following is (are) not true concerning malignant dysphagia?
   a. a risk factor for squamous cell cancer is Barrett's esophagus
   b. most esophageal cancers occur in the more distal parts of the esophagus
   c. malignant dysphagia usually can be distinguished from other dysphagias by the rapid progression of symptoms
   d. as a result of more sophisticated modes of diagnosis and treatment developed within the past 5 years, the overall 5-year survival rate is presently 50%
   e. a and d are false statements
   f. b and c are false statements

ANSWERS:

1. **f.** All choices should be considered.

2. **e.** It is most important to rule out myocardial ischemia with further testing, including blood analysis of cardiac enzymes and/or troponins and, perhaps, hospitalization and an exercise stress test. However, the most likely cause of the symptoms described is GERD complicated by anxiety brought about by job-related stress coupled with his fresh chest pain. When he awoke, his underlying anxiety was increased because of chest pain. This increased his blood pressure, inducing a feeling of heaviness in his chest, further raising his anxiety level to that of panic, which in turn further increased his blood pressure. The nitroglycerin helped break this vicious cycle, allowing him to calm down, to think more rationally, and to remember past symptoms (which included a history of probable GERD). Although a final diagnosis cannot be made on the basis of the described symptoms alone, the absence of abnormal cardiac examination findings and the normal ECG point away from heart problems. Moreover a number of factors point toward

GERD being an underlying cause: (1) the relatively high prevalence of GERD in the population (in one study, 25% to 40% of adults were found to be affected at least monthly and 7% to 10% daily), (2) his history of acid reflux symptoms relieved by antacids, and (3) his indulgence in "comfort eating" of GERD-inducing foods the previous night. In addition, the stress of being laid off and a night of poor sleep made conditions ripe for onset of his symptoms.

Although GERD usually manifests itself as heartburn, a sizable minority report chest pain with minimal or no burning sensation, making diagnosis more difficult. Others report hoarseness or even shortness of breath as the presenting symptom. Peptic ulcer can produce aching discomfort in the upper abdomen or lower chest and thus must be included in the differential. However, it rarely is described as retrosternal pain radiating to the neck; moreover, eating generally relieves, not worsens, symptoms.

3. **a.** The most common cause of acid reflux is a transient relaxation of the LES. However, permanent relaxation and increased abdominal pressure that overcomes the LES also may be causative factors. Transient relaxation may be caused by foods (chocolates, coffee, and other sources of caffeine; alcohol; fatty meals; peppermint or spearmint) or by drugs (beta blockers, nitrates, calcium, channel blockers, anticholinergics) and by smoking (nicotine).

In addition to relaxation of the LES, other potential precipitants are poor esophageal motility and delayed gastric emptying. Hiatal hernias also are found in high frequency in patients with symptoms of GERD.

Achalasia is characterized by dysphagia, not by acid regurgitation. Whereas excess gastric acid may exacerbate symptoms, GERD can occur with normal acid secretion. Esophageal spasm can cause acid reflux, but it is a relatively rare condition, not a major mechanism.

Although some of the symptoms described were the result of anxiety, it was described as an acute attack, not a chronic condition.

4. **d.** The prokinetic motility agents metoclopramide (Reglan) and cisapride (Propulsid) were once marketed as the drugs of choice to prevent GERD relapse. However, in July 2000 Jansen voluntarily withdrew cisapride from the market because of concern about possible adverse side reactions, and in March 2003 the U.S. Food and Drug Administration required metoclopramide to carry warnings concerning neuroleptic malignant syndrome as a possible adverse reaction and suggested limiting its use. Antacids and/or over-the-counter H_2 antagonists coupled with certain lifestyle changes is the most conservative treatment and is recommended as an initial line of treatment by the American College of Gastroenterology. Life-style changes include the following: (1) lose weight, if obese; (2) avoid lying down after meals; (3) avoid late night meals or midnight snacks; (4) elevate the head of the bed by about 6 inches; (5) avoid wearing tight-fitting clothes; (6) avoid dietary irritants such as fat, chocolate, caffeine, spearmint or peppermint, and alcohol; (7) avoid drugs that reduce the LES pressure, such as calcium channel blockers, beta blockers, and theophylline; (8) discontinue tobacco use; (9) avoid use of antiinflammatory drugs; and (10) eat slowly and chew thoroughly. These lifestyle changes treat the reflux component of acid reflux disease.

Should symptoms persist despite lifestyle changes, an H_2 receptor antagonist or a PPI can be added to increase the pH of the material being regurgitated. The H_2 receptor antagonist medications available include cimetidine (Tagamet), ranitidine (Zantac), nizatidine (Axid), and famotidine (Pepcid). The PPIs are omeprazole (Prilosec), lansoprazole (Prevacid), rabeprazole (Aciphex), esomeprazole (Nexium), and pantoprazole (Protonix). Although the PPIs are more effective and need only be taken once a day, the H_2 receptor antagonists cost less although they need be taken twice a day. Although these drugs effectively reduce symptoms, they do so by reducing the gastric acidity, which may in the long run lead to other problems such as reducing the ability to absorb vitamin B_{12} and/or reducing protection against ingested pathogens. Also, PPIs interfere with the bioavailability of many other drugs dependent on low gastric pH for absorption, such as digoxin and ketoconazole.

As in the case described, anxiety can provoke addition symptoms and can exacerbate the gastric reflux systems. Supportive counseling and possibly the temporary addition of an anxiolytic also can be considered.

Patients should be evaluated every 8 to 12 weeks, and if symptoms are alleviated the dosage of the drug used may be decreased with the aim of titrating to the lowest possible dose and, ideally, eventual discontinuation. Should a relapse occur treatment can be started again.

If patients do not have an adequate response to therapy, or for patients age 50 years old and older, endoscopy should be considered because of the higher incidence of gastric malignancies and peptic ulcer disease.

5. **d.** Esophageal varices are a byproduct of portal hypertension, not esophageal reflux disease.

The potential pathologic sequence of events associated with chronic GERD is as follows: (1) the acid irritates the esophageal lining causing inflammation and esophagitis; (2) the esophagitis can lead to ulcer and stricture formation causing difficulty in swallowing; (3) chronic inflammation also may induce metaplasia and transformation of the cells lining the esophageal lumen causing Barrett's esophagus; and (4) Barrett's esophageal cells can transform into malignant cells. Only about 5% of people with GERD develop Barrett's esophagus, but once diagnosed there is at least a 30-fold greater chance of developing a malignancy.

6. d. All listed choices are potential causes of dysphagia. An additional cause for consideration in this case is malignant dysphasia. Although not listed in this question, it is critical to always first rule out malignancy as a potential cause of even mild dysphagia because failure to diagnose and start treatment of esophageal cancer in a timely manner is almost a certain death sentence. Moreover the patient described in Clinical Case Problem 2 has several risk factors for esophageal cancer, including his age, sex, and smoking and drinking habits. (See Answer 7 for further discussion.)

However, among the five conditions listed, pharyngeal paralysis is the least likely cause of dysphagia in the case described. This condition is produced by weakness and incoordination of the muscles in the pharynx that propel food into the esophageus. Both liquids and solids are difficult to swallow and aspiration into the windpipe and regurgitation into the nose commonly occurs. It is a result of faulty transmission of nerve impulses to the pharyngeal muscles generally caused by an associated neuromuscular disease such as myasthenia gravis, amyotrophic lateral sclerosis, or stroke. No such neurologic condition was described.

Achalasia, meaning failure to relax, is a rare disorder with an incidence in the United States of about 1 per 100,000. It is caused by incoordination of the esophageal peristaltic muscles and the failure of the LES to relax because of a lack of inhibitory input from nonadrenergic, noncholinergic, ganglionic cells. As a consequence food cannot pass into the stomach. The cause is not known and swallowing liquids and solids are affected. The most effective treatment is endoscopic dilation, including injection of botulism toxin into the LES to block acetylcholine release, with the aim of restoring the balance between excitatory and inhibitory stimulation. A less effective but less abrasive treatment worth trying as the first line of treatment, particularly for elderly or other more fragile patients, are medications that relax the LES. Calcium channel blockers or nitrates are the drugs of choice. However, such treatment is successful in only some 10% of the cases. If all else fails the patient can be advised to hold his or her arms straight up in the air. This has been alleged to facilitate swallowing.

Diffuse esophageal spasm is characterized by multiple high-pressure, poorly coordinated esophageal contractions that usually occur after a swallow. The cause is unknown and symptoms mimic GERD, but if the cause is spasm the symptoms will continue intermittently over a period of years and may become progressively worse. Esophageal dilation may provide relief. If not, surgery might be necessary.

A Schatzki ring is a diaphragm-like mucosal ring that forms at the esophagogastric junction (the B ring). If the lumen of this ring gets too small symptoms occur. The cause is not clear, but such rings usually are found in older individuals and have been observed in 6% to 15% of patients undergoing a barium swallow; however, only 0.5% of those being examined have significant symptoms. Symptoms correlate with the size of the lumen of the ring: a lumen greater than 20 mm in diameter provides few if any symptoms, if less than 13 mm in diameter chronic and more severe symptoms occur. Most patients have an intermittent, nonprogressive dysphagia for solid foods that occurs while consuming a heavy meal with meat that was "wolfed down"—hence the pseudonym the "steakhouse syndrome." Sometimes the meal is regurgitated, relieving the block, and eating can be resumed. Patients with a Schatzki ring are also at risk for GERD. A diagnosis is confirmed by radiographic barium swallow or endoscopic means, and if symptoms are sufficiently troublesome, the treatment of choice is rupture of the ring by dilatation.

An esophageal stricture is a narrowing of the lumen of the esophagus preventing the passage of foods. Most typically it is at the distal end of the tube and is the result of scarring after chronic exposure to gastric juice resulting from GERD. Scarring and consequently stricture formation also can occur in response to other types of trauma, including swallowing caustic solutions, chronic swallowing of pills without water, or residual scarring after surgery. Usual treatment is dilation.

7. e. Prior to 1970 in the United States, and still in many parts of the world, squamous cell carcinoma accounted for 90% to 95% of the cases of esophageal cancer. However, since that time the relative incidence of adenocarcinoma has increased markedly in the United States, and by the early 1990s they accounted for about 50% of all cases. Currently the proportion of adenocarcinomas is probably even higher.

In the United States the incidence of all types of esophageal cancer is 3-6 cases per 100,000; it is more prevalent in males (male:female ratio = 7:1) and more prevalent in African American males than in white males. It generally is diagnosed in the sixth or seventh decade.

Nonkeratinizing stratified epithelial squamous cells line the esophagus. Irritations of these cells and/or exposure to carcinogens cause a malignant transformation inducing a squamous cell carcinoma. Tobacco use and excess alcohol consumption account for most squamous cell cases and are the major modifiable risk factors in the United States. Other potential factors include nitrosamines and other nitrosyl compounds, commonly found in smoked or pickled foods. In some environments there are nitrosyl compounds in the water, and certain mineral deficiencies lead to the accumulation of these compounds in certain food plants. Both events have been suggested to cause squamous cell carcinoma. It also has been reported that chronic ingestion of very hot liquids, very spicy foods, or other irritants promote squamous cell tumors. Longstanding cases of achalasia or strictures, radiation, and a host of other relatively uncommon factors also have been reported to induce squamous cell carcinomas, but squamous cell cancer does not arise from Barrett's esophagus. A diet rich in fruits and vegetable seems to protect against this malignancy.

In contrast to the multiple causes of the squamous cell malignancies, adenocarcinomas arise from a well-characterized sequence. In response to chronic exposure to acid reflux, the normal stratified epithelium first becomes inflamed, then metaplasia occurs, and these columnar epithelia cells are transformed into a specialized glandular epithelium called Barrett's epithelium. The Barrett epithelial cells then can undergo a progressive dysplasia, from low to high grade and ultimately to adenocarcinoma. Most adenocarcinomas occur in the more distal parts of the esophagus because this area is more likely to be exposed to regurgitated acid.

Because very early symptoms are only a very mild dysphagia, early cancers tend to be ignored. Unfortunately both squamous cell and adenocarcinomas are very aggressive, and by the time the tumors have grown large enough to obscure the lumen and produce severe symptoms, they also are likely to have grown through the esophageal wall and have invaded other tissues. The fact that the esophageal wall is thin, composed of only two tissue layers, facilitates this escape. Because of this tendency to overlook early symptoms, a great many patients have a stage IV cancer at the time of diagnosis with a 5-year survival rate of only 5%; the overall 5-year survival rate at all stages is 20% to 25% and is the same for both squamous cell and adenocarcinoma.

SUMMARY OF ESOPHAGEAL DISORDERS

A. Acid reflux disease (GERD):

The most common cause is a transient relaxation of the lower esophageal sphincter, the LES.

Permanent LES relaxation, increased abdominal pressure, and strictures are less common causes. Diagnosis usually can be made by a detailed history, confirmed if desired by a therapeutic challenge with an antacid (if symptoms immediately improve, the diagnosis is probable). In addition the diagnoses can be further tested and more importantly Barrett's esophagus or adenocarcinoma can be ruled in or out by barium swallow or endoscopy.

The first line of treatment should be lifestyle changes (see Answer 4) supplemented with over-the-counter antacids. Over-the-counter calcium carbonate antacids generally are effective and inexpensive and also increase the daily intake of calcium. If acid reflux continues, either an H_2 blocker or a PPI should be prescribed. There is no absolute agreement as to which; PPIs are more effective, but H_2 blockers are less expensive.

Potential long-term consequences include esophagitis, strictures, Barrett's esophagitis, and adenocarcinoma.

B. Dysphagia

1. Archetypal esophageal based causes include:
   a. *Achalasia* is characterized by the loss of peristalsis and constriction of the lower esophageal sphincter. Achalasia is diagnosed by esophageal manometry (to measure intraluminal pressure, pH, and transit time) and pneumatic dilatation of the esophagus. It is treated by endoscopic dilation with injection of botulism toxin or by LES relaxants (calcium channel blockers or nitrates).
   b. *Esophageal spasm* is characterized by an increased percentage of uncoordinated peristolic waves with some preserved peristalsis. It is diagnosed by esophageal manometry and treated with bougienage or calcium channel blockers or nitrates. Anxiolytics also may be prescribed to reduce anxiety induced by the spasms.
   c. *Esophageal stricture* is a narrowing in one or more parts of the esophagus, most often caused by chronic gastric reflux; very serious cases, however, are caused by ingestion of toxic liquids or solids. The latter most commonly occurs in children, and all family physicians have an obligation to inform parents about the danger of having easy access to corrosive substances. It is diagnosed by history and confirmed by barium swallow or endoscopy. The treatment of choice is progressive dilatation.

Continued

SUMMARY OF ESOPHAGEAL DISORDERS—cont'd

d. *Esophageal ring (Schatzki ring)* is a narrowing of the diameter of the esophageal lumen at the point of the ring, which is generally at the level of the LES. The degree of blockage is correlated with the diameter of the retained opening. As a rule symptoms are intermittent and are associated with swallowing solid foods without chewing them sufficiently; the larger chunks tend to get caught in the narrowed passageway. The diagnosis can be confirmed by barium swallow or endoscopy. The first line of treatment is behavioral modification—learning to eat more slowly. If symptoms are severe and/or occur often, treatment is dilatation and fracture of the ring.

e. *Acute foreign body obstruction* is a commonly experienced phenomenon—"food is felt to be going down the wrong pipe." Usually the offending particle is coughed up. However, on occasion a particle remains lodged. If this occurs high in the esophagus or in the lower pharynx, it may block the air passage, resulting in an inability to breathe or talk. The affected individual will turn blue and pass out within a matter of minutes; the "Heimlich maneuver" is a practical and effective way to dislodge the offending object quickly. More often the foreign body is lodged more deeply in the esophagus where it can best be removed by a fiberoptic endoscope. Small children are prone to put all sorts of foreign objects into their mouths. If one of these is swallowed, it too may become stuck in the esophagus. Although the basic principles remain the same, the swallowed object is more likely to be a hard, often sharp, object with the potential of perforating the esophagus or other parts of the gastrointestinal track.

f. Almost all *esophageal malignancies* are either squamous cell or adenocarcinomas. Adenocarcinoma of the esophagus occurs as a secondary response to Barrett's esophagus and recently has become the most common esophageal cancer in the United States. Squamous cell carcinoma was the most common form in the United States and still is in many parts of the world. It arises in response to many carcinogenic factors, the most modifiable ones being smoking and excess alcohol consumption. Diagnosis of either type is confirmed by endoscopy with biopsy. Unfortunately this is rarely done until dysphagia has become marked and weight loss has started; by that time prognosis has become poor. Endoscopy cannot be conducted on every patient with heartburn, but ongoing research is trying to develop newer diagnostic methods able to screen for early esophageal cancer in a practical way. However, treatment modalities have become more aggressive in recent years. Surgical resection is the procedure of choice supported by chemotherapy and radiotherapy.

Although the 5-year survival rate is still miserable, it actually has improved significantly over the past two decades.

2. Miscellaneous causes of dysphagia:

a. *Systemic sclerosis* is characterized by progressive muscle atrophy and fibrosis, leading to loss of peristalsis and reduction of sphincter pressure. This may lead to substantial GERD and its complications. Treatment is similar to that for GERD.

b. *Candidal esophagitis* associated with the acquired immune deficiency syndrome

c. *AIDS*

d. *Herpes simplex esophagitis*

e. *Cerebrovascular accidents and neurologic disorders* such as acute lateral sclerosis

f. *Pharyngeal paralysis and pharyngeal diverticula:* Although these are not esophageal problems, they should be considered in a differential diagnosis of dysphagia.

SUGGESTED READING

Blot WJ, McLauglin JK: The changing epidemiology of esophageal cancer. *Semin Oncol* 26 (5 suppl 15):2-8, 1999.

Heath EI, et al: Adenoma of the esophagus, risk factors and prevention. *Oncology* 4:507-514 and 518-520, 2000.

Kirby TJ, Rice TW: The epidemiology of esophageal cancer. The changing face of a disease. *Chest Surg Clin N Am* 4(2):217-225, 1994.

Lagergren J, et al: Symptomatic gastropharyngeal reflux as a risk factor for esophageal adenocarcinoma. *N Engl J Med* 340(11):825-831, 1999.

Scott M, Gelhot AR: Gastroesophageal reflux disease: diagnosis and management. *Am Fam Phys* 59:1170-1177, 1999.

Spechler SJ: American gastroenterological association medical position statement on the treatment of patients with dysphagia caused by benign disorders of the distal esophagus. *Gastroenterology* 117(1):229-233, 1999.

Patti MG, Way LW: Evaluation and treatment of primary esophageal motility disorders. *West J Med* 166(4):263-269, 1997.

Wilde SM, et al: Rapid food intake induces gastroesophageal reflux. Your mother was right. *Gastroenterology* 124:A72, 2003.

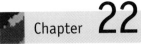

Chapter 22

Peptic Ulcer Disease

> "You don't really mean I have bacteria eating holes in my intestines, do you?"

CLINICAL CASE PROBLEM 1:

A 41-YEAR-OLD MALE WITH EPIGASTRIC PAIN

A 41-year-old male with a 4-month history of epigastric pain comes to your office. The pain is described as dull and achy and is intermittent. There is no radiation of the pain. Exacerbating factors include coffee intake. Infrequently, he is awakened at night from the pain. Temporary alleviating factors include eating a meal or drinking some milk. The baseline intensity of the pain is about a 6/10, but it can fluctuate in intensity to an 8/10. The pain has not changed since it began 4 months ago. No weight loss, vomiting, melena, or hematochezia have been noted, but nausea does occur at times. The patient denies any dramatic increase in his usually stressful career, and he describes his position as a "high-powered executive." He admits that he is a "workaholic." He has no prior history of chronic abdominal pain, and he takes no medications including any over-the-counter medicines.

On examination, the patient has some epigastric tenderness with no rebound or guarding. The remainder of the examination is unremarkable.

SELECT THE BEST ANSWER TO THE FOLLOWING QUESTIONS:

1. What is the most likely diagnosis in this patient?
   a. gastric carcinoma
   b. gastric ulcer
   c. duodenal ulcer
   d. cholecystitis/cholelithiasis
   e. irritable bowel syndrome

2. Which of the following statements regarding the patient described is (are) false?
   a. if you are going to investigate this patient, an upper endoscopy with antral biopsy for *Helicobacter pylori* are the diagnostic procedures of choice
   b. cigarette smoking may aggravate the condition
   c. drinking alcohol aggravates the condition
   d. this patient should be treated with a bland diet
   e. this condition may be aggravated by the ingestion of certain medications

3. The patient described is prescribed a combination of bismuth, metronidazole, and amoxicillin for his condition. His symptoms improve rapidly, and he is essentially pain free in 2 weeks. Which of the following statements is (are) true about this treatment?
   a. amoxicillin was prescribed because of a high probability of sepsis in his condition
   b. amoxicillin and metronidazole were prescribed because of the association between this condition and *H. pylori*
   c. the addition of omeprazole to the regimen of bismuth, metronidazole, and amoxicillin increases the cure rate of *H. pylori*-induced peptic ulcer disease (PUD)
   d. b and c
   e. a and c

4. Which of the following drugs has not been approved as an effective agent against *Helicobacter pylori*?
   a. bismuth subsalicylate
   b. metronidazole
   c. amoxicillin
   d. tetracycline
   e. azithromycin

5. What is the mode of action of omeprazole?
   a. an H_1 receptor antagonist
   b. an H_2 receptor antagonist
   c. a proton pump inhibitor (PPI)
   d. a cytoprotective agent
   e. an anticholinergic agent

6. The condition described should respond to treatment with complete healing within a maximum of how many weeks?
   a. 1-2
   b. 3-6
   c. 8-12
   d. 16-20
   e. 26-52

7. Which of the following drugs is classified as a cytoprotective agent?
   a. metoclopramide
   b. misoprostol
   c. bismuth subsalicylate
   d. ondansetron
   e. nizatidine

8. Which of the following statements regarding the role of drugs in the condition described is false?
   a. Cyclooxygenase type II (COX II) inhibitors do not cause this condition
   b. the use of dexamethasone is a risk factor for this condition

c. aspirin may precipitate this condition

d. some nonsteroid antiinflammatory drugs (NSAIDs) seem more likely than others to precipitate this condition

e. the incidence of this condition in patients taking indomethacin or other NSAIDs is increased

9. Which of the following statements regarding *H. pylori* is true?
   a. acute infection is self-limited and will resolve without antibiotics
   b. organisms are found in human feces but not saliva
   c. income and socioeconomic factors do not influence prevalence
   d. approximately 25% of adults are colonized by the age of 50 years
   e. prevalence of infection is higher in Hispanics and African Americans

10. Which of the following statements regarding the diagnosis and treatment of gastric ulcers is false?
    a. the pain of gastric ulcers, in contrast with duodenal ulcers, sometimes is aggravated rather than relieved by food
    b. gastric ulcers do not present with bleeding or perforation as the initial presentation
    c. endoscopy should follow the identification of a gastric ulcer on a gastrointestinal (GI) series
    d. the healing rate and the time to heal for gastric ulcers is generally longer than for duodenal ulcers
    e. anorexia, nausea, and vomiting are more common in patients with gastric ulcer than duodenal ulcer

11. Advantages of PPIs over H$_2$ blockers include all of the following except:
    a. superior acid suppression
    b. faster healing rates
    c. safe for use in hepatically impaired patients
    d. faster symptom relief
    e. lower and less frequent dosing requirement

12. Endoscopy is indicated for all of the following except:
    a. a 50-year-old male with new dyspepsia and weight loss
    b. a 35-year-old female with epigastric pain worse with eating and associated with anorexia and early satiety
    c. a 40-year-old female with a duodenal ulcer seen on upper GI (UGI) series

d. a 45-year-old male with *H. pylori* PUD with persistent symptoms after 3 weeks of acid suppression therapy

e. a 47-year-old male with a history of PUD with recurrence of symptoms soon after completion of treatment

13. *H. pylori* testing is indicated for all of the following except:
    a. patient with a history of PUD not previously treated with eradication therapy who develops dyspepsia
    b. a patient with nonulcer dyspepsia confirmed by endoscopy
    c. a patient with chronic gastroesophageal reflux disease (GERD)
    d. a and b
    e. b and c

14. Which of the following types of *H. pylori* testing is not useful for confirming eradication?
    a. stool antigen test
    b. urea breath test
    c. ELISA (enzyme-linked immunosorbent assay) serology
    d. culture
    e. Steiner's stain of gastric biopsy specimen

15. In the United States the most common cause of the condition described here is:
    a. drinking alcohol
    b. aspirin use
    c. Zollinger-Ellison syndrome
    d. *H. pylori*
    e. idiopathic

CLINICAL CASE MANAGEMENT PROBLEM

Discuss the pathophysiology of nonsteroidal antiinflammatory drugs (NSAID) and *H. pylori*-induced peptic ulcers.

ANSWERS:

1. **c.** This patient has a duodenal ulcer. Duodenal ulcer pain is characterized by a deep, aching, recurrent pain located in the mid-epigastrium. It often is relieved by food or antacid intake and is aggravated by aspirin, coffee, or other irritants. Nocturnal pain is common and may awaken the patient at night.

Anorexia, weight loss, and vomiting are infrequently associated symptoms of duodenal ulcer. The occurrence of these symptoms should lead one to suspect a gastric ulcer, which may be worse with food intake and is a risk for developing gastric carcinoma.

2. **d.** The diagnostic procedures of choice in this patient are an upper endoscopy with an antral biopsy for *H. pylori*. It is reasonable and safe, however, to treat patients with typical duodenal ulcer symptoms with no alarm signs for 6-8 weeks before investigating with endoscopy. Patients should be tested for *H. pylori* and treated if positive. Alarm signs include age older than 45 years, rectal bleeding or melena, weight loss, anorexia/early satiety, anemia, dysphagia, jaundice, family history of gastric cancer, and previous history of gastric cancer or complicated ulcer disease. If the symptoms improve with acid suppression and *H. pylori* eradication treatment, then no investigation is needed. If they do not, investigation with endoscopy should proceed.

Cigarette smoking has been shown to aggravate PUD and delay healing of peptic ulcers. Patients who smoke also have an increased probability of recurrence.

Aspirin and other NSAIDs may aggravate or produce a peptic ulcer. Alcohol is a strong stimulant of acid secretion.

Bland diets or other special diets should not be prescribed; they actually may increase acid production.

3. **d.** Initial studies identified *H. pylori* in 95% of duodenal ulcers and 80% of gastric ulcers, but more recent studies have shown the prevalence of *H. pylori* to be decreasing to 60% to 75% as a result of eradication treatment. After standard acid-blocking therapies, 75% of patients will have an endoscopically documented recurrence within 1 year. With the successful eradication of *H. pylori,* the recurrence rate is less than 10% within a year. The addition of omeprazole to the regimen of metronidazole, bismuth, and amoxicillin increases the cure rate from 88% to 94% to 98%. The use of amoxicillin in the treatment of PUD has nothing to do with sepsis.

4. **e.** The eradication of *H. pylori* is difficult, and multiple drugs are required. Triple and quadruple therapies are recommended and provide eradication rates of at least 90%. Single- and dual-drug combination therapies are not recommended because of unacceptably low cure rates. The most frequently used combination is omeprazole 20 mg or lansoprazole 30 mg plus clarithromycin 500 mg and amoxicillin 1 g, all taken twice a day. Treatment regimens should last at least 10 to 14 days. A recent concern in the treatment of *H. pylori* ulcer disease is the development of antibiotic resistance associated with their increased use. Antibiotic resistance to amoxicillin and tetracycline is not common. There has not been any resistance reported to bismuth. Metronidazole resistance is from 30% to 48% and clarithromycin resistance is increasing to more than 8%. Erythromycin and azithromycin are much less effective and should not be used for *H. pylori* eradication.

5. **c.** Omeprazole binds to the proton pump of the parietal cell, inhibiting secretion of hydrogen ions into the gastric lumen. In doses of 20 mg to 40 mg/day, it inhibits more than 90% of total 24-hour gastric acid secretion, a significant improvement when compared with the 50% to 80% inhibition achieved with a H_2 blocker. This greater inhibition of gastric acid secretion results in greater pain relief and a decrease in healing time for the peptic ulcer.

6. **b.** A duodenal ulcer, treated appropriately, should respond to treatment and heal completely within 3 to 6 weeks. *H. pylori* treatment should be 10 to 14 days. A course of acid suppression therapy following eradication treatment is no longer thought to be needed.

7. **b.** Misoprostol is a prostaglandin analogue and is a cytoprotective agent to GI mucosa. It is approved for the prevention of NSAID-induced ulcers in people at high risk; however, PPIs are better at preventing duodenal ulcers and are as good as misoprostol in preventing gastric ulcers. Metoclopramide is a prokinetic and may be useful as an adjunct therapy for GERD; however, in March 2003, the U.S. Food and Drug Administration required labels to carry warnings concerning the neuroleptic malignant syndrome as a possible adverse reaction. Bismuth is an agent available as part of the combination therapies used for *H. pylori* eradication. Ondansetron is a $5HT_3$ antagonist that is used to prevent nausea and vomiting in patients undergoing chemotherapy. Nizatidine is an H_2 receptor antagonist. H_2 receptor antagonists inhibit the action of histamine at the histamine H_2 receptor of the parietal cell, decreasing both basal and food-stimulated acid secretion. All H_2 receptor antagonists are equally efficacious. At this time, the treatment of choice for PUD not associated with *H. pylori* is either a PPI or an H_2 receptor antagonist. The PPIs omeprazole and lansoprazole have the advantage of inducing a shorter healing time with a lower chance of recurrence.

8. **a.** COX-II specific NSAIDs still have a risk of causing PUD but at a reduced rate than typical NSAIDs. NSAIDs including indomethacin are well

known to be causative agents in both gastritis and PUD. There is a 10% to 20% prevalence of gastric ulcers and a 25% prevalence of duodenal ulcers in chronic NSAID users.

Dexamethasone (a potent corticosteroid) is used extensively in palliative care to reduce cerebral edema and inhibit centrally mediated nausea and/or vomiting. It is, however, a potent stimulator of gastric acid secretion and must be used with an H_2 receptor antagonist or a PPI to prevent gastritis or peptic ulcer formation.

Aspirin is the most ulcerogenic NSAID. The risk appears to be dose related and is present even at doses of 325 mg every other day. Risks of PUD/gastritis with NSAID increases with age, prior GI disease, steroid use, anticoagulant use, female sex, and increased dose.

9. e. Infection with *H. pylori* is a chronic infection that will last throughout a person's life if left untreated. By the age of 50 years approximately 40% of those in the United States will be colonized with *H. pylori*. Transmission is through oral–oral and fecal–oral routes, and organisms can be found in infected individuals' feces and saliva. There is a strong association between socioeconomic class and the risk of infection. Prevalence of infection in African Americans and Hispanics is on average one-third higher than in whites.

10. b. NSAID-induced gastric ulcers can be asymptomatic, and initial presentation can be perforation or bleeding. A gastric ulcer identified endoscopically must be followed by another endoscopy to confirm that healing has occurred. The pain of gastric ulcer disease is aggravated rather than relieved by food. Anorexia, nausea, and vomiting are more common in patients with gastric ulcers than in patients with duodenal ulcer. Also, the healing rate for gastric ulcers generally is slower than for duodenal ulcers.

11. c. Several of the PPIs, namely lansoprazole and rabeprazole, need to be used with caution in patients with hepatic impairment. PPIs do provide better acid suppression, healing rates, and symptom relief than the H_2 blockers. The dose and frequency of dosing is also less for PPIs.

12. c. It is acceptable to empirically treat a patient with documented duodenal or suspected duodenal ulcer who has no alarm signs, as was reviewed in Answer 2.

13. e. There is no convincing evidence that eradication therapy for *H. pylori* improves nonulcer dyspepsia or GERD. Patients with history of PUD who were never tested or treated for *H. pylori* who develop symptoms again should be tested and treated as needed.

14. c. ELISA serology testing, although very convenient and commonly used, is not reliable to determine successful eradication of *H. pylori*. Antibody titers are slow to decline and therefore can lead to many false-positive results even after successful treatment. Serology testing is appropriate for patients never treated for the organism in the past. Steiner's stain of gastric biopsy and culture require invasive endoscopy but are sensitive and specific for detecting persistence of *H. pylori* after treatment. Stool antigen and urea breath tests are also accurate tests to check for persistence of infection. Stool tests are more convenient because they are office-based, compared to the urea breath test that needs to be collected in a hospital outpatient setting.

15. d. *H. pylori* continues to be the number-one cause of PUD, followed by NSAIDs. Zollinger-Ellison syndrome is not common but causes multiple duodenal and gastric ulcers. Idiopathic ulcers are on the increase as *H. pylori* prevalence declines.

 ## SOLUTION TO THE CLINICAL CASE MANAGEMENT PROBLEM

NSAIDs can cause acute mucosal injury with submucosal hemorrhages and erosions with gross bleeding as a topical effect. Chronic use leads to ulceration from systemic effect by inhibiting prostaglandins that protect against injury in the GI tract.

H. pylori infection causes gastric inflammation. Infected persons have increased gastric acid secretion, and in patients with ulcers this may be sixfold higher than in normal individuals. There are also interactions between NSAIDs and *H. pylori*. NSAID users are more prone to developing an ulcer if they are *H. pylori*-positive; in fact, they have a twofold higher risk of having a bleeding peptic ulcer with concomitant *H. pylori* infection.

SUMMARY OF PEPTIC ULCER DISEASE

A. Symptoms:
1. Duodenal ulcer: mid-epigastric pain, relieved by ingestion of food or antacids
2. Nocturnal pain is present
3. Gastric ulcer: midepigastric pain, relieved by antacids but often aggravated by food;
4. Anorexia, weight loss, nausea, and vomiting frequently are associated

B. Differential diagnosis:
cholecystitis, pancreatitis, appendicitis, carcinoma of the stomach, ischemic bowel disease in the elderly, inflammatory bowel disease

C. Investigations:
1. No endoscopy may be needed if the symptoms suggest duodenal ulcer without alarm signs and symptoms resolve within a maximum of 8 weeks of acid suppression therapy. *H. pylori* testing can be done noninvasively, and treatment can be provided if positive.

2. Gastroscopy must be used for both the assessment and the reassessment of gastric ulcers.

D. Treatment:
1. NSAID-associated peptic ulcer:
   a. H_2 receptor antagonist
   b. proton pump inhibitor (such as omeprazole)
2. Non–NSAID-associated peptic ulcer: associated with *H. pylori*; see treatment protocols
3. Limited role at this time for antacid therapy, sucralfate, or misoprostol, which has as its chief function the possible prevention of gastric ulcers

SUGGESTED READING

Meurer LN: Management of *Helicobacter pylori* infection. *Am Fam Phys* 65(7):1327-1336, 2002.
Peptic ulcer disease @ www.guideline.gov.
Smoot DT: Peptic ulcer disease. *Primary Care* 28(3):487-503, 2001.
Talley N: Peptic ulcer. In: Rakel R, ed. *Conn's current therapy, 2003*, Elsevier, 2000, Philadelphia.
Vanderhoff BT: Proton pump inhibitors—an update. *Am Fam Phys* 6(2): 273-280, 2002.

Chapter 23

Inflammatory Bowel Disease

"I must have picked up a super bug. It has been tearing my gut apart for months."

CLINICAL CASE PROBLEM 1:
A 32-YEAR-OLD FEMALE WITH FEVER, WEIGHT LOSS, AND CHRONIC DIARRHEA

A 32-year-old female comes to your office with a 6-month history of loose bowel movements, approximately eight per day. Blood has been present in many of them. She has lost 30 lb. For the past 6 weeks she has had an intermittent fever. She has had no previous gastrointestinal (GI) problems, and there is no family history of GI problems.

On examination, the patient looks ill. Her blood pressure is 130/70 mm Hg. Her pulse is 108 and regular. There is generalized abdominal tenderness with no rebound. A sigmoidoscopy reveals a friable rectal mucosa with multiple bleeding points.

SELECT THE BEST ANSWER TO THE FOLLOWING QUESTIONS:

1. What is the most likely diagnosis in this patient?
   a. irritable bowel syndrome
   b. Crohn's disease
   c. ulcerative colitis
   d. Crohn's colitis
   e. bacterial dysentery

2. At this time which of the following represents the investigation of choice?
   a. colonoscopy
   b. barium enema
   c. upper GI series and follow-through
   d. a and c
   e. a, b, and c

3. Which of the following may be indicated in the management of the acute phase of the condition described?
   a. steroid enemas
   b. oral corticosteroids
   c. parenteral corticosteroids

d. a and b
e. all of the above

4. Which of the following statements regarding the use of sulfasalazine in the condition described is (are) false?
   a. sulfasalazine is structurally related to both aspirin and sulfa drugs
   b. sulfasalazine is effective in maintaining remission in this condition and in the acute treatment of mild disease
   c. sulfasalazine may impair folic acid metabolism
   d. all of the above are false
   e. a, b, and c

5. Which of the following completions regarding the long-term prognosis of the patient described in the case history is false? Following an initial attack:
   a. 10% of patients go into remission lasting up to 15 years
   b. 75% of patients experience intermittent exacerbations for many years
   c. 10% of patients continue to have active disease until surgical intervention is undertaken
   d. 5% of patients die within a year
   e. none of the above are false

6. Which of the following complications occur in the disease described?
   a. toxic megacolon and strictures
   b. colonic cancer
   c. iritis
   d. a and b
   e. a, b, and c

CLINICAL CASE PROBLEM 2:

A 25-YEAR-OLD MALE PRESENTS WITH AN 18-MONTH HISTORY OF CHRONIC ABDOMINAL PAIN

A 25-year-old male presents with an 18-month history of chronic abdominal pain. The patient has seen several physicians and has been diagnosed as having "nervous stomach," irritable bowel syndrome, and "depression." Associated with this abdominal pain for the last 3 months have been nonbloody diarrhea, anorexia, and a weight loss of 20 lb. He has developed a painful area around the anus.

On examination, the patient has diffuse abdominal tenderness. He looks thin and unwell. He has a tender, erythematous area in the right perirectal area.

7. What is the most likely diagnosis?
   a. irritable bowel syndrome
   b. Crohn's disease
   c. ulcerative colitis
   d. bacterial dysentery
   e. amebiasis

8. Pathologically, what is the difference between the patient in this case and the patient described in Clinical Case Problem 1?
   a. inflammation in this case involves all layers of the bowel; the former involves only the mucosa
   b. inflammation in the former case involves all layers of the bowel; the latter involves only the mucosa
   c. inflammation in the former case involves the first two layers of the bowel (mucosa and submucosa); the latter involves only the mucosa
   d. inflammation in this case involves the first two layers of the bowel (mucosa and submucosa); the former involves only the mucosa
   e. the two diseases are essentially identical on a pathophysiologic basis

9. Which of the following investigations is the most sensitive test for confirming the diagnosis in this patient?
   a. sigmoidoscopy
   b. colonoscopy
   c. barium enema
   d. computed tomography (CT) scan of the abdomen
   e. magnetic resonance imaging (MRI) scan of the abdomen

10. Which of the following drugs is (are) appropriate initial therapy in the acute phase of the condition described in Clinical Case Problem 2?
    a. budesonide
    b. sulfasalazine
    c. metronidazole
    d. 6-mercaptopurine
    e. all of the above

11. Metronidazole is effective in which of the following subtypes of Crohn's disease?
    a. mild Crohn's disease
    b. perianal disease
    c. Crohn's disease of the small bowel
    d. a and b
    e. a, b, and c

12. Which of the following is (are) not associated with Crohn's disease?
    a. skip lesions on x-ray
    b. thumbprinting on x-ray
    c. anti-*Saccharomyces cerevisiae* antibodies
    d. perinuclear-staining anti-neutrophil cytoplasmic antibodies
    e. a and c

13. Which of the following statements regarding complications of the condition described in Clinical Case Problem 2 is false?

a. rectal fissures, rectocutaneous fistulas, and perirectal abscesses are common complications of this condition
b. arthritis sometimes is seen as a complication of this condition
c. erythema nodosum and pyoderma gangrenosum sometimes are found with this condition
d. patients with this condition are not at increased risk of colorectal cancer
e. none of the above statements are false

CLINICAL CASE PROBLEM 3:

A Thin, Anemic-Appearing, 31-Year Old Female

A 31-year-old female comes to your office with a 6-month history of GI problems including abdominal distention, excessive flatus, foul-smelling stools, weight loss, and nonspecific complaints of weakness and fatigue. The patient describes the symptoms as being especially severe after the intake of cereal grains and bread of any kind. The patient has not traveled to any specific area in the recent past. She has not left the country.

She is thin and looks anemic. Vital signs are normal. The patient is in no acute distress, but her abdomen reveals active bowel sounds, mild distention, and diffuse discomfort to palpation.

14. On the basis of this information, what is the most likely diagnosis in this patient?
    a. lactase deficiency
    b. acute pancreatitis
    c. celiac sprue
    d. tropical sprue
    e. bacterial overgrowth syndrome

15. What is the pathophysiology of this disease?
    a. an immunologic disorder of the small bowel mucosa
    b. a disaccharide deficiency of the small intestinal mucosa
    c. a deficiency of pancreatic exocrine
    d. secondary contamination of the small intestine by coliform bacteria
    e. none of the above

CLINICAL CASE PROBLEM 4:

A 15-Year-Old Female Who Can No Longer Drink Milk

A 15-year-old female presents to your office with a 1-month history of abdominal cramping, abdominal bloating, and increased flatulence following the ingestion of milk or milk products. The patient drank three glasses of milk 2 hours ago.

On examination, the abdomen is tympanic and appears to be slightly distended. No other abnormalities are found on examination.

16. What is the most likely diagnosis in this patient?
    a. tropical sprue
    b. celiac sprue
    c. lactase deficiency
    d. regional enteritis
    e. chronic pancreatitis

CLINICAL CASE MANAGEMENT PROBLEM

Discuss the relationship between inflammatory bowel disease (ulcerative colitis and Crohn's disease) and the risk of acquiring carcinoma of the colon.

ANSWERS:

1. **c.** This patient almost certainly has ulcerative colitis. Ulcerative colitis usually presents with: (1) abdominal pain; (2) diarrhea; (3) passage of blood via the rectum; (4) tenesmus; (5) fever; (6) chills; (7) malaise and fatigue; and (8) weight loss. Sigmoidoscopy usually reveals friability (with easy bleeding) and granularity. Crohn's disease (regional enteritis) is usually not associated with rectal bleeding, although it may be. Crohn's disease will be discussed in a subsequent question. Bacterial dysentery would not be as long-lasting as this illness. Irritable bowel syndrome is a diagnosis of exclusion and does not present with systemic symptoms.

2. **a.** Barium enema or colonoscopy may be performed in this patient. However, colonoscopy is preferable to barium enema because it identifies the extent of disease and at the same time allows biopsies to be taken. Again, friability is the hallmark finding, as is involvement of the rectum. Radiographic findings in ulcerative colitis include the following: (1) continuous involvement of the colon; (2) superficial ulcerations; and (3) "backwash ileitis."

   Although the rectum and the distal colon are the most common sites of involvement, patients with more severe disease may have involvement of the entire colon. A GI series and follow-through would not add any useful information to the investigation of a patient strongly suspected of having ulcerative colitis.

3. **e.** Therapy of ulcerative colitis depends on the site and severity of the disease. Corticosteroids remain the cornerstone of management of patients with severe acute ulcerative colitis. They are not, however, efficacious in the maintenance of remission. Patients with severe, acute disease are usually severely ill and

require hospitalization and close monitoring for the potential development of toxic megacolon and silent perforation. Current treatment for mild and moderate, severe, refractory, and remission states of illness are listed as follows for distal (rectal) and extensive (entire colon) forms of the disease.

A. DISTAL DISEASE
   1. Mild to Moderate
      a. Oral or rectal aminosalicylates (Sulfasalazine, mesalamine, or olsalazine remain the initial therapy of choice in the treatment of patients with mild to moderate acute disease and in the maintenance of remission. Sulfasalazine is structurally related both to aspirin and to sulfa drugs. It inhibits folic acid, and patients taking it thus need a supplement of at least 1 mg of folic acid per day.)
      b. Rectal corticosteroids (given as a retention enema, hydrocortisone 100 mg once or twice/ day)
   2. Severe
      a. Oral or parenteral corticosteroids (They usually are given as prednisone in the range of 20 to 60 mg/day as a single oral dose for 2 weeks to 4 weeks or methylprednisolone intravenously. When the relief of symptoms has been attained, the dose can be tapered gradually.)
      b. Rectal corticosteroids
   3. Refractory
      a. Oral or intravenous (IV) corticosteroids, plus
      b. Oral azathioprine or mercaptopurine (The purine analogues, azathioprine [Imuran] and 6-mercaptopurine, have corticosteroid-sparing effects and are useful in the induction and maintenance of remission.)
   4. Remission
      a. Oral or rectal aminosalicylates
      b. Oral azathioprine or mercaptopurine
B. EXTENSIVE DISEASE
   1. Mild to moderate; oral aminosalicylates
   2. Severe:
      a. Oral or parenteral corticosteroids
      b. Intravenous cyclosporine (an immunosuppressant that works by inhibiting the production of cytokine by helper T cells)
   3. Refractory Disease:
      a. Oral or IV corticosteroids, plus
      b. Oral azathioprine or mercaptopurine
   4. Remission:
      a. Oral aminosalicylates
      b. Oral azathioprine or mercaptopurine

4. **e.** Sulfasalazine, like the other aminosalicylates, has a proven efficacy in the management of patients with ulcerative colitis. It is the therapy of choice in the treatment of patients with mild to moderately severe active disease. It is the treatment of choice for the maintenance of remission in patients with established ulcerative colitis.

5. **e.** All of the statements are true. Following an initial attack of ulcerative colitis, 10% of patients go into remission lasting up to 15 years. Of patients, 75% have intermittent exacerbation, 10% have continually active disease, and 5% die within 1 year of the initial attack. Of all patients with ulcerative colitis of any severity, 25% of patients will undergo total proctocolectomy within 5 years of the first attack. The risk of colonic cancer increases with time. By 15 years after initial diagnosis, patients with colonic disease are at a risk significant enough to consider prophylactic colectomy.

6. **e.** Complications of ulcerative colitis include the following: (1) toxic megacolon; (2) perforation; (3) colorectal carcinoma; (4) colonic stricture; and (5) hemorrhage.

Extracolonic complications include the following: (1) skin disease (erythema nodosum and pyoderma gangrenosum); (2) aphthous ulcers; (3) iritis; (4) arthritis; and (5) hepatic disease.

7. **b.** This patient has Crohn's disease (regional enteritis).

8. **a.** Pathologically, Crohn's disease involves an inflammation of all layers of the bowel, in contradistinction to ulcerative colitis, which involves just the mucosa.

Associated anorectal complications include the following: (1) fistulas; (2) fissures; and (3) perirectal abscesses.

The peak incidence of Crohn's disease is at 30 years of age; most cases occur between the ages of 20 and 40 years. Crohn's disease may follow an indolent course resulting in diagnostic delay. The signs and symptoms include the following: (1) mild chronic abdominal pain; (2) mild nonbloody diarrhea; (3) anorexia; (4) weight loss, and (5) fatigue.

Pain often is confined to the lower abdomen and is "aching" or "cramping." A misdiagnosis of irritable bowel syndrome often is made.

9. **b.** In most cases, no one test is sufficient for diagnosis, but endoscopy does allow for biopsy of abnormal tissue and pathologic confirmation of the disease. Colonoscopy is more sensitive than sigmoidoscopy, but it will not show the transmural involvement. Sigmoidoscopy alone will miss Crohn's disease

in 30% to 50% of patients. Barium air-contrast enema and upper-GI series with small bowel follow-through are also valuable diagnostic procedures in the evaluation for diagnosis of Crohn's disease in this patient. Crohn's disease often presents as segmental involvement of two or more colonic areas; between these areas the colon is normal. The transmural involvement often is suggested by radiologic features including the protrusion of a defect into the lumen (thumbprinting). CT scanning and MRI scanning often are performed in Crohn's disease, but they can miss many subtle lesions. Gadolinium-enhanced MRI with oral dilute barium sulfate and rectal water depicts intestinal and extraintestinal changes of Crohn's disease and shows promise as a diagnostic aide.

10. **e.** The drug of choice for the treatment of patients with Crohn's disease varies according to the severity of illness. Mild to moderate disease often is treated with a combination of oral aminosalicylates, oral antibiotics (metronidazole and ciprofloxacin), and oral corticosteroids (budesonide). Oral azathioprine or mercaptopurine also have been used. In severe disease, oral or systemic corticosteroids are used with subcutaneous or IV methotrexate and the anti-tumor necrosis factor infliximab, a monoclonal antibody. The latter drug has been particularly useful in refractory disease. As in ulcerative colitis, steroid dosage should be tapered after a few weeks of therapy. Maintenance of remission has been a challenge in Crohn's disease. The 5-aminosalicylates have been, at best, variable in effectiveness. Azathioprine and mercaptopurine have been used extensively with satisfactory results, although the long-term use of immunosuppressants is always a concern. The use of probiotics seems effective in subgroups of patients with Crohn's disease, and antibiotics, especially metronidazole, have been useful in all forms of disease, and particularly for patients with perianal fistulas. Attention to maintenance of proper nutrition is a constant job in all inflammatory bowel diseases.

11. **d.** Metronidazole is effective in the management of Crohn's colitis and Crohn's perianal disease. It is not, however, effective in the treatment of Crohn's disease of the small bowel.

12. **d.** Radiographic manifestations of Crohn's disease include skip lesions on x-ray (normal and abnormal alternating sections of bowel) and thumbprinting (characteristic defect protruding into the lumen). Anti-*Saccharomyces cerevisiae* antibodies are seen in more than 50% of patients with Crohn's disease and only occasionally in patients with ulcerative colitis.

Perinuclear-staining anti-neutrophil cytoplasmic antibodies are seen in more than 70% of patients with ulcerative colitis and only occasionally in patients with Crohn's disease.

13. **d.** Rectal fissures, rectocutaneous fistulas, or perirectal abscesses occur in up to 50% of patients with Crohn's disease at some time during their illness. Extracolonic manifestations of Crohn's disease occur in 10% of patients with the disease. These include arthritis (which in fact may precede the GI symptoms), iritis, erythema nodosum, pyoderma gangrenosum, and aphthous ulcers. The risk of colorectal cancer is less in patients with Crohn's disease than in patients with ulcerative colitis. Patients who have had the disease for more than 15 years are still, however, at increased risk for this malignancy.

14. **c.** This patient most likely has celiac sprue (gluten enteropathy).

15. **a.** Gluten enteropathy is an immunologic disorder of the small bowel observed in both children and adults. Exposure of the small intestine to antigenic components of certain cereal grains in susceptible people causes subtotal or total villous atrophy with reactive crypt hyperplasia.

Common GI complaints include the following: (1) abdominal distention; (2) excessive flatus; (3) large, bulky, foul-smelling stools; and (4) weight loss.

Other nonspecific complaints that commonly occur are weakness or fatigue. Patients may present with anemia from either an iron-deficiency anemia or a megaloblastic anemia (folic-acid deficiency). Other patients suffer from deficiency of a fat-soluble vitamin or vitamin B_{12}.

Therapy consists of a gluten-free diet (avoiding any products containing wheat, rye, barley, or oats). Cereals such as corn, rice, buckwheat, sorghum, and millet are not pathogenic and may be substituted. Clinical improvement generally is seen after several days on a gluten-free diet. Restoration of normal histologic architecture takes weeks to months.

16. **c.** This patient has a lactase deficiency in the small intestine. Thus symptoms characteristic of malabsorption (bloating, diarrhea, crampy abdominal pain, foul-smelling stools) occur when milk or milk products are ingested. The treatment of choice for these patients is replacement of the deficient enzyme with an enzyme supplement such as Lactaid tablets and/or replacement of lactose-rich dairy products with low-lactose products, such as yogurt, lactose-reduced milk and most hard (fermented) cheeses.

SOLUTION TO THE CLINICAL CASE MANAGEMENT PROBLEM

Inflammatory bowel disease, which includes ulcerative colitis and Crohn's disease, is directly related to the risk of acquiring carcinoma of the colon. The risk is related to the following:

1. Which disease: Ulcerative colitis has a greater risk than Crohn's disease; but both have increased risk.
2. Severity of the disease: The more severe the disease, the greater is the risk of carcinoma of the colon.
3. The length of time with the disease: The longer the patient has had the disease, the greater the risk.

4. The site of the disease: The risk of cancer of the colon is much higher in patients who have ulcerative colitis than ulcerative proctitis.

Patients with ulcerative proctitis, ulcerative colitis, and Crohn's colitis should be screened by endoscopy (colonoscopy) every 1 to 2 years depending on the factors listed. For ulcerative colitis, the screening process may indicate the appropriate time for a prophylactic hemicolectomy (average 15 years since disease onset).

SUMMARY OF INFLAMMATORY BOWEL DISEASE

A. Ulcerative colitis:

1. Pathophysiology involves the mucosa only.
2. Local symptoms include the following: (a) diarrhea (bloody); (b) mucus from the rectum; (c) tenesmus; (d) constipation (may alternate with diarrhea); and (e) abdominal pain. Complications such as toxic megacolon and perforation are uncommon.
3. Systemic symptoms include fever, chills, anorexia, weight loss, malaise, fatigue, erythema nodosum, pyoderma gangrenosum, aphthous ulcers, iritis, arthritis; and hepatic disease.
4. Investigations include sigmoidoscopy, colonoscopy, and air-contrast barium enema. If there is danger of perforation (megacolon), barium enema is contraindicated. Perinuclear-staining anti-neutrophil cytoplasmic antibodies are seen in more than 70% of patients with ulcerative colitis.
5. Therapy of ulcerative colitis depends on the site and severity of the disease. See Answer 3.

B. Crohn's disease:

1. Pathophysiology involves all layers of the bowel wall
2. Local symptoms include abdominal pain, non-bloody diarrhea, mucus from the rectum
3. Systemic symptoms include fever, chills, anorexia, malaise, fatigue, weight loss, erythema nodosum, pyoderma gangrenosum, aphthous ulcers, arthritis, and iritis
4. Other features include rectal fistulas, rectal fissures, and perirectal abscesses
5. Investigations include endoscopy and biopsy, barium enema, and GI series and follow-

through; anti-*Saccharomyces cerevisiae* antibodies are seen in more than 50% of patients with Crohn's disease.

6. The drug of choice for the treatment of patients with Crohn's disease varies according to the severity of illness. See Answer 10.

C. Other diseases that may resemble inflammatory bowel disease

1. Celiac sprue:
   a. Pathophysiology is gluten-sensitive enteropathy. It is an immunologic reaction of the small bowel wall that causes villous atrophy and crypt hyperplasia.
   b. Symptoms include bloating; diarrhea; foul-smelling stools; and weight loss, especially after eating gluten-containing products (breads, pasta, etc.)
   c. Treatment involves elimination of gluten from the diet.
2. Lactase deficiency:
   a. Pathophysiology is deficiency of the disaccharide enzyme lactase.
   b. Symptoms include crampy abdominal pain, bloating, foul-smelling stools, and diarrhea after the ingestion of milk or dairy products.
   c. Treatment involves replacement enzymes, such as lactase supplements before ingesting milk and milk products.

SUGGESTED READING

Bengmark S: Pre-, pro- and symbiotics. *Curr Opin Clin Nutr Metab Care* 4(6):571-579, 2001.

Crohn's and Colitis Foundation of America website with useful information for patients and professionals is at http://www.ccfa.org/.

Farthing MJ: Severe inflammatory bowel disease: medical management. *Dig Dis* 21(1):46-53, 2003.

Podolsky DK: Inflammatory bowel disease. *N Engl J Med* 347(6):417-429, 2002.

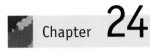

Chapter 24

Irritable Bowel Syndrome

> "I have to strain too hard, and I find
> a lot of mucus on the toilet paper."

CLINICAL CASE PROBLEM 1:
A 38-YEAR-OLD FEMALE WITH LOWER ABDOMINAL PAIN AND CONSTIPATION

A 38-year-old female comes to your office with a 1-year history of lower abdominal pain associated with constipation (one hard bowel movement every 3 days) and the passage of mucus per rectum on a regular basis. She has never passed blood per rectum to her knowledge. She describes no fever, chills, weight loss, jaundice, or any other symptoms. There is no relationship between the abdominal pain and food intake.

On physical examination, the abdomen is scaphoid, and no hepatosplenomegaly or other masses are palpated. There is a very mild generalized abdominal tenderness, but it does not localize.

■ **SELECT THE BEST ANSWER TO THE FOLLOWING QUESTIONS:**

1. What is the most likely diagnosis in this patient?
   a. *Yersinia enterocolitis*
   b. Crohn's disease
   c. ulcerative colitis
   d. lactose intolerance
   e. none of the above

2. Which of the following statements regarding the condition described is (are) false?
   a. the typical location of the abdominal pain is the lower abdomen
   b. defecation frequently relieves the pain
   c. there is often a perception of incomplete emptying of the rectum
   d. bowel movements are often irregular
   e. very severe abdominal tenderness is a hallmark of the disease

3. What is the most likely cause of the disorder described?
   a. a mass lesion in the area of the sigmoid colon
   b. a food allergy
   c. an autoimmune phenomenon
   d. a decreased ability to digest certain foods
   e. none of the above

4. Which of the following would be most unlikely in a patient with the condition described?
   a. alternating diarrhea and constipation
   b. increased pain at times of stress
   c. pain on awakening from sleep
   d. abdominal bloating
   e. increased passage of flatus

5. Which of the following investigations is not indicated in the condition described?
   a. a complete blood count
   b. liver function tests
   c. electrolytes
   d. abdominal ultrasound
   e. thyroid function studies

6. Which of the following has to be considered in the differential diagnosis of the condition described?
   a. colonic adenocarcinoma
   b. fecal impaction
   c. lactase deficiency
   d. endometriosis
   e. all of the above

7. Which of the following conditions (symptoms) is not associated with the condition?
   a. fibromyalgia
   b. cholelithiasis
   c. interstitial cystitis
   d. depression
   e. fatigue

8. Which of the following statements concerning the condition described is (are) true?
   a. this condition is the most common reason for referral from a family physician to a gastroenterologist
   b. this condition is slightly more common in men
   c. the symptoms associated with this condition are more common in young adults than in older adults
   d. this condition has been associated with a specific biochemical abnormality in some patients
   e. all of the above statements are true

9. Which of the following is the most important component of management of the condition described?
   a. single-agent pharmacologic therapy
   b. multiple-agent pharmacologic therapy
   c. a therapeutic physician–patient relationship
   d. a focused diet
   e. a diet elimination trial: eliminating one food at a time until the responsible food is found

10. Which of the following medications should not be used in the treatment of the condition described above?
    a. psyllium
    b. loperamide

    c. cholestyramine
    d. codeine phosphate
    e. desipramine

■ ANSWERS:

1. e. The most likely diagnosis is irritable bowel syndrome (IBS). IBS is characterized by (Rome criteria) abdominal pain or discomfort present for at least 12 weeks (not necessarily consecutive) in the past year that cannot be explained by structural or biochemical abnormalities and two of the following three features: (1) pain relieved with defecation; (2) onset associated with a change in the frequency of bowel movements (diarrhea or constipation); and/or (3) onset associated with a change in the form of the stool (loose, watery, or pelletlike).

Yersinia is one of several bacteria (others include *Campylobacter, Shigella,* and *Salmonella*) that can produce a diarrheal syndrome. *Yersinia* has been associated with a more chronic enterocolitis, but this usually is seen in children aged 1-4 and can mimic appendicitis. Occasionally, young adults can present with a syndrome that includes low-grade fever, crampy abdominal pain, nausea and vomiting, hematochezia, and a generalized maculopapular rash.

Crohn's disease is unlikely in the absence of systemic symptoms including nonbloody diarrhea, anorexia, weight loss, fever, and fatigue.

Ulcerative colitis is unlikely in the absence of weight loss, tenesmus, and the passage of bright red blood per rectum.

Lactose intolerance is linked specifically to the intake of milk and milk products.

2. e. The perception of incomplete emptying of the rectum, irregular bowel action, and the relief of the abdominal pain with defecation are common in IBS. Abdominal pain is confined to the lower abdomen, with the most common location being in the area of the sigmoid colon. Although abdominal tenderness may be present, it is usually not very severe and is not a hallmark of the disease.

3. e. The exact cause of IBS is unknown. Altered bowel motility, visceral hypersensitivity, psychosocial factors, an imbalance in neurotransmitters, and infection all have been proposed as playing roles in the development of IBS. Psychiatric disorders, such as somatization, depression, or anxiety, are seen in as many as 60% of patients with IBS. A history of physical or sexual abuse should be considered.

4. c. Pain on awakening from sleep is suggestive of an organic etiology. In addition to this symptom, pain that interferes with normal sleep patterns, diarrhea that awakens the patient from sleep, visible or occult blood in the stool, weight loss, and fever also suggest organic disease.

5. d. The investigations recommended in a patient with IBS include complete blood count, chemistry panel, flexible sigmoidoscopy (colonoscopy in patients 50 years or older), and thyroid function studies.

6. e. Diagnoses that may need to be considered in patients with symptoms of IBS include lactase deficiency, colonic adenocarcinoma, ulcerative colitis, Crohn's disease, ischemic colitis, diverticulitis, drugs, mechanical obstruction of the colon or small intestine, malabsorption, endometriosis, depression, somatization, and panic disorder.

7. b. Patients with IBS are at increased risk for such functional disorders as fibromyalgia and interstitial cystitis. Conditions that are more common in patients with IBS include fatigue and depression. Cholelithiasis is not associated with irritable bowel syndrome.

8. a. IBS is the most common reason for referral by a family physician to a gastrointestinal specialist. IBS is more common in women than in men. It affects three times as many women. Although symptoms typically begin in young adulthood, the prevalence is similar in elderly and younger adults. No specific biochemical abnormality has been found in patients with IBS.

9. c. The most important component of treatment in IBS is establishing a therapeutic, communicative, and trusting physician–patient relationship and educating the patent regarding the benign nature of the condition and favorable long-term prognosis.

The important components of the physician–patient relationship that should be emphasized include a nonjudgmental attitude, concern regarding the patient's understanding of the illness, expectations and consistent limits, and involvement of the patient in treatment decisions. Because of the long-term nature of IBS, primary management by a family physician is essential. Although consultants may be needed in some cases for both patient and family physician reassurance, this should be the exception rather than the rule.

Diet therapy and pharmacologic therapy will be discussed in a subsequent question.

10. d. Treatment of IBS includes the following:
    1. Eliminating certain foods including gas-forming foods such as legumes, caffeine, alcohol, fatty foods, and products containing sorbitol. Patients

should keep a diary to identify foods that exacerbate symptoms.
2. Supplementing with high-fiber foods such as bran.
3. Engaging in supportive therapy, relaxation exercises, hypnosis, cognitive behavioral therapy, and psychodynamic interpersonal psychotherapy.

Other agents used in the treatment of IBS include the following:
1. Psyllium (another bulking agent)
2. Antispasmodic or anticholinergic agents
3. Antidiarrheal agents such as diphenoxylate, loperamide, or cholestyramine in cases in which diarrhea is the predominant symptom
4. Tricyclic antidepressants such as amitriptyline or desipramine
5. Osmotic laxatives such as milk of magnesia when constipation is the predominant symptom. Tegaserod, a 5-HT$_4$ receptor agonist, is used for the short-term treatment of IBS in women whose primary bowel symptom is constipation.

Long-term benzodiazepines are not recommended, although treatment for short periods may be indicated. Codeine phosphate or other narcotic agents are contraindicated in the treatment of IBS because of the potential for abuse or tolerance.

In the management of a patient with IBS consider doing and not doing the following:

A. YOU SHOULD:
1. Do a complete history including a psychosocial history, a family history, and a marital history.
2. Attempt to ascertain the patient's understanding and concerns about the condition.
3. Establish a strong, trusting family physician–patient relationship. This forms the basis for the therapy (supportive psychotherapy) that follows.
4. Have the patient ask all of his or her questions in an unhurried atmosphere.
5. Perform a complete or relatively complete physical examination to reassure yourself that nothing significant has been missed and to reassure the patient that you are truly interested in the problem.
6. Ascertain what dietary and drug therapies have been tried, and decide on those therapies that may be indicated at this time.

B. YOU SHOULD NOT:
1. Repeat investigations, nor should you order other, more costly investigations.
2. Criticize your colleagues for failure to completely investigate this problem until a cause was found; you will find yourself in the same situation someday.

3. Promise what you cannot deliver, which is a cure for IBS. Also, do not let the patient transfer ownership of the problem to you. It is the patient's problem, and your job is not to solve it; your job is to provide the empathic support necessary to help the patient understand and deal with the illness.
4. Rely on a polypharmacy approach to achieve a better result. Use the suggested drugs with prudence and caution.
5. Use narcotic analgesics as a treatment for IBS.

SUMMARY OF IRRITABLE BOWEL SYNDROME

1. IBS is extremely common; prevalence estimates suggest that 15% of the population have symptoms compatible with this diagnosis.
2. IBS is the most common condition that gastroenterologists see in referral or consultation practice.
3. Consider IBS as a diagnosis of inclusion rather than exclusion. Base your diagnosis on the positive criteria discussed previously.
4. Consider the minimal investigations that have been suggested as sufficient; do not overinvestigate.
5. After establishing a strong physician–patient relationship, consider dietary manipulation as primary therapy.
6. Antispasmodics, anticholinergics, tricyclic antidepressants, antidiarrheal agents, and osmotic laxatives and 5-HT$_4$ receptor agonist agents are drugs that can be used for the treatment of IBS. Use caution combining them.
7. Reassurance regarding the benign nature of the condition and the provision of hope for eventual resolution of the symptoms are likely the most important therapy for this condition (supportive psychotherapy).
8. Identification and treatment of psychosocial stressors (stressors of some kind are almost invariably associated with this condition) are paramount.

SUGGESTED READING

Horwitz BJ, Fisher RS: Current concepts: the irritable bowel syndrome. *N Engl J Med* 344(24):1846-1850, 2001.
Jailwala J, et al: Pharmacologic treatment of the irritable bowel syndrome: a systematic review of randomized, controlled trials. *Ann Intern Med* 133(2):136-147, 2000.
Silk D: Management of irritable bowel syndrome: start of a new era? *Eur J Gastroenterol Hepatol* 15(6):679-696, 2003.

Chapter 25

Diagnosis and Treatment of Hepatitis and Cirrhosis

> "My husband's beer belly is really expanding."

CLINICAL CASE PROBLEM 1:
A 50-Year-Old Male with Ascites

A 50-year-old male is brought into your office by his wife. His wife states that for the past several months he has experienced extreme weakness and fatigue. In addition, he has gained 20 lb in the past 3 weeks. During the last few weeks she states the patient has eaten virtually nothing. When you question the patient he states that his wife is overreacting. The patient's wife is extremely concerned about his alcohol intake. When you question the patient, he states that he is a social drinker. When you pursue this line of questioning further and ask him what he means by being a social drinker, you find out that he means that he drinks a few drinks before and after most meals plus a few drinks before he goes to bed.

You decide to pursue the question of drinking even further. When you ask him what he drinks, he says vodka. When you ask him if he drinks two 26-oz bottles a day, he says, "Heck, no! I would never put away more than a bottle a day."

On physical examination, the patient has a significantly enlarged abdominal girth. There is a level of shifting dullness present. The patient's liver edge is felt 6 cm below the right costal margin. It has a nodular edge. In addition, spider nevi are present over the upper part of the patient's body. Palmar erythema is noted, and a flapping tremor is elicited.

■ SELECT THE BEST ANSWER TO THE FOLLOWING QUESTIONS:

1. Which of the following statements regarding this patient's condition is false?
   a. the most likely diagnosis is cirrhosis of the liver
   b. this condition probably is associated with alcohol abuse
   c. jaundice is an uncommon sign in the disorder described
   d. approximately 33% of patients with a history of alcohol abuse will develop alcoholic hepatitis
   e. approximately 50% of patients with this condition (in an advanced stage) will die within 2 years

CLINICAL CASE PROBLEM 2:
A 25-Year-Old Male with Abdominal Pain for the Past 3 Weeks

A 25-year-old male with a history of heavy alcohol intake comes to your office for a periodic health assessment. He states that his appetite has been off and he has had generalized abdominal pain for the past 3 weeks.

On examination, there is no clinical jaundice. There is tenderness present in the right upper quadrant of the abdomen. The liver edge is palpable 5 cm below the right costal margin. You suspect alcoholic hepatitis.

2. Which of the following statements regarding alcoholic hepatitis is false?
   a. alcoholic cirrhosis develops in approximately 10% of patients with alcoholic hepatitis
   b. serum bilirubin often may be 10 to 20 times what is normal in this condition
   c. serum alanine aminotransferase (ALT) is almost always lower than serum aspartate aminotransferase (AST; formally SGOT)
   d. hepatomegaly is seen in 80% to 90% of patients with alcoholic hepatitis
   e. a mortality rate of 10% to 15% is seen in acute alcoholic hepatitis

3. What is the most common cause of cirrhosis in the United States?
   a. hepatitis A
   b. hepatitis B
   c. hepatitis C
   d. alcoholism
   e. cytomegalovirus hepatitis

4. The ascites associated with cirrhosis generally should be treated by which of the following?
   a. sodium restriction
   b. water restriction
   c. spironolactone
   d. a and c
   e. a, b, and c

CLINICAL CASE PROBLEM 3:
A Nauseated 25-Year-Old Schoolteacher with Icteric Sclera and Right Upper Quadrant Pain

A 25-year-old schoolteacher presents with nausea, vomiting, anorexia, aversion to her usual 2 packs a day tobacco habit, and right upper quadrant pain. She has been sick for the past 3 days. Two of the students in her class have come down with similar symptoms. She has had no exposure to blood products and has no significant risk factors for sexually transmitted disease. On examination, she looks acutely ill. Her pulse is 100/min, BP 110/70, respirations 18, temperature 101° F. Her sclera are icteric, and her liver edge is tender.

5. What is the most likely diagnosis in this patient?
   a. hepatitis A
   b. hepatitis B
   c. hepatitis C
   d. atypical infectious mononucleosis
   e. none of the above

6. Which of the following tests is the most sensitive in confirming the diagnosis suspected in the patient presenting in the preceding question?
   a. anti-hepatitis A virus (HAV)-immunoglobulin G (IgG)
   b. anti-HAV-IgM
   c. HAV core antigen
   d. anti-hepatitis B core antigen (HBcAg)
   e. anti-hepatitis C virus

7. Initial screening for hepatitis B should include which of the following?
   a. anti-hepatitis B surface antigen (HBsAg) and anti-hepatitis B core antibody (anti-HBc)
   b. hepatitis B early antigen (HBeAg) and anti-HBe
   c. HBsAg and anti-HBs
   d. HBsAg and anti-HBc
   e. anti-HBe and anti-HBc

8. Which of the following laboratory tests is (are) usually abnormal in a patient with acute viral hepatitis?
   a. serum AST
   b. serum bilirubin
   c. serum ALT
   d. serum alkaline phosphatase
   e. all of the above

9. Clinical manifestations of cirrhosis include which of the following?
   a. fatigue
   b. jaundice
   c. splenomegaly
   d. hypoalbuminemia
   e. all of the above

10. Indications for the use of hepatitis B vaccine include which of the following?
    a. health care personnel
    b. patients undergoing hemodialysis
    c. all children
    d. all previously unvaccinated adults
    e. all of the above

11. Which of the following types of viral hepatitis is (are) associated with the development of chronic active hepatitis?
    a. hepatitis B
    b. hepatitis C
    c. hepatitis A
    d. a and b only
    e. all of the above

12. The pathophysiology of alcoholic cirrhosis includes which of the following?
    a. macronodular and micronodular fibrosis
    b. nodular regeneration
    c. increased portal vein pressure
    d. increase in hepatic size followed by a decrease
    e. all of the above

13. Which of the following is (are) appropriate treatment for cirrhosis of the liver?
    a. cessation of alcohol use
    b. propranolol
    c. maintenance of proper nutrition
    d. liver transplantation
    e. all of the above

14. Which of the following is (are) a complication(s) of alcoholic cirrhosis?
    a. hypersplenism
    b. hepatic encephalopathy
    c. congestive gastropathy
    d. spontaneous bacterial peritonitis
    e. all of the above

CLINICAL CASE MANAGEMENT PROBLEM

Describe the relationship between cirrhosis of the liver and right-sided heart failure.

ANSWERS:

1. **c.** This patient has alcoholic hepatitis with cirrhosis of the liver. Alcohol abuse is thought to be related to one in five hospitalizations in the United States. Many cases of cirrhosis of the liver are directly attributable to alcohol abuse, although infectious agents, particularly hepatitis C, are an emerging cause. Cirrhosis is an irreversible inflammatory disease that disrupts liver structure and function. Alcoholic hepatitis is seen in approximately 20% of heavy drinkers. Men with alcoholic hepatitis usually consume at least 70 g of alcohol daily and have done so an average of 10 years. In women, a lower threshold of 20 to 40 g for the same period is average for the development of hepatitis.

Cirrhosis is the disorganization of hepatic tissues caused by diffuse fibrosis and nodular regeneration. Nodules of regenerated tissue form between fibrous bands, giving the liver a cobbled appearance.

Symptoms of early alcoholic liver disease include weakness, fatigue, and weight loss. In advanced disease the patient develops anorexia, nausea and vomiting, swelling of the abdomen and the lower extremities, and central nervous system symptoms related to the cirrhotic liver disease. Other symptoms that may occur include loss of libido in both sexes, gynecomastia in men, and menstrual irregularities in women.

The liver of patients with alcoholic hepatitis and cirrhosis usually is enlarged, palpable, and firm. In advanced cirrhosis, the liver actually may shrink. Dermatologic manifestations include spider nevi, palmar erythema, telangiectases on exposed areas, and occasional evidence of vitamin deficiencies. Although jaundice is rarely an initial sign, it usually develops later. Other later developing signs include ascites, lower-extremity edema, pleural effusion, purpuric lesions, asterixis, tremor, delirium, coma, fever, splenomegaly, and superficial venous dilatation on the abdomen and thorax. There appears to be a genetic predisposition to the development of these complications. Of patients with advanced cirrhosis, 50% will be dead in a period of 2 years; 65% will be dead in 5 years. Hematemesis, jaundice, and ascites are unfavorable signs.

2. **a.** The first clinical stage of alcoholic liver disease is termed alcoholic hepatitis. Alcoholic hepatitis is a precursor of cirrhosis that is characterized by inflammation, degeneration, and necrosis of hepatocytes and infiltration of polymorphonuclear leukocytes and lymphocytes.

During the last 10 years in the United States, deaths from alcohol-related liver disease have increased. The incidence is greatest in middle-aged males, and mortality from cirrhosis is higher in blacks than in whites. Although alcoholic cirrhosis is a prevalent type of cirrhosis, only about 15% of alcoholics actually develop the disease. There appears to be a genetic predisposition to its development. The amount and duration of alcohol consumption are correlated directly with the extent of damage to the liver.

The symptoms of alcoholic hepatitis include anorexia, nausea, vomiting, weight loss, emesis, fever, and generalized abdominal pain. Hepatomegaly is found in 80% to 90% of these patients. Other signs include jaundice, ascites, splenomegaly, and spider angiomas.

Laboratory abnormalities in alcoholic hepatitis include hyperbilirubinemia and elevated serum transaminase. The ratio of serum AST/ALT is often 2:1 or greater. This can help differentiate alcoholic hepatitis from viral hepatitis. Other laboratory abnormalities include elevated alkaline phosphatase, hypoalbuminemia, and a prolonged prothrombin time.

The prognosis of alcoholic hepatitis is variable; many patients develop only a mild illness. There is, however, a 10% to 15% mortality rate from the acute event.

The treatment of alcoholic hepatitis involves cessation of alcohol consumption, increased caloric and protein intake, and vitamin supplementation (especially thiamine).

Alcoholic cirrhosis develops in approximately 50% of patients surviving alcoholic hepatitis. In the other 50%, various degrees of hepatic fibrosis develop.

3. **c.** The most common cause of cirrhosis in the United States is now hepatitis C, surpassing alcohol-induced cirrhosis. Hepatitis C (HCV) is also the most common cause of hepatocellular carcinoma. There are more than 4 million Americans infected with hepatitis C, and the yearly incidence is 35,000. Patients with hepatitis C go on to develop chronic active hepatitis and subsequent cirrhosis in approximately 20% to 40% of cases. HCV is also the leading cause of liver transplantation. Hepatitis A does not progress to chronic active hepatitis. Hepatitis B progresses to chronic active hepatitis and subsequently to cirrhosis in up to 50% of cases. Cytomegalovirus infection does not produce cirrhosis.

4. **d.** The treatment of ascites and the edema associated with ascites includes the following: (1) sodium restriction to 800 mg of Na^+/day (or 2 g of NaCl); (2) spironolactone (Aldactone) 25 mg to 100 mg qid (effective in 40% to 75% of cases); (3) paracentesis; (4) combination diuretic therapy in those patients who do not respond, with either spironolactone plus hydrochlorothiazide or spironolactone plus furosemide; and (5) paracentesis with albumin (or dextran) infusion in refractory cases.

The 1-year survival rate of patients with cirrhosis with ascites is 50%, compared with 90% in patients with uncomplicated cirrhosis. Formation of ascites results from a combination of portal hypertension, hypoalbuminemia, lymphatic leakage, and sodium retention. The management of ascites in patients with cirrhosis is complicated. Diagnostic paracentesis should be performed in any patient with cirrhosis who undergoes clinical deterioration. Defined indications for the treatment of ascites include significant patient discomfort, respiratory compromise, a large umbilical hernia, and recurrent bacterial peritonitis.

Sodium restriction is considered the cornerstone of therapy for ascites. Patients with cirrhosis require significant curtailment of sodium intake (800 mg/day) to obtain clinical benefit. Approximately 10% to 20% of patients who maintain a strict low-salt diet achieve complete resolution of ascites without additional therapy. However, hyponatremia may accompany sodium restriction, and severe hyponatremia (serum Na less than 125 mEq) is a reason to begin fluid restriction as well. The vast majority of patients also will require diuretics.

Spironolactone (Aldactone), an aldosterone antagonist, is the first-line diuretic of choice in the treatment of cirrhotic ascites. It is effective in controlling up to 50% of patients with cirrhosis. Other potassium-sparing diuretics may be substituted for spironolactone, including triamterene (Dyrenium) and amiloride (Midamor). The addition of loop diuretics (such as furosemide) sometimes is needed to achieve maximum benefit. Alternatives to furosemide include bumetanide (Bumex) and torsemide (Demadex). Watch for hypokalemia with diuretics. Up to 90% of patients with cirrhosis and ascites will respond to diuretics and salt restriction. For those who do not, periodic paracentesis with albumin replacement is an alternative, as are portocaval shunts and transjugular intrahepatic portosystemic shunts (TIPS), the latter for those requiring frequent large-volume paracenteses.

5. a. This patient most likely has hepatitis A. Hepatitis A occurs either spontaneously or in epidemics. Transmission is via the oral–fecal route. The presenting signs and symptoms of hepatitis A include the following: (1) general malaise and fatigue; (2) general myalgias; (3) arthralgias; (4) abdominal pain; (5) nausea and vomiting; (6) severe anorexia, out of proportion to the degree of illness; and (7) aversion to smoking (if the patient smokes).

Hepatitis B and hepatitis C are unlikely in this case because risk factors are absent. Although infectious mononucleosis may involve the liver and present with some of the same signs and symptoms, hepatitis A is much more likely.

6. b. Acute infection with hepatitis A is confirmed by the demonstration of IgM antibodies to HAV (IgM-anti-HAV). These antibodies persist for approximately 12 weeks after appearance. IgG antibodies to HAV follow and simply indicate exposure at some time in the past.

HAV core antigen is incorrect because hepatitis A does not possess a recognizable core antigen; the tests using core antigen apply to hepatitis B only, and antibodies to HB core antigen have nothing to do with hepatitis A. Choice e, anti-hepatitis C virus, is not correct because anti-non-A, non-B hepatitis antigen does not exist.

7. d. There are so many antigens and antibodies associated with hepatitis virology that it is difficult to figure out what is what. However, it can be simplified considerably.

Initial screening for hepatitis B should include HBsAg and anti-HBc (HBcAb, the antibody to the core antigen). These two tests will identify most cases of acute hepatitis B. There is a period between the clearance of HBsAg and the appearance of anti-HBs (HBsAb). This period lasts for 4-6 weeks, and during this time the only marker for hepatitis B that can detect the infection with any certainty is anti-HBc (HBcAb). If acute hepatitis B is suggested from the initial screening, then further laboratory tests should be ordered. These include the following:

1. HBeAg: the e antigen indicates the presence of a highly infectious or contagious state or a chronic infection.
2. anti-HBe (HBeAb, the antibody to the previously listed antigen): the presence of this antibody indicates low infectivity and predicts the later seroconversion or resolution of hepatitis B.
3. anti-HBs (HBsAb, the antibody to the surface antigen): the presence of this antibody indicates past hepatitis B infection and current immunity.

8. e. In acute viral hepatitis, the serum transaminases (serum AST and serum ALT) are elevated, along with serum bilirubin and serum alkaline phosphatase.

9. e. The clinical manifestations of cirrhosis were discussed earlier. Another common finding in cirrhosis is ascites resulting from hypoalbuminemia.

10. e. Hepatitis B vaccine should be offered to all people not previously immunized and is particularly important for those at high risk and those with continued exposure to hepatitis B infection. Those at high risk for acquiring hepatitis B include the following: (1) all health care personnel; (2) patients undergoing hemodialysis; (3) patients requiring frequent blood transfusions; (4) employees and residents of institutions for people with developmental disabilities; (5) men who have sex with men and all of their contacts; (6) intravenous drug users; (7) sexual contacts of chronic HBsAg carriers; and (8) children born to mothers who have chronic hepatitis B.

The Centers for Disease Control and Prevention (CDC) recommend all children be immunized with hepatitis B vaccine.

11. d. Chronic active hepatitis (which may lead to cirrhosis of the liver, liver failure, and hepatocellular carcinoma) is associated with hepatitis B, hepatitis C, and hepatitis D (delta virus hepatitis, which occurs only in patients who are also chronically infected with hepatitis B).

Chronic active hepatitis is not associated with hepatitis A or hepatitis E.

12. e. Cirrhosis is an irreversible inflammatory condition of disordered and disrupted liver structure and function. Cirrhosis results from the disorganization of hepatic tissues caused by diffuse fibrosis and nodular regeneration. Micronodular and macronodular fibrosis occurs. Nodules of regenerated tissue form between the fibrous bands, giving the liver a cobbled appearance. The liver is initially larger than normal in size and then usually becomes smaller than normal. The changes in the liver result in increased portal vein pressure, which leads to the formation of ascites and to esophageal varices.

13. e. In uncomplicated cirrhosis, treatment includes cessation of alcohol use, maintenance of proper nutrition, and use of beta blockers to reduce portal hypertension. Patients with uncomplicated cirrhosis may have a relatively benign course of illness for many years. Once the patient has an episode of decompensation, such as fluid retention, variceal bleeding, encephalopathy, spontaneous bacterial peritonitis, or hepatorenal syndrome, mortality is high without transplantation.

14. e. Complications of cirrhosis include the following: (1) portal hypertension, leading to esophageal varices, congestive gastropathy, and hypersplenism; (2) hepatic encephalopathy; (3) ascites, leading to spontaneous bacterial peritonitis and umbilical hernia (spontaneous rupture); (4) hepatorenal syndrome; (5) coagulation abnormalities; (6) hepatocellular carcinoma; (7) pulmonary dysfunction; (8) hepatic osteodystrophy; (9) cholelithiasis; (10) pericardial effusion; and (11) impaired reticuloendothelial system function.

SOLUTION TO THE CLINICAL CASE MANAGEMENT PROBLEM

Briefly, the relationship between cirrhosis of the liver and right-sided heart failure is that micronodular fibrosis, macronodular fibrosis, and nodular regeneration eventually lead to portal hypertension with all of its complications, one of which can be right-sided heart failure.

SUMMARY OF HEPATITIS AND CIRRHOSIS

A. Infectious forms of hepatitis:
   1. **Hepatitis A:** (a) the etiologic agent is an RNA hepatovirus; (b) sporadic or epidemic infections are spread by fecal–oral route; (c) the primary symptoms are anorexia, nausea, vomiting, malaise, and aversion to smoking; (d) the clinical signs are fever, enlarged tender liver, and jaundice; (e) the relevant laboratory findings are normal to low white blood cell count and abnormal ALT, AST, bilirubin, and alkaline phosphatase values; and (f) diagnostic clues include elevated transaminase levels and the presence of serum IgM–anti-HAV.

   The only treatment required is symptomatic, namely rest; it is rarely fulminating and does not become chronic.

   Prevention is meticulous hand washing because the oral–fecal route is the main route of spread. Although important for all, it is essential for food handlers. Hepatitis A vaccine is now available for patients at risk.

   2. **Hepatitis B:** (a) the etiologic agent is a DNA hepadnavirus; (b) it usually is transmitted sexually or by blood or blood products and is particularly common in intravenous drug users and in patients with acquired immune deficiency syndrome (AIDS); (c) up to 30% of infected individuals may be carriers; and (d) it is diagnosed by finding an elevation of liver transaminases and HBsAg and anti-HBc in the serum.

   The treatment is symptomatic unless it becomes fulminating—as it will in 0.1% to 1% of the cases—or chronic—as it will in 1% to 10% of infected adults and 90% of neonates.

The recommended treatment of symptoms is with interferon, which has a 40% success rate.

Hepatitis B hyperimmunoglobulin is used to prevent symptoms after known or suspected exposure and prevention is obtained via hepatitis B vaccine, administration of which is now recommended for all children and adults by the CDC.

3. **Hepatitis C:** (a) the etiologic agent is a single-stranded virus belonging to the *Flaviviridae* family; (b) there are more than 100 strains belonging to six major "genotypes"; (c) the disease usually is transmitted by blood or blood products, and sexual transmission is also possible; (d) the development of a screening test in 1990 virtually eliminated spread via transfusions, and it is thought that sharing of contaminated needles is the main route of transfer.

The disease course is very variable. Some 15% to 25% of infected individuals recover spontaneously. The remaining individuals become chronically infected, of whom some 10% to 20% will develop cirrhosis and another 1% to 5% will develop hepatocellular cancer.

Hepatitis C is the most common chronic bloodborne infection in the United States, with an incidence of some 35,000 cases per year. About 4 million of the U.S. population is infected, and as the population ages hepatitis C–related deaths, now about 8,000 to 10,000 per year, will increase. Presently it is the most common cause of cirrhosis and liver transplantation.

Treatment of hepatitis C is symptomatic and depends on liver biopsy staging and viral genotyping. As mentioned it often progresses to become a chronic disease, which can be treated with pegylated interferon and ribavirin. Factors associated with successful treatment include genotypes other than 1, lower baseline levels, less fibrosis on biopsy, and lower body surface area and weight. Major side effects include flulike symptoms, neuropsychiatric symptoms, and cytopenias. Sustained responses (absence of viral HCV-RNA in serum) of 55% in carefully selected individuals are typical.

4. **Delta hepatitis (hepatitis D):** Found only in association with chronic hepatitis B. This combination is particularly likely to lead to chronic active hepatitis and its complications, including cirrhosis, liver cell failure, and hepatocellular carcinoma.

5. **Hepatitis E:** An enterically transmitted form of hepatitis. Like hepatitis A, it never leads to chronic infection.

B. Alcoholic hepatitis:

The signs and symptoms of alcoholic hepatitis closely resemble the symptoms of viral hepatitis. In alcoholic hepatitis, the ratio of AST to ALT is usually 2:1.

Patients who develop alcoholic hepatitis are at high risk for developing cirrhosis of the liver. The symptoms and sign of cirrhosis are weakness, fatigue, weight loss, anorexia, hepatomegaly, spider nevi, palmar erythema, asterixis, tremor, and ascites. Patients with cirrhosis often develop portal hypertension with its complications and hepatic encephalopathy.

The treatment is supportive. The use of glucocorticoids in acute alcoholic hepatitis is controversial. Colchicine may slow disease progression. Treatments for ascites include sodium restriction, diuretics (especially spironolactone) with or without thiazides or loop diuretics, paracentesis, and shunts.

Cirrhotic liver complications include uppergastrointestinal bleeding from varices, hemorrhagic gastritis, or gastroduodenal ulcers; liver failure; hepatic encephalopathy; hepatorenal syndrome; and hepatocellular carcinoma.

SUGGESTED READING

Flamm SL: Chronic hepatitis C virus infection. *JAMA* 289(18):2413-2417, 2003.

Iredale JP: Cirrhosis: new research provides a basis for rational and targeted treatments. *BMJ* 327(7407):143-147, 2003.

Madhotra R, Gilmore IT: Recent developments in the treatment of alcoholic hepatitis. *QJM* 96(6):391-400, 2003.

Marsano LS: Hepatitis. *Prim Care* 30(1):81-107, 2003.

Russo MW, Fried MW: Side effects of therapy for chronic hepatitis C. *Gastroenterol* 124(6):1711-1719, 2003.

Ryder SD, Beckingham IJ: ABC of diseases of liver, pancreas, and biliary system: Acute hepatitis. *BMJ* 322(7279):151-153, 2001.

Schiff ER: Update in hepatology. *Ann Intern Med* 132(6):460-466, 2000.

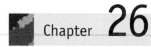

Chapter 26

Diabetes Mellitus

> "I must've gotten up 10 times last night to go to the bathroom."

CLINICAL CASE PROBLEM 1:

A 17-Year-Old Female with Weight Loss, Polyuria, and Polydipsia

A 17-year-old female comes to your office with her mother. Her mother tells you that her daughter has lost 10 lb in the last 2 months. As well, she has been increasingly thirsty and has been experiencing a significantly increased frequency of urination. The patient has been feeling generally well, but she complains that her breath smells "funny."

On examination, the patient is well below the 5th percentile for weight. She looks thin and pale. Her blood pressure is 100/70 mm Hg. She has a few anterior cervical and axillary nodes measuring 1.0 cm. Her abdomen is slightly tender. No other abnormalities are found.

■ SELECT THE BEST ANSWER TO THE FOLLOWING QUESTIONS:

1. If you could order only one test, which would it be?
   a. urine for protein and glucose
   b. finger-stick blood sugar
   c. serum electrolytes
   d. blood gases
   e. complete blood count (CBC)

2. You perform your one test. The result is 250 mg/dl. Which of the following statements is (are) false?
   a. the diagnosis of the disorder described should be confirmed with a 3-hour test
   b. dietary modifications are necessary in the treatment of this disorder
   c. candidal vaginitis is a frequent presentation of this condition in females
   d. insulin likely will be required to manage this patient's illness
   e. hospital inpatient management may not be necessary to begin treatment of this disorder

3. Which of the following statements regarding the diagnosis of the disorder described is (are) true?
   a. this disorder is confirmed if the fasting level of the particular substance exceeds 125 mg/dl on two occasions
   b. this disorder is confirmed if the venous plasma level of the particular substance exceeds 200 mg/dl on one occasion in the presence of symptoms
   c. this disorder is confirmed if the asymptomatic patient has a measurement of the particular substance that exceeds 200 mg/dl
   d. all of the above
   e. none of the above

4. Which of the following conditions is most closely associated with the described disorder?
   a. hypercholesterolemia
   b. hypothyroidism
   c. hypertriglyceridemia
   d. obesity
   e. cholelithiasis

5. What is (are) the best measure(s) of long-term control of the disease described?
   a. urine sugar levels
   b. daily fasting blood sugar levels
   c. hemoglobin A_{1C}
   d. hemoglobin F
   e. no microvascular or macrovascular complications

6. The hemoglobin A_{1C} should be below what value to be of use in predicting the development of microvascular and macrovascular complications?
   a. 3.5%
   b. 5.0%
   c. 7.0%
   d. 9.0%
   e. 10.0%

7. Which of the following statements is true?
   a. microvascular complications are associated with type 1 diabetes; macrovascular complications are associated with type 2 diabetes
   b. macrovascular complications are associated with type 1 diabetes; microvascular complications are associated with type 2 diabetes
   c. microvascular and macrovascular complications are associated with type 1 diabetes; neither is associated with type 2 diabetes
   d. microvascular and macrovascular complications are associated with both type 1 and type 2 diabetes
   e. none of the above

8. An example of a macrovascular complication of diabetes is:
   a. myocardial infarction
   b. gastroparesis
   c. loss of vision
   d. renal failure
   e. peripheral neuropathy

9. Which of the following treatments does not decrease the risk of macrovascular disease in diabetes?
   a. advise the patient to stop smoking
   b. prescribe simvastatin
   c. prescribe vitamin E
   d. prescribe low-dose aspirin
   e. prescribe enalapril

10. Which statement is false regarding the treatment of diabetic nephropathy?
    a. if the patient has evidence of nephropathy, he or she also should be checked for likely retinopathy
    b. amitriptyline is useful in the treatment of nephropathy
    c. enalapril is useful in the treatment of nephropathy
    d. metoprolol is useful in the treatment of nephropathy
    e. improving glycemic control will decrease the progression of nephropathy

CLINICAL CASE PROBLEM 2:
A 64-Year-Old Woman with Burning Feet

A 64-year-old woman with type 2 diabetes is complaining of a burning sensation in her feet at night. On your physical examination you note decreased sensations in her toes and calluses on her lateral 5th digits.

11. Appropriate care of this patient's neuropathy includes:
    a. referral to podiatry
    b. topical capsaicin
    c. improved glycemic control
    d. a and c
    e. all of the above

12. Which one of the following statements is true regarding diabetic nephropathy in the United States?
    a. the prevalence of diabetic nephropathy is contributed to mainly by people with type 1 diabetes
    b. the prevalence of diabetic nephropathy is contributed to mainly by people with type 2 diabetes
    c. the ratio of people with type 2 diabetes to people with type 1 diabetes in the United States is 10 to 1
    d. the ratio of people with type 1 diabetes to people with type 2 diabetes in the United States is 2 to 1

    e. a and d
    f. b and c

CLINICAL CASE PROBLEM 3:
A 27-Year-Old Patient with Type 1 Diabetes with Protein in Her Urine

A 27-year-old patient with type 1 diabetes presents to your office for her regular 3-month checkup. Her urine microalbumin is in the 80s on three spot samples. A 24-hour urine test produces a protein reading of 150 mg.

13. What should your next management step be?
    a. do nothing—this is microalbuminuria
    b. do nothing—this is still considered normal
    c. start the patient taking an angiotensin-converting enzyme (ACE) inhibitor
    d. change the patient's diet—decrease protein by 10% a day
    e. refer the patient to a diabetologist

14. Which one of the following statements regarding dietary recommendation to the patient described in Clinical Case Problem 1 is false?
    a. make an effort to distribute carbohydrate intake evenly throughout the day
    b. eating a high-fiber diet improves glycemic control, allowing the patient to consume more carbohydrate
    c. total fat intake should be limited to reduce total caloric consumption
    d. a prudent diabetic diet limits high-sugar foods
    e. high-protein diets should be avoided in patients with longstanding diabetes

15. Which statement is false regarding insulin therapy in diabetes?
    a. human insulin is the only available insulin in the United States
    b. average insulin doses are 0.6 to 0.8 units/kg of body weight per day
    c. Glargine insulin should be given within 30 minutes of starting a meal
    d. insulin can be coadministered with oral sulfonylureas
    e. in long-time type 2 diabetes, insulin can be added at bedtime to improve control

16. A newly diagnosed patient with type 1 diabetes is diagnosed and started taking a total insulin dose of 18 units. Which of the following is likely to be the correct morning/evening: AM/PM: regular/intermediate insulin dose?

a. morning: total 12 units: regular 6 units, intermediate 6 units
   evening: total 6 units: regular 3 units, intermediate 3 units
b. morning: total 9 units: regular 6 units, intermediate 3 units
   evening: total 9 units: regular 6 units, intermediate 6 units
c. morning: total 12 units: regular 4 units, intermediate 8 units
   evening: total 6 units: regular 2 units, intermediate 4 units
d. morning: total 6 units: regular 4 units, intermediate 2 units
   evening: total 12 units: regular 4 units, intermediate 8 units
e. morning: total 6 units: regular 3 units, intermediate 3 units
   evening: total 12 units: regular 8 units, intermediate 4 units

17. What is the most likely explanation for the "abnormal gas in the stomach" seen in upright abdominal radiographs of many patients with diabetes?
    a. gastroparesis as a result of diabetic autonomic neuropathy
    b. gastroparesis as a result of sympathetic dysfunction
    c. associated with diabetic ketoacidosis
    d. associated with hyperosmolar coma
    e. none of the above

18. Regarding the pathophysiology of the disorder described in Clinical Case Problem 1, which of the following statements is (are) true?
    a. environmental factors are likely involved in the pathology of this condition
    b. human leukocyte antigen (HLA-DR4) is strongly associated with this condition
    c. this disorder may be associated with other autoimmune disorders
    d. all of the above
    e. none of the above

CLINICAL CASE PROBLEM 4:
A 65-Year-Old Female with a Fasting Sugar of 240 mg/dl

A 65-year-old asymptomatic obese female has a routine fasting sugar drawn at the time of her annual physical examination. The level comes back at 240 mg/dl. Her urine is negative for ketones. The test is repeated the following day and comes back at the same level.

19. Which of the following statements about this patient is (are) incorrect?
    a. the patient has type 2 diabetes mellitus
    b. insulin is the agent of first choice in the management of this condition
    c. a diabetic diet forms the cornerstone of therapy in this condition
    d. increased physical activity is indicated
    e. monitoring of this condition is best done by home glucose monitoring

20. The described patient returns to discuss her condition with you. At this time, you should:
    a. check her serum creatinine
    b. check her fasting lipid profile
    c. check her CBC
    d. a and b
    e. all of the above

21. She returns in 3 months after unsuccessfully trying diet and weight loss. Her HbA_{1C} is 7.3%. What do you do at this time?
    a. prescribe glyburide
    b. prescribe metformin
    c. continue diet therapy only
    d. prescribe enalapril
    e. prescribe pioglitazone

22. Which of the following statements regarding type 2 diabetes is false?
    a. impaired glucose tolerance is defined by a fasting blood sugar range of 100–125
    b. elevated fasting blood sugar provides the first evidence of loss of glucose control
    c. lifestyle changes of increased physical activity and improved nutrition can decrease the risk of developing diabetes by 50% or more.
    d. metformin may be effective in decreasing the risk of developing diabetes
    e. lifestyle changes are more effective than treatment with metformin

23. Which of the following statements regarding type 2 diabetes mellitus is true?
    a. most patients present to their physicians with symptoms
    b. most patients are essentially asymptomatic at diagnosis (apart from being obese)
    c. most patients can control the diabetes by diet and exercise
    d. most patients will not manifest complications
    e. most patients are younger than age 40

CLINICAL CASE MANAGEMENT PROBLEM

A patient who you had been treating for type 2 diabetes and who has been struggling to adhere to a sensible diet comes to your office for a follow-up appointment and tells you he has great news: "I found a new simple way to design a diet that will keep my HbA1c values below 7% by only eating low glycemic index foods." What should your response be? How do you explain what the glycemic index (GI) is? Is there any value to the GI concept? What can you tell your patient about the GI that may help him develop better eating habits?

■ ANSWERS:

1. **b.** A finger-stick blood sugar test is the one to order.

2. **a.** The diagnosis of the described disorder need not be confirmed with a 3-hour test.

3. **d.** This patient has diabetes mellitus type 1. Diabetes mellitus type 1 is also known as insulin-dependent diabetes and must be managed with a combination of a diabetic diet using "exchanges," human insulin, and exercise. Unless the patient has diabetic ketoacidosis, there is no reason that both diagnosis and initial management cannot take place on an outpatient basis.

The diagnosis of diabetes mellitus type 1 is very important. The criteria that have been adopted by the American Diabetes Association are as follows: (1) one fasting plasma glucose value exceeding 125 mg/dl, or (2) one random plasma glucose value exceeding 199 mg/dl in the presence of symptoms, or (3) a 2-hour postglucose value exceeding 199 mg/dl in an oral glucose tolerance test.

Each must be confirmed on a subsequent day by a different method for diagnosis to occur. In the patient described, criterion 2 can be used to make the diagnosis of diabetes mellitus. A random nonfasting glucose of 160 mg/dl or greater is considered a positive screen and warrants further testing as mentioned to determine if the diagnostic criteria can be met.

4. **c.** The disease of those listed that is most closely associated with diabetes mellitus is hypertriglyceridemia. Triglyceride levels of two to three times normal are often the first sign of undiagnosed diabetes mellitus. All individuals with a significantly elevated serum triglyceride level should be screened for diabetes mellitus.

5. **c.** The best measure of long-term control of diabetes mellitus (type 1 and type 2) is hemoglobin A_{1c}.

6. **c.** Recent studies have shown that "tight control" (i.e., maintenance of the mean plasma glucose at less than 155 mg/dl and hemoglobin A_{1c} at 7.0% or less) produces at least a 60% reduction in microvascular and macrovascular complications.

7. **d.** One very important and underappreciated fact is that both macrovascular (atherosclerotic heart disease, coronary artery disease, peripheral vascular disease, cerebrovascular disease) and microvascular disease (retinopathy, nephropathy, peripheral neuropathy, autonomic neuropathy) are associated with both types of diabetes.

Patients with type 2 diabetes are not immune to diabetic complications; quite the contrary is true.

8. **a.** Retinopathy, nephropathy and neuropathy are all examples of microvascular disease. Gastroparesis is a form of autonomic neuropathy.

9. **c.** Recent studies have not been able to demonstrate a positive effect of vitamin E on macrovascular complications. Macrovascular complications are large-vessel disease and are best treated with approaches that decrease risk for heart attack. These include lowering blood pressure, stopping smoking, lowering hyperglycemia and hyperinsulinemia, losing weight and exercising, lowering cholesterol, and undergoing aspirin therapy.

10. **b.** Amitriptyline is for symptomatic chronic pain management of diabetic peripheral neuropathy. Peripheral neuropathy can present in various ways including fatigue, muscle weakness, chronic pain, paraesthesia (pins and needles, electriclike shocks, burning, cold), dysaesthesia (strange feeling on touching objects), hypothesia, or anesthesia (numbness, loss of feeling), ataxia, and paralysis. It often acts bilaterally in a "glove and sock manner" causing lose of manual dexterity, difficulty in walking, or inability to react to pain, resulting in diabetic foot ulcers and eventually possible amputation.

Usually retinopathy and nephropathy coexist; therefore if one is found, the other needs to be evaluated for. Lowering blood pressure and good glycemic control are cornerstones of treatment.

11. **d.** The best management of diabetic foot problems involves podiatric care for careful debridement of corns and calluses that might predispose to foot

ulcers. Improved glycemic control is the primary available treatment for the pathology underlying neuropathy. Medications such as gabapentin and amitriptyline may be used to help relieve neuropathy-associated chronic pain. Although topical capsaicin cream is used to help relieve pain, it does so by creating a burning sensation itself and is not recommended to relieve a burning sensation such as that described in this case.

12. f. Because there are at least 10 patients with type 2 diabetes for each patient with type 1 diabetes, the prevalence of complications resulting from type 2 diabetes is higher than for type 1 diabetes.

13. c. The patient with diabetes who presents with microalbuminuria already has a problem. The probability of this individual developing overt nephropathy is quite high. It has been demonstrated that progression to overt nephropathy can be prevented by the prophylactic administration of an ACE inhibitor or angiotensin receptor blocker.

14. b. Diet is an essential component of treatment in all patients with diabetes. It is especially important, however, for the patient with insulin-dependent type 1 diabetes. In the patient with insulin-dependent diabetes the rate at which insulin enters the blood from an injection site is fixed, and the patients must match meals to the pattern of insulin absorption. A high-fiber diet slows the rate of glucose or fructose absorption, which decreases the initial insulin surge from the beta cells, a fact of importance to the patient with type 2 diabetes. However, in the long run the same amount of glucose will be accessible and the total insulin demand will be the same. Thus to the patient with type 1 diabetes who has nonfunctional beta cells and is taking a set amount of insulin, the fiber content is not a relevant factor.

During the past several years the avoidance of sweets and foods that contain simple carbohydrates has been challenged by the concept of the glycemic index that proposes the rate at which a substance is converted to glucose is also important. However, as was the case with fiber, this concept is only applicable to the patient with type 2 diabetes; until further information is presented it seems reasonable to instruct all patients with diabetes to avoid beverages with sucrose and desserts that are highly sweetened.

The patient with diabetes undergoing insulin therapy must have three meals at fixed times each day, with a fixed distribution of calories. Frequent snacks, also with a fixed distribution of calories, also are recommended.

If a patient with diabetes is overweight, a weight-reducing program should be initiated. This may be facilitated by substituting complex carbohydrates with high residue for simple sugars. As well, saturated animal fats should be replaced with polyunsaturated vegetable fats. One-fifth of the daily caloric intake should be consumed at breakfast and about two-fifths at each of lunch and supper. These percentages may be reduced to allow for small snacks, such as crackers or fruit, in mid-afternoon and bedtime. A reasonable exercise program is fundamental to the treatment of all patients with diabetes. Also the patient with diabetes should moderate sugar and alcohol consumption and limit intake of high-sugar foods. Because carbohydrate has the greatest impact on blood glucose, its effect can be minimized by spreading out carbohydrate consumption evenly throughout the day. Discourage the use of high-protein fad diets in all people with longstanding diabetes and with particular emphasis to those with impaired renal function.

15. c. Human insulin is the only available insulin in the United States. The average insulin doses are 0.6–0.8 units/kg of body weight per day.

Glargine insulin is very long acting and should be given once daily, often in the evening or at bedtime. Lispro insulin is quick acting and should be given within 30 minutes of starting a meal.

Insulin can be coadministered with oral sulfonylureas. In long-time type 2 diabetes, long-acting or intermediate-acting insulin can be added at bedtime to improve control.

16. c. The starting dose of insulin is usually as follows: (1) morning—two-thirds of total daily dose; (2) evening—one-third of total daily dose; (3) morning—two-thirds intermediate, one-third regular; and (4) evening—two-thirds intermediate, one-third regular.

17. a. The "abnormal gas in the stomach" is most likely the result of diabetic gastroparesis, an autonomic neuropathy variant. This is a very common complaint, and it is best treated by a prokinetic agent, such as metoclopramide or domperidone, or by macrolide antibiotics.

18. d. Two distinct types of type 1 diabetes have been identified. In type 1A, the environmental factors combined with genetic factors are thought to result in cell-mediated destruction of pancreatic beta cells. Human leukocyte antigen (HLA-DR4) is strongly associated with this phenomenon.

Type 1B is an uncommon primary autoimmune condition that occurs in individuals with other autoimmune conditions, such as Hashimoto's disease, Graves' disease, pernicious anemia, and myasthenia gravis. This condition is associated with histocompatibility antigen HLA-DR3 and occurs later in life, typically between the ages of 30 and 50.

Specific environmental factors linked to type 1 diabetes mellitus include the following: (1) drugs and chemicals (streptozocin and pentamidine); and (2) viruses (mumps, coxsackie, rubella [40% of patients with congenital rubella develop type 1 diabetes late], and cytomegalovirus.

19. b. This patient has type 2 diabetes mellitus, in which insulin is not used as the initial treatment.

20. d. Because nephropathy is often an early development in type 2 diabetes her serum creatinine level should be checked; similarly, because dyslipidemia is also an early complication, her fasting lipid profile should be ascertained.

21. b. As mentioned earlier, this patient has type 2 diabetes mellitus, which accounts for 90% of all cases of diabetes; it is characterized by both an impairment of beta-cell function and a decreased sensitivity to insulin in the cells of the body.

Type 2 diabetes mellitus often is discovered in asymptomatic patients by finding an elevated blood sugar. It also may present with nonspecific symptoms including fatigue, weakness, blurred vision, vaginal and perineal pruritus and candidiasis, impotence, and paresthesias. Unlike the patient with type 1 diabetes, weight loss is uncommon in these patients. In fact, the majority of patients with type 2 diabetes mellitus are obese and many have a strong family history of obesity and diabetes.

A reasonable workup for the diagnosis of type 2 diabetes includes laboratory evaluation of fasting or random plasma glucose; HbA$_{1C}$; fasting lipid profile; serum creatinine; and urinalysis for ketone, glucose, protein and microalbumin.

A diabetic diet plus weight management plus exercise should be pushed to the maximum. If these are not effective, the oral hypoglycemic agent metformin should be the next step. Oral hypoglycemic agents currently available include sulfonylureas, alpha-glucosidase inhibitors, biguanides, meglitinides and thiazolidinediones. The first-generation sulfonylurea agents include tolbutamide, chlorpropamide, acetohexamide, and tolazamide. The second-generation agents include glyburide, glipizide, and glimepiride. These sulfonylureas work by stimulating the secretion of insulin in the pancreas. One member of this class glimepiride (Amaryl) is claimed to also increase insulin sensitivity in the peripheral tissue. All sulfonylureas tend to induce weight gain and like insulin itself can induce hypoglycemia.

Biguanides inhibit gluconeogenesis; thus they decrease the production of glucose. They also decrease the rate of glucose absorption and increase its uptake in the periphery. Because of the rare complication of lactic acidosis, biguanides should be used with caution, particularly in patients with renal insufficiency. Despite these precautions, biguanides have become the recommended first line of therapy for adult patients with type 2 diabetes. The only biguanide available is metformin, sold as Glucophage and Glucophage XL, a slow-release variant. Two advantages of metformin are it should not induce hypoglycemia and it does not promote weight gain.

Meglitinides are nonsulfonylurea benzoic acid derivatives that work by stimulating insulin release from the pancreas but by a different mechanism than the sulfonylureas; they have a short half-life and have a reduced effectiveness at normal fasting glucose levels. Therefore they are to be taken shortly before a meal (1 to 30 minutes) to reduce the postprandial hyperglycemic surge, which has been shown to play an important role in causing secondary complications. Postmeal serum glucose levels should not regularly be greater than 162 mg/dl and levels higher than 180 mg/dl are grounds for action. Prandin (repaglinide) and Starlix (nateglinide) are U.S. Food and Drug Administration–approved meglitinides. Drug interactions have been reported to enhance the activity of these drugs, possibly creating a risk of hypoglycemia. The manufacturer warns that nateglinide should not be used in the presence of other drugs that enhance insulin secretion; similarly a Finnish study has shown that gemfibrozil (Lopid) increases the circulating concentration of repaglinide; this effect is enhanced if itraconazole (Sporanox) also is being used.

Thiazolidinedione (TZD) derivatives, such as pioglitazone (Actos) and rosiglitazone (Avandia), decrease insulin resistance and also inhibit liver gluconeogenesis. TZDs can cause elevations in hepatic enzymes, jaundice, and in rare instances hepatic failure. They are also contraindicated in severe cardiac heart failure because they facilitate fluid retention.

The alpha-glucosidase inhibitors, acarbose (Precose) or miglitol (Glyset), work by slowing the rate of disaccharide and polysaccharide hydrolysis, thereby reducing the rate of glucose absorption and the peak glucose levels. They have been associated with gastrointestinal discomfort.

Oral hypoglycemic therapy should begin with the lowest effective dose; this then should be increased every few days to achieve maximal control. Self-monitoring of blood glucose is the key to the evaluation of efficacy of an oral hypoglycemic–mediated treatment program.

About 25% to 30% of patients with type 2 diabetes mellitus fail to respond to sulfonylurea drugs. These patients are called primary failures. In addition, about 5% of patients who initially responded to these drugs will lose their responsiveness. These patients are termed secondary failures. Sometimes a combination of a morning oral hypoglycemic and an evening intermediate-acting insulin can be beneficial in lowering blood sugar to normal.

With the several classes of agents now available, other combination therapies are available besides combination with insulin. Sulfonylureas maybe combined with several different classes of agents. Sulfonylureas may be combined with metformin, acarbose, and troglitazone. Sulfonylureas also may be combined with the meglitinides. Repaglinide may be used in combination with metformin. All combination therapies require the same careful attention to side-effect profiles and outcomes that monotherapies do. Nevertheless, with the increased variety and range of agents available, patients with type 2 diabetes now have more options for effective pharmacotherapy.

22. b. Although rarely measured in the usual clinical setting, postprandial glucose abnormalities, not elevated fasting blood glucose levels, usually provide the first evidence of such impaired glycemic control.

The pre–type 2 diabetic condition sometimes is called the insulin resistance syndrome or syndrome X and is marked by obesity, dyslipidemia, hypertension, and increased resistance to the action of circulating insulin. The pancreatic beta cells compensate by increasing the secretion of insulin until eventually glucose levels increase and a diagnosis of type 2 diabetes can be made. This syndrome may exist for decades before a diagnosis of frank diabetes can be made and may initiate some of the common diabetic complications. Therefore it is important to identify and treat the patient with prediabetes.

The patient with pre-type 2 diabetes may be diagnosed with reasonable certainty by either (1) a 2-hour postprandial glucose level greater than 140 mg/dl and less than 200 mg/dl (because there is no such thing as a standard meal, this usually is done via a 75-g oral glucose tolerance test ([OGTT]); or

(2) at least two consecutive fasting plasma glucose values greater than 100 mg/dl and less than 126 mg/dl. Because neither of these test are done routinely, they should be done because of a strong clinical suspicion made on the basis of the simultaneous presence of several of the following criteria: race (Mexican-American, some Native American tribes [mainly the Southwestern pueblo tribes]); family history; and personal history, including age (older than age 45 years), dyslipidemia, obesity [body mass index of 30>kg/m², abdominal in particular], history of gestational diabetes, history of polycystic ovary syndrome, and hypertension.

Treatment of prediabetes can reduce the risk of type 2 diabetes in this population by about 58%. The following treatments are recommended for patients suspected of having prediabetes: (1) an intensive lifestyle behavioral change including a nutrition and activity plan by a registered dietitian, health educator, or other qualified health professional. (Because motivation often is lacking in the patient with prediabetes, ongoing support of behavioral change is necessary.); (2) cardiovascular risk reduction appropriate to the needs of the individual; and (3) regular follow-up and reassessment of risks including rescreening for diabetes every 1-3 years.

There also is some evidence supporting the value of diabetes prevention during the prediabetic state through pharmacotherapy with biguanides (metformin), alpha-glucosidase inhibitors, ACE inhibitors, and thiazolidinediones. However, none of these treatments have been extensively studied and represent off-label usage of these drugs.

23. b. Patients with type 2 diabetes demonstrate the following: (1) except for being obese, most patients are asymptomatic (identification most often occurs by screening); (2) most patients are older than age 40; (3) most patients develop the same complications (microvascular and macrovascular complications) as in patients with type 1 diabetes; and (4) most patients have motivational difficulties in relation to diet and exercise.

SOLUTION TO THE CLINICAL CASE MANAGEMENT PROBLEM

1. What is the glycemic index? The GI is a comparison of the ability of various foods, administered one at a time, to raise postprandial glucose values, their

so-called glycemic response. This glycemic response is compared to a control, usually 50 g of glucose given a GI value of 100, or alternately to an equivalent amount

SOLUTION TO THE CLINICAL CASE MANAGEMENT PROBLEM—cont'd

of white bread also set at 100 (using the white bread standard, the GI value of glucose is 140). The lower the GI value of the food tested, the lower the post-prandial glucose peak and presumably the better for the patient with type 2 diabetes. It sounds simple, yet it has raised a great deal of controversy. It sounds simple, yet it has raised a great deal of controversy. Both the American Diabetic Association (ADA) and the American Heart Association (AHA) have come out against it, feeling the older system of carbohydrate counting and the food exchange system are simpler to understand and provide a more reliable guide and that the GI system is popularized by commercial diet programs as a way to sell their products. However, the GI system is endorsed, to a greater or lesser degree, by the Australian and Canadian Diabetic Associations and by the World Health Organization and now is advocated by your patient.

2. Is there any value to the GI concept? Obviously avoiding those food that raise the postprandial glucose peak to a great degree would be of value to the patient with type 2 diabetes. This is the same rational as used in prescribing Acarbose; in fact a meta-analysis reported by Brand-Miller and colleagues in 2003 indicates that using the GI as a dietary guide provides a small but clinically usefully reduction in HbA1c values, about as much as use of Acarbose.

As rightly stressed by the ADA and AHA, one of the greatest faults of the GI system is its inherent complexity. In large part this is because the comparisons are made on the basis of glucose equivalents in a food and ignore the total amount of carbohydrate. Thus, for example, the GI value of carrots is 131; at face value eating carrots is a greater risk to the patient with diabetes than consuming glucose. This might be true if the patient with diabetes ate the 50 pounds or so of carrots required to ingest the 50 g of glucose the index is based on. To circumvent this problem, GI advocates have devised a new index, the glucose load (GL). The GL is determined by multiplying the GI by the percent carbohydrate (about 4% for carrots); thus the GL for carrots is only 5 ($131 \times 0.04 = 5$), and carrots are returned to the status of an acceptable food. In essence the GL index is similar to the old concept of glucose load; both systems advise patients to eat vegetables and other low-carbohydrate foods.

The real potential value of the GI and its offspring (the GL system) is in uncovering differences in the rate of digestion and absorption of foods. Once again for the most part the GI and the older systems arrive at the same conclusions, namely unprocessed foods and foods with fiber are better for a person because the carbohydrate they contain is digested and absorbed more slowly. However, the GI system does provide a few surprises. For instance, the GI/GL value for mashed potatoes is higher than for baked potatoes because presumably mashing speeds up digestion.

Another surprise of the GI/GL systems is that simple sugars have lower index values than complex carbohydrates. Although mechanisms (based on digestive enzyme levels and different modes of absorption and metabolism of fructose) can be devised to explain why complex carbohydrates may be broken down and absorbed more quickly than simple ones, the truth still is sugar lacks the fiber, vitamins, and minerals found in potatoes (i.e., a person can't live on empty calories alone); no sane clinician would recommend sugar as a significant part of anybody's diet, let alone for a person with diabetes. However, fruits can be eaten in significant quantities because they provide many valuable nutrients besides fruit sugar (fructose); moreover, the fact that fructose provides a smaller postprandial peak than an equivalent amount of glucose, as demonstrated by the GI, is an added bonus.

3. What can you tell your patient about the GI that may help him develop better eating habits? Because he is already hooked on the GI diet, it would be best not to simply pooh-pooh it; instead, work with him and try to get the maximum benefit. It probably would be a good idea to advise him about the GL index; following this may be easier for him and psychologically more acceptable than trying to adhere to the carbohydrate exchange system, and, as discussed earlier, both arrive at similar conclusions. Also you should explain that table sugar should be avoided, although its GI value is lower than that of many other foods. Another shortcoming of the GI/GS system is that it only considers one food at a time; thus, it is important to point out the value of a balanced diet, of proteins, and even of the essentially fatty acids. With these thoughts in mind, in the long run the major difference in his GI/GL-based diet as compared to one based on the exchange system is that he might be substituting whole-wheat bread for white bread,

Continued

SOLUTION TO THE CLINICAL CASE MANAGEMENT PROBLEM—cont'd

whole-wheat spaghetti for ordinary spaghetti, and so on (i.e., substituting foods with a lower GI/GL value for a similar food having the same exchange value), adding more fruit, and making other similar small changes. Moreover, he may find the new system more psychologically satisfying, at least until he tires of it. Thus, at least for this patient, with the caveats mentioned, the GI/GL system may be used to help him reduce his HbA1c value a fraction of a percent, a small but significant advantage.

SUMMARY OF DIABETES MELLITUS

A. Type 1 diabetes:
1. **Epidemiology:** 10% of all cases of diabetes
2. **Signs/symptoms:** Polyuria, polydipsia, nocturia, weight loss
3. **Etiology:** Genetics plus environment:
   a. Most common: HLA-DR4 plus viral exposure
   b. Less common: associated with other autoimmune diseases.
4. **Diagnosis:**
   a. Two fasting values of 126 mg/dl or greater
   b. One random blood sugar 200 mg/dl plus symptoms
   c. Two blood sugars 200 mg/dl in a 3-hour 75-g glucose tolerance test (GTT) (one value at 2-hours)
5. **Self-monitoring:** Home blood sugar monitoring, emphasizing strict control reduces complications. When there is a risk of hypoglycemia, recommend 4 values 3 times a week.
6. **Long-term control (every 3 months; red cell turnover is 102 days):** Hemoglobin A_{1c} (HbA$_{1c}$) less than 7.0%. Fructosamine analysis is a newer measure (based on glycated serum protein turnover [average about 17 days]) that can be used to measure intermediate control (2–4 weeks). It is particularly useful to monitor changes in patients in which control is deteriorating and in patients with hemoglobinopathies (abnormal HB turnover times) in which HbA$_{1c}$ values are not reliable.
7. **Treatment:**
   a. Diet
   b. Exercise
   c. Insulin (regular/intermediate): The total initial insulin dose is 15-20 units using the rule of two-thirds (i.e., two-thirds total dose in the morning (split 2:1, regular:intermediate) and one-third total dose in the evening (split 2:1, regular:intermediate)

8. **Complications:** Both macrovascular and microvascular. Both in type 1 and type 2 diabetes mellitus macrovascular and microvascular complications are present. Because the ratio of type 2/type 1 diabetics is 10/1, of 100 cases of diabetic nephropathy, more than 80% of the secondary complications are the result of type 2 diabetes.

B. Type 2 diabetes mellitus:
1. **Epidemiology:** 90% of all cases of diabetes mellitus are type 2.
2. **Signs/symptoms:** Because a minority of patients with type 2 diabetes present with symptoms, most patients are discovered when undergoing screening in a medical setting.
3. **Risk factors:**
   a. Race (such as Native American)
   b. Type 2 diabetes in a first-degree relative
   c. Obesity
4. **Diagnosis:** Diagnosis of type 2 diabetes is the same as type 1.
5. **Self-monitoring:** Same as type 1. However for the patient with type 2 diabetes, also recommend at least a 2-hour postprandial determination after meals containing newer foods; in this way the patient can self-estimate what and/or how much he or she can or cannot eat and help monitor diet.
6. **Long-term control:** Same as type 1.
7. **Treatment:**
   a. Weight control absolutely essential
   b. Exercise almost daily
   c. Oral hypoglycemics: second- or first-degree oral agents as summarized in Table 26-1.
   d. A small percentage (15% to 20%) of patients with type 2 diabetes need insulin in the evening in addition to oral hypoglycemics (Glyburide/Glipizide) in the morning.
8. **Complications:** Same as type 1 diabetes mellitus.

Table 26-1 Classes of Oral Hypoglycemic Agents

Class	Example	Mechanism of action	Comments
Sulfonylureas	Many, see A21, for several	Increases insulin secretion	Sulfonylureas have the potential of causing hypoglycemia and tend to cause weight gain.
α-Glucoside inhibitors	Acarbose miglitol	Reduces post-meal glucose surge by delaying CHO absorption, when taken with the first bite of a meal	Tends to cause gas, bloating and diarrhea, thus not to be used by patients with intestinal disease. Since it slows CHO absorption, any advent of hypoglycemia should be treated with glucose not a more complex CHO. However, when used alone it will not induce hypoglycemia or weight gain.
Biguanides	Metformin	Decreases gluconeogenesis and intestinal absorption and increases peripheral uptake	Doesn't promote weight gain or hypoglycemia when used alone. In rare cases it can cause lactic acidosis.
Meglitinides	Repaglinide nateglinide	Increases insulin secretion after meals and thereby reduces the level of the postprandial surge	To be taken within 30 minutes before meals and CHO rich snacks. Can cause hypoglycemia, particularly if taken without a meal containing CHO.
Thiazolindinediones	Rosiglitazone pioglitazone	Decreases insulin resistance and inhibits gluconeogenesis	Potential of liver damage. Takes 4-6 weeks to show an effect. May induce ovulation.

SUGGESTED READING

American Diabetes Association at http://www.diabetes.org.

American Diabetes Association: Implications of the diabetes control and complications trial. *Diabetes Care*: 23(suppl 1) S24-S76, 2000.

Bastry EJ III, et al: Therapy focused on postprandial glucose, not fasting glucose may be superior for lowering HbA1c. IOEZ study group. *Diabetes Care* 23(9):1236-1241, 2000.

Brand-Miller J, et al: Low-glycemic index diets in the management of diabetes: A meta-analysis of randomly controlled trials. *Diabetes Care* 26:2261-2267, 2003.

Dunstan DW, et al: The rising prevalence of diabetes and impaired glucose tolerance: the Australian Diabetes, Obesity and Lifestyle Study. *Diabetes Care* 25(5):829-834, 2002.

Institute for Clinical Systems Improvement (ICSI). *Management of type 2 diabetes mellitus.* Bloomington, MN: Institute for Clinical Systems Improvement, 2002 Sep.

Liu S, et al: A prospective study of dietary glycemic load, carbohydrate intake and risk of coronary heart disease. *Am J Clin Nutr* 76(6):1455-1461, 2000.

National Institute of Diabetes, Digestive Disorders, and Kidney Disease at http://www.niddk.nih.gov.

Rao G: Insulin resistance syndrome. *Am Fam Phys* 63:1159-1163, 1165-1166, 2001.

Sherwin RS, et al: American Diabetes Association and the NIH Institute of Diabetes and Digestive and Kidney Disease Workgroup on Diabetes. The Prevention or Delay of Type 2 Diabetes. *Diabetes Care* 25:742-749, 2002.

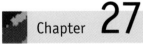

Chapter 27

Thyroid

"You are giving me radioactive iodine. Isn't that the same stuff that causes cancer after a nuclear plant accident?"

CLINICAL CASE PROBLEM 1:

A 38-YEAR-OLD FEMALE WITH SWEATING, PALPITATIONS, NERVOUSNESS, IRRITABILITY, AND TREMOR

A 38-year-old female comes to your office with a 3-month history of sweating, palpitations, weight loss, nervousness, irritability, insomnia, hand tremors, and diarrhea. She has had no significant past illnesses. One of her sisters has rheumatoid arthritis. The patient, a stockbroker, is finding it harder and harder to perform her job because of profound fatigue and inability to concentrate.

On examination, her blood pressure is 110/70 mm Hg. Her pulse is 120 and regular. She demonstrates mild proptosis; you feel a smooth, diffusely enlarged, and nontender thyroid gland. Cardiovascular examination reveals a loud S1 and a loud S2 with an ejection systolic murmur heard loudest along the left sternal edge. This murmur does not radiate. No other abnormalities are noted.

■ SELECT THE BEST ANSWER TO THE FOLLOWING QUESTIONS:

1. What is the most likely diagnosis in this patient?
   a. toxic multinodular goiter
   b. Graves' disease

c. Hashimoto's thyroiditis
d. pheochromocytoma
e. panic disorder

2. What is the etiology of the disorder described?
   a. idiopathic
   b. an autoimmune disease
   c. a hereditary disease
   d. the result of an as-yet-undetermined interaction between genetic and environmental factors
   e. iatrogenic in most cases

3. What is the best test to diagnose this condition?
   a. 24-hour radioiodine uptake test
   b. thyroid scan
   c. free serum T4
   d. serum thyroid-stimulating hormone (TSH)
   e. thyroid antibodies

4. What is the treatment of choice for the patient presented in Clinical Case Problem 1?
   a. propylthiouracil
   b. methimazole
   c. radioactive iodine
   d. subtotal thyroidectomy
   e. propranolol

5. What medications are curative in the disease presented in Clinical Case Problem 1?
   a. methimazole
   b. propranolol
   c. levothyroxine
   d. prednisone

6. The recommended treatment of choice is undertaken in this patient. Which of the following will be the end result of this treatment?
   a. complete cure: no further medication or other treatments necessary
   b. complete cure: hyperthyroid medication should be started immediately and continued for life
   c. complete cure: patient should be monitored every 6 months for the development of hypothyroidism
   d. partial cure: hypothyroid medication needed for 5 years
   e. partial cure: hyperthyroid medication needed for 5 years

7. Untreated hyperthyroidism can lead to:
   a. increased bone density
   b. amenorrhea
   c. atrial fibrillation
   d. dry skin
   e. thyroid nodules

8. The patient tells you that she would like to get pregnant in 2 years. Which statement is false regarding the treatment of hyperthyroidism in women of childbearing age?
   a. propylthiouracil is recommended for use in pregnant women
   b. women treated with radioactive iodine before pregnancy have children with a higher incidence of birth defects
   c. thyroidectomy is indicated for pregnant women who cannot tolerate antithyroid medications
   d. radioactive iodine treatment is contraindicated in pregnant women because it may destroy fetal thyroid tissue
   e. in pregnant women, propylthiouracil is preferred over methimazole

CLINICAL CASE PROBLEM 2:
A 25-YEAR-OLD FEMALE WITH A HIGHER-THAN-NORMAL T4 LEVEL

A 25-year-old female is seen for her periodic health examination. Her past history is unremarkable; she is feeling well at present and currently is taking the oral contraceptive pill.

On physical examination, her blood pressure is 130/75 mm Hg. Examination reveals that the head and neck are completely normal; specifically, no abnormalities of the thyroid gland are noted. A routine serum T4 level done is elevated at 13 mg/dl (169 nmol/l).

9. What is the most likely explanation for the elevated T4 level in this patient?
   a. Graves' disease
   b. thyrotoxicosis
   c. toxic nodular goiter
   d. an elevated thyroid binding globulin (TBG) secondary to the oral contraceptive pill
   e. laboratory error

10. To confirm your diagnosis in the patient just described, which of the following would you order?
    a. the all-out, all-inclusive, miss-nothing workup
    b. serum T3
    c. serum TBG
    d. serum free T4
    e. serum TSH
    f. d or e

11. Which of the following statements about the category of disorders labeled as thyroiditis is true?
    a. Hashimoto's thyroiditis can present as a hyperthyroid condition
    b. lymphocytic thyroiditis is the least common form

c. granulomatis thyroiditis is an autoimmune condition

d. suppurative thyroiditis is associated with viral infections

e. Reidel's thyroiditis commonly is seen in young men

CLINICAL CASE PROBLEM 3:
A "WONDERFULLY HEALTHY" 38-YEAR-OLD-FEMALE

A 38-year-old female is seen in your office for a complete baseline health assessment. You have never seen this patient before. She feels well and tells you that she is "wonderfully healthy." She has had no weight loss or gain; no sweating, no tremors, no diarrhea or constipation; no anxiety or depression; no irritability; and no other symptoms.

On examination she is found to have a 2-cm nodule in the left lobe of the thyroid gland. Her blood pressure is 120/70 mm Hg. Her pulse is 90 and regular.

12. What is the most important investigation to be carried out in a patient with this finding?
    a. a serum T4
    b. a thyroid radionuclide scan
    c. a fine-needle aspiration of the nodule
    d. a thyroid ultrasound
    e. a computed tomography (CT) scan of the thyroid

13. Which of the following statements regarding "warm (hot) nodules" and "cold nodules," found on radionuclide scan, is (are) true?
    a. cold nodules are more likely to be benign than warm nodules
    b. cold nodules need not be investigated any further
    c. cold nodules are more likely to be associated with signs and symptoms of hyperthyroidism than warm nodules
    d. cold nodules require further investigation to differentiate benign from malignant status
    e. none of the above statements are true

14. A fine-needle aspiration showed that the mass is benign. What would you do now?
    a. perform a radionuclide thyroid scan
    b. refer the patient to a surgeon for excision
    c. give a trial of suppressive levothyroxine and reevaluate in 6 months
    d. reassure the patient and give no further therapy
    e. obtain an magnetic resonance imaging (MRI) scan of the head and neck to look for further disease

15. Her sister has a similar thyroid nodule. Her fine-needle aspiration showed a follicular carcinoma. Which of the following choices is (are) true?
    a. management of thyroid cancer involves regular follow-up of thyroglobulin in patients that have had total thyroidectomy and postsurgical radioactive iodine ablation
    b. papillary carcinoma without lymph-node spread has a better prognosis than papillary carcinoma with spread to the lymph nodes
    c. management of thyroid cancer involves treatment with levothyroxine to keep the TSH between 2 and 3
    d. a and b
    e. all of the above

CLINICAL CASE PROBLEM 4:
A LETHARGIC 65-YEAR-OLD MALE

A 65-year-old male presents with a 6-month history of lethargy, weakness, psychomotor retardation, cold intolerance, constipation, hair loss, and weight gain. You suspect hypothyroidism.

16. Which of the following investigations will provide the most useful information for diagnosing hypothyroidism in this patient?
    a. serum T4
    b. serum T3
    c. free serum T4
    d. serum TSH
    e. serum TBG

17. Which of the following statements is (are) consistent with the diagnosis of hypothyroidism in this patient?
    a. his total cholesterol has been climbing along with his weight for the past year
    b. he began amiodarone therapy 1 year ago for recalcitrant atrial fibrillation
    c. it can be difficult to separate hypothyroidism from depression in the elderly
    d. a and c
    e. all of the above

18. Which of the following statements regarding the treatment of the patient described in Clinical Case Problem 4 is (are) false?
    a. optimal therapy for this condition can be determined by measurement of the serum TSH level
    b. the average replacement dose of levothyroxine is 1.6 mg/kg/day
    c. patients with significant cardiac disease and elderly patients should be treated cautiously

d. desiccated thyroid is the treatment of choice
e. coadministration of iron with levothyroxine does not alter absorption of either medication

19. After starting the appropriate medication in this patient, when should his TSH be reassessed?
    a. 2-4 weeks
    b. 6-8 weeks
    c. 10-12 weeks
    d. about 6 months
    e. about 1 year

20. What is the most common cause of hypothyroidism in the United States?
    a. autoimmune thyroiditis
    b. post I^{131} hypothyroidism
    c. iodine deficiency
    d. idiopathic hypothyroidism
    e. postthyroidectomy hypothyroidism

21. Which of the following statements is (are) true regarding Hashimoto's thyroiditis?
    a. Hashimoto's thyroiditis is more common in females than in males
    b. antithyroid antibodies are found in 80% of individuals with this condition
    c. this condition is also known as chronic lymphocytic thyroiditis
    d. symptoms of hyperthyroidism often precede symptoms of hypothyroidism
    e. a, b, and c
    f. all of the above

CLINICAL CASE MANAGEMENT PROBLEM

List the most common contributory relationships for the following: (1) hyperthyroidism; (2) hypothyroidism; (3) a thyroid antibody-associated condition; (4) thyroid carcinoma; and (5) elevated total serum T_4 and elevated TBG levels.

 ANSWERS:

1. **b.** This patient has Graves' disease. Graves' disease is the most common cause of hyperthyroidism in the United States. It usually presents with symptoms of sweating, palpitations, nervousness, irritability, tremor, diarrhea, heat intolerance, and weight loss.

Physical signs of Graves' disease include a diffuse, nontender thyroid gland enlargement (goiter); tachycardia; loud heart sounds; and a cardiac murmur. A bruit sometimes is heard over the thyroid gland itself. Proptosis, with a straight-ahead stare and lid lag, is seen frequently. Occasionally patients present with severe exophthalmos accompanied by ophthalmoplegia, follicular conjunctivitis, chemosis, and even loss of vision.

Toxic nodular goiter and toxic adenoma are other causes of hyperthyroidism. Their presentation, however, is distinguished on physical examination with the presence of a nodule or several nodules, whereas the thyroid examination in Graves' disease shows a diffusely enlarged gland.

Hashimoto's thyroiditis is a cause of hypothyroidism rather than hyperthyroidism. Its presentation is usually that of hypothyroid symptoms but can less commonly present as an initial short-lived hyperthyroid condition. It is also of an autoimmune origin.

Pheochromocytoma and panic disorder are not really serious considerations with this presentation history.

2. **b.** Graves' disease is thought to be the result of an autoimmune process, and antibodies are present in the serum.

3. **d.** The serum TSH level now is used to measure and detect hyperthyroidism and hypothyroidism. Indeed, the *sine qua non* of hyperthyroidism at this time is a low serum TSH level. That is the screening test that should be used. The T4 should be measured; the laboratory will measure a total T4 and a calculated free T4. If the free T4 comes back normal, then a serum T3 should be ordered; 10% to 15% of the cases of hyperthyroidism are actually the result of a T3 toxicosis rather than a T4 problem. Radioactive iodine uptake will be elevated. An I^{123} scan will show a diffuse uptake in Graves' disease. Thyroid antibodies will be present in Graves' disease.

4. **c.** See Answer 8.

5. **a.** See Answer 8.

6. **c.** See Answer 8.

7. **c.** See Answer 8.

8. **b.** The two basic treatments for Graves' disease are antithyroid drugs (propylthiouracil or methimazole) and radioiodine therapy.
   1. Antithyroid drugs:
      a. Advantage: These drugs provide the opportunity for the patient to experience a spontaneous remission and avoid lifelong medication (e.g., levothyroxine).
      b. Disadvantages: remissions are attained in fewer than 50% of patients, and continuous or repeated courses of drug therapy are usually necessary.
   2. Radioiodine therapy:

a. Advantages: radioiodine is curative, and managing postradiation hypothyroidism is simpler than managing most patients undergoing long-term antithyroid drug therapy.

b. Disadvantage: iatrogenic hypothyroidism is produced in the majority of patients within 10 years.

On the basis of weighing advantages versus disadvantages for both, the recommendation has been made that radioiodine is the treatment of choice for adult patients. In children and adolescents, the antithyroid drug therapy remains first-line treatment, with radioiodine being second-line treatment. Radioiodine is contraindicated in pregnant women. Women treated with radioactive iodine before pregnancy have children with no higher incidence of congenital malformation or childhood cancers than controls and no difference in fertility.

Beta-adrenergic antagonists provide symptomatic relief and can be administered prior to radioactive iodine treatment.

Untreated hyperthyroidism can cause atrial fibrillation, osteoporosis, hypermenorrhea, diarrhea, and sweating. It does not cause thyroid nodules but may result from hyperfunctioning thyroid nodules.

9. d. The most likely explanation for the elevated serum T4 in this patient is an elevated TBG secondary to the estrogen component of the oral contraceptive pill.

TBG is increased in patients taking the oral contraceptive pill, patients taking estrogen supplementation, and patients with infectious hepatitis.

TBG is decreased in patients with chronic liver disease, patients with nephrotic syndrome, patients with hypoproteinemia from other causes, and patients undergoing androgen therapy.

10. f. To confirm your diagnosis of the patient described in Clinical Case Problem 2, you would order either a serum free T4 level or a TSH level. As stated before, the serum TSH level now is being used to diagnose hyperthyroidism and hypothyroidism. Thus, in this patient, you would expect to find a normal TSH level, rather than a low TSH level.

11. a. The group of disorders labeled as thyroiditis encompasses a diverse group of thyroid disorders of various causes. Hashimoto's thyroiditis can present as a hyperthyroid condition and is also known as lymphocytic thyroiditis and is the most common form. Granulomatous thyroiditis is associated with viral infections and is self-limiting, with full return to normal thyroid function. Suppurative thyroiditis is associated with bacterial infections usually associated with postradiation treatment. Reidel's thyroiditis is not common and usually is seen in older women.

12. c. The initial procedure of choice in most patients is fine-needle aspiration for cytology.

13. d. Cold nodules require further investigation to differentiate benign from malignant status because they have a greater risk of being malignant.

14. c. Give a trial of suppressive levothyroxine and reevaluate in 6 months to determine if the nodule regresses, indicating that it is not malignant.

15. a. Thyroid papillary carcinoma is the most common type of thyroid cancer and also is the thyroid cancer with the best prognosis. Moreover, its spread to regional lymph nodes does not necessarily influence the prognosis. Patients are managed with levothyroxine suppression to keep the TSH <1.0, and thyroglobulin is a useful test to monitor tumor recurrence in patients that have had total thyroidectomy and remnant thyroid tissue ablation with radioactive iodine.

16. d. The most useful test for diagnosing hypothyroidism is the serum TSH level. Serum TSH is elevated in almost all cases of primary hypothyroidism. If hypothyroidism is suspected, the serum TSH will provide definite proof for or against the condition.

17. e. All of the above.

18. d. The serum TSH level will determine optimal thyroid replacement therapy. With adequate replacement, the serum TSH should return to normal. Levothyroxine is the preferred therapeutic agent, although both desiccated thyroid and triiodothyronine can return the TSH to normal.

19. b. It is appropriate to check the TSH in 6-8 weeks after making a dosage adjustment.

20. a. The most common cause of hypothyroidism is the autoimmune thyroiditis, Hashimoto's thyroiditis. The patient with Hashimoto's thyroiditis initially may be hyperthyroid but always progresses to a hypothyroid state. Symptoms of hypothyroidism include fatigue, lethargy, constipation, cold intolerance, dry skin, hair loss, weight gain, edema, headache, arthralgias, hoarseness, amenorrhea, bradycardia, and hypotension.

21. f. Hashimoto's thyroiditis is also known as chronic lymphocytic thyroiditis. It is much more common in females than in males. Antithyroid antibodies are present in up to 80% of patients. In the acute thyroiditis stage of the disease, symptoms of hyperthyroidism precede symptoms of hypothyroidism.

SOLUTION TO THE CLINICAL CASE MANAGEMENT PROBLEM

The most common contributory relationships in thyroid conditions are as follows: (1) Hyperthyroidism: Graves' disease; (2) hypothyroidism: Hashimoto's thyroiditis; (3) thyroid antibody-associated condition: Hashimoto's thyroiditis; (4) thyroid carcinoma: papillary carcinoma; and (5) elevated total serum T$_4$ and elevated TBG levels: oral contraceptive pill.

SUMMARY OF THYROID

A. Important epidemiology:
1. Hypothyroidism is one of the most commonly underdiagnosed conditions, particularly in the elderly.
2. Hypothyroidism is significantly more common than hyperthyroidism. All elderly patients admitted to a long-term care facility or nursing home probably should have a serum TSH performed.

B. Hyperthyroidism:
1. **Causes:** The most common cause is Graves' disease. Toxic nodular goiter and toxic adenoma are less common.
2. **Signs/symptoms:** The most common signs and symptoms include tremor; anxiety, nervousness, or irritability, diarrhea; weight loss; sweating; palpitations; insomnia; proptosis or exophthalmosis; and loud cardiac sounds or cardiac murmur.
3. **Investigations:** A simplified initial investigation approach is to directly measure free serum T4 and serum TSH. (Note: This is becoming more important in diagnosis of hyperthyroidism and hypothyroidism.) If directly measured free serum T4 is normal, then serum T3 should be measured as well. Also perform a thyroid scan followed by a thyroid ultrasound to identify and categorize thyroid nodules (cold/warm).
4. **Treatment:** Radiation is the treatment of choice for Graves' disease in adults. Antithyroid drugs are the treatment of choice in children and adolescents. The drugs of choice are propylthiouracil and methimazole. Subtotal thyroidectomy may be the most appropriate treatment for a toxic or solitary adenoma (nonmalignant). Radiation sometimes may be a reasonable alternative.

C. Hypothyroidism:
1. **Causes:** The most common cause is Hashimoto's thyroiditis (chronic lymphocytic thyroiditis). Other common causes include hypothyroidism induced by thyroid surgery or radiation ablation.
2. **Investigations:** Serum TSH is the most sensitive test in diagnosing primary hypothyroidism. For the elderly patient who has become depressed and is losing interest in life in general, think of hypothyroidism and screen for it. Screen all elderly patients entering a long-term care facility for clinical hypothyroidism.
3. **Treatment:** Levothyroxine 50-200 mg/day (start at 50 mg and work up)

D. Thyroid carcinoma:
The most common type is papillary carcinoma. It is minimally invasive even after it has spread to regional lymph nodes.

SUGGESTED READING

AACE Thyroid Task Force: American Association of Clinical Endocrinologists medical guidelines for clinical practice for the evaluation and treatment of hyperthyroidism and hypothyroidism. *Endocr Pract* 8(6):457-469, 2002.

Davidson A, Diamond B: Advances in immunology: autoimmune diseases. *N Engl J Med* 345:340-350, 2001.

Kamradt T, Mitchison N: Tolerance and autoimmunity. *N Engl J Med* 344:655-664, 2001.

Pearce EN et al: Thyroiditis. *N Engl J Med* 348:2646-2655, 2003.

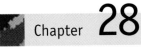

Chapter 28

Diagnosis and Some Features of Certain Endocrine Diseases

> Too much or too little messenger or, perhaps, poor reception.

CLINICAL CASE PROBLEM 1:
A 45-YEAR-OLD MALE WITH "VISUAL PROBLEMS," HEADACHES, WEIGHT GAIN, SWEATING, AND "HANDS AND FEET THAT ARE CHANGING"

A 45-year-old male come to your office with his wife. He is very concerned about some "bizarre symptoms" that he has been experiencing. He is the chief executive officer of a major manufacturing company and is "really embarrassed to go out in public any longer." He tells you that about 6 months ago he began to experience the following symptoms: headaches, visual spots or defects, weight gain, an appearance of his forehead growing, enlarging hands and feet (he could no longer get his gloves and shoes on), and increased sweating.

On examination, the apical impulse is felt in the 5th intercostal space, midclavicular line. His blood pressure is 170/105 mm Hg. He does have a protruding brow, and three discrete visual field defects are noted (two in the left eye and one in the right eye). His tongue appears enlarged, and he is sweating profusely.

■ SELECT THE BEST ANSWER TO THE FOLLOWING QUESTIONS:

1. What is the most likely diagnosis in this patient?
   a. adrenocorticotropin hormone (ACTH) excess
   b. acromegaly
   c. prolactinoma
   d. primary hypopituitarism
   e. primary hyperparathyroidism

2. The pathophysiologic lesion resides in which of the following?
   a. adrenal gland: adenoma
   b. hyperparathyroid glands: adenoma in one or more of the four glands
   c. pituitary gland: adenoma
   d. gastrointestinal ectopic tumor: adenoma
   e. none of the above

3. The treatment(s) for this patient may include which of the following?
   a. surgery: transsphenoidal
   b. pituitary radiation
   c. bromocriptine
   d. somatostatin analogues
   e. all of the above
   f. none of the above

CLINICAL CASE PROBLEM 2:
A 24-YEAR-OLD MALE WITH WEAKNESS AND HYPERPIGMENTATION

A 24-year-old male comes to your office with the following symptoms: an extreme feeling of weakness, a 20-lb weight loss, a change in the color of his skin (his skin has become very hyperpigmented), and lightheadedness and dizziness.

On examination, the patient has definite skin hyperpigmentation since you last saw him 9 months ago. His blood pressure is 90/70 mm Hg. He looks acutely ill.

On laboratory examination, his serum Na^+ is low (115 mEq/L); his serum potassium is high (6.2 mEq/L); his serum urea is elevated at 9.0 mg/dl; and his serum calcium is elevated (12.0 mg/dl).

4. On the basis of his history, physical examination, and laboratory findings, what is the most likely diagnosis of the patient in Clinical Case Problem 2?
   a. Conn's syndrome
   b. Cushing's syndrome
   c. Addison's syndrome
   d. primary hyperparathyroidism
   e. primary pituitary failure

5. What is the most likely cause for this patient's symptoms?
   a. overstimulation of the adrenal gland
   b. an adrenal adenoma
   c. autoimmune destruction of the hyperparathyroid glands
   d. autoimmune destruction of the adrenal gland
   e. a pituitary adenoma

6. What is the acute treatment of choice for this patient?
   a. prednisone orally
   b. dexamethasone orally
   c. hydrocortisone intravenously (IV)
   d. ACTH IV
   e. Depo-Provera intramuscularly

7. This patient will need chronic treatment with which of the following?
   a. hydrocortisone
   b. fludrocortisone acetate
   c. a or b
   d. a and b
   e. none of the above

CLINICAL CASE PROBLEM 3:
A 25-Year-Old Female with Increased Thirst and Urination

A 25-year-old female presents with the sudden onset of increased thirst and increased urination. This began abruptly 1 week ago and has not abated since. She states that since that time she has been thirsty all the time. The only significant illness in her life has been the recent diagnosis of bipolar affective illness subtype I that was made 6 weeks ago. She started taking lithium carbonate and currently is taking 1200 mg/day. Her serum lithium levels have been normal since the beginning.

On examination, her blood pressure is 110/70 mm Hg. She has lost 5 lb during the last week and looks somewhat dehydrated.

8. What is the most likely diagnosis in this patient?
   a. psychogenic polydipsia
   b. diabetes mellitus type 1
   c. central diabetes insipidus
   d. nephrogenic diabetes insipidus
   e. adverse drug reaction to lithium

9. What is the treatment of choice in this patient?
   a. hospitalization and complete psychiatric assessment
   b. insulin: beginning at 10-20 units/day
   c. glyburide
   d. discontinuation of lithium carbonate
   e. substitution of carbamazepine for lithium carbonate

CLINICAL CASE PROBLEM 4:
An Overly Tired 37-Year-Old Female with Hypertension

A 37-year-old female comes to your office because she was found to be "hypertensive" by a nurse in a shopping mall screening program. She tells you that when she thinks about it, she really has not felt well for a couple of months. Her major complaint has been profound generalized fatigue and weakness. She also has been increasingly thirsty, urinating more frequently, and having to urinate frequently at night.

On physical examination, her blood pressure is 190/110 mm Hg. Laboratory abnormalities include a mildly increased serum Na^+ (150 mEq/L), hypokalemic metabolic alkalosis, a low renin level, and increased urine potassium.

10. What is the most likely diagnosis based on the information presented in Clinical Case Problem 4?
    a. Conn's syndrome
    b. Cushing's syndrome
    c. Addison's syndrome
    d. Bartter's syndrome
    e. diabetes insipidus

11. What is the most likely pathophysiologic cause of this syndrome?
    a. benign adenoma of the adrenal gland
    b. malignant adenoma of the adrenal gland
    c. pituitary adenoma
    d. bilateral hyperplasia of the adrenal gland
    e. none of the above

12. What is the treatment of choice for the condition described in Clinical Case Problem 4?
    a. bromocriptine
    b. transsphenoidal surgery
    c. clomiphene
    d. spironolactone
    e. surgical removal of the adenoma

CLINICAL CASE PROBLEM 5:
A 22-Year-Old Female with Breast Secretions, Amenorrhea, and Decreased Libido

A 22-year-old female, married for 18 months, has been trying to get pregnant without success. Approximately 9 months ago, she developed breast secretions, amenorrhea, and decreased libido. No other symptoms are present.

On examination, there is definite galactorrhea present. Her blood pressure is 140/80 mm Hg. No abnormalities are found on physical examination.

13. From the information provided, what is the most likely diagnosis?
    a. anorexia nervosa
    b. stress-induced amenorrhea
    c. "I want to have a baby but can't" syndrome
    d. prolactinoma
    e. hypopituitarism

14. If you could order only one test, what would that test be?
    a. serum estrogen
    b. serum progesterone
    c. serum luteinizing hormone (LH)
    d. serum follicle-stimulating hormone (FSH)
    e. serum prolactin

15. What is the treatment of choice for this condition?
    a. transsphenoidal resection
    b. bromocriptine
    c. clomiphene
    d. lithium carbonate
    e. thyroxine

CLINICAL CASE PROBLEM 6:
A 42-Year-Old Female with Increased Body Hair and Purple Streaks on Her Abdomen

A 42-year-old female comes to your office with the following signs and symptoms: obesity (she has gained 40 lb in the last 6 months), elevated blood pressure at her last walk-in clinic visit, increased body hair, purple streaks on her abdomen, "a fat face" (her description), and pains in her bones and joints.

She is taking no medication at present, nor has she been on any medication for the past year.

On examination, her body mass index (BMI) is 35 kg/m². Her blood pressure is 160/110 mm Hg; she has obvious hirsutism over her entire body, and her abdomen (which is obese) has purple stria. Her face is not only plethoric but also demonstrates a double chin. Her thoracic spine shows evidence of what is known as a buffalo hump.

16. Based on the information provided, what is the most likely diagnosis in this patient?
   a. Conn's syndrome
   b. Cushing's syndrome
   c. Addison's syndrome
   d. primary hyperparathyroidism
   e. prolactinoma

17. Of all possible causes for the condition in this patient, which of the following is the most common?
   a. adenoma of the adrenal gland
   b. adenoma of the pituitary gland
   c. hyperplasia of the adrenal gland
   d. corticosteroid therapy for suppression of inflammation
   e. small-cell carcinoma of the lung

18. Which of the following tests is (are) appropriate screening test(s) for the patient presenting in Clinical Case Problem 6?
   a. serum cortisol
   b. low-dose dexamethasone (cortisol analogue) suppression test
   c. 24-hour urine for free cortisol
   d. all of the above
   e. none of the above

19. The patient in Clinical Case Problem 6 has an imaging study that confirms she has the most common cause of Cushing's syndrome. Which of the following is the recommended treatment?
   a. surgery to remove the adenoma of the pituitary gland
   b. surgery to remove the adenoma of the adrenal gland
   c. surgery to remove the carcinoma of the adrenal gland
   d. chemotherapy to kill as much abnormal tissue as possible
   e. none of the above

20. Which of the following conditions is metastatic malignancy most likely to mimic?
   a. Cushing's syndrome
   b. primary hyperparathyroidism
   c. Conn's syndrome
   d. Addison's syndrome
   e. Nelson's syndrome

CLINICAL CASE MANAGEMENT PROBLEM

For hyperparathyroidism: (1) define the condition; (2) provide the sex predilection; (3) provide the age predilection; (4) explain the pathogenesis; (5) provide the clinical symptoms; (6) explain the mnemonic "stones, bones, abdominal groans, and psychic moans"; (7) explain the changes in blood and serum levels that characterize the condition; (8) discuss treatment; and (9) identify the most characteristic laboratory abnormality.

ANSWERS:

1. **b.** The condition is acromegaly, which often goes undiagnosed for many years. Acromegaly produces many signs and symptoms, including the following:
1. General symptoms: (a) fatigue; (b) increased sweating; (c) heat intolerance; and (d) weight gain.
2. Changes in peripheral and general appearance: (a) enlarging hands and feet; (b) coarsening facial features; (c) oily skin; and (d) hypertrichosis.
3. Head: (a) headaches; (b) parotid enlargement; and (c) frontal bossing.
4. Nose-throat: (a) sinus congestion; (b) voice change; (c) obstructive sleep apnea; and (d) goiter.
5. Cardiovascular system: (a) hypertension; (b) congestive cardiac failure; and (c) left-ventricular hypertrophy.
6. Genitourinary system: (a) kidney stones; (b) decreased libido/impotence; (c) infertility; and (d) oligomenorrhea.
7. Neurologic system: (a) paresthesias; (b) hypersomnolence; and (c) carpal tunnel syndrome.
8. Muscular system: (a) weakness; and (b) proximal myopathy.
9. Skeletal system: (a) joint pains; and (b) osteoarthritis.

2. **c.** Acromegaly is the result of a growth hormone excess caused by a pituitary adenoma.

3. e. Treatments include transsphenoidal surgery, heavy-particle pituitary radiation, conventional pituitary radiation, bromocriptine, somatostatin analogues such as octreotide and its longer-acting "cousin" Sandostatin LAR depot, and growth hormone receptor blockers such as Pegvisomant (not yet available in the United States).

4. c. This patient has Addison's disease or primary adrenocortical insufficiency. The prominent clinical features of Addison's disease include weakness (100%), weight loss (100%), hyperpigmentation (95%), and hypotension.

The pertinent laboratory findings include hyponatremia, hyperkalemia, increased blood urea nitrogen (BUN), hypercalcemia, increased plasma ACTH, and decreased serum cortisol level.

In Addison's disease both the short ACTH stimulation test and the prolonged ACTH stimulation test yield no cortical response.

5. d. Most commonly, Addison's disease results from an autoimmune destruction of the adrenal gland. At least 50% of patients with Addison's disease have antiadrenal antibodies. Other potential causes of adrenocortical insufficiency include tuberculosis, disseminated meningococcemia, and metastatic cancer.

6. c. Because of the acutely ill state of this patient, dexamethasone sodium phosphate 4 mg q12h or hydrocortisone 100 mg IV q6h for 24 hours should be administered acutely. If the patient shows adequate clinical response, the dose may be tapered gradually and changed to oral prednisone.

7. d. The chronic treatment of Addison's disease is a combination of hydrocortisone (10 mg to 30 mg/day) and 9-alpha-fluorocortisol (50-100 mg/day). This combination is based on the need for a combination of glucocorticoid replacement and mineralocorticoid replacement.

8. d. This patient has nephrogenic diabetes insipidus. This has resulted from the lack of renal response to antidiuretic hormone (ADH); in this case the diabetes insipidus is of the nephrogenic subtype and caused by the drug lithium carbonate.

There are two basic types of diabetes insipidus: (1) central (the central type is usually idiopathic) and (2) nephrogenic (the collecting tubules of the kidney are not responsive to the ADH that is produced). The nephrogenic type of diabetes is usually the result of either a drug (lithium carbonate, amphotericin B) or severe hypokalemia (which makes the renal tubules resistant to ADH).

9. e. The treatment for central diabetes insipidus is intramuscular ADH; nephrogenic diabetes insipidus is best treated by discontinuation of the offending drug (if the drug is the cause, as is the most common scenario). In the case of this patient, who was started taking lithium carbonate to treat bipolar affective disorder, a switch to carbamazepine would be most appropriate.

10. a. This patient has Conn's syndrome.

11. a. Conn's syndrome is primary aldosteronism that results from an excess mineralocorticoid production from (in most cases) an adenoma of the adrenal cortex. If not the result of an adenoma, hyperplasia of the adrenal cortex is found. The benign adenoma usually is present in the zona glomerulosa.

The clinical signs/symptoms of Conn's syndrome are weakness (as a result of the effect of hypokalemia); hypertension; carbohydrate intolerance (as a result of increased insulin release from hypokalemia); and polyuria, polydipsia, and nocturia as the result of either hypokalemic nephropathy or nephrogenic diabetes insipidus.

Laboratory abnormalities include mild hypernatremia; hypokalemic metabolic alkalosis; low renin; increased urine potassium; and an inability to suppress aldosterone with isotonic saline load, captopril, or use of another mineralocorticoid.

12. e. The treatment of choice for the patient described in Clinical Case Problem 4 who most probably has a benign adenoma is surgical removal of the adenoma. If a case of Conn's syndrome were the result of a bilateral hyperplasia of the adrenal glands, spironolactone would be the treatment of choice.

13. d. This patient has hyperprolactinemia, most likely from a pituitary adenoma. The combination of galactorrhea, amenorrhea, infertility, and decreased libido is almost certainly the result of a prolactinoma.

14. e. A prolactinoma can be confirmed by performing a serum prolactin level test. A level of serum prolactin of 300 ng/ml or greater is always the result of a pituitary adenoma (in the absence of pregnancy).

A magnetic resonance imaging (MRI) scan of the pituitary gland will confirm the diagnosis. It should be mentioned that a prolactinoma is the most common overall pituitary tumor in women.

15. b. Treatment is controversial, but because of a high rate of recurrence with surgery, initial therapy with bromocriptine is the best choice. Treatment with bromocriptine is not curative; it does, however, reduce the prolactin level, reduce the tumor mass, and increase fertility. Side effects include nausea and vomiting, an increase in liver enzymes, and an increase in serum uric acid.

16. b. This patient has Cushing's syndrome. The definition of Cushing's syndrome is "a manifestation of hypercorticalism due to any cause."

17. b. The most common cause of Cushing's syndrome is corticosteroid therapy. If steroids are excluded, the three major causes are as follows: (1) pituitary Cushing's disease (60% to 70%) as a result of an adenoma; (2) adrenal Cushing's (15%) may be from an adenoma, hyperplasia, or malignancy; and (3) ectopic Cushing's (15%) from a malignancy (small-cell carcinoma of the lung).

Thus the most likely cause of Cushing's syndrome in the patient described, who has not been taking any medication for over a year, is a pituitary adenoma.

18. d. The clinical features of Cushing's syndrome consist of the following: (1) truncal obesity (90%); (2) hypertension (85%); (3) decreased glucose tolerance (80%); (4) hirsutism (70%); (5) wide, purple, abdominal stria (65%); (6) osteoporosis (55%); (7) plethoric face; (8) easy bruising; (9) mental aberrations; and (10) myopathy.

In terms of laboratory tests, the best overall screening tests are serum cortisol level, low-dose (1 mg) dexamethasone suppression test (in Cushing's syndrome there is no suppression), and 24-hour urine for free cortisol. Confirmation tests include high-dose (8 mg) dexamethasone suppression test (suppresses pituitary Cushing's but will not suppress adrenal or ectopic Cushing's) and plasma ACTH (normal to slightly increased in pituitary Cushing's, markedly increased in ectopic Cushing's, and very low in adrenal Cushing's; suppressed by cortisol).

19. a. The correct answer is surgery to remove the pituitary adenoma.

20. b. Metastatic malignancy is most likely to produce hypercalcemia. Hypercalcemia is most likely to mimic primary hyperparathyroidism. (Hyperparathyroidism is discussed in the Clinical Case Management Problem.)

SOLUTION TO THE CLINICAL CASE MANAGEMENT PROBLEM

Hyperparathyroidism:
1. Definition: Overactivity of the parathyroid glands (one or more of the four glands)
2. Sex predilection: females > males
3. Age predilection: age 40-70 years
4. Pathology:
   a. 82% of cases of hyperparathyroidism are the result of adenomas;
   b. 15% of cases of hyperparathyroidism are the result of hyperplasia of the glands
   c. 3% are malignant
5. Clinical symptoms:
   a. Renal stones (calcium oxalate): most common symptomatic presentation
   b. Peptic ulcer disease: calcium stimulates gastrin release
   c. Acute pancreatitis: calcium activates phospholipases
   d. Constipation: most common gastrointestinal complaint
   e. Band keratopathy: metastatic calcification in the limbus of the eye
   f. Nephrocalcinosis: polyuria, loss of concentrating ability, and diluting capability the result of metastatic calcification of the renal tubules
   g. Pruritus: metastatic calcification in the skin
   h. Short QT interval; bradycardia
   i. Hypertension: calcium increases muscular contraction in the resistance vessels
   j. Osteitis fibrosa cystica: late finding, commonly found in jaw, called "brown tumor" because of hemorrhage into cysts
   k. Pseudogout: calcium pyrophosphate; positively birefringent crystals
   l. Mental changes: personality changes, psychosis, depression
   m. X-ray changes:
      i. "salt and pepper skull" on x-ray
      ii. subperiosteal resorption of bone from the second and third middle phalanges and lamina dura around the teeth
      iii. distal resorption of clavicle
6. The mnemonic "stones, bones, abdominal groans, and psychic moans"
   a. Stones: calcium oxalate renal stones
   b. Bones: osteitis fibrosa cystica, salt and pepper skull, resorption of clavicle, subperiosteal resorption of bone from the second and third phalanges and the lamina dura around the teeth
   c. Abdominal groans: abdominal pain resulting from acute pancreatitis
   d. Psychic moans: psychosis, depression

Continued

SOLUTION TO THE CLINICAL CASE MANAGEMENT PROBLEM—cont'd

7. Changes in blood and serum:
   a. hypercalcemia (most common characteristic)
   b. hypercalciuria
   c. hypophosphatemia
   d. hyperphosphaturia
   e. normal anion gap metabolic acidosis

8. Treatment:
   a. Adenoma: surgery to locate and remove adenoma (biopsy second gland to see if atrophic)
   b. Hyperplasia: subtotal parathyroidectomy, monitor for tetany postoperatively

9. Most common laboratory abnormality: hypercalcemia

 SUMMARY OF THE DIAGNOSIS AND SOME FEATURES OF CERTAIN ENDOCRINE DISEASES

A. Acromegaly:
1. **Signs/symptoms:** enlarged hands, feet, and head; hypertension; cardiomegaly; weight gain
2. **Pathology:** results from pituitary adenoma, growth hormone
3. **Treatment:** transsphenoidal surgery, radiation, bromocriptine, somatostatin analogues, growth hormone receptor blockers

B. Addison's disease:
1. **Signs/symptoms:** weakness, hypotension, hyperpigmentation
2. **Pathology:** autoimmune destruction of adrenal glands
3. **Acute treatment:** acutely ill: intravenous hydrocortisone or dexamethasone
4. **Chronic treatment:** replacement with glucocorticoid (hydrocortisone) plus mineralocorticoid (9-alpha-fluorocortisol)
5. **Results:** adrenocortical insufficiency

C. Diabetes insipidus:
1. **Signs/symptoms:** polyuria, polydipsia as a result of deficiency of antidiuretic hormone
2. **Subtypes:** central and nephrogenic
3. **Differential diagnosis:** psychogenic polydipsia
4. **Most common cause:** nephrogenic subtype most commonly from lithium use
5. **Treatment:** intramuscular ADH for treatment of central subtype

D. Prolactinoma:
1. **Signs/symptoms:** galactorrhea, amenorrhea, infertility, decreased libido
2. **Frequency:** most common pituitary tumor
3. **Investigation and confirmation:** serum prolactin of 300 or more; MRI pituitary.

4. **Differential diagnosis:** rule out pregnancy, hyperthyroidism, and drugs (major tranquilizers, oral contraceptive pills, IV cimetidine, opiates)
5. **Treatment:** transsphenoidal surgery, bromocriptine

E. Conn's syndrome:
1. **Signs/symptoms:** weakness (as a result of hypokalemia), hypertension, carbohydrate intolerance (polyuria, polydipsia)
2. **Most common cause:** adenoma of the adrenal
3. **Pathology:** excess mineralocorticoid production
4. **Laboratory investigations:** mild hypernatremia, hypokalemic metabolic alkalosis
5. **Treatment:** adenoma removal; spironolactone for hyperplasia

F. Cushing's syndrome:
1. **Signs/symptoms:** truncal obesity, carbohydrate intolerance, moon face, buffalo hump, abdominal stria, osteoporosis, psychic changes (depression and euphoria), easy bruising, myopathy, plethoric face
2. **Pathology:** pituitary adenoma, adrenal adenoma, steroid therapy
3. **Most common cause:** corticosteroid therapy
4. **Laboratory investigation:** lab tests (screen): serum cortisol; 24-hour urine for cortisol; dexamethasone suppression test (1 mg). Confirmation and differentiation between pituitary Cushing's, adrenal Cushing's, and ectopic Cushing's syndrome; plasma ACTH; high-dose dexamethasone (8 mg) suppression test
5. **Treatment:**
   i. Exogenous Cushing's: stop steroids, decrease dose, or use steroids every other day with a drug holiday
   ii. Endogenous Cushing's: removal of adenoma in pituitary and adrenal Cushing's syndrome

G. Primary hyperparathyroidism:
1. **Signs/symptoms:** mnemonic: stones, bones, abdominal groans, psychic moans; renal colic

(Ca oxalate); acute pancreatitis; constipation; x-ray: bone resorption, salt and pepper skull

2. **Pathology:** most commonly adenoma of the parathyroid gland

3. **Laboratory abnormalities:** hypercalcemia, hypophosphatemia, hypocalciuria, hyperphosphaturia. Hypercalcemia is most common metabolic abnormality; also may occur in metastatic carcinoma.

4. **Treatment: adenoma:** removal; hyperplasia: subtotal parathyroidectomy

SUGGESTED READING

Bornstein, SR, et al: Adrenocortical tumors: recent advances in basic concepts and clinical management. *Ann Intern Med* 130(9):750-771, 1999.

Boscaro M, et al: Cushing's syndrome. *Lancet* 357(9258):783-791, 2001.

Melmed S, et al: Guidelines for acromegaly management. *J Clin Endocrinol Metab* 87(9):4054-4058, 2002.

Singer I, et al: The management of diabetes insipidus. *Arch Intern Med* 157(12):1293-1301, 1997.

Ten S, et al: Clinical review 130: Addison's disease 2001. *J Clin Endocrinol Metab* 86(7):2909-2922, 2001.

Veznedaroglu E, et al: Diagnosis and therapy for pituitary tumors. *Curr Opin Oncol* 11(1):27-31, 1999.

 Chapter **29**

Immune-Mediated Inflammatory Disorders and Autoimmune Disease

"Just look at these gnarled hands and I am only 26 years old."

CLINICAL CASE PROBLEM 1:
A 32-Year-Old Female with Pain in Her Hands and Wrists

A 32-year-old female comes into the office with complaints of fatigue and pain in her hands and wrists for the past 4 months. Recently she also developed swelling in her knees. After a thorough history and physical examination you diagnose rheumatoid arthritis. She tells you she is not surprised because her sister has rheumatoid arthritis, and she asks if there are any "new" medications to treat this condition.

■ **SELECT THE BEST ANSWER TO THE FOLLOWING QUESTIONS:**

1. Which of the following conditions is considered an immune-mediated inflammatory disorder (IMID)?
   a. asthma
   b. Crohn's disease
   c. psoriasis
   d. diabetes
   e. all of the above

2. Which of the following medications have been approved by the U.S. Food and Drug Administration for the treatment of rheumatoid arthritis, Crohn's disease, and psoriatic arthritis?
   a. etanercept
   b. infliximab
   c. nedocromil sodium
   d. a and b
   e. all of the above

CLINICAL CASE PROBLEM 2:
A 29-Year-Old Female with Fatigue, Weight Loss, and Generalized Muscle Weakness

A 29-year-old female comes into your office with fatigue, weight loss, and generalized muscle weakness. She has not had her menses in more than 6 months and has noticed darkening of her skin in certain areas. She also has noticed that she has not had to shave her underarms as frequently as she has had to in the past. Her past medical history is unremarkable.

Examination is as follows: blood pressure 90/60; pulse 95 beats/min; respiration 18 breaths/min; temperature 98.0° F; height 66 inches; weight 108 lbs; cardiovascular, normal; lungs, normal; abdomen, normal; and skin, hyperpigmentation noted at palmar creases, buccal mucosa, elbows, and knees.

Lab results are as follows: Na^+ = 135, K^+ = 5.6, glucose = 71, blood urea nitrogen/creatinine (BUN/Cr) = 34/1.3; white blood cell count (WBC) = 2.8; hemoglobin = 10.4 g/dl; tuberculin PPD (purified protein derivative) test, negative; pregnancy test, negative.

3. What is the most likely diagnosis?
   a. hypothyroidism
   b. Lyme disease
   c. anorexia nervosa
   d. Addison's disease
   e. hemochromatosis

4. Which of the following infectious diseases is responsible for up to 15% of cases of the condition described?
a. tuberculosis
b. Lyme disease
c. syphilis
d. mycoplasma pneumonia
e. streptococcal pharyngitis

CLINICAL CASE PROBLEM 2:
A 39-YEAR-OLD FEMALE WITH JOINT PAINS AND A RASH

A 39-year-old female consults with you regarding joint pains and a rash on her face. She tells you that her knees and hands have been very sore and sometimes swollen over the past few months. She has always had "excellent skin," and she is upset about this "breakout" on her cheeks. Her past medical history is negative, and she takes no prescription or over-the-counter medications.

Examination reveals tenderness over the hands and wrists with no palpable swelling, erythema, or increased warmth. There is an erythematous, macular rash on her cheeks with no involvement of the nasolabial folds.

Lab tests reveal a thrombocytopenia (85,000/mm^3), leukopenia (2200/mm^3), and proteinuria.

5. The most likely diagnosis is:
a. rheumatoid arthritis
b. progressive systemic sclerosis
c. ankylosing spondylitis
d. Lyme disease
e. systemic lupus erythematosus

► ANSWERS:

1. e. An IMID is in a group of conditions characterized by abnormal immune function leading to acute or chronic inflammation. The conditions share common inflammatory pathways. There are a broad range of diseases referred to as IMID that include inflammatory bowel disease, inflammatory skin conditions, cancer, allergies, cardiovascular diseases, endocrine diseases, asthma, and chronic obstruct-pulmonary disease (COPD).

Inflammatory proteins, called cytokines, are involved in these immune-mediated inflammatory conditions. Tumor necrosis factor-alpha (TNF-α), a cytokine, plays an especially important role in the inflammation and pathogenesis.

In rheumatoid arthritis, TNF-α has been identified in the rheumatoid fluid and synovial membranes and is involved in leukocyte recruitment, synovial inflammation, and cartilage degradation. In Crohn's disease, TNF-α and other proinflammatory cytokines are responsible for inflammation of the intestinal mucosa.

2. d. Etanercept (Enbrel) and infliximab (Remicade) are anti-TNF-α agents that are approved for the treatment of rheumatoid arthritis, Crohn's disease, and psoriatic arthritis. Adalimumab (Humira), also an anti-TNF-α agent, is approved for the treatment of rheumatoid arthritis.

Anti-TNF-α agents also have been shown to be effective in the treatment of ankylosing spondylitis. Anti-TNF therapies may prove to be effective in many more conditions in which TNF-α is involved in the pathogenesis. Such conditions may include Still's disease, Behçet's disease, Alzheimer's disease, congestive heart failure, cancer, asthma, diabetes, Felty's syndrome, multiple sclerosis, organ transplant, Parkinson's disease, trauma, Wegener's granulomatosis, vasculitis, and uveitis.

Interleukin-1 is another proinflammatory cytokine associated with inflammatory joint destruction seen in rheumatoid arthritis. Anakinra is an interleukin-1 receptor antagonist that has been approved for the treatment of rheumatoid arthritis.

Nedocromil (Kineret) sodium is an antiinflammatory medication used in the treatment of asthma.

3. d. This patient has Addison's disease. Autoimmune destruction of the adrenal glands accounts for most cases of the disease. Tuberculosis is responsible for 15% of cases. The symptoms of adrenal insufficiency usually begin gradually. Chronic fatigue, muscle weakness, loss of appetite, and weight loss are characteristic. Hypotension, amenorrhea, and loss of axillary hair in females are common. Hyperpigmentation is noted especially in palmar creases, in buccal mucosa, at pressure points such as at the elbows and knees, in perianal mucosa, and around the nipples. Addison's disease can cause depression and irritability.

In some cases, onset can be sudden. This is known as an addisonian crisis. Symptoms include penetrating pain in the low back, abdomen, or legs; vomiting; diarrhea; hypotension; dehydration; and eventual loss of consciousness. This is a medical emergency.

Abnormal laboratory tests include hyperkalemia, hyponatremia, decreased chloride and glucose, increased BUN/Cr, neutropenia, and anemia.

If the diagnosis of adrenocortical insufficiency is suspected, a rapid adrenocorticotropic hormone (ACTH; Cortrosyn) test can be performed.

Treatment involves replacement of corticosteroid and mineralocorticoid hormones. If an addisonian crisis is suspected, do not delay treatment while waiting for confirming laboratory results.

4. a. As discussed previously, tuberculosis is responsible for up to 15% of cases of Addison's disease. Therefore, in patients with suspected Addison's disease, a PPD test should be part of the workup.

5. e. This patient has systemic lupus erythematosus (SLE), a multisystem autoimmune disease. Patients with SLE have been shown to have autoantibodies in their blood years before the symptoms of SLE appear. SLE is much more prevalent in females and usually presents in the childbearing years.

According to the American Rheumatism Association, the diagnosis of SLE is made when four or more of the following eleven criteria are present: (1) malar (butterfly) rash; (2) discoid rash; (3) photosensitivity (especially leg ulcerations); (4) oral ulcers; (5) polyarthritis; (6) serositis (pleuritis, pericarditis); (7) renal disorder (persistent proteinuria, cellular casts); (8) neurologic disorder (seizures, psychosis); (9) hematologic disorder (hemolytic anemia with reticulocytosis, leukopenia, thrombocytopenia); (10) anti-DNA, anti-Sm positive, false-positive STS (syphilis); and (11) antinuclear antibody titer (ANA) positive.

In addition to laboratory tests the workup should include radiographs of the chest and an echocardiogram to screen for pleural effusions, pulmonary infiltrates, and valvular heart disease.

Treatment options include nonsteroidal antiinflammatory drugs, antimalarials such as hydroxychloroquine, corticosteroids, and cytotoxic drugs. Newer treatments, such as antibodies against interleukin-10, may prove effective.

SUMMARY OF IMMUNE MEDIATED INFLAMMATORY DISORDERS AND AUTOIMMUNE DISEASE

IMIDs are conditions characterized by abnormal immune function leading to acute or chronic inflammation. The conditions in this group share common inflammatory pathways. A broad range of diseases can be referred to as IMID, including inflammatory bowel disease, inflammatory skin conditions, cancer, allergies, cardiovascular diseases, endocrine diseases, asthma, and COPD.

Inflammatory proteins, called cytokines, are involved in these immune-mediated inflammatory conditions. Tumor necrosis factor-alpha (TNF-α), a cytokine, plays an especially important role in the inflammation and pathogenesis.

A broad range of medications, including anti-TNF-α, monoclonal antibodies, and agents targeting specific aspects of the inflammatory cascade have been developed and are being tried in the conditions listed. In many ways this revolution makes this the decade of antiinflammatory medications.

SUGGESTED READING

Arbuckle M, et al: Development of autoantibodies before the clinical onset of systemic lupus erythematosus. *N Engl J Med* 349(16): 1526-1533, 2003.

Davidson A, Diamond B: Advances in immunology: autoimmune diseases. *N Engl J Med* 345(5):340-350, 2001.

Shanahan, JC, et al: Upcoming biologic agents for the treatment of rheumatic diseases. *Curr Opin Rheumatol* 15(3):226-236, 2003.

Taylor PC: Anti-tumor necrosis factor therapies. *Curr Opin Rheumatol* 13(3):164-169, 2001.

Ten S, et al: Addison's disease 2001. *J Clin Endocrinol Metab* 86(7): 2909-2922, 2001.

Chapter 30

Multiple Sclerosis

"I'm so clumsy and I can hardly see out of my left eye. Why, oh why?"

CLINICAL CASE PROBLEM 1:
A 27-Year-Old Female with Weakness, Visual Loss, Ataxia, and Sensory Loss

A 27-year-old female comes to your office for assessment of symptoms including weakness; visual loss; bladder incontinence; sharp, shooting pain in the lower back; clumsiness when walking; and sensory loss. These symptoms have occurred during three episodes (different combinations of symptoms each time) approximately 3 months apart, and each episode lasted approximately 3 days.

The first episode consisted of weakness, bladder incontinence, and sharp shooting pains in the lower back (in both hip girdles). The second episode consisted of visual loss, clumsiness when walking, and sensory loss. The third episode (last week) consisted of sharp, shooting pains in the lower back and sensory loss (bilateral) in the upper extremities.

On neurologic examination, you find the following: swelling of the optic disc on funduscopy, inability to walk heel to toe, and slight objective weakness of both hip girdles. She has no symptoms today.

■ **SELECT THE BEST ANSWER TO THE FOLLOWING QUESTIONS:**

1. Given this information, what is the most likely diagnosis in this patient?
   a. amyotrophic lateral sclerosis
   b. multiple sclerosis (MS)
   c. vitamin B_{12} deficiency
   d. hysterical conversion reaction
   e. tertiary syphilis

2. There are four clinical categories of this disease. Which of the following subtypes does the patient presented fit into?
   a. relapsing-remitting
   b. secondary progressive
   c. primary progressive
   d. progressive relapsing
   e. none of the above

3. If you had the opportunity to do only one diagnostic test, which of the following would you choose?
   a. computed tomography (CT) scan of the head/spinal cord
   b. magnetic resonance imaging (MRI) scan of the brain/spinal cord
   c. serum vitamin B_{12} levels
   d. Beck's depression scale
   e. venereal disease research laboratory (VDRL) test for syphilis

4. The disease described is most correctly described as which of the following?
   a. an uncommon neurologic disease that can be corrected by the administration of subcutaneous vitamin B_{12}
   b. the number-one cause of disabling disease of young adults in the United States
   c. a very common psychiatric condition in which psychologic symptoms are manifested by physical symptoms
   d. a fatal neurologic condition that results in continual deterioration to the point of respiratory depression and the cessation of respiration
   e. none of the above

5. The disease described is associated with which of the following?

   a. racial predilection: whites > African Americans
   b. sex predilection: females > males
   c. high socioeconomic status
   d. environmental exposure
   e. all of the above

6. Which of the following statements regarding the behavior of the disease described is (are) true?
   a. in 80% to 90% of all cases, the first episode is followed by a cycle of relapses and remissions
   b. 50% of those with relapsing-remitting cases switch to a progressive course approximately 5 years after the onset of the first symptoms
   c. 10% of patients have progressive disease from the onset of symptoms
   d. up to 10% of patients with this disease have a relatively "benign" course
   e. all of the above

7. The disease, if diagnosed as a central nervous system (CNS) disease, has to involve how many different areas of the central nervous system?
   a. one
   b. two
   c. three
   d. four
   e. not applicable: not primarily a neurologic disease

8. Which of the following clinical findings support the diagnosis?
   a. a cerebrospinal fluid (CSF) mononuclear cell pleocytosis
   b. an increase in CSF immunoglobulin G (IgG)
   c. oligoclonal banding of CSF IgG (two or more bands)
   d. abnormalities in evoked-response testing (any type)
   e. all of the above

9. The target of this disease process is an attack on which of the following?
   a. the neurotransmitter balance in the CNS
   b. the "oligodendrocytes" of the CNS
   c. the peripheral nerves in the posterior columns of the spinal cord
   d. the cerebral hemispheres
   e. the cerebellum

10. What is (are) the treatment(s) of choice for the disease process described?
    a. adrenocorticotropic hormone (ACTH)
    b. corticosteroids

c. cytotoxic immunosuppressive agents
d. interferon beta
e. all of the above

11. Which of the following statements is true regarding the use of interferon in this disorder?
a. interferon has been shown to reduce the rate of relapse
b. interferon may delay the progression to disability
c. interferon reduces the development of new lesions as seen by MRI
d. interferon delays the increase in volume of lesions as seen by MRI
e. all of the above

12. Which of the following symptoms is the least common?
a. optic neuritis
b. ataxia
c. vertigo
d. loss of bladder control
e. impotence

CLINICAL CASE MANAGEMENT PROBLEM

What causes MS, and what cell type is the primary target?

■ ANSWERS:

1. b. This patient has MS. Although no laboratory test, symptom, or physical finding necessarily means a person has MS, the diagnosis relies on two broad criteria: (1) there must have been two attacks that were defined as the sudden appearance or worsening of an MS symptom or symptoms that last at least 24 hours and are at least 1 month apart; and (2) there must be more than one area of damage to CNS myelin, the damage having occurred at more than one point in time and not being attributed to any other disease process.

The differential diagnosis includes ruling out metabolic diseases such as B_{12} deficiencies; other autoimmune disorders such as Behçet's disease, lupus erythematosus, and Sjögren's syndrome; infections such as human immunodeficiency virus (HIV) myelopathy; genetic disorders such as hereditary ataxias; psychiatric disorders such as conversion reaction; and malignancies such as spinal cord tumors.

2. a. The most common pattern or clinical category of MS is the relapsing-remitting category. In relapsing-remitting MS, episodes of acute worsening are followed by recovery and a stable course between relapses.

In the secondary progressive category, gradual neurologic deteriorating occurs with or without superimposed acute relapses in patients who previously have relapsing-remitting MS.

In primary progressive MS, gradual continuous deterioration occurs from the onset of symptoms.

In progressive relapsing MS, gradual neurologic deterioration occurs from the onset of symptoms but with subsequent superimposed relapses.

A small fraction of patients have a relatively benign form that never becomes debilitating.

The patient described most likely has relapsing-remitting MS.

3. b. The most sensitive and specific investigation for this disorder is an MRI of the brain and/or spinal cord scan. The MRI scan will reveal plaque formation (a subsequent stage that results from the loss of the myelin sheath in different parts of the CNS) and spotty and irregular demyelination in the affected areas in a patient with MS.

4. b. MS is the number-one disabling disease of young adults, primarily women. It is more common at northern latitudes than at southern latitudes. Other risk factors will be addressed in Answer 5.

5. e. The documented risk factors for MS include the following: (1) white race > African American race; (2) female > male (2:1); (3) environmental influences (latitude north > south) and suspected but unidentified environmental toxins; (4) genetic (common human leukocyte antigen [HLA] histocompatibility antigen patterns); (5) viral infections are suspect but none has yet been identified; and (6) high socioeconomic status.

6. e. The clinical categories are described in Answer 2. All of the following are correct: (1) 80% to 90% of all cases after the first symptom have relapses followed by remissions; (2) 50% of those who have relapsing-remitting cases switch to a progressive course approximately 5 years after the onset of the first symptoms; (3) 10% have progressive disease from the onset; and (4) 10% of patients have clinical courses that are benign. These patients have one or two relapses and then recover or have episodes of mild nondebilitating relapses with long-lasting remissions. These individuals have multifocal plaques at autopsy with-out evidence of an inflammatory demyelinating reaction.

There is a very rare type termed acute multiple sclerosis of the Marburg type with rapid progression of symptoms.

7. b. For a patient to be diagnosed as having MS, two separate areas of the CNS must be involved.

8. e. The following are laboratory findings that support the diagnosis of MS: (1) CSF mononuclear cell pleocytosis (5 cells/mL); (2) CSF IgG is increased in the absence of a normal concentration of total protein; (3) oligoclonal banding of CSF IgG is detected by agarose gel electrophoresis techniques (two or more oligoclonal bands are found in 75% to 90% of patients with MS); (4) metabolites from myelin break-down may be detected in the CSF; and (5) evoked-response testing may detect slowed or abnormal conduction in visual, auditory, somatosensory, or motor pathways. (One or more evoked potentials are abnormal in 80% to 90% of patients with MS.)

MRI scans of the brain are abnormal in a proportion of patients with MS at presentation; this is associated with more severe disease.

MRI imaging of the brain and spinal cord is the most useful imaging method available, and abnor-mal MRI scans are seen in 90% of patients with definite MS.

9. b. The targeted cells in the MS disease process are the oligodendrocytes of the CNS. These cells fabricate and maintain the myelin sheaths, the material covering the axons that is necessary for the normal conduction of nerve impulses. Destruction of oligodendrocytes occurs in clusters and is accompanied by loss of oligodendrocytes and their myelin sheath appendages with axon sparing (primary demyelination).

The cluster destruction of oligodendrocytes-myelin sheaths forms multifocal plaques, the pathologic hallmark of the disease. The vast majority of these plaques are in the white matter.

10. d. The treatments of choice for MS are as follows:
1. Corticosteroids are the mainstay of treatment for initial and acute relapses of MS. Although cor-ticosteroid therapy can shorten the duration of a relapse, it is uncertain whether the long-term

course of the disease will be altered with their use. ACTH has been replaced by high-dose intra-venous methylprednisolone.
2. Interferon beta remains the long-term treatment of choice for patients with relapsing-remitting MS. Interferon beta is available in two forms: 1A and 1B. Both types are generally well tol-erated by most patients. Flulike symptoms are common after each injection, and questions about different responses in different people remain. Therefore interferon beta doses should be individualized.
3. Glatiramer acetate is an alternative to beta inter-feron for those who have failed the latter therapy.
4. Azathioprine and other cytotoxic immunosup-pressant agents may reduce the rate of relapse in MS, but they have no effect on the progression of the disability. Nevertheless, in progressive MS, cytotoxic immunosuppressant agents have been shown to be of moderate benefit.

11. e. Interferon beta 1B and 1A are used in the treatment of MS. Both interferons have been shown to reduce the rate of clinical relapse, reduce the number of new lesion seen on MRI, and delay the increase in volume of new lesions seen on MRI. Interferon beta 1A also may delay the progression to disability in some patients. Glatiramer acetate, mitoxantrone, and immunoglobulins also have been shown to reduce the rate of relapse, although much uncertainty still remains about their precise usage.

12. e. The initial symptoms of MS and their fre-quency are outlined in the table.

Symptom	Percentage of Patients
Fever	98-100
Lymphadenopathy	98-100
Tonsillopharyngitis	80-90
Splenomegaly	50
Eyelid edema	35
Hepatomegaly	30
Palatal petechiae	25

Thus, of the symptoms listed in the question, the most common is optic neuritis, and the least common is impotence/other sexual dysfunction.

SOLUTION TO THE CLINICAL CASE MANAGEMENT PROBLEM

The etiologic agent(s) producing MS is (are) unknown. There is reasonable evidence that it results from an interaction between the individual (immunology) and his or her environment. The basic target of MS is the oligodendrocyte, the cell that fabricates and maintains myelin. Destruction of oligodendrocytes occurs in clusters and is accompanied by loss of the oligodendrocyte and the myelin sheaths. The cluster destruction of oligodendrocytes-myelin sheaths produces plaques, the pathologic hallmark of MS. This destruction of oligodendrocytes and myelin is patchy, leaving more areas unaffected. The axons invariably are spared.

SUMMARY OF MULTIPLE SCLEROSIS

1. Prevalence:
   It is a major disabling condition of young adults in the United States; in 2000, 250,000 to 350,000 people in the United States had physician-diagnosed MS.
2. Epidemiology:
   a. Almost all patients fit into one or more of the following categories:
      i. 80% to 90% of patients have after their first symptom a cycle of relapses and remissions.
      ii. 50% of the 80% to 90% switch to a progressive course about 5 years after the first symptom.
      iii. 10% of patients have progressive disease from the onset.
      iv. Up to 10% of patients have a benign course, with one or two relapses and then a good recovery.
   b. Risk factors for MS:
      i. Race: white > African American
      ii. Sex: females > males (2:1)
      iii. High socioeconomic status
      iv. Northern latitudes
      v. Other environmental factors as yet not identified such as toxins and viruses
      vi. HLA histocompatible antigens
3. Symptoms: most common symptoms are the following:
   a. Sensory loss
   b. Optic neuritis
   c. Weakness
   d. Paraesthesias

4. Diagnosis: criteria:
   a. Two episodes, or attacks, of symptoms
   b. Two different areas of the CNS involved
5. Testing for MS:
   a. MRI scan of the brain and spinal cord: This will show the areas of demyelination better than any other test.
   b. CSF pleocytosis
   c. Increased CSF IgG
   d. Oligoclonal banding of IgG in the CSF
   e. Evoked potentials: visual, auditory, somatosensory, and motor
6. Treatment:
   a. Pharmacotherapy:
      i. Methylprednisolone for acute attacks
      ii. Long-term medication include interferon beta 1A and 1B, glatiramer acetate, anti-integrin monoclonal antibodies, and mitoxantrone
   b. General supportive treatments:
      i. A regular exercise program
      ii. The pursuit of wellness and a positive attitude
      iii. Education regarding the disease
      iv. Support: family/support groups

SUGGESTED READING

Lublin FD: The diagnosis of multiple sclerosis. *Curr Opin Neurol* 15(3):253-256, 2002.

National Multiple Sclerosis Society at http://www.nmss.org.

Noseworthy JH: Treatment of multiple sclerosis and related disorders: what's new in the past 2 years? *Clin Neuropharmacol* 26(1):28-37, 2003.

Noseworthy JH, et al: Multiple sclerosis. *N Engl J Med* 343(13):938-952, 2000.

O'Connor P: The Canadian Multiple Sclerosis Working Group. Key issues in the diagnosis and treatment of multiple sclerosis. An overview. *Neurology* 59(6 Suppl 3):S1-33, 2002C.

Chapter **31**

Acne, Rosacea, and Other Common Dermatologic Conditions

> "Those zits are ruining my life.
> Please hit that zit."

CLINICAL CASE PROBLEM 1:

A 15-Year-Old Distressed Adolescent with "The Zits"

A 15-year-old female comes to your office with a complaint of the "zits." She has been attempting to treat these with frequent washings with a buff puff and avoidance of cosmetics and other facial products. She is very distressed and breaks down crying. She is afraid that "no boys will ever go out with someone with such an ugly face." Her past history is unremarkable. She is taking no medications at present. She has no allergies. Her family history is unremarkable.

On physical examination the patient has multiple maculopapular-pustular lesions with comedones on her face and back. No other abnormalities are found on examination.

■ SELECT THE BEST ANSWER TO THE FOLLOWING QUESTIONS:

1. What is the diagnosis in this patient?
   a. acne vulgaris
   b. polycystic ovary syndrome
   c. acne cystica
   d. rosacea
   e. folliculitis

2. What is the treatment of first choice in this patient at this time?
   a. topical tretinoin
   b. intralesional corticosteroids
   c. topical benzoyl peroxide
   d. topical erythromycin
   e. oil-based antiacne moisturizers

3. The patient returns. There has been an improvement of about 20% in the skin lesions since her first visit. She gradually has increased the strength of the preparation you gave her. What would you do at this time?
   a. discontinue the first agent and treat her with topical benzoyl peroxide
   b. discontinue the first agent and treat her with topical tretinoin
   c. continue the first agent and add topical tretinoin
   d. discontinue the first agent and treat her with topical clindamycin

   e. continue the first agent and add topical erythromycin

4. The patient returns again in another 8 weeks. She now has sustained an improvement of about 35% in the lesions since her first visit, and she continues to execute your instructions faithfully. However, she is still not satisfied, and neither are you. What would you do at this time?
   a. discontinue the first and second agents and substitute a systemic antibiotic
   b. continue the first and second agents and add a systemic antibiotic
   c. continue the first and second agents and add topical clindamycin or erythromycin
   d. continue the first and second agents and add oral isotretinoin
   e. continue the first and second agents, and add a new "oil-free" product that through your local pharmaceutical detail agent you have learned "kills acne bugs dead"

5. The patient returns again in 4 weeks. She now has sustained an improvement of about 50% but is still not satisfied. What would you do at this time?
   a. refer her for psychiatric counseling for distorted body image perception
   b. refer her to a dermatologist
   c. tell her to "hang in there" for a little longer and if she is not satisfied then, she will start taking an oral antibiotic
   d. stop all the medication and try something else
   e. continue all three agents and add a systemic antibiotic

CLINICAL CASE PROBLEM 2:

A Case of Nodular-Pustular Acne

An 18-year-old male comes to your office with moderately severe nodular-pustular acne on his face and back.

6. What would be your agent of first choice in this case?
   a. topical benzoyl peroxide
   b. topical tretinoin
   c. systemic tetracycline
   d. penicillin
   e. isotretinoin

7. The patient described in Clinical Case Problem 2 returns in 6 weeks with only moderate improvement. What would you now prescribe?
   a. systemic tetracycline
   b. systemic erythromycin
   c. cyproterone acetate
   d. isotretinoin
   e. none of the above

8. Choose the correct statement:
   a. a closed comedone is also known as a black-head
   b. an open comedone is a noninflamed follicular opening containing a keratotic plug that appears black
   c. an open comedone also is known as a white-head
   d. a papule is a round elevation of skin with a central pocket of pus
   e. mild acne is characterized by comedones, papules, and cysts

9. Acne is the result of a pathophysiologic process in the pilosebaceous unit that stems from abnormalities in:
   a. sebum production
   b. follicular hyperkeratization
   c. proliferation and colonization of *Propionibacterium acnes*
   d. release of inflammatory mediators
   e. all of the above

10. Which of the following statements regarding acne is (are) true?
    a. chocolate can exacerbate acne vulgaris
    b. acne medications initially may worsen acne
    c. acne is a result of poor hygiene
    d. it is not necessary to use sunscreen with topical retinoid products but it is with oral retinoid products
    e. all of the above

11. Which of the following bacteria is associated with the condition described?
    a. *Staphylococcus aureus*
    b. *Streptococcus viridans*
    c. *Propionibacterium acnes*
    d. all of the above
    e. none of the above

12. Which of the following is (are) essential for a good skin-care program specifically designed for patients with the described disorder?
    a. oil-free products
    b. thorough, frequent cleansing of skin with exfoliants
    c. manual manipulation of skin lesions
    d. use of gels and solutions for dry skin
    e. applying all of topical medications at bedtime

13. On further questioning you learn that the patient in Clinical Case Problem 1 has missed several periods, but that isn't unusual for her. Her skin looks a little worse. You now would:
    a. inquire about excessive hair growth
    b. check a pregnancy test

   c. if no contraindications exist, prescribe an oral contraceptive
   d. after confirmatory testing, consider an anti-androgen
   e. all of the above

14. The patient in Clinical Case Problem 1 is started taking oral contraceptives and tetracycline. Important information about these medications and acne are:
    a. because she is taking an oral contraceptive, no risk for pregnancy exists with concomitant tetracycline therapy
    b. tetracycline is more photosensitizing than doxycycline
    c. vaginal yeast infections are seen rarely with tetracycline
    d. isotretinoin may be prescribed only by physicians enrolled in a program monitored by Roche Pharmaceutical Company
    e. adapalene is more irritating than tretinoin

15. What is (are) the absolute contraindication(s) to the use of oral isotretinoin for the treatment of acne vulgaris?
    a. children younger than age 14
    b. women of childbearing potential who are not adequately protected against pregnancy
    c. allergy to topical tretinoin
    d. all of the above
    e. none of the above

16. Which of the following is (are) true concerning rosacea?
    a. rosacea occurs in middle-aged individuals
    b. rosacea consists of papules and pustules on the face
    c. rosacea produces a background erythema and telangiectasias on the face
    d. all of the above
    e. none of the above

17. What is the first-line treatment of rosacea?
    a. topical benzoyl peroxide
    b. topical tretinoin
    c. topical erythromycin or clindamycin
    d. topical metronidazole
    e. none of the above

18. What is the second-line treatment of rosacea?
    a. topical metronidazole
    b. oral metronidazole
    c. oral tetracycline
    d. oral 13-cis-retinoic acid
    e. oral erythromycin

19. Other treatments for rosacea include:
    a. avoidance of alcoholic beverages to reduce flushing
    b. use of permethrin cream to reduce papules and erythema
    c. use of isotretinoin in nonpregnant women
    d. use of laser therapy to eradicate telangiectasias
    e. all of the above

20. Which of the following conditions sometimes is associated with rosacea?
    a. rhinophyma
    b. cellulitis
    c. multiple carbuncle formation
    d. cavernous sinus thrombosis
    e. anaerobic septicemia

CLINICAL CASE MANAGEMENT PROBLEM

Describe the pathophysiology of acne vulgaris.

ANSWERS:

1. **a.** This patient has acne vulgaris. Acne vulgaris primarily affects teenagers but continues to affect many patients into their 20s and 30s.

2. **c.** See Answer 7 for explanation.

3. **c.** See Answer 7 for explanation.

4. **c.** See Answer 7 for explanation.

5. **c.** See Answer 7 for explanation.

6. **c.** See Answer 7 for explanation.

7. **d.** The treatment of choice for acne can take many forms, but a recommended approach is outlined here. In this approach, only one drug is added at a time; this allows you to evaluate clearly the efficacy of that agent. Allow 6-8 weeks for treatment to work before deciding to try another regimen or add another agent. This approach may need to be amended if the patient presents with a nodular-pustular acne (as in Clinical Case Problem 2, Answer 6 and 7).
    1. Treatment protocol for mild to moderate acne:
       a. Begin with topical benzoyl peroxide 2.5%. Increase to 5% and 10% rapidly. Benzoyl peroxide usually is applied twice a day.
       b. Add topical tretinoin or adapalene. These are applied at bedtime. Remember to tell your patient to expect redness and irritation of the face, especially in the initial period. Urge them not to discontinue the product because of this side effect.
       c. Add topical erythromycin or topical clindamycin. This should be used in combination with 1 and 2. If there are significant lesions on the back that are difficult for the patient to reach (even at the beginning of treatment) you may need to prescribe a systemic antibiotic from the beginning.
       d. Add systemic tetracycline to the topical benzoyl peroxide and topical tretinoin. Continue the topical antibiotic.
    2. Moderate to severe nodular pustular acne:
       a. The choices for systemic antibiotic therapy include tetracycline, minocycline, doxycycline, erythromycin, clindamycin, and trimethoprim-sulfamethoxazole.
       b. In severe cystic acne an oral retinoid, isotretinoin, may be necessary.

8. **b.** An open comedone is a noninflamed follicular opening containing a keratotic plug that appears black (i.e., a blackhead).

9. **e.** Acne vulgaris is the result of the obstruction of sebaceous follicles by sebum and desquamated epithelial cells. An anaerobic organism, *Propionibacterium acnes* will proliferate, which leads to inflammation. Clinically these pathophysiologic events will lead to noninflammatory open and closed comedones and in more severe cases, inflammatory papules, pustules, and nodules. Most patients will have a mixture of both noninflammatory and inflammatory lesions. Closed comedones also are known as whiteheads, and open comedones are also known as blackheads. Mild acne is characterized by comedones and papules. Cystic acne is moderate to severe.

The pathophysiology of acne vulgaris involves the following six steps: (1) the androgen stimulation of sebum production; (2) keratinous obstruction of the sebaceous follicle outlet; (3) accumulation of keratin and sebum with the formation of open and closed comedones (blackheads and whiteheads); (4) bacterial colonization of the trapped sebum with *Propionibacterium acnes*; (5) inflammatory reaction to the colonization of the trapped sebum; and (6) production of inflammatory papules, pustules, nodules, and cysts.

10. **b.** Acne medications can cause an initial worsening of symptoms. There is no indication that the intake of certain foods is associated with acne. This includes chocolate, nuts, and shellfish. A common acne myth is that acne is the result of poor hygiene. Retinoid products of any kind are photosensitizing, and sunscreen is mandatory with the concurrent use of these products.

11. **c.** Acne vulgaris is associated with the bacterium *Propionibacterium acnes*.

12. a. A good skin-care program includes the following: cleansing gently and nonabrasively, using oil-free products, and leaving the skin lesions alone. It is also important to match the vehicle (lotion, cream, gel, or solution) with the skin type. Gels and solutions tend to be more drying, whereas lotions and creams are somewhat more emollient.

13. e. This patient exhibits two of the three characteristics of polycystic ovarian syndrome (PCOS). The triad consists of acne, hirsutism, and irregular periods. Obesity and the metabolic syndrome also may be features of this condition. Oral contraceptives can be beneficial for acne treatment and restoration of menses to prevent endometrial proliferation. Antiandrogens (spironolactone) are useful in the management of the acne and hirsutism. Last, a pregnancy test must be checked in a woman with amenorrhea because pregnancy is the primary cause of amenorrhea. PCOS is the second leading cause of amenorrhea.

14. d. Broad-spectrum antibiotics may reduce the effectiveness of oral contraceptives. Certain estrogen-containing oral contraceptives may be used in the treatment of moderate acne vulgaris in females 15 years of age or older who desire contraception, have achieved menarche, and are unresponsive to topical antiacne medications. Doxycycline is slightly more photosensitizing than tetracycline. An advantage of adapalene over tretinoin is that it is less irritating. In April 2002, Roche Laboratories released the System to Manage Accutane Related Teratogenicity (SMART) program aimed at preventing pregnant women from receiving isotretinoin. The prescriber must be enrolled in this program.

15. d. The single most important absolute contraindication to the use of 13-cis-retinoic acid (Accutane) is women in the reproductive years. Accutane is teratogenic and never should be used in this age group. Children younger than age 14 years and individuals with allergic reactions (not the redness that is characteristic of topical isotretinoin) also should not be given 13-cis-retinoic acid.

16. d. Rosacea is an acneiform condition that affects middle-aged or older patients. It is characterized by papules and pustules occurring on a background of erythema and telangiectasia of facial skin. The main area affected is the middle third of the face, from the forehead to the chin. With rosacea, comedones are typically absent. There is, however, a tendency for the facial skin of patients affected by rosacea to become thickened and to produce enlarged sebaceous glands. When this happens in the area of the nose, the condition is known as rhinophyma. Rosacea is more common in women, but affected men seem more prone to develop severe cases of rhinophyma. W.C. Fields' nose was a classic example.

17. d. The first-line treatment for rosacea is a topical antibiotic. The antibiotic of choice is metronidazole (MetroGel) applied twice daily. Topical tretinoin and topical benzoyl peroxide preparations aggravate the erythema and are usually not helpful. Topical corticosteroids also aggravate the condition.

18. c. The second-line treatment for rosacea is a systemic antibiotic. Tetracycline is the drug of choice. After the first month, the dosage often can be lowered and then ultimately discontinued. Recurrences are common, however, and repeated courses of antibiotics often are needed. Systemic antibiotics are also useful in treating the associated keratitis and blepharitis that occasionally are associated with rosacea.

Systemic therapy with erythromycin, minocycline, doxycycline or metronidazole is effective if tetracycline is ineffective.

Rosacea that fails to respond to the treatment alternatives just outlined may respond to oral isotretinoin.

19. e. There are many lifestyle recommendations for the treatment of rosacea. Many involve avoidance of substance that may be vasoactive, such as hot beverages, cold beverages, caffeine, alcohol, or spicy foods. A recent study found efficacy with the use of permethrin cream to reduce papules and erythema. Laser treatments can eradicate telangiectasias.

20. a. Rhinophyma is hypertrophy of the soft tissue of the nose. Patients have a large, bulbous, ruddy appearance of the nose. Seen in men, usually over 40 years of age, it is considered a severe form of rosacea. Treatment is usually surgical, often with lasers, although Accutane has been used with good results.

SOLUTION TO THE CLINICAL CASE MANAGEMENT PROBLEM

The pathophysiology of acne vulgaris involves the following six steps: (1) the androgen stimulation of sebum production; (2) keratinous obstruction of the sebaceous follicle outlet; (3) accumulation of keratin and sebum with the formation of open and closed comedones (blackheads and whiteheads); (4) bacterial colonization of the trapped sebum with *Propionibacterium acnes*; (5) inflammatory reaction to the colonization of the trapped sebum; and (6) production of inflammatory papules, pustules, nodules, and cysts.

SUMMARY OF ACNE, ROSACEA, AND OTHER COMMON DERMATOLOGIC CONDITIONS

A. Acne vulgaris:

1. **Prevalence:** 75% of teenagers and young adults (up to and including patients in their 20s and 30s)
2. **Pathophysiology:** see the Clinical Case Management Problem box
3. **Causative organism:** *Propionibacterium acnes*
4. **Classification of acne vulgaris:**
   a. Obstructive acne:
      i. closed comedones (whiteheads);
      ii. open comedones (blackheads)
   b. Inflammatory acne: formation of lesions generally follows the following order: papules, pustules, nodules, cysts, and scars.
5. **Treatment measures:**
   a. Nonpharmacologic: gentle face washing; avoidance of manipulation of acne lesions; using water-based cosmetics only; and using oil-free moisturizers only.
   b. Pharmacologic: the treatment of acne vulgaris can be seen as a series of discrete steps:
   Step 1: Begin with benzoyl peroxide gel.
   Step 2: Add topical tretinoin or adapalene. (Consider using step 1 in the morning and step 2 in the evening.)
   Step 3: Add topical antibiotic (erythromycin, clindamycin). (Consider using step 3 along with a combination of steps 1 and 2.)
   Step 4: Add systemic antibiotics, such as tetracycline, minocycline, doxycycline, erythromycin, clindamycin, or trimethoprim–sulfamethoxazole. (Consider using a combination of steps 1, 2, 3, and 4.)
   Step 5: For severe nodular-cystic acne only, use oral isotretinoin (associated with serious, dose-related side effects).
6. **Common myths believed by patients:**
   a. Acne is caused by failure to wash away dirt and oil with sufficient zeal. Not true—acne can be made worse by washing too vigorously and causing irritation. Gentle washing with normal soap is sufficient.
   b. Too much junk food causes acne. Not true—no connection between diet and acne has ever been established.
   c. "Unhealthy" sex habits, including masturbation, same-sex play, or even simple indulgence can cause acne. Not true—sex with the wrong person can cause rashes but it will not be acne.
   d. Stress can cause acne. Not true—however, stress can increase a nervous tendency to pick, squeeze, and/or rub pimples and make them worse.
   e. Acne is a normal adolescent problem of no consequence that should be allowed to run its course. Not true—the physical and psychologic consequences of acne can be cataclysmic. Prompt treatment can prevent severe outbreaks and avoid physical and emotional scarring.
   d. Acne vulgaris always clears up after adolescence. Not true—more than 10% of individuals continue to have this form of acne well into adulthood.

B. Rosacea:

1. **Definition:** acneiform eruption that affects middle-aged patients. It is characterized by papules and pustules occurring on a background of erythema and telangiectasia of facial skin.
2. **Complications:** Thick skin forms on face (especially on nose). This condition is called rhinophyma.
3. **Treatment:**
   a. Step 1: topical metronidazole
   b. Step 2: systemic therapy: tetracycline, erythromycin, minocycline, doxycycline, metronidazole, or isotretinoin

SUGGESTED READING

American Academy of Dermatology at http://www.aad.org.

Blount BW, Pelletier AL: Rosacea: A common, yet commonly overlooked, condition. *Am Fam Phys* 66(3):435-440, 2002.

Institute for Clinical Systems Improvement: *Health Care Guidelines, Acne Management*. www.icsi.org, 2002

Liao D: Management of Acne. Research findings that are changing clinical practice. *J Fam Pract* 52(1):43-51, 2003.

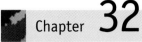

Chapter 32

Headache

"Acetaminophen is just not strong enough anymore!"

CLINICAL CASE PROBLEM 1:
A 45-YEAR-OLD MALE WITH A HEADACHE

A 45-year-old male comes to your office with a 4-week history of recurrent headaches that wake him up in the middle of the night. The headaches have been occurring every night and have been lasting approximately 1 hour. The headaches are described as a deep burning sensation centered behind the left eye. The headaches are excruciating (he rates them as a 15 on a 10-point scale) and are associated with watery eyes, "a sensation of heat and warmth in my face," nasal discharge, and redness of the left eye.

Before the onset of these headaches 4 weeks ago, the patient describes no more than the occasional tension headache. Headaches were certainly never a problem.

The patient describes no recent life changes and no major life stresses. He is happily married, has three children, and has a secure job that he enjoys.

On examination, his blood pressure is 120/70 mm Hg. His pulse is 82 and regular.

■ **SELECT THE BEST ANSWER TO THE FOLLOWING QUESTIONS:**

1. What is the most likely cause of this patient's headache?
   a. subarachnoid hemorrhage
   b. tension-migraine syndrome
   c. atypical migraine headache
   d. cluster headache
   e. classic migraine headache

2. How would you best treat his acute headache?
   a. oral ergotamine
   b. high-flow oxygen
   c. subcutaneous sumatriptan
   d. b and c
   e. all of the above

3. He returns 3 days later and tells you that the medicine you gave him works, but he still keeps getting these awful headaches. What medication listed here would not help prevent his headaches?
   a. verapamil
   b. lithium
   c. Valium
   d. prednisone
   e. methysergide

CLINICAL CASE PROBLEM 2:
A 32-YEAR-OLD FEMALE WITH A 2-YEAR HISTORY OF RECURRENT HEADACHES

A 32-year-old female comes to your office with a 2-year history of recurrent headaches. These headaches occur between three and four times per month and last 12-24 hours. The headaches almost always are confined to the left side of the head and are associated with malaise, nausea, vomiting, photophobia, and phonophobia. The patient has been using acetaminophen without significant relief.

On examination, the patient's blood pressure is 100/70 mm Hg. Her neurologic examination is within normal limits. The optic fundi are normal, as is the rest of the neurologic examination.

4. What workup would you perform to determine the etiology of this headache?
   a. complete blood count (CBC)
   b. erythrocyte sedimentation rate (ESR)
   c. magnetic resonance imaging (MRI) scan of the brain
   d. careful history and physical
   e. c and d

5. This patient's headache is most likely a:
   a. migraine headache without aura (common migraine)
   b. migraine headache with aura (classic migraine)
   c. complicated migraine
   d. tension-migraine syndrome
   e. nervous headache

CLINICAL CASE PROBLEM 3:
A 38-YEAR-OLD FEMALE WITH A 6-YEAR HISTORY OF RECURRENT HEADACHES

A 38-year-old female comes to your office with a 6-year history of recurrent headaches. These headaches occur approximately once per week. She is concerned that she may be having some kind of stroke because before the headache, nausea, and severe vomiting begin she sees a "type of odd visual feeling or sight—flashing lights, almost like a pattern in front of my eyes." With respect to the headache itself, it usually lasts for 24-36 hours. It is throbbing in nature and often "switches from one side to the other" with each attack. She needs to be in a dark room and finds noise bothersome when she has these headaches. She is otherwise healthy and taking no medications.

On physical examination, the patient's blood pressure is 110/70 mm Hg. Examination of the optic fundi is completely normal as is the rest of the neurologic examination.

6. What is the most likely type of headache in this patient?
   a. migraine headache without aura (common migraine)
   b. migraine headache with aura (classic migraine)
   c. basilar migraine
   d. tension-migraine syndrome
   e. complicated migraine headache

7. What is the best acute treatment for this patient's headaches?
   a. subcutaneous sumatriptan
   b. intramuscular Demerol
   c. dihydroergotamine
   d. naratriptan
   e. ketorolac

8. The appropriate treatment you prescribed did not work and she goes to the emergency room (ER) 12 hours later. The ER doctor is asking what to treat her with next. You recommend:
   a. intravenous Demerol
   b. zolmitriptan
   c. dihydroergotamine
   d. Fiorinal with codeine
   e. morphine

CLINICAL CASE PROBLEM 4:
A 24-YEAR-OLD FEMALE PATIENT WITH CHRONIC HEADACHES PRECEDED BY NAUSEA AND VOMITING

A 24-year-old patient comes to your office for assessment of headache. She describes the onset of, characteristics of, duration of, and associated features of a migraine headache that is preceded by nausea and vomiting, confined to the left side of the head, and characterized by a throbbing pain lasting approximately 48 hours. The unusual feature of this headache is that it always begins approximately 2 days before menstruation, and it always ends with the onset of menstruation.

On physical examination, the patient's blood pressure is 120/70 mm Hg. Her optic fundi are clear, and her neurologic examination is completely normal.

9. What is the most likely type of headache in this patient?
   a. migraine without aura: premenstrual syndrome
   b. menstrual migraine
   c. migraine without aura: premenstrual dysphoric disorder
   d. migraine-tension syndrome: premenstrual symptom complex
   e. complicated migraine syndrome

10. Which statement regarding preventive treatment of menstrual is false?
    a. prophylactic use of naproxen reduces migraine frequency
    b. prophylactic use of triptans is safe and effective
    c. prophylactic use of sertraline is safe and effective
    d. prophylactic use of low-dose estrogen is recommended
    e. none of the above statements are false

11. Which of the following statements regarding migraine headache is (are) true?
    a. migraine headache is more common in men than in women
    b. migraine headache is more common in patients who have a family history of migraine headache
    c. migraine headache is more common in patients in lower socioeconomic groups than in higher socioeconomic groups
    d. migraine headache is more common in urban dwellers than in rural dwellers
    e. all of the above

12. What is the prevalence of migraine headache in adult women?
    a. 1%
    b. 4%
    c. 14%
    d. 19%
    e. 31%

13. Which of the following is (are) a recognized trigger(s) of migraine headache?
    a. stress, worry, and anxiety
    b. excessive sleep
    c. certain foods and alcohol
    d. weather changes
    e. all of the above

14. Which of the following has not been recommended as a prophylactic agent for the prevention of migraine headache?
    a. riboflavin
    b. propranolol
    c. amitriptyline
    d. fluoxetine
    e. methysergide

CLINICAL CASE PROBLEM 5:
A 35-YEAR-OLD MALE WITH A 6-MONTH HISTORY OF RECURRENT STEADY, ACHING, "VISELIKE" HEADACHES

A 35-year-old male comes to your office with a 6-month history of recurrent daily headaches, usually in the late afternoon. The headaches are described by the patient as "a vice around my head."

The headaches are not associated with nausea, vomiting, or malaise. The patient does, however, describe some light-headedness with these headaches. He smokes one pack of cigarettes per day and says he does not drink alcohol.

On examination, the patient's blood pressure is 130/70 mm Hg. His optic fundi are normal. There are no neurologic abnormalities.

15. What is the likely type of headache in this patient?
    a. chronic daily headache: tension type
    b. episodic tension-type headache
    c. migraine without aura
    d. migraine tension-type headache complex (mixed or combined headache)
    e. cluster headache

16. What is (are) the treatment(s) of first choice for the patient described in Clinical Case Problem 5?
    a. a nonsteroidal antiinflammatory drug (NSAID)
    b. acetaminophen
    c. codeine
    d. a tricyclic antidepressant
    e. all of the above
    f. a, b, and/or d

17. The patient returns to your office a few months later complaining of daily headaches and constant heartburn since he started taking ibuprofen for his headaches. Which of the following statements best represents the current problem?
    a. he has developed *Helicobacter pylori*-associated headache syndrome
    b. his smoking will make it more difficult to treat his condition successfully
    c. his headaches will improve with daily Valium use
    d. he has developed analgesic rebound headache
    e. b and d
    f. c and d

CLINICAL CASE PROBLEM 6:
A 75-Year-Old Female with a Severe Left-Sided Temporal Headache

A 75-year-old female comes to your office with a severe left-sided temporal headache. She describes a tender area in the left temple. She also describes pain in the area of the jaw while chewing her food. This headache has been present for the past 3 days.

On physical examination, the patient's blood pressure is 170/100 mm Hg. Her neurologic examination is normal. There is moderate tenderness in the area of the left temple.

18. Which of the following statements regarding this patient's symptoms is (are) true?
    a. this probably represents a late-onset migraine syndrome
    b. simple analgesics should be prescribed before embarking on any extensive investigation of these symptoms
    c. this headache is unlikely to be associated with any significant complications
    d. an ESR should be ordered on this patient
    e. all of the above

19. What is the appropriate treatment for this headache?
    a. acetaminophen
    b. sumatriptan
    c. cyclobenzaprine
    d. prednisone
    e. verapamil

20. Which of the following statements regarding the investigation of headaches is (are) true?
    a. patients with migraine with aura or migraine without aura rarely require more than a careful history and physical examination
    b. patients with episodic tension-type headaches rarely require more than a careful history and physical examination
    c. electroencephalography (EEG) rarely is useful in the diagnosis of headache (other than when headache may indicate a brain tumor)
    d. radiographic brain imaging is not routinely indicated in the investigation of a patient with a headache syndrome
    e. all of the above

CLINICAL CASE PROBLEM 7:
A 35-Year-Old Female with Almost Constant Migraine Headaches

A 35-year-old female comes to the ER with another "migraine headache." She has had migraine headaches for the past 20 years, and during the last 4 years they have been almost constant.

Her headaches have required intramuscular Demerol and Dilaudid injections approximately twice per week for the last 3 years. She has made 157 trips to the ER with the same symptoms during the past year.

This patient categorically tells you that she has "tried every abortive agent and every prophylactic agent and nothing has worked."

21. Which of the following statements regarding this patient's headaches is (are) true?

a. this headache most likely is an example of status migrainous
b. the major component of this headache is likely an analgesic rebound headache
c. the scenario presented here is uncommon
d. the majority of the patients with this headache type are female
e. all of the above

22. What is the treatment of choice for the headache described in Clinical Case Problem 7?
   a. continue the present treatment plan: repeated injections of Demerol and Dilaudid
   b. change the treatment plan to regular injections of dihydroergotamine and metoclopramide
   c. seek immediate psychiatric consultation
   d. change the treatment plan to one that uses nonnarcotic analgesics (in fairly large doses) in place of the narcotic analgesics
   e. none of the above

CLINICAL CASE PROBLEM 8:

A 62-Year-Old Male Patient with Headaches That Have Been Getting Progressively Worse

A 62-year-old patient comes to the ER with headaches that have been getting progressively worse over the last 7 days. He has not had previous problems with headache, and his only significant illness was a lobectomy and radiation therapy for carcinoma of the lung 3 years ago. He has not had any recurrence and is feeling well.

The significant features of this headache include the following: the headache appears to be significantly worse every day; the headache is absolutely constant (it never goes away and never decreases in severity to any extent); and the headache is described as a "terrible pressure within my head."

23. What is the most likely cause of this patient's headache?
   a. migraine without aura: status migrainous type
   b. migraine without aura: complex etiology
   c. secondary headache: cerebral edema
   d. secondary headache: primary brain tumor resulting from previous radiation therapy
   e. none of the above

24. What is the drug of choice for this patient at this time?
   a. sumatriptan
   b. ergotamine
   c. meperidine and Dilaudid
   d. dexamethasone
   e. chlorpromazine

CLINICAL CASE PROBLEM 9:

A 17-Year-Old Male with a Headache from Hell

A 17-year-old male comes to the ER with "a headache like I've never had before." He is brought to the ER by his mother. The patient has been completely well, healthy, and active prior to this episode (which began last night). Nausea and vomiting began shortly after the headache onset.

On examination, there is significant neck stiffness. The patient is unable to move his neck without extreme pain. You are just about to continue with the neurological examination when a patient with a cardiac arrest is wheeled through the ER doors.

25. At this time, with this information you have to this point, what is the most likely diagnosis?
   a. acute subdural hematoma
   b. acute epidural hematoma
   c. subarachnoid hemorrhage
   d. migraine headache without aura: severe
   e. glioblastoma multiforme

26. With the provisional diagnosis you have made on the patient in Clinical Case Problem 9, what should you do now?
   a. perform a lumbar puncture
   b. perform a computed tomography (CT) or MRI scan of the brain
   c. observe the patient for 12 hours before doing anything
   d. sedate and medicate the patient in an effort to alleviate the headache, and sort things out later
   e. none of the above

CLINICAL CASE MANAGEMENT PROBLEM

Discuss the classification of primary headache disorders that has been proposed by the International Headache Society. Distinguish between primary headache and secondary headache.

ANSWERS:

1. **d.** This patient has developed a typical cluster headache. Although we can diagnose with considerable confidence, it is too early to predict which of the two subtypes of cluster headache the patient ultimately will develop. These subtypes are episodic cluster headache and chronic cluster headache.

The typical cluster headache awakens a patient from sleep, although both daytime clusters and nighttime clusters are well described. Multiple daily episodes usually lasting between 45 minutes and 1 hour may occur on a regular basis for periods of 2-3 weeks. Remissions may last from several months to several years. Episodic cluster headaches constitute 90% of cases. In the other 10% of patients, the headaches do not remit (chronic cluster headache). The typical description of cluster headache is a headache that has the properties of a "deep, burning, or stabbing pain." It very often is described by the patient as "excruciating" or "the worst pain I have ever had." It is almost exclusively unilateral in nature. The pain may become so bad that the patient actually becomes suicidal. Cluster headache is associated with lacrimation, facial flushing, and nasal discharge. The affected eye often becomes red, conjunctival vessels become dilated, and a Horner's-type syndrome including both ptosis and pupillary constriction develops.

2. d. Cluster headache is thought by many authorities to be a migraine variant. Sumatriptan (Imitrex) is the drug of choice for acute episodes of cluster headache. Also, oxygen inhalation is very beneficial in an acute cluster attack. Ergotamine preparations also have been shown to be effective, but oxygen and subcutaneous sumatriptan have a faster onset of action and are the first line in treatment.

3. c. Prophylactic medications that are indicated in the treatment of cluster headache include verapamil, ergotamine, lithium, methysergide, prednisone and other corticosteroids, indomethacin, beta blockers, tricyclic antidepressants, and selective serotonin reuptake inhibitors (SSRIs). Valium is not indicated as a prophylactic agent in cluster headache.

4. d. At this time a careful history and physical is the most important diagnostic step to take. See Answer 5.

5. a. This patient has migraine headache without aura (common migraine headache). Migraine headache is a type of headache that is typically episodic, usually occurring 1 or 2 times per month. More frequent episodes of migraine, such as migraine headache every day, second day, or third day, should make you suspicious regarding the true diagnosis. The most common alternative diagnosis would be rebound analgesic headaches, and many patients who are labeled as having migraine headaches actually have analgesic rebound headaches.

The prodromal phase of migraine consists of symptoms of excitation or inhibition of the central nervous system (CNS), including elation; excitability; irritability; increased appetite and craving for certain foods, especially sweets; depression; sleepiness; and fatigue. This phase occurs in approximately 30% of patients. These symptoms may precede the migraine attack by up to 24 hours. The headache phase of the cycle is certainly the most prominent. Migraine headache is unilateral in more than 50% of patients, but bilateral migraine is more common than previously thought. In addition, it is not uncommon for a migraine headache to begin on one side and switch to the other. The character of the pain is also much more variable than previously thought: "pulsating or throbbing" in only 50% of cases, and a "dull, achy" pain in the other 50%. The headache phase itself usually lasts between 4 and 72 hours but is occasionally longer. Migraine headache almost invariably is associated with other symptoms including nausea, vomiting, and diarrhea. Heightened sensory perceptions such as photophobia, phonophobia, and increased sensitivity to smell occur during the attacks.

Although a mixed headache syndrome (mixed migraine and tension headaches) and tension headaches themselves often are confused with migraine, pure migraine headache usually can be distinguished by moderate to severe intensity and aggravation by activities including coughing, running, or bending down. Those two characteristics, plus one of nausea, vomiting, photophobia, or phonophobia, establish the diagnosis as migraine headache.

The workup of a migraine is basically a careful history and physical and focused neurologic examination to rule out other causes of headache (secondary headache). Blood testing and radiographic imaging are not necessary with the secure diagnosis of migraine headache.

6. b. This patient has migraine headache with aura. The visual symptoms that this patient describes follow the classical description for what is called an aura. An aura is usually visual, although neurologic auras consisting of hemisensory disturbances, hemiparesis, dysphasia, and change in memory or state of consciousness can occur occasionally. Only approximately 20% of migraine headaches can be classified as migraine with aura. Also, it is quite frequent for a patient to alternate between migraine with aura and migraine without aura. Migraine with aura and migraine without aura are, other than the aura itself, similar in characteristic features.

7. a. The first-line treatment for a moderate to severe migraine headache in the absence of contraindications is subcutaneous sumatriptan. Its nonoral route is essential in effective treatment of a patient who is vomiting.

8. c. If subcutaneous sumatriptan fails and the patient comes to the emergency department, intravenous dihydroergotamine and intravenous metachlorpropamide is an underused but highly effective treatment. There is no place for the use of Demerol in the treatment of a patient with migraine.

9. b. Although migraine headache without aura can occur at any time during the menstrual cycle, this patient's description of a cyclic repeatable headache that occurs between 2 days prior to menstruation and the last day of menses clearly establishes this headache as what is referred to as menstrual migraine. Estrogen withdrawal is likely the trigger for migrainous attacks.

10. c. Therapy for an acute attack is similar to that for a menstrual migraine. Prophylaxis for menstrual migraine includes low-dose estrogen supplementation, NSAIDs, and ergot and triptan use premenstrually. The SSRIs do not have a role in prophylaxis of migraine headaches.

11. b. Migraine headache is significantly more common in individuals who have a family history of migraine headache, particularly women whose mother had migraine headache.

Migraine headache prevalence does not vary among the populations of the world; the prevalence is the same in rural Nigeria as it is in cosmopolitan Los Angeles. Moreover, contrary to what is commonly believed, migraine headache is not more common among lower socioeconomic groups than among higher socioeconomic groups unless there are triggering factors (see Answers 9 and 13) that may be more common in a certain segment of the population.

12. d. Migraine headache is more common in women than in men. In the general population the prevalence of migraine headache is approximately 19% in women.

13. e. Common triggers of migraine are as follows: (1) stress, worry, or anxiety; (2) menstruation; (3) oral contraceptive use; (4) certain foods (aged cheese, chocolate); (5) alcohol; (6) lack of sleep; (7) glare or dazzle; (8) weather or ambient temperature changes; and (9) caffeine withdrawal.

Less common triggers of a migraine are as follows: (1) high humidity; (2) excessive sleep; (3) high altitude; (4) excessive vitamin A; (5) drugs such as nitroglycerin, reserpine, estrogens, hydralazine, or ranitidine; (6) pungent odors; (7) fluorescent lighting; (8) allergic reactions; (9) cold foods; and (10) refractory errors.

14. d. The drugs of first choice for the abortive treatment of acute severe to very severe migraine headache are the 5-HT1 receptor agonists. Sumatriptan is the prototype. These drugs activate serotonin receptors. Oral, subcutaneous, and intranasal preparations are available. There are extremely effective in more than 80% of cases.

Additionally, dihydroergotamine mesylate (DHE) given intravenously (1 mg) and ergotamine (rectal suppositories, sublingual tablets, and oral tablets) also are used to abort acute migraine headache in moderately severe cases of migraine.

Phenothiazines (such as chlorpromazine) and nonsteroidal antiinflammatory agents are useful as alternative agents in the treatment of migraine headaches and can be thought of as an alternative to the abortive agents just mentioned.

Fluoxetine and SSRIs have not been shown to be beneficial in migraine prophylaxis.

15. a. This patient has chronic tension-type headache. Chronic tension-type headaches often are described as a steady, aching, "viselike" sensation that encircles the entire head. Chronic tension-type headaches often are accompanied by tight and tender muscles at the site of maximal pain, often in the posterior cervical, frontal, or temporal muscles. Tension headaches are recurrent and often are brought on by stress.

The pathogenesis of tension-type headaches is unclear. It may be related to the release of vasoactive substances that also explain migraine headaches. Often it is very difficult to separate the two syndromes.

16. f. Chronic daily headaches (either tension type or migraine tension type) usually are related to causal factors that include stress and worry, depression, overwork, lack of sleep, incorrect posture, and marital and family dysfunction.

Treatment approaches for the relief of tension-type headaches should center on the following principles: (1) attempt to identify the causal factor(s); (2) attempt to modify or eliminate the stressor with behavior modification, biofeedback, relaxation therapy, yoga, exercise, and so on; (3) consider the use of mild analgesics such as acetaminophen, NSAIDs, or aspirin for acute, less frequent headaches; and (4) tricyclic antidepressants and SSRIs are beneficial when headache frequency is greater than 15 days per month and prophylactic medication is required.

Codeine or other narcotic agents should be avoided.

17. e. This patient has analgesic rebound headache and has developed gastritis as a side effect of frequent NSAID use. This condition requires prophylactic treatment. Tricyclic antidepressants are helpful in treating analgesic rebound. The patient also needs to minimize his use of simple analgesics. Patients who smoke are harder to treat successfully for chronic daily headache and analgesic rebound headache and have a higher chance of success if they quit smoking.

18. d. This patient has temporal arteritis (giant cell arteritis) until proved otherwise. When an elderly patient presents with a new-onset headache, temporal arteritis must be excluded. This patient presents with a unilateral headache with a tender temporal area. This probably represents the inflamed temporal artery.

The most significant complication of temporal arteritis is sudden unilateral blindness resulting from occlusion of the terminal branches of the ophthalmic artery. This is a completely preventable complication.

Temporal arteritis often is associated with polymyalgia rheumatica.

The ESR is a highly sensitive test in a patient you suspect of having temporal arteritis. The ESR usually is elevated higher than 50 mm/hr and may exceed 100 mm/hr.

19. d. The treatment of choice for a patient with temporal arteritis is high-dose prednisone. When temporal arteritis is diagnosed or even suspected, treatment should be started immediately with at least 50 mg of prednisone. If the diagnosis is confirmed, treatment should be continued for at least 4 weeks before any gradual reduction is instituted. If ocular complications have occurred, treatment should continue for 1-2 years.

20. e. Because headache is such a common disorder and the excessive application of expensive and highly technical laboratory procedures to the diagnosis and management of benign headache is expensive and epidemiologically unsound, the following principles should apply to the investigation of headache:

1. Patients with migraine headache with or without aura or tension-type headache rarely require more than a careful history and physical examination.
2. Headaches of recent origin or progression deserve investigation. This is especially true of headaches that have a consistently focal distribution, headaches that follow trauma, or headaches that begin after the age of 40 years. CT or MRI scanning is recommended.
3. The EEG is almost never helpful in the diagnosis of primary headache.
4. Skull x-rays are useful only when abnormalities involving the base of the brain are suspected or immediately following head trauma.
5. Diagnostic lumbar puncture should be performed in any patient with a headache that is accompanied by fever or is explosive in nature. Lumbar puncture should, if possible, be deferred until after CT scanning in other forms of acute headache, especially if the patient has a stiff neck.
6. CT scanning and MRI scanning are the diagnostic modalities of choice in the evaluation of

acute headache in which serious pathology is suspected.

21. b. This is an extremely common scenario that is repeated thousands of times daily in ERs across North America. When these patients come through the ER doors we all feel like "heading for the nearest exit." This patient is an excellent example of the mistakes made in treating this type of headache pattern.

1. These patients should not be started taking narcotic analgesics in the first place. Although there is a place in the rare patient for a one- or two-time dose of Demerol, that should be the limit.
2. When a patient with migraine headache tells you that "no abortive or prophylactic agent has ever worked," they are essentially telling you that they do not have a migraine headache. We now realize the importance of the neurotransmitter serotonin in the pathogenesis of migraine headache. If none of the abortive prophylactic agents work, then you can draw the reasonable conclusion that the major headache component is not dependent on serotonin. In this patient, there is no doubt that migraine headache was the beginning of the problem, but now rebound analgesic headache with migraine underlay is the most likely diagnosis and the treatment problem to be faced.
3. Status migrainous indicates a prolonged migraine attack usually lasting for more than 72 hours that does not resolve spontaneously.

22. e. The treatment of this patient must include both an empathetic physician who takes the time to explain what is happening to the patient and a physician who is prepared to do what needs to be done: gradual reduction (suggested 10% a week) of the total narcotic dosage.

It would be very unwise to use large doses of nonnarcotic analgesics in this patient. The most common cause of rebound analgesic headaches is, in fact, acetaminophen.

23. c. This patient has a secondary headache (a headache resulting from a secondary disease or process). The description is a classic presentation of the headache of cerebral edema. In this case, the cerebral edema is the result of metastatic deposits related to the carcinoma of the lung that was previously resected and radiated. The classic symptoms in this case are fairly acute onset, constant headache, pressurelike sensation, and a progressively more severe headache every day.

24. d. The treatment of choice for this patient is dexamethasone. The correct starting dose is 4 mg qid with ranitidine or omeprazole to protect the gastric mucosa and prevent peptic or stress ulceration.

25. **c.** This patient has the classic description of a subarachnoid hemorrhage ("headache like I've never had before" and acute onset). This is subarachnoid hemorrhage until proved otherwise.

26. **b.** This patient should have an immediate CT scan or MRI scan, and this should be followed by angiography or special MRI technique imaging to localize the blood vessel. The most common pathogenesis of subarachnoid hemorrhage is rupture of a berry aneurysm in the circle of Willis.

SOLUTION TO THE CLINICAL CASE MANAGEMENT PROBLEM

The reclassification of primary headache disorders (according to the International Headache Society) is as follows: (1) migraine; (2) migraine without aura (common migraine); (3) migraine with aura (classic migraine); (4) complicated migraine (migraine with prominent neurologic symptoms); (5) basilar migraine; (6) hemiplegic migraine; (7) ophthalmoplegic migraine; (8) cluster headache; (9) episodic headache; (10) chronic headache; (11) episodic tension-type headache; (12) chronic daily headache; (13) chronic tension-type headache; (14) migraine-tension-type headache complex (mixed or combined headache) usually evolved from migraine; (15) analgesic/ergotamine rebound headache; (16) secondary headache defined as a headache resulting from a disease or condition that is initially unrelated to the headache. (The most common cause of secondary headache probably is related to side effects or adverse reactions produced by any number of pharmaceutical products.)

SUMMARY OF HEADACHE

The reclassification of primary headache disorders (according to the International Headache Society) is outlined in the Clinical Case Management Problem and Solution boxes.

This chapter has outlined completely the important points of the diagnosis and treatment of headache; therefore the summary will take the form of a list of dos and don'ts in headache diagnosis and management.

1. Take a complete history and perform a complete physical (especially neurologic) examination.
2. Do not rely on CT or MRI scans to make the majority of your headache diagnoses.
3. Recognize that migraine headache in the same patient may have different presentations on different occasions.
4. Do not label a headache as tension headache unless the criteria for its diagnosis are met.
5. Attempt to discover the triggers or stresses that bring on both migraine-type headache and tension-type headaches.
6. Remember that the pathophysiology of migraine is related to serotonin depletion.

7. Recognize the contraindications to 5-HT-1 agonists: (a) ischemic heart disease/angina pectoris (b) previous myocardial infarction; (c) uncontrolled hypertension; (d) basilar artery migraine; (e) hemiplegic migraine; and (f) patients taking monoamine oxidase inhibitors (MAOs), SSRIs, or lithium.
8. Avoid narcotics for the treatment of migraine headaches.
9. Recognize the underdiagnosis of rebound analgesia headache.
10. Beware of the patient with "migraine headache" for whom no abortive agent and no prophylactic agent works. The probability of that patient having migraine headache as the primary headache diagnosis is very low.

SUGGESTED READING

Dalessio DJ: Relief of cluster headache and cranial neuralgias: Promising prophylactic and symptomatic treatments. *Postgrad Med* 109(1):69-78, 2001.
Fettes I: Menstrual migraine. *Postgrad Med* 101(5):67-77, 1997.
Institute for Clinical Systems Improvement. Health Care Guideline: Migraine Headache, 5th edition. www.icsi.org, July 2003.

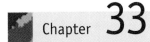

Chapter 33

Seizures

Seize the moment.

CLINICAL CASE PROBLEM 1:
A 65-YEAR-OLD MALE WITH A NEW-ONSET SEIZURE

A 65-year-old male is brought to the emergency room (ER) after suffering a seizure while eating a meal in a restaurant. His wife states that he has never had anything like this before. Apparently, the patient developed convulsive jerking in his right arm and leg that lasted approximately 5 minutes. In addition, the patient lost consciousness for a short interval. This patient's history includes 80 pack-years of cigarette smoking and chronic bronchitis.

On examination, his blood pressure is 150/100 mm Hg, his pulse is 96 and regular, his respirations are 16, and he is afebrile. He is in no acute distress, and his neurologic examination is normal except for some increased somnolence. The rest of his examination also is completely normal.

■ SELECT THE BEST ANSWER TO THE FOLLOWING QUESTIONS:

1. Which of the following is the most correct statement regarding his seizure and history of smoking and symptoms of bronchitis?
   a. there is probably no association between these conditions
   b. the nicotine in the cigarette smoke lowered his seizure threshold
   c. chronic hypoxemia increases the risk of seizure activity
   d. a complication of chronic cigarette smoking may manifest first as seizures
   e. chronic aspiration resulting bronchitis increases the risk of seizure activity

2. What is the type of seizure described in this patient?
   a. a simple partial seizure
   b. a complex partial seizure
   c. an absence seizure
   d. a tonic-clonic (grand mal) seizure
   e. a myoclonic seizure

3. What is the most common cause of a new-onset seizure in a patient of this age?
   a. idiopathic
   b. alcohol withdrawal
   c. head trauma
   d. brain tumor
   e. an old stroke

4. Which of the following medications would not be a drug of first choice for the prevention of further seizures in this patient?
   a. phenytoin
   b. carbamazepine
   c. phenobarbital
   d. valproic acid
   e. ethosuximide

5. Which of the following investigations is the most important investigation to be performed on this patient at this time?
   a. an magnetic resonance imaging (MRI) scan of the brain
   b. an electroencephalograph (EEG) of the brain
   c. angiography of the cerebral vessels
   d. auditory and brainstem-evoked potentials
   e. a computed tomography (CT) scan of the chest

CLINICAL CASE PROBLEM 2:
A 22-YEAR-OLD MALE WHO SUDDENLY LOST CONSCIOUSNESS, BECAME RIGID, AND FELL TO THE GROUND

A 22-year-old male is brought to the ER by his wife. While he was raking leaves in the backyard, he suddenly lost consciousness, became rigid, and fell to the ground. His respirations temporarily ceased. This lasted for approximately 45 seconds and was followed by a period of jerking of all four limbs lasting 2 to 3 minutes. The patient then became unconscious for 3 to 4 minutes.

On examination, the patient is drowsy. There is a large laceration present on his tongue and a small laceration present on his lip. The neurologic examination is otherwise normal. The vital signs are normal.

6. What type of seizure is patient in Clinical Case Problem 2 suffering from?
   a. simple partial seizure
   b. complex partial seizure
   c. absence seizure
   d. grand-mal (tonic-clonic) seizure
   e. myoclonic seizure

7. Which of the following medications would not be a drug of first choice for the prevention of further seizures in the patient described?
   a. phenytoin
   b. carbamazepine
   c. phenobarbital
   d. primidone
   e. ethosuximide

CLINICAL CASE PROBLEM 3:

A 12-Year-Old Girl Who Stares into Space

A mother comes to your office with her 12-year-old daughter. The mother states that for the past 6 months she (and the girl's teacher) frequently have noted the child staring into space. This lack of concentration usually lasts only 30 to 45 seconds. Sometimes there appears to be brief twitching of all limbs during this time. The child's neurologic examination is normal.

8. What is the most likely cause of the symptoms described in Clinical Case Problem 3?
   a. simple partial seizures
   b. complex partial seizures
   c. absence seizures
   d. myoclonic seizures
   e. none of the above

9. All of the following may be useful in the treatment of the patient in Clinical Case Problem 3 except:
   a. valproic acid
   b. clonazepam
   c. ethosuximide
   d. phenytoin
   e. none of the above are useful

10. Which of the following statements regarding beginning and stopping antiepileptic therapy is (are) true?
    a. antiepileptic therapy can be discontinued safely after a seizure-free interval of one year
    b. every patient who has a seizure should be started taking antiepileptic medication
    c. antiepileptic medication should be started with a combination of two or more antiepileptic agents
    d. the decision to stop antiepileptic medication should be guided by the results of the EEG
    e. none of the above are true

11. Which of the following investigations is (are) useful in the initial evaluation of a patient with new-onset seizures?
    a. EEG
    b. MRI scan of the brain
    c. serologic test for syphilis
    d. carotid ultrasound
    e. a, b, and c
    f. a, b, c, and d

12. Which of the following statements regarding the diagnosis and treatment of status epilepticus is (are) true?

a. poor compliance with the anticonvulsant drug regimen is the most common cause of tonic-clonic status epilepticus
b. the mortality rate of status epilepticus may be as high as 20%
c. the establishment of an airway is the first priority in the management of status epilepticus
d. intravenous (IV) diazepam is the drug of first choice in the immediate management of status epilepticus
e. all of the above statements are true

13. Which of the following is (are) causes of non-epileptic seizures?
    a. hypocalcemia
    b. hypomagnesemia
    c. pyridoxine deficiency
    d. thyrotoxic storm
    e. a, b, and c
    f. all of the above

14. Which of the following most often is confused with petit-mal seizures (absence seizures) in adults?
    a. benign rolandic epilepsy
    b. complex partial seizures
    c. myoclonic seizures
    d. simple partial seizures
    e. clonic seizures

15. Which of the following is the most common neurologic disorder?
    a. epilepsy
    b. multiple sclerosis
    c. stroke
    d. myasthenia gravis
    e. Bell's palsy

16. Which of the following primary brain tumors is most likely responsible for a new-onset seizure in a 68-year-old male?
    a. meningioma
    b. schwannoma
    c. ependymoma
    d. glioblastoma
    e. pituitary adenoma

CLINICAL CASE MANAGEMENT PROBLEM

Discuss the pathophysiology and treatment of febrile seizures in children.

ANSWERS:

1. There is a high probability of association between this patient's smoking and his seizures. This is because in a patient older than 40 years of age the most common cause of a new-onset seizure is a

brain tumor (primary or secondary), and a history of chronic bronchitis and an 80 pack/year history of cigarette smoking suggests a significant probability of bronchogenic carcinoma. Consequently, seizure plus cigarette smoking suggests a probability of primary bronchogenic cancer with secondary metastases to the brain. Overall, about 8% of patients with a first seizure may have a brain tumor. This drops to 1% among patients with a normal history and physical examination. Among the elderly, seizures are most often the result of primary or secondary brain tumors or are secondary to ischemic or hemorrhagic stroke.

2. a. The seizure described in this patient is a simple seizure. The symptoms of simple seizures include focal motor symptoms and somatosensory symptoms that spread or "march" to other parts of the body. Other symptoms include special sensory symptoms that involve visual, auditory, olfactory, or gustatory regions of the brain and autonomic symptoms or signs. Psychologic symptoms, often accompanied by impaired level of consciousness, also can occur.

3. d. As discussed in Answer 1, the most common cause of a new-onset seizure in patients in this age group is a brain tumor. As in this case, a primary bronchogenic carcinoma with secondary brain metastases would be the most likely cause of a new-onset seizure in a 65-year-old heavy cigarette smoker with chronic obstructive pulmonary disease (COPD). The common causes of new onset seizures by age are as follows:
1. Younger than 10 years: (a) idiopathic; (b) congenital; (c) birth injury; (d) metabolic; and (e) febrile.
2. 10 to 40 years of age: (a) idiopathic; (b) head trauma; (c) preexisting focal brain disease; and (d) drug withdrawal.
3. Older than 40 years of age: (a) brain tumor; (b) stroke; and (c) trauma.

4. e. Partial seizures can be treated effectively with phenytoin, carbamazepine, phenobarbital, primidone, and valproic acid. Treatment with one drug is preferable to combination therapy.

Ethosuximide is not a good choice for the treatment of partial seizures. It is primarily indicated in petit-mal (also known as absence) seizures.

5. a. The most important investigation in this patient at this time is an MRI scan of the brain, which will identify any cerebral or leptomeningeal mass that may be associated with the new-onset seizure. A CT scan would be a reasonable alternative. An EEG will identify the type of abnormal discharge and the location of same. It, however, would be a poor second choice.

6. d. This patient has had a grand-mal (tonic-clonic) seizure. Tonic-clonic seizures often are associated with a sudden loss of consciousness. The tonic phase is followed by a clonic phase characterized by generalized body musculature jerking. Following this is a stage of flaccid coma. Associated manifestations include tongue or lip biting, urinary or fecal incontinence, and other injuries. An aura may precede a generalized seizure.

7. e. As in partial (focal) seizures, the drugs of choice are phenytoin, carbamazepine, phenobarbital, primidone, and valproic acid. Ethosuximide is not an effective drug in the treatment of grand mal seizures.

8. c. This patient presents with typical absence (petit-mal) seizures. Petit-mal seizures may present with impairment of consciousness, sometimes accompanied by mild clonic, tonic, atonic, or autonomic symptoms. These seizures, often very brief in duration, interrupt the current activity and are characterized by a description of the patient "staring into space."

Petit-mal seizures that begin in childhood are terminated by the beginning of the third decade of life. A bilaterally synchronous and symmetric 3-Hz "spike-and-wave" pattern is seen on EEG.

9. d. Petit-mal seizures can be treated effectively with ethosuximide, valproic acid, or clonazepam. Phenytoin is not an effective treatment for petit-mal seizures.

10. d. The criteria for decision to treat or not to treat an initial seizure should include details of the seizure; adequate laboratory data including measurement of glucose, electrolytes, alcohol, and other toxins; and the presence of EEG evidence of epileptic activity at least 2 weeks after the seizure. Careful reevaluation and monitoring are essential.

A consideration of discontinuation of medication can be made after a seizure-free period of 2 to 4 years. This decision should be confirmed by a lack of seizure activity on EEG.

11. e. Laboratory investigations for a patient with an initial seizure should include a complete blood count, blood glucose determination, liver and renal function tests, and a serologic test for syphilis. Initial and periodic EEG is mandatory. CT scanning or MRI scanning should be performed in patients with focal neurologic symptoms and/or signs, focal seizures, or EEG findings indicating a focal disturbance.

A chest x-ray should be performed in all patients who are cigarette smokers; a primary lung neoplasm with secondary brain metastases producing cerebral edema and seizures is not uncommon. However, a plain x-ray of the skull or a skull series is unlikely to produce any useful diagnostic information.

12. e. Status epilepticus is a medical emergency, with a mortality rate of up to 20% and a high incidence of neurologic and mental sequelae in survivors.

Status epilepticus may be caused by poor compliance with medication, alcohol withdrawal, intracranial infection, neoplasm, a metabolic disorder, or a drug overdose. Prognosis depends on the length of time from the onset of the seizure activity to effective treatment.

The management of status epilepticus includes establishing an airway, giving 50% dextrose in case of hypoglycemia, giving IV diazepam, giving IV phenytoin, and treating resistant cases with IV phenobarbital.

13. **f.** There are many causes of nonepileptic seizures. These are divided into the following categories:
1. Cardiogenic: (a) simple syncope; (b) transient ischemic attacks; (c) arrhythmias; and (d) sick sinus syndrome
2. Electrolyte imbalance: (a) hypocalcemia; (b) hyponatremia and water intoxication; and (c) hypomagnesemia
3. Metabolic: (a) hypoglycemia; (b) hyperglycemia; (c) thyrotoxic storm; and (d) pyridoxine deficiency
4. Acute drug withdrawal: (a) alcohol; (b) benzodiazepines; (c) cocaine; (d) barbiturates; and (e) meperidine
5. Drug intoxication: (a) cocaine; (b) dextroamphetamine; (c) theophylline; (d) isoniazid; (e) lithium; (f) nitrous oxide anesthesia; and (g) acetylcholinesterase inhibitors
6. Metals: (a) mercury and (b) lead
7. Infections: (a) gram-negative septicemia with shock; (b) viral meningitis; and, bacterial meningitis (gram-negative or syphilitic)
8. Hyperthermia
9. Pseudoseizures (psychogenic)
10. Malignancies
11. Idiopathic (isolated unprovoked seizure)

14. **b.** Absence (petit-mal) seizures often are confused with complex partial seizures in adolescents and adults. An accurate diagnosis often can be made on the basis of history, the duration of the seizure, the presence of an aura and/or postictal confusion, the pattern of autonomic behavior, and the EEG.

In absence seizures, minor clonic activity (eye blinks or head nodding) is present in up to 45% of cases; the mean duration is seconds; and the EEG shows the typical bilateral symmetric three-cycle second spike and wave that may be easily provoked by hyperventilation. There is no aura or postictal confusion.

In contrast, complex partial seizures may be preceded by an aura, are followed by postictal confusion, last longer (1-3 minutes), and are associated with more complex automatisms and less frequent clonic components. The EEG tends to show focal slow or sharp and slow wave activity. The differentiation between these two types of seizures is important. Absence seizures tend to disappear in adulthood, but complex partial seizures do not. Furthermore, phenytoin (Dilantin) and carbamazepine (Tegretol) are effective in treating complex partial seizures but not absence attacks.

15. **c.** The most common neurologic disorder is stroke. Epilepsy is the second most common disorder, with the prevalence ranging anywhere between 0.6% and 3.4% in the general population.

16. **d.** The most common primary brain tumor in elderly patients is a glioma. Of the gliomas, the glioblastomas and the astrocytomas are by far the most common.

SOLUTION TO THE CLINICAL CASE MANAGEMENT PROBLEM

Febrile Seizures in Children:
1. Age of risk: age 6 months to age 5 years
2. Risk factors for febrile convulsions:
   a. Previous febrile convulsion: the risk of a subsequent febrile convulsion is 30% when the first seizure occurred between the ages of 1 and 3 years; 50% when it occurred first at other ages; and 50% after a second febrile seizure.
   b. Family history of febrile convulsion (25%)
3. Prognosis: The prognosis for normal school progress and for seizure remission is excellent in children with febrile seizures.
4. Chances of progression of febrile seizures to epilepsy are very small: 98% of children with febrile seizures will have no further seizures after 5 years of age.
5. Factors that increase the chance of progression of febrile seizures to epilepsy:
   a. Presence of developmental delay
   b. Cerebral palsy
   c. Abnormal neurologic development
   d. History of epilepsy in a parent or sibling
   e. A seizure that has a focal onset, lasts more than 15 minutes, or recurs in the same febrile illness.
6. Treatment: usually no treatment necessary
   a. Usually not indicated. If you do use prophylactic anticonvulsants it will be only to treat the febrile seizure, not to prevent later epilepsy.
   b. Drug of choice when indicated: rectal or oral diazepam.

SUMMARY OF SEIZURES

1. Absolute rules concerning seizures:
   a. *Not all that seizes is epilepsy.*
   b. *Not all epilepsy seizes.*
   c. Many "seizures" are associated with other systemic disorders.
2. Major classification causes of nonepileptic seizures:
   a. Metastases to the brain
   b. Cardiogenic
   c. Electrolyte imbalance
   d. Metabolic causes
   e. Acute drug withdrawal
   f. Drug intoxication
   g. Heavy metal poisoning
   h. Infections
   i. Hyperthermia
   j. Pseudoseizures
3. Greatly simplified classification of epileptic seizures:
   a. Partial seizures:
      i. simple partial seizures
      ii. complex partial seizures
   b. Generalized seizures:
      i. petit-mal (absence seizures)
      ii. tonic-clonic (grand mal) seizures.
   c. Myoclonic seizures
   d. Tonic, clonic, or atonic seizures
4. Diagnosis and investigations:
   a. History (from a relative or bystander)
   b. Physical examination
   c. EEG
   d. CT and/or MRI
   e. Blood profile including CBC, blood glucose, liver function tests, renal function tests, human immunodeficiency virus serology (in high-risk groups), serum calcium, serologic test for syphilis
5. Treatment:
   a. Carefully evaluate whether the patient needs treatment after the first seizure. In both adults and children, risk of recurrence is increased from 33% to 50% by the presence of a focal seizure, abnormalities on neurologic examination, a preexisting neurologic disorder, and focal spikes or generalized spike-waves on EEG.
   b. Monotherapy suffices for most seizure disorders. As Blume (CMAJ, 2003) states, "Severity of the seizure disorder, not the laboratory numbers, determines the therapeutic range." Whatever serum drug level renders the patient seizure free is adequate for that patient, even if it is below the laboratory range.
   c. Both effectiveness and side effects are dependent on dosage, with small changes often having major effects. There are currently no studies to suggest that newer antiepileptic drugs are more effective than older ones. The most common side effect of most antiepileptic drugs is fatigue.
   d. Drugs for generalized tonic-clonic (grand-mal) seizures or partial seizures include the following:
      i. Phenytoin (drug of choice). Phenytoin also is the only antiepileptic drug that can be started at full dose.
      ii. Carbamazepine
      iii. Phenobarbital
   e. Once antiepileptic drug therapy is initiated, it should be maintained for a time period measured in years, not months. Patients must be considered carefully for discontinuation of therapy.
   f. Febrile seizures are not necessary to treat; diazepam can be taken every 8 hours for prevention, if that has been evaluated carefully.
   g. Status epilepticus: treatment is IV diazepam; alternatively, IV phenytoin or IV phenobarbital.
   h. Newer non-pharmacologic treatments: implantable vagal nerve stimulation for intractable seizures.

SUGGESTED READING

Blume WT: Diagnosis and management of epilepsy. *CMAJ* 168(4): 441-448, 2003.

Diaz-Arrastia R, et al: Evolving treatment strategies for epilepsy. *JAMA* 287(22):2917-2920, 2002.

Riviello JJ: Classification of seizures and epilepsy. *Curr Neurol Neurosci Rep* 3(4):325-331, 2003.

Schachter SC: Vagus nerve stimulation therapy summary: five years after FDA approval. *Neurology* 59(6 Suppl 4):S15-20, 2002.

So EL: Role of neuroimaging in the management of seizure disorders. *Mayo Clin Proc* 77(11):1251-1264, 2002.

Chapter 34

Anemia

> "I hardly have enough energy to get out of bed."

CLINICAL CASE PROBLEM 1:
A 35-YEAR-OLD FEMALE WITH FATIGUE

A 35-year-old female comes to your office with a 4-month history of fatigue. Her history is unremarkable; she has had no major medical illnesses. She has noticed that during the past 12 months her menstrual periods have become heavier and longer; instead of lasting for only 4 days with bleeding that was "light to moderate," she now has a 7- to 9-day period with "very heavy flow." She is the mother of three healthy children.

On examination, the patient appears pale. Her lower eyelids are pale and so is her skin. Her blood pressure is 100/70 mm Hg. Her pulse is 86 beats per minute. Physical examination, including a pelvic examination, is otherwise normal. Her blood smear reads as follows: red blood cells (RBCs) are microcytic and appear to be hypochromic. Her platelet count is 175,000/mm³. Her hemoglobin is 9.5 g/dl.

■ SELECT THE BEST ANSWER TO THE FOLLOWING QUESTIONS:

1. What is the most likely cause of this patient's anemia?
   a. iron-deficiency anemia
   b. hemolytic anemia
   c. folic acid–deficiency anemia
   d. pernicious anemia
   e. anemia of chronic disease

2. What treatment(s) is (are) therapeutic in this patient's condition?
   a. naproxen 375 mg bid (or a similar nonsteroidal antiinflammatory drug [NSAID]) during the last 2 weeks of the menstrual cycle
   b. a low-dose oral contraceptive pill (OCP) given either continuously or in a cyclic manner
   c. ferrous sulfate 300 mg od to 300 mg tid
   d. all of the above
   e. none of the above

3. The patient comes later in the week to the emergency room. Now her hemoglobin is 6.0 g/dl. She is tachycardic and hypotensive. Of the treatments listed, which will be most beneficial?
   a. Intramuscular (IM) medroxyprogesterone acetate
   b. Intravenous (IV) conjugated estrogen
   c. cryoprecipitate

   d. fresh frozen plasma
   e. high-dose OCPs given every hour

4. The patient follows up in your office a week after hospitalization. Her hemoglobin is now 9.6 g/dl. She says she has black stools, constipation, and nausea with the Fem-Iron (ferrous fumarate) medication. Your next suggestion is:
   a. prescribe Slow Fe (ferrous sulfate)
   b. prescribe an enteric-coated iron preparation
   c. prescribe weekly IM injections of iron
   d. advise her to continue her current medication with concomitant antacid use
   e. admit to the same day unit for IV iron administration

5. Which statement about the treatment of iron-deficiency anemia is false?
   a. treatment goals should be for 150-200 mg of elemental iron per day
   b. tea drinkers may show decreased iron absorption
   c. concurrent vitamin C administration may decrease iron absorption
   d. reticulocyte count should increase in 1 week
   e. iron therapy should continue for 6 months after hemoglobin level goal is reached

6. Which of the following investigations should be performed in this patient to rule out a secondary cause?
   a. pelvic ultrasound plus or minus pelvic laparoscopy
   b. coagulation profile
   c. computed tomography (CT) scan of the abdomen/pelvis
   d. a and b
   e. a, b, and c
   f. none of the above

7. What is the most sensitive test for the detection of the anemia described in Clinical Case Problem 1?
   a. serum iron
   b. serum iron binding capacity
   c. serum ferritin
   d. serum transferrin
   e. reticulocyte count

8. Based on a complete blood count (CBC) and peripheral smear only, how can iron-deficiency anemia be differentiated from thalassemia?
   a. thalassemia is normochromic, normocytic and iron deficiency is microcytic, hypochromic
   b. previous CBCs are normal in patients with thalassemia
   c. thalassemia shows a high to normal RBC count, whereas iron deficiency shows a low RBC count

d. b and c
e. a, b, and c

CLINICAL CASE PROBLEM 2:

A Pregnant Woman with a Hemoglobin Level of 10.8 g/dl

A pregnant woman at 22 weeks of gestation comes to your office for her regular checkup. Her hemoglobin level is 10.8 g/dL.

9. Which of the following statements regarding anemia and pregnancy is false?
   a. iron supplementation is necessary in pregnancy to prevent microcytic anemia
   b. a "false" anemia is seen as a result of the relative expansion of the plasma volume relative to the RBC mass
   c. folic-acid supplementation is necessary in pregnancy to prevent macrocytic anemia
   d. hemoglobinopathies often are first diagnosed when a woman comes for prenatal care
   e. iron deficiency is the most common anemia in pregnancy

CLINICAL CASE PROBLEM 3:

A Fatigued 55-Year-Old Male

A 55-year-old male comes to your office for a periodic health assessment. His only complaint is that he has been feeling quite fatigued during the last 3 months. He does not smoke and rarely drinks.

On physical examination the patient appears pale. His blood pressure is 100/80 mm Hg. His pulse is 96 and regular. No other abnormalities are found. A CBC reveals a hemoglobin value of 10.0 g/dl. His blood smear also shows a decreased mean corpuscular hemoglobin count (MCHC) and a decreased mean corpuscular volume (MCV).

10. Until proved otherwise, what is the most likely cause of his low hemoglobin level?
    a. lymphoma
    b. gastrointestinal malignancy
    c. lack of intrinsic factor
    d. dietary deficiency of folic acid
    e. dietary lack of iron

CLINICAL CASE PROBLEM 4:

A 78-Year-Old Female Complaining of a "Lack of Energy"

A 78-year-old female with osteoarthritis comes to your office complaining of a "lack of energy" that began 8 months ago. On examination, the patient has marked pallor. Her hemoglobin level is 7.5 g/dl at this time. A peripheral blood smear reveals hypochromasia and microcytosis. One year ago her hemoglobin was 13.0 g/dl.

11. What is the most likely cause of this patient's anemia?
    a. malnutrition
    b. pernicious anemia
    c. folic-acid deficiency
    d. gastrointestinal bleeding
    e. hypothyroidism

12. The anemia of chronic disease is most often which of the following?
    a. hypochromic and normocytic
    b. hypochromic and microcytic
    c. normochromic and macrocytic
    d. normochromic and normocytic
    e. hyperchromic and macrocytic

13. What is the most common cause of anemia of chronic disease?
    a. chronic hepatic failure
    b. chronic renal failure
    c. congestive cardiac failure
    d. autoimmune disease
    e. chronic neurologic disease

14. What are acceptable treatments for anemia of chronic disease?
    a. iron therapy
    b. erythropoietin
    c. treatment of the underlying condition
    d. b and c
    e. a, b, and c

15. Which of the following disorders is (are) associated with the anemia of chronic disease?
    a. rheumatoid arthritis
    b. non-Hodgkin's lymphoma
    c. chronic renal failure
    d. chronic hepatic failure
    e. all of the above

16. Which of the following is the most common type of anemia in the North American population?
    a. anemia of chronic disease
    b. iron-deficiency anemia
    c. macrocytic anemia
    d. autoimmune hemolytic anemia
    e. iatrogenic anemia

CLINICAL CASE PROBLEM 5:

A 75-Year-Old Female with Fatigue, Paresthesias, Weakness, and an Unsteady Gait

A 75-year-old female comes to your office with an 8-month history of increasing fatigue, paresthesias, weakness, and an unsteady gait. These are new symptoms. Her past medical history is significant for hemicolectomy for colon cancer of the terminal ileum 3 years ago.

On examination, her skin is pale, as are her lower conjunctival lids. She has a number of interesting neurologic findings on physical examination, including patchy impairment of the sensations of touch and temperature, loss of both vibration and position sense, a positive Romberg sign, hyperreflexia, and bilateral up-going Babinski signs. Her hemoglobin is 6.8 g/dl.

17. Which of the following statements regarding this patient's condition is (are) true?
    a. this patient has a hemolytic anemia
    b. a CT scan of the brain should be performed
    c. hyposegmented neutrophils will be seen on the blood smear
    d. the MCV value will be > 100 mm^3
    e. all of the above

18. If you could choose only one investigation to do next, what would it be in this patient?
    a. reticulocyte count
    b. serum folate
    c. serum vitamin B$_{12}$ level
    d. gastroscopy
    e. bone marrow biopsy

19. What is the probable etiology of this patient's condition?
    a. decreased dietary intake of vitamin B$_{12}$
    b. alcoholism
    c. surgical resection of the terminal ileum
    d. brain tumor
    e. chemotherapy with methotrexate

20. During the first 2 weeks of therapy for the condition described in Clinical Case Problem 5, which of the following is the most reasonable treatment regimen?
    a. folic acid 5 mg/day orally
    b. vitamin B$_{12}$ 100 mg/day orally
    c. vitamin B$_{12}$ 1000 mg/day intramuscularly
    d. ferrous sulfate 300 mg/day; folic acid 5 mg/day; vitamin B$_{12}$ 100 mg/day (all orally)
    e. none of the above

21. What is (are) the acceptable option for the long-term treatment of this condition?
    a. long-term treatment is not necessary
    b. oral B$_{12}$ at 100 mcg daily
    c. nasal B$_{12}$ gel weekly
    d. oral folate
    e. b and c

22. Which of the following statements regarding folic-acid deficiency is false?

a. folic-acid deficiency demonstrates a macrocytic anemia
b. hypersegmented neutrophils often are seen on the peripheral blood smear
c. the most common cause of folic-acid deficiency is an inadequate dietary intake of folic acid
d. folic-acid deficiency is uncommon in patients who demonstrate alcohol abuse
e. reduced folate levels usually are seen in red blood cells and in the serum

CLINICAL CASE PROBLEM 6:
A 38-YEAR-OLD MALE WITH A HEMOGLOBIN VALUE OF 10.0 G/DL

A 38-year-old male with a history of a gastric bypass for morbid obesity comes to your office with a hemoglobin of 10.0 g/dl. His MCV is 88 mm^3. His ferritin is 35 µg/L, and his red cell distribution width (RDW) is high. His reticulocyte count is high.

23. Which of the following statements about his clinical presentation is (are) true?
    a. his anemia is the result of iron deficiency
    b. his anemia is the result of vitamin B$_{12}$ deficiency
    c. his anemia is result of chronic disease
    d. a and b
    e. a and c

CLINICAL CASE PROBLEM 7:
AN 18-YEAR-OLD FEMALE WITH SEVERE FATIGUE AND LIGHTHEADEDNESS

An 18-year-old female you saw for a urinary tract infection last week comes to your office with severe fatigue and lightheadedness. She states that her last menstrual period was 3 weeks ago and that her flow was light, as usual. Her hemoglobin is 8.7 g/L, and her MCV is 84 mm^3. Last year her CBC was normal.

24. Which of the following statements describes her condition?
    a. this is iron-deficiency anemia
    b. this is folic-acid deficiency anemia probably resulting from anorexia
    c. this is hemolytic anemia secondary to Macrodantin
    d. this patient has sickle cell anemia
    e. none of the above

CLINICAL CASE MANAGEMENT PROBLEM

Distinguish between megaloblastosis and macrocytosis.

ANSWERS:

1. **a.** The patient in Clinical Case Problem 1 has an iron-deficiency anemia. This is the most common cause of anemia. In this patient, the most likely cause of the anemia is excessive blood loss during her menstrual periods.

Pernicious anemia, folic-acid deficiency anemia, hemolytic anemia, and anemia of chronic disease are not associated with the hypochromic, microcytic changes that characterize iron-deficiency anemia.

2. **d.** The OCP will accomplish the result of reducing menstrual blood flow and is the drug of choice. An NSAID drug such as naproxen may have a profound effect on decreasing the menstrual blood flow. For the patient in Clinical Case Problem 1, the appropriate symptomatic treatment to build up her iron stores is ferrous sulfate or ferrous gluconate. The initial dose of ferrous sulfate should be 300 mg tid. It may be necessary to use ferrous sulfate for only 1-2 months; at that time the patient can stop taking off iron and continue taking the OCP.

3. **b.** The patient has severe menorrhagia with hemodynamic compromise or impending hemodynamic compromise, and the treatment of choice is IV conjugated estrogen, 25 mg repeated every 4 hours until the menorrhagia subsides.

4. **a.** See Answer 5.

5. **c.** Iron therapy can be associated with many gastrointestinal side effects. To minimize side effects, iron supplements should be taken with food; this may decrease iron absorption somewhat. Changing to a different iron salt or to a controlled-release preparation also may reduce side effects. Enteric-coated preparations are ineffective because they do not dissolve in the stomach. Unpredictable absorption and local complications of IM administration make the IV route preferable when it is necessary to treat with parenteral iron. Antacids and caffeinated beverages, especially tea, will reduce iron absorption. Vitamin C therapy will facilitate iron absorption.

Treatment goals for iron administration should aim for 150-200 mg of elemental iron per day. Iron therapy should continue for 4-6 months when the serum ferritin level reaches 50, indicating adequate iron replacement. Reticulocyte count does increase within 1 week of starting iron therapy.

6. **d.** Pelvic ultrasound, laparoscopy, and a coagulation profile should uncover the potential presence of uterine fibroids, endometriosis, or von Willebrand's disease, respectively. A CT scan of the abdomen/pelvis is not indicated.

7. **c.** The most sensitive test for the diagnosis of iron-deficiency anemia is the serum ferritin level. In iron-deficiency anemia, the serum ferritin level usually decreases first. Thereafter, total iron binding capacity (TIBC) increases and serum iron levels gradually decrease. The transferrin saturation also will decrease at this time. The reticulocyte count is not useful in assessing the degree of iron-deficiency anemia.

8. **c.** Both thalassemia and iron-deficiency anemia are hypochromic, microcytic. Thalassemia tends to be more hypochromic and microcytic than iron deficiency. A quick way to differentiate the two anemias is to look at the RBC count. In iron deficiency the number will be low. In thalassemia, the number will be normal to high.

9. **c.** Folic-acid supplementation is necessary in pregnancy to prevent neural tube defects, not macrocytic anemia. Iron supplementation is necessary in pregnancy to prevent microcytic anemia. A "false" anemia is seen because of the relative expansion of the plasma volume relative to the RBC mass. Hemoglobinopathies often are first diagnosed when a woman comes to your office for prenatal care. Iron deficiency is the most common anemia in pregnancy.

10. **b.** Until proved otherwise, iron-deficiency anemia in a middle-aged or elderly male is the result of gastrointestinal blood loss, the most sinister cause of which is a gastrointestinal malignancy. Carcinomas of the colon or rectum are the most important and most common malignancies found in this situation. This patient should have fecal occult blood testing followed by colonoscopy. Air-contrast barium enema may or may not be indicated for further elucidation. If all of the investigations are normal, the upper gastrointestinal tract should be investigated by endoscopy.

Dietary iron deficiency or dietary folic-acid deficiency is extremely unusual in a male without alcoholism.

A lymphoma is more likely to produce a normochromic-normocytic blood smear rather than a hypochromic, microcytic picture.

Bleeding hemorrhoids also may produce iron-deficiency anemia in middle-aged males.

Vitamin B_{12} deficiency resulting from lack of intrinsic factor would present as a macrocytic rather than a microcytic anemia.

11. **d.** This patient's hypochromic, microcytic blood picture, coupled with a decrease in hemoglobin from 13.0-7.5 g/dl in 1 year, is almost certainly the result of blood loss from a gastrointestinal malignancy or other bleeding source. A good bet is that she has a gastrointestinal bleed secondary to NSAID use, but colon cancer needs to be seriously considered too. The discussion in Answer 10 regarding the iron-deficiency anemia in males also applies to females past menopause. The other common cause of iron-deficiency anemia in elderly patients is malnutrition.

In contradistinction to hypochromic, microcytic anemia, the most common causes of megaloblastic anemia are B_{12} and folic-acid deficiencies.

12. d. The anemia of chronic disease is most often normochromic and normocytic. It can present as a mild hypochromic, microcytic anemia also.

13. b. See Answer 15.

14. d. See Answer 15.

15. e. The anemia of chronic disease is associated most frequently with the following: (1) anemia of chronic inflammation that may be associated with infection; autoimmune connective tissue disorders; or malignancy (excluding malignancies where blood loss is a major factor, as in colon cancer); (2) anemia as a result of chronic renal failure (this is the most common cause of anemia of chronic disease); (3) anemia as a result of endocrine failure; or (4) anemia of hepatic disease.

Treatment of anemia of chronic disease is aimed at treating the underlying condition. In some cases, particularly when chronic renal disease or cancer is the causative source, erythropoietin injections are helpful in treating the anemia.

16. b. In North America the most common category of anemia is iron-deficiency anemia. In order of frequency, anemia prevalence is as follows:
1. Iron-deficiency anemia as a result of blood loss from (a) excessive menstrual flow and (b) the gastrointestinal tract.
2. Anemia of chronic disease: the most common causes are (a) chronic renal failure and (b) anemia resulting from connective tissue disorders.
3. Macrocytic anemia generally is caused by (a) pernicious anemia or (b) folic-acid deficiency anemia.
4. Hemolytic anemia caused by either (a) autoimmune hemolytic anemias or (b) nonautoimmune hemolytic anemias.

17. d. This patient has pernicious anemia. The signs and symptoms of pernicious anemia can be remembered well by the 5 Ps, namely: (1) pancytopenia; (2) peripheral neuropathy; (3) posterior spinal column neuropathy; (4) pyramidal tract signs; and (5) papillary (tongue) atrophy.

The blood smear of a patient with pernicious anemia will show the following: megaloblastic anemia as demonstrated by MCV > 100 mm^3, hypersegmented (not hyposegmented) neutrophils, and oval macrocytes.

18. c. The most significant single determination would be serum vitamin B_{12} level.

19. c. Pernicious anemia is defined as a deficiency of vitamin B_{12} resulting from lack of production of intrinsic factor by the gastric parietal cells or decreased absorption in the terminal ileum. Much less commonly vitamin B_{12} deficiency results from inadequate intake, such as a true vegan diet. Methotrexate is a folate inhibitor and is associated with macrocytic anemia as a result of folate deficiency. Alcoholism is associated with B_{12} and folate deficiency, but the surgical resection of the terminal ileum is the most likely cause of this patient's anemia.

20. c. The acute treatment of pernicious anemia that is recommended is 1000 mg/day for 1 week followed by 1000 mg/week for 4 weeks and then followed by maintenance therapy of 1000 mg/month. Because the root cause of the disease lies in an inability to absorb the vitamin, it cannot be administered orally.

21. c. The recommended treatments for maintenance therapy of vitamin B_{12} deficiency classically have been monthly injections of 1000 mcg of vitamin B_{12}. Recently a nasal gel formulation to be used once weekly has demonstrated success. There are even some studies that have shown successful treatment with daily large doses of oral vitamin B_{12} of 1000-2000 mcg, but because poor absorption is the underlying problem a dose of 100 mcg daily will be insufficient.

Because the underlying cause is a B_{12} deficiency, administration of folate is not the proper treatment. Nonetheless, folate will resolve the macrocytic anemia because the anemia itself is caused by an inhibition of nucleic acid synthesis resulting from an inability to regenerate active tetrahydrofolate, one of the two functions normally provided by vitamin B_{12}. However, administration of folate will not prevent the neurologic damage, which is a direct effect of a deficiency of vitamin B_{12}, because of its second normal function as a cofactor in the methylmalonyl CoA mutase reaction. This reaction is a necessary step in the catabolism of fatty acids with an odd number of carbons and branched-chained fatty acid formed during branched-chain amino acid catabolism. (Apparently when these unusual fatty acids are not effectively catabolized they are incorporated into myelin sheets and cause neuropathies.) As a consequence, administration of folate in cases of megaloblastic anemia will alleviate the hematologic symptoms but will permit the neurologic symptoms to progress. Thus megaloblastic anemia should never be treated with folate alone; it should be treated with a combination of folate and vitamin B_{12}.

22. d. The most common cause of folic-acid deficiency is inadequate intake. Folic-acid deficiency is most commonly seen in patients with alcoholism, patients with a malignancy, elderly patients, patients on a vegan diet, and pregnant patients.

Folic-acid deficiency anemia such as vitamin B_{12} deficiency also induces a megaloblastic anemia (see Answer 21). Patients with pure folic-acid deficiency usually have normal vitamin B_{12} levels. Patients with folic-acid deficiency anemia should be given 1-5 mg of folic acid/day.

23. d. This patient has a mixed-picture anemia, primarily because of his gastric bypass, which is preventing him from effectively absorbing iron and vitamin B_{12}. Anemia of chronic disease would not be associated with a high reticulocyte count.

24. c. This patient has hemolytic anemia resulting from the use of Macrodantin. It is unlikely to be iron deficiency without the history of heavy menses. Her MCV is not elevated, which makes a folic-acid deficiency anemia unlikely. Her CBC would have been abnormal last year if she had sickle cell anemia, which is a normochromic, normocytic anemia.

SOLUTION TO THE CLINICAL CASE MANAGEMENT PROBLEM

The difference between macrocytosis and megaloblastosis is that in megaloblastosis the macrocytes are oval, whereas in macrocytosis the macrocytes are round.

Megaloblastic anemias are only one cause of macrocytosis. The differential diagnosis of macrocytosis includes the following: (1) megaloblastic anemias; (2) liver disease; (3) reticulocytosis; (4) myeloproliferative diseases (leukemia, myelofibrosis); (5) multiple myeloma; (6) metastatic disease of bone marrow; (7) hypothyroidism; (8) aplastic anemia; (9) drugs (cytotoxic agents, alcohol); and (10) autoagglutination or cold agglutination disease.

SUMMARY OF ANEMIAS

1. Normal adult hemoglobin levels are 14.0-18.0 g/dl for males and 12.0-16.0 g/dl for females.
2. Classification of anemias on the basis of cause (production, destruction, loss).
   a. Production problems include the following: (i) hemoglobin synthesis disturbances as may be caused by iron deficiency, thalassemia, chronic disease, (ii) DNA synthesis disturbances that lead to megaloblastic anemia; (iii) bone marrow infiltration in malignancies; and (iv) stem-cell disease as in aplastic anemia and myeloproliferative disease.
   b. Destruction problems include the following: (i) intrinsic hemolysis as in spherocytosis, sickle cell, enzyme deficiencies and (ii) extrinsic hemolysis as in infection, immune complexes, thrombocytopenic purpura, hemolytic/uremic syndrome, or mechanical valves.
   c. Blood loss problems include the following: (i) excessive menstruation; (ii) bleeding in the gastrointestinal or genitourinary tracts; and (iii) trauma.

3. Classification of anemias on the basis of cell size and appearance (microcytic, macrocytic, normocytic, hypochromic, normochromic).
   a. Microcytic anemias may be the result of the following: (i) iron deficiency, potentially caused by blood loss or nutritional deficiencies; (ii) thalassemias; and (iii) chronic disease.
   b. Macrocytic anemias are either megaloblastic caused by folate or B_{12} deficiencies or nonmegaloblastic such as from chemotherapy.
4. Iron-deficiency anemia:
   a. Most common cause of anemia
   b. Most common cause in premenopausal women is excessive menstrual flow
   c. Iron-deficiency anemia in males or in postmenopausal females should be considered to be from gastrointestinal blood loss until proved otherwise; most common secondary cause is GI malignancy
   d. Iron-deficiency anemia is hypochromic, microcytic: microcytosis comes first; hypochromasia is seen in advanced cases
   e. Serum ferritin level is usually less than 12 mg/L and is the most sensitive test for iron deficiency

Continued

SUMMARY OF ANEMIAS—cont'd

f. Most pregnant women with decreased hemoglobin are not truly anemic; they simply have a greater increase in plasma volume than in RBC mass; true anemia in pregnancy has been defined by the Centers for Disease Control and Prevention as hemoglobin in first and third trimester less than 11.0 g/dL or by hemoglobin in second trimester less than 10.5 g/dL

g. Investigations in women with excessive menstrual flow include pelvic ultrasound/laparoscopy (uterine fibroids, endometriosis) and coagulation disorders (such as von Willebrand's disease)

h. Treatment for iron-deficiency anemia: (i) find the cause and correct if possible; (ii) administer ferrous sulfate 300 mg tid; provide menorrhagia: prophylaxis via OCP; and severe menorrhagia with unstable vital signs using IV conjugated estrogen

5. Anemia of chronic disease:
   a. Anemia of chronic disease is normochromic, normocytic.
   b. Causes of anemia of chronic disease are as follows: (i) chronic renal failure (most common); (ii) connective tissue disorders (autoimmune diseases); (iii) malignancies (except GI blood loss) such as multiple myeloma or lymphomas; (iv) inflammatory diseases, and (v) chronic hepatic disease.
   c. Make the diagnosis (find the cause) and treat the cause.

6. Megaloblastic anemia as the result a vitamin B_{12} deficiency:
   a. Pernicious anemia is the most common cause. It is from vitamin B_{12} deficiency caused by lack of intrinsic factor. Other causes of vitamin B_{12} deficiency are total or subtotal gastrectomy and a vegan diet.
   b. Blood smear: (i) MCV > 100 mm^3; (ii) hypersegmented neutrophils; and (iii) oval macrocytes.
   c. Confirming tests are determination of the serum vitamin B_{12} level and a Schilling test.
   d. The five defining Ps are as follows: (i) **p**ancytopenia; (ii) **p**eripheral neuropathy; (iii) **p**osterior spinal column neuropathy; (iv) **p**apillary (tongue) atrophy; and (v) **p**yramidal tract signs.
   e. Treatment: (i) vitamin B_{12} subcutaneously (sc) 1000 mg/day; (ii) vitamin B_{12} sc 1000 mg/week; and (iii) vitamin B_{12} sc 1000 mg/month.
   f. Remember that a vitamin B_{12} deficiency also may induce a neuropathy.

7. Megaloblastic anemia resulting from folic-acid deficiency:
   a. Diagnosis: blood smear with hypersegmented neutrophils and macroovalocytes
   b. Confirmation: decreased serum folate or RBC folate
   c. Most common cause of folic-acid deficiency is a dietary deficiency associated with alcoholism, vegan diet, and elderly patients on a "tea and toast" diet; Also results from medications such as methotrexate and OCPs, pregnancy, and malignancy
   d. Folic-acid supplementation is recommended for all pregnant women (1 mg).

8. Hemolytic anemias:
   a. Classification: (i) autoimmune hemolytic anemias and (ii) nonautoimmune hemolytic anemias
   b. Common causes are as follows: (i) drugs (iatrogenic disease), the most common cause of hemolytic anemia; (ii) lymphoproliferative disorders (chronic lymphocytic leukemia [CLL], non-Hodgkin's lymphoma); (iii) autoimmune connective tissue disorders (systemic lupus erythematosus (SLS), rheumatoid arthritis; (iv) infections (Ebstein-Barr virus, cytomegalovirus, mycoplasma pneumoniae, human immunodeficiency virus); (v) glucose 6-phosphate dehydrogenase (G6PDH) deficiency; and (vi) paroxysmal cold hemoglobinuria.
   c. Diagnosis: (i) Coombs test: direct and indirect and (ii) reticulocyte count (elevated)
   d. Treatment: (i) corticosteroids; (ii) splenectomy (in those who do not respond); and (iii) IV immunoglobulin

9. Miscellaneous disorders include the following: (a) aplastic anemias; (b) thalassemia; (c) sickle cell disease; (d) hemophilia; (e) platelet-associated bleeding disorders; and (f) disseminated intravascular coagulation.

SUGGESTED READING

Armas-Loughran B, et al: Evaluation and management of anemia and bleeding disorders in surgical patients. *Med Clin N Am* 87(1):229-242, 2003 Jan.

Balducci L: Epidemiology of anemia in the elderly: information on diagnostic evaluation. *J Am Geriatr Soc* 51(3 Suppl):S2-9, 2003 Mar.

Brill J, Baumgardner D: Normocytic anemia. *Am Fam Phys* 62:2255-2264, 2000.

Hermiston ML, Mentzer WC: A practical approach to the evaluation of the anemic child. *Pediatr Clin N Am* 49(5):877-891, 2002 Oct.

Means RT Jr: Recent developments in the anemia of chronic disease. *Curr Hematol Rep* 2(2):116-121, 2003.

Smith D: Anemia in the elderly. *Am Fam Phys* 62:1565-1574, 2000.

Tefferi A: Anemia in adults: a contemporary approach to diagnosis. *Mayo Clin Proc* 78(10):1274-1280, 2003.

Weiss G: Pathogenesis and treatment of anaemia of chronic disease. *Blood Rev* 16(2):87-96, 2002.

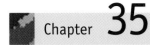

Chapter 35

Certain Hematologic Conditions

"You mean I got this disease
from a Mr. Hodgkin?"

CLINICAL CASE PROBLEM 1:

A 16-YEAR-OLD MALE WITH A SUPRACLAVICULAR MASS

A 16-year-old male is brought to your office by his mother. He has noticed a significant swelling in the left supraclavicular area that has been present for approximately 4 months. According to the patient, it has not changed significantly in size over that time. He has had no fever, chills, nausea, vomiting, fatigue/malaise, weight loss, or other symptoms.

On examination, vital signs are normal. A mass measuring 2.5 cm × 1.5 cm is felt to be attached to the muscle above the left scapula. His chest is otherwise normal to auscultation and percussion. The abdomen is soft. There is no hepatomegaly or splenomegaly. The skin is benign. No significant lymph-node enlargement is present in the cervical, axillary, or inguinal regions.

■ SELECT THE BEST ANSWER TO THE FOLLOWING QUESTIONS:

1. What is the most appropriate definitive diagnostic step for this patient?
   a. a complete blood workup
   b. a fine-needle biopsy
   c. an excisional biopsy
   d. a chest radiograph
   e. none of the above

2. The evaluation produces a report that reads as follows: "Reed-Sternberg cells present." What is the most likely diagnosis?
   a. reactive lymph-node enlargement
   b. acquired immune deficiency syndrome (AIDS)
   c. metastatic carcinoma
   d. Hodgkin's disease
   e. non-Hodgkin's lymphoma

3. What is the next step in the investigation of this patient?
   a. computed tomography (CT) scan of the abdomen
   b. radiation therapy
   c. combination chemotherapy
   d. bone scan
   e. a and d

4. In the staging of the disease from which this patient suffers, there are two distinct categories, A and B. To what do these two categories refer?
   a. the presence or absence of metastases
   b. the presence or absence of symptoms
   c. the presence or absence of bone marrow involvement
   d. the possibility or nonpossibility of cure
   e. the presence or absence of intraabdominal disease

5. The patient's disease is staged, and he is found to have disease throughout the mediastinum but not below the diaphragm. At this time, what kind of therapy is likely to be administered?
   a. no therapy is indicated at this time; await the development of symptoms
   b. combination chemotherapy
   c. radiation therapy
   d. combination chemotherapy plus radiotherapy
   e. radical surgery

6. The patient's mother asks you about his prognosis. Which of the following is not true regarding this patient's illness?
   a. most patients with this disease have an overall survival of between 80% and 90%
   b. he may be at risk for premature cardiovascular disease as a result of treatment
   c. he may be at increased risk for infertility
   d. he may be at increased risk for secondary malignancies
   e. once treated, he will have little risk of recurrence

CLINICAL CASE PROBLEM 2:

A 62-YEAR-OLD MALE WITH SWELLINGS IN HIS NECK AND ELBOWS AND CHEST PAINS

A 62-year-old male comes to your office to reassure himself about "some swellings in my neck, elbows, as well as some chest pain." The other symptom is profound fatigue (for the last 3 months). On examination, his vital signs are normal, but he looks pale and has lost 10 lb since a visit 1 year ago. He has multiple enlarged cervical lymph nodes (and bilateral epitrochlear nodes); they measure anywhere from 1.0 cm to 2.0 cm in diameter. His liver edge is palpated approximately 3 cm below the left costal edge, and the tip of the spleen can be felt when he lies on his side.

7. If you could select only one test to perform on this patient, which of the following would you select?
   a. Enzyme-linked immunosorbent assay human immunodeficiency virus (HIV) screening test

b. Immunoglobulin G-viral capsid antigen (IgG-VCA) antibody titer for cytomegalovirus
c. IgG-VCA antibody titer for toxoplasmosis
d. CT scan of the chest
e. excisional lymph-node biopsy

8. The test you ordered is performed. The result shows diffuse small cleaved cell (diffuse poorly differentiated lymphocytic) histology. Based on what you know at present, what is the most likely diagnosis?
   a. non-Hodgkin's lymphoma
   b. Hodgkin's disease
   c. systemic toxoplasmosis: systemic immune deficiency
   d. systemic cytomegalovirus: systemic immune deficiency
   e. AIDS

9. The patient turns out to have an advanced stage (III) of a follicular form of non-Hodgkin's lymphoma. The treatment of choice may include which of the following?
   a. Zidovudine (AZT)
   b. intensive chemotherapy and bone marrow transplantation
   c. interferon-alpha and monoclonal antibodies
   d. intensive chemotherapy and radiotherapy
   e. c and d

10. Which of the following statements is true regarding the illness seen in this patient?
    a. it is more common in younger individuals
    b. patients usually live a normal lifespan without treatment
    c. there appears to be a relationship with the Epstein-Barr virus in some forms of the disease
    d. it is less common than the Hodgkin's form of lymphoma
    e. there is no relationship between the disease's incidence and HIV disease

CLINICAL CASE PROBLEM 3:

A 62-Year-Old Male with "Bone Pain"
in His "Breast Bone" and Skull

A 62-year-old male comes to your office with a chief complaint of "bone pain" in "my breast bone and my head, Doc." He tells you that he is sure he is OK but is here only because "the wife kept bugging me until I gave in." The patient also appears somewhat pale and tells you that he has been feeling tired lately and a bit "weak, depressed, and maybe confused."

He had a "touch of the flu" a few months ago. His wife tells you that this "touch of the flu" was actually bacterial pneumonia (organism *Streptococcus pneumoniae*). On examination, the patient has a tender sternum, tender occipital area of the skull, and pale conjunctiva.

You perform a series of laboratory tests.

11. The laboratory test results are as follows: hemoglobin 8.5 g/dl; normochromic/normocytic anemia; erythrocyte sedimentation rate (ESR) 55 mm/h; platelets 15,000/mm³; serum calcium 14 mg/dl; Na$^+$ 151 mEq/L; and serum creatinine 5.3 mmol/L. Based on the information you now have for Clinical Case Problem 3, what is the most likely diagnosis?
    a. metastatic carcinoma: metastasized to bone
    b. chronic lymphocytic leukemia
    c. multiple myeloma
    d. chronic renal failure: secondary to macroglobulinemia
    e. chronic myelogenous leukemia

12. Further investigations substantiate your findings. What is the treatment of choice at this time?
    a. bone marrow transplantation
    b. total body radiotherapy
    c. adjuvant combination chemotherapy: adriamycin, vincristine, bleomycin
    d. melphalan plus prednisone
    e. none of the above

13. The patient's disease is the result of a proliferation of which of the following?
    a. myeloblasts
    b. lymphoblasts
    c. metastatic cancer cells
    d. plasma cells
    e. none of the above

MATCHING QUESTIONS

In Part A certain hematologic disorders are listed a. through z. Match each numbered question (Questions 14-23) describing a hematologic disorder in part B with a (the) appropriate disease(s) as listed in part A. Each disease may be used once, twice, three times, or not at all.

Part A: Diseases
a. Aplastic anemia
b. Secondary polycythemia
c. Hemolytic anemia
d. Drug-induced thrombocytopenia
e. Idiopathic thrombocytopenia purpura
f. Sickle cell disease

g. Sickle cell trait
h. Preleukemia
i. Acute lymphocytic leukemia
j. Disseminated intravascular coagulation
k. Hemophilia
l. Multiple myeloma
m. Chronic lymphocytic leukemia
n. Hemochromatosis
o. Acute myelogenous leukemia
p. Chronic myelogenous leukemia
q. Cutaneous t-cell leukemia
r. Neutrophilia
s. von Willebrand's disease
t. Thalassemia
u. Hairy cell leukemia
v. Acute intermittent porphyria
w. Polycythemia rubra vera
x. Secondary thrombocytopenia
y. Transfusion reaction
z. Myelofibrosis

PART B: DESCRIPTION

14. Clinical Case 4: Choice_____
    - Disease is associated with excessive proliferation of erythroid, granulocytic, and megakaryocytic precursors.
    - Splenomegaly is almost universal in this disease.
    - Disease has significantly elevated red blood cell mass.
    - Patient presents with plethora.
    - Disease characteristically has thrombocytosis.

15. Clinical Case 5: Choice_____
    - Disease produces a major disorder of the bone marrow.
    - Splenomegaly is present in all patients.
    - As the disease progresses, patients experience weight loss; skin and mucous membrane bleeding; and bone pain, jaundice, and lymphadenopathy.
    - Bone marrow tap is almost always unsuccessful: it is known as a "dry tap."
    - Bone marrow biopsy reveals fibrosis of marrow spaces and osteosclerosis.

16. Clinical Case 6: Choice_____
    - This disease has the presence of the Philadelphia chromosome.
    - When this disease is diagnosed, the total WBC often exceeds 200,000 cells/mm^3.
    - This disease usually follows the following course: (a) chronic phase of variable duration, (b) blastic transformation, with (c) some patients experiencing a distinct intermediate accelerated phase.

- The most consistent physical finding is splenomegaly.
- This is the most common serious hematologic disorder diagnosed in patients who survived the atomic bombs of Hiroshima and Nagasaki.

17. Clinical Case 7: Choice_____
    - This form of leukemia is the most common form of leukemia in the United States.
    - The disease usually is seen in patients older than 50 years of age.
    - The abnormal cells morphologically resemble mature, small lymphocytes of the peripheral blood and accumulate in the bone marrow, blood, lymph nodes, and spleen in large numbers.
    - This disease has an "indolent nature."
    - Median survival exceeds 10 years, and many patients require no treatment.

18. Clinical Case 8: Choice_____
    - This disease has characteristic cells that exhibit cytoplasmic projections on their surfaces.
    - This disease is the result of an expansion of neoplastic type B lymphocytes.
    - This disease usually presents in male patients older than age 40 years.
    - Approximately 30% of patients with this disease have a vasculitislike disorder.
    - The treatment of choice for this disease is very characteristic of the disease: cladribine.

19. Clinical Case 9: Choice_____
    - This disease is a disease of children and young adults.
    - This disease is characterized by the clonal proliferation of immature hematopoietic cells.
    - The most common abnormal cells seen on bone marrow biopsy are immature lymphoblasts.
    - Infection is a nearly universal complication.
    - Approximately 50% of patients either are cured or characterized as being in long-term remission.

20. Clinical Case 10: Choice_____
    - The incidence of this disease increases with increasing age.
    - The most common abnormal cells seen on bone marrow biopsy are immature myeloblasts or immature promyelocyte.
    - Some patients with this disease develop the disease after either a preleukemia syndrome or a myelodysplastic syndrome.
    - Between 10% and 30% of patients with this disease survive 5 years; most of these patients are likely to survive long term.

- Bone marrow transplantation from either an identical twin or human leukocyte antigen-identical sibling is a very important part of treatment.

21. Clinical Case 11: Choice_____
    - This disease usually follows recovery from either a viral exanthem or a viral upper-respiratory tract illness.
    - The acute form of this disease is caused by immune complexes containing viral antigens that bind to platelet receptors.
    - This disease produces a profound rapid decrease in the cell line in question.
    - Corticosteroids are the agents of choice in the treatment of this disease.
    - In severe cases of this disease, splenectomy may need to be performed.

22. Clinical Case 12: Choice_____
    - This is the most common inherited bleeding disorder.
    - The factor that is missing in this disease is responsible for platelet adhesion.
    - The factor that is missing in this disease also serves as a plasma carrier for factor VIII.
    - Women with this disorder initially may be diagnosed because of severe menorrhagia.
    - The treatment of choice for this disease is cryoprecipitate.

23. Clinical Case 13: Choice_____
    - This disease is associated most frequently with obstetric catastrophes.
    - Other major causes of this disease are major trauma, metastatic malignancies, and bacterial sepsis.
    - In this disease, the combination of potent thrombogenic stimuli causes the deposition of small thrombi and small emboli throughout the microvasculature.
    - Most patients with this disease have extensive skin and mucous membrane bleeding and hemorrhage from multiple sites.
    - Patients with bleeding as a major symptom should receive fresh frozen plasma as therapy for the disorder.

ANSWERS:

1. c. This patient should have an excisional biopsy of the mass performed as soon as possible. Although a piece of tissue could be removed (a fine-needle biopsy), an excisional biopsy makes more sense because the diagnosis of a malignant disease often requires histologic identification of cell types, usually detected by lymph-node biopsy. Fine-needle aspirate is often inadequate to detect certain of these types of cells. Excisional-node biopsy therefore is preferable to approaches that do not yield accurate and timely diagnosis. Although a chest radiograph and complete blood count (CBC) would not necessarily be incorrect things to do, even with a normal chest examination and CBC, the possibility of a malignancy must be ruled out by biopsy.

2. d. The anatomic pathology report of Reed-Sternberg cells present (these are large binucleate cells with a single distinct nucleoli) is pathognomonic of Hodgkin's disease. One or two unexplained, enlarged lymph nodes in a young person indicates Hodgkin's disease until proved otherwise. Hodgkin's disease most commonly presents with painless lymphadenopathy. The so-called classic symptoms of fever, weight loss, and night sweats are present in only a small number of patients and usually in those with more aggressive disease. Excisional biopsy always should be undertaken as the diagnostic procedure of choice. Fine-needle aspirate is often inadequate to detect Reed-Sternberg cells, and 20% of interventional radiologic procedures performed to diagnose Hodgkin's disease give false-negative results. Hodgkin's disease is one of the most important success stories of medical oncology. It was a disease that was once uniformly fatal, but now the vast majority of patients are cured.

3. e. After an anatomic diagnosis is made, the disease must be staged. Clinical staging of Hodgkin's disease includes physical examination of all lymph-node regions; chest x-ray; CT scan of the chest, abdomen, and pelvis; nuclear imaging with gallium scans or positive emission tomography (PET); bone scans; and bone marrow biopsy. Pathologic staging by open laparotomy also is done. The Ann Arbor Staging Classification of Hodgkin's disease is as follows: Stage I, single lymph node or single extralymphatic organ; Stage II, two or more lymph nodes on the same side of the diaphragm; Stage III, lymph nodes involved on both sides of the diaphragm or localized involvement of spleen or extralymphatic organ or both; and Stage IV, diffuse or disseminated disease or involvement of the liver or bone marrow.

4. b. The staging is added to further by the presence or absence of the following symptoms: fever, night sweats, and weight loss of more than 10% in the last 6 months. The presence of any of the symptoms indicates that the stage of the disease should be labeled B. The absence of any of these symptoms indicates that the stage of the disease should be labeled A.

5. d. Although extended radiation was very successful in the treatment of patients with early Hodgkin's disease, patients experienced an increased risk of cardiovascular disease and second cancers. To reduce these risks of therapy for early-stage disease, combined therapy now is preferred. This has resulted in improved tumor control with no obvious increased risk for death from any particular cause in long-term follow-up. Unfortunately, chemotherapy alone is slightly inferior to combined therapy in disease eradication, but chemotherapy is advancing, and the search continues for treatment that obviates the need for radiotherapy, particularly in children.

6. e. As mentioned, Hodgkin's disease is one of the major success stories in cancer treatment. Survival rates exceed 80%, and patients have the potential for cure regardless of initial stage of presentation. However, successful treatment has not been without associated down sides. Secondary cancers and coronary artery disease result in premature death for many patients, and infertility is not uncommon for many patients. Early recurrence is always a probability, but the vast majority of patients beat this cancer and go on to live productive lives.

7. e. The one test you should have done is excisional lymph-node biopsy.

8. a. This patient has a non-Hodgkin's lymphoma. The characteristics that suggest this diagnosis rather than Hodgkin's disease are the presence of lymph nodes draining Waldeyer's ring, the presence of epitrochlear lymph nodes, and the presence of chest pain suggesting involvement of lung tissue. The lymph-node histology involving non-Hodgkin's lymphoma will not be discussed in detail. However, the lymph-node pathology of diffuse small cleaved cell (diffuse poorly differentiated lymphocytic) suggests a high-grade lymphoma with extensive involvement including the liver, the spleen, and the bone marrow. Your physical examination confirms the possibility of the former two.

Staging is similar (although not identical) to the staging for Hodgkin's disease. Non-Hodgkin's lymphoma can be found in nodal sites, in viscera, or both. Extranodal disease is often solitary. Waldeyer's ring, upper gastrointestinal tract, testes, and bone are the most common extranodal sites. The staging of non-Hodgkin's lymphoma is divided into early and late stages of indolent (follicular) disease and aggressive

disease. Histologic grading differentiates tumors into low, intermediate, and high-grade neoplasia.

9. e. Treatment modalities are based on diagnosed staging and disease aggressiveness. Indolent disease in early stages (I or II) generally are given radiotherapy. Patients with advanced-stage (stages III and IV) follicular lymphoma have a median survival measured in years, and the natural history is variable, leading many asymptomatic patients to reasonably choose a watchful-waiting strategy. For patients with progressive or symptomatic disease, treatment approaches include radiotherapy, chemotherapy, or both. Most patients respond to chemotherapy, but duration of response is usually only 1 to 2 years. Fewer than one-third of patients remain in remission for more than 5 years. Interferon-alpha and monoclonal antibodies also have been demonstrated to be beneficial in primary therapy for follicular lymphoma. In aggressive disease, combined therapy is an accepted standard of care for patients with early-stage disease (I and II). Combined therapy also is used for late disease stages in aggressive non-Hodgkin lymphomas, but response rates are less than 50% despite aggressive treatment regimens. Bone marrow transplantation after aggressive chemotherapy shows promise as an effective treatment.

10. c. Non-Hodgkin's lymphoma is responsible for up to 80% of lymphomas, making it much more common than Hodgkin's lymphoma. Some 60,000 people in the United States will develop non-Hodgkin's lymphoma each year, leading to more than 26,000 deaths. The disease is more common in older individuals, and prognosis for a normal lifespan is poor with and without treatment. There appears to be a relationship with the Epstein-Barr virus in some forms of the disease, and the disease's incidence has increased partly as a result of HIV disease, which confers greater risk.

11. c. The critical elements of this patient's history/physical/laboratory data are as follows:
1. Signs of bone pain (sternum and skull) and anemia
2. Symptoms of weakness, depression, fatigue, and confusion
3. Recent history of bacterial pneumonia; possible immune suppression
4. Laboratory evidence of the following: (a) anemia, usually normocytic but rouleau formation is common; (b) hypercalcemia; (c) renal failure; (d) thrombocytopenia; (e) hyponatremia; and (f) elevated ESR.

The combination of bone pain (location specific), hypercalcemia, normochromic/normocytic anemia, renal failure, weakness/depression/confusion, and history of bacterial pneumonia points to the diagnosis of multiple myeloma. The diagnosis will be substantiated by skull x-ray (showing punched-out lesions), serum electrophoresis with monoclonal peak, and demonstration of Bence-Jones protein in the urine. Multiple myeloma is a disease of older patients, with the mean age being 68 years. It appears to be more common than average in farmers, petroleum workers, wood workers, and leather workers.

12. a. The treatment of choice for multiple myeloma used to be a standard combination of melphalan and prednisone; more recently chemotherapy with alkylating agents (vincristine, Adriamycin, dexamethasone) also is being used. The median survival rate with these regimens was 36 months.

Now, newly diagnosed patients with good performance status are being treated with autologous stem-cell transplantation, resulting in improved survival, particularly for patients younger than age 60 years. Thalidomide has been found to be effective in patients with refractory myeloma. Supportive care measures also have improved, including the use of bisphosphonates to prevent osteolytic lesions. Additional treatment with radiation for bone pain and aggressive treatment for hypercalcemia is important. With newer treatment regimens, patients may live long periods with virtually no symptoms.

13. d. Pathologically, multiple myeloma is a plasma-cell malignancy or proliferation.

14. w.

15. z.

16. p.

17. m.

18. u.

19. i.

20. o.

21. e.

22. s.

23. j.

SUMMARY OF CERTAIN HEMATOLOGIC CONDITIONS

A. **Most common solid hematologic malignancies are the lymphomas:**
1. **Disorders types and their prevalence:**
   a. Non-Hodgkin's lymphoma: most common (60,000 new cases per year in the United States)
   b. Hodgkin's lymphoma: second most common (7500 new cases per year in the United States)
2. **Signs and symptoms:**
   a. The most common sign/symptom is solitary or nonsolitary lymph-node enlargement.
   b. The presence or absence of systemic symptoms not only is a staging phenomenon (A or B) but is also prognostic.
   c. The most common systemic symptoms include weight loss, night sweats, fevers, and pain.
3. **Differentiation of Hodgkin's from non-Hodgkin's:**
   a. Reed-Sternberg cells are pathognomonic to the diagnosis of Hodgkin's lymphoma.
   b. Lymph-node enlargement in the supraclavicular area is very common for Hodgkin's disease.
   c. In non-Hodgkin's lymphoma the lymph nodes draining Waldeyer's ring and epitrochlear nodes most commonly enlarged.
   d. Non-Hodgkin's lymphoma often presents with mediastinal, abdominal, and extranodal symptomatology.
4. **Prognosis:**
   a. Hodgkin's lymphoma has a much better prognosis than non-Hodgkin's lymphoma, with treatment of the former resulting in cure up to 80% of the time.
   b. Prognosis depends on accurate staging.
5. **Treatment:** Hodgkin's and non-Hodgkin's are treated with combination of chemotherapy and

radiation. Monoclonal antibodies also are used. See Answers 5 and 9.

B. Multiple myeloma:
1. **Prevalence:** multiple myeloma is mainly a disease of the elderly
2. **Pathology:** plasma cell malignancy/plasma cell proliferation
3. **Signs and symptoms:** (a) bone pain (sternum, skull, ribs, and back); (b) anemia (normochromic/normocytic); (c) immune suppression (history of bacterial infections); (d) renal failure; (e) hypercalcemia; and (f) weakness/confusion/depression/fatigue
4. **Diagnosis:** (a) serum protein electrophoresis; (b) bone marrow biopsy; and (c) Bence-Jones protein in the urine

C. Miscellaneous important hematologic conditions:
1. **Polycythemia rubra vera:**
   a. Plethora, sometimes cyanosis
   b. Proliferation of all hematopoietic cell lines
   c. Elevated hemoglobin, red blood cell mass, thrombocytosis
2. **Myelofibrosis:**
   a. Weight loss
   b. Bleeding from skin and mucous membranes
   c. Bone marrow biopsy: dry tap, normal bone marrow is replaced by fibrotic material
3. **Chronic myelogenous leukemia:**
   a. Atomic bomb survivors (or other radiation victims)
   b. Philadelphia chromosome
   c. White blood cells at diagnosis often greater than 200,000/mm^3
   d. Chronic phase followed by blastic phase
4. **Chronic lymphocytic leukemia:**
   a. Most common leukemia in United States
   b. Disease of older patients
   c. Indolent nature; no treatment needed in many patients; median survival 10 years
5. **Hairy cell leukemia:**
   a. Cytoplasmic projections give disorder its name
   b. Remarkably effective treatment with cladribine usually presents with pancytopenia
6. **Acute lymphocytic leukemia:**
   a. Disease of children
   b. Immature lymphoblasts

   c. Infections very common
   d. Up to a 70% cure rate at present
7. **Acute myeloblastic leukemia:**
   a. Most common acute leukemia of adults
   b. Auer rods are pathognomonic
   c. Immature myeloblasts on smear
   d. Infections very common
   e. Bone marrow transplantation essential for survival (10% to 30%)
   f. May follow myelodysplastic disorder or preleukemia
8. **Idiopathic thrombocytopenic purpura:**
   a. Acute onset after viral exanthem or viral infection
   b. Rapid drop in platelet count
   c. Corticosteroids are treatment of choice: splenectomy in resistant cases
9. **von Willebrand's disease:**
   a. Most common inherited bleeding disorder
   b. Results from a factor VIII deficiency
   c. Often presents as severe menorrhagia in women
   d. Factor VIII concentrates are treatment of choice
10. **Disseminated intravascular coagulation:**
    a. Follows obstetric catastrophes, major trauma, metastatic malignancies, or bacterial sepsis
    b. Microemboli or microthrombi in vasculature
    c. Profuse bleeding from many sites
    d. Treatment: fresh frozen plasma for severe bleeding

SUGGESTED READING

Hauke RJ, Armitage JO: Treatment of non-Hodgkin lymphoma. *Curr Opin Oncol* 12(5):412-418, 2000.
Horwitz SM, Horning SJ: Advances in the treatment of Hodgkin's lymphoma. *Curr Opin Hematol* 7(4):235-240, 2000.
McCune SL, et al: Monoclonal antibody therapy in the treatment of non-Hodgkin lymphoma. *JAMA* 286(10):1149-1152, 2001.
Rajkumar SV, et al: Mayo Clinic Myeloma, Amyloid, and Dysproteinemia Group. Current therapy for multiple myeloma. *Mayo Clin Proc* 77(8):813-822, 2002.
Schwartz CL: The management of Hodgkin disease in the young child. *Curr Opin Pediatr* 15(1):10-16, 2003.
Staudt LM: Molecular diagnosis of the hematologic cancers. *N Engl J Med* 348(18):1777-1785, 2003.
Zweegman S, Huijgens PC: Treatment of myeloma: recent developments. *Anticancer Drugs* 13(4):339-351, 2002.

Chapter 36

Rheumatoid Arthritis

"I hurt a bit and am kind of stiff when I wake up, but it's not serious, is it?"

CLINICAL CASE PROBLEM 1:
A 35-YEAR-OLD FEMALE WITH MALAISE AND VAGUE PERIARTICULAR PAIN AND STIFFNESS

A 35-year-old female comes to your office with a 6-month history of malaise, paraesthesias in both hands, and vague pain in both hands and wrists. She also has felt extremely fatigued. She tells you that the pains in her joints are much worse in the morning. She also is beginning to notice pain and swelling in both knees.

The patient has a normal family history, with no significant diseases noted. She is taking no drugs and has no allergies.

On examination, vital signs are normal, and there is a sensation of "bogginess" and slight swelling in both hands, both wrists, and in the small bones of her hands. Both knees also feel somewhat "swollen and boggy." There are no other joint abnormalities, and the rest of the physical examination is normal.

■ SELECT THE BEST ANSWER TO THE FOLLOWING QUESTIONS:

1. What is the most likely diagnosis in this patient?
   a. nonarticular rheumatism
   b. synovitis
   c. gonococcal arthritis
   d. rheumatoid arthritis (RA)
   e. systemic lupus erythematosus

2. What is the most characteristic symptom of this disease?
   a. early-morning joint stiffness
   b. progressive joint pain
   c. predilection for the small joints
   d. joint swelling
   e. normal cartilage despite joint pain

3. What is the most characteristic sign of this disease?
   a. joint swelling
   b. bilateral (symmetric) joint involvement
   c. erythema surrounding the affected joints
   d. joint bogginess
   e. involvement of the glenohumeral joint in all cases

4. On what is the pathophysiology of this disease based?
   a. bone destruction
   b. bone spur formation
   c. bone sclerosis
   d. symmetric joint involvement
   e. synovial inflammation

5. In the course of the pathophysiology of this disease, which of the following is most characteristic of the disease?
   a. synovial proliferation with cartilage erosion stimulated by cytokines
   b. cartilage destruction stimulated by the proliferation of proteoglycans
   c. cartilage destruction stimulated by the enzymatic action of proteoglycans
   d. loss of the synovial membrane
   e. none of the above; the pathophysiology of the disease is not known with any certainty

6. The disease described affects one particular part of the spine. What is the affected part, and what are the affected vertebrae?
   a. cervical: C6-C7
   b. cervical: C1-C2
   c. thoracic: T7-T9
   d. lumbar: L1-L3
   e. lumbar: L4-L5

7. Which anemia usually accompanies this disease process?
   a. microcytic, hypochromic
   b. microcytic, normochromic
   c. normocytic, normochromic
   d. macrocytic, hyperchromic
   e. normocytic, hypochromic

8. Which of the following is (are) a systemic complication(s) of the disease process?
   a. vasculitis
   b. pericarditis
   c. pleural effusion
   d. diffuse interstitial fibrosis of the lung
   e. all of the above

9. Felty's syndrome is a complication of the described disorder. Which of the following is (are) part of Felty's syndrome?
   a. splenomegaly
   b. neutropenia
   c. positive rheumatoid factor
   d. a and b
   e. a, b, and c

10. For the described disorder, which of the following is a proven therapeutic agent?
    a. auranofin

b. hydroxychloroquine
c. methotrexate
d. D-penicillamine
e. all of the above

11. The patient develops a local flareup in her right knee. Her left knee is affected to a small degree but not nearly as severely as the right knee. Up to this time, remission had been induced, and she was taking antiinflammatory agents for suppression of inflammation. What is the treatment of choice for this local flareup?
a. methotrexate
b. hydroxychloroquine
c. intraarticular corticosteroid injection
d. oral prednisone
e. auranofin

12. What is the drug of choice for the suppression of inflammation in a patient with this disease?
a. auranofin
b. methotrexate
c. oral prednisone
d. naproxen
e. D-penicillamine

13. Which of the following is not a classical radiologic feature of RA?
a. loss of juxtaarticular bone mass
b. narrowing of the joint space
c. bony erosions
d. subarticular sclerosis
e. all of the above are radiologic manifestations

CLINICAL CASE MANAGEMENT PROBLEM

Clinic Case Problem Matching Questions 1–12.
Match the characteristic with the type of arthritis.

Type of Arthritis

1. ankylosing spondylitis
2. gonococcal arthritis
3. systemic lupus erythematosus
4. Lyme disease
5. rheumatic fever
6. gouty arthritis
7. juvenile rheumatoid arthritis
8. Reiter's disease
9. psoriatic arthritis
10. inflammatory bowel disease arthritis
11. calcium pyrophosphate (CPPD) arthritis
12. tuberculous arthritis

ANSWERS:

1. **d.** The most likely diagnosis is RA.

2. **a.** The most characteristic symptom of RA is early-morning stiffness. The total array of rheumatoid arthritic symptoms include the following: (1) morning stiffness (characteristic symptom) lasting more than 1 hour; (2) pain on motion of joints; (3) tenderness in joints; (4) swelling (soft-tissue inflammation of fluid, not bony overgrowth); (5) symmetric joint involvement; (6) subcutaneous nodules; (7) positive agglutination (RA) factor; and (8) characteristic histologic changes in the synovial membrane.

3. **b.** The most characteristic sign of RA is symmetric joint involvement.
   In most patients, RA starts out with a whimper and not a bang. The disease has an insidious start with nonspecific symptoms, such as fatigue and malaise, accompanied by arthralgias and low-grade fever. Later, polyarticular, symmetric joint swelling begins (usually with the proximal interphalangeal, metacarpophalangeal, wrist, elbow, shoulder, knee, ankle, and metatarsophalangeal joints involved) but sparing the distal interphalangeal joints. Cervical spine involvement is common at the region C1-C2, but the remainder of the spine usually is spared.

4. **e.** The pathophysiology of this disease is based on synovial inflammation.

5. **a.** The pathophysiology of RA begins with synovial membrane swelling and synovial membrane

Characteristic

a. Positively birefringent under the polarizing microscope
b. Negatively birefringent under the polarizing microscope
c. Most common cause of infective arthritis in young adults
d. Conjunctivitis and urethritis are other features
e. Erythema chronicum migrans
f. Bamboo spine
g. Streptococcal pharyngitis usually occurs first
h. Arthritis may precede abdominal symptoms
i. Renal failure is major cause of death in this disease
j. Arthritis may appear before classical "silver-scaled" skin lesions
k. Major cause of arthritis in children
l. Lung disease is major manifestation of this disease in most patients

proliferation. The synovium, which is normally only two cell layers thick, proliferates and erodes adjacent cartilage and adjacent bone. Macrophages secrete cytokines, particularly interleukin-1 and tumor necrosis factor-alpha (TNF-α), which induce chondrocyte and osteoclast stimulation, prostaglandin secretion, and endothelial activation. CD4-positive T lymphocytes promote the inflammation early in the disease and are abundant in the synovium and the synovial fluid. The macrophage/cytokine system also triggers systemic effects such as fever and anemia.

6. b. Instability of the cervical spine is a life-threatening complication of RA. The instability results from a cervical ligament synovitis in the region of the first two cervical vertebrae. This complication occurs in 30% to 40% of patients who develop RA. Of patients with RA, 5% eventually develop a myelopathy or cord injury as a result of this instability.

7. c. The anemia that most often accompanies RA is characterized as mild, normochromic, normocytic.

The characteristics at the cellular level of the anemia include the following: low to normal iron, low to normal iron-binding protein, and normal to low erythropoietin.

8. e. RA is a systemic disease. Some of the more important complications are as follows:
1. Vasculitis: from the very beginning of the synovial membrane thickening process, a microvascular vasculitis process is involved. This can progress to mesenteric vasculitis, polyarteritis nodosa, or other vascular syndromes.
2. Pericarditis: fibrinous pericarditis is present in 40% of patients with RA at autopsy. Although infrequent, this pericarditis occasionally can be of the constricting type with life-threatening tamponade.
3. Pleural effusions: rheumatic pleural effusions are extremely common.
4. Rheumatic nodules in the heart (affecting the conducting system): rheumatic nodules frequently may lead to conducting disturbances including heart block and bundle-branch blocks.
5. Rheumatic nodules in the lung can cavitate or become infected.
6. Diffuse interstitial fibrosis with a restrictive pattern on pulmonary function tests and with a honeycomb pattern on chest x-ray may occur.

9. e. Felty's syndrome usually occurs fairly late in the disease process. Felty's syndrome is manifested by splenomegaly, neutropenia, and a positive rheumatoid factor.

10. e. All of the medications listed are disease-modifying antirheumatic drugs used in the treatment of RA.

11. c. Because the flareup is limited to one joint, it is reasonable to treat with a localized approach. An intraarticular corticosteroid injection temporarily may help control local synovitis.

12. d. The drug(s) of choice for the suppression of inflammation in a patient with RA are the nonsteroidal antiinflammatory drugs (NSAIDs). Although aspirin is still theoretically the agent of first choice, patients are more likely to take 1-2 pills/day rather than the 10-12 required with aspirin therapy. Thus the answer to this question is naproxen. If an NSAID from a certain class does not work when given up to maximum dose, then try an agent from a second or different class. A cyclooxygenase-2 (COX-2) inhibitor may be preferable in long-term treatment because of decreased gastrointestinal side effects, although all NSAIDs can cause gastrointestinal bleeding.

13. d. In early RA, few radiologic findings are seen. Soft-tissue changes in synovial fluid or capsular thickening occasionally may be seen on the radiograph but are more readily detected by physical examination. Loss of juxtaarticular bone mass (osteoporosis) often is detected near the finger joints and may be seen early in the disease. Narrowing of the joint space, as a result of thinning of the articular cartilage, usually is seen late in the disease. Bony erosions are seen best at the margins of the joint. Subarticular sclerosis is a feature of osteoarthritis, not RA.

SOLUTION TO THE CLINICAL CASE MANAGEMENT PROBLEM

1. f	4. e	7. k	10. h
2. c	5. g	8. d	11. a
3. i	6. b	9. j	12. l

SUMMARY OF RHEUMATOID ARTHRITIS

1. **Prevalence:** RA occurs in 1% of the population. Clinical risk for developing RA is highly associated with HLA DR4 (human leukocyte antigen D-related antigen 4).
2. **Signs/symptoms:**
   a. Early-morning stiffness is the most common symptom, and symmetric joint swelling is the most common sign.
   b. Other signs/symptoms: (i) tenderness, swelling, and "bogginess of joints"; (ii) characteristic changes in the synovial membrane including microvascular changes; (iii) positive rheumatoid factor; (iv) subcutaneous nodules; and (v) radiographic changes including loss of juxtaarticular bone mass, joint space narrowing, and bony erosions.
3. **Sequence and order of pathophysiologic changes:** (a) macrophage activation; (b) product(s) of activation are production of interleukin and tumor necrosis factor cytokines; (c) synovial membrane thickening, proliferation, and local "microvasculitis"; (d) chondrocyte, osteoclast, CD4-positive T lymphocytes, and endothelial proliferation; (e) joint space narrowing; and (f) cytokines are also responsible for extraarticular symptoms such as fever and anemia.
4. **Systemic manifestations:** (a) normochromic, normocytic anemia; (b) fever; (c) pericarditis; (d) pleural effusion; (e) rheumatoid nodules in lung; (f) diffuse interstitial disease; (g) Felty's syndrome; (h) rheumatoid nodules in heart causing heart block and bundle-branch block; and (i) systemic vasculitis.
5. **Treatment:** early and aggressive treatment will yield better long-term outcomes.
   a. Nonpharmacologic treatment: (i) systemic rest; (ii) articular rest (splints, braces, canes); (iii) physiotherapy including heat, cold, joint range of motion, and exercise as tolerated; (iv) weight loss; and (v) education (describe disease course, patient and family support).
   b. Disease-modifying antirheumatologic drugs (DMARDs): The early use of DMARDs for RA is beneficial. The critical question of how combination DMARD therapy compares with methotrexate plus biologic therapy is unanswered. DMARDs include the following:
      i. Gold compounds: Gold compounds are contraindicated in patients with hepatic or renal disease or blood dyscrasia.
      ii. Hydroxychloroquine: Ophthalmologic screening is recommended before and routinely during the treatment with hydroxychloroquine.
      iii. Sulfasalazine
      iv. Penicillamine: CBC and urinalysis must be checked routinely while the patient is taking this medication.
      v. Azathioprine
      vi. Methotrexate: Methotrexate is one of the most widely prescribed disease DMARDs for RA. It has a rapid onset of action (3-4 weeks) and dependable clinical response and is well-tolerated long term. Side effects include reversible bone marrow suppression, hepatotoxicity, pulmonary hypersensitivity, and nephrotoxicity. Consider starting within 2 months of diagnosis to reduce the possibility of irreversible joint destruction.
      vii. Cyclosporine
      viii. Leflunomide
      ix. Minocycline
      It should be noted that many of the disease-modifying drugs have significant side-effect profiles, and these should be considered when prescribing. If you are not comfortable using these medications, consult and comanage with an appropriate specialist.
   c. Glucocorticoids can be use for refractory disease when NSAIDs and DMARDs have not been successful. Start at the lowest dose, and for chronic use consider Fosamax or Actonel. Injected corticosteroids are the first choice as local remitting agents. Some consultants now are using glucocorticoids earlier in the course of illness.
   d. Biologics: This class of new therapy for RA includes biologic response modulators that target specific cytokines (TNF-α and IL-1) involved in the perpetuation of the inflammatory cascade in RA. However, current recommendations are to start therapy with single, conventional DMARDs, followed by the addition of combination therapy or biologics.
   e. Acute inflammation
      i. First choice: NSAID or COX-2 inhibitors for those at risk for gastrointestinal toxicity or consider proton pump inhibitors to protect against gastrointestinal complaints if NSAIDs are used.
      ii. Alternative first choice: aspirin. Requires many tablets and may lead to gastrointestinal side effects.
      iii. Second choice: nonacetylated salicylates
      iv. Surgery in severe cases to relieve pain and provide stability to joint if possible.

SUGGESTED READING

Cannella AC, O'Dell JR: Is there still a role for traditional disease-modifying antirheumatic drugs (DMARDs) in rheumatoid arthritis? *Curr Opin Rheumatol* 15(3):185-292, 2003.

Furst DE, et al: Updated consensus statement on biological agents for the treatment of rheumatoid arthritis and other rheumatic diseases. *Ann Rheum Dis* 61 Suppl 2:ii2-7, 2002.

Jenkins JK, et al: The pathogenesis of rheumatoid arthritis: a guide to therapy. *Am J Med Sci* 323(4):171-180, 2002.

Jenkins JK, Hardy KJ: Biological modifier therapy for the treatment of rheumatoid arthritis. *Am J Med Sci* 323(4):197-205, 2002.

Pisetsky DS: Progress in the treatment of rheumatoid arthritis. *JAMA* 286:2787-2790, 2001.

 Chapter **37**

Osteoarthritis

| The "normal?" aches and pains of aging.

CLINICAL CASE PROBLEM 1:

AN 80-YEAR-OLD FEMALE WITH PAINFUL FINGER JOINTS

An 80-year-old female comes to your with a 6-month history of stiffness in her hands bilaterally. The stiffness is worst in the morning and subsides thereafter. She also has noticed increasing (but not severe) pain in the lower back, both hips, and both knees.

On examination, the patient is obese. She has significant swelling of both the proximal interphalangeal (PIP) joints and the distal interphalangeal (DIP) joints. There is also deformity of both knees on examination. The rest of her physical examination is within normal limits.

■ SELECT THE BEST ANSWER TO THE FOLLOWING QUESTIONS:

1. Which of the following statements regarding this patient's condition is (are) true?
   a. the swelling present at the DIP joint may represent Bouchard's nodes
   b. the swelling present at the PIP joint may represent Heberden's nodes
   c. this patient most likely will demonstrate an elevated erythrocyte sedimentation rate (ESR) and a positive rheumatoid factor
   d. synovial fluid analysis probably will demonstrate a low viscosity and normal mucin clotting
   e. none of the above are true

2. Which of the following statements regarding the symptomatology of the condition described is (are) false?
   a. pain is the chief symptom and it is usually deep and aching in character
   b. stiffness of the involved joint is common but of relatively brief duration
   c. the pain of osteoarthritis is characteristically dull and aching

   d. the major physical finding in osteoarthritis is bony crepitus
   e. the presence of osteophytes is sufficient for the diagnosis of osteoarthritis

3. Which of the following statements concerning the condition described is (are) false?
   a. this condition is the most common form of joint disease in the North American population
   b. 85% of the population have radiographic features of this condition in weightbearing joints after the age of 65 years
   c. this condition has both primary and secondary forms
   d. narrowing of the joint space is unusual
   e. pathologically, the articular cartilage is first roughened and then finally worn away

CLINICAL CASE PROBLEM 2:

A 65-YEAR-OLD FEMALE WITH AN ARTHRITIC HIP

A 65-year-old female with moderately severe osteoarthritis of her left hip comes to your office requesting an exercise prescription. She wishes to "get into shape."

4. Which of the following would you recommend to this patient at this time?
   a. exercise is not good for osteoarthritis; rest is much more appropriate
   b. a graded exercise program consisting of brisk walking gradually increasing the distance to 3-4 miles a day probably will not cause pain and will be good for her.
   c. a passive isotonic exercise program is preferable to an active isometric exercise program
   d. any exercise program probably will hasten her need for total hip replacements
   e. swimming is the best exercise prescription you can give her; it promotes cardiovascular fitness and at the same time keeps pressure off the weightbearing joints

5. Which of the following radiographic features usually is (are) seen with the condition just described?
   a. narrowing of the joint spaces
   b. bony sclerosis

c. osteophyte formation

d. subchondral cyst formation

e. all of the above

6. Which of the following treatment modalities is (are) useful in the treatment of the condition just described?
   a. weight loss in obese patients
   b. canes, crutches, and walkers
   c. the application of heat to involved joints
   d. nonsteroid antiinflammatory drugs (NSAIDs)
   e. all of the above

7. Which of the following statements concerning the incidence of the condition described in Cases 1 and 2 is (are) true?
   a. one-third of adults aged 25 to 75 years have radiographic evidence of osteoarthritis
   b. cartilaginous fraying is common
   c. mild synovitis may develop in response to crystals or cartilaginous debris
   d. the most common sites for this disease are in the small joints of the hand, the foot, and the knees and/or hips
   e. all of the above are true

8. What is (are) the major goal(s) of therapy in the disease described in Cases 1 and 2?
   a. minimize pain
   b. prevent disability
   c. delay progression
   d. a and b only
   e. all of the above

9. Which of the following statements regarding the use of NSAIDs in the condition described in Cases 1 and 2 and as given to an elderly patient is (are) true?
   a. NSAIDs are generally very safe for the treatment of the condition described in elderly patients
   b. NSAID toxicity in elderly patients is uncommon
   c. NSAID toxicity in elderly patients is unlikely to be associated with renal insufficiency
   d. the most common NSAID toxicity in elderly patients is gastrointestinal
   e. none of the above are true

10. What is (are) the drug(s) of choice for the treatment of primary osteoarthritis?
    a. acetaminophen
    b. naproxen sodium
    c. diclofenac
    d. indomethacin
    e. any of the above

CLINICAL CASE MANAGEMENT PROBLEM

Describe the nonpharmacologic and the pharmacologic management of the condition described.

■ ANSWERS:

1. **e.** This patient has obvious osteoarthritis. However, the location of Bouchard's nodes represents both overgrowth and significant osteoarthritic changes at the PIP joints (not the DIP joints), whereas Heberden's nodes represent bony overgrowth and significant osteoarthritic changes at the DIP (not the PIP) joints.

A significantly elevated ESR seldom is seen with osteoarthritis (except in the unusual cases in which there is a significant inflammatory component).

Synovial fluid analysis most likely will reveal a high (not low) viscosity and normal mucin clotting. The total leukocyte count in the synovial fluid likely will be less than 1000 cells/mm^3.

2. **e.** The most common symptom in osteoarthritis is pain. The pain is described as dull, aching, aggravated by joint use, and relieved by joint rest. Joint stiffness in weightbearing joints is common but usually is a very transient finding (especially in the morning). It also occurs after prolonged rest.

Osteoarthritis pain is the result of movement of one joint surface against another with both joint surfaces exhibiting characteristic articular cartilage damage including fraying and, ultimately, complete lack of cartilage. In addition, there are subchondral bone microfractures, irritation of the periosteal nerve endings, ligamentous stress, muscular strain, and soft-tissue inflammation such as bursitis and tendonitis.

Bony crepitus is the most common physical finding in osteoarthritis. Osteophytes are a common radiologic finding, especially with advanced age. The diagnosis of osteoarthritis, however, is clinical, and the mere presence of osteophytes on an x-ray is not sufficient for the diagnosis itself.

3. **d.** Joint space narrowing is common. It almost always is associated with osteoarthritis. The pathologic process involved in osteoarthritis is as follows:
   1. The primary defect in primary osteoarthritis and secondary osteoarthritis is loss of articular cartilage. In primary osteoarthritis this is the result of "normal" wear and tear. In secondary osteoarthritis the loss is the result of acute or chronic trauma; congenital deformities; metabolic disorders; septic and tubercular arthritis; and endocrine disorders such as acromegaly, obesity, or diabetes. The end result is that some 85%

of the population have evidence of osteoarthritis in weightbearing joints by the time they are 65 years old.

2. Cartilage changes progress as follows: (a) glistening appearance is lost; (b) surface areas of the articular cartilage flake off; (c) deeper layers of the articular cartilage develop longitudinal fissures (fibrillation); (d) the cartilage becomes thin and eventually absent in some areas, leaving the underlying subchondral bone unprotected; (e) the unprotected subchondral bone becomes sclerotic (dense and hard); (f) cysts develop within the subchondral bone and communicate with the longitudinal fissures in the cartilage; (g) pressure builds up in the cysts until the cystic contents are forced into the synovial cavity, breaking through the articular cartilage on the way; (h) as the articular cartilage erodes, cartilage-coated osteophytes may grow outward from the underlying bone and alter the bone contours and joint anatomy; (i) these spurlike bony projections enlarge until small pieces, called joint mice, break off into the synovial cavity; and (j) the process of loss of articular cartilage probably takes place through the enzymatic breakdown of the cartilage matrix (the proteoglycans, glycosaminoglycans, and collagen are involved).

4. e. Muscle spasm and muscle atrophy can be prevented in osteoarthritis by a graded exercise program. Active exercises are preferred to passive exercises; isometric exercises are preferred to isotonic exercises.

Because of minimal involvement of the weightbearing joints, swimming can be recommended as an ideal exercise.

A graded exercise program that includes walking 3-4 miles a day will result in trauma to the joints and should be discouraged. It very well may hasten the need for total joint replacement.

5. e. Radiographic changes in osteoarthritis include narrowing of the joint space as a result of loss of articular cartilage, bony sclerosis as a result of thickening of subchondral bone, subchondral bone cysts, and osteophyte (bone spur) formation.

6. e. The treatments for osteoarthritis includes nonpharmacologic measures and pharmacologic measures.

Nonpharmacologic measures include rest; the avoidance of overuse of the affected joint; walking aids such as canes, crutches, and walkers; weight loss; the application of heat; and other physiotherapy techniques. Exercises should be mainly isometric (nonmovement such as quadriceps strengthening, stretching, and range-of-motion exercises. Heat modalities such as hot packs, soaks, and warm pools

for aerobic exercise may decrease discomfort and facilitate the exercise program.

Pharmacologic measures include simple analgesics such as acetaminophen, NSAIDs, and local steroid injections. Newer concepts in the treatment of osteoarthritis include chondroprotective agents, which conserve cartilage or stimulate cartilage repair within the osteoarthritic joint. These agents include tetracyclines, glycosaminoglycans, hyaluronan preparations, and gene therapy. Over-the-counter topical preparations, such as capsaicin cream, are used for relief of pain. Other complementary approaches are under investigation. Nonnarcotic analgesics include acetaminophen, propoxyphene (Darvon), and tramadol (Ultram).

Antiinflammatory agents such as NSAIDs are very effective with limiting factors being gastric problems and problems with renal functions. Cyclooxygenase-2 (COX-2) inhibitors are very effective and do not have the degree of gastric side effects shared by conventional NSAIDs. There is still a risk of renal side effects, and cost may limit their use.

Orthopedic surgery is used in severe cases. Joint replacement, especially of the knee and hip, is the treatment of choice when more conservative therapy has failed to control pain and maintain function.

7. e. At least 33% of adults between the ages of 25 and 75 years have radiographic findings commonly seen in osteoarthritis. There are some studies that suggest that osteoarthritis begins as early as 15 or 16 years of age.

The cartilaginous fraying that is associated with cartilage degeneration has been described. Associated with this may be a mild synovitis that develops in response to cartilaginous fragments (joint mice) in the joint space itself.

The most common sites for osteoarthritis to develop are the small joints of the hands, the small joints of the feet, the hips, the knees, and the vertebral column where the cartilaginous degeneration is of a somewhat different type (the intervertebral discs) but nevertheless is the same basic pathologic process.

8. e. The goals for the patient with osteoarthritis are to minimize pain, prevent disability, and delay progression.

Some would argue that it is not possible to delay progression in osteoarthritis. However, this is false. Weight loss in an obese individual and decreased repetitive trauma or impact to a joint with osteoarthritis will delay progression.

9. d. The most common type of toxicity associated with NSAIDs in elderly patients is gastrointestinal. This may take the form of an acute or chronic gastritis, a peptic ulcer, or a perforated duodenal ulcer. This may result in secondary anemia and other complications.

10. **a.** NSAIDs (although a mainstay of treatment for osteoarthritis) have very significant toxicity, especially when used in elderly patients with renal impairment or any other disease. Thus ordinary acetaminophen is safer and must be considered a drug of first choice.

If a NSAID is used for the treatment of osteoarthritis in elderly patients it is suggested that (1) the dose be kept as low as possible and (2) the drug be given with food and preferably with a cytoprotective agent such as misoprostol.

Avoid NSAIDs with greater propensity to produce side effects (indomethacin, phenylbutazone, and the like). Celecoxib, rofecoxib, and valdecoxib (COX-2 inhibitors) should have less risk for gastrointestinal complications and may become preferred.

SOLUTION TO THE CLINICAL CASE MANAGEMENT PROBLEM

A. Nonpharmacologic treatment: (1) weight loss; (2) exercise prescription (strengthening; range of motion; and aerobic exercises including cycling, swimming, and cross-country training; (3) work modification (limit joint stress trauma); (4) regular physiotherapy (heat, cold, ultrasound); (5) TENS (transcutaneous electric nerve stimulation); and (6) walking aids and braces.

B. Pharmacologic treatment: (1) acetaminophen is the drug of first choice; (2) NSAIDs; (3) intraarticular steroid injection (improvement is usually only temporary); (4) chondroprotective agents; and (5) capsaicin cream.

SUMMARY OF OSTEOARTHRITIS

1. **Diagnosis:** a noninflammatory joint disease characterized by its lack of inflammatory signs and symptoms and characterized by the loss of articular cartilage and degeneration in synovial joints.

2. **Prevalence:** most common rheumatologic condition. Majority of people older than 65 years of age have radiographic evidence of osteoarthritis.

3. **Pathology:** proteolytic enzymes (proteoglycans, glycosaminoglycans) produce the characteristic changes in the articular cartilage just described.

4. **Subtypes:** idiopathic and secondary. Secondary osteoarthritis is related to acute or chronic trauma, congenital abnormalities, and certain common conditions including obesity and diabetes mellitus.

5. **Treatment:** divided into nonpharmacologic and pharmacologic. The keys of nonpharmacologic treatment include weight loss; physiotherapy; stretching leading up to a mild aerobic, active, isometric exercise program (swimming is the single best exercise); work modification to limit weight bearing on affected joints; and use of aids such as canes and walkers.

   The most important key of pharmacologic therapy is *primum non nocere* (first do no harm). Acetaminophen is the drug of choice because of its relative lack of toxicity in the elderly; if using NSAIDs, use cytoprotection or a COX-2 inhibitor.

Limit intraarticular corticosteroid injections to large joints that fail to respond to other measures. Intraarticular hyaluronate preparations are a valuable therapeutic intervention. In patients with moderate to severe osteoarthritis of the knee, intraarticular injections of sodium hyaluronate (Hyalgan) are effective and may prevent or delay total knee replacement. The use of sodium hyaluronate is being studied for use in osteoarthritis of the shoulders.

Alternative treatments for osteoarthritis include topical capsaicin, glucosamine sulfate, and chondroitin. These last two may act as antiinflammatory agents and substrates for proteoglycan synthesis. There has not been any evidence of cartilage regeneration, however. Additional interventions, such as S-adenosyl methionine (SAM), ginger, dimethyl sulfoxide (DMSO), boron, and cetyl myristoleate, are in need of further research to firmly establish efficacy.

Consider surgery if all therapies fail and/or osteoarthritis is very severe.

SUGGESTED READING

Easton BT: Evaluation and treatment of the patient with osteoarthritis. *J Fam Pract* 50(9):791-797, 2001.

Hinton R, et al: Osteoarthritis: diagnosis and therapeutic considerations. *Am Fam Phys* 65(5):841-848, 2002.

Morelli V, Naquin C: Alternative therapies for traditional disease states: Osteoarthritis. *Am Fam Phys* 67:339-344, 2003.

Sharma L: Nonpharmacologic management of osteoarthritis. *Curr Opin Rheumatol* 14(5):603-607, 2002.

Chapter **38**

Mononucleosis

"Oh, Doctor, why am I so tired?"

CLINICAL CASE PROBLEM 1:

A 20-Year-Old College Student
with a Fever and a Sore Throat

A 20-year-old college student comes to your office with a 3-week history of fatigue, malaise, fever, chills, and a sore throat. She was well prior to the onset of this illness and was taking part in many activities. She finds at this time that she has no energy and is barely able to make her university classes in the mornings. She also describes aches and pains all over.

On physical examination, the patient's temperature is 39° C. There is pharyngeal hyperemia, and edema and marked exudates are present in both tonsillar areas. There is significant cervical lymphadenopathy present. On abdominal examination, there is dullness over the left upper quadrant, and you can just feel the tip of the spleen. There is no hepatic enlargement. The rest of the examination is unremarkable.

■ SELECT THE BEST ANSWER TO THE FOLLOWING QUESTIONS:

1. Based on the history and the physical examination described, what is the most likely diagnosis?
   a. infectious hepatitis
   b. infectious mononucleosis
   c. chronic fatigue syndrome
   d. fibromyalgia
   e. acute lymphoblastic leukemia

2. Of the following clinical features of the disorder, what is the least common?
   a. splenomegaly
   b. hepatomegaly
   c. fever
   d. exudative tonsillitis
   e. lymphadenopathy

3. Which of the following statements regarding this condition is false?
   a. this condition is caused by the Epstein-Barr virus (EBV).
   b. kissing is thought to be the most common mode of transmission.
   c. greater than 90% of all adults are carriers of the virus that causes the disease.
   d. in young children, fever and pharyngitis may be clinically indistinguishable from upper-respiratory tract infections caused by other viral agents.
   e. bacterial throat culture is usually necessary in patients suspected of having this disease.

4. Which of the following statements concerning the serologic testing for the condition described is false?
   a. the heterophile antibody test is negative in up to 20% of adults.
   b. the heterophile antibody test will be negative 12 months after onset of symptoms.
   c. in acute primary infections, anti-EA (early antigen) titers are usually low.
   d. in acute primary infections, immunoglobulin M-viral capsid antigen (IgM-VCA) titers are high.
   e. after several months, the anti-Epstein-Barr nuclear antigen (EBNA) titers become high.

5. The infectious agent that causes most of the cases of this disease has been associated with other conditions. Which of the following condition has not been associated with the infection described?
   a. Burkitt's lymphoma
   b. T-cell lymphoma
   c. chronic fatigue syndrome
   d. anaplastic nasopharyngeal carcinoma
   e. Hodgkin's disease

6. Of the following clinical features of the acute infection described, which is most common?
   a. fever
   b. hepatomegaly
   c. eyelid edema
   d. palatal petechiae
   e. splenomegaly

7. What is the treatment of choice for an uncomplicated episode of this condition?
   a. penicillin
   b. prednisone
   c. acyclovir
   d. strict bed rest
   e. supportive treatment that includes acetaminophen

8. Which of the following is not a complication of this condition?
   a. splenic rupture
   b. myocarditis
   c. meningoencephalitis
   d. acute lymphocytic leukemia
   e. Bell's palsy

9. In patients with this condition and splenomegaly, which of the following is recommended?
   a. stool softeners
   b. prednisone
   c. acyclovir
   d. ampicillin
   e. splenectomy

10. The patient described in the initial presentation presents 1 week later with great difficulty swallowing solids or liquids. You notice a significant increase in the erythema of the pharynx, an increase in tonsillar hypertrophy, and increased exudates on the tonsils. What should you do at this time?
    a. repeat the throat culture
    b. start the patient taking ampicillin
    c. start the patient taking penicillin
    d. start the patient taking prednisone
    e. start the patient taking high-dose acetylsalicylic acid

11. The disease is an infection of which of the following?
    a. T-cell lymphocytes
    b. B-cell lymphocytes
    c. neutrophils
    d. basophils
    e. none of the above

12. In patients with a negative heterophile antibody test, other plausible etiologic agents for this syndrome include all of the following, except:
    a. human immunodeficiency virus (HIV)
    b. human herpes virus 6
    c. toxoplasmosis
    d. human herpes simplex virus 1 (HSV-1)
    e. cytomegalovirus (CMV)

13. The patient described in Clinical Case Problem 1 is a lacrosse player. Her coach requests clearance to return to play. The appropriate recommendation to the coach would be to:
    a. return to full contact play in 2 weeks after her fever has subsided
    b. be disqualified from all sports for 3 months until her fatigue has resolved
    c. return to play when any splenic and laboratory abnormalities have returned to normal
    d. return to noncontact practice in 2 weeks
    e. suspend any physical activity until she is cleared by an infectious disease specialist

14. Which of the following statements concerning this disease is true?

a. atypical lymphocytes are not specific for this kind of infection
b. agranulocytosis is common
c. infections are most common in the spring
d. the male:female ratio for this condition is 2:1
e. patients younger than age 15 years with this condition are easiest to diagnose because of the severity of the symptoms

15. Which of the following statements about the epidemiology of this disease is true?
    a. transmission does not require close personal contact
    b. the incubation period of this disease is 2-5 days
    c. the period of communicability is indeterminant
    d. endemic infection of this disease is uncommon in group settings such as colleges
    e. donation of blood during or soon after infection is not contraindicated

---

CLINICAL CASE MANAGEMENT PROBLEM

What is the relationship between the disease described and chronic fatigue syndrome?

▶ **ANSWERS:**

1. **b.** This patient has infectious mononucleosis. Infectious mononucleosis is caused by EBV and most commonly is seen in children and young adults, particularly college students and military recruits. The major symptoms of infectious mononucleosis are sore throat, fatigue, and malaise. The major signs of infectious mononucleosis include fever, pharyngeal erythema, pharyngeal edema, tonsillar exudates, lymphadenopathy, splenomegaly, palatal petechiae, eyelid edema, and hepatomegaly.

Fibromyalgia, although most characteristic for its description of "pain all over," is characterized by multiple trigger points on examination.

Infectious hepatitis, although it presents with fatigue and malaise, also presents with abdominal pain, jaundice, an aversion to cigarettes, and significantly elevated liver function test values.

Chronic fatigue syndrome shares certain characteristics with infectious mononucleosis. However, patients with chronic fatigue syndrome must meet specific criteria defined by the Centers for Disease Control and Prevention to be classified as such. These criteria are unexplained fatigue for more than 6 months time plus four or more of the following: (1) memory/concentration problems; (2) sore throat;

(3) enlarged or tender cervical or axillary nodes; (4) myalgias; (5) multijoint pain; (6) new headaches; (7) unrefreshing sleep, and (8) postexertion malaise. Also, chronic fatigue syndrome occurs predominately in middle-aged individuals, whereas infectious mononucleosis is primarily a disease of young adults.

Although acute lymphoblastic leukemia can present with very similar signs and symptoms, it is seen more commonly in children and is not the most likely diagnosis.

2. b. The least common clinical feature is hepatomegaly. It occurs in about 30% to 50% of cases. Splenomegaly occurs in more than 50% of cases. Fever, exudative tonsillitis, and lymphadenopathy are most common.

3. e. As stated earlier, infectious mononucleosis is caused by EBV. The usual mode of transmission of the virus is through infected saliva (kissing). Most adults (90%) have been infected with EBV and are carriers.

Infectious mononucleosis is usually distinguishable from other viral infections in older children and young adults. In younger children and older adults, however, it may be difficult to distinguish from other respiratory tract infections including those caused by other viruses, mycoplasma, or streptococci.

Bacterial throat culture should be done only in patients with significant pharyngitis to exclude coexisting group A beta-hemolytic streptococcal infection.

4. c. Acute infectious mononucleosis produces high anti-EA and anti-IgM-VCA titers and low anti-IgG-VCA and anti-EBNA titers. In recovering patients, the anti-IgG-VCA titer is high and the anti-EA, anti-IgM, and anti-EBNA titers are low. With time, the anti-EBNA titer also becomes high.

The heterophil antibody test can be negative in up to 20% of adults with EBV-associated infectious mononucleosis. Persistence of heterophile antibody for 3-12 months after onset of symptoms occurs in about 30% of patients. After 12 months the test is negative.

Serologic testing for EBV infection includes determining antibody titers to latently infected (anti-EBNA) viral proteins and determining antibody titers to early-replication-cycle (anti-EA) viral proteins or determining antibody titers to late-replication-cycle (anti-VCA) viral proteins.

5. c. EBV also has been associated with Burkitt's lymphoma, T-cell lymphoma, nasopharyngeal carcinoma, and Hodgkin's disease. Studies have not supported any association with chronic fatigue syndrome.

6. a. The major clinical features of acute symptomatic infectious mononucleosis are listed in the table:

Major Criteria	Minor Criteria
Carditis	Arthralgias
Polyarthritis	Fever
Chorea	Elevated erythrocyte sedimentation rate
Erythema marginatum	Elevated C-reactive protein
Subcutaneous nodules	Prolonged PR interval on electrocardiogram

7. e. Supportive treatment including rest, avoidance of strenuous exercise (because of the potential complication of splenic rupture), and analgesics are the only treatments necessary in acute uncomplicated infectious mononucleosis. There is no evidence that bed rest hastens recovery.

Antibiotics are unnecessary unless a streptococcal pharyngitis coexists. Ampicillin should be avoided. It will produce a skin rash in approximately 90% of patients with infectious mononucleosis.

8. d. The complications of acute infectious mononucleosis include meningoencephalitis, Guillain-Barré syndrome, Bell's palsy, pneumonitis, pericarditis, myocarditis, and splenic rupture.

9. a. To decrease the risk of splenic rupture, straining with bowel movements should be avoided. Therefore, increased fluids and/or stool softeners should be recommended. Prednisone, acyclovir, and ampicillin have not been shown to have any effect on the incidence of splenic rupture. There is no medical indication for splenectomy.

10. d. At this time, the single most important maneuver is to prescribe a corticosteroid to decrease the swelling and inflammation present in the airway. In severe cases of infectious mononucleosis, the swelling and inflammation of the airway may be so significant that airway compromise and respiratory distress may occur. A reasonable starting dose would be in the range of 40 mg to 60 mg of prednisone/day with gradual tapering of the dose over 10-14 days.

11. b. EBV, which causes infectious mononucleosis, is a B-cell lymphotropic human herpes virus. EBV is a ubiquitous agent that has been found in all population groups surveyed to date.

12. d. Mononucleosis-like syndromes can be caused by CMV, HIV, toxoplasmosis, human herpesvirus 6, and viral hepatitis species. These agents are included in the differential diagnosis of patients presenting with this syndrome but have negative serologies for EBV. A majority of HSV 1 infections are asymptomatic; however, gingivostomatitis and genital herpes are the common clinical manifestations and not mononucleosis.

13. c. There is no clear time-based consensus on return to play for athletes with mononucleosis. The chief concerns for athletes with mononucleosis are hepatomegaly and splenomegaly. Avoidance of contact sports is necessary until the liver and spleen are no longer palpable and have returned to normal size. For athletes who have no hepatosplenomegaly, fever, or laboratory abnormalities, noncontact practice and reconditioning can be resumed in 3 weeks and full contact sports can be restarted at 4-5 weeks after the onset of the illness.

14. a. Atypical lymphocytes are not specific for EBV infection but also can occur with rubella, viral hepatitis, and allergic rhinitis. Severe hematologic complications such as agranulocytosis and hemolytic anemia are rare. There is no seasonal pattern to infection, and the incidence is equal in males and females. Patients younger than age 15 years who acquire the infection often are asymptomatic or may have a mild "flulike" illness.

15. c. Respiratory tract viral shedding can occur for many months after symptoms have subsided; thus the period of communicability is indeterminate. The incubation period is estimated to be 30-50 days. Close contact usually is required for transmission, which may occur through the exchange of saliva. Infections in close groups such as educational settings can be endemic. Patients with recent mononucleosis or a similar syndrome should not donate blood.

SOLUTION TO THE CLINICAL CASE MANAGEMENT PROBLEM

Acute mononucleosis and chronic fatigue syndrome share symptomatology. However, no link has been established between the causative agent in mononucleosis and chronic fatigue syndrome. As yet, no causative agent or agents has been established for chronic fatigue syndrome. Serologic antibody levels against EBV are no more common in patients with chronic fatigue syndrome than in the general population. See Answer 1 for the criteria for diagnosing chronic fatigue syndrome.

SUMMARY OF MONONUCLEOSIS

1. **Identification:** EBV is the causative agent.
2. **Incubation period:** 2-5 weeks
3. **Symptoms:** malaise, fatigue, fever, chills, myalgias, and severe sore throat
4. **Signs:** pharyngeal erythema and edema, exudative tonsillitis, lymphadenopathy, splenomegaly, and hepatomegaly
5. **Laboratory diagnosis:** lymphocyte atypia, positive heterophil antibody titer, and antibodies to EBV antigens:
   a. Acute phase antibodies: anti-EA, anti-IgM-VCA
   b. Convalescent antibody: anti-IgG-VCA
   c. Recovered state: anti-IgG-VCA, anti-EBNA
6. **Treatment:**
   a. Symptomatic treatment: rest, fluids, mild analgesics
   b. Treatment of severe odynophagia and airway compromise: oral prednisone

SUGGESTED READING
AAP 2003 Red Book.
DeLee JC: Common Viral Infections in the Athlete. In: DeLee JC, et al, eds: *DeLee and Drez's Orthopaedic Sports Medicine: Principles and Practice*, 2nd ed. W.B. Saunders, 2003, Philadelphia.
Macsween KF: Epstein-Barr virus—recent advances. *Lancet Infect Dis* 3(3):131-140, 2003.

Chapter **39**

Fibromyalgia

"Oh, I ache all over."

CLINICAL CASE PROBLEM 1:
A 35-YEAR-OLD FEMALE WITH TOTAL BODY MUSCLE PAIN

A 35-year-old female comes to your office with a 1-year history of "aching and hurting all over." As well, she complains of a chronic headache, difficulty sleeping, and generalized fatigue. When questioned carefully, she describes "muscle areas tender to touch." Although the pain is "worse in the back," there really is no place where "it doesn't exist." She also describes headaches, generalized abdomen pains, and some constipation.

On examination, the most striking finding is the presence of 13 discrete "trigger points" (tender muscle areas when palpated). These include the trapezius muscle, the sternomastoid, the masseter muscle, the levator scapulae, the muscles inserting into the area of the greater trochanter, the muscles inserting into the upper border of the patellae, and six areas on the back that together cover almost the entire back area.

The rest of the physical examination is normal. Her blood pressure is 120/70 mm Hg, and her cardiovascular system, respiratory, and abdomen exams are normal.

■ SELECT THE BEST ANSWER TO THE FOLLOWING QUESTIONS:

1. What is the most likely diagnosis in this patient?
   a. polymyalgia rheumatica
   b. masked depression
   c. fibromyalgia
   d. diffuse musculoskeletal pain, not yet diagnosed (NYD)
   e. early rheumatoid arthritis

2. Which one of the following is not usually a site of tenderness in the disorder described?
   a. the rectus abdominis muscle
   b. the supraspinatus tendon
   c. the lateral epicondyle of the humerus
   d. the trapezius muscle
   e. the middle gluteus muscle

3. The differential diagnosis of the condition described includes which of the following?
   a. chronic fatigue syndrome
   b. hypothyroidism
   c. masked depression
   d. myofascial pain syndrome
   e. all of the above

4. The diagnostic criteria of the disorder described includes tenderness at how many of 18 specific sites?
   a. 5
   b. 7
   c. 9
   d. 11
   e. 13

5. What is the most characteristic symptom of the condition described?
   a. pain in at least three or four body quadrants
   b. "pain all over my body"
   c. pain in specific bursa and tendons
   d. pain in specific joints
   e. pain in both arms, the posterior neck, and the upper back

6. What is the most important condition that must be considered in the differential diagnosis of the condition described?
   a. generalized anxiety disorder
   b. panic disorder
   c. major depression
   d. rheumatoid arthritis
   e. osteoarthritis

7. What is the cause of this disorder?
   a. an autoimmune process
   b. a chronic inflammatory process
   c. an acute inflammatory process
   d. a slow or chronic virus infection
   e. idiopathic

8. Which of the following statements regarding sleep disorders and the condition described is true?
   a. there is no association between this condition and sleep disorders
   b. patients with this disorder have an abnormal sleep pattern
   c. patients with this disorder have difficult sleep induction, early-morning wakening, and nightmares
   d. patients with this disorder have profound insomnia
   e. patients with this disorder usually have profound hypersomnia

9. Regarding therapy for this disorder, which of the following statements is (are) true?
   a. Nonsteroidal antiinflammatory drugs (NSAIDs) have demonstrated a significant advantage over placebo
   b. antidepressants are superior to placebo
   c. muscle relaxants are superior to placebo
   d. b and c
   e. all of the above are true

10. Regarding the use of corticosteroids in the condition described, which of the following statements is (are) true?
    a. repetitive local injections with corticosteroids/lidocaine should be considered a first-line treatment option
    b. oral prednisone has been shown to be effective
    c. local injection of steroids/lidocaine should be reserved for resistant cases of this disorder
    d. no benefit from oral steroids has been demonstrated
    e. none of the above are true

CLINICAL CASE MANAGEMENT PROBLEM

Describe the criteria established by the American Rheumatological Society to establish a diagnosis of fibromyalgia.

■ ANSWERS:

1. **c.** This patient has fibromyalgia. Fibromyalgia is characterized by widespread musculoskeletal pain (defined as pain in the left and right side of the body, above and below the waist, plus axial pain) and the presence of 11 or more out of 18 specifically designated tender points or trigger points.

These musculoskeletal symptoms often are associated with total body pain, severe fatigue, nonrestorative sleep, postexertional increase in muscle pain, reduced functional ability, recurrent headaches, irritable bowel syndrome, atypical paraesthesia, cold sensitivity (Raynaud's phenomena), aerobic deconditioning, restless leg syndrome, sleep apnea, and nocturnal myoclonus.

Fibromyalgia is much more common in women than in men and usually is diagnosed between the ages of 20 and 50.

Rheumatoid arthritis is unlikely because of the lack of objective evidence of joint warmth, swelling, or deformity and the multiple soft-tissue areas. Laboratory evaluation, however, is necessary to exclude this inflammatory condition.

Polymyalgia rheumatica occurs in an older age group and is discussed in Chapter 134.

Diffuse musculoskeletal pain NYD is not a diagnosis.

A primary diagnosis of masked depression or a somatoform disorder always should be considered when vague, somatic complaints are accompanied by sleep disturbance and fatigue. The multiple tender areas, however, are not usually seen in masked depression.

2. **a.** Fibromyalgia is associated with tender points, or trigger points, at multiple characteristic locations. These locations include the following: (1) the supraspinatus tendon; (2) the costochondral junction; (3) the lateral epicondyle of the humerus; (4) the iliac crest; (5) the greater trochanteric bursa of the femur; (6) the medial fat pad of the knee; (7) the suboccipital region of the head; (8) the nuchal ligament; (9) the trapezius muscle; (10) the infraspinatus tendon; (11) the rhomboid muscle; (12) the erector spinae of the lumbar spine; (13) the middle gluteus muscle; and (14) the piriformis muscle.

An additional four less anatomically descriptive areas also are included. The rectus abdominous muscle is not included.

The sensitivity of the trigger points can be assessed by measuring the exact amount of pressure applied over a certain anatomic site. This can be measured by a dolorimeter.

3. **e.** Fibromyalgia certainly has some vague symptoms, and the trigger points are the most objective evidence of the disorder. Many health care professionals, however, still doubt its authenticity.

Hypothyroidism and chronic fatigue syndrome present with severe fatigue and share this major symptom with fibromyalgia.

Myofascial pain syndrome shares the symptom of trigger points with fibromyalgia and should be considered in the differential diagnosis.

4. **d.** The number of trigger points identified by the American College of Rheumatology as being diagnostic of fibromyalgia is 11 or more.

5. **b.** The most characteristic symptom of fibromyalgia is the symptom described by patients as "total body muscle pain." This is a symptom that from clinical experience appears to have reasonable sensitivity and specificity.

6. **c.** The most important differential diagnosis of fibromyalgia is major depression or a somatoform disorder. Depression is a very common correlate with fibromyalgia, and it appears that many patients actually meet the criteria for both disorders. In addition, the tricyclic antidepressants (TCAs) are recommended for both conditions. In many cases, the major depression that accompanies fibromyalgia is a masked depression, with many of the symptoms being somatic in origin.

7. **e.** The cause of fibromyalgia is unknown. There is no significant evidence that the process is an autoimmune process, the result of a true acute or chronic inflammatory process (although this is a possibility), or the result of any type of viral infection.

8. **b.** The many nonrheumatologic features of fibromyalgia include a pattern that is best described as a disorder of nonrestorative sleep (alpha nonrapid eye movement sleep anomaly). Although other sleep disorders, including sleep apnea in a small minority of patients, nocturnal myoclonus, and restless leg syndrome, are associated with fibromyalgia, a disorder of nonrestorative sleep (alpha-delta disorder) is the most common and the most diagnostic.

9. **e.** There is certainly considerable controversy regarding what pharmacologic medications (if any) work and which do not. Results have been mixed, but it is fair to say that at least some studies have demonstrated favorable results for NSAIDs, tricyclics,

fluoxetine, and cyclobenzaprine. Tramadol has a dual effect on both opiate and serotonin receptor systems and has become a popular alternative.

If the patient experiences sleep disturbances, which are often associated with fibromyalgia, serotonin reuptake inhibitors (particularly fluoxetine) should be used only with caution for the treatment of this condition.

10. **c.** It is recommended that local injections of corticosteroid/lidocaine combination be reserved for resistant trigger points because the risk:benefit ratio (especially for repeated injections) is questionable. Muscle atrophy, overlying skin atrophy, fibrosis, infection, abscess formation, and other complications may arise from repeated steroid injections.

SOLUTION TO THE CLINICAL CASE MANAGEMENT PROBLEM

American College of Rheumatology Diagnosis of Fibromyalgia:

1. Widespread musculoskeletal pain in the left and right sides of the body, above and below the waist, plus axial pain; typically described by patient as "total body muscle pain" or "I hurt all over."
2. The presence of 11 or more out of a total of 18 specifically designated tender points or trigger points.
3. The major clinical features of fibromyalgia include

the following: (a) total body pain; (b) multiple tender points on examination; (c) severe fatigue; (d) nonrestorative sleep (alpha nonrapid eye movement sleep anomaly); (e) postexertional increase in muscle pain; (f) reduced functional ability; (g) recurrent headaches; (h) irritable bowel syndrome; (i) atypical paresthesia; (j) cold sensitivity (often Raynaud's phenomenon); (k) restless leg syndrome; and (l) aerobic deconditioning.

SUMMARY OF FIBROMYALGIA

1. **Diagnosis:** See the Solution to the Clinical Case Management Problem.
2. **Treatment:**
   a. **Nonpharmacologic:** (i) physical therapy (heat, cold, ultrasound, TENS); (ii) massage therapy; (iii) psychologic counseling; (iv) biofeedback; and (v) cardiovascular fitness training program.
   b. **Pharmacologic:** (i) TCAs (low dose). Amitriptyline and Nortriptyline often are used. Selective serotonin reuptake inhibitors have been found to be helpful alone and as an adjunct therapy with TCAs; (ii) NSAIDs are of limited

usefulness in fibromyalgia. Cyclobenzaprine and a newer muscle relaxant tizanidine (Zanaflex) can be helpful. In other cases, response to tramadol or gabapentin has been noted. Many of the positive effects of the medications tend to diminish over time.

SUGGESTED READING

Buskila D: Fibromyalgia, chronic fatigue syndrome, and myofascial pain syndrome. *Curr Opin Rheumatol* 13(2):117-127, 2001.
Puttick MP: Rheumatology: 11. Evaluation of the patient with pain all over. *CMAJ* 164(2):223-227, 2001.
Sprott H: What can rehabilitation interventions achieve in patients with primary fibromyalgia? *Curr Opin Rheumatol* 15(2):145-150, 2003.

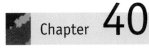

Chapter 40

Chronic Fatigue Syndrome

"I just can't get up, any time of day."

CLINICAL CASE PROBLEM 1:

A 25-Year-Old Female with
Chronic Fatigue

A 25-year-old female comes to your office with a 9-month history of "unbearable fatigue." Before the fatigue began 9 months ago, she worked as a high school chemistry teacher. Since the fatigue began she has been unable to work at all. She tells you that "one day it just hit me. I literally could not get out of bed."

Her past history is unremarkable. She has a husband and two children who have been very supportive during her 9-month illness. She has no history of any significant illnesses, including no history of any psychiatric disease. She has not expressed any signs of depression.

The other symptoms that the patient describes are difficulty concentrating, headache, sore throat, tender lymph nodes, muscle aches, joint aches, feverishness, difficulty sleeping, abdominal cramps, chest pain, and night sweats.

On physical examination, the patient has a low-grade fever (38.6° C), nonexudative pharyngitis, and palpable and tender anterior and posterior cervical and axillary lymph nodes.

▌ SELECT THE BEST ANSWER TO THE FOLLOWING QUESTIONS:

1. What is the most likely diagnosis in this patient?
   a. major depressive illness
   b. masked depression
   c. chronic fatigue syndrome
   d. fibromyalgia
   e. malingering

2. What is the etiology of the condition presented here?
   a. unequivocally related to a viral infection
   b. associated with an imbalance of neurotransmitters in the brain
   c. a factitious illness
   d. associated with major psychiatric pathology in almost all cases
   e. unknown

3. Which of the following statements regarding the condition described is (are) false?
   a. this condition is relatively new
   b. this condition also is known as epidemic neuromyasthenia
   c. this condition also is known as myalgic encephalomyelitis
   d. this condition also is known as multiple chemical sensitivity syndrome
   e. none of the above are false

4. Which of the following statements concerning the epidemiology of the condition described is (are) true?
   a. patients with this condition are twice as likely to be women as to be men
   b. the patients with this condition are likely to be in the 25 to 45 age bracket
   c. clusters of outbreaks of this condition have occurred in many countries over the last 60 years
   d. the primary symptom of this condition may be found in up to 20% of patients attending a general medical clinic
   e. all of the above are true

5. Which of the following best describes the onset of the condition described in the majority of patients?
   a. gradually increasing symptoms over a 3-month period
   b. gradually increasing symptoms over a 6-month period
   c. acute onset of symptoms in a previously healthy, well-functioning patient
   d. chronic onset of symptoms over 1-2 years
   e. the onset of symptoms is extremely variable; it is impossible to predict them with any degree of certainty

6. Which of the following is not a criterion in the diagnosis of the condition described?
   a. sore throat
   b. mild fever
   c. prolonged generalized fatigue following previously tolerable levels of exercise
   d. sleep disturbance
   e. anxiety or panic attacks

7. Regarding the laboratory diagnosis of the condition, which of the following statements is true?
   a. no laboratory test, however esoteric or exotic, can diagnose this condition or measure its severity
   b. a well-defined laboratory test that is sensitive but not specific exists for diagnostic purposes
   c. a well-defined laboratory test that is specific but not sensitive exists for diagnostic purposes
   d. a well-defined laboratory test that is both sensitive and specific exists for diagnostic purposes

e. a number of laboratory tests in combination are used for definite confirmation of the condition

8. Which of the following has been shown to be the most effective therapy for the condition described?
   a. a tricyclic antidepressant
   b. a nonsteroid antiinflammatory drug (NSAID)
   c. a sensitive, empathetic physician who is willing to listen
   d. cognitive psychotherapy
   e. none of the above

9. The disorder described is associated with all of the following except:
   a. hypothalamic dysfunction
   b. conversion disorder
   c. alpha-intrusion sleep disorder
   d. chronic immune activation
   e. myofascial pain

10. The disorder described is associated with which of the following symptoms?
    a. sleep disruption
    b. cognitive dysfunction
    c. anxiety and/or depression
    d. neurologic symptoms
    e. all of the above

11. Empiric evidence suggests that the best drug(s) to treat symptoms of the disorder is (are) which of the following?
    a. NSAIDs
    b. antidepressants
    c. clarithromycin
    d. tryptophan
    e. a and b

12. When using antidepressant medications to treat either the sleep disorder or the mood disorder associated with this condition, what should the dose be?
    a. the usual dose given to treat depression
    b. 1 and ½ times the usual dose given to treat depression
    c. ½ the usual dose given to treat depression
    d. ¼ or less of the usual dose given to treat depression
    e. twice the usual dose given to treat depression

13. What is the main therapeutic strategy used to reduce the symptoms of the disorder described?
    a. correct the sleep disorder
    b. provide psychotherapy for the conversion disorder

c. encourage the development of a support network
d. encourage the patient to return to work and full activity as soon as possible
e. none of the above

14. Most patients with the disorder:
    a. fully recover with 2 years
    b. partially recover with 2 years
    c. never recover
    d. are at risk for relapse following recovery
    e. b and d

CLINICAL CASE MANAGEMENT PROBLEM

Describe the relationship between the described disorder and fibromyalgia.

▶ ANSWERS:

1. **c.** This patient has the clinical manifestations that support a diagnosis of chronic fatigue syndrome. Clinically evaluated, unexplained chronic fatigue cases can be classified as chronic fatigue syndrome if the patient meets both of the following criteria:

   1. Clinically evaluated, unexplained persistent or relapsing chronic fatigue that is of new or definite onset (i.e., not lifelong); is not the result of ongoing exertion; is not substantially alleviated by rest; and results in substantial reduction in previous levels of occupational, educational, social, or personal activities.
   2. The concurrent occurrence of four or more of the following symptoms: substantial impairment in short-term memory or concentration; sore throat; tender lymph nodes; muscle pain; multijoint pain without swelling or redness; headaches of a new type, pattern, or severity; unrefreshing sleep; or postexertional malaise lasting more than 24 hours.

These symptoms must have persisted or recurred during 6 or more consecutive months of illness and must not have predated the fatigue.

The Centers for Disease Control and Prevention (CDC) in Atlanta established a working definition of chronic fatigue syndrome in 1988, which was revised in 1993: "A thorough medical history, physical examination, mental status examination, and laboratory tests (diagram) must be conducted to identify underlying or contributing conditions that require treatment. Diagnosis or classification cannot be made without such an evaluation." The complaint of chronic fatigue accounts for 10-15 million office visits per year in the United States. Depression and anxiety, along with overwork, are the most common causes of chronic fatigue encountered in primary care practice.

2. **e.** The etiology of chronic fatigue syndrome is unknown. There are several common themes underlying attempts to understand the disorder. It is often postinfectious, often is accompanied by immunologic disturbances, and commonly is accompanied by depression. Viral agents that have been implicated as being associated with chronic fatigue syndrome include the lymphotropic herpesviruses, the retroviruses, and the enteroviruses. The real etiology, however, is unknown.

3. **a.** Chronic fatigue syndrome is not a new disease; it has been around for centuries. Certain individuals in the past have been labeled with a variety of diagnoses such as neurasthenia, effort syndrome, hyperventilation syndrome, chronic brucellosis, epidemic neuromyasthenia, myalgic encephalomyelitis, hypoglycemia, multiple chemical sensitivity syndrome, chronic candidiasis, chronic mononucleosis, chronic Epstein-Barr virus infection, and postviral fatigue syndrome.

4. **e.** Patients with chronic fatigue syndrome are twice as likely to be women as men and are generally 25 to 45 years of age.

Cases are recognized in many developed countries. Most arise sporadically, but more than 30 clusters of similar illnesses have been reported. The most famous of such outbreaks occurred in Los Angeles County Hospital in 1934; in Akureyri, Iceland, in 1948; in the Royal Free Hospital, London, in 1955; in Punta Gorda, Florida, in 1945; and in Incline Village, Nevada, in 1985.

The prevalence of chronic fatigue syndrome is difficult to estimate because this is entirely dependent on case definition. Chronic fatigue itself is a ubiquitous symptom, occurring in as many as 20% of patients attending a general medical clinic; the syndrome itself is much less common.

5. **c.** The typical case of chronic fatigue syndrome arises suddenly in a previously active and healthy individual. An otherwise unremarkable flulike illness or some other acute stress is recalled with great clarity as the triggering event. Unbearable exhaustion is left in the wake of the incident. Other symptoms, such as headache, sore throat, tender lymph nodes, muscle and joint aches, and frequent feverishness lead to the belief that an infection persists. Then, over several weeks, the impact of reassurances offered during the initial evaluation fades as other features of the syndrome become evident such as disturbed sleep, difficulty in concentration, and depression.

6. **e.** Panic attacks and anxiety are not criteria in the CDC definition.

7. **a.** No laboratory test, however exotic or esoteric, can make the diagnosis of chronic fatigue syndrome. Elaborate, expensive laboratory workups should be avoided; they only make an already complicated picture even more so. However, it is reasonable to perform testing to exclude other causes of fatigue.

8. **c.** A sensitive, empathetic physician who is willing to listen is the most effective intervention that can be offered for chronic fatigue syndrome. NSAIDs alleviate headache and diffuse pain and feverishness. Nonsedating antidepressants (typically low-dose tricyclic agents) improve mood and disordered sleep and thereby attenuate the fatigue to some degree. The ingestion of caffeine and alcohol at night makes it harder to sleep, compounding fatigue, and should be avoided. Nothing, however, takes the place of an empathetic physician.

In terms of psychotherapy, the most effective therapy appears to be behavior-oriented therapy, not cognitive psychotherapy. If the patient is severely depressed and if tricyclic agents at full doses to treat depression have too many side effects, serotonin reuptake inhibitors (SSRIs) or the combination medication venlafaxine (Effexor) may be used. This medication is a combination of an SSRI and norepinephrine.

9. **b.** Chronic fatigue syndrome is not a conversion disorder, nor is it a psychosomatic illness. Current research describes immune dysfunction in which T cells are chronically activated and hypothalamic dysfunction occurs presumably as a result of cytokine penetration of the blood–brain barrier. Alpha-intrusion sleep disorder is also probably the result of cytokine penetration and may be worsened by myofascial pain, if present.

10. **e.** Chronic fatigue syndrome may be classified as mild, moderate, or severe, depending on the number of symptoms present. Severe chronic fatigue syndrome may include not only fatigue, myofascial pain, and sleep disruption but also numerous neurologic complaints such as blurred vision, migrating paresthesias, and tinnitus. Mood disruption may be present; either depression or anxiety or both are often endogenous, reflecting neurochemical dysequilibrium. Cognitive dysfunction may be severe, with complaints of poor memory, poor concentration, and the inability to read.

11. **e.** NSAIDs are often helpful in treating the symptoms of headache, diffuse pain, and feverishness. The nonsedating antidepressants may be useful in the treatment of depression, which is a predominant symptom in many patients.

12. **d.** Empiric evidence suggests that patients with chronic fatigue syndrome lose their tolerance to many

agents, including toxins such as secondhand cigarette smoke, certain fumes, alcohol, and medications. Antidepressants, such as amitriptyline, should be given initially to patients with chronic fatigue in a dose approximately one-fourth of the usual dose, although gradual tolerance may develop. When higher doses are used, physicians should watch carefully for symptoms of neurologic toxicity, which may, according to some, leave permanent deficits.

13. The main therapeutic strategy in treating chronic fatigue syndrome should be to correct the sleep disorder. If the sleep disorder can be reduced and a period with more stage 3, stage 4, or rapid eye movement sleep attained, the number of symptoms and their severity may be reduced greatly. This includes not only the symptoms of fatigue and pain but also the neurologic and mood/cognitive complaints. Patients required to return to work early when still symptomatic tend to suffer relapses and actually prolong their illness.

14. Most patients with chronic fatigue syndrome partially recover within 2 years, often to the extent that they can return to work and resume most of the normal activities of their previous life. They are, however, at risk for relapse at any time (especially at times where they experience immune activation or sleep disruption).

SOLUTION TO THE CLINICAL CASE MANAGEMENT PROBLEM

The relationship between chronic fatigue syndrome and fibromyalgia is fascinating. There certainly seems to be some connection between the two disorders. Some authorities believe that fibromyalgia and chronic fatigue syndrome are actually the same illness with different presentations. Clinicians see patients with more pain than fatigue, with more fatigue than pain, or with both fatigue and pain. Both fibromyalgia and chronic fatigue syndrome appear to share the alpha-intrusion sleep disorder.

SUMMARY OF CHRONIC FATIGUE SYNDROME

1. **Prevalence:** difficult to establish. One study suggests a prevalence of 37 cases/100,000 people. Chronic fatigue syndrome is not a new disease; it has been present for centuries. Most evidence for the disorder comes from outbreaks of the disorder, discussed earlier.
2. **Etiology:** the etiology of chronic fatigue syndrome is unknown. Chronic fatigue syndrome, does, however, appear to be related to infectious agents (although none that have been investigated have been found to be linked to the disease) and immunologic disturbances; T-cell activation may play a prominent role. Cytokines also appear to be involved. Alpha-intrusion sleep disorder appears to be related to cytokine involvement.
3. **Signs and symptoms:** the best diagnostic criteria at present have been set by the CDC. These criteria are listed in Answer 1. It is important to diagnose and treat other syndromes, including major depressive disorder, which may present with complaints of chronic fatigue, or others that otherwise complicate the picture. Growing evidence shows that it may have a biologic basis and that the central nervous system and immune system are involved.

4. **Course:** most patients partially recover within 2 years. All, however, are prone to relapse.
5. **Treatment:**
   a. Nonpharmacologic: an understanding physician who is prepared to spend time with the patient and listen and counsel in an empathetic fashion. The physician should help the patient reduce stress, develop a regular schedule, and maintain and gradually increase activity.
   b. Pharmacologic: NSAIDs can be used to treat headaches, myalgias, and arthralgias. Low-dose tricyclic antidepressants can be used to improve the quality of sleep. For severe depression, full antidepressant therapy should be used. Select the dose carefully, and begin at one-fourth the usual dose. Additional trials in steroid therapy, immunomodulation, and antimicrobial therapy (acyclovir) need further research and have not been found to be helpful at this time.

SUGGESTED READING

Afari N, Buchwald D: Chronic fatigue syndrome: a review. *Am J Psych* 160(2):221-236, 2003.
Sabin TD: An approach to chronic fatigue syndrome in adults. *Neurologist* 9(1):28-34, 2003.
Whiting P, et al: Interventions for the treatment and management of chronic fatigue syndrome: a systematic review. *JAMA* 86(11): 1360-1368, 2001 Sep 19.

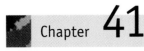

Chapter 41

Acute Gout and Pseudogout

| "Ouch, my big toe!"

CLINICAL CASE PROBLEM 1:
A 45-YEAR-OLD MALE WITH EXCRUCIATING PAIN IN HIS LEFT FOOT

A 45-year-old obese male presents to the emergency room (ER) in the middle of the night screaming and holding his left foot. He tells you that he thinks he has an "acute blood vessel blockage" in his left toe. He wakes up the entire ER observation unit with his screams. His past history is significant for essential hypertension, for which he has been treated with a thiazide diuretic for the past 5 years. He categorically relates to you that he has never had the symptoms that he is experiencing now (and further adds that instead of all these questions he would prefer if you just got on with treatment).

On examination the patient's temperature is 38° C and his blood pressure is 170/110 mm Hg. He has an inflamed, tender, swollen left great toe. There is extensive swelling and erythema of the left foot, and his whole foot is tender. No other joints are swollen. No other abnormalities are found on physical examination.

■ SELECT THE BEST ANSWER TO THE FOLLOWING QUESTIONS:

1. What is the most likely diagnosis?
   a. acute cellulitis
   b. acute gouty arthritis
   c. acute rheumatoid arthritis
   d. acute septic arthritis
   e. acute vasculitis

2. Which of the following statements regarding this man's condition is (are) false?
   a. the disease is more common in males than in females
   b. fever is unusual
   c. more than 50% of the initial attacks of this condition are confined to the first metatarsophalangeal joint
   d. peripheral leukocytosis can occur
   e. initial involvement is usually in several joints

3. What is the definitive diagnostic test of choice for this patient's condition?
   a. a plasma level
   b. a random urine determination
   c. a 24-hour urine determination
   d. a synovial fluid analysis
   e. a gram stain plus culture and sensitivity

4. What is the most common metabolic abnormality found in the condition described in this patient?
   a. increased production of uric acid
   b. decreased renal excretion of uric acid
   c. increased production of uric acid metabolites
   d. decreased renal excretion of uric acid metabolites
   e. none of the above

5. What is the pharmacologic agent of choice for the initial management of this patient's condition?
   a. indomethacin
   b. colchicine
   c. acetaminophen
   d. aspirin
   e. phenylbutazone

6. Regarding the prophylaxis recommended for the prevention of future attacks of the condition described in the patient, which of the following would describe most accurately the current recommendation (as applied)?
   a. this patient probably should not be treated with a prophylactic agent
   b. this patient should be treated with a uricosuric agent as prophylaxis against future attacks of this condition
   c. this patient should be treated with a xanthine oxidase inhibitor as prophylaxis against future attacks of this condition
   d. this patient could be treated with either a uricosuric agent or a xanthine oxidase inhibitor as prophylaxis against future attacks of this condition
   e. none of the above

7. The determination of the agent of choice for the prophylaxis of the condition described is made by which of the following?
   a. a serum blood level
   b. a joint fluid aspiration
   c. a 24-hour urine determination of uric acid
   d. a joint x-ray
   e. none of the above

8. Which of the following drug(s) increase(s) the excretion of uric acid?
   a. sulfinpyrazone
   b. probenecid
   c. allopurinol
   d. a and b only
   e. all of the above

9. In patients started on prophylactic therapy, which of the following statements regarding the use of prophylactic agents is (are) true?

a. the patient who is started taking a prophylactic agent also should start taking colchicine

b. colchicine should be added and maintained for 3-6 months

c. indomethacin can replace colchicine in this instance

d. none of the above statements are true

e. all of the above statements are true

10. Which of the following drugs would be most likely to provide significant relief in the case of an acute attack of the condition described?
    a. oral prednisone
    b. oral Decadron
    c. Intravenous (IV) Solu Cortef
    d. IV Solu Medrol
    e. intraarticular methylprednisolone acetate

11. Which of the following classes of drugs is most likely to precipitate the condition described?
    a. thiazide diuretics
    b. calcium-channel blockers
    c. angiotensin converting enzyme (ACE) inhibitors
    d. beta blockers
    e. alpha blockers

CLINICAL CASE PROBLEM 2:

A 55-Year-Old Male with Joint Pain

A 55-year-old male patient comes to your office complaining about joint pain. He states that he has had pain in both ankles for the past 4 months, and it has been getting progressively worse. He also states that, on occasion, he also has pain in his wrists. Although his blood pressure is now within high normal limits (138/75 mm Hg), he states that for the last 5 years he has been treated with 50 mg of hydrochlorothiazide per day for hypertension.

As part of a routine workup you find that he has a serum uric acid level of 12.4 mg/dl.

12. Should the condition described be treated to reduce the serum uric acid level?
    a. yes, vigorously to prevent an acute attack of gout
    b. yes, but cautiously to prevent a too-rapid release of feedback inhibition of purine synthesis
    c. no, the patient is not likely to develop gout
    d. a and c are true under certain conditions
    e. nobody really knows

CLINICAL CASE PROBLEM 3:

A 65-Year-Old Male with a Swollen, Painful Knee

A 65-year-old male comes to your office with pain in his right knee. He says he fell and "banged it up fairly bad"

some 6 or so months ago, but that it had since recovered spontaneously and provided no further trouble until now. He further said the pain did not become greater during the day, if anything it hurt more upon awakening. His past history showed no evidence of hypertension and he never had any other joint pain of significance.

On examination his temperature is 37.5° C and his blood pressure is 125/70 mm Hg. He has an inflamed, tender, swollen right knee. No other joints are affected. No other abnormalities are found on physical examination. A plain x-ray revealed streaking of the surrounding soft tissue with calcium deposits (chondrocalcinosis). You remove accumulated synovial fluid for polarized light microscopic analysis and also obtain a serum sample.

13. Which of the following possible results from these laboratory studies is most consistent with the symptoms described and will confirm a diagnosis?
    a. needlelike crystals with negative birefringence and a normal serum urate level
    b. needlelike crystals with negative birefringence and a high serum urate level
    c. rhomboidal crystals with weak positive birefringence and a high serum urate level
    d. rhomboidal crystals with weak positive birefringence and a normal serum urate level
    e. not any of the above

14. Which of the following condition(s) predispose(s) individuals toward the disease described in Clinical Case Problem 2?
    a. hemochromatosis
    b. hyperparathyroidism
    c. trauma
    d. surgery
    e. all of the above

CLINICAL CASE MANAGEMENT PROBLEM

Discuss the indications for the use of prophylactic agents in hyperuricemic states.

ANSWERS:

1. This patient has acute gouty arthritis. This is a very typical presentation for gout. With acute gout, the patient usually develops an acute pain in a single joint (monoarticular) of the lower extremity, with the most common joint being the metatarsophalangeal joint of the big toe. The pain of acute gout often wakes the patient from sleep, and the patient ends up in the ER with pain that is described as crushing or excruciating.

The joint rapidly becomes erythematous, swollen, warm, and extremely tender. The skin surrounding the joint is usually tense and shiny. The swelling in acute gout often extends well beyond the joint itself and may involve the entire foot (or other part of the extremity). This swelling, resulting from periarticular edema, makes the differentiation from septic arthritis particularly difficult. Often the patient is unable to bear weight on the affected foot.

2. **b.** Fever may occur in patients with gout, especially in patients with polyarticular disease. The temperature may reach 39.5° C (103-104° F).

Initial presentation is usually monoarticular, and more than 50% of patients experience their first acute attack in a metatarsophalangeal joint. However, gout can present in other joints, such as the knee. Acute gout also may involve the bursae or the tendon sheaths.

Leukocytosis also may be seen. In older patients tophi occasionally are seen with the first attack. Usually, however, there is a time interval (often 10 years or more) between the initial attack and the appearance of the complication of gouty tophi.

Gout is uncommon in people younger than age 30 years and is more common in men than in women until the age of 60 years when half of newly diagnosed cases are in women. In women gout most often occurs following menopause.

3. **d.** A definitive diagnosis of gout is made by demonstrating negatively birefringent, needle-shaped crystals under a polarizing microscope. Although an elevated serum uric acid concentration is seen often with acute gout, it is neither as sensitive nor as specific a test as the demonstration of uric acid crystals under the microscope from the synovial fluid. Serum uric acid levels can be normal or even low in patients with gout.

The diagnosis of septic arthritis can be ruled out by appropriate gram stains and cultures of the same specimen of synovial fluid as obtained for examination with the polarizing microscope.

4. **b.** The most common metabolic abnormality associated with gout is decreased renal excretion of uric acid. This may be a primary or a secondary event. Secondary causes, (such as chronic renal disease, acute ethanol ingestion, low-dose salicylates [at high doses salicylates are uricosuric], and diuretic [especially thiazide diuretics] therapy) are associated with the development of elevated serum uric acid levels and subsequent gout. The most common cause of overproduction of uric acid is a myeloproliferative or lymphoproliferative disorder. In addition, when a patient is undergoing cancer chemotherapy there is a very significant liberation of uric acid from dying cells.

The greater the responsiveness of the tumor to chemotherapy or radiotherapy, the quicker is the tumor breakdown and the more extensive the breakdown of uric acid.

5. **a.** Nonsteroidal antiinflammatory drugs (NSAIDs), such as indomethacin, are the drugs of choice in most settings. There is no evidence that one NSAID is superior to another in the treatment of gout.

Colchicine has many gastrointestinal side effects that limit its usefulness, especially with the frequency and dose needed in acute gout (hourly).

Aspirin taken in small doses actually can aggravate the problem. Acetaminophen has no antiinflammatory activity and is not indicated in the acute treatment of gout. Phenylbutazone is an excellent antiinflammatory agent but has been associated with bone marrow suppression and aplastic anemia.

Systemic corticosteroid therapy can be used to treat patients with acute, polyarticular gout who have not responded to other therapies and in patients in whom other therapies are contraindicated.

Intraarticular injections of a corticosteroid are usually very effective in patients with acute monoarticular gout.

6. **a.** From the history, you gather that this is the first attack of acute gout in this patient. It is not advisable to begin prophylactic therapy until the patient has had at least two attacks, or perhaps three. This recommendation is made for two reasons: (1) if there is a precipitating secondary cause (as in this patient the treatment of hypertension with a thiazide diuretic), it may very well be able to be eliminated and (2) because a second attack may not occur for years (if at all), the risk:benefit ratio for prophylactic medication is not favorable.

7. **c.** The choice of a prophylactic agent (if one is going to be used) is made by determining the 24-hour secretion of uric acid. This helps determine if a patient is an overproducer or underexcreter of uric acid. It is not always necessary to perform a 24-hour urine collection in older patients because most are underexcreters of uric acid.

8. **d.** If the patient excretes significantly more uric acid than 750 mg/24 hours, he is producing too much uric acid, and the production should be slowed by treatment with a drug that inhibits production. The rate determining step in the synthetic pathway depends on the enzyme xanthine oxidase. Allopurinol, the usual drug given, is an inhibitor of xanthine oxidase. If the patient excretes less than 750 mg/24 hours of

uric acid, then the metabolic problem rests with the failure to excrete the uric acid once it is produced. In this case, drugs that increase the excretion rate, known as uricosuric agents, should be used. The two most common drugs in this class are probenecid and sulfinpyrazone.

9. e. As previously discussed, the prophylactic agents for the prevention of gouty arthritis fall into two classes: the xanthine oxidase inhibitors (which inhibit the formation of uric acid) and the uricosuric agents (which increase the excretion of uric acid).

When prophylaxis against recurrent attacks is begun, either colchicine or a NSAID such as indomethacin should be added to the choice of the prophylactic agent for 3-6 months. The colchicine or indomethacin then can be discontinued, and the patient can remain on the uricosuric agent or the xanthine oxidase inhibitor indefinitely.

If the uricosuric agent is the preferred treatment because of the 24-hour urine uric acid determination, the following rules should be followed: (1) uricosuric agents should be used only in patients with normal renal function; (2) uricosuric agents should be used only in patients who have no history of renal stone formation; and (3) uricosuric agents should be used only in patients who are not overproducers of uric acid.

Allopurinol is indicated in patients with urate overproduction, history of renal stones, and renal impairment.

10. e. A local injection of a corticosteroid such as methylprednisolone acetate into an inflamed gouty joint reliably produces a resolution of the acute gouty condition. This treatment is most beneficial in patients with acute gouty monoarthritis and in patients with resistant attacks in whom coexistent infection has been excluded.

11. a. Diuretics in general, and thiazide diuretics in particular, elevate the serum uric acid level. Although the vast majority of patients who are receiving thiazide diuretics do not develop gout, those that do tend to be on relatively high doses of thiazide (greater than 25 mg) and have other coexistent reasons for the development of gout (such as acute ethanol intake).

The six metabolic side effects of thiazide diuretics are as follows: hyperuricemia, hyperglycemia, hyperlipidemia, hypokalemia, hyponatremia, and hypomagnesemia.

12. c. The condition described in Clinical Problem Case 2 is asymptomatic hyperuricemia. The symptoms described do not sound like gout and are unlikely to be related to the elevated uric acid level. The question that arises from this condition is "Should it be treated?" The answer is no.

Hyperuricemia is commonly the result of renal insufficiency or pharmacologic agent such as thiazide diuretics or low-dose salicylates. Ethanol consumption and obesity also can raise serum uric acid levels. Most patients with hyperuricemia are asymptomatic and never develop gout. Thus the treatment of asymptomatic hyperuricemia is not recommended.

13. d. The condition described is undoubtedly pseudogout, a common form of calcium pyrophosphate deposition disease (CPDD); the two terms often are used interchangeably. The symptoms are caused by calcium pyrophosphate deposition in nonosseous tissues in joints, most commonly in a knee. The differential includes the many factors that can cause swelling and pain in a knee. Considering the man's age and history the more likely conditions are osteoarthritis, gout, and pseudogout. The fact that the pain does not get worse in the evening points away from, but certainly does not exclude, osteoarthritis. Similarly, that the condition is in a knee and not a big toe points away from but does not exclude gout. The chondrocalcinosis found on x-ray is almost pathognomic for CPDD, and the presence of rhomboidal crystals with weak positive birefringence in the synovial fluid confirms this diagnosis. The serum urate level is not elevated.

14. e. CPDD can be caused by any condition that provides a local nucleation site for formation of a calcium pyrophospate crystals (likely via initial precipitation of apatite with subsequent conversion) or in conditions that increase the serum phosphate levels until precipitates form at vulnerable sites. Trauma and surgery are likely to create nucleation sites prone to such crystallization, whereas hemochromatosis and hyperparathyroidism tend to increase the serum phosphate level. Many cases appear not to be associated with any known risk factors but possibly are the result of some forgotten relatively mild trauma.

Prevalence increases with age, having been reported to be 3% to 4% in patients younger than age 60 years, as high as 25% in individuals in their 80s, and 50% in patients older than 90 years. It also is said to be seen about half as often as gout in the typical primary care office setting.

Symptoms tend to resolve with conservative treatment consisting of rest and use of antiinflammatory drugs. Intraarticular steroid injections are usually helpful in otherwise intractable cases, and on rare occasions surgery is used as a last resort; the crystals simply are scraped off of the soft tissues.

SOLUTION TO THE CLINICAL CASE MANAGEMENT PROBLEM

The prophylactic agents used in the prevention of recurrence of acute gout have been discussed in detail. In brief review, prophylactic agents should be used only if the patient has had more than one attack of gout, a gouty tophus develops, there is x-ray evidence of joint destruction from the gouty arthritis, or there is a history of urolithiasis.

SUMMARY OF ACUTE GOUT AND PSEUDOGOUT

1. Diagnosis of gout is firmly established by examination of joint aspirate under a polarizing microscope and finding needlelike, negatively birefringent uric acid crystals. In contrast the diagnosis of pseudogout (CPDD) is established by finding rhombic-shaped positively birefringent crystals in joint aspirates.
2. The primary symptom of gout is acute onset of pain in a joint of the lower extremity, most commonly the first metatarsophalangeal joint. Along with the pain there is associated tenderness, erythema, and swelling of the surrounding tissues.
3. The most important differential diagnosis in acute gout is septic arthritis.
4. Acute gout is associated most often with decreased renal excretion of uric acid (rather than an overproduction of uric acid).

5. Treatment of gout:
   a. Acute attack: (i) NSAIDs; (ii) corticosteroid injection; (iii) Colchicine; and (iv) corticosteroids, by mouth or intramuscularly.
   b. Prophylactic treatment of gout: (i) not given after only one attack; (ii) choose either a uricosuric agent or a xanthine oxidase inhibitor (choice is based on the results of the 24-hour urine uric acid determination plus other factors previously discussed); (iii) if prophylaxis is given, then use either NSAID or colchicine in low dose in addition to your prophylactic agent; (iv) do not treat asymptomatic hyperuricemia.
   c. Pseudogout symptoms tend to resolve with conservative treatment.

SUGGESTED READING
Concoff AL, Kalunian KC: What is the relation between crystals and ostearthritis? Curr Opin Rheumatol 11(5):436-440, 1999.
Rosenthal AK: Hyperuricemia and gout. In: Rakel RE, Bope ET, eds. Conn's Current Therapy 2003, 55th ed. WB Saunders, 2003, Philadelphia.
Rott KT, Agudelo CA: Gout. JAMA 289(21):2857-2860, 2003.

 Chapter **42**

Renal Diseases

"You are telling me that the blood in my urine came from my sore throat?"

CLINICAL CASE PROBLEM 1:
A 29-YEAR-OLD FEMALE WITH FATIGUE, ANOREXIA, AND BLOODY URINE

A 29-year-old female comes to your office with symptoms of extreme fatigue, no appetite, and bloody urine. She developed a very sore throat 3 weeks ago but did not have it examined or treated. Her 6-year-old daughter had a similar sore throat 1 week before her. Her doctor (over the phone) said, "You probably have a viral infection from your daughter. Don't worry about it."

Three days ago she began to have bloody urine and swelling of her hands and feet, and she felt terrible. Her past health has been excellent. There is no family history of significant illness. She has no allergies.

On examination, she has significant edema of both lower extremities. Her blood pressure is 170/105 mm Hg. Her blood pressure was last checked 1 year ago; at that time it was normal.

SELECT THE BEST ANSWER TO THE FOLLOWING QUESTIONS:

1. What is the most likely diagnosis in this patient at this time?
   a. hemorrhagic pyelonephritis
   b. immunoglobulin A (IgA) nephropathy (Berger's disease)
   c. poststreptococcal glomerulonephritis
   d. hemorrhagic cystitis
   e. membranous glomerulonephritis

2. Which of the following is (are) pathognomonic of the disorder described?
   a. macroscopic hematuria
   b. microscopic hematuria

c. eosinophils in the urine
d. red blood cell casts
e. protein 1.0 g/24 h

CLINICAL CASE PROBLEM 2:

A Girl with Joint Swelling Erythema and Pain

Approximately 4 weeks after the mother develops her symptoms, her daughter comes down with an illness characterized by swelling of a number of joints with erythema and pain, bumps on both of her elbows, significant fatigue, fever, and a skin rash covering her body.

On examination, the daughter has a grade III/VI pansystolic murmur. Her blood pressure is 100/70 mm Hg.

3. What is the most likely diagnosis in her daughter's case?
   a. juvenile rheumatoid arthritis
   b. Still's disease
   c. postviral arthritis syndrome
   d. rheumatic fever
   e. autoimmune complex disease

4. Which of the following statements regarding the prevention of the problems experienced by the patient and her daughter is (are) true, assuming both are treated with 10 days of penicillin?
   a. the mother's condition was preventable by penicillin; the daughter's condition was not
   b. the mother's condition was not preventable by penicillin; the daughter's condition was
   c. both the mother's condition and the daughter's conditions were preventable by treatment with penicillin
   d. neither the mother's condition nor the daughter's condition could have been prevented by treatment with penicillin
   e. prevention is variable with both conditions: penicillin may prevent both conditions, but it may not prevent either

5. What is the treatment of choice for the condition described in the mother?
   a. penicillin
   b. gentamicin
   c. prednisone
   d. a and b
   e. none of the above

6. Which of the following statements concerning prognosis of the condition described in the mother is (are) true?
   a. most patients with this disorder eventually develop end-stage renal failure
   b. the prognosis in the mother depends on how aggressively the antecedent streptococcal infection is treated
   c. most patients with the acute disease recover completely
   d. up to 20% of patients with this acute disease end up with chronic renal insufficiency
   e. c and d

7. Which of the following is (are) a complication(s) of the disease process described in the mother?
   a. hypertensive encephalopathy
   b. congestive cardiac failure
   c. acute renal failure
   d. a and b
   e. all of the above

8. Which of the following subtypes of the disease presented in the mother is associated with group A beta-hemolytic streptococcus?
   a. minimal change
   b. focal segmental sclerosis
   c. membranous
   d. diffuse proliferative
   e. crescentic

9. Which of the following subtypes of the disease presented in the mother is associated most closely with nephrotic syndrome?
   a. minimal change
   b. focal segmental sclerosis
   c. membranous
   d. diffuse proliferative
   e. crescentic

10. What is the most common cause of chronic renal failure?
    a. glomerulonephritis (acute to chronic)
    b. chronic pyelonephritis
    c. diabetes mellitus
    d. hypertensive renal disease
    e. congenital anomalies

11. What is the least common cause of chronic renal failure among the following causes?
    a. glomerulonephritis (acute to chronic)
    b. chronic pyelonephritis
    c. hypertensive renal disease
    d. diabetes mellitus
    e. congenital anomalies

12. Which of the following is true regarding angiotensin-converting enzyme (ACE) inhibitors?
    a. ACE inhibitors are contraindicated in patients with chronic renal insufficiency.

b. ACE inhibitors dilate the efferent arteriole of the kidney.
c. In patients with diabetes, ACE inhibitors prevent progression of microalbuminuria, even in patients with controlled blood pressure.
d. b and c
e. all of the above

13. What is the major cause of death in patients with chronic renal failure?
a. uremia
b. malignant hypertension
c. hyperkalemia-induced arrhythmias
d. myocardial infarction
e. subarachnoid hemorrhage

14. What is the anemia usually associated with chronic renal failure?
a. hypochromic
b. macrocytic
c. normochromic, normocytic
d. microcytic
e. hypochromic, microcytic

15. Which of the following classes of medications have been shown to slow the decline in glomerular filtration rate (GFR) in patients with chronic renal failure?
a. ACE inhibitors
b. nondihydropyridine calcium channel blockers
c. angiotensin receptor blockers (ARBs)
d. a and c
e. all of the above

16. Which of the following is (are) associated with nephrotic syndrome?
a. proteinuria, 3.5 g/day
b. edema
c. hypoalbuminemia
d. hypercholesterolemia
e. all of the above

17. Which of the following are causes of nephrotic syndrome?
a. diabetes mellitus
b. amyloidosis
c. Hodgkin's lymphoma
d. preeclamptic toxemia
e. all of the above

18. Which of the following statements regarding diabetes mellitus and chronic renal failure is (are) true?
a. diabetes mellitus is an uncommon cause of chronic renal failure
b. diabetes mellitus type 1 is a more common cause of chronic renal failure than diabetes mellitus type 2

c. diabetes mellitus type 2 is a more common cause of chronic renal failure than diabetes mellitus type 1
d. diabetes mellitus type 2 does not lead to chronic renal failure
e. diabetes mellitus type 1 does not lead to chronic renal failure

19. The treatment of nephrotic syndrome includes which of the following?
a. corticosteroids
b. loop diuretics
c. anticoagulant therapy
d. sodium restriction
e. all of the above

20. Comparing the recommended treatment of poststreptococcal glomerulonephritis (PSGN) with the recommended treatment on nonpoststreptococcal glomerulonephritis (NPSGN), which of the following statements is most accurate?
a. the treatment protocols are the same
b. corticosteroid treatment is indicated for both PSGN and NPSGN
c. corticosteroid treatment is generally not indicated for PSGN but it is for NPSGN
d. corticosteroid treatment is generally indicated for PSGN but not for NPSGN
e. the prognosis of neither PSGN nor NPSGN depends on the presence or absence of treatment

■ ANSWERS:

1. **c.** This patient has poststreptococcal glomerulonephritis. Poststreptococcal glomerulonephritis is the most common cause of acute glomerulonephritis. The syndrome may begin as early as 1 week after the initial streptococcal infection. Poststreptococcal glomerulonephritis predominantly affects children between the ages of 2 and 10 years. In patients with mild disease, there may be no signs or symptoms. In more severe disease, the symptoms of malaise, headache, mild fever, flank pain, edema, hypertension, and pulmonary edema may occur. Oliguria is common. The urine often is described as bloody, coffee colored, or smoky.

2. **d.** The pathognomonic clue concerning acute glomerulonephritis is red blood cell casts in the urine of patients. Other notable abnormalities include an elevated erythrocyte sedimentation rate (ESR) and an elevated antistreptolysin O (ASO) titer. Some strains of streptococci do not produce streptolysin, thereby limiting the usefulness of the ASO titer in patients with recent pharyngeal infections.

3. d. In this case, the daughter of the patient has developed rheumatic fever. The Jones criteria for the diagnosis of rheumatic fever are outlined in the table.

Symptom	Percentage of Cases (%)
Sensory loss	37
Optic neuritis	36
Weakness	35
Paresthesias	24
Diplopia	15
Ataxia	11
Vertigo	6
Paroxysmal symptoms	4
Bladder disorders	4
Lhermitte's sign	3
Pain	3
Dementia	2
Visual loss	2
Facial palsy	1
Impotence	1
Myokymia	1
Epilepsy	1
Falling	1

Two major criteria or one major criterion and two minor criteria are virtually diagnostic of rheumatic fever.

It is important to realize that in some parts of the United States, the incidence of rheumatic fever is increasing, not decreasing. The increase may be the result of more virulent strains of streptococci.

4. b. Poststreptococcal glomerulonephritis is not preventable by penicillin; rheumatic fever, however, is preventable. In both conditions, the cause of complications is group A beta-hemolytic streptococcus. Once the clinical or laboratory diagnosis of streptococcal pharyngitis is made, therapy with penicillin should be instituted and continued for a period of 10 days.

5. e. The primary treatment of acute glomerulonephritis associated with streptococcal infection is symptomatic. Although penicillin will eradicate the carrier state of group A beta-hemolytic streptococci, it will not influence the course of the glomerulonephritis.

Symptomatic treatment should include bed rest and protein restriction (if the blood urea nitrogen or creatinine level is elevated). Fluid overload and hypertension should be treated with diuretics and other antihypertensive medications as needed. Immunosuppressive treatment may be necessary if heavy proteinuria or rapidly decreasing GFR is present. If acute renal insufficiency develops and volume overload is unresponsive to diuretics, hemodialysis should be considered.

6. e. Most patients with PSGN recover completely. However, up to 20% of patients will end up with chronic renal insufficiency. As indicated earlier, the treatment of the antecedent streptococcal infection has no bearing on the prognosis.

7. e. Complications of acute PSGN include hypertensive encephalopathy, congestive cardiac failure, acute renal failure, chronic renal insufficiency, and nephrotic syndrome.

8. d. PSGN usually presents as a diffuse proliferative glomerulonephritis.

9. c. Membranous glomerulonephritis is the most common cause of nephrotic syndrome. The majority of children with nephrotic syndrome have minimal change disease.

10. c. The most common cause of chronic renal failure is diabetes mellitus, followed by hypertension and then glomerulonephritis.

11. b. Chronic pyelonephritis is the least likely cause of chronic renal failure of those listed. Chronic pyelonephritis rarely leads to chronic renal failure in the absence of obstruction.

12. d. The treatment of chronic renal failure is aggressive control of blood pressure and proteinuria. ACE inhibitors are a vital part of this treatment.

13. d. The major causes of death in patients with chronic renal failure are myocardial infarction and cardiovascular accidents (CVAs), secondary to atherosclerosis and arteriolosclerosis. Uremia itself can be controlled by dialysis or renal transplantation. Hypertension is usually controllable by individualized antihypertensive therapy. Arrhythmias, although they do occur in these patients, are not the major cause of death. Subarachnoid hemorrhage, as a subset of a CVA, does occur but is less common as a cause of death than myocardial infarction.

14. **c.** The anemia of chronic renal failure is usually normochromic, normocytic. Hematocrit often starts to decrease when the serum creatinine reaches 200-300 µmol/L (2-3 mg/dl) or when the GFR has decreased to about 20-30 ml/min. The etiology of the normochromic, normocytic anemia is probably a decreased synthesis of erythropoietin by the kidney.

15. **e.** Treatment of chronic renal failure may include the following: (1) ACE inhibitors, adrenergic receptor binders (ARBs), and nondihydropyridine calcium channel blockers (diltiazem or verapamil) slow the progression of chronic renal disease; (2) limitation of dietary protein (usefulness is controversial); (3) statins (HMG-CoA [3-hydroxy-3-methylglutaryl coenzyme A] reductase inhibitors; recent studies have shown that statins slow the decline in GFR); (4) erythropoietin; (5) diuretics if significant fluid overload is present; and (6) control of renal osteodystrophy with calcium and vitamin D supplementation.

16. **e.** Nephrotic syndrome, as previously mentioned, is associated most closely with membranous glomerulonephritis. Nephrotic syndrome is characterized by albuminuria (>3.5 g/day), hypoalbuminemia, hyperlipidemia, edema, hypertension, and renal insufficiency.

17. **e.** Causes of nephrotic syndrome include the following: (1) primary glomerular diseases (all subtypes); (2) secondary to infections (including poststreptococcal glomerulonephritis); (3) drugs (such as NSAIDs, penicillamine, and gold); (4) neoplasia (as in Hodgkin's lymphoma); (5) multisystem disease (systemic lupus erythematosus, Goodpasture's syndrome); (6) endocrine diseases (diabetes mellitus); and (7) miscellaneous (preeclamptic toxemia).

18. **c.** As stated before, diabetes mellitus is the most common cause of chronic renal failure. Although the prevalence is less common in type 2 (20%) as opposed to type 1 (40%) diabetes, the prevalence of type 2 diabetes is actually 10 times the prevalence of type 1 diabetes. The logical conclusion from this consideration is that type 2 diabetes mellitus is a more common cause of chronic renal failure than type 1 diabetes mellitus.

19. **e.** Nephrotic syndrome is treated with nonpharmacologic symptomatic therapies such as sodium restriction and fluid restriction and pharmacologic symptomatic therapies such as loop diuretics, ACE inhibitors (to reduce proteinuria), anticoagulant therapy (while patients have nephrotic proteinuria and/or albumin level <20g/L), prednisone, and in some cases cytotoxic drugs.

20. **c.** The most important difference in therapy between PSGN and NPSGN is corticosteroid therapy (useful in NPSGN but not in PSGN).

SUMMARY OF RENAL DISEASES

A. Glomerulonephritis:
1. **Classification (simplified):** (a) PSGN and (b) NPSGN with many subtypes
2. More than 50% of cases involve children younger than 13 years old
3. **Symptoms and signs:** (a) malaise; (b) headache; (c) anorexia; (d) low-grade fever; (e) edema; (f) hypertension; (g) gross hematuria with red blood cell casts; (h) proteinuria; and (i) impaired renal function.
4. **Treatment:**
   a. PSGN = symptomatic: protein restriction, fluid restriction, low salt intake, loop diuretics
   b. NPSGN = symptomatic (as described for PSGN) plus corticosteroids
5. **Prognosis:**
   a. 95% of patients with PSGN recover renal function within 8-12 weeks
   b. Excellent prognosis in patients with minimal change disease
   c. More than 70% of patients with mesangial capillary glomerulonephritis will develop chronic renal failure

B. Nephrotic syndrome:
1. **Etiology and prevalence:** (a) many and diverse causes and (b) membranous glomerulonephritis is most common cause of nephrotic syndrome.
2. **Signs/symptoms:** (a) edema; (b) hypoalbuminemia; (c) hypertension; (d) hyperlipidemia; and (e) renal insufficiency.
3. **Treatment:** (a) sodium restriction; (b) fluid restriction; (c) loop diuretics; (d) ACE inhibitors; (e) anticoagulant therapy; (f) prednisone; and (g) cytotoxic agents.

C. Chronic renal failure:
1. **Causation:** most common cause = diabetes mellitus
2. **Symptoms/signs/laboratory findings:** (a) weakness; (b) fatigue; (c) headaches; (d) anorexia; (e) nausea; (f) pruritus; (g) polyuria; (h) nocturia; (i) edema; (j) hypertension; (k) congestive heart failure; (l) pericarditis; (m) anemia; (n) azotemia; (o) acidosis; (p) hyperkalemia; (q) hypocalcemia; and (r) hyperphosphatemia

Continued

SUMMARY OF RENAL DISEASES
—cont'd

3. **Treatments:** (a) restrict protein (insufficient evidence for routine recommendation); (b) maintain careful fluid balance (may need to restrict fluids if edema is present); (c) restrict sodium, potassium, and phosphate; (d) avoid potentially renal toxic drugs, such as NSAIDs; (e) adjust certain drug doses to correct for prolonged half-lives; (f) prescribe ACE inhibitors, ARBs, and nondihydropyridine calcium channel blockers; (g) prescribe erythropoietin for anemia; (h) prescribe loop diuretics if fluid overload; (i) correct electrolyte abnormalities; (j) prescribe HMG-CoA reductase inhibitors (get low-density lipoprotein cholesterol to less

than 100 mg/dl); (k) prescribe calcium and vitamin D supplementation; (l) maintain hypertension control; (m) provide hemodialysis or peritoneal dialysis; and (n) perform renal transplantation

SUGGESTED READING

Hricik DE, et al: Medical progress: glomerulonephritis. *N Engl J Med* 339(13):888-899, 1998.
Madaio MP, Harrington JT: The diagnosis of glomerular diseases: acute glomerulonephritis and the nephrotic syndrome. *Arch Intern Med* 161(1):25-34, 2001.
Orth SR, Ritz E: Medical progress: the nephrotic syndrome. *N Engl J Med* 338(17):1202-1211, 1998.
Singri N, et al: Acute renal failure. *JAMA* 289(6):747-751, 2003.
Yu HT: Progression of chronic renal failure. *Arch Intern Med* 163(12):1417-1429, 2003.

Chapter 43

Urinary Tract Infections

"Let's avoid dialysis if we can."

CLINICAL CASE PROBLEM 1:
A 27-Year-Old Female with Spina Bifida and Bilateral Costovertebral Angle Pain

A 27-year-old female presents to the emergency room (ER) with a 4-day history of fever, chills, and bilateral costovertebral angle (CVA) pain. She has an indwelling urinary catheter and describes to you "at least 12 of these episodes before this current one." She has been seeing the same family physician since birth and has been diagnosed as having "nervous bladder and kidney syndrome." He has prescribed some over-the-counter "kidney pills" in the past for these symptoms. She tells you that they "never really worked," and she often has found herself bedbound with symptoms for several weeks before the fever broke.

You, the ER doctor on shift, are somewhat skeptical about the nervous bladder and kidney syndrome.

On examination, the patient is flushed. Her temperature is 40° C. She has intermittent shaking rigors. She has CVA tenderness bilaterally. Her abdomen is somewhat tender to palpation. There is blood in the catheter collection bag.

SELECT THE BEST ANSWER TO THE FOLLOWING QUESTIONS:

1. What is the most likely diagnosis in this patient?
   a. nervous bladder and kidney syndrome
   b. acute hemorrhagic cystitis
   c. acute urethritis
   d. acute pyelonephritis
   e. SBBSS (the newly named spina bifida bladder spasm syndrome)

2. What would be the most likely organism in this patient?
   a. a gram-positive coccus
   b. a gram-positive rod
   c. an anaerobic organism
   d. a fungal organism
   e. a gram-negative organism

3. Which of the following bacteria would not likely be considered as highly probable of causing this problem?
   a. *Pseudomonas aeruginosa*
   b. *Klebsiella pneumoniae*
   c. *Enterobacter*
   d. group A beta-hemolytic streptococcus
   e. *Proteus*

4. After obtaining a urinalysis and a urine specimen for culture and sensitivity, you now should treat the patient with which of the following?

a. the OTC kidney pills
b. ciprofloxacin 500 mg tid by mouth (po) (outpatient)
c. Septra DS two tabs bid po (outpatient)
d. intravenous (IV) antibiotics in a hospital
e. no medications are indicated at this time

5. Which of the following antibiotics would not be of first choice for this patient?
a. IV ceftriaxone (Rocephin) or cefotaxime (Claforan)
b. IV trimethoprim-sulfamethoxazole (TMP-SMX)
c. IV ciprofloxacin
d. IV ampicillin and gentamicin
e. IV piperacillin-tazobactam

6. The investigations that should be performed on this patient at this time include which of the following?
a. serum blood urea nitrogen (BUN) and creatinine
b. renal ultrasound
c. blood cultures
d. complete blood count (CBC) with differential
e. all of the above

7. The renal ultrasound shows small, shrunken kidneys, with no enlargement of the ureters and no stones. What is the most likely diagnosis in this patient?
a. chronic pyelonephritis
b. uterovesical reflux
c. hydronephrosis
d. vesicular diverticula
e. none of the above

8. Which of the following statements regarding chronic prophylaxis in this patient is true?
a. chronic prophylaxis is not indicated
b. chronic prophylaxis is unlikely to be of any benefit
c. chronic prophylaxis may make a significant difference in the preservation of this patient's renal function
d. chronic prophylaxis is unlikely to be difficult because of resistant organisms
e. none of the above are true

CLINICAL CASE PROBLEM 2:
A 34-YEAR-OLD FEMALE WITH HEMATURIA, DYSURIA, INCREASED URINARY FREQUENCY, AND NOCTURIA

A 34-year-old female presents with a 3-day history of hematuria, dysuria, increased urinary frequency, and nocturia. She has had no fever, no chills, and no back pain.

On examination, she does not look ill. Her temperature is 37.5° C. Her abdomen is nontender. There is no CVA tenderness.

9. What is the most likely diagnosis?
a. Berger's disease (immunoglobulin A nephropathy)
b. acute hemorrhagic cystitis
c. acute hemorrhagic urethritis
d. acute glomerulonephritis
e. acute cystitis with concomitant coagulation disorder

10. What is the treatment of choice for the patient described?
a. a 10-day course of ampicillin and probenecid
b. a 7-day course of ampicillin and probenecid
c. a 3-day course of TMP-SMX
d. a 1-day course of TMP-SMX
e. a single dose of ampicillin 3.5 g and probenecid 1 g

11. You have decided on your therapeutic plan for the patient described. At what time would you implement this plan?
a. right away: forget about the culture
b. right away: start therapy immediately after taking the urine specimen for culture and sensitivity (C and S)
c. tomorrow: send the urine culture stat and order the pathologist to call you with the result personally
d. tomorrow: send the urine culture and ask the pathology department for a report as soon as possible without aggravating the pathologist
e. whenever: send the urine culture and when you get it back call the patient. If the symptoms have not cleared up then consider starting the antibiotic

12. What is the most likely organism involved in the infection that has developed in the patient described?
a. *Pseudomonas aeruginosa*
b. *Providencia*
c. *Escherichia coli*
d. *Klebsiella*
e. *Enterococcus*

13. The quinolone antibiotics (such as ciprofloxacin and levofloxacin) are a very significant advance in antimicrobial treatment. They also work by a unique mechanism. The mechanism(s) of action is (are):
a. bactericidal mode of action
b. inhibition of DNA gyrase

c. blocks protein synthesis
d. inhibition of cell-wall synthesis
e. a and b

14. All of the following about asymptomatic bacteruria in women are false except:
a. risk is increased with sexual intercourse
b. risk is not increased in women who use diaphragms
c. it has been shown to lead to renal damage in normal hosts
d. prevalence in elderly women may be as high as 75%
e. treatment is never indicated

15. The patient in Clinical Case Problem 2 returns to your office 3 days after you start her treatment and states symptoms have not improved. What is the most appropriate next step?
a. change the antibiotic and add pyridium
b. check a urine culture and sensitivity and change therapy according to results
c. send the patient for a renal ultrasound to rule out obstruction and change antibiotic
d. collect a urine sample and check BUN and creatinine
e. c and d

CLINICAL CASE MANAGEMENT PROBLEM

Discuss a classification of UTIs in adult males and adult females.

ANSWERS:

1. d. This patient has acute pyelonephritis. First, she has very significant predisposing factors for urinary tract infections (UTIs), including an indwelling urinary catheter and a neurologic condition that increases the probability of same. Second, she seems to have had some less than optimal medical diagnoses. Third, she almost certainly has had recurrent episodes of pyelonephritis. This raises the possibilities of chronic pyelonephritis, reflux kidney damage, and resistant organisms. Fourth, the symptoms fit. Fever, chills, and CVA pain in a patient with a neurologic predisposing condition and an indwelling catheter equal acute pyelonephritis.

2. e. First, this patient is classified as having a complicated UTI. A complicated UTI occurs when any of the following are present in the patient: obstruction (stones), indwelling urinary catheter, high postvoid residual urine volume, anatomic or functional geni-

tourinary abnormalities, renal impairment, and renal transplantation.

Although the most common organism is a gram-negative organism, it is frequently an organism that would not occur in patients without urinary tract disease. Examples include *Proteus*, *Providencia*, *Serratia*, *Pseudomonas*, and *Klebsiella*. Overall, *E. coli* (one of many serotypes and one likely to be resistant to multiple antibiotics) is probably still the most common organism. Not as common but alternative causes of pyelonephritis would be gram-positive cocci including group B streptococci or enterococci (group D streptococci).

3. d. The only organism listed that is an unlikely candidate is group A beta-hemolytic streptococcus. Group A streptococci, *Streptococcus pneumoniae*, *Staphylococcus saprophyticus*, and *Staphylococcus aureus* do not cause acute pyelonephritis.

4. d. This patient has not had proper assessment, an accurate diagnosis, or proper treatment at any time in the past.

At this time, she should be hospitalized, should be treated with IV fluids and IV antibiotics, and should have a complete assessment of both urinary tract function and urinary tract damage. In addition, ways of preventing future infections should be considered.

5. b. Quinolones (such as ciprofloxacin or levofloxacin) are indicated for the treatment of complicated UTIs and will cover most if not all gram-negative organisms including *Proteus* and *Pseudomonas*. It also would be reasonable to use gentamicin, a combination of ampicillin and gentamicin, or a third-generation cephalosporin. Piperacillin-tazobactam also would be appropriate for complicated pyelonephritis.

TMP-SMX is not appropriate because resistance in uropathogenic *E. coli* is increasing.

6. e. At this time, a complete workup should be done. This should include the following (as a minimum): (1) blood: CBC with differential, serum BUN and creatinine, electrolytes, and blood cultures; (2) urine: a complete urinalysis; urine culture for bacterial sensitivity and examination for white blood cell casts and red blood cell casts; (3) diagnostic imaging: a renal and abdominal ultrasound or an intravenous pyelogram (IVP)

7. a. This patient's abnormal ultrasound shows small, shrunken kidneys secondary to repeated UTIs that have gone untreated, causing chronic pyelonephritis. It is important from this time onward to measure renal function regularly and do everything possible to preserve this patient's renal function.

Chronic pyelonephritis is treated with 4 weeks of oral antibiotics after acute pyelonephritis is treated.

8. c. First, repeated urine cultures must be done to determine the dominant organisms growing. Next, the susceptibility/resistance of these organisms needs to be determined to guide prophylactic therapy. It is difficult to say at this time what that therapy should be; it all depends on the results, but it certainly needs to be done.

9. b. This patient has acute hemorrhagic cystitis. Acute hemorrhagic cystitis is simply a variant of acute cystitis, and it is no more difficult to treat and does not have any more complications than other forms of acute cystitis. Hematuria does not signify a poor prognosis.

10. c. Patients with uncomplicated UTIs respond well to a 3-day treatment regimen. This abbreviated course of management is a good compromise between a 1-day course of therapy and the conventional 7- to 14-day regimens. The relapse rate with the 3-day regimen is comparable to longer courses of therapy. An abbreviated therapy is also more cost-effective and is associated with fewer adverse drug effects than the more prolonged courses of therapy.

TMP-SMX is certainly a drug of first choice for uncomplicated UTIs at the present time. The other drug of first choice would be a quinolone such as norfloxacin, ciprofloxacin, or levofloxacin.

11. b. You should not wait to begin therapy. Pretherapy urine culture in acute uncomplicated cystitis is not considered to be cost-effective. Culture is reserved instead for those that do not respond to therapy, those that have recurrent symptoms shortly after therapy, and those with complicated UTIs. Ask for the result as soon as possible, but do not aggravate the pathologist.

12. c. This is a case of uncomplicated UTI. Hemorrhagic cystitis cannot really be considered a complication. With an uncomplicated infection, you likely are going to be dealing with an uncomplicated organism. Therefore, *E. coli* is the most likely organism involved in the infection.

There are many serotypes of *E. coli* that can produce UTI. Some serotypes are more likely to produce hemorrhagic cystitis; others are more likely to produce nonhemorrhagic cystitis.

13. e. The quinolone antibiotics are a significant advance in antimicrobial therapy. They use a totally unique mechanism of action. These antibiotics are extremely effective against many gram-positive and especially gram-negative organisms. The quinolone antibiotics work essentially at a molecular genetic level.

The quinolone antibiotics are bactericidal in action. Action is achieved mainly by inhibition of the DNA gyrase. This is an essential component of the bacterial DNA replication system. The inhibition of the alpha subunit of the DNA gyrase blocks the resealing of the nicks on the DNA strands induced by this alpha subunit, leading to the degradation of the DNA by exonucleases.

14. a. Asymptomatic bacteruria has never been shown to lead to renal damage in those without anatomic abnormality or urinary obstruction. Sexual intercourse and diaphragm use both increase the risk for it (as well as for symptomatic UTI). Prevalence in postmenopausal elderly women approaches 20% to 50%. Treatment is indicated only in pregnancy.

15. b. Patients who do not respond to initial empiric 3-day treatment should have a urine culture with sensitivity done to guide change in antibiotic. Indication for renal ultrasound and laboratory tests other than culture would be a complicated infection.

SOLUTION TO THE CLINICAL CASE MANAGEMENT PROBLEM

A. Classification of UTIs in Adult Females:

1. With uncomplicated lower-tract infections, it is either acute cystitis or acute hemorrhagic cystitis.
2. With complicated upper-tract infections, it is either acute pyelitis or acute pyelonephritis.
3. Conditions that are likely to increase the risk of acquiring a complicated UTI include the following: diabetes mellitus, stone disease, chronic indwelling catheterization, immunosuppression, pregnancy, neuropathic bladder, congenital anomalies (reflux), urethral stenosis, and urinary tract obstruction.
4. Sexually transmitted UTIs: Acute urethritis can be caused by *Chlamydia trachomatis, Mycoplasma hominis, Ureaplasma urealyticum,* or *Neisseria gonorrhea.*

Continued

SOLUTION TO THE CLINICAL CASE MANAGEMENT PROBLEM—cont'd

B. Classification of UTIs in Adult Males:

1. Uncomplicated UTI is very rare in the absence of obstruction except for acute prostatitis and epididymitis.
2. Complicated UTIs include the following: acute cystitis (needs to be investigated with renal ultrasound), acute pyelitis, acute pyelonephritis, chronic prostatitis, or benign prostatic hypertrophy/ hyperplasia.

   The most common complicating factor in males is obstruction caused by benign prostatic hypertrophy/hyperplasia. However, all males with a UTI not resulting from STDs need to be investigated. The minimal investigation is a renal ultrasound.

3. STDs:
   a. Acute urethritis may be the result of infection by *Chlamydia trachomatis* (nongonococcal urethritis [NGU]), *Mycoplasma hominis* (NGU), *Ureaplasma urealyticum* (NGU), or *Neisseria gonorrhea* (gonococcal urethritis [GU])
   b. Acute epididymoorchitis is caused by *C. trachomatis*

SUMMARY OF URINARY TRACT INFECTIONS

1. **Classification:** see the Clinical Case Management Problem box
2. **Signs/symptoms:**
   a. Lower-tract dysuria: frequency, nocturia, hematuria, terminal dribbling, discharge (from sexually transmitted diseases [STDs])
   b. Upper tract: same as lower tract plus fever, chills, CVA pain/tenderness
3. **Laboratory:**
   a. Urinalysis, urinalysis for culture and sensitivity (lower tract)
   b. CBC, blood cultures, 24-hour urine for creatinine clearance and protein, renal ultrasound, IVP, computed tomography
4. To avoid complications, evaluate each patient in terms of risk factors and avoid indwelling catheterization whenever possible
5. **Treatment:**
   a. Lower-tract UTIs in females: a 3-day course of TMP-SMX plus Pyridium for analgesia
   b. Upper tract:
      i. Quinolone (such as ciprofloxacin or levofloxacin)
      ii. Ampicillin plus gentamicin
      iii. Third-generation cephalosporin with or without gentamicin
   c. Inpatient versus outpatient: acute pyelonephritis: hospitalize those with complications or complicating diseases; otherwise outpatient IV port therapy daily or high-dose oral therapy
   d. Prophylaxis: consider for high-risk patients: first choice, quinolones or Macrodantin
   e. STDs:
      i. Gonorrhea: Rocephin intramuscularly (250 mg) plus azithromycin (1-g single dose) or doxycycline for 7 days
      ii. Nongonococcal urethritis: azithromycin (1-g single dose) or doxycycline for 7 days

SUGGESTED READING

Arsdalen K: The urogenital tract. In: Rakel R, ed. *Conn's Current Therapy, 1995* 48th ed. W.B. Saunders, 1994, Philadelphia.

Bass PF: Urinary tract infections. *Primary Care* 30(1):41-61, 2003.

Bremnor JD: Evaluation of dysuria in adults. *Am Fam Phys* 65(8): 1589-1596, 2002.

Brown PD: Bacterial infections of the urinary tract in women. In: Rakel R, ed. *Conn's Current Therapy, 2003* 55th ed. W.B. Saunders, 2002, Philadelphia.

Cunha B: Urinary tract Infection in males. In: Rakel R, ed. *Conn's Current Therapy, 2003* 55th ed. W.B. Saunders, 2002, Philadelphia.

Hooton TM: The current management strategies for community-acquired urinary tract infection, *Infect Dis Clin N Am* 17(2):303-332, 2003.

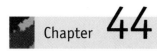

Chapter 44

Sleep Disorders

"Sweet sleep, where are you?"

CLINICAL CASE PROBLEM 1:

A 48-YEAR-OLD MALE WITH A 6-MONTH HISTORY OF SNORING, NOCTURNAL BREATH CESSATIONS, AND EXCESSIVE DAYTIME SLEEPINESS

A 48-year-old male comes to your office with his wife. His wife tells you that "he is constantly snoring" and she has put up with all she can. This has been going on for a number of years, but it has been getting worse lately. His wife also tells you that "sometimes he even stops breathing during the night." When you ask the patient directly, he says, "Well, I may snore a bit, but I think my wife is exaggerating." You somehow doubt the latter statement. There is a history of sleepiness during the day; he has fallen asleep at his desk at work.

On examination, the patient weighs 310 pounds. His blood pressure is 200/105 mm Hg (measured with a large cuff). Head, ears, eyes, nose, and throat (HEENT) examination shows boggy nasal mucosae but a normal pharynx. There is a grade III/VI systolic murmur present along the left sternal edge. You believe that there is elevated jugular venous pressure when he lies at a 45-degree angle. Chest is normal to auscultation and percussion. His abdomen is obese, and his extremities are without edema.

■ **SELECT THE BEST ANSWER TO THE FOLLOWING QUESTIONS:**

1. What is the most likely diagnosis in this patient?
   a. narcolepsy
   b. obstructive sleep apnea (OSA) syndrome
   c. generalized poor physical condition
   d. central sleep apnea syndrome
   e. adult-onset adenoid hypertrophy

2. To what is the pathophysiology of this condition related?
   a. collapse of the pharyngeal walls repetitively during sleep
   b. failure of upper airway dilator muscle activity
   c. sleep-related upper airway obstruction and cessation in ventilation (apneas)
   d. a and c
   e. all of the above

3. This condition is accompanied by which of the following?
   a. hypoxemia
   b. hypercarbia
   c. metabolic acidosis
   d. respiratory acidosis
   e. a, b, and d
   f. a, b, c, and d

4. What is (are) the major symptom(s) of this disorder?
   a. loud snoring
   b. daytime hypersomnolence
   c. disturbed nonrefreshing sleep
   d. weight gain
   e. a, b, and c
   f. a, b, c, and d

5. What is (are) the clinical feature(s) associated with the condition described?
   a. systemic hypertension
   b. inhibited sexual desire
   c. depression
   d. a and b
   e. a, b, and c

6. What is (are) the factor(s) that predispose to this condition?
   a. alcohol intake
   b. benzodiazepines
   c. hyperthyroidism
   d. a and b
   e. a, b, and c

7. What is the treatment of first choice for this disorder?
   a. uvulopalatopharyngoplasty surgery (UPP)
   b. tracheostomy
   c. continuous positive airway pressure (CPAP)
   d. nortriptyline
   e. alprazolam

8. Which of the following drugs is contraindicated in the treatment of the disturbed, nonrefreshing sleep that is associated with the condition described?
   a. fluoxetine
   b. sertraline
   c. alprazolam
   d. phenelzine
   e. paroxetine

CLINICAL CASE PROBLEM 2:

A 35-YEAR-OLD MALE WITH WEAK MUSCLES AFTER LAUGHING

A 35-year-old male presents to your office with a chief complaint of "weak muscles," especially after laughing. On further questioning you discover that the patient has excessive daytime sleepiness and "weird imaginings" just before going to sleep at night. The patient appears anxious and tense.

9. What is your tentative diagnosis?
   a. narcolepsy
   b. hysterical conversion reaction
   c. psychosomatic symptoms secondary to chronic anxiety
   d. hypochondriasis
   e. obstructive sleep apnea

10. Which of the following is not a symptom of the disorder described in Clinical Case Problem 2?
    a. catalepsy
    b. hypnagogic hallucinations
    c. sleep paralysis
    d. restless and disturbed sleep
    e. persistent daytime sleepiness

11. The "daytime symptoms" of the disorder described are treated well with which of the following medications?
    a. methylphenidate
    b. dextroamphetamine
    c. mazindol
    d. a and b only
    e. all of the above

12. The "nighttime symptoms" of the disorder described are best treated by which of the following?
    a. alprazolam
    b. nortriptyline
    c. protriptyline
    d. b or c
    e. all of the above

13. The diagnosis for the problem described is best established by which of the following?
    a. nocturnal polysomnogram (NPSG)
    b. multiple sleep latency test (MSLT)
    c. either a or b
    d. a and b together
    e. neither a nor b

14. What percentage of adult Americans experience significant sleep difficulties in any given year?
    a. 5%
    b. 10%
    c. 15%
    d. 25%
    e. 50%

15. People with insomnia often compensate for lost sleep by delaying their morning awakening time or by napping, which actually may have the effect of further fragmenting their nocturnal sleep. What is this disorder known as?

   a. mixed-up insomniac syndrome
   b. insufficient sleep syndrome
   c. inadequate sleep hygiene
   d. adjustment sleep disorder
   e. psychophysiologic insomnia

16. People with insomnia who voluntarily curtail their time in bed, usually in response to social and/or occupational demands, are best diagnosed as having which of the following?
    a. workaholic sleep loss syndrome
    b. inadequate sleep hygiene
    c. insufficient sleep syndrome
    d. adjustment sleep disorder
    e. psychophysiologic insomnia

17. Developing anticipatory anxiety over the prospect of another night of sleeplessness followed by another day of fatigue in response to a previously resolved stressor is known as which of the following?
    a. adjustment sleep disorder
    b. psychophysiologic insomnia
    c. inadequate sleep hygiene
    d. insufficient sleep syndrome
    e. generalized anxiety disorder insomnia

18. A 73-year-old male is admitted to the hospital for a transurethral resection of the prostate (TURP) procedure. The procedure is postponed because of some abnormal test results. The patient tells you that he has had extreme difficulty in sleeping since coming into the hospital. What is the most likely diagnosis in this patient?
    a. adjustment sleep disorder
    b. psychophysiologic insomnia
    c. inadequate sleep hygiene
    d. insufficient sleep syndrome
    e. sudden-onset central sleep apnea

19. What is the major difference between idiopathic hypersomnolence and narcolepsy?
    a. daytime somnolence
    b. frequent daytime naps
    c. awakening unrefreshed versus awakening refreshed from these frequent daytime naps
    d. significant differences in treatment
    e. none of the above

20. What is the difference between periodic limb movement disorder (nocturnal myoclonus) and restless legs syndrome?
    a. kicking of the lower extremities in nocturnal myoclonus versus sensory loss in restless legs syndrome

b. patient awareness with nocturnal myoclonus versus patient unawareness with restless legs syndrome
c. kicking of the lower extremities in restless legs syndrome versus sensory loss in nocturnal myoclonus
d. patient awareness with restless legs syndrome versus patient unawareness in nocturnal myoclonus
e. none of the above

CLINICAL CASE MANAGEMENT PROBLEM

Discuss the principles of the use of hypnotic agents in the management of sleep disorders.

■ ANSWERS:

1. b. This patient has OSA. The major symptoms of OSA syndrome are as follows: (1) loud snoring; (2) reports of prolonged pauses in respiration during sleep; (3) daytime hypersomnolence; (4) disturbed nonrefreshing sleep; and (5) weight gain.

Polysomnography will demonstrate disordered sleep with periods of apnea and hypopnea and will confirm the diagnosis.

2. e. The pathophysiology of OSA syndrome includes the following: (1) the pharyngeal walls collapse repetitively during sleep, causing intermittent sleep-related upper airway obstruction and cessation in ventilation (apneas); (2) the cessation of ventilation is related to a concomitant loss of inspiratory effort; and (3) upper airway closure in OSA occurs as a result of a failure of the genioglossus and other upper airway dilator muscles and apnea results.

3. e. OSA produces the following acid–base balance situation: (1) apnea causes hypercarbia, hypoxemia, and a resulting respiratory acidosis and (2) only if there is another preexisting condition associated with OSA will metabolic acidosis be produced.

4. f. See Answer 1.

5. e. Associated clinical features of OSA include systemic hypertension; inhibited sexual desire; impotence; ejaculatory impairment; depression; deficits in attention, motor efficiency, and graphomotor ability; deterioration in interpersonal relationships; marital discord; and occupational impairment.

6. d. Factors that predispose to OSA include sedating pharmacologic agents including alcohol and benzodiazepines (all are contraindicated in OSA); nasal obstruction; large uvula; low-lying soft palate; retrognathia, micrognathia, and other craniofacial abnormalities; pharyngeal masses such as tumors or cysts; macroglossia; tonsillar hypertrophy; vocal cord paralysis; obesity; hypothyroidism; and acromegaly.

7. c. Polysomnography demonstrates that CPAP devices reverse apnea and hypopnea. In randomized controlled trials, CPAP devices also reduce daytime somnolence and improve mood and alertness. Compliance ranges from 50% to 80%. Although a CPAP is the best choice of these listed, always recommend weight reduction in obese individuals.

8. c. The most established management options, in addition to weight loss, in order of preference are as follows: (1) CPAP, (2) UPP, and (3) tracheostomy. Additional measures are: antidepressants that are stimulating, such as protriptyline, fluoxetine, sertraline, and paroxetine, particularly with coexistent depression. Chronic anxiety, which may complicate the OSA picture, should not be managed with benzodiazepines. Instead, the nonbenzodiazepine buspirone, which does not appear to aggravate OSA, should be used, along with behavioral treatments. Thus alprazolam is contraindicated.

9. a. This patient has narcolepsy.

10. a. The major symptoms of narcolepsy are as follows: (1) persistent daytime sleepiness; (2) cataplexy (not catalepsy); (3) hypnagogic or hypnopompic hallucinations; (4) sleep paralysis; and (5) restless and disturbed sleep.
Definitions:
1. Cataplexy is defined as an abrupt paralysis or paresis of skeletal muscles that usually follows emotional experiences such as anger, surprise, laughter, or physical exercise.
2. Hypnagogic (or hypnopompic) hallucinations are hallucinations that are vivid and often frightening dreams occurring after falling asleep (or on awakening).
3. Sleep paralysis is a global paralysis of voluntary muscles that usually occurs shortly after falling asleep and lasts a few seconds or minutes.
Cataplexy, hypnagogic hallucinations, and sleep paralysis are thought to be manifestations of an underlying aberration in the control of the timing of rapid eye movement (REM) sleep that in turn results in "attacks" of REM sleep during wakefulness.

11. e. Commonly used medications used to control excessive daytime sleepiness include the central nervous system stimulants, methylphenidate and dextroamphetamine. Long-term compliance is poor, especially in those with severe excessive daytime sleepiness. Modafinil (Provigil), approved for excessive daytime sleepiness associated with narcolepsy, has a more favorable side-effect profile. Unfortunately, stimulants do not treat cataplexy very well. For cataplexy, tricyclics (imipramine, protriptyline) and selective serotonin uptake inhibitors (SSRIs, such as fluoxetine, paroxetine) are used, usually at lower doses than for depression. Tolerance may be minimized by prescribing the lowest effective dose and asking patients to take regular drug holidays on days when their need for alertness is lowest.

12. d. The REM-related symptoms of cataplexy (hypnagogic hallucinations and sleep paralysis) can be controlled with REM-suppressant medications such as the tricyclic antidepressants protriptyline, imipramine, or nortriptyline. Sodium oxybate (Xyrem), a putative brain neurotransmitter that increases REM sleep efficiency, shows promise as a new treatment for narcolepsy. Patients with narcolepsy also require emotional support through group and individual counseling.

13. b. Other than the obvious behavioral manifestations of excessive daytime sleepiness (yawning, drooping eyelids, psychomotor retardation), physical examination is typically unrevealing in narcolepsy. If the diagnosis is suspected, it must be confirmed by a multiple sleep latency test (MSLT), which is the primary test for narcolepsy. The test assesses two major components of narcolepsy: hypersomnolence and sleep-onset REM periods, which occur in narcolepsy but are otherwise uncommon. Time to sleep onset provides evidence for hypersomnolence (falling asleep in 5 minutes or less), and patients with narcolepsy also will have sleep-onset REM periods. A polysomnogram usually also is performed to rule out other forms of disordered sleep.

14. d. Approximately 25% of all American adults express sleep-related complaints over the course of a 1-year period.

15. c. Many individuals unknowingly engage in habitual behaviors that harm sleep—they have poor or inadequate "sleep hygiene." People with insomnia, for example, often compensate for lost sleep by delaying their morning awakening time or by napping. These behaviors actually have the effect of further fragmenting nocturnal sleep. Instead, patients with insomnia should be advised to adhere to a regular awakening time regardless of the amount of sleep that they have gotten and to avoid naps.

16. c. Individuals who voluntarily curtail their time in bed, usually in response to social and occupational demands, have what is best termed insufficient sleep syndrome. Although sleep reduction may be as little as 1 hour per night, over long periods such a pattern may lead to daytime hypersomnolence and result in impairment.

17. b. Patients who develop anticipatory anxiety over the prospect of another night of sleeplessness followed by another day of fatigue have what is known as psychophysiologic insomnia. Anxiety typically increases as bedtime approaches and reaches maximum intensity following retirement. Sufferers often spend hours in bed awake focused on and brooding over their sleeplessness, which in turn aggravates their insomnia even further. Persistent psychophysiologic insomnia often complicates other insomnia disorders.

18. a. This patient has adjustment sleep disorder. This common disorder is caused by acute emotional stressors such as job loss or hospitalization. The result is insomnia, typically difficulty in falling asleep, mediated by tension and anxiety. Symptoms usually remit shortly after abatement of the stressors. Treatment is warranted if daytime sleepiness and fatigue interfere with functioning or if the disorder lasts for more than a few weeks.

19. c. Idiopathic hypersomnolence is a lifelong and incurable disorder that has a variable age of onset. The most prominent symptom of this disorder is unrelenting daytime somnolence. Patients spend lengthy periods sleeping at night only to awaken feeling more sleepy. They take frequent and lengthy daytime naps. However, unlike patients with narcolepsy, they awaken from these naps feeling unrefreshed.

20. d. Periodic limb movement disorder (nocturnal myoclonus) is characterized by the repetitive (usually every 20-40 seconds) twitching or kicking of the lower extremities during sleep. Patients usually present with the complaint of unrelenting insomnia, most often characterized by repeated awakenings following sleep onset.

Restless legs syndrome is a creeping, crawling sensation in the lower extremities manifested by irresistible leg kicks that affect patients on reclining prior to falling asleep. Unlike periodic limb movement disorder, however, the patient is very aware of this phenomenon and resorts to moving the affected extremity by stretching, kicking, or walking to relieve symptoms. Many patients are depressed, irritable, and angry. Psychosocial impairment such as job loss and relationship difficulties are quite common.

SOLUTION TO THE CLINICAL CASE MANAGEMENT PROBLEM

The use of hypnotic agents in sleep disorders is a subject of great controversy (mainly because of their very wide and sometimes very inappropriate use). There are many factors that influence the decision of whether to prescribe a hypnotic agent and which hypnotic agent to prescribe.

The disadvantages of prescribing a hypnotic agent include the following:

1. There is a propensity for daytime somnolence with the use of an agent that has either a medium half-life or a long half-life.
2. A second factor is the propensity for the development of drug tolerance; larger and larger quantities of the drug are needed to produce the same effect.

3. Hypnotics may produce symptoms of autonomic hyperactivity and irritability the following day. This is a particular problem with those hypnotics that have a very short half-life. Next-day tremors and nervousness are very good examples of this phenomenon.
4. In the vast majority of cases, although hypnotics are specifically indicated for only short periods, they are used for longer and longer time periods The result of this is that after approximately 3 weeks, the hypnotic agents begin working in the opposite manner to which they were intended: instead of helping sleep, they actually hinder sleep.

SUMMARY OF SLEEP DISORDERS

1. **Prevalence:** the overall prevalence of sleep disorders and sleep difficulties in the American population is estimated to be approximately 25% in any given year. This includes, of course, all forms of sleep disturbance, both long and short.
2. **Sleep phases and laboratory investigation:**
   a. Human sleep: human sleep is made up of basically two types of sleep patterns: non-REM sleep and REM sleep. Non-REM sleep has four stages and accounts for approximately 75% of total sleep. REM sleep occupies approximately 25% of total sleep.
   b. Sleep investigations: all sleep investigations should be performed in a proper, accredited sleep laboratory. The two basic tests indicated in sleep disorders are the NPSG and the MSLT.
3. **Specific sleep disorders:**
   a. OSA: consists of loud snoring; prolonged pauses in breathing during sleep; daytime hypersomnolence; disturbed, nonrefreshing sleep; and weight gain
      i. Pathophysiologic abnormalities produce apnea.
      ii. Associated conditions include obesity, systemic hypertension, sexual dysfunction, depression, and anxiety. Confirmatory test: polysomnogram
      iii. Treatment of choice for OSA is CPAP. Second and third management choices include UPP surgery and tracheostomy.
      iv. Weight loss should be encouraged in all overweight patients with OSA; alcohol should be discouraged; benzodiazepines should be prohibited; and systemic hypertension should be treated.
      v. Depression should be treated with a nonsedating antidepressant (SSRIs) or protriptyline.
   b. Central sleep apnea (CSA): a rare syndrome and is characterized by cessation of ventilation related to a concomitant loss of inspiratory effort
   c. Narcolepsy:
      i. Symptoms: cataplexy, hypnagogic or hypnopompic hallucinations and sleep paralysis.
      ii. Associated conditions include persistent daytime sleepiness and restless and disturbed sleep. Confirming test: MSLT
      iii. Treatment: medications used to combat excessive sleepiness include pemoline, methylphenidate, and dextroamphetamine. Mazindol is used in resistant cases. The REM-related symptoms of cataplexy and hypnagogic hallucinations are best treated with a stimulating tricyclic antidepressant such as nortriptyline or protriptyline.
   d. Idiopathic hypersomnolence: a lifelong and incurable disorder that has, as its most prominent feature, unrelenting daytime somnolence. Patients spend lengthy periods sleeping at night only to awaken feeling more sleepy. Unlike the patient with narcolepsy, they awaken from their frequent daytime naps feeling unrefreshed.

Continued

SUMMARY OF SLEEP DISORDERS —cont'd

e. Periodic limb movement disorder (nocturnal myoclonus): characterized by repetitive (usually every 20-40 seconds) twitching or kicking of the lower extremities during sleep. Patients usually present with the complaint of unrelenting insomnia, most often characterized by repeated awakenings following sleep onset. Baclofen, clonazepam, and carbidopa-levodopa may relieve these symptoms.

f. Restless legs syndrome: the hallmark of this disorder is a "creeping sensation" in the lower extremities and irresistible leg kicks that affect patients on reclining prior to falling asleep. Unlike periodic limb movement disorder, the patients are very well aware of these symptoms

and resort to moving the affected extremity by stretching, kicking, or walking to relieve the symptoms.

4. **Hypnotic agents:** in most primary care practices, the distinct disadvantages described in the solution to the Clinical Case Management Problem outweigh any possible benefit, especially on a long-term basis include UPP surgery and tracheostomy.

SUGGESTED READING

Anders TF, Eiben LA: Pediatric sleep disorders: a review of the past 10 years. *J Am Acad Child Adol Psychiatr* 36(1):9-20, 1997.
Feldman NT: Narcolepsy. *South Med J* 96(3):277-282, 2003.
Flemons WW: Clinical practice. Obstructive sleep apnea. *N Engl J Med* 347(7):498-504, 2002.
Qureshi A, Ballard RD: Obstructive sleep apnea. *J Allergy Clin Immunol* 112(4):643-651; quiz 652, 2003.
Shamsuzzaman AS, et al: Obstructive sleep apnea: implications for cardiac and vascular disease. *JAMA* 290(14):1906-1914, 2003.

Chapter 45

Fluid and Electrolyte Abnormalities

> "You mean that even though orange juice is acidic it increases the alkalinity of my body."

CLINICAL CASE PROBLEM 1:

A 72-YEAR-OLD MALE WITH CHRONIC OBSTRUCTIVE PULMONARY DISEASE

A 72-year-old male with chronic obstructive pulmonary disease (COPD) is seen in the emergency room. Over the past 2 days he has experienced a worsening cough with yellow-brown sputum production and fever to 101° F. On examination, his respiratory rate (RR) is 26/min using accessory muscles. His acid/base gas (ABG) values on room air are pH, 7.24; PaO_2, 54 mm Hg; SaO_2, 88%; $PaCO_2$, 60 mm Hg; and HCO_3^-, 27 mEq/L.

SELECT THE BEST ANSWERS TO THE FOLLOWING QUESTIONS

1. Which process is disturbing the acid–base balance?
   a. metabolic acidosis
   b. respiratory alkalosis
   c. metabolic alkalosis
   d. respiratory acidosis
   e. none of the above

CLINICAL PROBLEM CASE 2:

A 22-YEAR-OLD FEMALE WHO IS DIZZY AND HAS TINGLING AROUND HER MOUTH AND FINGERTIPS

A 22-year-old female comes into the emergency room with dizziness and tingling around her mouth and fingertips. Her blood pressure (BP) is 140/70, pulse (P) is 110 beats/min, RR is 30, and temperature is 98.6° F. Her ABG values on room air are pH, 7.52; PaO_2, 90 mm Hg; SaO_2, 97%; $PaCO_2$, 25 mm Hg; and HCO_3^-, 18 mEq/L.

2. Which process is disturbing the acid–base balance?
   a. metabolic acidosis with respiratory compensation
   b. respiratory alkalosis with metabolic compensation
   c. metabolic alkalosis without respiratory compensation
   d. respiratory acidosis with metabolic compensation
   e. none of the above

CLINICAL PROBLEM CASE 3:

A 28-YEAR-OLD PREGNANT FEMALE WITH PERSISTENT VOMITING

A 28-year-old female in the first trimester of pregnancy comes into the emergency room with several days of morning sickness with persistent vomiting. She is now lethargic. Her BP is 90/60, P is 120, RR is 16, and temperature is 99.0° F. Her ABG values on room air are pH, 7.50; PaO_2, 80 mm Hg; SaO_2, 94%; $PaCO_2$, 49 mm Hg; and HCO_3^-, 38 mEq/L.

3. Which process is disturbing the acid–base balance?
   a. metabolic acidosis with respiratory compensation
   b. respiratory alkalosis without metabolic compensation
   c. metabolic alkalosis with respiratory compensation
   d. respiratory acidosis with metabolic compensation
   e. none of the above

CLINICAL CASE PROBLEM 4:
A 60-Year-Old Male Resuscitated In the Cardiac Care Unit

A 60-year-old male, admitted to the Cardiac Care Unit for chest pain, suddenly becomes unresponsive in cardiac arrest. He is resuscitated after a 20-minute code. His ABG values on 100% O_2 are pH, 7.28; PaO_2, 211; SaO_2, 100%; $PaCO_2$, 28; and $HCO_3^- = 14$. His blood test values are Na^+, 140 mEq/L; K^+, 5.6 mEq/L; Cl^-, 100 mEq/L; CO_2, 14 mEq/L; glucose, 130 mg/dl; creatinine (Cr), 1.2 mg/dl; and blood urea nitrogen (BUN) = 25 mg/dl.

4. Which process is disturbing the acid–base balance?
   a. metabolic acidosis with respiratory compensation
   b. respiratory alkalosis with metabolic compensation
   c. metabolic alkalosis with respiratory compensation
   d. respiratory acidosis with metabolic compensation
   e. none of the above

5. What is the calculated anion gap?
   a. 8
   b. 12
   c. 16
   d. 26
   e. none of the above

► ANSWERS:

1. d. Cellular function is dependent on adequate oxygenation and a normal acid–base ratio. Any deviation in acid–base balance or blood pH can be life threatening. Whereas the body's ability to correct for inadequate oxygenation is limited, its compensatory mechanisms and ability to maintain normal blood pH are not.

Normal values for an ABG are pH, 7.38-7.42 (average 7.4); PaO_2, 80-100 mm Hg (average 90); SaO_2, >95%; $PaCO_2$, 38-42 mm Hg (average 40); HCO_3^-, 22-26 mEq/L (average 24).

Clinical Case Problem 1 is an example of acute respiratory acidosis. The pH is <7.38 and the $PaCO_2$ is >42 mm Hg. Respiratory acidosis is the result of either decreased alveolar ventilation or increased carbon dioxide production. Decreased alveolar ventilation is seen in COPD, acute respiratory failure, neuromuscular disorders that result in peripheral muscle weakness (i.e., myasthenia gravis), and central nervous system (CNS) depression (i.e., narcotics, general anesthetics). Increased CO_2 production occurs in hypermetabolic states such as sepsis or fever.

Renal compensation requires several hours to develop and is maximal after 4 days. In an acute respiratory acidosis the HCO_3^- increases 1 mEq/L per 10 mm Hg increase in $PaCO_2$. In chronic respiratory acidosis the HCO_3^- increases 4 mEq/L per 10 mm Hg increase in $PaCO_2$. In an acute respiratory acidosis for every 10 mm Hg increase in the $PaCO_2$, the pH falls by 0.08.

In Clinical Case Problem 1, the $PaCO_2$ is increased by 20 mm Hg and the pH is decreased by 0.16. The HCO_3^- has increased by three. This is an acute respiratory acidosis.

2. b. This is a respiratory alkalosis with metabolic compensation. The pH is >7.42 and the $PaCO_2$ is <38. The HCO_3^- is <22.

Respiratory alkalosis results from hyperventilation. Specific causes include a catastrophic CNS event such as a hemorrhage, drugs such as salicylates, pregnancy (especially during the third trimester), interstitial lung diseases, and anxiety.

In respiratory alkalosis, a decrease in HCO_3^- compensates for the decrease in $PaCO_2$. Acutely, HCO_3^- decreases 2 mEq/L for every 10 mm Hg decrease in $PaCO_2$. In chronic cases, HCO_3^- decreases 4 mEq/L for every 10 mm Hg decrease in $PaCO_2$. In acute respiratory alkalosis, for every 10 mm Hg decrease in the $PaCO_2$, the pH increases by 0.08.

In Clinical Case Problem 2, the $PaCO_2$ has decreased by 15 and the pH has increased by 12. The HCO_3^- has compensated.

3. c. This is a metabolic alkalosis with respiratory compensation. The pH is >7.42 and the HCO_3^- is >26.

Metabolic alkalosis is a common metabolic disturbance in hospitalized patients related to loss of H^+ seen in vomiting, nasogastric suction, and hypokalemia as a result of diuretics.

In metabolic alkalosis the $PaCO_2$ increases 6 mm Hg for every 10 mEq/L increase in HCO_3^-.

In Clinical Case Problem 3, the HCO_3^- is increased by 15 mEq/L. To compensate, the $PaCO_2$ has increased by 9.

4. a. This is metabolic acidosis with respiratory compensation. The pH is <7.38 and the HCO_3^- is <22.

Metabolic acidosis can be divided into anion gap acidosis and non–anion gap acidosis. The anion gap is $Na^+ - (Cl^- + HCO_3^-)$. A normal anion gap is 12. Anion gap acidosis results from accumulation of acidic metabolites. Examples of anion gap acidosis anion gap >14 are ketoacidosis, lactic acidosis, renal failure, and toxic doses of salicylates. Non–anion gap acidosis (anion gap <10) results from loss of bicarbonate or external acid infusion. Examples of non–anion gap acidosis are diarrhea, renal tubular acidosis, and hyperalimentation.

In metabolic acidosis the $PaCO_2$ decreases 1.2 mm Hg for every 1 mEq/L the HCO_3^- decreases.

5. d. Anion gap is $Na^+ - (Cl^- + HCO_3^-)$. In this case, $140 - (100 + 14) = 26$. This is an elevated anion gap (>14), a result of lactic acidosis secondary to the cardiac arrest.

SUMMARY OF FLUID AND ELECTROLYTE ABNORMALITIES

A. Approach to analysis of arterial blood gases:

1. Is the pH elevated or decreased? Acidemic (pH <7.38) or alkalemic (pH >7.42)? Normal arterial pH is 7.40 ± 2.
2. Is the primary disturbance respiratory or metabolic? Does the problem affect primarily the $PaCO_2$ or the HCO_3^-?
   a. $PaCO_2$ (normal value 40, range 38-42)
   b. HCO_3^- (normal value 24, range 22-26)
3. If a respiratory disturbance, is it acute or chronic?
   a. In acute respiratory acidosis bicarbonate increases 1 mEq/L per 10 mm Hg increase in $PaCO_2$
   b. In chronic respiratory acidosis the bicarbonate increases 4 mEq/L per 10 mm Hg increase in $PaCO_2$
   c. In acute respiratory acidosis the bicarbonate decreases 2 mEq/L per 10 mm Hg decrease in $PaCO_2$
   d. In chronic respiratory acidosis the bicarbonate decreases 4 mEq/L per 10 mm Hg decrease in $PaCO_2$
4. For a metabolic acidosis, determine whether an anion gap is present.
   a. Anion gap = $Na^+ - (Cl^- + HCO_3^-)$
   b. Normal anion gap = 12 ± 2
5. Assess the normal compensation by the respiratory system for a metabolic disturbance.
   a. In metabolic acidosis the $PaCO_2$ decreases 1.2 mm Hg per 1 mEq/L decrease in bicarbonate
   b. In metabolic alkalosis the $PaCO_2$ increases 6 mm Hg per 10 mEq/L increase in bicarbonate

B. Specific acid–base disorders and diagnoses

1. Respiratory acidosis results from either decreased alveolar ventilation or increased CO_2 production. Decreased alveolar ventilation can be caused by COPD, acute respiratory failure, neuromuscular disorders, and CNS depression.
2. Respiratory alkalosis results from hyperventilation as might be caused by a catastrophic CNS event; certain drugs, such as salicylates; pregnancy, especially in the third trimester; interstitial lung disease; anxiety; or liver cirrhosis.
3. Anion gap acidosis results from accumulation of acidic metabolites as may be induced by ketoacidosis, lactic acidosis, renal failure; or toxic doses of salicylates.
4. Non–anion gap acidosis results from loss of bicarbonate or external acid infusion as occurs in diarrhea, renal tubular acidosis, or hyperalimentation.
5. Metabolic alkalosis results from elevation of serum HCO_3^- and can be caused by vomiting, hypokalemia, nasogastric suction, excess glucocorticoids or mineralocorticoids, or Bartter's syndrome.

SUGGESTED READING

Adrogue HJ, Madias NE: Medical progress: management of life-threatening acid-base disorders: First of two parts. *N Engl J Med* 338(1):26-34, 1998.

Hornick DB: An approach to the analysis of arterial blood gases and acid-base disorders. *University of Iowa, Virtual Hospital,* 2003.

Sirker AA, et al: Acid-base physiology: the "traditional" and the "modern" approaches. *Anaesthesia* 57(4):348-356, 2002.

Chapter 46

Developmental Disabilities

"I just wanted to be treated like you."

CLINICAL CASE PROBLEM 1:

A 55-Year-Old Female with a 6-Month History of "Acting Out," Increased Moodiness, and Weight Loss

A new patient, a 55-year-old female with Down syndrome, is brought to your office by her caretaker for a health maintenance visit. She lives in a residential group home with three other individuals and is cared for by in-home staff provided by a residential care company under contract with the state Department of Human Services, Division of Developmental Disabilities. The caretaker reports that for the past 6 months the patient has become increasingly "moody." She normally is quite active; she works part-time at a local supermarket and participates in activities such as hiking and arts and crafts at home. However, slowly she has become withdrawn, refusing to go out, and sometimes "acts out" by throwing things at staff when encouraged to participate in meals and laundry chores. She recently has had to be coached to perform activities of daily living in which she was formerly independent. Her appetite has diminished, and her clothes are loosely fitting, whereas before they were snug.

■ SELECT THE BEST ANSWER TO THE FOLLOWING QUESTIONS:

1. Appropriate areas of particular inquiry regarding this behavior should include:
   a. any recent changes in staff or residents in the home
   b. any recent changes at work or in her family
   c. new and current medications and recent health care events
   d. any other declines in normal functioning
   e. all of the above

2. You are unable to obtain records of her previous health care. If you were, particular areas of interest might include:
   a. previous residential history
   b. immunization record
   c. sexual history
   d. a and b
   e. a, b, and c

3. You call her legal guardian for additional information. Appropriate issues to discuss with the guardian at this time include:
   a. sterilization and contraception
   b. any advance directives
   c. the appropriateness of the patient's deinstitutionalization
   d. any suspicion of neglect or abuse in the residential setting
   e. b and d

4. You attempt to examine the patient, but she refuses. At this time, an appropriate method to deal with this behavior is:
   a. physically restrain the patient so you can perform the examination
   b. reschedule several more brief visits before performing an examination
   c. give the patient chloral hydrate
   d. administer a dose of haloperidol
   e. give the patient a short-acting benzodiazepam

5. You see the patient at a later date to finish the evaluation. Appropriate health maintenance interventions at this time would include:
   a. vision and hearing screening
   b. obtaining a serum thyroid stimulating hormone (TSH) measurement
   c. obtaining an osteoporosis assessment
   d. colon cancer screening
   e. a, c, and d
   f. a, b, c, and d

6. Despite no obvious findings of illness and behavioral intervention by the group home staff and clinical psychologists, the patient's behavior deteriorates. She is now very withdrawn and refusing most meals. She has little interest in and interaction with those around her, including her good friend and housemate of 10 years. At this time, you decide to give a trial of which of the following medications:
   a. risperidone
   b. valproic acid
   c. carbamazepine
   d. Depo-Provera
   e. sertraline

CLINICAL CASE MANAGEMENT PROBLEM

Discuss the principles of the use of psychotropic medications in the management of behavioral disorders in the developmentally disabled.

■ ANSWERS:

1. **e.** Developmental disability (DD) is a chronic mental or physical impairment that results in the delay or failure to achieve normal developmental

milestones. By federal statute, developmental disabilities are defined as a group of conditions that include mental retardation, autism, cerebral palsy, spina bifida, and others. Individuals with mental retardation make up the largest group of those with DD. In the past 30 years, many individuals with DD have been deinstitutionalized to group residential settings. Family physicians often are called to care for these individuals in community settings. There can be many challenges and rewards in rendering care to patients with DD. Among them is the challenge of interpreting and diagnosing behavioral changes. Changes in behavior in the developmentally disabled are a form of communication and a clue to an underlying disturbance. The disturbance can range from something as small as a social or environmental change to a major physiologic event such as illness. Appropriate areas of particular inquiry regarding acute behavior change should include the search for social, physical, and temporal clues:

1. Any recent changes in staff or residents in the home. Residents of group homes, like all of us, are sensitive to changes in the social order. This includes not just other residents in the home but also changes in staff who could have become like family to the resident.
2. Any recent changes at work or in the family. Likewise, the patient's work environment or birth family can be a source of stress. Deaths are particularly difficult events in the developmentally disabled. Usual methods of sense-making may be absent or impaired, and cause behaviors that are a reflection of insecurity, fear, and all the other emotions concomitant with loss.
3. Medications are a frequent cause of behavioral change in DD. Similarly, recent or past health care events or experiences can be a cause of trauma and result in behavioral change.
4. Any other declines in normal functioning are also clues to what may be causing the behavioral change. Staff and family should be listened to for key insights into what they believe has contributed to the behavioral change in patients with DD.
5. Changes in vital signs. Although crude measures, they point to underlying illnesses and always should be attended to carefully.

2. e. The past history in initial data collection is of major importance and unfortunately is often unavailable or limitedly available. If available, particular areas of interest might include previous residential history' past medical, surgical, and reproductive history; immunization record including hepatitis, tetanus, and varicella status; guardianship; history of tuberculosis testing; and current medications and allergies.

3. e. Legal guardians vary according to circumstance and can range from family members to state professionals, but in all states, a court-appointed guardian for individuals with DD should exist. Clinicians should not presume that caretakers are necessarily the legal guardians of the patient. Appropriate issues to discuss with guardians include, at a minimum, all health status-related issues, acute and crisis care anticipation, advanced directives in the event of life-threatening illness, and any concerns about abuse or neglect. Physicians should be careful about fostering prejudices about the quality of life for patients with DD. Issues such as reproductive rights, if relevant, should be approached sensitively and with respect for the patient and probably after a relationship has been established with both the patient and guardian.

4. b. An appropriate approach is to schedule a series of brief visits to familiarize the patient with the routine and thereby desensitize the patient to the potential trauma of the examination and visit. The use of restraints is inappropriate in most situations but may be used briefly in situations of potential self-harm. The use of medications is a last resort, and short-acting anxiolytics are used most often, often administered just before the visit. Occasionally, the patient must be examined under general anesthesia, but this is necessarily limited in frequency. Given sufficient time and patience, most examinations, including pelvic examinations, can be accomplished in the office.

5. f. In this patient, given her age appropriate health maintenance interventions at this time would include vision and hearing screening; dental screening; thyroid screening via a serum TSH; an osteoporosis assessment; breast, cervical, and colon cancer screening; alcohol, tobacco, and drug use counseling; safe sex counseling; diet and exercise counseling; and immunization updates including tetanus, hepatitis, varicella, and influenza as needed.

6. e. This patient more than likely is suffering from depression. Factors that point to this include the many behavioral changes during the past 6 months, age older than 50 years, loss of interest in daily activities that formerly gave pleasure, withdrawn behavior, and loss of appetite. Behavioral disorders are common in patients with DD, particularly depression in the aging patient. Patients with Down syndrome are particularly susceptible; they can experience age-related declines in functioning seen much later in patients with Alzheimer's disease. Consultation with a psychiatrist and a psychologist experienced with treating behavioral disorders in patients with DD is often helpful.

SOLUTION TO THE CLINICAL CASE MANAGEMENT PROBLEM

The use of psychotropic agents in DD is a subject of great controversy (mainly because of their wide and sometimes inappropriate use). There are many factors that influence the decision of whether to prescribe a pharmacologic agent and which agent to prescribe. In general, nonpharmacologic measures should be tried first unless there is clear and present danger to the patient or those in the vicinity. Positive reinforcement of desirable behaviors is effective; punishment or limit setting is best accomplished by "time outs" or privilege restriction. However, should medication become necessary, the general rule is to start low and titrate slowly. The following medications may be considered as alternatives to traditional neuroleptics: (1) selective serotonin reuptake inhibitors (SSRIs) can help reduce self-injurious and aggressive behaviors; (2) buspirone is effective in mild chronic agitation and generally free of most side effects; (3) trazodone can be used for moderate agitation and irritability; (4) beta blockers can help with aggressive behaviors and tremulousness; (5) newer anticonvulsants (valproic acid, carbamazepine) may control mood swings and impulsivity; and (6) risperidone is preferred over older antipsychotics because of less incidence of tardive dyskinesias.

SUMMARY OF DEVELOPMENTAL DISABILITIES

DD is a chronic mental or physical impairment that results in the delay or failure to achieve normal developmental milestones. By federal statute, DD is defined as a group of conditions that include mental retardation, autism, cerebral palsy, spina bifida, and others. Individuals with mental retardation make up the largest group of those with DD.

In the past 30 years, many individuals with DD have been deinstitutionalized to group residential settings. Family physicians often are called to care for these individuals in community settings. There can be many rewards and challenges in caring for patients with DD.

Changes in behavior in the developmentally disabled are a form of communication and a clue to an underlying disturbance. The disturbance can range from something as small as a social or environmental change to a major physiologic event such as illness.

In general, health maintenance protocols are identical to other adults and children, but the problems associated with aging are being seen more often now as adults live longer, and aging effects occur earlier in particular in patients with Down syndrome.

Psychotropics must be used with particular caution and with careful attention to their effects. They can be overprescribed and generally should be used after a trial of behavior modification. However, behavioral illnesses are seen more often in patients with DD, and a trial of medications often is indicated. See the solution to the Clinical Case Management Problem for a discussion of agents.

SUGGESTED READING

Messinger-Rapport BJ, Rapport DJ: Primary care for the developmentally disabled adult. *J Gen Intern Med* 12(10):629-636, 1997.

Chapter 47

Breast, Lung, and Brain Cancer Updates

"I've been told I have a bad gene and should have my breasts removed. I don't know what I should do."

CLINICAL CASE PROBLEM 1:

A 38-YEAR-OLD WOMAN WITH BRCA 1 AND 2 MUTATIONS AND THREE FIRST-DEGREE RELATIVES WITH BREAST CANCER

A 38-year-old woman comes to the office for counseling regarding news she received from the geneticist. She has been told that she has breast cancer susceptibility genes BRCA 1 and 2, which are responsible for up to 10% of all breast cancers, and that women with these mutations have a cumulative risk of developing breast cancer of 55% to 85% up to the age of 70. She is at a loss of what to do and is coming to you for information and advice.

■ SELECT THE BEST ANSWER TO THE FOLLOWING QUESTIONS:

1. Regarding the use of chemoprevention in patients with these genes, you tell her which of the following:
   a. there is nothing that can be done to prevent her from developing breast cancer
   b. her first-degree relatives are of no bearing on her risk
   c. reduction of exposure to estrogen through oophorectomy reduces risk
   d. use of tamoxifen reduces risk
   e. c and d

2. Regarding prophylactic mastectomy, which of the following is (are) true?
   a. this is a barbaric procedure of no proven value
   b. minimal benefit is gained in performing this procedure after age 60 years
   c. unilateral surgery for the right breast is recommended because incidence is highest in this location
   d. reduction in breast cancer incidence following surgery approaches 90%
   e. b and d

CLINICAL CASE PROBLEM 2:

A 62-YEAR-OLD FEMALE WITH A SOLITARY PULMONARY NODULE

A 62-year-old woman comes to your office with her chest radiograph performed at her place of employment. She was not told the results but that she needed to see her primary care physician "pronto." She feels fine, but you know she has been a one-pack-per-day smoker for 20 years. The film reveals a 1.5-cm nodule completely surrounded by lung normal parenchyma in her right upper lobe.

3. Which of the following, if present, is suggestive of a malignancy?
   a. the presence of "corona radiata" linear strands extending out from the nodule
   b. calcifications within the lesion
   c. smooth borders to the nodule
   d. presence of the nodule on previous films
   e. dimensions greater than 3 cm

4. Which of the following is (are) true regarding non-surgical approaches to diagnosis?
   a. computed tomography (CT) densitometry measures attenuation values that are higher in malignant lesions.
   b. contrast enhanced spiral CT has a sensitivity of 95% and specificity of between 70% and 90%
   c. specificity of transthoracic fine-needle aspiration biopsy is virtually 100%
   d. bronchoscopy sensitivity for lesions 1.5 cm or less is about 40%
   e. b and c

5. Which of the following is not true regarding video-assisted thoracoscopic surgery (VATS)?
   a. VATS lowers morbidity in resection of nodules
   b. all patients with solitary nodules are candidates for VATS
   c. VATS shortens hospital length of stay in nodule resection
   d. VATS is especially successful for treatment of peripheral lung lesions
   e. VATS allows for intraoperative decision about whether to proceed to lobectomy

6. Which of the following is (are) true regarding lung cancer?
   a. non–small-cell carcinoma is less common than small-cell cancers
   b. surgery plays the major role of managing stage 1 and 2 non–small-cell lung cancers
   c. adjuvant radiation increases survival time in non–small-cell cancer
   d. surgery is the treatment of choice in small-cell cancer
   e. single-drug chemotherapy is effective in patients with extensive small-cell carcinoma

CLINICAL CASE PROBLEM 3:

A 79-YEAR-OLD MALE WITH
A BAD HEADACHE

A 79-year-old farmer presents to your office complaining of bad headaches. They have been worsening during the past several months, and lately he has developed accompanying nausea and vomiting. He was seen in a local emergency room 2 months ago and was told he has migraines. He awakes with headaches, and yesterday he walked into a partially opened barn door. He has a big lump on the side of his head. Vital signs show blood pressure 140/89, pulse 89, and respirations 17. He is afebrile. Neurologic examination shows a partial visual field loss on the right. The rest of his examination is normal. You are concerned about the possibility of serious intracranial pathology.

7. Which of the following is the best test to perform at this time?
   a. no testing is indicated at this time
   b. CT scan of the head without contrast
   c. CT scan of the head with and without contrast
   d. magnetic resonance angiography (MRA) of the head
   e. contrast-enhanced magnetic resonance imaging (MRI) of the head

8. Which of the following is (are) true regarding brain tumors?
   a. ionizing radiation is an identified risk factor for glial neoplasms
   b. use of cellular telephones is a risk factor for meningiomas
   c. headache occurs in about 90% of all patients with brain tumors
   d. postictal hemiparesis or aphasia known as Todd's phenomenon is helpful in localizing tumors
   e. a and d

9. The patient in Clinical Case Problem 3 is found to have a brain glial malignancy. Based on his history, he is likely to have which of the following?
   a. anaplastic astrocytoma
   b. glioblastoma
   c. meningioma
   d. anaplastic oligodendroglioma
   e. primary central nervous system lymphoma

10. The described patient is started with the appropriate therapy. He experiences difficulty with the chemotherapy and radiotherapy and schedules an appointment to ask you about using various mind–body interventions (MBIs) including contingency management counseling, relaxation therapy, and guided imagery to help with side effects. Regarding various MBIs, you can tell him which of the following?
   a. MBIs have not scientifically been proved to work
   b. MBIs have been effective in reducing acute pain from therapeutic procedures
   c. MBIs have been ineffective in treating anticipatory nausea and vomiting from therapeutic procedures
   d. MBIs have no effect on mood and can worsen coping capacity
   e. MBIs are extremely effective in postchemotherapy nausea reduction

■ ANSWERS:

1. **e.** BRCA 1 and 2 genes are responsible for 10% of breast cancers, and women who have these mutations have a cumulative risk of developing breast cancer up to age 70 of 55% to 85%. Women with first-degree relatives with breast cancer are additionally at increased risk. What to do with this information is the challenge faced by patients and their primary care physicians. Strategies for surveillance and chemoprevention are in transition, but the efficacy of tamoxifen chemoprevention and prophylactic mastectomy now is proven. Tamoxifen in the National Adjuvant Breast and Bowel Project Prevention Trial reduced the risk in high-risk women by 49%. Reducing exposure to estrogen by oophorectomy also seems to reduce risk in the population. Because stakes are high, confirmation of testing is recommended.

2. **e.** Prophylactic mastectomy reduces the risk of breast cancer by approximately 90% in women at high risk. However, minimal survival gains are seen in women older than age 60. Some physicians and patients find this procedure unacceptable; however, psychologic functioning in women who choose to have this procedure seems to be well-maintained. The decision to undertake any prophylactic measures, be it chemoprevention or surgery, should rest with a well-informed patient aware of all the risks, benefits, and alternatives.

3. **a.** An estimated 150,000 solitary pulmonary nodules are discovered each year, and their evaluation represents a thorny clinical problem. Lesions that are greater than 3 cm have a high probability of malignancy. Although there can be many causes for a pulmonary nodule, carcinoma must be ruled out. Several characteristics seen on plain films increase the likelihood of a nodule being a malignancy: a "corona

radiata" sign of fine linear strands or spiculated rays radiating out from the nodule, an irregular or scalloped border to the nodule, lack of calcification, or growth in size of the nodule within 2 years. High-resolution CT can be used to follow nodules over time for changes in appearance.

4. b. Several nonsurgical approaches to diagnosis are useful in distinguishing benign from malignant lesions in high-risk patients such as long-term smokers. CT densitometry involves the measurement of attenuation values, which are higher in benign lesions. Local expertise varies with this technique, and it has not been widely adopted. Contrast-enhanced spiral CT is widely available and has a sensitivity of 95% and specificity of between 70% and 90%. Specificity of transthoracic fine-needle aspiration biopsy is 55% to 88%, and sensitivity is 80% to 95%. However, nodules must be in the periphery to be accessible. Bronchoscopy sensitivity for lesions 1.5 cm or less is only about 10% but increases to 60% in larger lesions. Positron emission tomography (PET) scanning uses measures of glucose metabolism to distinguish between benign and malignant lesions, and sensitivities of 96% and specificities of 78% have been attained. However, the procedure is not widely available and requires further study. The approach to diagnosis will be guided by risk assessment, location of the lesion, and available technologies.

5. b. VATS has been shown to reduce morbidity in resection of nodules compared to open thoracotomy. Although available to most patients with solitary nodules, the procedure requires anesthesia with double lumen tubes for separate ventilation of each lung followed by discontinuation of ventilation and induced partial pneumothorax on the side of the nodule. VATS shortens hospital length of stay in nodule resections and is especially successful for treatment of peripheral lung lesions. The procedure allows for intraoperative frozen-section diagnosis to aid in the decision of full lobectomy. Mortality and morbidity are in part a function of volume of procedures performed, with better outcomes in high-volume centers.

6. b. Lung cancer is one of the most common malignancies, and primary lung cancers can be broadly classified into two forms: non–small-cell and small-cell carcinomas. Non–small-cell carcinomas account for up to 75% of all lung cancers. Surgery plays a major role of managing stages 1 and 2 non–small-cell lung cancers, whereas patients with advanced non–small-cell disease are treated with combination chemotherapy. Adjuvant radiation reduces local recurrence and, when combined with chemotherapy, may confer a small survival advantage in non–small-cell cancer. Surgery has only a limited role in the treatment of small-cell cancer. Patients with limited small-cell disease are treated with a platinum-based chemotherapeutic regimen plus radiation. Extensive small-cell disease is treated with combination chemotherapy. Unfortunately, most lung cancers at the time of diagnosis are incurable.

7. e. The best test to confirm the diagnosis of a brain malignancy is the gadolinium contrast-enhanced MRI of the brain.

8. e. Approximately 17,000 new brain tumors are diagnosed each year, and 14,000 people die each year of primary cancers of the central nervous system. Ionizing radiation is an identified risk factor for glial neoplasms, whereas use of cellular telephones has not been identified as a risk factor for any brain malignancies. Headache occurs in about half of all patients with brain tumors, and seizures occur in up to 60% in some studies. Headache is usually diffuse, often is noticeable on awakening in the morning, and can be confused with migraines or cluster headaches. In seizures related to brain malignancy, postictal hemiparesis or aphasia known as Todd's phenomenon is helpful in localizing tumors. Other symptoms or signs that help localize tumors include hemiparesis, aphasia, and visual field losses, as is seen in this patient.

9. b. Brain tumors are a heterogenous group of neoplasms. Glial tumors are divided into two main categories: astrocytic and oligodendroglial. Astrocytomas are seen predominately in young patients, and most astrocytomas progress to high-grade malignant lesions within 5 years and ultimately cause death. Malignant astrocytomas are made up of anaplastic astrocytomas and glioblastomas. Glioblastomas tend to be a disease seen later in life, usually in the sixth or seventh decades (mean age 55). Oligodendrogliomas, like astrocytomas, can be low grade or anaplastic. Most of the former eventually progress to the latter. Meningiomas are not strictly brain tumors because they arise from the meninges, which cover the brain, and occur primarily at the base of the skull. Primary central nervous system lymphomas have tripled in incidence in the last two decades and often are associated with immunosuppression, particularly human immunodeficiency virus (HIV).

10. b. MBIs include a wide range of interventions including contingency management counseling, stress reduction and relaxation therapy, meditation and guided imagery, hypnosis, and traditional behavioral counseling. After many years, studies finally have subjected these treatments to the scientific method. There is now considerable evidence that a wide range of mind–body therapies can be used as effective adjuncts for several common clinical conditions related to cancer treatment. For example, MBIs have been effective in reducing acute pain from therapeutic procedures and have been effective in treating anticipatory nausea and vomiting from therapeutic procedures. MBIs have had positive effects on mood and can enhance coping capacity. They are mildly effective in postchemotherapy nausea reduction. The clinician should keep an open mind regarding these and other adjunctive therapies for the cancer patient, while relying on the scrutiny of the scientific method to examine their effects.

SUMMARY OF BREAST, LUNG, AND BRAIN CANCER UPDATES

Breast Cancer–Associated Gene Mutations

BRCA 1 and 2 genes are responsible for 10% of breast cancers, and women with these mutations have a cumulative risk of breast cancer up to age 70 of 55% to 85%. Because stakes are high, confirmation of testing is recommended.

Strategies for surveillance and chemoprevention are in transition, but efficacy of tamoxifen chemoprevention and prophylactic mastectomy is proven.

Tamoxifen in the National Adjuvant Breast and Bowel Project Prevention Trial reduced risk in women at high risk by 49%. Reducing exposure to estrogen by oophorectomy also seems to reduce risk in the population.

Prophylactic mastectomy reduces risk of breast cancer by approximately 90% in high-risk women. However, survival gains are minimal after age 60 years.

Decisions to undertake any prophylactic measures, be it chemoprevention or surgery, should rest with a well-informed patient aware of all the risks, benefits, and alternatives.

Solitary Lung Nodules

Each year, 150,000 solitary pulmonary nodules are discovered. Although there are many causes, carcinoma must be ruled out. Approach to diagnosis is guided by risk assessment, location of the lesion, and available technologies.

Characteristics on plain films associated with malignancy are as follows: lesions > 3 cm, "corona radiata" sign of spiculated rays, irregular or scalloped border, lack of calcification, and growth in size within 2 years. High-resolution CT should be performed to follow over time for changes in appearance.

Nonsurgical approaches to distinguish benign from malignant lesions in high-risk patients (such as long-term smokers) include the following:

1. CT densitometry: measures attenuation values, which are higher in benign lesions. Local expertise varies; not widely adapted.
2. Contrast-enhanced spiral CT: widely available, sensitivity 95% and specificity 70% to 90%.
3. Transthoracic fine-needle aspiration biopsy: specificity 55% to 88% and sensitivity 80% to 95%. However, must be in periphery to be accessible.
4. Bronchoscopy: sensitivity (lesions 1.5 cm or smaller) 10%, but 60% in larger lesions
5. PET scanning: measures glucose metabolism to distinguish between benign and malignant lesions; sensitivity 96%, specificity 78%. However, not widely available, and requires further study.
6. VATS: reduces morbidity, shortens hospital length of stay, and is very successful for peripheral lung lesions. Allows for intraoperative frozen-section diagnosis to aid decision of full lobectomy. Mortality and morbidity are a function of number performed; better outcomes in high-volume centers.

Brain Tumors

Each year, 17,000 brain tumors are newly diagnosed and there are 14,000 deaths from primary central nervous system cancers.

Brain tumors are heterogenous; the best test to confirm diagnosis contrast-enhanced MRI.

There are two main categories of glial tumors: astrocytic and oligodendroglial. Astrocytomas are seen in young patients, and most progress to high-grade malignant lesions within 5 years and are fatal. Malignant astrocytomas are made up of anaplastic astrocytomas and glioblastomas. Glioblastomas occur in the sixth or seventh decades (mean age 55). Oligodendrogliomas, like astrocytomas, are low grade or anaplastic. Most of the former progress to the latter.

Meningiomas are not strictly brain tumors (arise from meninges); they occur primarily at the base of the skull.

Primary central nervous system lymphomas have tripled in incidence in the last two decades; they often are associated with immunosuppression, particularly HIV disease.

Continued

SUMMARY OF BREAST, LUNG, AND BRAIN CANCER UPDATES —cont'd

Ionizing radiation is a risk factor for glial neoplasms; cellular telephones are not confirmed as a risk factor.

Headache occurs in 50% of all patients, and seizures occur in up to 60%. Headache is diffuse, often confused with migraines or cluster headaches. In seizures related to brain malignancy, postictal hemiparesis or aphasia known as Todd's phenomenon helps localize tumors.

Other symptoms or signs include hemiparesis, aphasia, and visual field losses.

Mind–body interventions (MBIs) include contingency management counseling, stress reduction and relaxation therapy, meditation and guided imagery, hypnosis, and traditional behavioral counseling. MBIs can be used as effective adjuncts for reducing acute pain from therapeutic procedures, for treating anticipatory nausea and vomiting from procedures, for positive effects on mood, and for enhancing coping capacity.

SUGGESTED READING

Astin JA, et al: Mind-body medicine: state of the science, implications for practice. *J Am Board Fam Pract* 16(2):131-147, 2003.

Cersosimo RJ: Lung cancer: a review. *Am J Health Syst Pharm* 59(7): 611-642, 2002.

DeAngelis LM: Brain tumors. *N Engl J Med* 344(2):114-123, 2001.

Morrow M, Gradishar W: Breast cancer. *BMJ* 324(7334):410-414, 2002.

Ost D, et al: Clinical practice. The solitary pulmonary nodule. *N Engl J Med* 348(25):2535-2542, 2003.

Tacon AM: Meditation as a complementary therapy in cancer. *Fam Community Health* 26(1):64-73, 2003.

Chapter 48

Cancer Pain Management

When not to say no to drugs.

CLINICAL CASE PROBLEM 1:
A 75-Year-Old Male with Metastatic Bone Pain Secondary to Advanced Prostate Cancer

A 75-year-old male diagnosed with stage D cancer of the prostate 6 months ago comes to your office. He has been asymptomatic for the past 6 months, but last week he began to develop severe pain in the lower lumbar spine. He also appears quite pale.

On examination his prostate is rock hard. He has tender lumbar vertebrae L2 to L5. Your suspicions of metastatic bone disease are confirmed when a technetium-99 bone scan shows increased uptake of radionuclide in L2-5 and in both femurs, both tibias, and both humeri.

■ **SELECT THE BEST ANSWER TO THE FOLLOWING QUESTIONS:**

1. What is the treatment of first choice at this time?
   a. high-dose morphine sulfate
   b. high-dose hydromorphone
   c. transdermal fentanyl
   d. palliative radiotherapy to the lumbar spine
   e. acetaminophen–hydrocodone

2. You institute appropriate therapy for this patient. He quickly becomes pain free and remains that way for 6 months. He then returns with cervical, thoracic, and lumbar back pain; bilateral thigh pain; bilateral knee and leg pain; and pain in both shoulders and both arms (diffuse). Therapeutic options at this time include which of the following?
   a. intravenous (IV) chlorinate
   b. IV radioactive strontium
   c. morphine sulfate
   d. hydromorphone
   e. naproxen
   f. all of the above

3. Which of the following pharmacologic agents is the drug of first choice for the treatment of mild metastatic bone pain?
   a. morphine sulfate
   b. hydromorphone
   c. fentanyl
   d. a nonsteroid antiinflammatory drug (NSAID)
   e. carbamazepine

4. Which of the following drug(s) should not be used in the management of chronic pain?
   a. codeine
   b. meperidine
   c. levorphanol
   d. methadone
   e. a and b
   f. b and d

CLINICAL CASE PROBLEM 2:
A 52-Year-Old Male with Metastatic Renal Cell Carcinoma

A 52-year-old male with metastatic renal cell carcinoma presents for assessment of a pain beginning in the buttocks and traveling down the left leg. It has a sharp, stabbing, burning, or "zingerlike" quality, according to the patient. The patient indicates that the baseline pain is 5 on a 10-point scale increasing up to 7/10 and decreasing down to 3/10.

5. What is (are) the drug(s) of first choice for the management of this patient's cancer pain?
   a. carbamazepine
   b. hydromorphone
   c. morphine sulfate
   d. amitriptyline
   e. desipramine

CLINICAL CASE PROBLEM 3:
A 66-Year-Old Female with Metastatic Renal Cell Carcinoma

A 66-year-old female patient with metastatic renal cell carcinoma presents for assessment of a pain also beginning in the buttocks and traveling down the left leg. The only difference between this patient's pain and that of the patient in Clinical Case Problem 2 is that this patient describes her pain as dull and throbbing. The baseline level is 4/10 increasing up to 8/10 and decreasing down to 2/10.

6. What is (are) the drug(s) of first choice for the management of this patient's cancer pain?
   a. carbamazepine
   b. hydromorphone
   c. morphine sulfate
   d. desipramine
   e. valproic acid

7. The location of the lesions described in the two patients presented in cases 2 and 3 is best portrayed as which of the following?
   a. retroperitoneal
   b. lumbar-sacral plexopathy
   c. intraabdominal-visceral
   d. a and b
   e. b and c

8. What percentage of patients with cancer pain responds well to first-line analgesic therapy such as acetaminophen or NSAIDs?
   a. 1%
   b. 5%
   c. 10%
   d. 15%
   e. 20%

9. Which of the following agents would be classified as second-line analgesic therapy for the management of cancer pain?
   a. hydrocodone
   b. acetaminophen
   c. morphine sulfate
   d. levorphanol
   e. hydromorphone

10. Which of the following agents is not classified as a third-line pharmacologic agent in the management of cancer pain?
    a. methadone
    b. morphine sulfate
    c. hydromorphone
    d. fentanyl
    e. codeine

11. A patient comes to your office with moderately severe cancer pain. You prescribe the third-line agent (because of the description of the pain as moderately severe). Which of the following best describes the preferred approach to managing this patient's cancer pain?
    a. begin with a twice-daily oral (po) dose of long-acting morphine
    b. begin with a twice daily po dose of long-acting morphine plus short-acting po morphine for breakthrough pain
    c. begin with a q4h dose of short-acting po morphine
    d. begin with a transdermal fentanyl analgesic patch
    e. begin with a dose of 200 mg morphine/day in any form

12. A patient who is maintained on long-acting morphine with short-acting morphine for breakthrough presents with a 1-week history of an increasing need for short-acting morphine. He is now taking three times the number of short-acting tablets as previously. What should you do at this time?
    a. prescribe more short-acting morphine; keep the amount of long-acting morphine the same
    b. transfer the increased requirement into long-acting morphine and maintain a supply of short-acting morphine
    c. transfer the increased requirement into both increasing amounts of long-acting morphine and increased amounts of short-acting morphine
    d. switch to another third-line oral agent
    e. switch to a transdermal delivery system

13. What is the average starting daily dose of morphine sulfate in the treatment of a patient with moderately severe cancer pain?

a. 10-15 mg
b. 15-30 mg
c. 30-60 mg
d. 60-120 mg
e. 120-240 mg

14. Which of the following statements regarding the use of morphine in the treatment of terminal cancer pain is (are) relevant to the patent in question?
    a. morphine produces rapid tolerance
    b. morphine produces euphoria
    c. morphine produces respiratory depression
    d. none of the above
    e. all of the above

15. When starting a patient taking a narcotic analgesic, what is the single most important agent that should be started at the same time?
    a. an agent to prevent constipation
    b. an agent to prevent nausea and vomiting
    c. an agent to enhance sedation
    d. an agent to prevent drowsiness
    e. an antidepressant

16. Which of the following is (are) essential to cancer pain management?
    a. a collaborative, interdisciplinary approach to care
    b. an individualized pain-control plan developed and agreed on by the patient
    c. ongoing assessment and reassessment of the patient's pain
    d. the use of both pharmacologic and nonpharmacologic therapies to prevent or control pain
    e. all of the above

17. Which of the following is (are) an aim(s) of pain management in palliative care?
    a. to identify the cause of the pain
    b. to prevent the pain from recurring
    c. to maintain a clear sensorium
    d. to maintain a normal effect
    e. all of the above

18. Which of the following factors modify the pain threshold in patients with cancer pain?
    a. insomnia
    b. fear
    c. anxiety
    d. sadness
    e. all of the above

19. Which of the following statements concerning the use of narcotic analgesics in the treatment of cancer pain is (are) true?
    a. most patients with cancer pain can be treated effectively with oral agents

b. narcotic analgesics may be administered effectively by the rectal route
c. the subcutaneous infusion of narcotic analgesics has become the delivery method of choice in patients who cannot, for whatever reason, tolerate oral analgesics any longer
d. intramuscular narcotic administration on a regular basis is a reasonable alternative for pain control in terminally ill patients with cancer
e. all of the above
f. a, b, and c only

20. A patient develops severe nausea and vomiting as the dose of morphine being used for terminal cancer pain (endometrial) is increased. The patient is undergoing triple antinauseant therapy. Triple antinauseant therapy includes dimenhydrinate, metoclopramide, and prochlorperazine. Which of the following statements regarding this situation is (are) true?
    a. you should add a fourth antinauseant to the regimen at this time, preferably a corticosteroid or ondansetron
    b. you should put an IV line in place and make sure the input equals the output; do not change drugs
    c. decrease the dose of the morphine by 10% for 24 hours
    d. switch to another narcotic analgesic; no further investigations are necessary or desired
    e. none of the above

21. A patient is switched from morphine sulfate to hydromorphone. You are aware that the oral equianalgesic equivalent dose is 6/1 (6 parts morphine to 1 part hydromorphone). What should you do at this time?
    a. start oral hydromorphone at the equianalgesic dose
    b. start oral hydromorphone at 1/5 of the equianalgesic dose
    c. start oral hydromorphone at twice the equianalgesic dose
    d. start oral hydromorphone at 1/2 the equianalgesic dose
    e. start oral hydromorphone at 1/3 the equianalgesic dose

22. A patient who is being treated for terminal cancer (esophageal adenocarcinoma) pain with oral morphine requires increased morphine doses daily. Six weeks ago his morphine dose was 180 mg/day; it is 600 mg/day now. Which of the following statements regarding this increased dose of morphine is (are) true?
    a. the dosage increase most likely represents tolerance to the morphine

b. the dosage increase most likely represents increased requirements as a result of tumor growth

c. both of the above statements are true

d. either a or b could be true, but not both

e. neither a nor b

23. A patient is being treated for breast cancer with adjuvant chemotherapy following a lumpectomy. One of the drugs she is taking is cisplatin. She develops intractable nausea and vomiting while taking this drug. Which of the following antiemetics is the drug of first choice for this patient?

a. prochlorperazine

b. ondansetron

c. dimenhydrinate

d. metoclopramide

e. dexamethasone

24. A patient develops intractable nausea and vomiting secondary to carcinoma of the colon with partial bowel obstruction. She has been taking both morphine and hydromorphone by mouth but is having great difficulty keeping anything down. What would you do at this time?

a. switch to levorphanol for the pain

b. switch to methadone for the pain

c. switch from the oral medication route to a subcutaneous infusion

d. switch from the oral route to the suppository route

e. switch from the oral route to the intravenous route

CLINICAL CASE MANAGEMENT PROBLEM

Discuss the following statement: "Overdosing cancer patients with narcotic analgesics is much more of a problem than underdosing cancer patients with narcotic analgesics."

ANSWERS:

1. **d.** This patient, who was diagnosed with stage D cancer of the prostate 6 months ago, was treated in a responsible way. When a man with metastatic cancer has no symptoms, it is probably better to wait and save the limited weapons available until needed.

A very important point in this case is that although his bone scan shows more diffuse skeletal disease, his clinical status suggests symptoms only in the lumbar spine. Thus radiation therapy to the lumbar spine is the most reasonable course of action. Again, the reasoning is that local symptoms should receive local therapy. (This applies to palliative situations only.)

Although it would not be wrong to start with morphine sulfate or hydromorphone, it would be wrong to start high-dose morphine sulfate or high-dose hydromorphone. These narcotics will be discussed in great length in subsequent questions.

2. **f.** The therapeutic options for the treatment of metastatic bone disease are increasing rapidly. The following treatment options have been shown to be effective: bisphosphonates, radioactive strontium, NSAIDs, and narcotic analgesics.

A reasonable treatment plan at this time would be to begin with a NSAID (naproxen) plus short-acting morphine sulfate or short-acting hydromorphone for breakthrough pain. Then ask the patient to call you within 24 hours to ensure that pain has begun to decrease. On his next visit (in perhaps a week if you are beginning to get his pain under control) you could (1) switch him to a long-acting morphine preparation or a longer-acting hydromorphone preparation, plus (2) continue the nonsteroidal antiinflammatory agent, plus (3) continue to supply him with short-acting narcotics for breakthrough pain, plus (4) decide on either clodronate or radioactive strontium as adjuvant therapy.

3. **d.** The drug class of first choice for the management of mild to moderate metastatic bone pain is the NSAID agents. If this does not work, then opioids can be added to NSAIDs for mild to moderate pain.

4. **b.** Meperidine (Demerol) is contraindicated in the management of chronic pain (both malignant and nonmalignant). The reasons for its contraindication are its relatively short half-life and its lack of efficacy.

The other drugs, levorphanol (oral) and methadone (oral), are all very reasonable agents to use in the management of chronic cancer pain, as is fentanyl (transdermal, subcutaneous, or IV). Note the words "cancer pain." From experience and the opinions of world authorities on this issue, it is best (in almost all cases) not to use narcotic analgesics to manage chronic nonmalignant pain.

5. **a.** See Answer 6.

6. **d.** These two cases illustrate the use of adjuvant analgesics in the treatment of neuropathic pain. Neuropathic pain is the most common type of cancer pain and presents diagnostic and therapeutic challenges. It basically is described as being either a sharp, stabbing, burning, ("zingerlike" pain) or as a dull, aching pain. Both types of neuropathic pain respond better to adjuvant analgesics than to narcotic analgesics. However, in response to typical adjuvant agents, the sharp, stabbing, burning pain responds better to anticonvulsant medications; the first choice

is carbamazepine, and the second choice is valproic acid. In contrast, the dull, "aching" pain responds better to two tricyclic antidepressants; the first choice is desipramine, and, unless sedation also would be of benefit to the patient, the second choice is amitriptyline.

7. d. The greatest number of neuropathic pains seen in cancer pain management result from retroperitoneal lesions either infiltrating or pressing on the lumbar-sacral plexus.

8. e. See Answer 10.

9. a. See Answer 10.

10. e. The World Health Organization (WHO) has developed an analgesic ladder for the treatment of cancer pain. Although it is not necessarily always in the patient's best interest to start with a first-line agent (the pain may be too severe), many patients can be managed with first-line agents such as acetaminophen or NSAIDs. In fact, 20% to 25% of patients with cancer pain can have their pain totally or almost totally controlled with these agents.

The WHO's analgesic ladder is summarized as follows: (1) first-line agents are acetylsalicylic acid (ASA; aspirin), other NSAIDs, or acetaminophen; (2) second-line agents are hydrocodone or codeine; and (3) third-line agents are morphine sulfate, hydromorphone, fentanyl, levorphanol, or methadone.

11. c. The best approach to the management of moderately severe cancer pain is to begin with an every-4-hour dose of short-acting morphine sulfate (the drug of first choice in the third-line group) and have the patient use the analgesic as needed to attain complete pain control. Once the dose is established you may switch to a longer-acting preparation (bid) and maintain for the patient a supply of short-acting morphine for breakthrough pain.

12. b. What the patient needs at this time is an increased supply of long-acting morphine as well as the maintenance of a supply of short-acting morphine for breakthrough pain.

13. c. The average daily starting dose of morphine sulfate (oral) in a patient with moderately severe cancer pain is 30-60 mg.

14. d. Although the use of morphine may cause tolerance, euphoria, and respiratory depression, these statements do not apply to patients who are in the terminal or palliative phase of their illness.

There is no maximum morphine or other analgesic equivalent dose. Each patient requires the dose to be individualized. This should be done by starting at lower doses and increasing the dose until you have achieved total pain control and are able to prevent further pain.

15. a. Any patient who is started taking a narcotic analgesic also should be started on a regimen to prevent constipation. The drugs most commonly used at this time include lactulose, an osmotic agent, and a combination of a stool softener and a peristaltic stimulant (such as docusate sodium and senna). An antiemetic such as dimenhydrinate, prochlorperazine, or metoclopramide may be indicated for the first 2 or 3 weeks to prevent nausea and vomiting that sometimes accompanies the initiation of a narcotic.

16. e. Clinical practice guidelines have been issued by the Agency for Healthcare Research and Quality (formerly the Agency for Health Care Policy and Research), a branch of the Department of Health and Human Services. The purpose of these guidelines is to correct the problem of inadequate treatment (or underdosing) pain treatment for cancer. These guidelines call for the following: (1) a collaborative, interdisciplinary approach to the care of patients with cancer pain; (2) an individualized pain-control plan developed and agreed on by the patient (the patient must be regarded as the head of the health care team); (3) an ongoing assessment and reassessment of the patient's pain; (4) the use of both nonpharmacologic and pharmacologic therapies to prevent or control pain; and (5) explicit institutional policies on the management of cancer pain, with clear lines of responsibility for pain management and for monitoring its effectiveness.

17. e. The aims of pain management in palliative care are as follows: (1) to identify the cause of the pain; (2) to prevent the pain from occurring again; (3) to erase the memory of the pain; and (4) to maintain a clear sensorium and a normal effect.

Remember that palliative care is active treatment, not passive treatment.

18. e. Cancer pain is a complex entity that requires treatment of not only the somatic source(s) but also the other aspects, including depression, anxiety, anger, and isolation. Pain threshold is raised by relief of symptoms, sleep, rest, empathy, understanding, diversions, elevation of mood, effective analgesic therapy, anxiolytic therapy, and antidepressant therapy.

Pain threshold is lowered by discomfort, insomnia, fatigue, anxiety, fear, anger, sadness, depression, mental isolation, introversion, and past painful experiences.

Cancer pain should be considered as a complex consisting of a physical component, a psychologic component, a social component, and a spiritual component.

Unless each one of these areas is addressed in the overall cancer pain management strategy, therapy will not be effective.

19. f. The following facts or treatments should be considered in cancer pain management: (1) cancer pain can be controlled in 90% of patients with oral medication; (2) the subcutaneous infusion of opioid analgesics by a programmed subcutaneous pump is the treatment of choice in patients who, for whatever reason, cannot tolerate the oral route; and (3) the rectal route is an acceptable alternative in patients who cannot tolerate the oral route. However, regular intramuscular injections to control cancer pain should be discouraged because of associated pain, inconvenience, and unreliable drug absorption.

20. e. At this time, the first priority is to determine the cause of the nausea. The narcotic analgesic may not be the cause. A thorough search for all other serious and potential causes of the nausea must be undertaken. In this case, a likely cause is hypercalcemia. Another common cause is the production by the tumor of emetic substances. Once causes such as these are ruled out, it is then reasonable to switch to another narcotic analgesic (such as hydromorphone) and/or to institute effective antiemetic therapy.

21. b. When a patient is switched from one narcotic analgesic to another, a major adjustment has to be made in equianalgesic dose. A common mistake made is to begin the patient on the exact equivalent (in mg) of the previously used narcotic. An equianalgesic dose no greater than one-fifth should be the starting dose of the next opioid. This is because of different types of opioid receptors in the brain.

For example, a switch from oral morphine to oral hydromorphone should be as follows:

1. The patient is currently taking 120 mg of oral morphine/day.

2. The equianalgesic dose is 120 mg/6 = 20 mg hydromorphone.
3. Starting the patient at one-fifth of the equianalgesic dose will be 20 mg/5 = 4 mg hydromorphone.

The pain control should be assessed frequently, and the dose should be increased as needed.

22. c. The increase in the dose of morphine over the 6-week period most likely represents a combination of tolerance to morphine and increased requirements resulting from growth of the tumor. As pointed out earlier, rapid tolerance usually is not seen when the patient is being given a narcotic for cancer pain. However, tolerance can be developed over time and must be considered.

23. b. Chemotherapy that includes the drug cisplatin is very likely to produce very severe nausea and vomiting. It is mandatory, therefore, to treat this aggressively. Ondansetron, a serotonin antagonist, has been found to be extremely useful for the control of chemotherapy-induced nausea and is recommended (other serotonin antagonist include granisetron and dolasetron). In other cases in which control is difficult despite combination antinauseant therapy, ondansetron also should be used.

24. c. Cancer pain can be controlled by oral medications in the vast majority of cases (90%). When control with oral medications becomes impossible, however, it is necessary to switch to another route. Four possible routes are available: the suppository route, the intravenous route, the subcutaneous route, and the transdermal route.

With a patient in severe discomfort, the subcutaneous route is the route of choice. This is best accomplished with the use of a computer-controlled subcutaneous infusion pump. This provides a constant infusion rate and boluses whenever needed.

SOLUTION TO THE CLINICAL CASE MANAGEMENT PROBLEM

This statement—"overdosing cancer patients with narcotic analgesics is much more of a problem than underdosing cancer patients with narcotic analgesics"—is completely false. Exactly the opposite is true. Patients with cancer pain often are treated very ineffectively. The ineffectiveness of treatment equates to significant undertreatment. It is estimated that 50% of patients with cancer pain die in significant pain. The major reasons for this appear to be fear on the part of physicians: (1) of using "too much" narcotic; (2) that the cancer patients will

become addicted to the narcotics; and (3) that they personally will get in trouble with their state medical board for prescribing strong narcotics to anyone. Underlying these fears is a lack of knowledge regarding cancer pain management, the drugs that need to be used, and the doses of those drugs.

All of these contribute to the significant undertreatment described. Consequently, many patients suffer needless pain in the final stages of life.

SUMMARY OF CANCER PAIN MANAGEMENT

A. The Ten Commandments of cancer pain management:

1. Thou shalt not assume that the patient's pain is a result of the malignant process. Always begin with steps aimed at making a specific, anatomic, and pathologic diagnosis.

2. Thou shalt consider the patient's feelings. Pain threshold varies with mood and morale. Given the opportunity to express fears, the patient should experience less pain.

3. Thou shalt not use the abbreviation "prn" (*pro re nata*, as required). Achieving balanced pain control means avoiding the return of pain resulting from gaps in medication administration. Less medication will be required if given around the clock.

4. Thou shalt prescribe adequate amounts of medication. The right dose of medication is not dictated by recommendations from a book, but rather by the patient's level of pain. Use what it takes to relieve the pain, titrating for effect.

5. Thou shalt always try nonnarcotic medications as the first step unless your clinical judgment deems the patient to be in moderately severe or severe pain. Mild to moderate pain in many cases will respond to acetaminophen or NSAIDs. NSAIDs are particularly useful for bony metastases.

6. Thou shalt not be afraid of narcotic analgesics. When nonnarcotic agents fail, move to a narcotic agent quickly.

7. Thou shalt not limit thyself to using only drug therapies. Nondrug therapies such as hypnosis, imagery techniques, biofeedback, physiotherapy, individual psychotherapy, group psychotherapy, and family psychotherapy are very beneficial.

8. Thou shalt not be reluctant to seek a colleague's advice. If you have exhausted your skills or run out of ideas, ask someone else to evaluate your patient.

9. Thou shalt provide support for the entire family. Treatment of anticipatory grief experienced by the family will help to prevent isolation and loneliness. Be able to intervene quickly when a crisis arises.

10. Thou shalt maintain an air of quiet confidence and cautious optimism. Aim for "graded relief," choosing small goals that can be accomplished to build the patient's trust and hope. Exhibit a determination to succeed.

B. The World Health Organization analgesic ladder:

1. Step 3: morphine sulfate, hydromorphone, fentanyl, levorphanol, or methadone

2. Step 2: codeine (with or without acetaminophen) or hydrocodone (with or without acetaminophen or ASA).

3. Step 1: acetaminophen, ASA or other NSAIDs Selective cyclooxygenase-2 (COX-2) inhibitors such as celecoxib (Celebrex), rofecoxib (Vioxx), and valdecoxib (Bextra) have gained popularity because of a decrease in gastrointestinal side effects. (Note: in 2002 Pharmacia added a warning indicating use of valdecoxib has a slight chance of inducing Stevens-Johnson syndrome, and Merck Inc. cited small studies indicating use of rofecoxib may cause increased risk of heart attack, stroke, blood clots, and aseptic meningitis.)

C. Classification of cancer pain:

1. Somatic pain (including bone pain)

2. Neuropathic pain:
   a. Type I is a sharp, stabbing, burning, "zinger" pain. Adjuvant analgesics to use are anticonvulsants, such as carbamazepine (Tegretol), oxcarbazepine (Trileptal), and gabapentin (Neurontin).
   b. Type II is a dull, aching pain. Adjuvant analgesics of choice are tricyclic antidepressants such as amitriptyline or desipramine.

3. Visceral pain: corticosteroids are used as adjuvant therapy especially in visceral pain where there is swelling around a visceral capsule (e.g., the hepatic capsule). These also can provide antiinflammation activity, stimulate appetite, and decrease cerebral or spinal cord swelling.

4. NSAIDs are used for somatic pain (metastatic bone).

5. Benzodiazepines have very little utility in pain management, but muscle relaxants may help muscle spasms and neuralgias.

D. Pathophysiology of cancer pain:

1. Physical (biologic) component: 25%
2. Psychologic (emotional) component: 25%
3. Social component: 25%
4. Spiritual component: 25%

Unless all four components are addressed, the treatment of cancer pain will be unsuccessful.

E. Routes of administration:

1. Oral (90% of cancer cases)
2. Subcutaneous (5% of cancer cases)
3. Rectal (5% of cancer cases)

F. Conversion of one narcotic analgesic to another:
1. Calculate equianalgesic doses between drug 1 (the drug about to be discontinued) and drug 2 (the drug to be started).
2. Begin drug 2 at no more than 20% of equianalgesic dose. The reasons for this are that there is tolerance built up to the first drug and that different narcotics react on different receptors in the brain.

G. Method of beginning narcotic analgesic for moderate to severe cancer pain is: (1) choice drug is usually morphine sulfate; (2) begin morphine sulfate with short-acting morphine (morphine 5- or 10-mg tabs); (3) the daily starting dose is 30-60 mg/day; (4) after a week, switch total daily dose to long-acting morphine, and continue short-acting morphine for breakthrough; (5) begin a bowel-regulating regimen at the same time as narcotic is begun using lactulose or a stool softener (Colace) plus peristaltic stimulant (senna alkaloid); and (6) consider antiemetic therapy for the first few weeks of narcotic therapy (prochlorperazine, dimenhydrinate, metoclopramide).

H. Cancer pain: Optimal management combines pharmacologic management with nonpharmacologic management: Nonpharmacologic therapies include relaxation techniques, support groups, biofeedback, mental imagery, physiotherapy, transcutaneous electrical nerve stimulation (TENS), physical activity, individual psychotherapy, group psychotherapy, and, family psychotherapy.

I. Other forms of palliative cancer pain therapy are: (1) palliative radiotherapy, which is especially useful for metastatic bone pain and neuropathic pain (lumbosacral plexopathy and brachial plexopathy); (2) palliative surgery; and (3) palliative chemotherapy.

SUGGESTED READING

Braunwald E, et al: Pain management. In: *Harrison's Manual of Medicine 15th ed.* McGraw-Hill Professional, 2001, Philadelphia, pgs 1-28.
Herr K: Pain management. In Reuben D, ed. *Geriatrics at your finger tips 2003.* Blackwell Publishers, 2002, Oxford, England, pgs 115-120.
Stillman MJ: Pain, nausea and vomiting. In: Rakel RE, Bope ET, eds.: *Conn's Current Therapy 2003.* WB Saunders, 2002, Philadelphia, pgs 1-10.

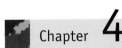

Chapter **49**

Palliative Care

When relief is the best you can hope for.

CLINICAL CASE PROBLEM 1:

A 51-Year-Old Female with Severe Nausea, Vomiting, and Anorexia in Severe, Advanced Ovarian Cancer

A 51-year-old female patient with advanced ovarian cancer has terminal disease. She is constantly nauseated, vomiting, and anorexic. You are called to see her at home. In addition to the symptoms mentioned, the patient complains of a "sore abdomen," and she is having significant difficulty breathing. She also has a "sore mouth."

The patient has gone through chemotherapy with cisplatinum. This therapy ended 8 months ago. Her ovarian cancer first was discovered 12 months ago. Since that time her condition has deteriorated to the point where she has lost 40 pounds and is feeling "weaker and weaker" every day.

On examination, the patient's breathing is labored. Her respiratory rate is 28 beats per minute. The breath sounds heard in both lungs are normal. Her mouth is dry, and there are whitish lesions that rub off with a tongue depressor. She looks significantly cachectic. Her abdomen is significantly enlarged. There is a level of shifting dullness, and there is a large abdominal mass that is approximately 8 cm by 35 cm.

■ SELECT THE BEST ANSWER TO THE FOLLOWING QUESTIONS:

1. What is (are) the drug(s) of choice for the management of cancer-associated cachexia and anorexia?
   a. prednisone
   b. prochlorperazine
   c. megestrol acetate
   d. cyproheptadine
   e. a or c

2. The nausea and vomiting that this patient has developed may be treated with various measures or drugs. Which of the following could be recommended as first-line agents for this patient's nausea and vomiting?

a. prochlorperazine
b. dimenhydrinate
c. metoclopramide
d. all of the above
e. none of the above

3. The drug that you selected for the treatment of the nausea and vomiting unfortunately was not effective. What would you do at this time?
a. forget drugs and use a nasogastric (NG) tube
b. combine two or three of the previously mentioned drugs
c. forget treatment and attempt hydration with intravenous (IV) fluids
d. select ondansetron as an antiemetic
e. b or d

4. Based on the history of her "sore mouth" and white lesions that scrape off with a tongue depressor, what would you recommend treatment with?
a. ketoconazole
b. penicillin
c. amphotericin B
d. chloramphenicol
e. methotrexate

5. The patient described undergoes palliative radiotherapy for severe bone pain that develops 1 month after the problems described. Following this, significant diarrhea develops. Which of the following agents may be helpful in the treatment of this problem?
a. diphenoxylate hydrochloride
b. loperamide
c. codeine
d. all of the above
e. none of the above

6. What is the most prevalent symptom in patients with cancer?
a. anorexia
b. asthenia
c. pain
d. nausea
e. constipation

7. What is the most frequent cause of chronic nausea and vomiting in advanced cancer?
a. bowel obstruction
b. raised intracranial pressure
c. narcotic bowel syndrome
d. hypercalcemia
e. autonomic failure

8. The patient described in the question becomes increasingly short of breath. You suspect a pleural effusion. A chest x-ray confirms the diagnosis of a left pleural effusion. Which of the following is the treatment of first choice for the treatment of this complication?
a. a thoracocentesis
b. home oxygen
c. a hospital bed that is elevated at the head
d. decreased fluid intake
e. prochlorperazine

9. Which of the following treatments also may be useful in treating this symptom?
a. palliative radiotherapy
b. prednisone
c. morphine sulfate
d. dexamethasone
e. all of the above

10. You treat the patient's pleural effusion effectively. One week later she develops increasing abdominal distention, nausea, and vomiting. You suspect a partial bowel obstruction. On examination, there are increased bowel sounds. A plain film of the abdomen confirms a diagnosis of partial bowel obstruction. Which of the following is (are) generally recommended as a palliative measure(s) for this symptom?
a. decreased fluid intake
b. metoclopramide
c. chlorpromazine
d. all of the above
e. none of the above

CLINICAL CASE PROBLEM 2:
A 53-YEAR-OLD MALE WITH SUDDEN-ONSET LEFT-SIDED WEAKNESS

A 53-year-old male comes to the emergency room with the sudden onset of left-sided weakness. He has a history of chronic obstructive pulmonary disease (COPD) resulting from chronic bronchitis. He describes himself as "healthy as a horse," although he smokes three packs of cigarettes per day.

On examination, the patient has a left-sided hemiplegia. A chest x-ray shows a left-sided mass lesion and prominent hilar lymphadenopathy. You suspect a bronchogenic carcinoma.

11. Which of the following statements regarding this patient is (are) true?
a. there is likely no relationship between the hemiplegia and the chest x-ray findings
b. the chances of recovery from the hemiplegia are essentially zero
c. the cause of the hemiplegia is likely a cerebral embolus

d. dexamethasone may be used both as a diagnostic test and a therapeutic maneuver in this patient
e. none of the above are true

CLINICAL CASE PROBLEM 3:
A 42-Year-Old Female with Disseminated Breast Cancer

You are called to the home of a 42-year-old female with disseminated breast cancer. She has a fungating breast carcinoma that is emitting a very offensive odor. Her friends have stopped coming to see her because of the odor. The patient and her family have tried numerous remedies without success.

12. Which of the following may be useful in the treatment of the odor associated with this fungating growth?
a. frequent cleansings with saline
b. application of yogurt dressings
c. application of buttermilk dressings
d. charcoal briquettes strategically placed throughout the house
e. all of the above

CLINICAL CASE PROBLEM 4:
A 51-Year-Old Patient with Terminal Colon Cancer

You are called to the home of a 51-year-old patient with terminal colon cancer. He has become increasingly depressed and agitated and now is unable to sleep at night. As you talk to the patient and review in your head the Diagnostic and Statistical Manual of Mental Disorders, 4th edition (DSM-IV) criteria for depression, you realize that this patient has an agitated depression.

13. Which of the following may be indicated in the treatment of this patient's condition?
a. a sedating tricyclic antidepressant in the evening
b. an anxiolytic agent given on a *prn* (as needed) basis
c. fluoxetine
d. a and/or b
e. all of the above

14. With regard to narcotic-induced nausea and vomiting, which of the following statements is (are) true?
a. nausea and/or vomiting is common in the initial narcotic administration period
b. nausea and/or vomiting associated with narcotic analgesics usually subsides within 2 weeks of beginning therapy

c. nausea and/or vomiting associated with narcotic administration usually can be prevented by the prophylactic use of medication
d. all of the above are true
e. none of the above are true

15. What is the drug of choice for the medical management of malignant ascites?
a. hydrochlorothiazide
b. spironolactone
c. prednisone
d. dexamethasone
e. none of the above

16. What is the most common metabolic derangement associated with advanced malignancy?
a. hyponatremia
b. hypokalemia
c. hypercalcemia
d. hypomagnesemia
e. hyperkalemia

17. What is the drug of choice for the management of narcotic-induced constipation?
a. a senna preparation
b. a psyllium compound
c. sodium docusate
d. lactulose
e. Metamucil

18. Which of the following statements regarding the use of combination antinauseant therapy in cancer is true?
a. combination antinauseants should not be used
b. the combination of any two drugs is just as effective as the combination of any other two
c. combination drugs should have affinity for different therapeutic receptors
d. oral antinauseants, especially when given together, are rarely effective for resistant nausea and/or vomiting
e. none of the above are true

CLINICAL CASE MANAGEMENT PROBLEM

Asthenia is the most commonly encountered symptom in patients who are terminally ill. Describe what the term asthenia means to you.

ANSWERS:

1. **e.** Prednisone (a corticosteroid) and megestrol acetate (a progestational agent) are the pharmacologic treatments of choice in patients with advanced cancer who have significant anorexia.

In patients with anorexia, oral nutrition should be the first priority, with particular attention being paid to the timing of meals in relation to medical and nursing procedures and to the administration of drugs. Selected patients in whom oral nutrition or hydration is not possible may benefit from enteral nutrition or hypodermoclysis. Parenteral nutrition has shown no significant benefit in terms of improving survival or comfort, and its routine use is not indicated in palliative care.

Megestrol acetate in a dosage of 460 mg/day rapidly is becoming the pharmacologic agent of choice in the treatment of anorexia. An alternative to progestational agents is prednisone. Prednisone may be given in doses of approximately 10-15 mg/day. This may be increased if necessary. Dronabinol also has been effective in weight gain for younger adults with specific conditions such as acquired immune deficiency syndrome (AIDS) and cancer.

With anorexia, particular attention must be paid to the mouth to prevent candidiasis and other problems.

Other potential choices for the pharmacologic treatment of anorexia include cyproheptadine, hydrazine sulfate, and cannabinoids.

2. d. The nonpharmacologic treatment of nausea and vomiting should include (1) attempting to find the cause; (2) the avoidance of a supine position to prevent the dangers of aspiration of vomit; (3) a general assessment of the environment of the patient and how it could be improved; (4) attention to body odors; (5) small, frequent meals (that the patient likes; not a bland diet); and (6) attractive food presentation.

Antiemetics can be divided into several classes: (1) anticholinergics such as hyoscine and atropine, (2) phenothiazines such as prochlorperazine and chlorpromazine, (3) butyrophenones such as haloperidol and droperidol, (4) antihistamines such as cyclizine and promethazine, (5) gastrokinetic agents such as domperidone and metoclopramide, (6) 5-HT$_3$ receptor antagonists such as ondansetron, (7) corticosteroids such as prednisone and dexamethasone, and (8) miscellaneous agents such as ibuprofen, tricyclic antidepressants, benzodiazepines, and nabilone.

There are some specific indications for certain antinauseants, such as the treatment of a partial bowel obstruction with a gastrokinetic agent, cyclizine for vestibular associated emesis, and ondansetron for chemotherapy-induced emesis. In most cases, however, an antinauseant from any of the classes can be tried for any cancer-associated nausea.

Three general rules should be followed when prescribing antinauseants in cancer and palliative care management: (1) before prescribing an antinauseant on a long-term basis, conduct a vigorous search for the underlying cause; (2) if you are using combination antinauseant therapy, do not combine antinauseants from the same class of drugs; and (3) if you are using combination antinauseant therapy, remember that antinauseants that work on the same neurotransmitter (dopamine, muscarinic/cholinergic, histamine) tend to be less effective when combined than antinauseants that work on different receptors.

Although a discussion of the receptors involved in each antinauseant is too detailed for this book, the following approach to treating the nausea and vomiting associated with cancer and palliative care is suggested: (1) always consider nonpharmacologic therapy first; small, frequent meals with appropriate food presentation and consisting of foods that the patient likes; (2) begin with prochlorperazine, dimenhydrinate, or metoclopramide; (3) combine any two of the previously mentioned drugs or all three for resistant nausea; (4) consider adding a corticosteroid such as prednisone or dexamethasone to the treatment regimen; (5) consider ondansetron for chemotherapy-induced nausea and vomiting; and (6) if emesis continues despite the previous treatment suggestions, try the rectal, subcutaneous, or suppository route.

3. e. As mentioned, a combination of two or three of the antinauseants discussed in the choices in Question 2 would be appropriate. It is surprising that a few significant problems with extrapyramidal side effects occur with combination therapy.

Ondansetron is a 5-HT receptor antagonist. However, it is very expensive, and this certainly should be considered when selecting between this and a combination of older agents.

Try to avoid an NG tube in patients undergoing palliative care whenever possible. NG tubes are uncomfortable and thus tend to have a negative, rather than a positive, impact on symptom control in patients with cancer.

4. a. White lesions that scrape off with a tongue depressor are almost certainly oral thrush. Oral thrush is extremely common in patients undergoing palliative care, even with good mouth care. Treatment with clotrimazole troches or fluconazole is recommended.

5. d. The diarrhea in this case is likely the effect of the radiotherapy on the bowel. Diphenoxylate, loperamide, and codeine are all good treatment choices. In most patients, the diarrhea will settle down 1-2 weeks after the completion of the course of radiotherapy.

6. b. Asthenia (fatigue) is the most prevalent symptom in patients with advanced cancer. The prevalence of symptoms in patients with advanced cancer is as follows: (1) asthenia, 90%; (2) anorexia, 85%; (3) pain,

76%; (4) nausea, 68%; (5) constipation, 65%; (6) sedation, 60% (7) confusion, 60%; and (8) dyspnea, 12%.

7. a. Although autonomic failure, hypercalcemia, narcotic bowel syndrome, and raised intracranial pressure can cause nausea and vomiting, the most frequent cause is bowel obstruction from pressure of an intraabdominal tumor on the bowel itself, involvement of the bowel in the tumor process, associated gastric stasis, or other causes.

8. a. A large pleural effusion initially should be treated by thoracentesis. If it recurs at infrequent intervals, this technique can be used repeatedly and with a sclerosing agent, such as infused talc. This can reduce the reoccurrence of a malignant effusion but often is irritating to the patient.

9. e. However, if pleural effusion recurs frequently, you may decide to use other symptom-relieving measures, including elevating the head of the bed, providing oxygen, breathing fresh air, decreasing fluid intake, prescribing prednisone or dexamethasone, prescribing morphine, and conducting palliative radiotherapy.

10. d. A partial bowel obstruction may be treated effectively by gastrokinetic agents such as metoclopramide or domperidone; decreased fluid intake; antiemetic agents such as prochlorperazine, dimenhydrinate, metoclopramide, or ondansetron; or corticosteroids such as prednisone. A NG tube should be considered if surgery is a possibility. Percutaneous venting gastrostomy for a complete high-level obstruction not responding to pharmacotherapy should be considered.

11. d. This patient most likely has a primary lung carcinoma with metastatic disease to the brain. The metastatic disease has produced increased intracranial pressure, which has resulted in the neurologic symptoms.

The use of dexamethasone in this case can be both diagnostic and therapeutic. If the symptoms improve with dexamethasone, your suspicion of increased intracranial pressure as a cause of the symptoms is confirmed. An H_2 receptor antagonist such as ranitidine always should be used when a patient undergoing palliative care is being treated with dexamethasone.

12. e. Fungating growths, particularly carcinomas of the breast, can produce very unsightly lesions and very offensive odors that have psychologic and social implications in addition to medical implications. Often friends of the patient will stop coming because of the odor.

The most important aspects of treatment include proper cleaning of the fungating growth with saline compresses (not Dakin's solution or other solutions, which actually may make it worse, not better), the application of yogurt (not fruit flavored) or buttermilk dressings, and the placement of charcoal briquettes strategically throughout the patient's room. The latter are very effective in weakening the odor of the fungating growth.

13. d. An agitated depression is best treated by a combination of a sedating tricyclic antidepressant and/or an anxiolytic agent given on a *prn* basis. Fluoxetine, in this case, actually may make the situation worse. Although fluoxetine and other selective serotonin reuptake inhibitors have turned out to be a very important advances in the treatment of depressive disorders, fluoxetine has the potential to make an agitated depression worse. In this case, thus, it is safer to stick to the older, proven reliable tricyclic antidepressants (TCA), especially a TCA with sedating properties.

14. d. When starting a patient taking a narcotic analgesic, it is wise also to begin the patient taking an antiemetic agent. Nausea and/or vomiting is an extremely common initial side effect that quickly (within 2-3 weeks) disappears. The antiemetic then can be discontinued. A good initial choice is prochlorperazine or dimenhydrinate.

15. b. The drug of choice for the management of malignant ascites is the aldosterone antagonist spironolactone. Spironolactone has been shown to be effective in both malignant ascites and in the ascites associated with cirrhotic liver disease. Paracentesis may provide significant relief from malignant ascites and should be considered a method of first choice for the acute relief.

16. c. Hypercalcemia is the most common life-threatening metabolic disorder associated with cancer. It usually occurs in the context of advanced disseminated malignancy and produces a number of distressing symptoms. These include general symptoms such as dehydration, polydipsia, polyuria, and pruritus; gastrointestinal symptoms such as anorexia, weight loss, nausea, vomiting, constipation, and ileus; neurologic symptoms such as fatigue, lethargy, confusion, myopathy, hyporeflexia, seizures, psychosis, and coma; and cardiovascular symptoms such as bradycardia, atrial dysrhythmias, ventricular dysrhythmias; prolonged PR intervals; QT interval reductions; and wide T waves.

The primary treatment of hypercalcemia is IV fluid therapy. Other important treatments include corticosteroids, bisphosphonates, and calcitonin.

17. d. The treatment of choice for narcotic-induced constipation is lactulose. Lactulose is an osmotic agent that also has been shown to be extremely useful in the management of hepatic encephalopathy.

A very reasonable alternative would be a combination of a stool softener such as docusate sodium and a peristaltic stimulant such as senna.

The advantages of lactulose appear to be greater efficacy, especially in patients who are taking high-dose narcotics. It is a liquid rather than a pill, which is another advantage.

Metamucil is contraindicated in the treatment of constipation in patients taking narcotic analgesics. Metamucil appears, in many cases, to make things worse by absorbing water and actually increasing the mass of stool that has to be evacuated.

Always attempt to find out why the patient is constipated—do not assume that it is from taking narcotic analgesics.

18. c. Antinauseants have been discussed previously. It also was mentioned that there are various neurotransmitter receptor sites that have been identified for antiemetic drugs. These neurotransmitters include dopamine, muscarinic/cholinergic receptors, and histamine receptors. In brief, some of the common antiemetics and their predominant neurotransmitter receptor sites include the following:

Antiemetic	Receptor Site
Dimenhydrinate	Dopamine
Prochlorperazine	Muscarinic/cholinergic
Chlorpromazine	Muscarinic/cholinergic
Metoclopramide	Muscarinic/cholinergic
Hyoscine	Dopamine/muscarinic/cholinergic

SOLUTION TO THE CLINICAL CASE MANAGEMENT PROBLEM

Asthenia is the most prevalent symptom in patients with advanced cancer. Two symptoms usually are included in the term asthenia: (1) fatigue or lassitude, defined as easy tiring and decreased capacity to maintain adequate performance; and (2) generalized weakness, defined as the anticipatory subjective sensation of difficulty in initiating a certain activity.

SUMMARY OF PALLIATIVE CARE

A. Nausea and vomiting:
1. Eat small, frequent meals
2. Avoid bland foods. Give the patient what he or she wants to eat.
3. Take antiemetics: (a) prochlorperazine; (b) dimenhydrinate; (c) metoclopramide; (d) prednisone; (e) Hycosin/atropine; and (f) ondansetron.
4. Consider combination of antiemetics if one is not sufficient.
5. If vomiting continues, consider suppository or subcutaneous route.

B. Constipation:
1. Attempt to find the cause—do not automatically assume it is from taking narcotics.
2. Lactulose appears to be the agent of choice for the treatment of constipation in palliative care. A combination of a stool softener and a peristaltic stimulant is a good alternative.

C. Anorexia:
1. Eat small, frequent meals
2. Avoid blended, pulverized foods; give the patient what he or she wants to eat.
3. Megestrol acetate is most the most effective agent for treating anorexia and cachexia in patients who are terminally ill. Prednisone is a good alternative.

D. Dry mouth/oral thrush:
1. Mouth care is very important.
2. Avoid drying agents such as lemon-glycerine swabs.
3. Hydrogen peroxide at one-fourth strength, lemon drops, pineapple chunks, and tart juices are helpful.
4. Look for oral thrush every day; treat with clotrimazole troches. If treatment is resistant, prescribe Diflucan.

E. Dehydration: Dehydration is usually not symptomatic; that is, it usually does not have to be treated. Always base your decision to use fluids on whether you think it will make the patient feel better and improve the patient's quality of life. Remember, the most common occurrence from treating patients receiving palliative care with IV fluids is iatrogenic pulmonary edema.

F. Diarrhea:
1. Try to identify the cause.
2. Diphenoxylate, loperamide, and codeine are equally effective.

G. Dyspnea and pleural effusion: Open windows, supplementary oxygen, semi-Fowler's position, bronchodilators, prednisone, narcotic analgesics, anxiolytics, diuretics, and palliative radiotherapy may all be of help with recurrent pleural effusions. Treat first occurrence with thoracocentesis. How often you repeat this procedure depends on the patient's comfort level and how quickly the fluid reaccumulates.

H. Partial bowel obstruction:
1. Restrict fluids.
2. Antiemetics: consider prokinetic agents such as metoclopramide first
3. Corticosteroids: prednisone
4. Narcotic analgesics
5. Try to avoid the use of a NG tube if possible

I. Malignant ascites:
1. Paracentesis is often effective: how often you perform this procedure is again dependent on the reaccumulation of fluid.
2. Spironolactone alone or with thiazide and/or loop diuretics may be helpful.

J. Cerebral edema: Dexamethasone with an H_2 receptor antagonist is both diagnostic and therapeutic.

K. Fungating growths:
1. Frequent dressing changes; normal saline or hydrogen peroxide
2. Yogurt or buttermilk dressings
3. Charcoal briquettes around the house
4. Fresh air

L. Depression and anxiety:
1. Remember bio-psycho-social-spiritual model of pain and symptom control
2. Psychotherapy: "be there, be sensitive, be silent"
3. Antidepressant medication
4. Anxiolytics (sublingual especially effective)

M. Hypercalcemia:
1. Most common serious metabolic abnormality in palliative care
2. Think about the diagnosis: otherwise, you will not make it
3. Fluids will treat hypercalcemia effectively in most cases

SUGGESTED READING

National Cancer Institute, Cancer Net. Pain Management, 1999, http://www.nci.nih.gov.

Rakel RE, Bope ET, eds.: *Conn's Current Therapy 2003*. Pain Management. WB Saunders, 2002, Philadelphia, pgs. 1-10.

Rueben D, et al: *Geriatrics 2003. Palliative and end of life care*. American Geriatric Society, 121-125, 2003.

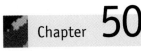

Chapter 50

Travel Medicine

> "Oh my stomach. I never thought about not using the local ice."

CLINICAL CASE PROBLEM 1:
A 42-YEAR-OLD MALE FILLED WITH TROPICAL DELIGHTS

A 42-year-old male and his life partner take a yachting vacation in the Caribbean. One night after a fabulous landside feast from the sea's bounty, including sea bass, red snapper, and a variety of tropical fish, the patient pays a visit to your dispensary complaining of nausea, vomiting, weakness, numbness and "lighteninglike" discomfort in his face and hands, and chills. His vital signs are as follows temperature 97° F orally, blood pressure 90/50 mm Hg, pulse 110 beats per minute, and respiration 20 breaths per minute. He appears ill. After supportive measures that you take, he improves in 24 hours.

SELECT THE BEST ANSWER TO THE FOLLOWING QUESTIONS:

1. Which of the following is the most likely cause of his symptoms?
   a. *Escherichia coli*
   b. *Vibrio cholera*
   c. ciguatoxin
   d. Norwalk virus
   e. giardiasis

CLINICAL CASE PROBLEM 2:
MORE TROPICAL DELIGHTS

He recovers, but several days later, his partner, who is 40 years old, drops by after another land excursion. He too has sampled the sea's bounty, but he carefully avoided eating what his friend had had the day he became sick. He stuck to mahimahi and yellow-fin tuna. After arriving back on board, he began to experience headache, flushing, hives, diarrhea, and vomiting. His physical examination reveals normal vital signs, urticarial wheals, and diffuse epidermal erythema. You take appropriate action, and he recovers.

2. The most likely cause of his symptoms is:
   a. ciguatoxin
   b. an insect bite
   c. scorpion bite
   d. histidine poisoning
   e. *E. coli*

CLINICAL CASE PROBLEM 3:

AN "ECOTOUR" WITH UNINTENTIONAL SAMPLING OF THE ECOSYSTEM

A 67-year-old female comes to your office 2 weeks after she returns from an "ecotour" to the Central American rainforest. She is an infrequent visitor to your office, and her health maintenance protocols are not up-to-date, nor did she consult you prior to her trip. She tells you that she "went native," which she explains means she ate and drank local foods and water, carefully not disturbing the local environment. Near the end of her trip, she developed nausea and vomiting, followed by persistent diarrhea, fever, and chills. All other symptoms have abated, but the diarrhea persists. The diarrhea is not bloody.

On examination, pulse is 80 beats per minutes, respirations are 16 per minute, blood pressure is 140/85 mm Hg, and temperature is 99.4° F. Aside for some increased bowel sounds and diffuse mild abdominal discomfort with deep palpation, the rest of her examination is normal. There is no blood or stool on rectal examination.

3. You order appropriate tests, which would include which of the following?
   a. complete blood count (CBC)
   b. stool culture
   c. stool for ova and parasites
   d. b and c
   e. no tests are necessary at this time

One week later she returns to your office complaining of passing tea-colored urine. Examination is normal. Previous tests have proved to be negative. You order blood work to confirm your hypothesis.

4. The most likely explanation of the patient's complaints is:
   a. *E. coli*
   b. hepatitis A
   c. giardiasis
   d. schistosomiasis
   e. shigella

CLINICAL CASE PROBLEM 4:

PLANNING A TRIP

A 35-year-old female comes for an office visit for advice regarding an upcoming trip overseas to the rural area of a developing country. She wonders what precautions she should take to avoid traveler's diarrhea.

5. Which of the following is (are) good advice to give her?
   a. avoid local sources of water that are not boiled
   b. avoid eating raw vegetables, salads, and unpasteurized milk
   c. do not use ice in drinks
   d. peel your own fruit
   e. all of the above

6. You review her immunizations. She has not received any since childhood. Which of the following would you recommend?
   a. tetanus and IPV
   b. hepatitis A
   c. hepatitis B
   d. a, b, and c
   e. a only

7. Which of the following are good traveler advice and precautions for trips to mosquito-infested areas?
   a. bring diethylmethyltoluamide (DEET)-based insect repellent
   b. do not use DEET on children older than age 2
   c. purchase permethrin impregnated bed netting if sleeping outdoors
   d. wear short-sleeve shirts and short pants sprayed with insect repellent
   e. a and c

CLINICAL CASE PROBLEM 5:

A 51-YEAR-OLD MALE WHO IS PLANNING ON TRAVELING TO AFRICA

A 51-year-old male comes to your office for a periodic health examination. He is planning on traveling to equatorial Africa in the near future and wishes to discuss immunizations and prophylaxis against malaria. He is feeling well. He has had no major medical problems in the past, nor has he had any surgeries. He has no known allergies. His examination is appropriate and normal for his age. You check the Centers for Disease Control and Prevention (CDC) Website, and there are no reports of drug resistance in the areas to which he is traveling.

8. What is the primary chemoprophylactic agent for the prevention of malaria in non-drug resistant areas of the world?
   a. chloroquine
   b. mefloquine
   c. pyrimethamine

d. dapsone

e. proguanil

9. The drug of choice you selected in Question 8 should be given for the following length of time:
    a. 1 week before travel and for a minimum of 4 weeks after return from travel
    b. 1 month before travel and for at least 1 month after return
    c. 2 weeks before travel and for at least 2 weeks after return
    d. 1 week before travel and for 1 week after return
    e. 6 weeks before travel and for at least 4 weeks after return

10. The drug of choice you selected in Question 8 was chosen primarily for its activity against which of the following?
    a. *Plasmodium falciparum*
    b. *P. vivax*
    c. *P. ovale*
    d. *P. malariae*
    e. none of the above

11. Which of the following symptoms is (are) common in clinical malaria?
    a. fever or chills
    b. diarrhea
    c. headache
    d. myalgias
    e. all of the above

■ ANSWERS:

1. c. This patient is exhibiting the classic features of the most common type of biotoxin in fish, ciguatoxin. Found in such commonly ingested tropical fish as red snapper, grouper, sea bass, and a wide range of reef fish, the potential for ciguatera poisoning exists in all subtropical and tropical insular areas of the Caribbean and the Pacific and Indian Oceans where these species thrive. Ciguatera poisoning is manifested by the following symptoms: gastroenteritis followed by neurologic problems such as weakness; paresthesias and dysesthesias; body temperature reversals; and, in severe cases, hypotension. Although the other choices are possibilities in gastrointestinal disturbances, the timing and history fits best with this explanation.

2. d. Another classical case of fish poisoning is exhibited by this patient; this time it is histidine poisoning, commonly seen after ingesting members of the Scombroid family of fish (tuna, mackerel, and bonito) and sometimes called Scombroid poisoning. Occurring after ingestion of fish that has been refrigerated or preserved improperly, histidine is converted to histamine and causes headache, flushing, nausea and vomiting, diarrhea, and hives. Other fish, particularly the popular bluefish, mahimahi, and herring, also can cause histidine poisoning; cases are distributed worldwide.

3. d. Given the patient's fever has resolved, but that it has been 2 weeks, it would be appropriate to culture the stool and check for ova and parasites. An argument might be made for watchful waiting because most domestic diarrheal illnesses resolve spontaneously, but this patient has been out of the country, which makes the possibility of parasites much more likely.

4. b. All prior tests are negative, and the tea-colored urine consistent with bilirubin cinches it, along with the incubation period, which is just about right for hepatitis A. Unfortunately, hepatitis A is often a common consequence of unimmunized travel to developing countries, the virus being spread via the fecal–oral route, most commonly through ingesting contaminated foods or water.

5. e. Ingestion of contaminated food and drink is the most common sources of infection during travel. The list of common infections occurring secondary to ingestion include *E. coli*, Shigella, giardiasis, cryptosporidiosis, Norwalk-like viruses (often seen in cruise ship outbreaks), and hepatitis A. Less common infections include typhoid fever (Salmonella), cholera, rotavirus infections, and a variety of parasites other than Giardia and cryptosporidium. To avoid illness, the CDC recommends selecting food with care. Avoid raw food such as salads and uncooked vegetables, sushi (raw fish), and unpasteurized milk and milk products such as cheese. Peel your own fruit. Avoid undercooked and raw meat and shellfish. Commercially available bottled water is safest, and do not use ice in drinks because it may be made from contaminated water sources. Bear in mind on trips home that food and water on commercial aircraft may be obtained in the country of departure where items may be contaminated.

6. d. Given this patient's age and immunization history, it is unlikely that she received hepatitis A, B, or tetanus prophylaxis. An inactivated polio vaccine booster now is recommended by the CDC committee on immunization practices for travel to many countries. Hopefully she has allowed sufficient time for more than the initial shots in the hepatitis series; nevertheless they all should be administered as soon as possible. In cases where poor planning or circumstance does not allow for the normal administration schedule, an accelerated schedule exists for administering hepatitis B vaccine with doses at days 0, 7, and 14. Hepatitis A immune globulin is also an option in such circumstances. The clinician also should check the CDC Website (http://www.cdc.gov) for the traveler's destination points to see if there are additional immunizations and precautions required. Many areas have cholera and yellow fever endemics, for which there are effective vaccines. Malaria is also common in many parts of the world, and it is a disease for which there is effective prophylaxis. Rabies prophylaxis is also available, given the need. The CDC Website also should be checked for the notification of possible communicable illness outbreaks.

7. **e.** Mosquito and other arthropod-borne illnesses are a serious concern for travelers. Malaria, Dengue fever, West Nile fever, and various encephalopathies are all capable of producing significant morbidity and mortality. Protecting oneself from the insect carriers of these diseases is important. Topical insect repellents containing DEET are most effective, but they should not be used in infants younger than age 2. Bed netting, proper clothing that covers skin surfaces as much as possible, and insect repellents for exposed areas are all good precautions.

8. **b.** Recommendations from the CDC are as follows: "For travel to areas of risk where chloroquine-resistant *P. falciparum* has NOT been reported, once-a-week use of chloroquine alone should be recommended for primary prophylaxis. Persons who experience uncomfortable side effects after taking chloroquine may tolerate the drug better by taking it with meals. As an alternative, the related compound hydroxychloroquine sulfate may be better tolerated. Travelers unable to take chloroquine or hydroxy-chloroquine should take atovaquone/proguanil, doxy-cycline, or mefloquine; these antimalarials are also effective against chloroquine-sensitive parasites." Generally, mefloquine 250 mg once a week is the drug of choice for travel to areas with chloroquine-resistant malaria.

9. **a.** The usual recommendation is that treatment begins 1 week before traveling to the malaria-infected area and continues for 4 weeks after the return home.

10. **a.** There are several strains of plasmodium that cause malaria. They are: *P. falciparum, P. ovale, P. vivax,* and *P. malariae.* Most of the concern arises over *P. falciparum;* it is crucial that treatment be directed to the most virulent and morbidity-producing strain. In addition, drug resistance has been seen primarily in *P. falciparum;* with only a few exceptions the others remain sensitive to chloroquine.

11. **e.** Typical symptoms of malaria include fever, chills, myalgia, arthralgias, and headache. Abdominal pain, cough, and diarrhea also may occur. Frequent clinical and laboratory findings include hepatospleno-megaly, anemia, and thrombocytopenia. Pulmonary or renal dysfunction (in the absence of dehydration) and changes in mental status may complicate *P. falciparum* malaria.

SUMMARY OF TRAVEL MEDICINE

"The world is getting smaller" is more than just a cliché. Infectious and communicable diseases respect no political boundaries, and increasingly mobile populations make the spread of once geographically limited or confined illnesses no longer unusual. The best medicine here is prevention.

Avoid areas of local epidemics and take precautions if this is unavoidable.

Travel insurance is important and less costly than the alternative, particularly if air transportation/ evacuation becomes necessary to access medical care.

Protection from arthropod-borne illnesses is key in warmer climates and primarily involves the use of protective clothing, protected sleep environment, and the application of the insect repellent DEET.

In rural or developing areas, avoid local drinking water supplies and food that is not thoroughly cooked.

Immunize against common infectious illnesses such as hepatitis A and B. Remember that seasonal differences may exist in travel to different hemi-spheres, necessitating influenza vaccination. If traveling to malaria endemic areas, begin prophy-laxis with appropriate medications.

Always check the CDC Website for the most up-to-date, geographically specific travel–related information.

SUGGESTED READING

The best and most up-to-date advice for health professionals and travelers may be found at the CDC's Traveler's Health Website at http://www.cdc.gov.

Kaplan DH: Holiday hazards: common stings from New World visits. *Clin Exp Dermatol* 28(1):85-88, 2003.

Katz BZ: Traveling with children. *Pediatr Infect Dis J* 22(3):274-276, 2003.

Moore DA, et al: Assessing the severity of malaria. *BMJ* 326(7393): 808-809, 2003.

Ryan ET, et al: Illness after international travel. *N Engl J Med* 347(7): 505-516, 2002.

Zuckerman JN: Recent developments: Travel medicine. *BMJ* 325(7358): 260-264, 2002.

WOMEN'S HEALTH

Chapter 51

Osteoporosis

> "I don't believe you, Doctor. How could me not drinking milk 50 years ago have anything to do with me breaking my hip yesterday?"

CLINICAL CASE PROBLEM 1:
A 61-Year-Old Postmenopausal Woman

A 61-year-old postmenopausal woman comes to your office for a routine health examination. She has a history of osteoarthritis and smokes one pack of cigarettes per day. Her blood pressure is 120/80, her height is 5 foot 3 inches, and her weight is 115 lb. The rest of her physical examination is normal. Her diet is low in calcium-rich foods, and she is not currently taking a calcium supplement.

■ **SELECT THE BEST ANSWER TO THE FOLLOWING QUESTIONS:**

1. You feel she is at risk for osteoporosis. You initially recommend that she:
   a. obtain a central dual-energy x-ray absorptiometry (DXA) scan
   b. start taking a bisphosphonate immediately
   c. order serum calcium, thyroid stimulating hormone (TSH), 25-hydroxyvitamin D
   d. obtain a lateral spine x-ray
   e. obtain a quantitative computed tomography (QCT) scan

2. The test of choice in the diagnosis of osteoporosis is:
   a. qualitative ultrasound densitometry
   b. peripheral DXA
   c. central DXA
   d. a QCT
   e. plain x-ray of the thoracic spine

3. Which of the following is not an established major risk factor for osteoporosis?
   a. weight less than 140 lb
   b. current smoking
   c. personal history of fracture without substantial trauma
   d. age older than 65
   e. chronic use of steroids

4. According to the National Osteoporosis Foundation (NOF), under what circumstances would primary screening for osteoporosis be appropriate?
   a. a 28-year-old female athlete with a 5-year history of amenorrhea
   b. a 40-year-old female with regular menses who smokes two packs of cigarettes per day
   c. a 68-year-old female with no risk factors
   d. a 35-year-old female with regular menses with multiple fractures after a motor vehicle accident
   e. a 40-year-old male who smokes two packs of cigarettes per day

5. According to the World Health Organization (WHO), osteoporosis is defined as:
   a. bone mineral density (BMD) between 1.5 to 2.0 standard deviations *below the mean* for young normal adults (T score)
   b. BMD is between 1.5 to 2.0 standard deviations *below the mean for* age-matched adults (Z score)
   c. BMD is less than 2.5 standard deviations *below the mean* for young normal adults (T score)
   d. BMD is less than 2.5 standard deviations *below the mean* for age-matched adults (Z score)
   e. osteoporosis is not defined by bone mineral density at all

6. Which of the following *is not* an associated risk factor associated with osteoporosis?
   a. impaired vision
   b. sedentary lifestyle
   c. cigarette smoking
   d. obesity
   e. excessive alcohol intake

7. What is the most common presenting fracture in osteoporosis?
   a. wrist fracture (Colles' fracture)
   b. vertebral compression fracture
   c. femoral neck fracture
   d. tibial fracture
   e. femoral head fracture

8. Which of the following sites for osteoporotic fracture is associated most commonly with morbidity and mortality?
   a. the head of the femur
   b. the neck of the femur

c. the thoracic vertebrae
d. the lumbar vertebrae
e. the distal radius

9. Which of the following conditions is not associated with an increased risk for osteoporosis?
   a. hyperparathyroidism
   b. Cushing's syndrome
   c. history of solid organ transplant
   d. chronic dilantin therapy
   e. history of osteoarthritis

10. You order a central DXA scan on the patient in Clinical Case Problem 1. The scan returns with a T score of –1.3 for the lumbar spine and a T score of –2.0 for the total hip. What do you recommend to the patient at this time?
    a. no action needed; her lumbar spine reading does not qualify her for treatment
    b. repeat a central DXA in 6 months
    c. recommend adequate calcium intake and weight-bearing exercise
    d. recommend adequate calcium intake, weight-bearing exercise, and starting alendronate
    e. recommend adequate calcium intake, weight-bearing exercise, and starting raloxifene

11. Which of the following is not a therapy approved by the U.S. Food and Drug Administration (FDA) for the prevention of osteoporosis?
    a. bisphosphonates
    b. selective estrogen receptor modulators (SERMS)
    c. calcium supplementation
    d. calcitonin
    e. combined estrogen and progestin hormone replacement therapy (HRT)

12. Which of the following statements regarding the use of calcium in the prevention and treatment of osteoporosis is true?
    a. calcium supplementation should begin at menopause
    b. calcium supplementation should begin after confirmed osteoporotic fracture
    c. calcium supplementation should consist of 1000-1500 mg a day with 400-800 IU of vitamin D
    d. calcium supplementation is not necessary in non-Asian, non-white women
    e. none of the above

13. Which of the following statements about calcium supplementation is true?
    a. calcium carbonate absorption is best in an acidic environment

b. calcium carbonate absorption is not dependent on pH
c. calcium citrate is not recommended in elderly patients
d. calcium citrate is not recommended in patients taking antacids
e. none of the above

14. Which of the following is not recommended for treatment of established osteoporosis?
    a. combined HRT
    b. calcium and vitamin D
    c. bisphosphonates
    d. SERMs
    e. calcitonin

15. All of the following studies may be indicated in an asymptomatic patient recently diagnosed with osteoporosis except:
    a. serum calcium
    b. serum 25-hydroxyvitamin D
    c. plain thoracic spine x-ray
    d. serum phosphate
    e. TSH

16. The following statements about BMD testing are true except:
    a. it is appropriate in patients who have evidence of osteopenia on plain x-ray
    b. Medicare does not cover BMD testing in any situation
    c. it is appropriate to repeat testing to monitor long-term treatment of osteoporosis
    d. it is appropriate to repeat testing every 1-2 years in at-risk patients
    e. none of the above

CLINICAL CASE PROBLEM 2:
A Concerned Patient

One of your patients with confirmed osteoporosis returns to your office after taking a bisphosphonate for 5 months. Her initial lab work was normal including TSH, serum calcium, and 25-hydroxyvitamin D. A baseline urine N-telopeptide level was done prior to the initiation of bisphosphonate therapy. The patient has followed your recommendations concerning weight-bearing exercises and calcium intake. She wants to know if the "treatments have worked."

17. Which of the following choices can you tell her may assess the effectiveness of her treatment at this time?
    a. repeat DXA
    b. plain x-ray of the hip
    c. repeat serum calcium level

d. repeat urine N-telopeptide level
e. there is no test that will reflect treatment efficacy at this time

CLINICAL CASE MANAGEMENT PROBLEM

Discuss nonpharmacologic measures that may be used in the prevention and treatment of osteoporosis.

■ ANSWERS:

1. a. A DXA is the gold standard for assessment of BMD. During this procedure two beams of different energy are directed at the patient. The difference in the absorption rate of the two energy beams by the patient's body is recorded to quantify the amount of bone mineral content. A BMD is computed at different sites including lumbar spine, femoral neck, greater trochanter, total hip, and Wards triangle (a computer-generated area that should not be used for diagnosis). Of all measurements, total hip BMD is the best predictor of future hip fracture. Advantages of central DXA include higher precision, minimal radiation exposure, and rapid scanning time. Disadvantages include cost and nonportability, which can make widespread screening in disadvantaged populations challenging.

QCT scans can selectively measure BMD and exclude extraosseous calcium deposits. However, QCT cannot assess BMD at the proximal femur and has relatively high doses of radiation. Central DXA BMD also has better correlation with fracture risk than QCT scan. A lateral spine x-ray may reveal evidence of vertebral compression fractures or osteopenia, which should make one suspicious of osteoporosis; but it is not a good screening tool in asymptomatic patients. Starting a bisphosphonate or laboratory assessment for secondary causes of osteoporosis is not appropriate until a diagnosis of osteopenia or osteoporosis has been established.

2. c. As discussed earlier, central DXA is the gold standard for assessment of BMD. QCT scan is discussed earlier as well. Peripheral bone densitometry devices use a variety of techniques including single-energy x-ray absorptiometry, DXA, and QCT. Peripheral quantitative ultrasound (QUS) is yet another method of assessing BMD. Measurement sites include the finger, forearm, and heel. Advantages of these modalities include less expense, easier portability, and relatively low to no radiation exposure. Although not considered equivalent to central DXA in terms of accuracy, recent research has indicated that peripheral site testing can predict short-term fracture risk. However, peripheral BMD devices should not be used for diagnosing osteoporosis or for monitoring patients receiving pharmacologic treatment for osteoporosis.

3. a. Of the major risk factors for osteoporosis, patient age is most consistently associated with increased risk of osteoporosis. Compared to women aged 50-54 years, there is a 5.9-fold higher risk of osteoporosis in women aged 65-69 and a 14.3-fold higher risk in women aged 75-79. Low body mass and hypoestrogenic state also consistently are associated with osteoporosis but less so than is age. A summary of established major risk factors for osteoporosis include the following: (1) age older than 65 years; (2) female sex; (3) postmenopausal status or hypoestrogenic state (menopause prior to age 45, bilateral oophorectomy); (4) low body weight (less than 127 lb [not less than 140 lb, as in question]); (5) white or Asian race; (6) personal history of fracture as an adult not associated with major trauma; (7) history of fragility fracture in a first-degree relative; (8) current cigarette smoking; and (9) oral corticosteroid therapy for more than 3 months.

4. c. The NOF expert panel recommends that all women age 65 years and older be screened for osteoporosis regardless of presence or absence of risk factors. Younger postmenopausal women with one or more risk factors (other than being white, postmenopausal and female) should also be screened for BMD (see major risk factors listed in A3). Although in practice these guidelines are extrapolated for all women and even men in some cases, the NOF's guidelines are based on studies done primarily on postmenopausal white women only. Data on men and women of other races are insufficient at this time to make definitive recommendations specific for these population groups. When deciding who to screen for osteoporosis, physicians should make recommendations that account for an individual's risk factors, willingness to start treatment, and preference. The United States Preventive Services Task Force (USPSTF) also recommends universal BMD screening for all women 65 and older. For women age 60 and older, the USPSTF recommends screening if there are risk factors for osteoporotic fractures. In contrast to the NOF, the USPSTF makes no recommendation for or against routine screening in postmenopausal women younger than age 60 or aged 60-64 without increased risk for osteoporotic fracture.

The patient described in choice a may suffer from the "female athlete triad," a condition commonly found in high-level competitive female athletes. The "triad" consists of an eating disorder, osteoporosis, and amenorrhea. Although this patient is certainly at risk for fracture later in adult life if this condition continues, there are no guidelines that recommend screening women at this young age. Medical attention should focus on correcting the underlying problem and encouraging adequate calcium intake. The patients described in choices b and d have risk factors associated with osteoporosis but are premenopausal and too young to recommend for screening. Of note, a "fragility" fracture is one not associated with major trauma such as a motor vehicle accident.

5. c. BMD measurements are reported as the number of standard deviations (SD) from the mean BMD in a young healthy female reference population (T score) or an age-matched reference population (Z score). WHO defines "normal" as a BMD T score above –1.0. Osteopenia is defined as a T score from –1.0 to –2.5. Osteoporosis is defined as a T score at or less than –2.5 (e.g., –2.6 to –4.0). Osteopenia and osteoporosis are not defined by Z scores.

6. d. The major risk factors for osteoporosis are discussed earlier in the chapter. Other associated risk factors for osteoporosis include impaired vision, frailty, poor health, heavy alcohol intake, and sedentary lifestyle. Chronic use of medications such as anticonvulsants (dilantin, phenobarbital), heparin, gonadotropin-releasing hormone (GnRH) agonists, immunosuppressants (tacrolimus, cyclosporine), and glucocorticoids is also a risk factor. Obesity appears to be protective against osteoporosis.

7. b. Vertebral compression fracture is the most common presenting fracture in osteoporosis. Wrist fracture is the second most common.

8. b. Femoral neck fracture is the most common cause of osteoporosis-related morbidity and mortality. Hip fractures in general can result in up to 10% to 20% of excess mortality within a year.

9. e. Many chronic medical conditions are associated with an increased risk of osteoporosis. Examples include hyperparathyroidism, hypogonadism, Cushing's syndrome, history of solid organ transplant (osteoporosis is secondary to chronic immunosuppression), multiple myeloma, and any malabsorptive syndromes (i.e., celiac sprue). A history of osteoarthritis may mimic symptoms of vertebral compression fracture pain but is not directly a risk factor for osteoporosis.

10. d. The decision to treat for osteoporosis should be based on the lowest T score measured. The NOF recommends treatment for patients with T scores below –2.0 by central DXA regardless of risk factors, for patients with T scores below –1.5 by central DXA if one or more risk factors are present, and for all patients who have had osteoporotic fractures. These guidelines are based on central DXA BMD measure-

ments and cannot be extrapolated to measurements made by other bone densitometry devices. The patient in this question should be considered for pharmacologic treatment of osteoporosis given her T score of –2.0 at the hip and her multiple risk factors (smoking, low body weight). Of note, central DXA BMD measurements may be falsely elevated in the lumbar spine secondary to osteoarthritic changes. The patient in this case does have a history of osteoarthritis, which may account for her higher vertebral BMD reading in comparison to her hip BMD.

Once the decision is made to initiate treatment, all patients should be counseled to engage in weight-bearing exercise and adequate calcium/vitamin D intake (1500 mg elemental calcium and 400-800 IU vitamin D in a postmenopausal female).

First-line therapy for treatment of established osteoporosis of hip should include bisphosphonates, such as alendronate and risedronate. Bisphosphonates work by inhibiting osteoclastic activity and binding to hydroxyapatite to decrease bone resorption. The FDA has approved bisphosphonates for prevention and treatment of osteoporosis. Both alendronate and risedronate have been shown to reduce risk of both vertebral and hip fractures by 30% to 50% in patients with established osteoporosis. Because a minority of patients may suffer from erosive esophagitis, the patient should be advised to take bisphosphonates with 8 oz of water on awakening, remain upright, and avoid food for 30 minutes afterward. Raloxifene is a SERM. SERMS have either agonist or antagonist effects on estrogen receptors depending on the target organ site. At the bone, raloxifene selectively binds to estrogen receptors and inhibits bone resorption. Raloxifene is FDA approved for both the prevention and treatment of osteoporosis. Although raloxifene decreases the risk of vertebral fracture, there is no evidence that it decreases the risk of nonvertebral fractures including the hip. Hence, raloxifene would not be the therapy of choice in this patient who has osteoporosis of the hip. SERMs do not increase the risk of endometrial carcinoma or breast cancer. Patients should be warned that use of SERMs carries the same risk of thromboembolic events as oral estrogen therapy and an increased incidence of vasomotor symptoms (hot flashes).

11. d. Bisphosphonates and SERMs are both approved for the prevention of osteoporosis and are discussed in the previous question. Preliminary data from the HRT arm of the Women's Health Initiative (WHI) reveals that 0.625 mg/day of conjugated equine estrogen and 2.5 mg/day of medroxyprogesterone acetate (Prempro) reduced the number of hip and spine fractures by 33% in postmenopausal women aged 50-79 with an intact uterus. Unfortunately, the HRT arm of the study was stopped early secondary to an observed increased risk of stroke, coronary artery disease (CAD) events, pulmonary embolism, and invasive breast cancers. Absolute excess risks and benefits per 10,000 person years attributable to HRT were as follows: seven more CAD events, nine more strokes, eight more pulmonary embolisms, eight more invasive breast cancers, six fewer colorectal cancers, and five fewer hip fractures. Although the absolute risks and benefits per year are small, the cumulative risks and benefits over time may be more significant. It is not known whether such outcomes would occur with a different formulation or route of HRT. Physicians need to counsel their patients about the known risks and benefits of HRT and individualize treatment plans accordingly. Calcitonin is delivered by nasal spray and works by inhibition of osteoclast activity. It is FDA approved for the treatment of osteoporosis, but it is not for prevention. It has been shown to reduce vertebral fracture risk, but there is no evidence demonstrating significant hip-fracture risk reduction. There are small trials that suggest that calcitonin may be helpful as analgesia for vertebral compression fractures. Combination therapy of two agents (i.e., bisphosphonate with nonbisphosphonate) may provide small additional gains in BMD, but it is unclear what long-term benefits are gained (i.e., fracture reduction). Cost and risk of side effects need to be considered before prescribing combination therapy. Adequate calcium intake is recommended for prevention of osteoporosis in all patients.

12. c. The NOF recommends that all individuals obtain at least 1200 mg of calcium per day. The specific age at which calcium supplementation should be started is unclear; however, it is reasonable to begin supplementation in the early to mid adult years to maintain bone mass later in life.

A general guideline is 1000-1200 mg for premenopausal patients and postmenopausal patients taking HRT, 1500 mg for postmenopausal patients not taking HRT, and 1500 mg for patients with established osteoporosis or who are older than 65 years old. The average postmenopausal woman consumes about 600 mg of dietary calcium a day, necessitating supplementation in most patients. The NOF recommends 400-800 IU of vitamin D a day to maximize calcium absorption in patients at risk for vitamin D deficiency (dark-skinned patients, patients living in northern locations). Approximately 10-30 minutes per day of sun exposure to the hands, face, and arms a few times a week is needed to receive the daily recommended allowance of vitamin D. Many calcium supplements already contain vitamin D, and most milk is fortified with vitamin D. There is no need to wait until menopause or after confirmed osteoporotic fracture before beginning calcium

supplementation. Calcium supplementation should be recommended in all women, not just those of white or Asian origin, because female gender is a universal risk factor for osteoporosis.

Studies conducted during the past decade also suggest that sufficient intake of vitamin K will increase bone density and reduce fractures. This vitamin is an essential cofactor in the gamma-carboxylation of osteocalcin—a bone protein believed to be involved in mineralization and also may affect calcium balance positively. Thus for optimal bone health and to reduce the risk of osteoporosis, throughout life diets should contain sufficient calcium, vitamin D, and vitamin K; a diet rich in leafy green vegetables should supply adequate amount of the latter. For optimal response, weight-bearing exercise, properly adapted for the state of health and age, also should be added to this regimen.

13. a. Calcium carbonate absorption is dependent on an acidic environment. Patients with chronic achlorhydria may not absorb calcium carbonate as effectively. Calcium citrate is effective regardless of pH and may be a better choice in patients with achlorhydria, such as the elderly or patients receiving proton pump inhibitors, H_2 blockers, or antacids.

14. a. As discussed earlier, bisphosphonates, SERMS (raloxifene), calcitonin, and calcium supplementation are recommended treatments for established osteoporosis. Parathyroid hormone therapy works by increasing bone formation and has been shown to decrease both vertebral and nonvertebral fractures. However, its use is limited given its cost and need for injection therapy. HRT is FDA approved for prevention of osteoporosis but not for treatment of osteoporosis.

15. c. An evaluation for secondary causes of osteoporosis may be appropriate in patients in whom vitamin D deficiency, renal insufficiency or other underlying pathology is suspected. Reasonable laboratory studies include serum calcium and phosphorus, parathyroid hormone level, 25-hydroxyvitamin D, and TSH. A plain thoracic spine x-ray in an asymptomatic patient is unlikely to yield useful information that will guide management.

16. b. An appropriate indication for BMD testing includes confirming suspicion of osteoporosis when a patient has an incidental finding of osteopenia noted on plain film x-ray. A patient must lose about one-third of bone mass to have evidence of osteopenia on plain film and is at high risk for osteoporosis. Central DXA testing is also appropriate to follow treatment for osteoporosis at 1-2 year intervals. It also is recommended to continue primary BMD screening in patients who are at risk for osteoporosis at 1-2 year intervals. Medicare *does* cover BMD testing for patients ages 65 and older under the following conditions: (1) hypoestrogenic women at risk for osteoporosis; (2) vertebral abnormalities; (3) chronic steroid therapy; (4) primary hyperparathyroidism; and (5) monitoring response to an approved osteoporosis drug therapy.

17. d. It generally is recommended that central DXAs be repeated no sooner than 1-2 years from initiation

or change in drug therapy to detect significant changes in BMD. It is also important to note that drug therapy may decrease fracture risk without an apparent increase in BMD. Plain x-rays of the hip are not recommended for monitoring treatment efficacy for osteoporosis. Some experts recommend using urine N-telopeptide levels to monitor drug treatment progress. N-telopeptide is a marker of increased bone turnover and may decline within 90 days of treatment and thus would be a measure of therapeutic success within the 5-month period indicated.

SOLUTION TO THE CLINICAL CASE MANAGEMENT PROBLEM

There are multiple nonpharmacologic strategies that should be used in conjunction with medical therapy to decrease a patient's risk of morbidity and mortality from osteoporosis. All patients should have adequate calcium and vitamin D intake. All patients should engage in weight-bearing exercise if possible. Other benefits of regular exercise include improved flexibility, strength, and agility. To minimize risk of falls, attention should be directed toward assessment of patient's vision and gait. Any visual deficits should be corrected as best as possible.

Physical therapy and/or referral to a physiatrist may be helpful for a comprehensive gait and fall risk evaluation. A home safety assessment may identify potentially correctable hazards that can lead to falls. "Hip protectors" are anatomically designed pads that can be worn in the patient's undergarment and have been shown to reduce the rate of hip fractures, particularly in frail, elderly patients. However, rates of compliance can be low because of patient concerns about comfort and appearance.

SUMMARY OF OSTEOPOROSIS

Major risk factors for osteoporosis include the following: (1) age older than 65 years; (2) female sex; (3) postmenopausal status or hypoestrogenic state (menopause prior to age 45, bilateral oophorectomy); (4) low body weight (less than 127 lb); (5) white or Asian race; (6) personal history of fracture as an adult not associated with major trauma; (7) history of fragility fracture in a first-degree relative; (8) current cigarette smoking; and (9) oral corticosteroid therapy for more than 3 months.

Other risk factors for morbidity associated with osteoporosis include the following: (1) impaired vision; (2) frailty/poor health; (3) excessive alcohol intake; (4) sedentary lifestyle; and (5) chronic use of certain medications (anticonvulsants, heparin, GnRH agonists, immunosuppressants, and glucocorticoids).

NOF guidelines for screening are as follows: (1) all women aged 65 and older and (2) younger postmenopausal women with one or more risk factors (other than being white, postmenopausal, and female). USPSTF guidelines for screening are as follows: (1) all women aged 65 and older; begin at

age 60 for women at increased risk for osteoporotic fractures (B recommendation); (2) no recommendation for or against screening in postmenopausal women younger than age 60 or in women aged 60-64 not at increased risk for osteoporotic fractures (C recommendation).

Other conditions in which BMD testing is appropriate are as follows: (1) evidence of osteopenia on x-ray; (2) to monitor response to treatment; and (3) to rescreen at-risk individuals every 1-2 years if initial testing is normal.

WHO criteria for osteoporosis and osteopenia based on central DEXA BMD testing are as follows: (1) normal = T score higher than –1.0; (2) osteopenia = T score from –1.0 to –2.5; (3) osteoporosis = T score at or less than –2.5; and (4) osteopenia and osteoporosis are not defined by Z scores.

NOF recommendations for treatment based on central DEXA BMD are as follows: (1) patients with a T score less than –2.0; (2) patients with a T score of less than –1.5 if one or more risk factors are present; and (3) patients who already have had osteoporotic fracture(s).

Recommended therapies for prevention and treatment of osteoporosis include the following:

a. for ALL patients: calcium supplementation (at least 1200 mg/day), vitamin D supplementation (400-800 mg in individuals at risk for deficiency), and weight-bearing exercise
b. only for prevention of osteoporosis: HRT
c. only for treatment of osteoporosis: nasal calcitonin spray (Miacalcin)
d. for prevention and treatment of osteoporosis: bisphosphonates (effective for vertebral and nonvertebral sites), SERMS (effective for vertebral sites only), and parathyroid hormone (effective for vertebral and nonvertebral sites)

SUGGESTED READING

American College of Obstetricians and Gynecologists: *Committee Opinion: Bone Density Screening for Osteoporosis.* Washington DC, 270:523-525, 2002.
Booth SL, et al: Vitamin K intake and bone mineral density in woman and men. *Am J Clin Nutr* 77:512-516, 2003.
Miller PD, et al: Prediction of fracture risk in postmenopausal white women with peripheral bone densitometry: Evidence from the National Osteoporosis Risk Assessment. *J Bone Miner Res* 17(12): 2220-2230, 2002.
National Osteoporosis Foundation: Clinical Guidelines. http://www.nof.org. Accessed 9/17/2003.
United States Preventive Services Task Force. Guidelines on Osteoporosis Screening. http://www.ahcpr.gov/clinic/uspstfix.htm. Accessed 9/16/2003.

 Chapter **52**

Vulvovaginitis and Bacterial Vaginosis

"Oh, Doctor! It's so embarrassing, but I am simply on fire down below."

CLINICAL CASE PROBLEM 1:
A 21-YEAR-OLD FEMALE WITH VAGINAL ITCHING AND DISCHARGE

A 21-year-old woman comes to your office complaining of severe vulvovaginal itching and discharge. She has no urinary or other symptoms. She has been sexually active with the same male partner for more than a year. They use latex condoms, and she has been taking oral contraceptive pills for the past 3 months. She has no medical problems or history of sexually transmitted diseases (STDs). Her annual Papanicolaou (Pap) tests all have been normal. On inspection of the external genitalia, you note vulvar erythema and swelling. On speculum examination you note a thick, white, curdy discharge adherent to the vaginal walls with no odor. She has no vulvovaginal or cervical lesions. You perform a gross and microscopic examination of the vaginal discharge: The pH is 4.0; the whiff test is negative; the wet mount (saline-prepped slide) reveals no evidence of clue cells or trichomonads; and the KOH prepped slide reveals several pseudohyphae noted.

∎ SELECT THE BEST ANSWER TO THE FOLLOWING QUESTIONS:

1. What is the most likely diagnosis in this patient?
   a. physiologic discharge
   b. bacterial vaginosis (BV)
   c. vulvovaginal candidiasis
   d. trichomoniasis
   e. an allergic vaginitis secondary to latex condoms

2. Which of the following has not been shown to increase the risk for recurrence of this condition?
   a. high-carbohydrate diets
   b. diabetes mellitus
   c. oral contraceptives
   d. frequent/prolonged antibiotic use
   e. immunodeficiency

3. Which of the following is an appropriate treatment for this patient?
   a. metronidazole (500 mg orally [PO] for 7 days)
   b. yogurt with live acidophilus cultures (8 oz PO or 1 tsp intravaginally, four times daily [qid] for 7 days)
   c. terconazole cream (5 g intravaginally qD [every day] for 3 days)
   d. fluconazole (one dose of 150 mg PO)
   e. c and d

4. This patient returns 2 weeks later stating that she has not responded to the treatment you prescribed. What should you do next?
   a. repeat the same treatment, but double the dose
   b. repeat the same treatment, but double the duration of use
   c. reconsider the diagnosis, and reevaluate the patient
   d. apply topical metronidazole gel to her vulvar and vaginal areas
   e. reassure the patient that it often takes several weeks for symptoms to resolve

5. Which of the following therapies has been shown to be useful in this patient if this condition is recurrent/chronic?

a. a high-potency topical steroid cream applied intravaginally
b. oral steroids
c. boric acid
d. Minocin (100 mg PO twice daily [bid] for 1 month)
e. vinegar and water douches

6. Which of the following statements regarding vulvovaginal candidiasis is true?
   a. *Candida albicans* is the most common cause of vulvovaginal candidiasis
   b. *Candida glabrata* is not associated with chronic/recurrent vulvovaginal candidiasis
   c. all *Candida* species are equally sensitive to imidazole antifungal agents
   d. Pap tests are reliable tests for candidiasis
   e. intestinal *Candida* is the major source of recurrent vulvovaginal candidiasis

CLINICAL CASE PROBLEM 2:

A 29-Year-Old Female with a Malodorous Vaginal Discharge

A 29-year-old female comes to your office with a 2-week history of a persistent, malodorous vaginal discharge. The unpleasant "fishy" odor appears to worsen after sex. She denies any vaginal itching, urinary symptoms, or any other complaints. She is in a longstanding monogamous relationship with her husband who is asymptomatic. She has no history of STDs or abnormal Pap test results. She has been douching weekly for the last several months. On examination, there is a thin, milky, off-white discharge present at the introitus without any evidence of vulvar irritation. On speculum examination, the discharge is homogeneous and pooling on the floor of the vagina with no signs of vaginal or cervical inflammation. You perform a gross and microscopic examination of the vaginal discharge: the pH is 6.0; the whiff test is strongly positive; the wet mount slide reveals the presence of several clue cells but no trichomonads or polymorphonuclear/white blood cells (WBCs); and the KOH slide reveals no evidence of pseudohyphae or budding yeast cells.

7. What is the most likely diagnosis in this patient?
   a. physiologic discharge
   b. trichomoniasis
   c. candidiasis
   d. atrophic vaginitis
   e. BV

8. Which of the following statement(s) regarding this patient's condition is (are) true?
   a. it is considered a STD
   b. the partner should be treated to reduce recurrence

c. it is a potential cause of preterm labor
d. it is the result of an overgrowth of lactobacilli in the vagina
e. a and b

9. Which of the following is not an acceptable treatment for this patient's condition?
   a. metronidazole (500 mg PO bid for 7 days)
   b. metronidazole (2 g PO for one dose)
   c. metronidazole gel 0.75% (5 g intravaginally every hour of sleep [qhs] bid for 5 days)
   d. miconazole cream 2% (5 g intravaginally qD for 7 days)
   e. clindamycin cream 2% (5 g intravaginally qhs for 7 days)

10. What is the most common class of organisms associated with this patient's condition?
    a. aerobic bacteria
    b. anaerobic bacteria
    c. virus
    d. fungi/yeast
    e. protozoa

CLINICAL CASE PROBLEM 3:

A 17-Year-Old Female with Severe Pruritus and Malodorous Vaginal Discharge

A 17-year-old female comes to your office with her partner complaining of severe vaginal itching and malodorous discharge. She denies any fevers, chills, nausea, weakness, abdominal or pelvic pain, vaginal bleeding, or urinary symptoms. She has been sexually active since she was 13 years old and has had at least 10 different male sexual partners in the past. She has been with the same partner for the past 3 months. She has never kept her appointments for an initial Pap test, but she was treated for chlamydia a year ago. She also has been treated for several yeast infections over the past year. She has used condoms in the past, but her current partner refuses to wear them and "pulls out" before ejaculating. He is noticeably angry and accuses her of cheating on him. He denies any symptoms or history of STDs. On inspection of her external genitalia you find some vulvar edema and erythema. Speculum examination reveals copious, frothy, yellow-green, malodorous discharge with petechial-like lesions on the cervix. A bimanual examination reveals no cervical motion tenderness and no uterine or adnexal masses or tenderness. You perform a gross and microscopic examination of the vaginal discharge: the pH is 6.0; the whiff test is slightly positive; the wet mount reveals several motile flagellated organisms and many WBCs (>10/HPF) but no clue cells; and there are no pseudohyphae or budding yeast cells noted on the KOH slide.

11. What is the most likely diagnosis in this patient?
   a. candidiasis
   b. trichomoniasis
   c. BV
   d. physiologic discharge
   e. atrophic vaginitis

12. Which of the following statements is not true regarding this patient's condition?
   a. it is an STD
   b. it is a potential cause of preterm labor
   c. males with this condition are usually symptomatic
   d. Pap tests are not reliable diagnostic tests for this condition
   e. the organism that causes this condition is a protozoa

13. Which of the following are acceptable treatments for her condition?
   a. clindamycin phosphate cream (5 g intravaginally qhs for 5-7 days)
   b. metronidazole gel (5 g intravaginally bid for 3-5 days)
   c. metronidazole (500 mg bid for 7 days)
   d. metronidazole (2 g PO for one dose)
   e. c and d

14. Which of the following patient recommendations are appropriate for her condition?
   a. her asymptomatic partner also should be treated now to reduce her risk of recurrence
   b. she must avoid alcohol while taking the medication you prescribed for this condition
   c. the patient and her partner also should be screened for other STDs promptly
   d. she also should be screened for a history of domestic violence and sexual abuse
   e. all of the above

15. Which of the following are potential noninfectious causes of vulvovaginitis?
   a. estrogen deficiency
   b. latex allergy
   c. nonoxynol-9
   d. local anesthetics
   e. all of the above

CLINICAL CASE MANAGEMENT PROBLEM

Describe the differences between the presentation of vulvovaginal candidiasis, bacterial vaginosis, and trichomoniasis based on the characteristics of vaginal discharge, pH, whiff test, and microscopic findings.

ANSWERS:

1. c. This patient has the classic symptoms, signs, and microscopic examination findings for vulvovaginal candidiasis. *Candida albicans* is a commensal organism in most women. When *Lactobacillus acidophilus* and specific fungal inhibitory factors are suppressed, infection can result. Vulvovaginal pruritus, irritation, and external dysuria are the most common symptoms. Vulvovaginal erythema is a common finding; vulvar scaling and fissures also may be present.

The vaginal discharge may be normal or increased and usually is described as thick, white, and curdy, like cottage cheese, with no odor. It is usually adherent to the vaginal walls. The vaginal pH is usually normal (3.8-4.2); the whiff test is negative for an amine ("fishy") odor; and the microscopic examinations of wet mount and KOH preparations are positive for pseudohyphae, mycelial tangles, and/or budding yeast cells in 50% to 70% of patients with vulvovaginal candidiasis.

2. a. Although high-carbohydrate and other diets have been suggested as causes of recurrent vulvovaginal candidiasis, most studies have not supported dietary factors as a significant risk factor nor dietary restrictions as effective prevention. Frequent antibiotic use decreases the protective flora that usually prevents the proliferation of *Candida* species. The risk of a yeast infection appears to increase with the duration of antibiotic use, regardless of the antibiotic type. Hyperglycemia (diabetes mellitus), increased glycogen production, pregnancy, and altered estrogen and progesterone levels (via oral contraceptive pills) enhance the ability of *Candida* to bind to vaginal epithelial cells and facilitate their proliferation. Patients with impaired or deficient cell-mediated immunity are susceptible to vulvovaginal and systemic candidal infections. Other potential risk factors for vulvovaginal candidiasis include tight fitting/poorly ventilated clothes, mechanical vulvovaginal irritation (e.g., sexual intercourse), diaphragm/spermicide use, and intrauterine devices (IUDs) use.

3. e. Both a single 150-mg dose of oral fluconazole (Diflucan) or a 3-7 day course of terconazole (Terazol) would be appropriate treatments. Other over-the-counter antifungal vaginal creams and suppositories are also appropriate. Metronidazole (Flagyl) is not indicated for yeast infections. Neither orally nor intravaginally administered *Lactobacillus acidophilus* has been proved to effectively prevent or treat vaginal yeast infections.

4. c. The patient typically should have responded to the previously mentioned treatments by this time. The most appropriate next step for this patient would be to reconsider the diagnosis and reevaluate the patient to rule out another etiology, concurrent infection, or partially treated candidiasis as a result of noncompliance or imidazole resistance. If your diagnosis is still vulvovaginal candidiasis, the patient may benefit from a different antifungal treatment.

5. **c.** Boric acid, administered in a 600-mg vaginal suppository, has been shown to be effective as treatment and prophylaxis for recurrent/chronic vulvovaginal candidiasis. However, its use is limited by significant local irritation. Oral and topical steroids, antibiotics (e.g., Minocin), and douching actually can worsen this condition.

6. **a.** *Candida albicans* is the most common pathogen identified in patients with vulvovaginal yeast infections. *Candida glabrata* often is associated with chronic/recurrent yeast infections. In fact, the number of cases of vulvovaginal candidiasis caused by non-*C. albicans* species is increasing and they are significantly less sensitive to imidazole antifungal agents. This is probably because of the inappropriate use of over-the-counter antifungal medications.

Pap tests are indicated for the screening of cervical dysplasia and malignancy, not vaginal infections. Pap tests provide no advantage over the microscopic examination of the wet mount and KOH preparations of the vaginal discharge. Patients should not be empirically treated for any vaginal infection based on the Pap test result alone. Studies have not found a strong association between recurrent vulvovaginal candidiasis and the presence of intestinal *Candida*.

7. **e.** This patient's symptoms, physical examination, and vaginal discharge findings are classic for BV, the most common cause of vaginitis in reproductive-aged women in the United States. Many women with BV are asymptomatic. BV appears to occur when something significantly reduces the number of vaginal hydrogen peroxide–producing *Lactobacillus acidophilus* organisms, altering the healthy normal vaginal pH (3.8-4.2), which subsequently facilitates the proliferation of organisms such as *G. vaginalis*, *M. hominis*, and *Mobiluncus* species, which usually are suppressed. These organisms produce metabolic byproducts, such as amines, which are responsible for the characteristic "fishy" odor. This process is intensified by the addition of KOH, indicating a positive "whiff test." Risk factors for BV include douching, antibiotic use, IUD use, and pregnancy. "Clue cells" are vaginal epithelial cells that are coated with coccobacilli. The presence of at least three of four of the following (Amsel's criteria) establish the accurate diagnosis of BV in 90% of affected women: presence of a thin, homogeneous, vaginal discharge; vaginal pH >4.5, positive "whiff" test; and microscopic identification of "clue cells."

8. **c.** BV is a risk factor for premature rupture of membranes and preterm labor. The role of sexual transmission for BV is unclear. Treating the male sexual partner of a woman with BV has not been shown to significantly reduce chronic or recurrent infection. BV is believed to result from a reduction of vaginal *L. acidophilus* organisms.

9. **d.** Miconazole cream is an antifungal treatment. The other options are all appropriate treatments for BV.

10. **b.** BV is believed to be caused by a proliferation of anaerobic bacteria, including *Gardnerella vaginalis*, *Mobiluncus* species, *Mycoplasma hominis*, and *Peptostreptococcus* species.

11. **b.** This patient's symptoms, physical examination, and vaginal discharge findings are classic for trichomoniasis.

12. **c.** The protozoan, *Trichomonas vaginalis*, is transmitted sexually. Trichomoniasis is associated with and may act as a vector for other STDs. Risk factors for trichomoniasis include multiple sexual partners, cigarette smoking, and IUDs. Trichomoniasis also may be associated with premature rupture of membranes and preterm delivery. Infected male partners are often asymptomatic.

13. **e.** Both metronidazole regimens are highly effective, but single-dose therapy is associated with better compliance.

14. **e.** Sexual partners should be treated and instructed to avoid sexual intercourse until both partners are cured. Alcohol should be avoided until 24 hours after completing metronidazole treatment. Trichomoniasis is associated with and may act as a vector for other STDs. Patients with trichomoniasis should be screened for other STDs. This patient presents with several "red flags," which warrant screening for domestic violence and sexual abuse.

15. **e.** As many as 90% of vaginitis cases are secondary to bacterial vaginosis, vulvovaginal candidiasis, and trichomoniasis. However, noninfectious causes can mimic infectious presentations (pruritus, vulvovaginal erythema and swelling, discharge) and should be excluded. They include vaginal atrophy, allergies, and chemical irritation. Patients with these conditions often are misdiagnosed initially as having candidiasis and are treated for it. Vaginal atrophy usually occurs in estrogen-deficiency states (i.e., menopause). An elevated vaginal pH (>4.5) usually is noted, and round "parabasal" cells may be found on wet mount. Patients usually improve with estrogen supplementation.

Vaginitis caused by either allergic reactions to latex condoms or other allergens or vaginal irritation from spermicides or other chemical agents do not typically demonstrate any classic physical findings or vaginal discharge characteristics. A thorough exposure history and examination to exclude infectious causes usually is required to make the proper diagnosis and to determine the offending agent.

SOLUTION TO THE CLINICAL CASE MANAGEMENT PROBLEM

	Vulvovaginal Candidiasis	Bacterial Vaginosis	Trichomoniasis
Vaginal discharge	Thick, white, curdy ("cottage cheese"); adherent, no odor	Thin, off-white, homogeneous; unpleasant "fishy" odor	Copious, frothy, yellow-green, adherent, malodorous
Vaginal pH	Normal (3.8-4.2)	Elevated (>4.5)	Elevated (>4.5)
Whiff test	Negative	Positive	Can be positive
Microscopic findings	Pseudohyphae, mycelial tangles, or budding yeast	Clue cells, no WBCs	Motile trichomonads, WBCs (>10/HPF)

SUMMARY OF VULVOVAGINITIS AND BACTERIAL VAGINOSIS

Diagnosis: See Table in the Clinical Case Management Problem for a summary of the diagnostic features.

Treatment options (based on 2002 Centers for Disease Control and Prevention treatment guidelines) for each condition are outlined as follows:

1. **Vulvovaginal candidiasis:** *Candida albicans* is the most common pathogen identified in patients with vulvovaginal candidiasis.
   Acute regimens are as follows:
   a. Various topical antifungal creams/tablets/suppositories (intravaginally for 1-14 days)
   b. Diflucan (150 mg PO for one dose)
   An alternative regimen is boric acid (600 mg vaginal suppository bid for 14 days).
   If the patient is pregnant, only use topical "azole" agents.
2. **Bacterial vaginosis:** Bacterial vaginosis is the most common cause of vaginitis among women of reproductive age in the United States.
   Recommended regimens are as follows:
   a. Metronidazole (500 mg PO for bid 7 days)
   b. Metronidazole 0.75% gel (5 g intravaginally qhs for 5 days)
   c. Clindamycin 2% cream (5 gm intravaginally qhs for 7 days)
   Alternative regimens include the following:
   a. Metronidazole (2 g PO for one dose)

   b. Clindamycin (300 mg PO bid for 7 days)
   c. Clindamycin ovules (100 g intravaginally qhs for 3 days)
   The regimen during pregnancy is as follows:
   a. Metronidazole (250 mg PO tid for 7 days)
   b. Clindamycin (300 mg PO bid for 7 days)
3. **Trichomoniasis:** Trichomoniasis is an STD. Sexual partners should be treated and instructed to avoid sexual intercourse until both partners are cured. Trichomoniasis is associated with and may act as a vector for other STDs. Patients with trichomoniasis should be screened for other STDs.
   The recommended regimen is metronidazole (2 g PO for one dose).
   An alternative regimen is metronidazole (500 mg PO bid for 7 days).
   The regimen during pregnancy is metronidazole (2 g PO for one dose). (Studies have not demonstrated a consistent association between use of metronidazole during pregnancy and teratogenic effects in infants.)

SUGGESTED READING

Centers for Disease Control and Prevention: Sexually transmitted diseases treatment guidelines. *MMWR* 51(RR-6): 7-61, 2002.

Egan ME, Lipsky MS: Diagnosis of vaginitis. *Am Fam Physician* 62:1095-1104, 2000.

Ringdahl EN: Treatment of recurrent vulvovaginal candidiasis. *Am Fam Physician* 61:3306-3312, 3317, 2000.

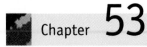

Chapter 53

Cervical Abnormalities

"Oh colposcopy. I thought you said colonoscopy."

CLINICAL CASE PROBLEM 1:
A 26-YEAR-OLD FEMALE WITH AN "ASC-US" PAP TEST RESULT

A 26-year-old woman comes to your office for her health maintenance examination. She is married, has two children, and has had no major medical illnesses. She has a 10 pack-year history of cigarette smoking. She has a lifetime history of 10 sexual partners but denies a history of sexually transmitted disease (STD). She always has had normal Papanicolaou (Pap) test results in the past. Her physical examination, including pelvic, is unremarkable. Her Papanicolaou (Pap) test comes back and is reported as "satisfactory for evaluation, ASC-US."*

■ **SELECT THE BEST ANSWER TO THE FOLLOWING QUESTIONS:**

1. Which of the following would be appropriate as initial management for this patient?
   a. repeat the Pap test in 1 year
   b. perform a dilation and curettage (D&C)
   c. perform human papilloma virus (HPV) DNA testing
   d. perform cryotherapy
   e. perform loop electrosurgical excision procedure (LEEP)

2. You perform an annual Pap test on another patient with liquid-based cytology (Thin Prep). It returns as *"satisfactory for evaluation, ASC-US, positive for high-risk HPV type."* Which of the following would be appropriate as initial management for this patient?
   a. repeat Pap test in 4-6 months
   b. cryotherapy or LEEP
   c. colposcopy
   d. continue annual Pap tests
   e. repeat HPV DNA testing in 4-6 months

*The 2001 Bethesda System for reporting cervical cytology and histology is used in the following questions:
ASC, atypical squamous cells
ASC-US, atypical squamous cells of undetermined significance
ASC-H, atypical squamous cells, cannot exclude HSIL
LSIL, low-grade squamous intraepithelial lesion
HSIL, high-grade squamous intraepithelial lesion
AGC, atypical glandular cells
CIN, cervical intraepithelial neoplasia

3. According to the 2003 United States Preventive Services Task Force (USPSTF) guidelines, which of the following regarding cervical cancer screening is correct?
   a. all women should begin cervical cancer screening at age 18 years
   b. all women who have had a total hysterectomy for benign disease should continue cervical cancer screening
   c. all women should begin cervical cancer screening within 3 years onset of sexual activity or age 21 years (whichever comes first)
   d. annual cervical cancer screening should continue past the age of 65 years
   e. pregnant women should not have Pap tests

4. According to the 2003 USPSTF guidelines, which of the following regarding cervical cancer screening intervals is correct?
   a. routine cervical cancer screening (via Pap test) should occur *at least* every 3 years
   b. women older than age 65 years with recent normal Pap tests and a low risk history still need to continue cervical cancer screening
   c. women that are heavy smokers should have more frequent Pap tests than nonsmokers
   d. pregnant women should have more frequent Pap tests than nonpregnant women
   e. HPV DNA testing alone can replace conventional Pap tests as a method of cervical cancer screening

5. Carcinoma of the cervix is associated with which subtype of HPV?
   a. 6, 11
   b. 16, 18, 31, 45
   c. 40, 42
   d. 53, 54
   e. all of the above

6. Which of the following is not a significant direct risk factor for carcinoma of the cervix?
   a. a partner who has had multiple sexual partners
   b. early age of first intercourse
   c. intercourse with more than three partners
   d. a history of genital warts
   e. a history of genital herpes

7. Which of the following statements is true?
   a. the risk of invasive carcinoma with ASC-US is extremely low
   b. AGC is associated with endometrial neoplasia, not cervical neoplasia
   c. approximately 75% of women with LSIL have histologically confirmed high-grade cervical lesions (CIN 2,3)

d. approximately 25% of women with HSIL have histologically confirmed high–grade cervical lesions (CIN 2, 3)

e. none of the above

8. Your nurse informs you that a patient of yours recently had a Pap test come back as *"satisfactory for evaluation, consistent with AGC, NOS."* You review her chart and note she is 40 years old and otherwise healthy. You bring the patient back to your office to discuss the results and advise that she:

a. repeat a Pap in 1 year

b. repeat a Pap in 4-6 months

c. undergo colposcopy and endocervical curettage

d. undergo colposcopy, endocervical curettage, and endometrial biopsy

e. undergo cryotherapy

9. Your colleague approaches you and asks whether you are using the "new Pap test." You explain that the advantages to liquid-based cytology (Thin Prep) include:

a. it is less expensive than conventional Pap tests

b. it permits reflex HPV testing

c. collection of cervical specimen is easier than with conventional Pap

d. the patient is more comfortable during cervical sampling than with conventional Pap

e. all of the above

CLINICAL CASE PROBLEM 2:

A 33-Year-Old Female with an "LSIL" Pap Test Result

A 33-year-old woman (gravida 2, para 2) comes to your office for a routine annual examination. She has never smoked and has no history of STDs. She is in a stable, monogamous relationship with her husband who is the only sexual partner she has had in her lifetime. Her previous Pap test results have been normal. Her physical examination is normal, including pelvic examination. You perform a Pap test at this time. Two weeks later, the Pap test results come back as *"satisfactory for evaluation, consistent with LSIL."*

10. Which of the following would be appropriate as initial management for this patient?

a. continue routine screening because she has no other risk factors for cervical dysplasia

b. repeat a Pap test in 4-6 months

c. have HPV DNA typing

d. perform colposcopy

e. perform LEEP or cryotherapy

11. If the routine Pap test results on this patient had come back as *"satisfactory for evaluation, negative for intraepithelial lesion or malignancy"* but also *"absence of an endocervical component,"* what would the most appropriate initial management have been?

a. perform an endocervical curettage

b. repeat the Pap test immediately

c. repeat the Pap test in 6 weeks

d. repeat the Pap test in 4-6 months

e. repeat the Pap test in 1 year

12. The patient in Clinical Case Problem 2 returns after having a colposcopy. Her cervical biopsy returns as *"CIN-I"* (cervical intraepithelial lesion), and her endocervical curettage (ECC) is *"negative for neoplasia."* You discuss the results with the patient, and she would like to proceed with treatment. Which of the following are acceptable methods of treatment?

a. total hysterectomy

b. D&C

c. cryotherapy

d. local application of trichloracetic acid (TCA)

e. interferon injections

13. Which part of the cervix is most vulnerable to dysplastic changes?

a. the squamous epithelium

b. the columnar epithelium

c. the squamocolumnar junction

d. the superior lip of the cervix

e. the inferior lip of the cervix

CLINICAL CASE PROBLEM 3:

A 26-Year-Old Pregnant Woman with a "HSIL" Pap Test Result

A 26-year-old woman (gravida 3, para 2) who is approximately 22 weeks pregnant recently moved to the area and would like to transfer her prenatal care to you. She brings her prenatal records with her. You note her prenatal history has been unremarkable except that her initial Pap test came back as "HSIL." She states that her last doctor recommended that she have colposcopy done but she never followed up because she thought it would "harm the pregnancy."

14. At this time, you should advise her that:

a. it is not safe for pregnant women to undergo colposcopy

b. it is safe for pregnant women to undergo colposcopy but not cervical biopsy

c. she should have a colposcopy 6 weeks postpartum

d. she should have a repeat Pap test 6 weeks postpartum

e. she should be scheduled for colposcopy now

CLINICAL CASE MANAGEMENT PROBLEM

Discuss the new 2001 Bethesda System for reporting results of cervical cytology. Correlate it with the cytopathologic findings and the histologic classification system.

■ **ANSWERS:**

1. **c.** The 2001 Bethesda System has revised terminology for reporting results of cervical cytology. This new system subdivides ASC (atypical squamous cells) into ASC-US (atypical squamous cells of undetermined significance) or ASC-H (atypical squamous cells, cannot exclude high-grade squamous intraepithelial lesion). The risk of a high-grade cervical lesion is higher for ASC-H (24% to 94%) than for ASC-US (5% to 17%). Women with ASC-H should be referred for colposcopy given the increased risk of cervical neoplasia.

According to the 2001 Consensus Guidelines for the Management of Women with Cervical Cytological Abnormalities, the management of ASC-US can involve either (1) repeat cytology at 4-6 month intervals until two consecutive negative Pap test results are obtained, with referral to colposcopy if repeat Pap is ASC-US or greater cytologic abnormality; or (2) testing for HPV DNA type, with referral to colposcopy if the patient tests positive for "high-risk" HPV.

In the past, clinicians have used repeat cytologic testing for management of ASC-US based on the fact that repeat consecutive Pap tests increase the sensitivity of detecting a high-grade cervical lesion. Disadvantages of this approach include potential added patient discomfort, risk of noncompliance secondary to multiple office visits, and possibly delayed diagnosis of high-grade cervical lesions or cancer.

Data have demonstrated that immediate HPV-based triage of ASC-US Pap tests has excellent sensitivity (90% to 96%) for the detection of high-grade cervical lesions, compared with 75% to 85% for a repeat Pap test. In fact, the negative predictive value for a single *negative* test for high-risk HPV DNA is at least 98%. The advent of sensitive HPV DNA tests (Hybrid Capture 2 system) allows for "triaging" women with ASC-US into those with high-risk HPV types from women with low-risk HPV types and women without HPV infection. Liquid-based cytology that permits reflex HPV testing for ASC-US also may be used.

Hence, the preferred approach to the management of ASC-US is to perform HPV DNA testing (Level A evidence). An acceptable alternative is repeat cytologic testing, as outlined earlier, if HPV DNA testing is not available (Level A evidence). There is less evidence supporting immediate referral to colposcopy for ASC-US (Level B evidence). Advantages to this approach include the immediate confirmation of the presence of absence of significant disease. However, several disadvantages exist, including creating unnecessary patient anxiety, discomfort, potential for overtreatment, and added expense.

2. **c.** There is a clear association between high-risk HPV DNA types and cervical neoplasia. As discussed earlier, those women with ASC-US who test positive for high-risk HPV should be referred for colposcopy. Women with ASC-US who test negative for high-risk HPV can return to routine screening.

3. **c.** The 2003 USPSTF guidelines recommend that cervical cancer screening begin within 3 years from the onset of sexual activity or age 21, whichever comes first. Data on the natural history of HPV infection suggest that there is a delay in incidence of high-grade lesions from onset of sexual activity, such that screening can safely occur within 3 years from onset of sexual activity. Other organizations have updated their guidelines to reflect similar recommendations for the initiation of cervical cancer screening, including the American Cancer Society (ACS) and the American College of Obstetricians and Gynecologists (ACOG).

The USPSTF recommends against routine Pap test screening in women who have had a total hysterectomy for benign disease because there is low yield for detecting significant disease. Women who have had a supracervical (cervix-sparing) hysterectomy should follow routine cervical cancer screening guidelines.

There is little evidence to support cervical cancer screening in women older than age 65 because the risk of high-grade cervical neoplasia decreases with age. In addition, cervical cancer in older women is not more aggressive than in younger women. Hence, those women older than age 65 with recent normal Pap test results and otherwise low-risk history may elect to stop screening.

4. **a.** The USPSTF did not find evidence to support that annual cervical cancer screening is more effective than screening every 3 years. Hence, the 2003 USPSTF guidelines recommend repeat Pap tests at least every 3 years. The American Academy of Family Physicians (AAFP) Recommendations for Periodic Health Exams makes the same recommendation. Other U.S. organizations recommend yearly screening until three consecutive negative Pap test results have been obtained, at which time screening can be lengthened out. Ultimately, the decision should be made on an individual basis based on the patient's risk factors, compliance, and personal preferences. Women older than 65 years of age who are otherwise low risk and

have had recent negative Pap test results may stop screening, as discussed in Question 3. Although cigarette smoking has been associated with an increased risk of cervical neoplasia, there is no evidence to support more frequent cervical cancer screening in these patients. The frequency of cervical cancer screening is the same for pregnant women as for non-pregnant women. There is insufficient evidence to recommend for or against using HPV testing as primary screening for cervical cancer.

5. b. There is a well-established association between persistent HPV infection and progressive cervical dysplasia. The type of the HPV involved is important in determining the malignant potential of the virus. HPV types 6 and 11 are associated with genital warts and are believed to be of low-risk malignant potential. In contrast, HPV types 16, 18, 31, and 45 are considered to be high risk. HPV 16 alone accounts for 68% of viral types found in squamous cell tumors. HPV 40 and 42 are low-risk subtypes.

6. e. It is now widely recognized that HPV is an STD necessary for the initiation and progression of cervical neoplasia. Risk factors for cervical carcinoma include early onset of intercourse, three or more sexual partners, a male sexual partner who has had other partners, a clinical history of condyloma acuminata (genital warts), and cigarette smoking. Herpes simplex virus (HSV) is not considered an identifiable risk factor for carcinoma of the cervix. Indirectly, of course, as an STD, an episode of HSV may be associated with the other risk factors for cervical dysplasia just discussed.

7. a. The risk of invasive carcinoma with ASC is extremely low (0.1% to 0.2%). Approximately 15% to 30% of women with LSIL will have a histologically confirmed high-grade cervical intraepithelial lesion (CIN 2/3). The risk of CIN 2/3 is *higher* with HSIL (70% to 75%), not lower. AGC is associated with cervical neoplasia, not just endometrial neoplasia.

8. d. The 2001 Bethesda System classifies glandular abnormalities into AGC-NOS (atypical glandular cells, not otherwise specified) and AGC ("favor neoplasia"). There is a higher risk of cervical neoplasia in women with AGC than with AGC-NOS. Regardless, all women with AGS should have colposcopy with endocervical sampling because the risk of cervical neoplasia is substantially higher than with ASC or LSIL. In addition, endometrial biopsy should be performed in conjunction with colposcopy in women older than age 35 years or in younger women with unexplained vaginal bleeding to rule out invasive disease. Repeat cytologic sampling is unacceptable as initial management of AGS. Cryotherapy is not appropriate as initial management without confirmation of absence or presence of disease.

9. b. Conventional Pap tests have been limited by inadequate sampling, obscuring elements, delays in fixation, and random distribution of cells. Liquid-based cytology involves mixing the specimen in a liquid fixative and then transferring a thin layer of evenly distributed cells on a slide. Liquid based cytology offers the opportunity to perform reflex HPV testing in cases of ASC-US (as discussed in Answer 2). There is good evidence that liquid-based cytology has improved sensitivity for detecting cervical dysplasia over conventional Pap tests. However, it is considerably more expensive and may have lower specificity. Collection of the cervical specimen is the same as for conventional Pap, using an Ayres spatula for collection of ectocervical cells and an endocervical brush for endocervical cells. Hence, patient comfort should not be any different than with conventional Pap.

10. d. According to the 2001 Consensus Guidelines, patients with LSIL should have colposcopy because 15% to 30% of these patients will have biopsy-confirmed CIN 2 or 3. Immediate referral for excisional or ablative procedures such as LEEP or cryotherapy without confirmation of disease via colposcopy is unacceptable. HPV DNA typing is not useful in patients with LSIL because 83% of these women are positive for high-risk subtypes. Repeating the Pap test in 4-6 months is not recommended because of the small but real risk of delaying diagnosis of invasive disease.

11. e. For Pap tests that are "satisfactory for evaluation" there is little evidence to suggest that lack of an endocervical component on Pap test increases the chance of missing significant disease. If endocervical cells are absent, the patient can repeat a Pap test in a year.

12. c. According to the 2001 Consensus Guidelines for the Management of Women with Cervical Intraepithelial Neoplasia, patients with CIN-1 may elect to be observed and followed with repeat cytology provided colposcopy was satisfactory (entire transformation zone was visualized), or they may opt for ablative or excisional treatment. Ablative treatment options include cryotherapy or laser ablation. Cryotherapy is a simple, minimally invasive method that can be performed easily in the office setting. Excisional modalities include LEEP or cold-knife conization. Total hysterectomy for localized disease is not recommended. Local application of TCA is used for treatment of genital warts, not confirmed CIN 1. Neither D&C nor interferon injections are treatments for cervical dysplasia.

13. **c.** The majority of the cervix is covered with stratified squamous epithelium. The area from the endocervix to the margin of the squamous cells is laid with columnar epithelium. At puberty, when estrogen levels increase and *Lactobacillus* species consequently colonize the vagina, the vaginal pH drops into an acidic range. Exposure of the fragile columnar epithelial cells around the cervical os to this acidic environment stimulates their transformation into squamous epithelium, a process referred to as *squamous metaplasia.* As this process proceeds over decades, the advancing edge of the squamous epithelium, also known as the *squamocolumnar junction* (SCJ), migrates centrally toward the cervical os and ultimately into the endocervical canal. Because of increased cell turnover, the SCJ is most vulnerable to dysplastic changes. There is no known anatomic preference for cervical dysplasia when comparing the superior lip to the inferior lip of the cervix.

14. **e.** Pregnancy is not a contraindication to colposcopy. The patient should be reassured that there is no increased risk of preterm labor or harm to the fetus with colposcopy or cervical biopsy. The most important goal of colposcopy in the pregnant patient is to rule out invasive carcinoma. Cervical biopsies may be performed during pregnancy, although the pregnant cervix is more vascular and may have increased incidence of minor (but not major) bleeding. Endocervical curettage is contraindicated during pregnancy because of potential risk of premature rupture of membranes, preterm labor, and bleeding. There is a high rate of spontaneous regression of cervical lesions postpartum. Hence, it is recommended that treatment for all but invasive carcinoma be delayed until postpartum reassessment.

SOLUTION TO THE CLINICAL CASE MANAGEMENT PROBLEM

Bethesda System	CIN Classification	Pap Test Findings
ASC ASC-US ASC-H	No direct histologic correlate	Variable
LSIL	CIN I	Mild dysplasia
HSIL	CIN II CIN III	Moderate dysplasia Severe dysplasia Carcinoma in situ

ASC, atypical squamous cells; ASC-US, atypical squamous cells of undetermined significance; ASC-H, atypical squamous cells, cannot exclude HSIL; LSIL, low-grade squamous intraepithelial lesion; HSIL, high-grade squamous intraepithelial lesion; CIN, cervical intraepithelial neoplasia.

SUMMARY OF CERVICAL ABNORMALITIES

2003 USPSTF Guidelines for Cervical Cancer Screening are as follows:
1. Cervical cancer screening should be initiated within 3 years of onset of sexual activity or at age 21, whichever comes first.
2. Cervical cancer screening should occur at least every 3 years in women age 21-65 years.
3. Women older than age 65 with recent normal Pap tests and low-risk history may stop cervical cancer screening.

4. Women who have had a total hysterectomy for benign disease do not need routine cervical cancer screening.
2001 Consensus Guidelines for the Management of Women with Cervical Cytological Abnormalities are as follows:
1. Women with ASC-US may be managed by either repeat cytologic testing or HPV DNA typing. Those women with either ASC or greater cytologic abnormality on repeat Pap, or who test positive for high-risk HPV, should be referred to colposcopy.
2. Women with ASC-H should be referred for colposcopy.

3. Women with LSIL should be referred for colposcopy.

4. Women with HSIL should be referred for colposcopy.

5. All women with AGC should be referred for colposcopy with possible endometrial biopsy if they are older than age 35 or younger with unexplained vaginal bleeding.

Risk factors associated with cervical neoplasia include the following: "high-risk" HPV types 16, 18, 31, and 45 acting along with cofactors, which include cigarette smoking, early first intercourse, three or more partners in a lifetime, partner who has had multiple sexual partners, and clinical history of condyloma acuminata.

Liquid-based cytology allows for "reflex" HPV testing in cases of ASC-US.

Acceptable treatments for confirmed CIN include cryotherapy or LEEP. Total hysterectomy is not acceptable for noninvasive disease.

The squamocolumnar junction of the cervix is most vulnerable to cervical dysplasia.

Pregnancy is not a contraindication for colposcopy. Abnormal descriptive diagnoses on Pap test reporting are as follows:

1. Infection: (a) fungus consistent with *Candida* species; (b) *Trichomonas vaginalis*; (c) predominance of coccobacilli consistent with shift in vaginal flora; (d) bacteria morphologically consistent with *Actinomyces* species associated with an intrauterine device (IUD); and (e) cellular changes consistent with HSV.

2. Reactive and reparative: (a) reactive cellular changes associated with inflammation; (b) atrophy with inflammation; (c) IUD; and (d) radiation.

3. Squamous cell abnormalities: (a) atypical squamous cells of undetermined significance (ASC-US); (b) atypical squamous cells, cannot exclude high-grade intraepithelial lesion (HSIL); (c) low-grade intraepithelial lesion (LSIL); (d) high-grade intraepithelial lesion (HSIL); and (e) squamous cell carcinoma.

4. Glandular cell abnormalities: (a) atypical glandular cells, favor neoplastic; (b) atypical glandular cells, not otherwise specified (NOS); (c) adeno-carcinoma; and (d) endocervical adenocarcinoma in situ (AIS).

SUGGESTED READING

Apgar B, et al: *Colposcopy principals and practice: an integrated textbook and atlas.* W.B. Saunders Company, 2002, Philadelphia.

Solomon D, et al: 2001 Bethesda System: terminology for reporting results of cervical cytology. *JAMA* 287:2114-2119, 2001.

U.S. Preventive Services Task Force: *U.S. Preventive Services Task Force guide to clinical preventive services, 3rd edition.* http://www.ahcpr.gov/clinic/uspstfix.htm Periodic Updates, accessed September 12th, 2003.

Wright TC, et al: Consensus guidelines for the management of women with cervical cytological abnormalities. *JAMA* 287:2120-2129, 2002.

 Chapter 54

Premenstrual Syndrome and Premenstrual Dysphoric Disorder

"I'm sorry I shot you. It's just my time of the month."

CLINICAL CASE PROBLEM 1:

A 23-YEAR-OLD FEMALE WITH CYCLIC PHYSICAL AND AFFECTIVE SYMPTOMS

A 23-year-old woman comes to your office with a 6-month history of fatigue, anxiety, emotional lability, difficulty concentrating, and insomnia. She also complains of breast tenderness, abdominal bloating, and food cravings. She denies any menstrual irregularities or prodromal life stressors. These symptoms recur on a regular basis during the week leading up to her menstrual period but completely resolve within the first 3 days of menses. She denies any suicidal ideations. However, she tearfully admits that she feels totally incapacitated when she is symptomatic and that these symptoms are adversely affecting her personal and professional life.

■ SELECT THE BEST ANSWER TO THE FOLLOWING QUESTIONS:

1. What is the most likely diagnosis in this patient?
   a. generalized anxiety disorder
   b. dysmenorrhea
   c. major depression
   d. panic disorder
   e. premenstrual dysphoric disorder syndrome (PMDD)

2. Which of the following is not a necessary Diagnostic and Statistical Manual of Mental Disorders, 4th edition (DSM IV) criteria for diagnosing this condition?
   a. symptoms must be present most of the time during the last week of the luteal phase

b. symptoms must remit a few days after the onset of the follicular phase (menses)
c. symptoms must be present in the week post menses
d. symptoms must occur in most menstrual cycles during the past year
e. symptoms must interfere with function

3. What is the main characteristic that differentiates this condition from major depression?
   a. the type of symptoms
   b. the severity of symptoms
   c. the duration of this condition
   d. the timing of the symptoms relative to the menstrual cycle
   e. occurs in reproductive-age women

4. What is the main characteristic that differentiates this condition from premenstrual syndrome (PMS)?
   a. the type of symptoms
   b. the severity of symptoms
   c. the duration of this condition
   d. the timing of the symptoms relative to the menstrual cycle
   e. occurs in reproductive-age women

5. Which of the following is a reliable aid in the diagnosis of this condition?
   a. patient completes a prospective daily symptom rating form for two consecutive cycles
   b. follicle stimulating to luteinizing hormone (FSH:LH) ratio
   c. progesterone withdrawal test
   d. an empiric 4-week trial of an selective serotonin reuptake inhibitor (SSRI)
   e. estradiol and progesterone levels obtained during the patient's late luteal phase

6. Which of the following statements comparing PMS and PMDD are true?
   a. PMDD is a more common condition than PMS
   b. PMS and PMDD both include physical symptoms
   c. early menopause often exacerbates the symptoms of PMS and PMDD
   d. symptoms have to interfere with normal function in PMDD but not PMS
   e. c and d

7. Which of the following is true regarding hormone levels in patients with PMS or PMDD?
   a. they have excess levels of female sex hormones (estrogen and progesterone)
   b. they have excess levels of male sex hormones (testosterone and dehydroepiandrosterone [DHEA])

   c. they have deficient levels of female sex hormones
   d. they have deficient levels of male sex hormones
   e. they have an abnormal response to normal female sex hormone fluctuations

8. Which of the following pharmacologic treatments has demonstrated the best evidence (level A) to support its effectiveness for the treatment of PMDD?
   a. SSRIs
   b. combined oral contraceptives (COCs), containing estrogen and progesterone
   c. progesterone vaginal suppositories
   d. transdermal estrogen patches
   e. oral medroxyprogesterone acetate (Provera)

9. Which of the following vitamins/minerals has demonstrated the best evidence to support its effectiveness for the treatment of PMDD?
   a. vitamin B_6
   b. calcium
   c. magnesium
   d. vitamin A
   e. vitamin E

10. Which of the following nonpharmacologic therapies have demonstrated the best evidence to support their effectiveness for the treatment of PMS/PMDD?
    a. dong quai and ginseng
    b. St. John's wort and kava kava
    c. evening primrose oil and chasteberry
    d. black cohosh and blue cohosh
    e. wild yams and soybeans

CLINICAL CASE MANAGEMENT PROBLEM

Compare the diagnostic criteria for PMS and PMDD.

ANSWERS:

1. **e.** The patient's presentation is most consistent with premenstrual dysphoric disorder (PMDD), a cyclic disorder of reproductive-aged women, characterized by a wide variety of severe emotional and physical symptoms that consistently occur during the luteal phase of the menstrual cycle. PMDD is a diagnosis of exclusion. Although the patient may have symptoms consistent with an affective disorder (anxiety, depression, panic), the cyclic onset and remission of her symptoms, in relation to her menstrual cycle, are classic for PMDD. Dysmenorrhea is a

condition characterized by pelvic pain that occurs just after the onset of menses and peaks with heaviest flow. This patient's symptoms precede the onset of menses and remit during menses.

2. **c.** The following are DSM IV diagnostic criteria for PMDD: (1) symptoms must be present most of the time during the last week of the luteal phase; (2) symptoms must remit a few days after the onset of the follicular phase (menses); (3) symptoms must be absent in the week post menses; (4) symptoms must occur in most menstrual cycles during the past year; (5) symptoms must interfere with function; and (6) symptoms must not be an exacerbation of an existing disorder.

3. **d.** The affective symptoms of PMDD can be indistinguishable from those of major depression. The recurrent onset and remission of these symptoms, in relation to the menstrual cycle, help distinguish PMDD from major depression.

4. **b.** Like PMDD, PMS is characterized by the cyclic recurrence of psychological and physical symptoms during the late luteal phase of the menstrual cycle. The variety of potential symptoms for both of these conditions is similar and generally begins between the ages of 25 and 35 years. Women who have more severe affective symptoms are classified as having PMDD. Both PMS and PMDD symptoms improve rapidly following the onset of menses.

5. **a.** PMS and PMDD can be diagnosed only after a variety of physical and psychiatric disorders have been excluded. PMS and PMDD are best distinguished from other conditions by the consistent occurrence of function-impairing symptoms only during the luteal phase of the menstrual cycle. This can be confirmed best by having the patient complete a prospective daily symptom rating form for at least two consecutive cycles. Although sensitivity to sex hormones may play a role in both of these conditions, patients with PMS and PMDD have normal estradiol, progesterone, FSH, LH, and other hormone levels. SSRIs often improve the symptoms of PMS and PMDD, although there is also a significantly high placebo effect when treating these conditions. SSRIs also alleviate the symptoms of several other similar conditions (depression, anxiety, panic), so the response to their empiric use is nondiagnostic.

6. **b.** PMS and PMDD have a variety of psychological and physical symptomatology in common, which interfere with normal function. PMS (20% to 40%) is a significantly more common condition than PMDD (2% to 10%) in menstruating women. As many as 85% of menstruating women report having one or more premenstrual symptoms. Menopause usually results in cessation of these conditions.

7. **e.** There is no consensus regarding the etiology of either PMS or PMDD. Patients with these conditions usually have normal hormone levels. However, they appear to have an abnormal response to normal female sex hormone fluctuations.

8. **a.** Although numerous treatment strategies are available, few have been evaluated adequately in randomized controlled trials (RCTs). Even the results of RCTs can be hard to apply because of the significant variability of inclusion criteria and outcome measures and the high response rate to placebo (25% to 50%). However, the systematic review of many of these RCTs has yielded some evidence-based recommendations. There is clear evidence that SSRIs can significantly improve the symptoms of severe PMS and PMDD (evidence level 1a). Fluoxetine and sertraline are the most extensively studied for the treatment of PMS and PMDD, but all SSRIs appear to be effective. SSRIs can be administered daily or only during the luteal phase. However, there are no definitive recommendations regarding how long to continue treatment because symptoms tend to return on discontinuation. Nonsteroidal antiinflammatory drugs (NSAIDs) can be helpful for symptoms of abdominal pain and headaches. Aldactone has been shown to relieve symptoms of fluid retention. Estrogen and/or progesterone/progestin containing products, administered via different routes (intravaginally, rectally, orally, transdermally), have been widely prescribed for the management of PMS and PMDD. However, none have been shown to be consistently effective and actually may exacerbate symptoms in some patients. Low-dose estrogen therapy may improve some physical symptoms, but it does not appear to have a positive effect on mood symptoms. The efficacy of estrogen therapy is limited by the need for progestin/progesterone opposition, which commonly exacerbates PMS and PMDD symptoms; however, it is required to prevent endometrial hyperplasia or carcinoma. Gonadotropin-releasing hormone (GnRH) agonists (e.g., Lupron) and androgens (e.g., Danazol) are somewhat effective in alleviating the physical and behavioral symptoms of PMS and PMDD. However, their short- and long-term side-effect profiles limit their use.

9. **b.** There is good evidence that calcium is effective for the treatment of PMS and PMDD (evidence level 1b). A large well-conducted RCT demonstrated that 1200 mg/day of calcium carbonate administered for

three consecutive menstrual cycles resulted in significant symptom improvement in 48% of women with PMS, compared with 30% of women treated with placebo. Although there is some evidence suggesting that vitamin B_6 may improve PMS/PMDD symptoms, most of the RCTs were of poor quality. Magnesium has only been shown to have minimal benefit in alleviating PMS-related bloating. Studies of vitamin A do not support its use for PMS or PMDD. The result of one RCT suggests that vitamin E, administered at 400 IU/day, during the luteal phase, may improve both affective and somatic symptoms (especially mastalgia) in women with PMS. However, larger, better-quality studies are needed.

10. **c.** Two herbal therapies, chasteberry and evening primrose oil, may be effective in alleviating breast tenderness in patients with PMS/PMDD (evidence level 1c). The other options either have been shown to be likely ineffective (dong quai) or lack enough data to support their use. Some even have potential severe side effects—such as kava kava (liver damage), blue cohosh (peripheral vascular constriction), and St. John's wort (decreased oral contraceptive pill efficacy). One also should keep in mind the following: (1) none of the therapies listed are approved by the U.S. Food and Drug Administration for PMS or PMDD; (2) their safety in pregnancy and lactation has not been established; and (3) the manufacturing standards for herbal products are not uniform. Recommended nonpharmacologic interventions for patients with PMS/PMDD include the following: (1) patient education regarding the biologic basis and prevalence of their condition; (2) keeping a daily symptom diary; (3) adequate rest/structured sleep schedule; (4) sodium and caffeine restriction; and (5) aerobic exercise.

SOLUTION TO THE CLINICAL CASE MANAGEMENT PROBLEM

PMS

National Institute of Mental Health Criteria

A 30% increase in the intensity of symptoms of PMS (measured using a standardized instrument) from cycle days 5 to 10 as compared with the 6-day interval before the onset of menses *and* documentation of these changes in a daily symptom diary for at least two consecutive cycles.

University of California at San Diego Criteria

At least one of the following affective and somatic symptoms during the 5 days before menses in each of the three previous cycles.
Affective symptoms: depression, angry outbursts, irritability, anxiety, confusion, withdrawal
Somatic symptoms: breast tenderness, abdominal bloating, headache, swelling of the extremities
  Symptoms relieved from days 4 through 13 of the menstrual cycle.

PMDD

DSM IV Research Criteria

A. In most menstrual cycles during the past year, five or more of the following symptoms were present for most of the time during the last week of the luteal phase, began to remit within a few days after the onset of the follicular phase, and were absent in the week after menses, with at least one of the symptoms being 1, 2, 3, or 4:
  1. Markedly depressed mood, feelings of hopelessness, or self deprecating thoughts
  2. Marked anxiety, tension, or feelings of being "keyed up" or "on edge"
  3. Marked affective lability
  4. Persistent and marked anger or irritability, or increased interpersonal conflicts
  5. Decreased interest in usual activities
  6. Subjective sense of difficulty concentrating
  7. Lethargy, easy fatigability, or marked lack of energy
  8. Marked change in appetite, overeating, or specific food cravings
  9. Hypersomnia or insomnia
  10. A subjective sense of being overwhelmed or out of control
  11. Other physical symptoms such as breast tenderness or swelling, headaches, joint or muscle pain, a sensation of "bloating," or weight gain

B. The disturbance markedly interferes with work or school, or with usual social activities and relationships with others.

C. The disturbance is not merely an exacerbation of symptoms of another disorder.

D. Criteria A, B, and C must be confirmed by prospective daily ratings during at least two consecutive symptomatic cycles.

SUMMARY OF PREMENSTRUAL SYNDROME AND PREMENSTRUAL DYSPHORIC DISORDER

For diagnostic criteria, see the Solution to the Clinical Case Management Problem.

Treatment options include the following:

1. **Nonpharmacologic:** (1) patient education; (2) daily symptom diary; (3) adequate rest/structured sleep schedule; (4) sodium restriction; (5) caffeine restriction; and (6) aerobic exercise.

2. **Pharmacologic:** (1) SSRIs (evidence level 1a); (2) estrogen therapy/COCs (mixed outcomes; may exacerbate symptoms); (3) androgen therapy (e.g., Danazol; use limited by side effects); (4) GnRH agonists (e.g., Lupron; use limited by side effects); (5) NSAIDs (effective for physical symptoms except breast tenderness); and (6) diuretics (i.e., spironolactone; effective for breast tenderness and bloating).

3. **Supplements and herbal therapies:** (1) calcium carbonate 1200 mg/day (evidence level 1b); (2) vitamin B_6 100 mg/day; (3) vitamin E 400 IU/day; (4) chasteberry (level 1c); and (5) evening primrose oil.

SUGGESTED READING

American College of Obstetricians and Gynecologists: ACOG Practice Bulletin. Clinical management guidelines for obstetrician-gynecologists. Premenstrual syndrome. *Obstet Gynecol* 95:1-9, 2000.

American Psychiatric Association: *Diagnostic and statistical manual of mental disorders,* 4th edition. 715-718, 1994.

Bhatia SK, Bhatia SK: Diagnosis and treatment of premenstrual dysphoric disorder. *Am Fam Physician* 66:1253-1254, 2002.

Dickerson LM, et al: Premenstrual syndrome. *Am Fam Physician* 67:1743-1752, 2003.

Evidence-Based Systemic Review Sources

Clinical Evidence Mental Health (BMJ Publishing) (http://www.bmjjournals.com).

Cochrane database (http://www.cochrane.org).

Medical Inforetriever/infopoems (http://www.medicalinforetriever.org).

Natural Medicines Comprehensive Database (http://www.naturaldatabase.com).

Chapter 55

Postmenopausal Symptoms

> "Darling, please open the windows and remove that blanket. I am sweating."

CLINICAL CASE PROBLEM 1:

A 51-Year-Old Female with Hot Flashes

A 51-year-old woman has been experiencing progressive symptoms of profuse night sweats and frequent hot flushes occurring both day and night. She finds her emotional state increasingly labile. She also is experiencing sleep disturbances and anxiety. She denies any other complaints. Her last period was about 12 months ago. She has no history of medical problems or affective disorders. Her pulse is 78, and her blood pressure is 122/74. Her pelvic examination reveals atrophic external genitalia, a small anteverted uterus, and no adnexal masses. The rest of her examination is completely normal.

▶ SELECT THE BEST ANSWER TO THE FOLLOWING QUESTIONS:

1. What is the most likely diagnosis in this patient?
   a. pheochromocytoma
   b. hyperthyroidism
   c. menopause
   d. generalized anxiety disorder
   e. depression or panic attacks

2. What is the most effective treatment option for this patient?
   a. thyroid replacement
   b. estrogen with progestin (hormone replacement therapy [HRT])
   c. antidepressants
   d. estrogen alone (ERT)
   e. progestin alone

3. Alternative therapies for this patient's condition might include:
   a. black cohosh
   b. soy products
   c. biofeedback
   d. clonidine patches
   e. all of the above

4. If this patient also was complaining of vaginal dryness, reasonable treatment options would include:
   a. estrogen creams
   b. an estrogen ring (Estring)
   c. vaginal moisturizers
   d. increased foreplay and intercourse
   e. all of the above

5. The HRT arm of the Women's Health Initiative (WHI) randomized controlled trial was stopped prematurely primarily because patients the treatment group demonstrated an increased relative risk for what condition?
   a. breast cancer
   b. endometrial cancer
   c. colon cancer
   d. osteoporotic fractures
   e. all of the above

6. What conclusions can be accurately made based on the findings of the WHI HRT trial?
   a. estrogen appears to cause breast cancer
   b. estrogen appears to cause coronary heart disease (CHD)
   c. progesterone appears to cause breast cancer
   d. progesterone appears to cause CHD
   e. daily combined use of 0.625 mg conjugated equine estrogen (CEE) and 2.5 mg medroxy-progesterone acetate progesterone (MPA) does not appear to prevent CHD

7. Potential limitations of the HRT arm of the WHI include:
   a. average age of the patients at start of the trial was 63 years
   b. patients with significant vasomotor symptoms were excluded from the trial
   c. only one dose, combination, and route of estrogen/progestin were studied
   d. quality-of-life indicators were not assessed
   e. all of the above

8. Current Food and Drug Administration (FDA) indications for ERT/HRT include:
   a. urge incontinence
   b. prevention of dementia
   c. prevention of osteoporosis
   d. treatment of osteoporosis
   e. treatment of hyperlipidemia

9. Which of the following statements regarding postmenopausal osteoporosis is true:
   a. the most rapid loss of bone density occurs within the first 5 years of menopause
   b. surgical menopause is a lower risk factor for osteoporosis than natural menopause
   c. the protective effects of ERT on bone density is maintained after discontinuation
   d. all women should undergo bone density testing at menopause
   e. the United States Preventive Services Task Force (USPSTF) recommends against bone density testing for women older than age 65 years old

10. Your patient also complains of chronic urinary urgency and frequency. She admits that she needs to wear a pad and also notes leakage of urine whenever she coughs, laughs, or sneezes. She has no history of urinary tract infections (UTIs), diabetes, or kidney problems. The most likely diagnosis for this patient is:
    a. urge incontinence
    b. stress incontinence
    c. mixed incontinence
    d. overflow incontinence
    e. neurogenic bladder

11. Initial workup for this patient would include all but the following:
    a. urinalysis
    b. postvoid residual
    c. voiding diary
    d. urine culture
    e. bladder ultrasound

 CLINICAL CASE MANAGEMENT PROBLEM

Discuss the latest USPSTF recommendations for HRT.

■ **ANSWERS:**

1. **c.** The most likely diagnosis in this patient is menopause. Menopause is a retrospective diagnosis based on 12 or more months of amenorrhea occurring at a mean age of 51 years. The diagnosis is based on the appropriate age of a female patient for menopause (range 45-55 years), symptoms of frequent classic "hot flashes," night sweats, and the association of these symptoms with the cessation of menses. Although the patient does have some symptoms associated with the other conditions listed, her lack of other complaints (hair loss, diarrhea, palpitations) or previous history of an affective disorder (depression, anxiety, panic) along with her normal vital signs and essentially normal physical examination make the diagnosis of these other conditions less likely. The findings of vulvo-vaginal atrophy are also consistent with menopause.

2. **b.** The most effective treatment for this patient's vasomotor symptoms is HRT (estrogen combined with a daily or cyclic progestin/progesterone). A progestin alone may alleviate some of this patient' symptoms, but the patient's symptoms are related primarily to estrogen deficiency and thus respond best to estrogen replacement. However, because this patient still has her uterus, ERT is not recommended because of the significantly increased risk of endometrial hyperplasia/ cancer with prolonged unopposed estrogen use.

Antidepressants might help alleviate some of this patient's symptoms if she was also clinically depressed. However, this patient's symptoms are most likely hormonally related, and HRT/ERT alone often alleviates both the affective and somatic symptoms of menopause. There is no strong evidence that this patient has hypothyroidism, and there is certainly no indication for empiric use of thyroid hormone without objective evidence of hypothyroidism (i.e., thyroid stimulating hormone [TSH], thyroid function test [TFT]).

3. **e.** Although ERT/HRT remains the most effective therapy for this patient's vasomotor symptoms, many women will not or cannot use estrogen. All of the therapies listed have shown some benefit in alleviating hot flushes and night sweats associated with menopause. Black cohosh is derived from a root. Its mechanism of action is not clearly understood. Soy contains isoflavones (plant sterols), which appear to bind to estrogen receptors. Biofeedback appears to help patients maintain their body's thermoregulatory control. Clonidine patches, traditionally used for blood pressure control, appear to help reduce the peripheral vascular changes associated with vasomotor symptoms. However, side effects (lightheadedness, fatigue) often limit its use, especially in normotensive patients. Several small randomized control trials (RCTs) have demonstrated the potential effectiveness of various serotonin reuptake inhibitors (SSRIs) in alleviating some menopausal-related symptoms. All of these therapies lack large, good-quality RCTs to support their use, and none of them are FDA-approved for menopausal symptoms.

4. **e.** Symptoms of urogenital atrophy related to menopause (estrogen deficiency) include vaginal dryness, vaginitis, dyspareunia, dysuria, urinary incontinence, and recurrent UTIs. Estrogen creams (usually applied intravaginally 3 times per week every hour of sleep [QHS]) and the estrogen-embedded vaginal ring (Estring; changed every 3 months) are highly effective for reducing both the signs and symptoms of urogenital atrophy, with significantly less systemic estrogen absorption compared to oral or transdermal estrogen therapy. Although this minimizes the risk of venous thromboembolic events (VTEs), there is no strong evidence that they are less likely to increase the risk of other cardiovascular events (i.e., myocardial infarct [MI], cardiovascular accident [CVA]) or breast cancer. Vaginal moisturizers and increased vaginal sexual activity also help with vaginal lubrication and reduce atrophic symptomatology.

5. **a.** The WHI is the largest multicenter clinical investigation of postmenopausal women, having recruited more than 60,000 patients. The WHI includes a randomized double-blind, placebo-controlled set of three trials and one observational study to examine the effects of various interventions on the major causes of morbidity and mortality in postmenopausal women, namely CHD, breast cancer, colon cancer, and osteoporotic fractures. One arm of the WHI followed 16,608 healthy patients aged 50 to 79 years at baseline, with an intact uterus, taking either HRT (using 0.625 mg of CEE combined with 2.5 mg of MPA) or placebo. On July 9, 2002, 5.2 years after study initiation (intended duration: 8 years), the HRT portion of the trial was halted because of the findings that the overall health risks of treatment (observed increases in CHD, VTE, and breast cancer) outweighed its benefits, which were observed decreases in osteoporotic fractures and colon cancer (Table 55-1). However, these increases in adverse

Table 55-1 Results of the Women's Health Initiative's Hormone Replacement Therapy Randomized Clinical Trial

ABSOLUTE AND RELATIVE RISK OR BENEFIT OF CEE/MPA

Health Event	Overall Hazard Ratio	Nominal 95%	Adjusted 95%	Increased Absolute Risk per 10,000 Women/Year	Increased Absolute Benefit per 10,000 Women/Year
CHD	1.29	1.02-1.63	0.85-1.97	7	—
Strokes	1.41	1.07-1.85	0.86-2.31	8	—
Breast cancer	1.26	1.00-1.59	0.83-1.92	8	—
BTED	2.11	1.58-2.82	1.26-3.55	18	—
Colorectal cancer	0.63	0.43-0.92	0.32-1.24	—	6
Hip fractures	0.66	0.45-0.98	0.33-1.33	—	5
Total fractures	0.76	0.69-0.85	0.63-0.92	—	44

CEE, conjugated equine estrogen; MPA, medroxyprogesterone acetate; CHD, coronary heart disease; VTED, venous thromboembolic disease.
Writing Group for the Women's Health Initiative Investigators. *JAMA.* 2002; 288:321–322.

events in the treatment group were small, and there were no significant differences between groups regarding endometrial cancer and mortality from any causes. The estrogen-only arm (ERT versus placebo), in women without a uterus, is still ongoing, and its results should be available in 2005.

6. e. The HRT arm of the WHI RCT did demonstrate a higher relative risk of cardiovascular events (MI, CVA, VTE) and breast cancer in the HRT treatment group compared with the control group. However, the absolute risk of these events attributable to HRT is small and no cause and effect conclusions should be inferred. In addition, the ERT arm of the WHI RCT is ongoing. Thus, it is not possible to determine whether the estrogen (CEE) or progestin (MPA) component of HRT, or the combination of the two, is most closely associated with the increased relative risk for these conditions. In addition, these findings may not apply to other estrogen and/or progestin formulations, combinations, dosages, and routes of administration (i.e., transdermal, intravaginal). However, it is reasonable to infer from these data that the combination of 0.625 mg/day of CEE and 2.5 mg/day of MPA does not appear to prevent CHD. Thus, the authors of the WHI HRT trial data made the following recommendations in the Conclusion section of their paper: "*Results from WHI indicate that the combined postmenopausal hormones CEE, 0.625 mg/day, plus MPA, 2.5 mg/day, should not be initiated or continued for the primary prevention of CHD. In addition, the substantial risks for cardiovascular disease and breast cancer must be weighed against the benefit for fracture in selecting from the available agents to prevent osteoporosis.*"

7. e. To ensure that patients in the placebo arm of the WHI HRT trial would continue to participate for the entire study, patients with significant vasomotor symptoms were excluded. Thus, the average participant age at the start of the study was 63 years, with an average of 6 years since the onset of menopause. In addition, quality-of-life indicators, including menopausal symptom relief, were not measured in this trial. For obvious reasons of project cost, recruitment, and statistical power, only one dose and route of one combination formulation of HRT were evaluated in this study. All of this limitation may affect the generalizability of this RCT's results to other HRT formulations, dosages, and routes, and it may affect the applicability of these results to younger, symptomatic postmenopausal patients.

8. c. The current FDA indications for ERT/HRT include the following: (1) treatment of moderate to severe vasomotor symptoms; (2) treatment of moderate to severe symptoms of vulvar and vaginal

atrophy (dryness and irritation) associated with menopause; and (3) prevention of postmenopausal osteoporosis. Despite recent studies, including the WHI HRT trial, supporting the effectiveness of ERT/HRT for preventing osteoporotic fractures, it is not indicated for the treatment of osteoporosis. Although Postmenopausal Estrogen/Progesterone Interventions (PEPI) trials and other RCTs have demonstrated the overall favorable lipid effects of ERT/HRT, it is not indicated for the treatment of hyperlipidemia. ERT/HRT may benefit urinary symptoms related to urogenital atrophy, but it is not indicated for urge incontinence.

On January 8, 2003, the FDA issued a statement advising women and health care professionals about important new safety changes to labeling of all estrogen and estrogen with progestin products for use by postmenopausal women. These changes reflected the FDA's analysis of data from the WHI that raised concern about risks of using these products. The FDA's new labeling changes include a new boxed warning that reflects new risk information and changes to the approved indications to emphasize individualized decisions that appropriately balance the potential benefits and risks of these products.

The new boxed warning, the highest level of warning information in labeling, highlights the increased risks for heart disease, heart attacks, strokes, and breast cancer. This warning also emphasizes that these products are not approved for heart disease prevention. The FDA also has modified the approved indications for Premarin, Prempro, and Premphase to clarify that these drugs should be used only when the benefits clearly outweigh risks. Of the three indications, two have been revised to include consideration of other therapies. The three indications are as follows:

1. Treatment of moderate to severe vasomotor symptoms (such as "hot flashes") associated with menopause. (This indication has not changed.)
2. Treatment of moderate to severe symptoms of vulvar and vaginal atrophy (dryness and irritation) associated with menopause. It now is recommended that when these products are being prescribed solely for the treatment of symptoms of vulvar and vaginal atrophy, topical vaginal products should be considered.
3. Prevention of postmenopausal osteoporosis, when these products are being prescribed solely for the prevention of postmenopausal osteoporosis. The current recommendation is that approved nonestrogen treatments should be considered carefully and estrogens and combined estrogen–progestin products should be considered only for women with significant risk of osteoporosis that outweighs the risks of the drug.

To minimize the potential risks and to accomplish the desired treatment goals, the new labeling also advises health care providers to prescribe estrogen and combined estrogen with progestin drug products at the lowest dose and for the shortest duration for the individual woman. Women who choose to take estrogens or combined estrogen and progestin therapies after discussing their treatment with their doctor should have yearly breast examinations by a health care provider, perform monthly breast self-examinations, and receive periodic mammography (scheduled based on their age and risk factors). Women also should talk to their health care provider about other ways to reduce their risk factors for heart disease (e.g., high blood pressure, poor diet, tobacco use) and osteoporosis (e.g., an appropriate diet, use of vitamin D and calcium supplements, weight-bearing exercise).

9. a. Osteoporosis is a systemic skeletal disease characterized by low bone mass and microarchitectural deterioration of bone tissue, with a consequent increase in bone fragility and susceptibility to fracture. There is a clear causal relationship between estrogen deficiency and osteoporosis. A woman's bone density tends to peak by ages 30-35 years, whereas her most rapid loss of bone tends to occur during the first 5 years of menopause. Postmenopausal status, regardless of the etiology (natural, surgically/hormonally induced), or estrogen deficiency at any age significantly increases a patient's risk for osteoporosis and subsequent fragility fractures. Estrogen appears to inhibit bone resorption by reducing the production of bone-resorbing osteoclasts, while promoting the activation of bone-forming osteoblasts. Estrogen deficiency leads to a rapid increase in osteoclast formation and activity, leading to accelerated bone resorption. Studies also suggest that bone loss is accelerated when ERT/HRT is discontinued. Therefore, ERT/HRT simply may postpone the rapid bone loss associated with menopause. This is a very important point when counseling patients about ERT/HRT compliance and the long-term prevention of osteoporosis.

The National Osteoporosis Foundation (NOF) expert panel recommends that all women age 65 and older be screened for osteoporosis regardless of presence or absence of risk factors. NOF also recommends screening younger postmenopausal women with one or more major risk factor (personal history of atraumatic fracture, family history of osteoporotic fracture, smoking, body weight less than 127 lb). The USPSTF also recommends universal bone mineral density (BMD) screening for all women 65 and older. For women from age 60 and older, the USPSTF recommends screening if there are risk factors for osteoporotic fracture. The USPSTF makes no recommendation for or against routine screening in postmenopausal women younger than age 60 or aged 60-64 without increased risk for osteoporotic fracture.

10. c. This patient's history is most consistent with mixed urinary incontinence. However, she requires further evaluation to confirm the diagnosis and rule out other causes. Urge incontinence usually is caused by irritability and/or instability of the detrusor muscle in the bladder. Patients with this condition often present with almost constant urinary urgency, frequency, and the sensation of incomplete emptying with voiding. Patients with more severe symptoms may have frequent incontinent episodes. Patients with stress incontinence often note that they "leak urine" whenever they cough, laugh, or sneeze (Valsalva). Patients with a neurogenic bladder (e.g., patients with paraplegia or severe diabetes) have no neurologic control of their bladder and are susceptible to overflow incontinence.

11. e. An appropriate initial workup for this patient would include the following: (1) a urinalysis (to assess for proteinuria, glucosuria); (2) a postvoid residual (to assess for incomplete emptying or overflow incontinence); (3) a urine culture (to rule out an infection); and (4) a daily fluid intake and voiding diary (to assess potential contributing factors to patients symptoms). A bladder ultrasound would not be indicated at this point in the evaluation, based on the patient's presenting complaints.

SOLUTION TO THE CLINICAL CASE MANAGEMENT PROBLEM

USPTF published their latest recommendations for HRT in September 2002. They recommend against the routine use of estrogen and progestin for the prevention of chronic conditions in postmenopausal women (a D recommendation), and they concluded that the evidence is insufficient to recommend for or against the use of unopposed estrogen for the prevention of chronic conditions in postmenopausal women who have had a hysterectomy (an I recommendation).

SUMMARY OF POSTMENOPAUSAL SYMPTOMS

Review the WHI HRT RCT results summarized in Table 55-1.

Symptoms are as follows:

1. Vasomotor: (a) hot flushes/hot flashes (occur in up to 85% of postmenopausal women) and (b) night sweats
2. Urogenital: (a) dyspareunia; (b) vaginitis; (c) vaginal dryness; (d) dysuria/urgency; (e) urinary incontinence; and (f) recurrent/chronic UTIs
3. Behavioral: (a) sleep disturbances; (b) irritability; (c) emotional lability; (d) decreased libido; (e) memory loss; and (f) problems concentrating

Treatments are as follows:

1. FDA indicates use of ERT/HRT for (a) treatment of moderate to severe vasomotor symptoms; (b) treatment of moderate to severe symptoms of vulvar and vaginal atrophy; and (c) prevention of postmenopausal osteoporosis
2. ERT/HRT Options
   a. Routes: oral, transdermal, intravaginal (cream/ring)
   b. Estrogen formulations: CEE, estradiol, estrone sulfate, ethinyl estradiol
   c. Progestin/progesterone formulations:* MPA, norethindrone, Prometrium, Aygestin
3. Alternative therapies: (a) black cohosh; (b) soy products (with active isoflavones); (c) biofeedback; (d) clonidine patches; and (e) SSRIs

*Patients with an intact uterus should receive an estrogen combined with a daily/cyclic progestin/progesterone (HRT) that is FDA-approved for the prevention of endometrial hyperplasia.

Screening tests for postmenopausal women are as follows: (1) height/weight (periodically); (2) blood pressure (periodically); (3) vision (periodically); (4) mammogram/clinical breast examination (after 40 years; annually); (5) Papanicolaou (Pap) test (every 1-3 years until age 65; stop if postabdominal hysterectomy, not because of malignancy); (6) colorectal (after 50 years; frequency depends on method; fecal occult blood test, flexible sigmoidoscopy, or colonoscopy); (7) BMD (see USPSTF and NOF screening guidelines); and (8) fasting lipid profile (after 45 years; every 5 years, if previous results were normal).

SUGGESTED READING

American College of Obstetricians and Gynecologists: *Questions and answers on hormone therapy.* August 30, 2002. Washington DC.

Morelli V, Naquin C: Alternative therapies for traditional disease states: menopause. *Am Fam Physician* 66:129-134, 2002.

National Osteoporosis Foundation. *Physician's guide to prevention and treatment of osteoporosis.* Excerpta Medica, Inc., 1998, Belle Mead, NJ.

Nelson HD, et al: Screening for postmenopausal osteoporosis: a review of the evidence for the U.S. Preventive Services Task Force. *Ann Intern Med* 137(6):529-541, 2002.

U.S. Department of Health and Human Services. U.S. Food & Drug Administration approves new labels for estrogen and estrogen plus progestin therapy for postmenopausal women following review of WHI. *FDA News* P03-01, Washington, DC, January 8, 2003.

U.S. Preventive Services Task Force: Postmenopausal hormone replacement therapy for primary prevention of chronic conditions: recommendations and rationale. USPSTF Guide to Clinical Preventive Services. *Ann Intern Med* 137(10):834-839, 2002.

Writing Group for the Women's Health Initiative Investigators. Risks and benefits of estrogen plus progestin in healthy postmenopausal women. *JAMA* 288(3):321-333, 2002.

Chapter 56

Dysmenorrhea

"Mama, I don't want to grow up.
This monthly thing hurts too much."

CLINICAL CASE PROBLEM 1:

A 14-Year-Old Female with Painful Menses

A 14-year-old female comes to your office with a 6-month history of lower midabdominal pain. The pain is colicky in nature, radiates to the back and upper thighs, begins with onset of menses, and lasts for 2-4 days. She has missed several days of school during the last 2 months because the pain was so severe. Menarche began 18 months ago, and her menses became regular 6 months ago. The patient is not sexually active. Physical examination, including abdomen and pelvis, is normal. The patient has normal secondary sexual development.

■ SELECT THE BEST ANSWER TO THE FOLLOWING QUESTIONS:

1. What is the most likely etiology of this patient's pain?
   a. primary dysmenorrhea
   b. pelvic inflammatory disease (PID)
   c. secondary dysmenorrhea
   d. endometriosis
   e. premenstrual syndrome

2. The etiology of this patient's conditions is related to:
   a. increased levels of prostaglandin
   b. decreased levels of prostaglandin
   c. increased levels of cyclic adenosine monophosphate (cAMP)
   d. decreased levels of cAMP
   e. none of the above

3. What would you recommend as initial treatment of choice?
   a. nonsteroidal antiinflammatory drugs (NSAIDs)
   b. oral contraceptive pills (OCPs)
   c. gonadotropin-releasing hormone (GnRH) agonist
   d. acetaminophen
   e. intrauterine device (IUD) placement

4. The pathophysiology of this patient's pain is associated with:
   a. vasodilation of the uterine arteries
   b. vasoconstriction of the uterine arteries
   c. vasodilation of the pelvic veins
   d. vasodilation of the uterine veins
   e. none of the above

5. When does the disorder described usually begin?
   a. 13-16 years of age
   b. within 3 years of onset of thelarche (breast development)
   c. within 5 years of onset of thelarche
   d. within 3 years of onset of menarche (first menses)
   e. within 5 years of onset of menarche

6. Which of the following is not usually associated with primary dysmenorrhea?
   a. pain beginning with onset of menses
   b. pain peaking during heaviest flow
   c. pain responsive to NSAIDs
   d. endometriosis
   e. pain responsive to OCPs

7. Which of the following is more consistent with premenstrual syndrome (PMS) than with primary dysmenorrhea?
   a. symptoms that interfere with patient's daily function
   b. symptoms that are cyclic in nature
   c. abdominal symptoms associated with menses
   d. symptoms with onset during late luteal phase
   e. diagnosis based generally on history alone

8. The patient in Clinical Case Problem 1 returns 6 months later. She has tried several different NSAIDs, using the correct doses and regimens you prescribed. She had partial relief of her pain but still experiences such bothersome symptoms that she still misses school occasionally. At this time, you recommend that she:
   a. continue the NSAIDs only
   b. discontinue the NSAIDs and begin oxycodone
   c. add OCPs
   d. switch to danazol
   e. undergo laparoscopic presacral neuroectomy

CLINICAL CASE PROBLEM 2:
A 24-YEAR-OLD FEMALE WITH INFERTILITY AND PAINFUL MENSES

A 24-year-old nulligravida woman comes to your office with an 18-month history of cyclic, debilitating pelvic pain related to menses. Her menses is regular and heavy, requiring 10-15 thick pads on the days of heaviest flow. She denies ever being diagnosed with a sexually transmitted disease (STD). She and her husband have been engaging in regular intercourse without contraception for 1 year in attempt to conceive. On pelvic examination, you find a normal-sized, immobile, retroverted uterus with nodularity and tenderness on palpation of the uterosacral ligaments.

9. You inform the patient that the most likely diagnosis is:
   a. uterine fibroid
   b. endometriosis
   c. adenomyosis
   d. PID
   e. endometrial carcinoma

10. You further explain that her pain is described most accurately as:
    a. primary dysmenorrhea
    b. secondary dysmenorrhea
    c. premenstrual syndrome
    d. psychogenic pain
    e. none of the above

11. Which of the following studies would establish a diagnosis in this condition?
    a. hysteroscopy
    b. ultrasound
    c. laparoscopy
    d. hysterosalpingogram (HSG)
    e. magnetic resonance imaging (MRI) scan

12. Which of the following is *not* an appropriate medical therapy for this condition?
    a. danazol
    b. GnRH agonist
    c. continuous OCPs
    d. Depo-Provera
    e. clomiphene

13. Which of the following is least consistent with secondary dysmenorrhea?
 a. normal pelvic examination
 b. onset of pain after the age of 25
 c. onset of pain during adolescence
 d. pain relief with NSAIDs
 e. pain relief with OCPs

14. Other causes of secondary dysmenorrhea include all of the following except:
 a. PID
 b. chronic use of OCPs
 c. uterine fibroids
 d. IUD
 e. adenomyosis

CLINICAL CASE MANAGEMENT PROBLEM

Discuss proposed etiologies of endometriosis.

■ **ANSWERS:**

1. a. This young woman has primary dysmenorrhea. Primary dysmenorrhea is the most common gynecologic complaint of young women, with reported prevalence rates as high as 90%. It is one of the leading causes of absenteeism in young women. Primary dysmenorrhea usually begins within 6-12 months of menarche. The pain is described as sharp spasms in the lower abdomen and suprapubic area. Associated symptoms include nausea, vomiting, diarrhea, headache and fatigue. The timing of the pain in relation to menses is key to the diagnosis. The onset of pain is usually within hours of menstrual flow onset and peaks on the day of heaviest flow. Secondary dysmenorrhea is defined as dysmenorrhea with identifiable pelvic etiology. PID and endometriosis are two causes of secondary dysmenorrhea. Premenstrual syndrome is characterized by symptoms of bloating, fatigue, and breast tenderness just *prior* to menses.

2. a. Women with primary dysmenorrhea have ovulatory cycles and produce progesterone during the luteal phase. Progesterone stimulates prostaglandin production in the endometrium. After progesterone withdrawal, the endometrium sloughs and releases prostaglandins. Prostaglandins stimulate myometrial contractions, leading to decreased blood flow and local ischemia. These physiologic changes result in increased production of vasoconstrictive prostaglandins, causing uterine hypoxia and pain. Women with primary dysmenorrhea have been found to have elevated levels of prostaglandin, particularly $PGF_{2\alpha}$

Hence, first-line therapy for dysmenorrhea is nonsteroidal antiinflammatory therapy, which decreases prostaglandin levels.

3. a. NSAIDs are the treatment of choice. They inhibit cyclooxygenase, thus decreasing prostaglandin levels. Oral contraceptives may be used in conjunction with NSAIDs for the treatment of dysmenorrhea and are particularly ideal in women who desire contraception. However, OCPs are not considered first-line treatment because they do not address directly the problem of elevated prostaglandin levels. The other answers listed are not first-line treatment for primary dysmenorrhea.

4. b. Primary dysmenorrhea is mediated pathologically by an increase in the level of the enzyme prostaglandin synthetase. Elevated levels of the enzyme produce vasoconstricting prostaglandins that are responsible for uterine hypoxia, or uterine angina, which produces the pain of dysmenorrhea. The vasoconstriction itself takes place in the branches of the uterine artery. Venous vasodilation is not responsible for dysmenorrhea.

5. d. Primary dysmenorrhea almost always begins within 3 years of the onset of menstruation. Exact age of onset for primary dysmenorrhea will vary depending on the age of menarche. If dysmenorrhea begins at a later time, one should suspect secondary dysmenorrhea. The definition of primary dysmenorrhea is related to menarche, not thelarche (breast development).

6. d. As discussed earlier, primary dysmenorrheal is painful menses coinciding with onset of menses, peaking during heaviest flow, and is responsive to NSAIDs and OCPs. Endometriosis is associated with secondary dysmenorrhea.

7. d. Both PMS and primary dysmenorrhea may involve abdominal symptoms associated with menses and are cyclic in nature. Both conditions may be so severe that they interfere with quality of life and daily function. However, PMS is characterized by symptoms occurring in the late luteal phase, just prior to the onset of menses, and resolve shortly after menstrual flow begins. PMS symptoms include abdominal bloating, breast tenderness, irritability, and fatigue.

8. c. NSAIDs are the drugs of choice for the treatment of primary dysmenorrhea. If there is no significant change in pain after a reasonable duration (approximately 3 months) of one NSAID regimen, it is sometimes helpful to try an NSAID from a different category. With each prescribed regimen, it is important to assess patient compliance, such that maximum daily frequency and dose has been reached. NSAIDs should not be given to patients who have nasal polyps, angioedema, and bronchospasm related to aspirin or other NSAIDs. If the patient has only partial relief from NSAIDs, switching directly to a narcotic is not appropriate until other alternatives have been explored. Second-line treatment for primary dysmenorrhea includes a trial of oral contraceptives. The use of OCPs is particularly advantageous if the patient also desires a method of birth control. OCPs help alleviate symptoms of dysmenorrhea by both reducing menstrual flow and inhibiting ovulation and have been shown to be 90% effective within 3-4 months of use. Continuous use of oral contraceptives can be very helpful by reducing the number of menstrual cycles. During continuous OCP use, the patient takes "active" hormone pills for 6-9 weeks straight, eliminating the placebo pills and subsequent withdrawal bleeding. An alternative treatment is Depo-Provera, which induces amenorrhea in half of all patients by the third injection and thus eliminates dysmenorrhea. Danazol, a synthetic androgen, also can induce amenorrhea but is associated with unpleasant side effects including acne, hirsutism, and virilizing symptoms. Laparoscopic presacral neuroectomy is reserved for refractory cases of dysmenorrhea and is not appropriate until conservative measures have been exhausted.

9. b. Endometriosis is a condition in which ectopic endometrial tissue implants are found in extrauterine sites, most commonly the ovaries, fallopian tubes, cul-de-sac, and uterosacral ligaments. Patients with endometriosis complain of dysmenorrhea that often begins years after pain-free cycles. Other associated symptoms include dyspareunia (painful intercourse), dyschezia (painful defecation), and low back pain. A history of infertility is also common. Pelvic examination can reveal a fixed, retroverted uterus and masses or nodularity along the uterosacral ligaments. A normal-sized uterus is less supportive of a diagnosis for uterine fibroid or adenomyosis. PID and endometriosis both could cause infertility and painful menses. However, the negative history for STDs makes PID less likely. Endometrial carcinoma is more closely associated with irregular bleeding than with painful menses.

10. b. Secondary dysmenorrhea is defined as dysmenorrhea with an identifiable pelvic abnormality.

Dysmenorrhea, whether primary or secondary, is not psychological in origin as once was believed.

11. c. The diagnosis of endometriosis can be strongly suspected on the basis of a careful history and physical examination. However, confirmation of the diagnosis requires direct surgical visualization of lesions, which usually is performed by laparoscopy. Hysteroscopy and HSG are not helpful diagnostically because they assess only the internal uterine anatomy, not the external pelvic cavity and peritoneal surfaces. Ultrasound and MRI may give useful information in differentiating solid from cystic lesions, but they cannot be used for primary diagnosis of endometriosis.

12. e. The primary goal of hormonal treatment of endometriosis is to reduce pain or dyspareunia because medical therapy has not been shown to restore fertility. Medical therapy is directed at induction of amenorrhea, which hopefully will result in atrophy of the ectopic endometrial tissue. Combination OCPs reduce menstrual volume and theoretically decrease retrograde flow. Symptoms of endometriosis are relieved in three-fourths of patients. Continuous use of OCPs as described in Question 8 can be used to achieve longer periods of amenorrhea. OCPs are an optimal choice in patients who also desire a method of contraception. Progestins (oral or injectable) also are effective at reducing the symptoms of endometriosis. Other therapies include GnRH agonists (i.e., Lupron), which suppress gonadotropin secretion with a secondary decrease in ovarian estrogen production. A pseudomenopausal state is effectively induced such that patients may experience hypoestrogenic side effects (i.e., vasomotor symptoms, decrease in bone density). Danazol, a synthetic androgen that inhibits luteinizing hormone and follicle-stimulating hormone, is also effective in the treatment of endometriosis. Like GnRH agonists, danazol has a problematic side-effect profile, which includes both hypoestrogenic symptoms (hot flushes, night sweats) and androgenic symptoms (acne, hirsutism, weight gain). The response rate is about 90% for both GnRH and danazol. The only answer listed that is not medical treatment for pain related to endometriosis is clomiphene, which is used for ovulation induction in patients being treated for infertility. Surgical therapy is reserved for patients with symptoms refractory to medical treatment or for patients who are infertile with advanced disease.

13. c. Primary dysmenorrhea usually begins within 6-12 months of menarche and thus is likely to be associated with onset of pain during adolescence. Answers a, b, d, and e are more consistent with a patient presenting with secondary dysmenorrhea. Presentation of pain later in adulthood or pain completely unresponsive to NSAIDs or OCPs should make you suspect secondary amenorrhea. The next step is to determine the etiology of the patient's secondary amenorrhea.

14. **b.** Secondary dysmenorrhea can be caused by any condition that affects the pelvic region. Commonly associated disorders include PID, endometriosis, and adenomyosis or the presence of an IUD. OCPs are beneficial in some cases and are not a cause of secondary dysmenorrhea.

SOLUTION TO THE CLINICAL CASE MANAGEMENT PROBLEM

The etiology of endometriosis is not completely understood and is likely multifactorial. The classic theory links endometriosis to "retrograde menstruation." According to this theory, fragments of endometrium are passed in a retrograde fashion through the fallopian tubes, into the pelvic cavity, and subsequently implant onto various uterine and extrauterine structures. These tissue implants have the ability to respond to hormonal cues, such that cyclic proliferation and sloughing occurs just as in native endometrial lining. Although an attractive explanation, it does not completely explain how endometrial tissue has been found in remote sites such as lung and brain.

Some have proposed that endometrial tissue travels via hematogenous or lymphatic spread to distal sites. The theory of "coelomic metaplasia" is based on the fact that peritoneal tissue shares the same origin as endometrial tissue in the primitive coelomic wall. It is hypothesized that peritoneal tissue has the potential to transform into endometrial tissue via "metaplasia" under the influence of certain environmental triggers. A third theory suggests that remnants of Müllerian cells in the pelvis retain their ability to differentiate into endometrial tissue under hormonal stimulation. Finally, alterations in cell-mediated and humoral immunity may play a role in the pathogenesis of endometriosis.

SUMMARY OF DYSMENORRHEA

A. Diagnosis:

1. **Primary dysmenorrhea:** Begins within 3 years of the onset of menarche. Presents with mid to lower abdominal pain, spasmodic in nature, starting within hours of menstrual flow onset and usually lasting for 2-4 days.
2. **Secondary dysmenorrhea:** Dysmenorrhea associated with pelvic pathology. Onset is usually later in relation to menarche.

B. Etiology:

1. **Primary dysmenorrhea:** Caused by increased levels of prostaglandin.
2. **Secondary dysmenorrhea:** Causes include endometriosis, adenomyosis, endometrial polyps, myomas, cervical stenosis, PID, and presence of an IUD.

C. Treatment:

1. **Primary dysmenorrhea:** First line are NSAIDs. If a drug from one class is not effective, try a drug from the other class. If this is not successful, proceed to an OCP. Although an

OCP is considered a second-line option it may be used as an initial treatment in conjunction with NSAIDs if patient desires contraception.
2. Secondary dysmenorrhea: Establish and treat the cause.

ENDOMETRIOSIS is (1) is classically associated with dyspareunia, dyschezia, lower back pain, and infertility; (2) a definitive diagnosis based on laparoscopy; and (3) medical treatment options include OCPs, progestins, danazol, or GnRH agonists.

SUGGESTED READING

Coco AS: Primary dysmenorrhea. *Am Fam Physician* 60:489-496, 1999.
Dickerson LM, et al: Premenstrual syndrome. *Am Fam Physician* 67:1743-1752, 2003.
Hatcher RA, et al: *Contraceptive technology*: Ardent Media, Inc., 1998, New York.
Lu PY, Ory SJ: Endometriosis: current management. *Mayo Clin Proc* 70:453-463, 1995.
Wellbery C: Diagnosis and treatment of endometriosis. *Am Fam Physician* 60:1753-1768, 1999.

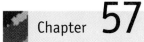

Chapter 57

Dysfunctional Uterine Bleeding

"How can an itty bitty cyst make me
weigh so much? Is it made of lead?"

CLINICAL CASE PROBLEM 1:

A 32-Year-Old Female with
Heavy Menses

A 32-year-old female comes to your office with concerns about heavy menstrual periods occurring at irregular intervals for the past year. She explains that sometimes her menses comes twice a month, but other times they will skip 2 months in a row. Her menses may last 7-10 days and require 10-15 thick sanitary napkins on the heaviest days. She admits having some fatigue but denies lightheadedness. She is does not smoke. She has had normal Papanicolaou (Pap) test results in the past. She is in a stable, monogamous relationship with her husband and denies a history of sexually transmitted disease (STD). On physical examination, her blood pressure is 120/80 mm Hg and her weight is 170 pounds. Her physical examination including a pelvic examination is normal.

■ **SELECT THE BEST ANSWER TO THE FOLLOWING QUESTIONS:**

1. The patient's bleeding pattern is best described as:
   a. menometrorrhagia
   b. polymenorrhea
   c. menorrhagia
   d. metrorrhagia
   e. oligomenorrhea

2. Which of the following should be considered in the differential diagnosis of this patient's problem?
   a. dysfunctional uterine bleeding (DUB)
   b. pelvic inflammatory disease (PID)
   c. endometrial carcinoma
   d. bleeding dyscrasia
   e. all of the above

3. All of the following are appropriate as initial work-up except:
   a. complete blood count (CBC)
   b. assessment for history of bleeding dyscrasia
   c. determination of free testosterone and dehydroepiandrosterone sulfate (DHEAS)
   d. urine pregnancy test
   e. all of the above

4. The most likely diagnosis is:
   a. DUB
   b. PID
   c. endometrial carcinoma
   d. bleeding dyscrasia
   e. all of the above

5. What is the most likely underlying mechanism for this patient's abnormal bleeding?
   a. a coagulation defect
   b. anovulation
   c. uterine pathology
   d. cervical pathology
   e. none of the above

6. Your patient returns to discuss test results. Her hemoglobin is 10.8 g/dL. She does not desire future fertility and has no method of birth control at this time. Appropriate medical management options for her include all *except*:
   a. iron supplementation
   b. cyclic progestin
   c. medroxyprogesterone acetate injection (Depo-Provera)
   d. combined oral contraceptives
   e. levonorgestrel intrauterine system (LNG-IUS)

CLINICAL CASE PROBLEM 2:

A 25-Year-Old Female
with Amenorrhea

A 25-year-old female (gravida 0, para 0) comes to your office complaining of not having her period for the last 6 months. She previously had regular cycles since menarche at age 13. Her blood pressure is 100/70, and her weight is 98 pounds. Her physical examination is unremarkable, including pelvic examination. She has normal secondary sexual development. On further questioning, she reveals that she has been training for a marathon and has lost about 10 lb in the last 2 months. She does not have an eating disorder. She is currently sexually active with one partner and desires contraception.

7. Which of the following best describes her bleeding pattern?
   a. primary amenorrhea
   b. secondary amenorrhea
   c. dysmenorrhea
   d. oligomenorrhea
   e. polymenorrhea

8. Common causes for this patient's bleeding pattern include all of the following *except*:
   a. pregnancy
   b. hypothyroidism
   c. hypothalamic amenorrhea
   d. hyperprolactinemia
   e. Turner's syndrome

9. You perform a urine pregnancy test, which is negative. Which of the following laboratory studies should be done as initial workup for this patient?
   a. thyroid stimulation hormone (TSH)
   b. free testosterone and DHEAS
   c. CBC
   d. comprehensive metabolic panel
   e. all of the above

10. What is the most appropriate initial step in the evaluation of this patient's condition?
    a. progestin challenge
    b. hysteroscopy
    c. pelvic ultrasound
    d. Depo-Provera shot
    e. none of the above

11. The patient's laboratory studies come back normal. She had a positive response to a progestin challenge. At this time, what would be most beneficial medical therapy for this patient?
    a. combined oral contraceptive pills (OCPs)
    b. monthly progestin pills on days 1-10
    c. monthly progestin pills on days 18-28
    d. nonsteroidal antiinflammatory drugs (NSAIDs)
    e. all of the above are acceptable

CLINICAL CASE PROBLEM 3:
A 55-YEAR-OLD POSTMENOPAUSAL WOMAN WITH IRREGULAR BLEEDING

A 55-year-old postmenopausal woman with a history of type 2 diabetes comes to your office for her annual gynecologic examination. She experienced menopause about 3 years ago. She mentions to you that she has had irregular menstrual bleeding for the last 8 months She describes the bleeding as lasting anywhere from 1-7 days, requiring 5-8 pads a day. The patient is not taking hormone replacement therapy (HRT). She complains of some fatigue but is otherwise feeling well. Her Pap test results always have been normal. Sexual history is significant for a new sexual partner for the last 6 months. Her blood pressure is 130/80, and her weight is 200 lb. The rest of her physical examination, including pelvic, is normal.

12. You perform a Pap test and a gonorrhea/chlamydia screen. You also check a CBC and TSH. What else do you recommend to the patient at this time?
    a. transvaginal ultrasound
    b. dilation and curettage (D&C)
    c. OCPs

    d. oral progestin challenge
    e. any of the above

13. A transvaginal ultrasound is performed and is read as *"no structural abnormalities, normal sized uterus and ovaries, 7 mm endometrial stripe noted."* The next step in management should be:
    a. repeat the ultrasound in 6 months
    b. give cyclic progestin
    c. perform endometrial biopsy
    d. give cyclic oral contraceptives
    e. observation only

CLINICAL CASE PROBLEM 4:
A 27-YEAR-OLD FEMALE WITH OLIGOMENORRHEA

A 27-year-old nulligravida female presents to your office for routine examination. On taking gynecologic history you discover that she has a 5-year history of oligomenorrhea, with only about 2-3 menses a year. She denies intercycle spotting or premenstrual symptoms. Her last menses was 3 months ago. Her blood pressure is 120/75, and her weight is 220 lb. Her physical examination reveals moderate amount of facial hair and inflammatory acne. Pelvic examination is unremarkable.

14. What condition do you suspect in this patient?
    a. adrenal tumor
    b. polycystic ovary syndrome (PCOS)
    c. hypothyroidism
    d. hyperprolactinemia
    e. none of the above

15. All of the following laboratory studies are appropriate for initial evaluation *except*:
    a. TSH
    b. luteinizing hormone (LH)
    c. follicle stimulating hormone (FSH)
    d. pregnancy test
    e. transvaginal ultrasound

16. The patient returns after 2 weeks to discuss her blood test results. Her pregnancy test is negative, and her prolactin, TSH, and 17 hydroxyprogesterone levels are normal. Her LH:FSH ratio is 4:1, and her testosterone level is mildly elevated. All of the following treatment options have been found to be beneficial in the treatment of PCOS except:
    a. weight loss
    b. oral contraceptives
    c. metformin
    d. ovarian wedge resection
    e. spironolactone

■ **ANSWERS:**

1. a. This patient has menometrorrhagia, which is defined as excessive menstrual bleeding (>80 cc per cycle) that occurs at irregular intervals. Metrorrhagia is defined as irregular, frequent bleeding of varying amounts but not excessive. Menorrhagia is excessive bleeding (>80 cc per cycle) that occurs at regular intervals. Polymenorrhea is regular bleeding at intervals less than 21 days. Oligomenorrhea is bleeding at intervals greater than every 35 days.

2. e. All of the listed answers could be causes of the patient's bleeding. DUB refers to uterine bleeding for which no specific genital tract lesion or systemic cause is found. If there is a secondary cause, it should be corrected if possible. The secondary causes that should be considered include the following: (1) uterine fibroids; (2) submucous fibroids; (3) endometriosis; (4) adenomyosis; (5) chronic PID; (6) endometrial polyps; (7) coagulation defects; (8) morbid obesity; (9) ovarian abnormalities; (10) severe hypothyroidism; (11) adenomatous hyperplasia; and (12) endometrial carcinoma.

3. c. The first and most important condition to rule out is pregnancy. A urine pregnancy test is quick and inexpensive to perform and should be done as part of initial evaluation. Once pregnancy has been ruled out, one can proceed with a further workup. A pelvic examination should be performed to assess for structural lesions such as a cervical polyp or uterine fibroid. A CBC should be done to assess for anemia. Other labs such as chemistry panel and liver function tests can be done if there is suspicion for systemic hepatic or renal disease. Routine performance of these studies in otherwise healthy patients generally does not reveal useful information. TSH and/or serum prolactin should be considered in women deemed anovulatory. A thorough history should be sought for bleeding dyscrasia (history of easy bruising, epistaxis, bleeding gums, family history), particularly in adolescents presenting with menorrhagia. Bleeding disorders have been demonstrated in up to 10.7% of women presenting with menorrhagia, the most common being von Willebrand's disease. Laboratory assessment for an inherited coagulation disorder should be done if indicated by history. A transvaginal ultrasound is not necessary in the initial evaluation unless pelvic examination reveals abnormalities or an adequate pelvic examination was unable to be performed (patient habitus or discomfort). Testosterone and DHEAS levels should be considered if there is evidence of androgen excess (hirsutism or acne) or virilization (male-pattern baldness, deepening voice, and clitoromegaly) but is not routinely indicated in the evaluation of irregular bleeding.

4. a. The most likely cause for bleeding in this patient is DUB. Her history of normal Pap test results and low-risk sexual history makes PID and cervical carcinoma unlikely. Given her age (younger than age 35 years), endometrial carcinoma is unlikely but always should be considered in the differential diagnosis. There should be a low threshold to perform endometrial biopsy if her bleeding is not responsive to medical therapy.

5. b. The most common cause of DUB is anovulatory bleeding. Ovulatory DUB accounts for less than 10% of all DUB. When the uterine lining is sequentially proliferated by estrogen, then it is ripened with progesterone (secretory phase); the endometrium is structurally stable. Sloughing of the endometrium does not occur unless progesterone withdrawal takes place. When progesterone is withdrawn, the tissue breakdown is orderly and progressive. Bleeding is limited in both amount and duration by spiral arteriolar vasoconstriction. Menstrual shedding is simultaneous in all endometrial segments. This is why ovulatory cycles are regular and predictable from month to month. When the uterine lining is proliferated by estrogen alone without progesterone to stabilize it, the endometrium continues to thicken. When the endometrial proliferation reaches a given thickness, it starts to shed, but this bleeding is not accompanied by spiral arteriolar vasoconstriction. Therefore it is not limited in either amount or duration and can occur at any time. Endometrial shedding occurs at random times from random sites within the uterus. This is why anovulatory bleeding is irregular and unpredictable.

In the evaluation of abnormal uterine bleeding, it is often helpful to consider the patient's reproductive status:

1. Premenopausal women: The majority of abnormal bleeding in patients of this age group with otherwise normal examinations is DUB and anovulation. A careful history and physical examination is usually all that is required in the

evaluation. OCPs and NSAIDs are of particular therapeutic benefit.

2. Perimenopausal and postmenopausal women: Endometrial carcinoma must be excluded early in the investigation in this age group. Endometrial sampling and/or transvaginal ultrasound are recommended.

6. b. Progestins in various forms directly address the problem of an inadequate luteal phase in those women with anovulatory cycles. Oral progestins may be administered in a cyclic fashion. However, although cyclic progestins may control her bleeding effectively, they are not indicated for contraception. Initial medical therapies for DUB may include the following: (1) Iron therapy for excessive blood loss. (2) NSAIDs can be beneficial in patients with menorrhagia. (3) Combined OCPs to shorten menses, decrease blood flow, impose a cycle in patients with irregular menses, and provide effective contraception. (4) Intramuscular injections of medroxyprogesterone acetate (Depo-Provera) eventually will induce amenorrhea, which can decrease anemia and provides highly effective contraception. (5) A LNG-IUS has been shown to be efficacious in the treatment of menorrhagia, with up to 96% of women reporting reduction in blood loss at 12 months. (The IUD releases a low level of levonorgestrel into the uterine cavity inducing gland atrophy and decreased menstrual flow. Approximately 50% of users become amenorrheic at 12 months of use. [Of note, clinical experience with LNG-IUD is limited to women with ovulatory abnormal uterine bleeding (AUB)]. LNG-IUS also provides up to 5 years of highly effective contraception.); (6) Tranexamic acid, an antifibrinolytic, reduces bleeding volume by 40% to 60%. (Although not a standard treatment for menorrhagia in the United States, tranexamic acid is widely used in Europe.); (7) Danazol, a synthetic androgen directly suppresses ovulation and has been shown to decrease menstrual flow more effectively than NSAIDs. (However, its adverse side effect profile [i.e., weight gain, acne] may limit its use); (8) GnRH agonists, which effectively induce a hypoestrogenic pseudomenopausal state, resulting in amenorrhea and has been shown to be effective treatment of ovulatory and anovulatory AUB. (Side effects include vasomotor symptoms and an increased risk of osteopenia, which often are treated with "add-back" cyclic estrogen/progestin therapy.)

For cases of DUB refractory to medical treatment, surgical intervention may be necessary (endometrial ablation, D&C, hysterectomy).

7. b. This patient has secondary amenorrhea, which is defined as either (1) absence of menses for 6 months in women with previous regular cycles or (2) absence of menses for three consecutive cycles in women with prior oligomenorrhea. Primary amenorrhea is defined as either (1) no menses by age 14 in the absence of secondary sexual development or (2) no menses by age 16 in the presence of secondary sexual development. Secondary amenorrhea is much more common, with a prevalence of 1% to 3%. Dysmenorrhea is defined as painful menses that occurs with onset of menstrual flow. Oligomenorrhea and polymenorrhea are defined in Answer 1.

8. e. Pregnancy is the most common cause of secondary amenorrhea and should be excluded first. Once pregnancy has been excluded, a TSH and prolactin should be done to assess for hypothyroidism or hyperprolactinemia. If there is evidence of thyroid disease, it should be treated appropriately. Signs and symptoms of hyperprolactinemia (i.e., galactorrhea, headache, or visual field deficits) should be sought. Medications that cause hyperprolactinemia (e.g., metoclopramide, antidepressants, or methyldopa) should be excluded as potential causes. It is recommended to order pituitary imaging, if prolactin levels are elevated, to exclude pituitary adenoma. Some experts recommend ordering magnetic resonance imaging (MRI) of the head with any degree of prolactin elevation. Others recommend a plain film screening view of the sella if prolactin is less than 100, and an MRI of the head if prolactin level is more than 100.

This patient most likely suffers from hypothalamic amenorrhea secondary to her recent weight loss and increased level of exercise. Functional hypothalamic amenorrhea is characterized by abnormal secretion of GnRH, resulting in low LH levels and absence of a mid-cycle LH surge. This leads to anovulation and low estradiol levels. There are multiple causes of hypothalamic amenorrhea including stress, weight loss, anorexia nervosa, poor nutrition, and strenuous exercise. This patient should be counseled that her amenorrhea may correct with gaining weight and returning to routine levels of exercise. She also should be advised that prolonged amenorrhea may put her at risk for accelerated bone loss and osteopenia later in life. Turner's syndrome is a cause of primary amenorrhea, not secondary amenorrhea. It is associated with delayed puberty, short stature, and the 45 XO karyotype.

9. a. Thyroid function should be evaluated in patients presenting with amenorrhea, as discussed earlier. The other answer choices are not appropriate as initial evaluation.

10. a. For a woman to have regular menses, the following factors must be present: (1) an unobstructed outflow tract; (2) a mature and intact hypothalamic–pituitary–ovarian (HPO) axis; (3) functional ovaries; and (4) a functional uterus with a responsive endometrium. Disruption at any of these levels can result in amenorrhea or irregular menses. Once the initial evaluation has excluded pregnancy, thyroid dysfunction, and hyperprolactinemia, one should assess the previously listed factors in a logical, stepwise fashion. First, assessment of estrogen status is accomplished with a progesterone challenge test. A standard protocol is to administer 10 mg of medroxyprogesterone (Provera) daily for 10 days. A positive test is indicated by presence of menses within 2-7 days of progestin withdrawal. If there is no menses, there is either an obstructed outflow tract or inadequate estrogen stimulation of the endometrium. At this time a challenge of combined estrogen and progesterone should be offered. A typical regimen consists of 1.25 mg of conjugated equine estrogen on days 1-21, followed by 5-10 mg of progesterone on the last 7 days of the 21-day cycle. Alternately, a standard cycle and dose of combined OCPs may be used. If the patient has withdrawal bleeding within 2-7 days of the last dose of progestin (or OCPs), it confirms a competent outflow tract and a responsive endometrium. If a patient fails to have menses, outflow tract obstruction should be suspected. Asherman's syndrome (extensive scarring of the uterine cavity) usually can be suspected by history (uterine infection, obstetric complication, repeated D&C). Congenital vaginal and uterine anomalies should be suspected in all patients presenting with primary amenorrhea. Outflow tract obstruction can be confirmed with imaging and/or hysteroscopic evaluation. Initial evaluation with ultrasound and hysteroscopy in this patient presenting with secondary amenorrhea is not indicated. The workup as outlined earlier is more appropriate because it is less invasive and likely to confirm the suspected diagnosis of hypothalamic amenorrhea. Depo-Provera would not be helpful in evaluating the cause of this patient's amenorrhea because it is likely to promote amenorrhea, not correct it.

11. a. Cyclic progestins will help establish regular menses but do not address any contraceptive needs. In this patient, a combined OCP may be more appropriate because it will regulate her cycles and also address her desire for contraception. She also should be encouraged to maintain normal body weight and levels of exercise because this usually will correct the underlying problem. NSAIDs have no role in the management of amenorrhea.

12. a. Evaluation of AUB is tailored specifically to age group and reproductive status of the woman. The evaluation of AUB in a reproductive-age women younger than age 35 years is outlined in Clinical Case Problem 1. In this case the patient is postmenopausal and does not need a pregnancy test, unless there is a suspicion that the history is unreliable and the postmenopausal status is questionable. Checking a CBC and TSH is reasonable in this patient given the duration of her irregular bleeding and complaints of fatigue. A prolactin level can be considered if indicated by history, although hyperprolactinemia usually presents as amenorrhea and not as irregular or excessive bleeding. Other routine tests include a Pap test to evaluate for cervical dysplasia as a cause for bleeding. Infection also can cause abnormal bleeding as in active cervicitis caused by gonorrhea or chlamydia. Given the patient's recent new sexual partner, checking cervical cultures would be prudent. Ultimately, the most serious condition to assess for is endometrial carcinoma. Of all postmenopausal women with bleeding, 5% to 10% are found to have endometrial carcinoma. A transvaginal ultrasound is a reasonable first step in this evaluation. An ultrasound may reveal structural abnormalities such as submucous fibroids, adenomyosis, or polyps. In a postmenopausal woman, an endometrial stripe of less than 5 mm on transvaginal ultrasound has a high negative predictive value such that endometrial biopsy can be avoided. In a meta-analysis comparing transvaginal ultrasound to endometrial biopsy in postmenopausal women presenting with vaginal bleeding, 96% of women with endometrial cancer had an endometrial stripe thickness greater than 5 mm. Based on this information, it has been recommended that postmenopausal women with irregular bleeding undergo a transvaginal ultrasound first to determine endometrial stripe thickness. An endometrial stripe less than 5 mm can exclude endometrial disease in the majority of women. If the endometrial stripe is greater than 5 mm, the patient should have an endometrial biopsy to confirm the presence of absence of atypia.

In general, an ultrasound is less specific for endometrial carcinoma in women taking HRT and in perimenopausal women. Hence, endometrial biopsy is recommended in premenopausal women older than age 35 (some sources cite age 40) who present with irregular bleeding or in postmenopausal women taking HRT for longer than 6 months with irregular bleeding. Risk factors for endometrial cancer include a history of chronic anovulation, obesity, diabetes, and infertility. A D&C would not be part of the initial evaluation given its greater expense and invasiveness. Cyclic progestins or oral contraceptives should not be administered until a complete evaluation for endometrial cancer has been undertaken. Hysterectomy is never accepted as first-line treatment without confirmation of invasive disease.

13. **c.** Endometrial biopsy should be performed on all postmenopausal patients with an endometrial stripe greater than 5 mm on transvaginal ultrasound. Administering hormonal therapy without confirming the presence or absence of disease is not appropriate. Repeating the ultrasound in 6 months will only delay the diagnosis. Observation is not appropriate.

14. **b.** The most likely diagnosis in this patient is PCOS. This condition is characterized by chronic anovulation and hyperandrogenism. PCOS is a diagnosis of exclusion and based largely on history and physical examination. Classic presentation includes amenorrhea, signs of androgen excess (i.e., hirsutism, acne), and polycystic ovaries. Other common findings include obesity and a history of infertility. Of patients, 20% are asymptomatic. Physical examination should focus on assessment for obesity (increased waist-to-hip ratio >0.85), hirsutism, acne, virilizing signs (i.e., male-pattern baldness, deepening voice, clitoromegaly, increased muscle mass), stigmata of Cushing's disease, a pelvic examination for ovarian enlargement, and a breast examination to assess for galactorrhea. This patient has classic features of PCOS. An androgen-secreting tumor is unlikely given that the patient has no virilizing symptoms or signs. Adult-onset congenital adrenal hyperplasia may cause oligomenorrhea and hirsutism but is much less common than PCOS. Although it is reasonable to evaluate for hyperprolactinemia given this patient's history of anovulatory cycles, her presentation is far more consistent with PCOS than prolactinoma. Of note, prolactin levels may be mildly elevated in patients with PCOS. Hypothyroidism may cause irregular bleeding but should not cause signs of androgen excess.

15. **e.** PCOS is a diagnosis that generally can be made based on a careful history and examination. The National Institutes of Health have proposed that diagnostic criteria include the following: (1) chronic anovulation and (2) signs of hyperandrogenism (i.e., acne, hirsutism, elevated testosterone) in women in whom secondary causes have been excluded. A summary of recommended initial testing in patients with amenorrhea/oligomenorrhea and signs of androgen excess include the following: (1) urine or serum pregnancy test; (2) TSH; (3) prolactin; (4) LH, FSH (the LH:FSH ratio in PCOS patients is classically 3:1 or higher); (5) a testosterone level is normal to moderately elevated in PCOS (a serum testosterone level of more than 200 should make one suspicious of a virilizing tumor).

Some sources recommend testing for adult-onset congenital hyperplasia only in select cases. The American College of Obstetricians and Gynecologists

(ACOG) recommends testing for this condition in all women (based on expert opinion). If screening is to be performed, a morning serum 17-hydroxyprogesterone level should be obtained; basal levels greater than 5 ng/ml suggest adult-onset congenital adrenal hyperplasia. A serum DHEAS level may be checked to evaluate for a virilizing tumor in selected patients with rapid onset of virilizing symptoms. Polycystic ovaries are present in more than 90% of women with PCOS, but they also are found in up to 25% of women in the general population. Polycystic ovaries are a sign of PCOS as a result of chronic anovulation; they are not a cause of this condition. Hence, a pelvic ultrasound is not routinely indicated in patients suspected to have PCOS unless there is persistent pelvic pain or an abnormal pelvic finding.

16. **d.** The etiology of PCOS is complex and not completely understood. There is emerging evidence that the underlying mechanism is insulin resistance, with resultant high insulin levels stimulating excessive ovarian androgen production. The increased level of ovarian androgens is believed to be responsible for chronic anovulation. The long-term sequela of chronic anovulation includes unopposed estrogen stimulation of the endometrium, putting women with PCOS at a three times higher risk for endometrial carcinoma than normal women. In addition, PCOS has been associated with a higher risk of lipid abnormalities, cardiovascular disease, and diabetes. All women identified to have PCOS should be screened for hyperlipidemia and diabetes. ACOG recommends that screening for diabetes should consist of a fasting glucose followed by a 2-hour glucose level after a 75-g glucose load. Treatment for women with PCOS ultimately should address the following: (1) chronic anovulation; (2) androgen excess; (3) insulin resistance; and (4) lipid abnormalities if present. Weight loss and exercise should be emphasized in all patients. Up to 70% of patients with PCOS are overweight, and it has been shown that even a modest weight reduction can decrease insulin resistance and improve menstrual regularity. Combined OCPs are inherently antiandrogenic and will impose regular cycles, addressing both the problems of chronic anovulation and androgen excess. OCPs are an ideal first-line treatment for patients who also desire contraception. Clomiphene ovulation induction is recommended for patients with PCOS suffering from infertility. Spironolactone, in a dose of 25-100 mg/day, commonly has been used for problematic hirsutism. There has been evidence that metformin, a second-generation biguanide, is a promising treatment for PCOS because it addresses the underlying problem of insulin resistance. Clinical studies have shown that women taking metformin (500 mg three times a day or 850 mg twice a day) have increased frequency of ovulation, normalization of menses, and ovulatory response to clomiphene. Universal use of metformin as first-line treatment in all patients with PCOS with or without infertility is still controversial, especially in women with no evidence of insulin resistance. Some have expressed concern about effects of metformin during first-trimester pregnancy, although there has been no reported association with fetal anomalies in obser-vational human trials or controlled animal trials. Ovarian wedge resection, a surgical technique more widely used in the past to induce ovulation, has fallen out of favor secondary to risks of postsurgical adhesion and the availability of medical ovulation-induction agents. Laparoscopic ovarian "drilling" is a surgical technique that in small trials has shown improvement in the spontaneous rate of ovulation in patients with PCOS.

SOLUTION TO THE CLINICAL CASE MANAGEMENT PROBLEM

Attention first should be directed at the patient's vital signs and symptoms and assessment of whether transfusion or surgical intervention is needed. Provided the patient is stable without significant symptoms and her pregnancy test is negative, the treatment of choice for this type of heavy DUB is intravenous (IV) estrogen (Premarin 25 mg IV q4h for 3-4 doses). In this patient the endometrial lining that is remaining (the basal layer) will be less responsive to progestin therapy. The high-dose estrogen rapidly proliferates the thinned basal endo-metrium, stopping the bleeding. The estrogen adminis-tration must be followed by 10 days of a progestin to allow a normal withdrawal bleed to occur. As an alter-native to IV Premarin, a standard-dosed OCP can be given four times per day for 5-7 days. This therapy may be limited by significant nausea.

SUMMARY OF DYSFUNCTIONAL UTERINE BLEEDING

A. AUB:
1. **Definitions:**
   a. Metrorrhagia: irregular, frequent bleeding of varying amounts, but not excessive
   b. Menorrhagia: excessive bleeding (>80 cc per cycle) that occurs at regular intervals
   c. Menometrorrhagia: excessive menstrual bleeding (>80 cc per cycle) that occurs at irregular intervals
   d. Polymenorrhea: regular bleeding at intervals less than 21 days
   e. Oligomenorrhea: regular bleeding at intervals greater than every 35 days
2. **Initial evaluation of abnormal uterine bleeding:** (a) thorough history and physical examination; (b) urine pregnancy test; (c) CBC if heavy bleeding suspected; (d) TSH/prolactin if indicated by history; (e) pituitary imaging if elevated prolactin; (f) evaluation for coagu-lation disorder if indicated by history; (g) trans-vaginal ultrasound if abnormal pelvic exami-nation or inadequate pelvic examination; (h) endometrial biopsy in perimenopausal patients or postmenopausal patients taking HRT for more than 6 months with irregular bleeding to exclude endometrial carcinoma; (i) transvaginal ultrasound in postmenopausal patients with irregular bleeding; and (j) endo-metrial biopsy if endometrial stripe >5 mm.
3. **Secondary causes of AUB:** fibroids, endo-metriosis, adenomyosis, chronic PID, coagula-tion defects, severe hypothyroidism, renal failure, liver failure, endometrial carcinoma.
4. **DUB:** AUB that cannot be attributed to any specific genital tract lesion or systemic disease. Usually anovulatory, although less than 10% of DUB is ovulatory.
5. **Treatment for DUB:** NSAIDs, OCPs, proges-tins, tranexamic acid, danazol, GnRH agonists, LNG-IUS. Surgical intervention for refractory cases endometrial ablation, hysterectomy.

B. Amenorrhea
1. **Primary amenorrhea:** (a) no menses by age 14 in the absence of secondary sexual develop-ment or (b) no menses by age 16 in the pres-ence of secondary sexual development.
2. **Secondary amenorrhea:** (a) absence of menses for 6 months in women with previous regular cycles or (b) absence of menses for three cycles in women with prior oligomenorrhea.
3. **Causes of primary amenorrhea:** Turner's syndrome, outflow tract obstruction.
4. **Causes of secondary amenorrhea:** preg-nancy, thyroid disfunction, hyperprolactine-mia, hypothalamic amenorrhea (stress, weight loss, excessive exercise)

Continued

SUMMARY OF DYSFUNCTIONAL UTERINE BLEEDING—cont'd

5. **Evaluation of secondary amenorrhea:** history and examination, pregnancy test, TSH, prolactin. If preliminary evaluation is unrevealing, administer progestin challenge. If no response to progestin challenge, give combined estrogen and progestin to exclude outflow tract obstruction.
6. **Treatment:** Correct underlying cause. Administer cyclic progestins or OCPs if contraception is desired and there are no contraindications.

C. PCOS
1. **Definition:** Condition characterized by chronic anovulation and hyperandrogenism. PCOS is a diagnosis of exclusion.
2. **Laboratory evaluation:** pregnancy test, TSH, prolactin, LH, FSH (LH:FSH ratio classically >3:1), 17-hydroxyprogesterone, testosterone. DHEAS if a virilizing tumor is suspected. Evaluation for diabetes and hyperlipidemia if

diagnosis of PCOS is confirmed. Transvaginal ultrasound is not routinely indicated unless there is pelvic pain or abnormality.
3. **Treatment options:** OCPs, spironolactone, metformin, clomiphene for patients with infertility. Surgical interventions include laparoscopic "drilling."

SUGGESTED READING

Crosignani PG, et al: Releasing intrauterine device versus hysteroscopic endometrial resection in the treatment of dysfunctional uterine bleeding. *Obstet Gynecol* 90(2):257-263, 1997.

Hunter MS, Sterrett JJ: Polycystic ovary syndrome: it's not just infertility. *Am Fam Physician* 62:1079-1088, 1090, 2000.

Munro, MG: Dysfunctional uterine bleeding: advances in diagnosis and treatment. *Curr Opin Obstet Gynecol* 13(5):475-489, 2001.

Oriel KA, Schrager S: Abnormal uterine bleeding. *Am Fam Physician* 60:1371-1382, 1999.

Prentice A: Medical management of menorrhagia. *West J Med* 172:253-255, 2000.

Smith-BR, et al: Endovaginal ultrasound to exclude endometrial cancer and other endometrial abnormalities. *JAMA* 280:1510-1517, 1998.

Smith MA, et al, eds: Twenty common problems in women's health care. In: *Menstrual Disorders*. McGraw-Hill, 2000, New York.

Chapter 58

Ectopic Pregnancy

> "You mean my baby is in the wrong part of my stomach?"

CLINICAL CASE PROBLEM 1:
A 37-YEAR-OLD FEMALE WITH PELVIC PAIN AND VAGINAL SPOTTING

A 37-year-old nulliparous female comes to your office with a 3-day history of progressive pelvic pain. She notes some vaginal spotting but no frank bleeding. She denies any fevers, chills, diarrhea, vaginal discharge, or urinary symptoms. She is married and has been trying to conceive for the past 6 months. Her menstrual periods always have been regular, but she is now several weeks past the date at which she would have expected her period. She is afebrile, and her pulse and blood pressure are normal. On speculum examination, her os appears closed and there is a small amount of dark brownish-red blood pooled in the fornix. On bimanual examination, her uterus feels slightly enlarged and boggy. Her left adnexa is tender without any obvious mass. She has no cervical motion tenderness.

SELECT THE BEST ANSWER TO THE FOLLOWING QUESTIONS:

1. At this time, what is the most important diagnosis to exclude?
   a. ruptured corpus luteum cyst
   b. acute pelvic inflammatory disease (PID)
   c. ectopic pregnancy
   d. threatened abortion
   e. incomplete abortion

2. Which of the following questions would be most relevant to ask this patient now?
   a. do you have a history of fever within the last 24 hours
   b. do you have a history of dysmenorrhea
   c. do you have a history of menorrhagia
   d. when did you have your last menstrual period
   e. do you have a history of infertility

3. What is the most appropriate initial test to support your diagnosis of this patient?
   a. urine or serum beta-human chorionic gonadotropin (β-hCG)
   b. hysterosalpingogram
   c. culdocentesis
   d. pelvic/transvaginal ultrasound
   e. laparoscopy

4. The patient's urine pregnancy test is positive. Because the patient is hemodynamically stable, you order a serum quantitative β-hCG test. Which of the following statements, regarding this patient's serum test results, is true?
   a. if <1500 IU/L, serial quantitative β-hCG testing should be performed
   b. if <1500 IU/L, a transvaginal ultrasound should be obtained
   c. if >1500 IU/L, a pelvic/abdominal ultrasound can be obtained
   d. if >6500 IU/L, a culdocentesis should be performed
   e. serum quantitative β-hCG testing is not indicated in a hemodynamically stable patient

5. A transvaginal ultrasound confirms a mass in the adnexa. Which of the following medical treatments is appropriate for this condition?
   a. intravenous estrogen
   b. combined oral contraceptives (contain estrogen and progestin)
   c. progestin only pills
   d. intramuscular (IM) medroxyprogesterone acetate
   e. IM methotrexate

6. Which of the following is not a risk factor for ectopic pregnancy?
   a. intrauterine devices (IUDs)`
   b. previous ectopic pregnancy
   c. PID
   d. endometriosis
   e. cigarette smoking

7. In which anatomic site do most ectopic pregnancies occur?
   a. the ampulla of the fallopian tube
   b. the isthmus of the fallopian tube
   c. the interstitial portion of the fallopian tube
   d. the interstitial portion of the ovary
   e. the endometrial lining

8. Which of the following is not a common presenting symptom of ectopic pregnancy?
   a. abdominal pain
   b. vaginal spotting
   c. fever
   d. amenorrhea
   e. all of the above

9. Major complication(s) of ectopic pregnancy include which of the following?
   a. intraabdominal hemorrhage
   b. hypovolemic shock
   c. fetal death
   d. a and b
   e. a, b, and c

10. Which of the following statements are true regarding ectopic pregnancy?
    a. the number of cases has markedly increased in the United States over the past 20 years
    b. the incidence decreases with age
    c. it occurs more commonly in nulligravida women
    d. there is no significant difference in incidence between different ethnic groups
    e. all of the above

CLINICAL CASE MANAGEMENT PROBLEM

Discuss the reason(s) for the marked increase in number of ectopic pregnancies in the United States for the past two decades.

ANSWERS:

1. **c.** The most important diagnosis to exclude at this time in this patient is ectopic pregnancy. An ectopic pregnancy is any pregnancy in which the fertilized ovum implants outside the intrauterine cavity. A ruptured ectopic pregnancy is a true medical emergency. It is the leading cause of maternal mortality in the first trimester and accounts for 10% to 15% of all maternal deaths. In a patient of childbearing age, any of the three As (amenorrhea, abdominal pain, and abnormal uterine bleeding) should suggest the possibility of an ectopic pregnancy. Ectopic pregnancy is more common in women older than 35 years old and in nonwhite ethnic groups.

The differential diagnosis of ectopic pregnancy includes the following: spontaneous abortion, molar pregnancy, ruptured corpus luteum, acute PID, adnexal torsion, degenerating leiomyoma, acute appendicitis, pyelonephritis, diverticulitis, regional ileitis, and ulcerative colitis.

2. **d.** The most important question to ask the patient at this time is as follows: "When was your last menstrual period (LMP)." The patient already had mentioned that her periods had been regular but that her period was now several weeks late. An accurate LMP aids in the early diagnosis and subsequent management of an ectopic pregnancy. The most

common presentation of ectopic pregnancy in symptomatic patients is abdominal pain with spotting, usually occurring 6-8 weeks after the LMP.

3. **a.** Based on this patient's history and physical examination, the probability of an ectopic pregnancy is very high. Therefore, a qualitative urine or serum β-hCG is the most important investigation to perform at this time. If the qualitative β-hCG is negative, ectopic pregnancy is ruled out. If the qualitative β-hCG is positive, it is vital to establish whether the pregnancy is intrauterine or extrauterine. This is accomplished by a combination of quantitative serum β-hCG and pelvic/transvaginal ultrasonography.

4. **a.** The discriminatory threshold is the critical serum quantitative β-hCG titer above which a normal gestational sac should be seen in the uterus by ultrasonography. The discriminatory threshold is 1500 mIU/ml when using transvaginal ultrasonography or 6500 mIU/ml with abdominal ultrasonography. Failure to find a gestational sac in the uterus when either of these thresholds is reached is presumptive evidence of an ectopic pregnancy. If the serum β-hCG titer does not exceed the threshold and no intrauterine gestational sac is seen, it is impossible to differentiate a normal pregnancy from an ectopic pregnancy. Because the serum quantitative β-hCG titer should double in 48 hours, repeat the β-hCG titer every 2 days until the discriminatory threshold is reached, then repeat the ultrasound. If the β-hCG titer fails to double in 48 hours, consider a diagnostic curettage to determine the presence (nonviable intrauterine pregnancy) or absence (probable ectopic pregnancy) of chorionic villi. Culdocentesis rarely is performed when ultrasonography is readily available.

5. **e.** The medical management of choice for ectopic pregnancy is IM methotrexate. Methotrexate is a folic-acid antagonist that destroys rapidly growing tissue including chorionic villi. It does have the potential for serious toxicity. A single dose is successful in resolving 90% of ectopic pregnancies. Declining serum β-hCG titers indicate success. Failure of titers to decrease at least 15% by day 4 to 7 posttreatment indicates the need for an additional dose or surgery. The cumulative success rate is 95% with subsequent evidence of tubal patency in 80% and fertility in almost 70%. These rates are similar to those reported with treatment of unruptured tubal pregnancy by salpingostomy. Methotrexate is optimal for small, unruptured ectopic pregnancies and should be considered only if the following conditions apply:

(a) early gestation (preferably <8 weeks); (b) patient desires future fertility; (c) nonlaparoscopic diagnosis; (d) patient is hemodynamically stable without signs of hemoperitoneum; (e) patient has normal hemoglobin, liver function, and renal function; and (f) patient is able to return for follow-up care.

6. **a.** Major risk factors for ectopic pregnancy include previous ectopic pregnancy; PID; endometriosis; previous tubal surgery; previous pelvic surgery; infertility and infertility treatments; uterotubal anomalies; history of in utero exposure to diethylstilbestrol (DES); and cigarette smoking. These risk factors all interfere with fallopian tube function. Other possible indirect risk factors include multiple sexual partners; early age at first intercourse; and vaginal douching. Contraceptive IUDs do not increase the risk of ectopic pregnancy.

7. **a.** The most frequent site of extrauterine implantation is the ampulla of the fallopian tube (78%), where most fertilizations occur. The isthmus of the fallopian tube is the next most common site of implantation (12%). Cornual pregnancies are uncommon, representing only 2.5% of the total. Abdominal, ovarian, and cervical pregnancies are rare.

8. **c.** There are no absolutely pathognomonic signs or symptoms of an early ectopic pregnancy. The most common symptoms noted are the three As (abdominal pain, abnormal vaginal bleeding, and amenorrhea). Between 96% and 100% of patients with ectopic gestation complain of pain, even before rupture. No specific type of pain is diagnostic. With tubal rupture, the pain becomes more severe. Amenorrhea or a history of abnormal menses is reported in 75% to 95% of patients with ectopic pregnancy. A careful history with respect to the character and timing of the last two or three menstrual cycles (amount of flow and number of days of flow) is important. Initially patients often will state that they have not missed a period; however, when questioned carefully, they may describe the period as being different (lighter than usual or irregular in timing). This bleeding may, in fact, represent bleeding from an endometrial slough. Profuse bleeding is uncommon. Common symptoms of early pregnancy such as nausea and breast tenderness are present in only 10% to 25% of patients with ectopic pregnancies. Vasovagal symptoms (dizziness and fainting) are present in 20% to 35% of patients. Abdominal tenderness is present in most patients (80% to 95%). Rebound tenderness may or may not be present. A mass is palpable in 50%

of patients with ectopic pregnancy. If there is uterine enlargement, it is not to the degree that would be expected for the duration of amenorrhea. A few patients will state that they, in fact, passed tissue (a decidual cast). Most patients are afebrile.

9. **d.** The major complications of ectopic pregnancy are intraabdominal hemorrhage and hypovolemic shock secondary to rupture. Rupture of the ectopic pregnancy is responsible for almost all maternal morbidity and mortality. Fetal death cannot be classified as a major complication because of its inevitability in ectopic pregnancy.

10. **a.** There has been a fivefold increase in the number of ectopic pregnancies in the United States over the past two decades. There is a marked increase in the rate of ectopic pregnancies with increasing age. Most ectopic pregnancies occur in multigravida women, with only 10% to 15% occurring in nulligravida women. Rates of ectopic pregnancies are up to 30% higher in nonwhite women.

SOLUTION TO THE CLINICAL CASE MANAGEMENT PROBLEM

The significant increase in the number of ectopic pregnancies in the United States during the last 20 years is mainly the result of improved early diagnosis, including some ectopic pregnancies that previously would have resolved spontaneously without detection. Increases in certain risk factors (e.g., PID) also may contribute to the increase in cases of ectopic pregnancy. However, the case-fatality rate also has declined dramatically in the past 20 years.

SUMMARY OF ECTOPIC PREGNANCY

1. **Incidence:** There has been a fivefold increase in the past 20 years. The increasing numbers appear to be mainly the result of improved early diagnosis. Maternal death rates have declined almost tenfold during the same time period.

2. **Pathogenesis:**
   a. Strong association: (i) previous ectopic pregnancy; (ii) PID; (iii) endometriosis; (iv) previous tubal surgery; (v) previous pelvic surgery; (vi) infertility and infertility treatments; (vii) uterotubal anomalies; (viii) history of in utero exposure to DES; and (ix) cigarette smoking.
   b. Weaker association: (i) multiple sexual partners, (ii) early age at first intercourse; and (iii) vaginal douching.

3. **Signs and symptoms:**
   a. The three As—abdominal pain, amenorrhea, and abnormal vaginal bleeding—indicate an ectopic pregnancy until proved otherwise.
   b. Vasovagal attacks and orthostatic hypotension are strong indicators of tubal rupture.

4. **Major complications:** Tubal rupture is indicated by intraabdominal hemorrhage or hypovolemia and shock.

5. **Investigations:** Perform qualitative urine or serum β-hCG; if positive, obtain quantitative serum β-hCG, abdominal/transvaginal ultrasound, and diagnostic curettage.

6. **Treatment:**
   a. Medical management: Methotrexate should be used only in patients who are hemodynamically stable with a normal hemoglobin, normal liver function tests, and normal renal function and in whom follow-up is probable.
   b. Surgical management: Laparotomy with salpingectomy, tubal sterilization, and fallopian tube conservative surgery, which can include salpingostomy, segmental resection and anastomosis, and fibril evacuation, can be performed.

SUGGESTED READING

American College of Obstetricians and Gynecologists: *Medical management of tubal pregnancy*. Practice Bulletin No. 3. ACOG, 1998, Washington, DC.
Tay JI, et al: Ectopic pregnancy. *West J Med* 173:131-134, 2000.
Tenore JL: Ectopic pregnancy. *Am Fam Physician* 61:1080-1088, 2000.

Chapter **59**

Contraception

> "Doctor, I've been married for 10 years and have seven kids. Is there any way I can stop from getting pregnant every year. Please?"

CLINICAL CASE PROBLEM 1:
A 23-Year-Old Female Presents for Her Annual Examination and Pap Test

A 23-year-old female comes to your office for her annual physical and Papanicolaou (Pap) test. She says that she has migraine headaches (without an aura) about twice a month, and they usually are relieved by nonsteroidal antiinflammatory drugs (NSAIDs) and rest. She has never had an abnormal Pap test result. She was treated for chlamydia about 2 years ago. She denies any other medical problems. She has never been pregnant. She has had a total of 10 male sexual partners but has been sexually active with only one male partner for the past 4 months. He has no known history of a sexually transmitted disease (STD). They only use the "withdrawal method" for contraception and STD protection. She has smoked about a pack of cigarettes a day for the past 5 years. On examination, her blood pressure is 120/80 mm Hg, her weight is 160 lb, and she is 5 feet 5 inches tall. The rest of her examination is unremarkable except for some mild facial acne. You perform a Pap test.

■ **SELECT THE BEST ANSWER TO THE FOLLOWING QUESTIONS:**

1. What would you tell her regarding the use of the "withdrawal method?"
   a. it is an effective method of contraception but not STD protection
   b. it is an effective method of STD protection but not contraception
   c. it is neither an effective method of contraception nor STD protection
   d. it is an effective method of contraception and STD protection
   e. it has only been shown to prevent viral STD transmission

2. Which of the following methods would offer this patient both effective contraception and STD protection?
   a. nonlatex male condoms made from animal products
   b. nonlatex female condoms made from polyurethane
   c. a diaphragm
   d. oral contraceptive pills (OCPs)
   e. the sponge

3. Which of the following statements is true regarding the use of any estrogen-containing hormonal contraceptive method for this patient?
   a. they are contraindicated because of her common migraines
   b. they are contraindicated because she smokes cigarettes
   c. they are contraindicated because of her history of chlamydia
   d. they are contraindicated because of her weight
   e. they all may improve her acne

4. Which of the following contraceptive methods would not be appropriate for this patient?
   a. combined oral contraceptives (COCs; contain both estrogen and progestin)
   b. Depo-Provera
   c. Mirena Intrauterine System (IUS)
   d. OrthoEvra patch
   e. NuvaRing

5. Your patient decides that she wants to start taking OCPs because she would like to have regular and predictable menstrual cycles. Which OCP option would not be ideal for this patient?
   a. progestin-only pills (POPs)
   b. COCs containing 35 mcg of ethinyl estradiol
   c. COCs containing 20 mcg of ethinyl estradiol
   d. monophasic COCs
   e. triphasic COCs

6. You counsel your patient about starting COCs. Which of the following statements regarding COC use and this patient is true?
   a. she must start the COCs on the first Sunday after her period begins
   b. nausea and breast tenderness are uncommon side effects of COCs
   c. if she develops any breakthrough bleeding, she should stop the COCs immediately
   d. weight gain is not a likely and unavoidable consequence of COC use
   e. if she misses taking a pill, she must wait until her next menses, then start a new pack

7. Your patient contacts you about 6 weeks after starting her COCs. She is complaining about some midcycle spotting and is concerned. Which of the following statements is true regarding COC use and breakthrough bleeding (BTB) in this patient?

a. smoking and cervicitis are potential causes of her BTB
b. BTB is rare after the first cycle of COCs
c. use of NSAIDs likely will exacerbate her BTB
d. BTB is a reliable indicator of noncompliance
e. BTB is a sign of inadequate contraceptive protection

8. Which of the following statements regarding long-term COC use is true?
a. there is strong evidence that long-term COC use increases ovarian cancer risk
b. there is strong evidence that long-term COC use increases breast cancer risk
c. there is strong evidence that long-term COC use decreases cervical cancer risk
d. there is strong evidence that long-term COC use decreases osteoporotic fracture risk
e. there is strong evidence that long-term COC use decreases endometrial cancer risk

9. Which of the following is not a potential non-contraceptive side effect or benefit of estrogen-containing hormonal contraceptives?
a. iron-deficiency anemia
b. cholelithiasis
c. dysmenorrhea
d. ectopic pregnancy
e. mittelschmerz

CLINICAL CASE PROBLEM 2:
A 40-Year-Old Postpartum Female

A 40-year-old female (gravida 2, para 2) comes to your office for her 6-week postpartum visit. She had an uncomplicated pregnancy, normal spontaneous vaginal delivery, and routine postpartum course. She and her baby are doing well. She is breastfeeding intermittently with formula, and she has not gotten her period yet. She does not want to get pregnant again, at least not for another few years. She is healthy, has had no major medical problems, is a nonsmoker, and already is back to her aerobics class. She has no history of STDs or abnormal Pap test results, and she has been monogamous with her husband for the past 20 years. She cannot remember to take her multivitamin everyday, so she wants a reliable birth control method that she does not have to remember to take everyday or remember to use every time she has sex with her husband. Her examination is completely normal.

10. What contraceptive method(s) would be most appropriate for this patient at this time?
a. bilateral tubal ligation (BTL) or vasectomy
b. OrthoEvra Patch or NuvaRing
c. Depo-Provera or Mirena IUS
d. continue with just the lactation amenorrhea method (LAM)
e. Norplant

11. Which of the following statements is true regarding the use of estrogen-containing hormonal contraceptives in this patient?
a. they are contraindicated in women older than 40 years of age
b. they may increase the patient's breast milk production
c. they will delay her age of onset of menopause
d. they will cause her to develop fibroids and/or increase their size
e. they may help regulate menses and/or reduce perimenopausal symptoms

12. Which of the following statements is true regarding the use of Depo-Provera in this patient?
a. it likely will provide her with a rapid return to fertility following its cessation of use
b. it will not adversely affect her quantity or quality of breast milk
c. it is contraindicated if she has a seizure disorder
d. it will accelerate her age of onset of menopause
e. it will increase her risk of postmenopausal osteoporosis

13. Which of the following statements is true regarding the use of a ParaGard T 380A (Copper IUD) in this patient?
a. it will increase her risk of ectopic pregnancy
b. there is usually a long delay in return to fertility following their removal
c. it is contraindicated in breastfeeding mothers
d. it may increase her symptoms if she suffers from dysmenorrhea or menorrhagia
e. it should not be inserted until she begins menstruating again

14. Your patient asks you about sterilization options in the future. Which of the following statements about vasectomies and tubal ligations is true?
a. vasectomies usually are performed in an outpatient office under local anesthesia
b. current vasectomy and tubal ligation procedures are easily reversible
c. vasectomies increase prostate cancer risk
d. tubal ligations increase the risk of ectopic pregnancy
e. vasectomies reduce libido, erectile function, and penile sensation

CLINICAL CASE PROBLEM 3:

A 16-Year-Old Female Who Had Unprotected Sex More than 2 Days Ago

A very tearful 16-year-old female (gravida 0, para 0) walks in to your office on a Monday afternoon after school. She tells you that she had sexual intercourse with her boyfriend (of 2 months) Friday night. They used a condom, but it broke. They previously had intercourse with a condom the week before. Her last menstrual period (LMP) was about 3 weeks ago and was normal in flow and duration. She had been given a sample pack of Ortho-Tri-Cyclen during her initial gynecologic examination 2 weeks ago, but she did not have a chance to start them yet. She would be devastated if she got pregnant. She has no medical problems, denies bleeding or other symptoms, and her examination is normal. Her Pap test and gonococcus/chlamydia results from her last visit are all normal. A urine pregnancy test in your office is negative.

15. Which of the following statements regarding the use of emergency contraceptive pills (ECP) in this patient is true?
   a. ECPs are contraindicated because it has been longer than 48 hours
   b. ECPs are contraindicated because she also had sex a week before
   c. ECPs could have been prescribed to this patient over the phone without an examination
   d. ECPs are not necessary because her LMP was more than 2 weeks ago
   e. ECPs would be contraindicated if either her Pap or gonococcus/chlamydia test was abnormal
   f. ECPs are contraindicated in pregnancy because they are abortifacients

16. Which of the following ECP options is not appropriate for this patient?
   a. Ovral: two white pills now; repeat 12 hours later
   b. Plan B: one pill now; repeat 12 hours later
   c. Preven: two pills now; repeat 12 hours later
   d. a ParaGard (copper IUD) inserted within 5 days
   e. all of the above options are appropriate

CLINICAL CASE MANAGEMENT PROBLEM

List the important user characteristics to assess to help a patient select the most appropriate contraceptive method for them.

ANSWERS:

1. c. The withdrawal method (coitus interruptus) offers neither an effective method of contraception nor protection from any type of STD. With "perfect use" of the withdrawal method, the failure rate is 4% within the first year of use. However, the average user has a significantly higher risk of pregnancy because the "typical use" failure rate for the withdrawal method is 19% within the first year of use.

2. b. The female condom is an effective "barrier" method of contraception, and it also provides excellent protection against STDs. It is made of polyurethane, but it does not contain a spermicide, which can be added. Male condoms made from animal products (usually lamb cecum) have pore sizes too large to prevent STD transmission (especially viral: human immunodeficiency virus [HIV], human papilloma virus [HPV], herpes simplex virus, or hepatitis B). Although the sponge is embedded with the spermicide nonoxynol-9, it does not provide effective STD protection alone. Diaphragms, with or without nonoxynol-9, may reduce the risk of cervicitis, pelvic inflammatory disease (PID), and cervical dysplasia, but they are not effective at preventing STD transmission (especially viral). Nonoxynol-9 alone may reduce the risk of cervicitis, HPV transmission, and cervical dysplasia. However, it does not decrease the risk of STD transmission. In fact, the World Health Organization (WHO) recommends that nonoxynol-9 not be used for protection against STDs because some studies have shown an increased risk of HIV infection in high-risk women (sex workers, women at STD clinics). The theory behind this finding is that nonoxynol-9 may have a disruptive, irritative effect on the vaginal/cervical mucosa, allowing for increased risk of HIV infection. These findings have not been demonstrated in average- to low-risk women. Although oral contraceptives may reduce the risk of PID, they do not significantly reduce the risk of STD transmission.

3. e. Estrogen-containing oral contraceptives offer several potential noncontraceptive benefits, which may improve patient satisfaction and compliance. All COCs may reduce acne vulgaris, mainly through the estrogen-mediated increase in sex hormone binding globulin (SHBG), which binds free testosterone. COCs are not contraindicated in patients with common migraines. Although some migraine patients may note an increase or decrease in their headache frequency and/or intensity with COC use, most patients will have no associated change. Patients with common migraines should keep a symptom diary before and after starting COCs to objectively record any changes in headache quality, frequency, intensity, or duration and to determine if they are associated with menses (menstrual migraines). Patients who suffer from "classic migraines," especially those with focal (asymmetric) neurologic symptoms, may be at an increased risk for embolic stroke and should avoid all estrogen-containing hormonal contraceptive methods. Estrogen-containing hormonal contraceptives are not recommended for women older than age 35 years who smoke because of the increased risk of premature cardiovascular disease. COCs are not contraindicated of women younger than age 35 who smoke. However, they are at an increased risk for venous thromboembolic events (VTEs) and should be encouraged to quit. Chlamydial cervicitis is more common in women taking OCPs. OCPs can cause cervical ectopy, a broadening of the area on the ectocervix covered by the mucus-secreting columnar cells that normally lines the cervical canal (ectropion), which ostensibly makes the OCP user more vulnerable to *Chlamydia trachomatis* infection. However, OCP use also is associated with a significant decreased risk of PID, probably because of cervical mucus thickening. This patient's previous history of a chlamydial infection is not a contraindication to OCP use, although she should be offered STD screening and strongly encouraged to use an effective method of STD protection (i.e., male latex, polyurethane condoms, female condoms) in addition to OCPs. Obesity itself is not a contraindication to COC use, although you may consider screening these patients for diabetes and hyperlipidemia. There is no evidence that overweight women need to be prescribed a higher-dose OCP to ensure contraceptive efficacy. However, women with a body weight of more than 198 lb should not be prescribed the OrthoEvra Patch because of the increased associated risk for contraceptive failure. There is no evidence supporting the common claim that estrogen-containing hormonal contraceptives themselves cause significant weight gain. However, all COC users should be encouraged to exercise and eat a well-balanced diet.

4. c. The Mirena IUS and the ParaGard T 380A (copper IUD) are not recommended in women who are nulliparous; not in a long-term monogamous relationship, or have a recent history of PID. They offer highly effective, long-term reversible contraception (Mirena 5 years; ParaGard 10 years). However, they do not provide any effective STD protection. Depo-Provera, the OrthoEvra Patch, and NuvaRing may be appropriate contraceptive options for this patient, depending on other user characteristics (e.g., desire for amenorrhea, comfort using an intravaginal device, affordability). These methods also should be combined with an effective means of STD protection in this patient. The only established advantage of the weekly OrthoEvra Patch and the monthly NuvaRing over COCs is the potential for improved compliance, especially in younger patients.

5. a. All COC pill types usually provide most users with regular and predictable menstrual cycles within the first 3 months of use. POPs often reduce the frequency, duration, and amount of menses in most users and may cause amenorrhea. They also have a higher potential for contraceptive failure with typical use than COCs. They should be reserved for women who (1) cannot or will not use an estrogen-containing hormonal contraceptive method; (2) do not require/desire regular and predictable menstrual cycles, and (3) have no problems with taking a pill the same time every day.

6. d. There is no evidence supporting the common claim that estrogen-containing hormonal contraceptive themselves cause significant weight gain. However, all COC users should be encouraged to exercise and eat a well-balanced diet, and their weight should be monitored during periodic follow-up visits. The best time to start any hormonal contraceptive method is actually on the first day of a woman's menses. COCs should be initiated within the first 7 days of the onset of menses. A "Sunday start" can be offered to women who would prefer not to get their menses during the weekend. Nausea and breast tenderness are common side effects of estrogen-containing hormonal contraceptive methods, which usually subside within the first 3 months of use. Using a lower estrogen dose COC and/or having the patient take their pill after dinner may reduce these side effects. BTB is one of the most common side effects of all hormonal contraceptive methods and one of the most common reasons for discontinuation. The most common cause of BTB in new COC users is noncompliance. Patients should be counseled about common side effects of COCs, including BTB, and the importance of compliance. They should be provided with verbal and written instructions on proper use, compliance tips, and what to do if they miss a pill and or develop side effects (including BTB). Patients should be instructed not to stop taking their COC pill if they develop BTB or miss a pill without speaking with their health provider first.

7. a. Smoking and cervicitis are potential causes of BTB and should be considered, especially in COC users with persistent BTB or who develop BTB after having had regular bleeding cycles while taking them. Although BTB usually decreases after the first cycle of proper COC use, it is not uncommon for it to occur until after the third cycle use. NSAIDs are actually an effective first-line therapy for reducing BTB for all methods of hormonal contraception. Although noncompliance is the most common cause of BTB in COC users, there are other potential causes that health providers also should consider, especially if the BTB is persistent or develops after the COC user previously had regular bleeding cycles while taking them. Pregnancy should be ruled out in patients with persistent BTB. However, the presence of BTB itself is not an indicator that any hormonal contraceptive method is subtherapeutic or ineffective.

8. e. There is strong evidence that long-term COC use is associated with a significant reduction of both endometrial and ovarian cancer risk and that this protective effect is sustained years after use. This is thought to be the result of the effect of COCs on reducing endometrial hyperplasia and incessant ovulation. Although some studies have suggested a potential association between COC use and breast cancer, there is no strong evidence to support this. In fact, one large study found no significant increased risk in long-term COC users, including women older than 40 years of age. However, COCs are contraindicated in women with a history of estrogen-dependent malignancies. There is some evidence to suggest that COC use may be associated with an increased risk for cervical cancer, but several potential confounding variables exist, including lack of condom use in COC users compared with nonusers. However, COCs do not provide adequate protection against STD transmission (including HPV). COCs may be associated with higher bone densities in users than aged-matched nonusers, but there is no evidence that this provides protection against postmenopausal osteoporosis and subsequent fractures later in life.

9. b. Although COCs are not associated with the development of gallstones, they actually may accelerate the progression of cholelithiasis in patients who are already susceptible. However, COCs do not increase the risk for gallbladder cancer. COCs promote regular, predictable menses and often reduce menstrual duration and blood loss. This may help prevent or correct iron-deficiency anemia, especially in patients with excessively heavy menses (i.e., menorrhagia). COCs are an effective treatment for primary and secondary causes of dysmenorrhea, especially when given continuously (without a pill-free/placebo period). Because the primary mechanism of action for COCs is ovulation suppression, they are highly effective for preventing ectopic pregnancies and for eliminating ovulatory symptoms (mittelschmerz). Other noncontraceptive benefits of COCs include the following: (1) prevention of functional ovarian cysts; (2) improvement of acne; (3) improvement of hirsutism; (4) decreased incidence of benign breast disease (fibrocystic disease, fibroadenoma); and (5) reduced risk of endometrial and ovarian cancer.

10. c. Depo-Provera and the Mirena IUS are progestin-only hormonal birth control methods. Both methods provide highly effective contraception, are safe to use while breastfeeding, do not require active daily use, and are preferable for patients who desire long-term contraception. WHO recommends waiting until patients who are breastfeeding are at least 6 weeks postpartum before starting progestin-only contraception to allow for milk let-down. Estrogen-containing hormonal methods (e.g., OrthoEvra or NuvaRing) can decrease milk production and flow and should be initiated only once the patient begins weaning their infant off breast milk. Depo-Provera provides up to 3 months of protection with every injection; however, it may take up to 1 year or more for patients to return to fertility after cessation of use. The Mirena IUS provides up to 5 years of contraception after insertion and is therefore most cost-effective for patients who desire contraception for at least several years, despite its high upfront cost. Fertility should return rapidly after its removal. Sterilization procedures (bilateral tubal ligation or vasectomy) should be recommended only for patients who desire permanent/irreversible methods of contraception; are in a stable, monogamous relationship; and already have children. Sterilization reversals are rarely successful, are expensive, and are susceptible to complications (e.g., ectopic pregnancy). LAM may provide up to 6 months of effective contraception but only in mothers who are breastfeeding their babies exclusively. It is not ideal for patients who are supplementing their infant with formula and who desire long-term contraception. Norplant, comprising of six implantable progestin-only rods, which provided at least 5 years of highly effective reversible contraception, has been withdrawn from the U.S. market. A single-rod implantable progestin-only contraceptive device, Implanon, which provides up to 3 years of contraception, is awaiting approval from the U.S. Food and Drug Administration.

11. e. Estrogen-containing hormonal contraceptives may help regulate menses and reduce other perimenopausal symptoms (i.e., hot flashes, night sweats) in women older than 40 years of age. They also may reduce the risk of endometrial and ovarian cancer later in life. However, they will neither delay nor accelerate the age of onset of menopause. Estrogen-containing hormonal contraceptives are not contraindicated in nonsmoking women older than 40 years of age unless they have an estrogen-dependent malignancy; undiagnosed abnormal vaginal/uterine bleeding; an undiagnosed breast mass; cardiovascular disease; a history of or high risk for VTE; uncontrolled hypertension or diabetes; significant hypertriglyceridemia; gallbladder disease; active liver disease; headaches with focal neurologic symptoms; or known or suspected pregnancy. However, estrogen-containing hormonal contraceptives should not be used in breastfeeding women until they begin weaning their infant off breast milk. Estrogen-containing hormonal contraceptives actually may be effective treatments for abnormal uterine bleeding or dysmenorrhea caused by uterine fibroids. All estrogen-containing hormonal contraceptives are combined with a progestin, which helps prevent or retard endometrial hyperplasia and fibroid growth.

12. **b.** Depo-Provera and other progestin-only methods of contraception are safe and effective for breastfeeding patients. It can take up to a year or more for a patient to return to fertility following cessation of Depo-Provera use, even after only one injection. It is very important to counsel all patients about this, especially if they desire a rapidly reversible contraceptive method. Depo-Provera appears to actually increase seizure thresholds, and thereby reduce seizure frequency, in patients with seizure disorders, possibly because of its sedative effect on the brain. Depo-Provera is administered via an intramuscular injection and does not require first-pass metabolism for activity, so, unlike COCs, its effectiveness is not compromised by drugs (i.e., anticonvulsants, antifungals) that are actively metabolized by the liver. Neither Depo-Provera nor any other hormonal contraceptive method will alter significantly a patient's age of onset of menopause. Although Depo-Provera has been shown to reduce bone density in users, bone density appears to be regained following cessation of use. In addition, there is no evidence that Depo-Provera users are at a higher risk for postmenopausal osteoporosis and subsequent fractures later in life.

13. **d.** The ParaGard T 380A (copper IUD) contains no hormones. It does not significantly affect menstrual flow or pain in most patients. However, it does create a sterile inflammatory reaction in the uterus, which may exacerbate bleeding and pain in patients who already suffer from significant dysmenorrhea or menorrhagia. Because the Copper IUD appears to act primarily as a spermicide, it actually can decrease the risk of ectopic pregnancy, as long as it remains properly inserted. The ParaGard T 380A provides up to 10 years of highly effective contraception, with a rapid return to fertility following its removal. It does not interfere with breast milk and may be inserted immediately postpartum or postabortion.

14. **a.** One of the advantages of vasectomies over BTLs is that they usually are performed in an out-

patient office with local anesthesia. Neither procedure is easily reversible, so patients need to be counseled to ensure that they desire and are prepared for permanent contraception. Despite many studies on this subject, there is no convincing significant evidence that vasectomies increase the risk of prostate cancer or reduce male libido, erectile dysfunction, or penile sensation. Properly performed BTLs actually may reduce the risk of ectopic pregnancy. However, reversal attempts can lead to narrowed and scarred fallopian tubes, increasing the risk of ectopic pregnancy.

15. **c.** Emergency contraception (EC) is defined as any method of preventing pregnancy after unprotected intercourse. Methods include oral combination pills (estrogen and progestin), POPs, and the placement of an IUD. The "Yuzpe regimen" involves two doses of 100 mcg of ethinyl estradiol and either 1.0 mg of norgestrel or 0.5 mg of levonorgestrel administered 12 hours apart. The Yuzpe regimen decreases the risk of pregnancy by about 75% when taken properly. Up to one-third to one-half of all patients experience some nausea or vomiting with this regimen, and coadministration of an antiemetic can be helpful. The progestin-only or "POPs EC regimen" involves the administration of two doses of 1.5 mg of norgestrel or 0.75 mg of levonorgestrel 12 hours apart. The POPs regimen is associated with much less nausea and vomiting than the Yuzpe method and can decrease the risk of pregnancy by up to 85%, with proper use. The mechanism of action of EC likely is related to inhibition of ovulation, although alterations in endometrial receptivity also may be involved. ECPs have not been shown to adversely affect or disrupt an implanted embryo and are thus not considered abortifacients by FDA standards.

The efficacy of both regimens is best when ECPs are initiated as soon as possible after unprotected intercourse, with standard protocols citing effectiveness up to 72 hours postintercourse. An international WHO trial demonstrated that a single combined dose of 1.5 mg of levonorgestrel showed excellent efficacy up until 120 hours after unprotected intercourse. Widespread use of this regimen has the potential for increased patient compliance. This same trial also demonstrated that a single low dose of 10 mg of mifepristone appears to be at least as safe and effective as currently approved ECPs. A ParaGard T 380A can be inserted within 5 days of unprotected intercourse, then left in to provide up to 10 years of effective contraception in appropriate patients.

ECPs can be prescribed safely to the majority of patients over the phone without an examination. According to WHO, the only contraindication for use of ECPs is known pregnancy. The main reason pregnancy is a contraindication is that ECPs will not be effective in an established pregnancy. There are no known associated teratogenic effects from ECPs administered inadvertently during pregnancy. The American College of Obstetricians and Gynecologists (ACOG) also adds known hypersensitivity to the ECP being prescribed and undiagnosed genital bleeding as contraindications to ECP use in addition to known pregnancy. Common contraindications for OCP use (smoking, hypertriglyceridemia, etc.) are not believed to be significant concerns with ECP given its short duration of use. Cervical dysplasia and STDs are not contraindications to ECP use. However, an IUD should not be used in such cases. Some experts suggest that history of thromboembolic disease should be a relative contraindication to ECP use, but to date there has been no reported cases of thromboembolic events resulting from ECP use. In fact, women who become pregnant are at far greater risk of thromboembolic event than nonpregnant women.

All sexually active women should be counseled about the availability of EC. Patients can be provided with an advance prescription for ECPs or the EC Hotline number (888-NOT-2-LATE) to have available if needed. Advance provision of ECPs can help overcome barriers to access (pharmacy not open late hours/weekends, not able to get a doctor's appointment) and allow patients to start EC in a timely manner. Advance provision of ECPs has not been shown to increase promiscuity or discourage regular contraception. Several states now allow pharmacists to dispense ECPs directly to patients without a prescription. However, patients should be encouraged to come into the office whenever possible so that they can be counseled on proper contraceptive use and other effective contraceptive options and to be screened for possible sexual abuse.

16. **d.** There are two FDA-approved dedicated EC products available: Preven (combined estrogen and progestin) and Plan B (progestin only). The Preven EC Kit includes a urine pregnancy test and easy-to-follow directions. In addition to Preven and Plan B, several commonly used COC and POP brands also can provide effective EC when administered in the correct doses (see the Table in the Summary section). Ovral administered as described (using the active pills) is an appropriate option. However, only the COC and POP combinations listed have been shown to be effective. Thus, the use of her Ortho-Tri-Cyclen sample pills for EC would not be appropriate. A ParaGard IUD is neither necessary nor appropriate EC for this patient given that she is (1) being seen within 72 hours of unprotected intercourse; (2) is nulliparous; and (3) is not in a long-term stable monogamous relationship.

SOLUTION TO THE CLINICAL CASE MANAGEMENT PROBLEM

Important user characteristics for contraceptive selection include the following:
- Gender preference
- Frequency of intercourse
- Number of past/current partners
- Problems with past/current methods
- Method of STD prevention
- Partner's willingness to participate in pregnancy/STD prevention
- Ability to cope with contraceptive failure
- Ability to use method correctly and consistently
- Personal beliefs about methods
- Contraindications to certain methods
- Medical conditions that may be adversely affected by certain methods
- Medical conditions that may be improved by certain methods
- Risk factors that may be modified by certain methods
- Desire for future fertility (long term versus short term)
- Financial ability to pay for contraception

SUMMARY OF CONTRACEPTION

1. Latex or polyurethane male condoms and the polyurethane female condom offer the most effective means of STD prevention, next to abstinence. The withdrawal method offers neither effective pregnancy nor STD protection.
2. Estrogen-containing hormonal contraceptives are only contraindicated in patients who have an estrogen-dependent malignancy, classic migraines,

known or suspected pregnancy, a history of VTEs, or unexplained vaginal bleeding or who are older than 35 years of age and smoke. Common migraines and obesity are not contraindications.

3. All hormonal contraceptives offer several potential noncontraceptive benefits including a reduction in dysmenorrhea, ovulatory pain (mittelschmerz), and iron-deficiency anemia. COCs also have been shown to help regulate menses and to reduce acne vulgaris and the risk of ovarian and endometrial cancers. There is no convincing evidence that COCs increase the risk of breast, cervical, or liver cancer.

4. BTB, nausea, and breast tenderness are common side effects of estrogen-containing hormonal contraceptive methods and usually resolve within the first three cycles of use. BTB is the most common cause of discontinuation from COCs and is most often the result of noncompliance. Health care providers can improve patient satisfaction and compliance significantly by discussing potential COC side effects with their patients before prescribing them and managing these side effects promptly as they occur.

5. Progestin-only hormonal contraceptives (Depo-Provera, Mirena, and POPs) may be used safely in breastfeeding women. Depo-Provera offers up to 3 months of highly effective contraception per injection, whereas the Mirena IUS can be used for up to 5 years. POPs must be taken at almost the same time daily for contraceptive efficacy. The Mirena IUS permits a rapid return to fertility, whereas it may take a woman using Depo-Provera at least a year or more to conceive following its cessation, even after only one injection. Depo-Provera also may decrease seizure frequency in patients with seizure disorders.

6. The ParaGard (Copper-T) IUD should be reserved for patients who desire a long-term (up to 10 years), rapidly reversible, nonhormonal contraceptive method and who already have children; are in a stable, monogamous relationship; and have no recent history of PID, no allergies to copper, and no significant menstrual disorders.

7. Sterilization procedures (vasectomies and bilateral tubule ligations) should be limited to patients who truly desire permanent contraception and who already have children and are in a long-term, stable relationship. Reversals are extremely difficult, are expensive, and can lead to severe complications (e.g., ectopic pregnancy). There is no conclusive evidence that vasectomies are associated with prostate cancer, cardiovascular disease, decreased libido, erectile dysfunction, or decreased penile sensitivity.

8. All sexually active female patients should be counseled about the availability of EC and provided with either a prescription for ECPs or the number for the EC Hotline (888-NOT-2-LATE). ECPs can be used within at least 72 hours of unprotected intercourse and have very few contraindications. The table contains a list of appropriate emergency contraceptive methods:

Brand Name	Instructions
Preven Kit	Follow kit instructions (2 pills now; repeat 12 hours later)
Plan B Kit	Follow kit instructions (1 pill now; repeat 12 hours later)
Ovral	Take 2 "white" pills now with 8 oz of water; repeat 12 hours later
LO/Ovral	Take 4 "white" pills now with 8 oz of water; repeat 12 hours later
Nordette	Take 4 "orange" pills now with 8 oz of water; repeat 12 hours later
Levlen	Take 4 "orange" pills now with 8 oz of water; repeat 12 hours later
Triphasil	Take 4 "yellow" pills now with 8 oz of water; repeat 12 hours later
Trilevlen	Take 4 "yellow" pills now with 8 oz of water; repeat 12 hours later
Alesse	Take 5 "pink" pills now with 8 oz of water; repeat 12 hours later
Ovrette	Take 20 "yellow" pills now with 8 oz of water; repeat 12 hours later
Copper-T intrauterine device	Insert within 5 days of unprotected intercourse

9. Health care providers should assess the user characteristics listed earlier to help patients select the most appropriate contraceptive and STD protection methods for them. Patients should receive both verbal and written information regarding the benefits, risks, proper use, and common side effects of the method, along with instructions on what to do if they have a problem. These steps will significantly improve patient satisfaction and compliance with their contraceptive method.

SUGGESTED READING

Hatcher RA: *Contraceptive technology, 17th ed.* Ardent Media, Inc., 1998, New York.

Knowles J: *Facts about birth control,* Planned Parenthood Federation of America, Inc., 1998, New York.

Levine JP: *Contraception textbook of family practice, 6th ed.* W.B. Saunders, 2001, Orlando, FL.

Schrager S: Abnormal uterine bleeding associated with hormonal contraception. *Am Fam Physician* 65:2073-2083, 2002.

Technical Guidance/Competence Working Group and WHO Scientific Group. Family planning methods: new guidance. *Population Reports, Series J,* no. 44, vol XXIV, no. 2., 1996.

Thomsen K, et al: *Management of women's health: contraception.* The Foundation for Better Health Care, 1999, New York.

Trussell J: The economic value of contraception. *The Contraception Report* 9(1):4-14, 1998.

Trussell J, Stewart F: An update on emergency contraception. *Dialogues in Contraception* 5(6):1-4, 1998.

Wertheimer RE: Emergency postcoital contraception. *Am Fam Physician* 62:2287-2292, 2000.

 Chapter **60**

Sexually Transmitted Diseases

> "My last lover was a real toad. He sure did give me a case of warts."

CLINICAL CASE PROBLEM 1:

A 24-YEAR-OLD FEMALE WITH DIFFUSE ABDOMINAL PAIN

A 24-year-old female comes to the emergency room with a 2-day history of lower abdominal pain, fever, chills, and malaise. The patient also complains of nausea and multiple episodes of vomiting in the last 24 hours. On physical examination, there is bilateral adnexal tenderness, mucopurulent cervical discharge, and cervical motion tenderness. The patient has a temperature of 40° C. Her last menstrual period was 4 weeks ago, and her pregnancy test is negative. She admits to being sexually active but denies a history of any sexually transmitted diseases (STD). She is not currently using birth control.

■ **SELECT THE BEST ANSWER TO THE FOLLOWING QUESTIONS:**

1. What is the most likely diagnosis in this patient?
   a. acute appendicitis
   b. acute pelvic inflammatory disease (PID)
   c. uncomplicated cervicitis
   d. ectopic pregnancy
   e. threatened abortion

2. What is the most appropriate intervention for this patient?
   a. hospitalize the patient for parenteral treatment
   b. begin outpatient treatment with follow-up within 24 hours
   c. begin outpatient treatment with follow-up in a week
   d. begin outpatient treatment with follow-up if condition worsens
   e. none of the above are acceptable

3. If hospitalization was chosen for this patient, which of the following regimens is first-line treatment for her condition?

   a. intravenous (IV) ampicillin and gentamicin
   b. IV cefotetan and doxycycline
   c. IV ceftriaxone
   d. IV ciprofloxacin
   e. IV ampicillin

4. If outpatient management was chosen for this patient, which of the following regimens is first-line treatment for her condition?
   a. Oral (per os [by mouth] [PO]) ofloxacin with or without PO metronidazole
   b. Intramuscular (IM) cefoxitin, PO probenecid, and PO doxycycline
   c. IM ceftriaxone, PO doxycycline with or without PO metronidazole
   d. any of the above
   e. none of the above

5. Which of the following statements regarding the relationship between combined oral contraceptive pills (OCPs) and this patient's condition is true?
   a. OCPs decrease the risk of this condition
   b. OCPs increase the risk of this condition
   c. OCPs do not influence this condition at all
   d. OCPs are contraindicated in patients with this condition
   e. none of the above

6. Which of the following organisms is not associated with this condition?
   a. *Neisseria gonorrhea*
   b. *Chlamydia trachomatis*
   c. *Gardnerella hominis*
   d. *Bacteroides fragilis*
   e. *beta-hemolytic streptococcus*

7. What is the current Centers for Disease Control and Prevention (CDC) recommendation for the treatment of uncomplicated cervical, urethral, or rectal gonococcal infection?
   a. PO cefixime and PO doxycycline
   b. IM ceftriaxone and PO doxycycline
   c. PO levofloxacin and PO doxycycline
   d. a, b, or c
   e. b or c

CLINICAL CASE PROBLEM 2:

A 24-YEAR-OLD MALE WITH DYSURIA

A 24-year-old sexually active male comes to your office with complaints of a 2-day history of dysuria. He denies fever, urgency, frequency, or hematuria. Physical examination reveals no suprapubic or costovertebral tenderness. Urologic examination reveals nontender testes, normal prostate, and no penile lesions but mucopurulent urethral discharge. Urine analysis is positive for leukocyte esterase, but it is negative for nitrite and blood. Microscopic examination of urine reveals >10 to 15 white blood cells (WBCs) per high field. You send a swab of his urethral discharge for gram stain.

8. The patient's urethral gram stain reveals WBCs per oil immersion field. There are no intracellular gram-negative diplococci seen. What is the most likely diagnosis in this patient?
   a. gonorrhea
   b. acute prostatitis
   c. epididymitis
   d. nongonococcal urethritis (NGU)
   e. bacterial cystitis

9. What is the most likely organism causing the condition described in Clinical Case Problem 2?
   a. *Chlamydia trachomatis*
   b. *Ureaplasma urealyticum*
   c. *Trichomonas vaginalis*
   d. *Neisseria gonorrhea*
   e. *Herpes simplex virus*

10. What is first-line treatment for the condition described in Clinical Case Problem 2?
    a. PO levofloxacin
    b. PO doxycycline
    c. PO erythromycin
    d. PO ampicillin and PO probenecid
    e. PO ofloxacin

11. You prescribe an appropriate antibiotic regimen for the patient in Clinical Case Problem 2 and also for his current sexual partner. Both he and his partner completed the recommended regimen. He states that they have been in a monogamous relationship since then. His symptoms have resolved completely. He wants to know if the "infection is gone" and if he should have a test of cure. Which of the following statement can you tell the patient?
    a. he should have a test of cure 2 weeks after treatment
    b. he should have a test of cure 6 months after treatment
    c. he and his partner should have a test of cure 2 weeks after treatment
    d. he and his partner should have a test of cure 6 months after treatment
    e. he and his partner do not need a test of cure

12. Which of the following is (are) a complication(s) of disseminated gonococcal infection (DGI)?
    a. arthritis
    b. tenosynovitis
    c. bacteremia
    d. endocarditis
    e. all of the above

CLINICAL CASE PROBLEM 3:

A 24-YEAR-OLD FEMALE WITH GENITAL LESIONS

A 24-year-old female comes to your office with a 2-day history of dysuria accompanied by painful genital lesions that have coalesced to form ulcers. The patient also has fever, malaise, myalgias, and headache. There is no previous history of this condition. She has had three sexual partners in the past and inconsistently uses barrier contraceptive methods.

13. You tell the patient the most likely diagnosis is:
    a. herpes simplex infection
    b. chancroid
    c. human papillomavirus (HPV) infection
    d. granuloma inguinale
    e. primary syphilis

14. Which of the following statements concerning the patient's condition is false?
    a. transmission of infection can occur during asymptomatic periods
    b. duration of viral shedding may be reduced with appropriate therapy
    c. time needed to heal lesions may be reduced with appropriate therapy
    d. frequency of recurrent episodes can be reduced with appropriate suppressive therapy
    e. subclinical viral shedding can be eliminated with appropriate suppressive therapy

CLINICAL CASE PROBLEM 4:

A 25-YEAR-OLD FEMALE WITH VULVAR "GROWTHS"

A 25-year-old sexually active female comes to your office with a 2-week history of "growths" in the vulvar region. On examination, you find multiple "cauliflower" verrucous lesions on the labia majora and minora.

15. What is the most likely diagnosis in this patient?
    a. condyloma lata
    b. condyloma acuminatum
    c. herpes simplex type 1

d. herpes simplex type 2
e. none of the above

16. All of the following are acceptable treatments for genital warts except:
a. podophyllin
b. trichloracetic acid
c. carbon dioxide laser
d. interferon
e. acyclovir

17. Which of the following statements about syphilis is true ?
a. primary syphilis is associated with a single, painful chancre
b. secondary syphilis is associated with skin lesions and lymphadenopathy
c. latent syphilis is associated with constitutional symptoms
d. treatment for primary syphilis is oral penicillin
e. the recommended treatment for early-latent and late-latent syphilis is the same

18. Which of the following statements about syphilis testing is true?
a. dark-field microscopy of lesion exudates is the most convenient way to confirm *Treponema pallidum*
b. nontreponemal tests (i.e., rapid plasma reagin [RPR]) can be falsely positive in certain medical conditions
c. treponemal-specific test (i.e., fluorescent treponemal antibody-absorption test [FTA-ABS]) titers decline after syphilis treatment
d. RPR titers can be used interchangeably with Venereal Disease Research Laboratory (VDRL) titers
e. none of the above

19. What is the treatment of choice in patients who are not allergic to penicillin for primary or secondary syphilis?
a. IM benzathine penicillin G in a single dose
b. IM benzathine penicillin G once a week for 3 weeks
c. IV aqueous crystalline penicillin G for 10-14 days
d. PO probenecid for 10-14 days
e. PO doxycycline

20. Which of the following statements about human immunodeficiency virus (HIV) is false?
a. HIV testing should be offered to all patients seeking evaluation for STDs
b. the HIV-2 strain is endemic to the United States
c. HIV testing is available through urine, oral mucosal, and blood samples
d. initial positive screening test should be followed by a more specific confirmatory test

e. repeat serologic testing should not be done prior to 3 months after exposure

CLINICAL CASE MANAGEMENT PROBLEM
Discuss risk factors for hepatitis B and preventive strategies to reduce transmission.

■ **ANSWERS:**

1. **b.** This patient meets diagnostic criteria for acute PID. The clinical diagnosis of acute PID is imprecise, and often episodes of PID go unrecognized. Clinicians need to maintain a low threshold of suspicion and account for epidemiologic factors when diagnosing PID. Patients who are young, have multiple sexual partners, live in high prevalence areas for gonorrhea or chlamydia, do not use barrier contraception, and have a history of prior PID are at highest risk. According to the 2002 CDC STD guidelines, minimal diagnostic criteria for acute PID includes uterine/adnexal tenderness or cervical motion tenderness in women at risk for STDs. Supportive criteria include the following: (1) oral temperature higher than 101° F (>38.3° C); (2) abnormal cervical or vaginal mucopurulent discharge; (3) presence of WBCs on wet prep; (4) elevated erythrocyte sedimentation rate (ESR); (5) elevated C-reactive protein (CRP); and (6) documentation of cervical infection with *N. gonorrhea* or *C. trachomatis*. More invasive studies such as endometrial biopsy to document endometritis, laparoscopy, or transvaginal ultrasound to document tubal disease are sometimes necessary in select cases to confirm diagnosis.

The differential diagnosis of acute PID is broad and includes disorders of any of the three organ systems within the pelvis: (1) reproductive tract (adnexal torsion, ectopic pregnancy, threatened abortion); (2) gastrointestinal tract (appendicitis, diverticulitis, regional ileitis); and (3) urinary tract (cystitis and pyelonephritis). The patient in Clinical Case Problem 1 is most likely to have acute PID than any other diagnosis given her history and examination. The presence of vaginal discharge and pelvic findings makes acute appendicitis less likely. Uncomplicated cervicitis does not present with systemic symptoms. The negative pregnancy test makes ectopic pregnancy or threatened abortion unlikely. Pregnancy should be excluded in all women of reproductive age presenting with abdominal and pelvic symptoms.

2. **a.** Early treatment of acute PID decreases the probability of tubal scarring and subsequent infertility. The incidence of infertility is 15% after one episode of untreated or inadequately treated PID. In the past, it generally was advocated to hospitalize all patients for parenteral antibiotics to ensure successful eradication

of infection. However, there are no data available to support that inpatient treatment results in better outcomes than outpatient treatment or that benefits exceed cost. In practice, the decision for hospitalization is made on an individual basis depending on severity of disease and patient factors, such as compliance. The CDC suggests the following guidelines for hospitalization: (1) observation for potential surgical emergencies that cannot be excluded (i.e., appendicitis); (2) pregnant patients; (3) failed outpatient treatment; (4) severe illness such as high temperature, nausea, or vomiting; and (5) presence of a tuboovarian abscess

In this patient's case, her high fever, nausea, and vomiting would be an indication for her to be hospitalized for parenteral antibiotics.

3. b. The treatment for acute PID is broad-spectrum coverage for *N. gonorrhea, C. trachomatis,* anaerobes, gram-negative bacteria, and streptococci. The CDC 2002 guidelines recommend as first-line treatment (1) cefotetan 2 g IV q 12 hours or cefoxitin 2 gm IV q 6 hours plus doxycycline 100 mg orally or IV q 12 hours or (2) clindamycin 900 mg IV q 8 hours plus a gentamicin loading dose IV or IM (2 mg/kg of body weight) followed by a maintenance dose (1.5 mg/kg) q 8 hours.

Less studied *alternative* regimens include the following: (1) ofloxacin or levofloxacin IV with or without metronidazole IV and (2) ampicillin/sulbactam IV plus doxycycline.

Parenteral therapy should continue for at least 24 hours after clinical improvement, at which time the transition can be made to oral antibiotics.

4. d. The recommended outpatient treatment regimen for patients with PID includes the following:

1. Oral ofloxacin 400 mg PO twice a day (bid) for 14 days or
2. Oral levofloxacin 500 mg PO bid for 14 days
3. Cefoxitin 2 g IM in a single dose and probenecid 1 gm PO in a single dose plus doxycycline 100 mg PO bid for 14 days
4. Ceftriaxone 250 mg IM in a single dose plus doxycycline 100 mg PO bid for 14 days

These regimens may be given with or without metronidazole (500 mg PO bid for 14 days). The choice to add metronidazole to these regimens is based on the assumption that PID involves a broad spectrum of organisms, including anaerobes. Empiric treatment should be initiated in all male sexual partners of women with PID.

5. a. Past epidemiologic studies have demonstrated that OCPs have a protective effect against PID. The proposed mechanism is believed to be multifactorial: (1) progestin-induced thickening of cervical secretions

inhibit bacterial ascent into the upper genital tract; (2) decreased menstrual blood flow, with menstrual blood potentially acting as a culture medium; (3) decreased cervical dilation at mid-cycle and menstruation; and (4) decreased strength of uterine contractions. It is interesting that OCPs do not decrease the risk of lower genital tract disease against chlamydia but in fact may increase the risk of cervicitis. OCPs may promote cervical ectopy, a process in which the delicate columnar cells that normally line the endocervical canal and surround the os evert onto the portio of the cervix. This ectropion of columnar cells may be more vulnerable to infection with chlamydia. All OCP users need to be advised that OCPs alone do not prevent transmission of STDs. Counseling should focus on consistent condom use; abstinence; or engaging in a stable, monogamous relationship to minimize risk.

6. e. The most common organisms associated with acute PID are *N. gonorrhea* and *C. trachomatis.* Many episodes of PID are polymicrobial and involve anaerobic organisms such as *Bacteroides fragilis* and *Peptostreptococcus.* Microorganisms that include vaginal flora such as *Gardnerella vaginalis* and *Streptococcus agalactiae* also have been associated with PID. Beta-hemolytic streptococcus (the streptococcus associated with bacterial pharyngitis) is not associated with acute PID.

7. d. The preferred treatment of uncomplicated adult gonococcal urethritis, cervicitis, or proctitis is as follows: (1) ceftriaxone 125 mg IM in a single dose or (2) cefixime 400 mg PO in a single dose or (3) an oral quinolone (such as levofloxacin, ofloxacin, or ciprofloxacin).

If chlamydia infection is not ruled out, azithromycin 1 g orally in a single dose or doxycycline 100 mg PO bid for 7 days should be added.

Ceftriaxone provides excellent cure rates for uncomplicated gonorrhea, eradicating 99% of infections in clinical trials. Cefixime has excellent efficacy as well (97.4%), but less than that of ceftriaxone. The advantage of cefixime is that it can be orally administered. The addition of fluoroquinolones to the treatment regimen for uncomplicated gonococcal infection expands the choice of oral therapies available. However, quinolone use is not advised in areas with quinolone-resistant *N. gonorrhea* (Asia, Pacific Coast regions including Hawaii and California). Patients with gonorrhea often have coinfection with chlamydia; this has led to the recommendation that dual treatment therapy be performed. The CDC 2002 guidelines recommend that decisions to cotreat for chlamydia be based on (1) geographic prevalence of coinfection; (2) availability of sensitive, rapid chlamydia testing; and (3) likelihood the patient will return for test results. All treatment regimens as noted earlier should include either azithromycin or doxycycline if chlamydial infection is not ruled out.

8. d. This patient has NGU. Urethritis can be associated with dysuria or mucopurulent discharge or can be completely asymptomatic. Patients presenting with urethritis should be investigated thoroughly for other urologic etiology such as cystitis or prostatitis. The patient's normal testicular and prostate examinations make epididymitis and prostatitis less likely.

A diagnosis of urethritis can be made on any of the following signs: (1) mucopurulent or purulent urethral discharge; (2) gram stain of urethral secretions revealing five or more WBCs per oil immersion field; and (3) positive leukocyte-esterase test on first-void urine or microscopic examination revealing 10 or more WBCs per high-power field. Testing for both *N. gonorrhea* and *C. trachomatis* is recommended to confirm the diagnosis. NGU can be diagnosed if a patient has urethritis with no evidence of gonorrhea infection (absence of gram-negative diplococci on urethral gram stain).

9. a. *C. trachomatis* is the most frequent cause of NGU (15% to 55% of cases), although the prevalence varies by age groups. Other organisms that may be associated with NGU include *U. urealyticum* and *M. genitalium*. Less frequent causes of NGU include *Trichomonas vaginalis* and herpes simplex virus. All partners of patients identified with NGU should be referred for evaluation and treatment.

10. b. First-line treatment for uncomplicated urethral *C. trachomatis* infection includes doxycycline 100 mg PO bid for 7 days or azithromycin 1 g PO in a single dose. The advantage of azithromycin is that a single-dose regimen enhances patient compliance. If taken as directed, azithromycin and doxycycline have equal efficacy. Alternative second-line treatments include oral erythromycin ethylsuccinate, levofloxacin, or ofloxacin for 7 days. Female patients with chlamydial cervicitis should undergo the same treatment regimen as for males with NGU.

11. e. The CDC does not recommend routine "tests of cure" in patients who have completed recommended regimens for uncomplicated gonorrhea or chlamydia infections unless symptoms persist or reinfection is suspected. Most post-treatment infections are a result of re-infection and not failed therapy. A test of cure may be considered if patients were treated with alternative regimens such as erythromycin. Tests of cure should be done no less than 3 weeks from the time of treatment, as false positives are more likely. Rescreening patients who are high risk for repeat infections (partner never treated, history of

prior infection) may be prudent and decision to do so should be individualized.

12. e. Gonococcal arthritis-dermatitis syndrome is the most common clinical manifestation of disseminated gonococcal infection (DGI) and consists of tenosynovitis, arthritis, and a pustular or papular rash. Meningitis and endocarditis are rare complications of bacteremic gonococcal infection. Gonococcal infection at other sites in adults includes gonococcal conjunctivitis and gonococcal epididymitis.

13. a. The patient's symptoms are consistent with herpes simplex virus (HSV) type 2 infection. Given her systemic symptoms, it is likely a primary infection. Classic symptoms of genital herpes infection include a prodrome of tingling or itching, followed by eruption of painful vesicular or ulcerative genital lesions. Systemic symptoms such as fever, malaise and inguinal adenopathy may occur. Most recurrent genital herpes cases are caused by HSV-2, although HSV-1 has been identified in genital lesions in up to 30% of first-episode cases. Culture of genital ulcers can confirm diagnosis, although the sensitivity of culture declines as lesions start to heal. False-negative HSV cultures are common, and serologic HSV type-specific antibody tests can be done to confirm diagnosis.

The genital lesions of chancroid caused by *Haemophilus ducreyi* are characterized by painful ulcer and tender inguinal adenopathy. The presence of suppurative inguinal adenopathy is almost pathognomonic for *H. ducreyi* infection. The CDC recommends that diagnosis of chancroid be based on: (1) presence of painful ulcer(s); (2) negative serologic tests for syphilis; and, (3) negative HSV testing of ulcer exudates. Genital lesions caused by primary syphilis and HPV infection are usually painless. Granuloma inguinale is a genital ulcerative infection caused by *Calymmatobacterium granulomatis*. It is characterized by painless, progressive ulcerative genital lesions without regional lymphadenopathy. The disease is extremely rare in the U.S.

14. e. Patients and their partners should be educated about the natural history of HSV with emphasis on the possibility of recurrent episodes and transmission of virus during asymptomatic shedding. Barrier contraceptive methods should be encouraged to prevent transmission. Physicians should inform patients that treatment of the first episode of genital herpes can shorten duration of viral shedding and time for lesion healing. Recommended regimens for first clinical episodes include: (1) acyclovir 400 mg PO tid; (2) acyclovir 200 mg PO five times a day; (3) famciclovir 250 mg PO tid; or; (4) valacyclovir 1gm PO bid. Treatment should continue for 7-10 days. Patients can be treated for recurrent episodes either with continuous suppressive therapy (for >6 episodes a year) or episodically for less frequent occurrences. Episodic treatment initiated within a day of lesion onset can reduce the severity and duration of lesions. Chronic, suppressive therapy can decrease the number of symptomatic outbreaks a year, but subclinical viral shedding is not completely eliminated.

15. b. This patient has condyloma acuminatum, or "genital warts." External genital warts are caused by HPV, most commonly types 6 and 11. These HPV subtypes are considered "low risk" and rarely are associated with cervical neoplasia. HPV types 16, 18, 31, 33, and 45 are considered "high-risk" types associated with cervical cancer precursors. Patients with external condyloma likely are infected with multiple subtypes of HPV and need to be counseled about the importance of routine cervical cancer screening. Patients with condyloma acuminatum should be screened for other STDs. Condyloma lata are painless genital lesions associated with primary syphilis. This patient's genital lesions are not consistent with genital herpes.

16. e. The primary goal of treatment for genital warts is removal of visible and symptomatic warts. There is no known definitive cure for genital warts. The treatment that has been reported to have the highest cure rate is carbon dioxide laser. Cure rates with this form of therapy approach 90%. Current treatments probably do not significantly affect the natural history of HPV infections or prevent the development of cervical carcinoma. Other treatment options include topical therapy, which can be patient applied (podofilox and imiquimod) or provider administered (podophyllin resin in benzoin or trichloroacetic acid). Destructive procedures include cryotherapy, electrodesiccation, and surgical excision for recalcitrant or larger lesions. Immunotherapy with intralesional injection of interferon is reserved as second-line therapy. Acyclovir is treatment for primary or recurrent genital herpes infection, not genital warts.

17. b. The causative agent of syphilis is the spirochete *T. pallidum.* Primary syphilis is characterized by a single, painless genital ulcer that develops an average of 3 weeks after exposure. Secondary syphilis is associated with skin lesions (maculopapular rash that may involve palm and soles), lymphadenopathy, condyloma latum (soft verrucous plaques), and involvement of other organ systems (renal, hepatic, musculoskeletal). Tertiary syphilis involves gummatous syphilis, cardiovascular syphilis, or neurosyphilis. Latent syphilis by definition is serologic evidence of syphilis without any clinical manifestations. Early-latent syphilis is defined as latent syphilis that was acquired within the preceding year. Early-latent syphilis cannot be distinguished reliably from late-latent syphilis by serologic testing alone and often requires documentation of prior seroconversion or a consistent history. The significance of making this distinction is that treatment therapy differs for early-latent versus late-latent syphilis. The treatment for syphilis is IM benzathine penicillin G, not oral penicillin.

18. b. Although dark-field microscopy is the most specific technique for diagnosing syphilis, it is not convenient to perform in the typical office setting. It involves the collection of exudate from an active chancre or condyloma lata and examining it under a microscope with a dark-field condenser. The characteristic shape of *T. pallidum* is a corkscrew appearance. Given the need for an active lesion, the proper equipment, and sufficient experience to interpret specimens, most clinicians turn to serologic tests to confirm the diagnosis. Nontreponemal tests such as VDRL and RPR test for a nonspecific antibody reaction to *T. pallidum.* VDRL and RPR titers cannot be used interchangeably. Quantitative nontreponemal titers should be repeated at 6 and 12 months after treatment for primary and secondary syphilis. Nontreponemal titers are used to monitor response to treatment, with a fourfold reduction in titers indicating treatment response. False-positive nontreponemal tests often can occur in the elderly, pregnant women and in patients with autoimmune disorders. Positive nontreponemal titers should be confirmed with treponemal-specific tests, which detect antibodies specific to *T. pallidum,* such as FTA-ABS or TPHA (*T. pallidum* hemagglutination test). Treponemal-specific tests tend to remain reactive for life, whereas nontreponemal test titers decline after treatment.

19. a. The treatment of choice for primary, secondary, and early-latent syphilis is benzathine penicillin G 2.4 million units IM in a single dose.

For late-latent syphilis and tertiary syphilis the treatment of choice is benzathine penicillin G 7.2 million units total, administered as three doses of 2.4 million units IM at 1-week intervals

For neurosyphilis the treatment of choice is aqueous crystalline penicillin G 18-24 million units per day divided q 4 hours or continuous infusion for 10-14 days or an alternative regimen of probenecid 500 mg PO four times daily (QID) for 10-14 days.

Oral doxycycline (100 mg PO twice daily [bid] for 14 days) is preferred for patients allergic to penicillin.

All patients should be warned of a possible localized "Jarisch-Herxheimer reaction" after treatment for syphilis. It is characterized by an acute febrile illness with headache and myalgia and occurs within the first 24 hours of initiating therapy. This phenomenon should be treated with salicylates (acetaminophen in pregnant women) or, in severe cases, with prednisone.

20. b. HIV testing should be offered to all patients seeking evaluation for STDs and to patients with risk factors. Urine and oral mucosal tests are available but need to be confirmed with more specific serologic testing if positive. In the United States, the HIV-1 strain is responsible for most HIV infections. The HIV-2 strain is endemic to West Africa, and patients from this region or who have sex partners from this region should have testing that will include HIV-2 detection. Standard serum screening tests (enzyme immunoassay [EIA]) detect both HIV-1 and HIV-2 antibodies. Positive EIA tests should be followed with more specific tests (Western blot) to confirm HIV. If testing was done within 3 months of exposure and there is concern about a false-negative result, repeat serologic testing may be performed at least 3 months after the time of exposure. Of patients with HIV, 95% will seroconvert within 3 months of infection. However, there have been rare documented cases of seroconversion 6-12 months after infection.

SOLUTION TO THE CLINICAL CASE MANAGEMENT PROBLEM

Hepatitis B is an STD caused by hepatitis B virus (HBV). Patients with chronic HBV infection are at risk for cirrhosis or hepatocellular carcinoma (15% to 25% chance). An effective vaccination exists for hepatitis B, yet the majority of patients diagnosed with hepatitis B were not offered immunization prior to infection. The CDC's national immunization strategy focuses on (1) preventing perinatal transmission through universal maternal screening and postexposure prophylaxis of at-risk infants (with hepatitis B immune globulin [HBIG]); (2) universal infant immunization; (3) universal immunization of previously unvaccinated children aged 11-12 years; and (4) vaccinations of at-risk adolescents and adults. High risk groups who should receive vaccination include the following: (1) sexually active adolescents and adults; (2) patients with a history of other STDs; (3) IV drug users; (4) household contacts or partners of patients with hepatitis B; (5) health care workers; (6) staff and residents at long-term care facilities and institutions; (7) patients undergoing hemodialysis; (8) recipients of clotting-factor concentrates; (9) persons from HBV endemic areas; and (10) international travelers. Vaccination consists of three doses at 0, 1, and 6 months. If a dose has been missed, there is no need to start the series over. Other preventive measures include counseling on barrier contraceptive use, practicing universal precautions (health care workers), and not sharing toothbrushes/razor blades with infected individuals (or household contacts). In addition, postexposure prophylaxis with HBIG should be administered when appropriate.

SUMMARY OF SEXUALLY TRANSMITTED DISEASES

A. PID:

1. Signs and symptoms supportive of diagnosis are as follows: (a) uterine/adnexal tenderness; (b) cervical motion tenderness; (c) oral temperature >101° F (>38.3° C); (d) abnormal cervical or vaginal mucopurulent discharge; (e) presence of WBCs on wet prep; (f) elevated ESR; (g) elevated CRP; and (h) documentation of cervical infection with *N. gonorrhea* or *C. trachomatis.*
2. Causative agents include *N. gonorrhea, C. trachomatis,* anaerobes, gram-negative bacteria and streptococci.
3. Risk factors for PID include young age, multiple sexual partners, living in high-prevalence areas for gonorrhea or chlamydia, not using barrier contraception, and having a history of prior PID.

4. Treatment of PID involves the following:
   a. Inpatient treatment: (i) IV cefoxitin or IV cefotetan plus doxycycline (PO or IV) or (ii) IV clindamycin and IV gentamicin
   b. Outpatient treatment: (i) PO ofloxacin or PO levofloxacin with or without PO metronidazole; (ii) IM cefoxitin and PO probenecid plus PO doxycycline with or without PO metronidazole; or (iii) IM ceftriaxone plus PO doxycycline with or without PO metronidazole

B. Uncomplicated gonococcal infection:

1. The organism is *N. gonorrhea*
2. Symptoms include dysuria, frequency, and discharge. It may be asymptomatic in women.
3. Treatment includes IM ceftriaxone or PO cefixime plus either PO doxycycline or PO azithromycin IF CHLAMYDIA INFECTION IS NOT RULED OUT.

C. NGU:

1. The organism is *C. trachomatis* or *U. urealyticum.*
2. Symptoms include dysuria, frequency, and mucopurulent or purulent urethral discharge.
3. Diagnosis involves the following: (a) mucopurulent or purulent urethral discharge; (b) gram stain of urethral secretions revealing five or more WBCs per oil immersion field; (c) positive leukocyte-esterase test on first-void urine or microscopic examination revealing 10 or more WBCs per high-power field; and (d) absence of intracellular diplococci on urethral gram stain.
4. Treatment includes PO doxycycline or PO azithromycin.
5. A "test of cure" is not routinely indicated. Rescreening can be performed if reinfection is suspected.

D. Genital herpes:

1. The majority of organisms are herpes simplex virus type 2.
2. Symptoms and signs include a prodrome of tingling, itching, followed by eruption of painful vesicular ulcers in genital area. Primary infection may be associated with systemic symptoms.
3. Laboratory diagnosis includes viral culture and serologic HSV type-specific antibody tests.
4. Treatment includes acyclovir, famciclovir, and valacyclovir.
5. In patient counseling, emphasize risk of recurrence and asymptomatic shedding.
6. Episodic treatment can decrease severity and duration of lesions. Suppressive therapy can decrease frequency of outbreaks.

E. Genital warts:

1. The most common organisms are HPV types 6 and 11.
2. Sign and symptoms include cauliflowerlike lesion in the genital area.
3. External condyloma is not directly associated with cervical dysplasia.
4. Patients with genital warts are at risk for infection with multiple HPV subtypes and need routine cervical cancer screening.
5. Treatment includes the following:
   a. Topical: Podofilox and imiquimod (patient applied) or Podophyllin resin in benzoin or trichloroacetic acid (provider administered).
   b. Surgical: Cryosurgery, surgical excision, electrodesiccation, carbon dioxide laser therapy, and immunotherapy.

F. Syphilis:

1. The organism is *T. pallidum.*
2. Definitions are as follows:
   a. Primary syphilis: single, *painless* genital ulcer
   b. Secondary syphilis: skin lesions, lymphadenopathy, condyloma latum, may be multisystem involvement.
   c. Tertiary syphilis: gummatous syphilis, cardiovascular syphilis, or neurosyphilis
   d. Latent syphilis: serologic evidence of syphilis *without* any clinical manifestations
   e. Early-latent syphilis: latent syphilis that was acquired within the preceding year
3. Laboratory diagnosis involves the following: (a) dark-field microscopic confirmation of *T. pallidum;* (b) nontreponemal tests, such as VDRL and RPR; and (c) treponemal-specific tests, such as FTA-ABS and TPHA.
4. Treatment is IM benzathine penicillin.
5. Retest nontreponemal test titers at 6 and 12 months; should see at least fourfold reduction in titer.
6. Treponemal-specific tests generally remain reactive for life.
7. With Jarisch-Herxheimer reaction, acute febrile illness occurs within 24 hours of treatment.

G. HIV:

1. The organism is the human immunodeficiency virus.
2. EIA serum testing, followed by more specific Western blot test if initially positive, should be done. Urine and oral mucosal testing also is available.
3. HIV-1 strain is responsible for the majority of HIV cases in the United States.
4. The HIV-2 strain is endemic to West Africa.
5. If repeat serologic testing is to be performed, it should occur no sooner than 3 months after exposure.

SUGGESTED READING:

Brown DL, Frank JE: Diagnosis and management of syphilis. *Am Fam Physician* 68:283-280, 297, 2003.
Centers for Disease Control and Prevention. Hepatitis B: a comprehensive strategy for eliminating transmission in the United States through universal childhood vaccination: Recommendations of the Immunization Practices Advisory Committee (ACIP). *MMWR* 40(RR-13):1-19, 1991.
Centers for Disease Control and Prevention. Sexually transmitted diseases treatment guidelines. *MMWR* 51(RR-6):7-61, 2002.
Miller KE, Graves JC: Update on the prevention and treatment of sexually transmitted diseases. *Am Fam Physician* 61:379-386, 2000.

Chapter 61

Infertility

> "Doctor, I'm 39 years old, and I'll just die if I can't have a baby."

CLINICAL CASE PROBLEM 1:
A 27-YEAR-OLD FEMALE COMES TO YOUR OFFICE WITH HER HUSBAND

A 27-year-old nulligravida female comes to your office with her husband. They are concerned about not having conceived after a year of regular, unprotected intercourse.

The patient denies any major medical illnesses, and she takes no medications. The husband reports he is healthy but has never fathered a child. Both the patient and her husband are visibly upset and somewhat tearful while discussing their frustrations about not being pregnant yet. They express that they are anxious to begin "all the tests necessary" as soon as possible so they can have a child without further delay.

■ **SELECT THE BEST ANSWER TO THE FOLLOWING QUESTIONS:**

1. What is the most appropriate diagnosis for this couples' condition?
   a. primary sterility
   b. secondary sterility
   c. primary infertility
   d. secondary infertility
   e. diminished fecundity

2. Infertility is defined as failure to conceive with unprotected regular sexual intercourse after:
   a. 1 month
   b. 3 months
   c. 6 months
   d. 1 year
   e. 2 years

3. What is the most appropriate initial step in this couple's evaluation?
   a. basal body temperature charting
   b. history and physical examination of both partners
   c. semen analysis
   d. referral to a reproductive specialist
   e. urine ovulation predictor kit testing

4. The patient reveals that menarche occurred at age 12. Her periods always have been irregular, with menses occurring every 2-3 months and lasting 5 days with normal flow. Her last menstrual period was 2 months ago. Her sexual history is significant for six total sexual partners, although she has been monogamous with her husband for the last 3 years. She has had no pelvic surgeries, and her Pap test results always have been normal. Physical examination reveals she is normal height for weight. She has normal secondary sexual characteristics, and there are no signs of androgen excess. Physical examination is normal including thyroid, breast, and pelvic examination. Appropriate initial workup in the patient may include all of the following except:
   a. gonorrhea and chlamydia screen
   b. serum thyroid stimulating hormone (TSH)
   c. serum prolactin level
   d. pelvic/transvaginal ultrasound
   e. urine pregnancy test

5. The patient's initial evaluation does not reveal any abnormalities. You discuss with the patient that the next step is to confirm the presence of ovulation. All of the following are acceptable methods for assessing ovulation except:
   a. basal body temperature charting
   b. urine luteinizing hormone (LH) levels
   c. urine follicle stimulating hormone (FSH) levels
   d. midluteal phase progesterone serum levels
   e. cervical mucus changes

6. All of the following may be direct causes of female infertility except:
   a. previous uncomplicated abortion
   b. pelvic inflammatory disease (PID)
   c. endometriosis
   d. polycystic ovarian syndrome (PCOS)
   e. hyperprolactinemia

7. Evaluation for tubal patency or "pelvic factor" is best accomplished by:
   a. transvaginal ultrasound
   b. hysteroscopy
   c. hysterosalpingogram (HSG)
   d. pelvic magnetic resonance imaging (MRI)
   e. pelvic computed tomography (CT) scan

8. The postcoital test is performed to assess which of the following:
   a. interaction of sperm with cervical mucus prior to ovulation
   b. interaction of sperm with cervical mucus after ovulation
   c. interaction of sperm with cervical mucus anytime during the cycle
   d. interaction of sperm with cervical mucus in midluteal phase
   e. none of the above

9. Which of the following statements about the etiology of infertility is true?
   a. male factor is associated with up to 40% of cases
   b. male factor is associated with only 5% of cases
   c. no etiology is found in the majority of cases
   d. ovulatory dysfunction is more common than pelvic etiology
   e. none of the above

10. Which of the following is not considered a cause of male infertility?
    a. varicocele
    b. obstructive azoospermia
    c. hypogonadism
    d. testicular cancer
    e. tight-fitting underwear

11. Appropriate initial screening for male infertility includes which of the following?
    a. two semen analyses done at least 1 month apart
    b. serum testosterone and FSH levels
    c. postejaculatory urinalysis
    d. scrotal ultrasonography
    e. transrectal ultrasonography

12. It is appropriate to initiate an infertility evaluation after 6 months of trying to conceive in which of the following conditions?
    a. the woman is older than 35 years old
    b. the man is older than 40 years old
    c. the woman has used Depo-Provera within the previous year
    d. the woman had used oral contraceptive pills for at least 10 years
    e. the woman has a history of recurrent vaginitis

CLINICAL CASE MANAGEMENT PROBLEM

Discuss and define the various treatments in reproductive technology available for infertile couples.

▸ ANSWERS:

1. **c.** This couple's condition is most consistent with primary infertility. Secondary infertility refers to couples who currently are experiencing infertility but have conceived in the past. Sterility is defined as an intrinsic inability to conceive, whereas infertility implies a decreased ability to conceive. Fecundity is a term used to express the likelihood of pregnancy per month of exposure and is not generally used as a diagnostic term. The average fecundity of a young, healthy couple having frequent intercourse is approximately 20% in a given month.

2. **d.** Infertility is defined as failure to conceive after 1 year of unprotected regular sexual intercourse.

3. **b.** Couples with infertility ideally should be assessed together, if possible. A woman who comes to your office with concerns about infertility should be encouraged to bring her partner for evaluation as well. During a couple's first office visit for infertility, reasonable and realistic goals regarding evaluation and timeline should be discussed. Emotional support should be provided by the physician because couples often experience significant anxiety and frustration when coping with infertility. Referral to infertility resource groups may be appropriate for couples looking for additional support. Couples should be questioned about timing and frequency of sexual intercourse. History of the female partner can be extensive but should focus on the following: (1) general medical health (diet, weight, tobacco use, caffeine use); (2) medications; (3) detailed menstrual history (onset, length, frequency, flow); (4) history of pubertal development; (5) history of in utero diethylstilbestrol (DES) exposure; (6) contraceptive history; (7) history of pelvic surgery; (8) history of sexually transmitted disease (STD) or PID; (9) history of abnormal Pap test results and treatments (i.e., cold knife conization); and (10) prior pregnancies and outcomes. Physical examination of the female should search for secondary sexual characteristics, signs of androgen excess (hirsutism, acne), galactorrhea; and thyroid enlargement. Body mass index also should be noted. Pelvic examination should look for signs of infection, congenital anomalies (e.g., absent vagina or uterus), uterine size, and signs of endometriosis (e.g., nodularities or fixed uterus).

History of the male patient also should include general medical health, history of STDs, health habits, surgical history, and medications. Additional history about the male partner should include (1) history of congenital abnormalities; (2) toxin exposure; (3) prior paternity history; and (4) history of infection (e.g., mumps/prostatitis) or trauma to the genitals. Examination of the male should assess for endocrine stigmata consistent with hypogonadism (e.g., small testes, gynecomastia). Testicular examination should assess size, firmness, masses (e.g., varicoceles, hydroceles) and confirm presence of both testes. Choices a, c, and e are reasonable steps to perform once a history and physical examination of both partners have been completed. The initial evaluation for infertility can be managed by a primary care physician, and direct referral to a specialist should be reserved for women older than 35 years or those at high risk for infertility based on medical history.

4. d. This patient has oligomenorrhea defined as cycles greater than every 35 days. Approach to this patient initially should be the same as for other patients with oligomenorrhea. A urine pregnancy test should be done. If pregnancy is excluded, serum TSH and prolactin levels should be measured to detect thyroid disfunction and/or hyperprolactinemia. An assessment for PCOS should be completed (i.e., LH, FSH, fasting glucose, insulin levels) if indicated by history or physical examination. Patients with evidence of androgen excess may have additional testing such as dehydroepiandrosterone sulfate and free testosterone to rule out virilizing tumor. Given the patient's past sexual history, occult PID should be ruled out with a gonorrhea/chlamydia screen. A pelvic ultrasound should be reserved for patients in which pelvic examination is difficult to interpret (e.g., body habitus) or to evaluate any abnormal pelvic examination findings.

5. b. The presence of ovulation can be confirmed a number of ways. Basal body temperature (BBT) is an inexpensive and simple method but requires careful patient instruction and compliance. Patients record their temperature in the resting state, just before rising in the morning. An increase in body temperature of 0.5-0.8° F (0.3° C) occurs just after ovulation. BBT is not useful in predicting ovulation and can confirm ovulation only in retrospect. BBT is not sensitive in all women because some women will not have a temperature change. BBT measurements can be combined with cervical mucus assessment (also inexpensive) for greater accuracy. At the time of ovulation, cervical mucus becomes thin, clear, and abundant under the influence of estrogen. Right after ovulation, cervical mucus becomes thick and scant under the influence of progesterone.

BBT and cervical mucus assessment can be time consuming and may not be ideal for some women. Another method of confirming ovulation is to measure midluteal phase serum progesterone level, with serum levels of more than 15 ng/ml providing presumptive evidence of ovulation. Commercial over-the-counter ovulation predictor kits can be used to detect LH surge. A "positive test" (usually indicated by a double line) indicates that ovulation will occur in 24-36 hours. Although use of ovulation predictor kits is convenient, cost of repeated testing can limit its utility. Urine FSH levels are not used for predicting ovulation.

6. a. Common causes of female infertility may be classified in the following manner:
1. Ovulatory dysfunction: amenorrhea, oligomenorrhea (secondary to PCOS, hyperprolactinemia etc.)
2. "Pelvic factor": PID, tubal scarring, endometriosis, congenital abnormalities
3 "Cervical factor": history of conization, DES exposure, infection, inhospitable cervical mucus
4. Other: immunologic, systemic disease (e.g., diabetes, neurologic disease).

History of previous uncomplicated abortion has no known direct associated with infertility.

7. c. Evaluation of tubal patency is best accomplished by HSG. During this procedure, radiographic liquid dye is injected into the uterine cavity and multiple x-rays are taken. Spillage of dye into the pelvic cavity confirms tubal patency.

Hysteroscopy involves the use of a light, flexible telescope that is passed through the vagina and into the uterine cavity. Hysteroscopy is useful to visualize anatomic defects such as fibroids and polyps and often is used to complement HSG. However, it cannot directly determine tubal occlusion or patency. Transvaginal ultrasound, pelvic MRI, and pelvic CT scan do not directly assess tubal patency.

8. a. The postcoital test commonly is used to assess what role the "cervical factor" plays in a couple's infertility. The postcoital test determines the quality of interaction between sperm and cervical mucus just prior to ovulation. The couple engages in intercourse at midcycle and then presents to the office 12-24 hours later to evaluate cervical mucus collected from the female partner. The cervical mucus then is examined under a microscope to determine the number of sperm and the quality and extent of motility. A satisfactory test reveals large numbers of forward-moving sperm. The test is inaccurate if performed after ovulation because cervical mucus thickens postovulation and is inherently inhospitable to sperm at this time.

9. a. A male factor is associated with up to 40% of infertility cases. Therefore it is imperative that male factors be assessed early in the evaluation of infertility. Pelvic conditions (such as PID, endometriosis) account for 35% of cases, whereas ovulatory dysfunction and cervical factors account for 10% to 15% of cases. Approximately 10% to 15% cases will have no identified etiology.

10. **e.** Male infertility can result from a variety of conditions. Causes of male infertility may be divided into the following categories:

1. Possibly reversible conditions: varicocele, obstructive azoospermia (complete absence of sperm from ejaculate)
2. Irreversible conditions but in which viable sperm are available: inoperable obstructive azoospermia, ejaculatory dysfunction
3. Irreversible conditions in which there are inadequate or no viable sperm available (i.e., hypogonadism)
4. Serious potentially life-threatening conditions: testicular cancer, pituitary tumor
5. Genetic abnormalities that affect fertility: cystic fibrosis, chromosome abnormalities

Although environmental exposures, such as prolonged heat exposure, may cause male infertility, there is no strong evidence that wearing tight-fitting underwear adversely affects sperm production.

11. **a.** The initial screening of the male should include (1) a comprehensive reproductive history; (2) general physical examination, including the genitalia; and (3) two semen analyses performed at least 1 month apart. Patients should abstain from sexual activity for 2-3 days prior to collection. The specimen should be kept at room or body temperature and examined within an hour of collection. The semen is analyzed for the following parameters: volume, sperm concentration, motility, and morphology. Specific additional procedures should be considered if abnormalities are noted during the initial evaluation. A postejaculatory urine analysis is used to evaluate for presence of retrograde ejaculation. A transrectal ultrasound may assess for ejaculatory duct obstruction. A scrotal ultrasound is performed if examination of the scrotum is limited or to evaluate testicular masses.

12. **a.** An infertility evaluation should be performed earlier than 1 year if (1) female infertility risk factors exist (e.g., including age older than 35 years); (2) male infertility risk factors (e.g., a history of bilateral cryptorchidism) exist; and (3) the couple questions the man's fertility potential. Additionally, men who are concerned about the fertility status and who do not have a current partner should undergo an evaluation.

SOLUTION TO THE CLINICAL CASE MANAGEMENT PROBLEM

Detailed discussion of the full range of reproductive technology options and indications are beyond the scope of this chapter. A brief summary of the most common treatments are noted as follows:

1. **Ovulation induction with clomiphene citrate:** For patients with anovulation, clomiphene citrate therapy is usually a standard first-line approach for ovulation induction. Clomiphene citrate acts by binding to estrogen receptors in the hypothalamus, resulting in decreased perception of endogenous estrogen by the hypothalamus. In response, the hypothalamus increases secretion of gonadotropin-releasing hormone, facilitating FSH release and ovarian follicular development.
2. **Human menopausal gonadotropins:** Injection of gonadotropins can be used in sequential combination with clomiphene for those women who do not generate or sustain adequate FSH in response to clomiphene alone.
3. **In vitro fertilization (IVF):** This technique involves retrieval of eggs via ultrasound-guided transvaginal aspiration. The eggs then are fertilized with sperm under laboratory conditions, and the fertilized egg then is placed in the uterus. To increase the success of IVF, "superovulation" is attempted with ovulation-induction agents to allow for retrieval of multiple eggs.
4. **Intrauterine insemination (IUI):** IUI is less invasive than IVF because it does not involve retrieval of eggs. In IUI, washed sperm are deposited directly in the uterus, bypassing cervical mucus and placing the sperm at closer proximity to the fallopian tubes. Patients with history of tubal damage are not good candidates for IUI.
5. **Gamete intrafallopian transfer (GIFT):** As in IVF, sperm and egg are retrieved from the couple. GIFT differs from IVF in that fertilization takes place *in vivo*, not *in vitro*. Egg and sperm then are transferred into the fallopian tubes in the hopes that natural fertilization will take place.
6. **Intracytoplasmic sperm injection (ICSI):** A new technique that directly addresses male infertility factors, ICSI involves the direct injection of a single sperm into a collected egg. If successful fertilization takes place, the fertilized egg is implanted into the female patient.

SUMMARY OF INFERTILITY

1. **Definitions:**
   a. Infertility: failure to conceive after 1 year of regular, unprotected intercourse
   b. Primary infertility: refers to couples who have never conceived
   c. Secondary infertility: refers to couples who may have conceived in the past
   d. Fecundity: likelihood of pregnancy in a given cycle

2. **Evaluation—female partner:**
   a. History and physical examination
   b. Evaluation of ovulatory status: basal body temperature, cervical mucus changes, ovulation predictor kits, midluteal phase progesterone
   c. Complete workup of amenorrhea or oligomenorrhea if necessary: TSH, prolactin, evaluation for PCOS if indicated
   d. Evaluation of "cervical factor": postcoital test
   e. Evaluation of "pelvic factor" or tubal patency: HSG

3. **Evaluation—male partner:**
   a. History and physical examination
   b. Semen analysis twice, 1 month apart
   c. Referral for further testing if abnormal semen analysis or abnormal physical examination findings

4. **Causes of infertility—female:**
   a. Pelvic factor: PID, tubal scarring, endometriosis, congenital abnormalities
   b. Ovulatory dysfunction: PCOS, hyperprolactinemia, hypothyroidism
   c. Cervical factor: history of conization, DES exposure, infection
   d. Other: immunologic, systemic disease

5. **Causes of infertility—male:**
   a. Possibly reversible: varicocele, obstructive azoospermia
   b. Irreversible conditions, possibly with viable sperm: inoperable obstructive azoospermia, ejaculatory dysfunction
   c. Irreversible conditions, no viable sperm: hypogonadism
   d. Testicular cancer, pituitary tumor
   e. Genetic abnormalities: cystic fibrosis, chromosome abnormalities

6. **Indications for referral:**
   a. Women older than age 35 years
   b. Identified infertility risk factor in male or female
   c. Abnormal semen analysis in men

SUGGESTED READING

Adamson D, et al: A model for initial care of the infertile couple. *J Reprod Med* 46(4):409-417, 2001.

Cahill DJ, Wardle PG: Management of infertility. *BMJ* 325:28-32, 2002.

Kolettis PN: Evaluation of the subfertile male. *Am Fam Physician* 67:2165-2173, 2003.

Sharlip ID, et al: Best practice policies for male infertility. *Fertil Steril* 77:873-882, 2002.

Whitman-Elia GF, Baxley EG: A primary care approach to the infertile couple. *J Am Board Fam Pract* 14(1):33-45, 2001.

MATERNITY CARE

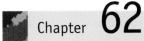 Chapter **62**

Family-Centered Maternity Care

"Doctor, will you help me make this a family affair?"

CLINICAL CASE PROBLEM 1:
A 26-YEAR-OLD PRIMIGRAVIDA WHO WISHES TO DISCUSS A BIRTH PLAN

A 26-year-old woman comes to your office at 14 weeks of gestation for her initial prenatal visit. You have been referred to her by friends who are your patients. She would like you to assume her prenatal care and deliver her child. Her uterus feels 14 weeks by size, and her blood pressure is 100/70 mm Hg. All other aspects of the initial complete physical examination are normal.

■ **SELECT THE BEST ANSWER TO THE FOLLOWING QUESTIONS:**

1. The patient asks you about birth plans during her initial visit and inquires as to your attitudes toward pregnant couples who wish to participate in decision making regarding the conduct of labor and delivery. How would you respond?
   a. birth plans are not a good idea; usually something goes wrong and the couple is disappointed
   b. birth plans are not a good idea; they frequently lead to unresolved guilt in the couple
   c. birth plans should be avoided; perinatal morbidity and mortality usually is increased
   d. birth plans are an excellent idea; everything always goes according to plan
   e. birth plans are a good idea; they involve the couple in the planning for their baby's delivery and can be a very important part of the prenatal, postnatal, and postpartum care

2. On the next prenatal visit, the couple wishes to discuss your feelings concerning a number of issues. The first issue is electronic fetal monitoring (EFM) The couple is aware that, in some hospitals and with some physicians, continuous EFM during labor is standard procedure. Which of the

following statements regarding continuous routine EFM is true?
   a. the perinatal mortality rate in laboring patients who undergo continuous EFM is lower than in those who do not
   b. the perinatal morbidity rate in laboring patients who undergo EFM is lower than in those who do not
   c. the incidence of cesarean section in laboring patients undergoing EFM is not statistically different from those who do not
   d. there is no significant difference in perinatal outcomes between those patients who undergo EFM and those who do not
   e. the incidence of admission to the intensive care nursery is greater in those babies who do not undergo EFM

3. The couple then asks you about routinely ordering ultrasound in pregnancy. Which of the following statements regarding the use of routine ultrasound in pregnancy is false?
   a. routine prenatal ultrasound has been shown by U.S. studies to be justified from a cost–benefit standpoint
   b. repetitive studies by independent researchers have not found any consistently adverse effects of obstetric ultrasound on perinatal outcome
   c. first-trimester ultrasound gestational age assessment should be performed on patients scheduled for elective repeat cesarean section
   d. vaginal bleeding in pregnancy should be assessed by ultrasound examination
   e. a size–date discrepancy in fundal height of 3 cm or more is an indication for obstetric ultrasound

4. The couple inquires about the routine administration of intravenous (IV) fluids during labor. Concerning this issue, which of the following statements is false?
   a. the use of routine IV fluids does not limit ambulation in the first stage of labor
   b. if epidural analgesia is to be administered, an IV line must be in place
   c. if the first stage of labor is prolonged, an IV line should be in place to prevent dehydration

d. if a patient has a history of a severe post-partum hemorrhage, an IV line should be established

e. none of the above statements are false

5. When you mention the words "epidural analgesia," the couple becomes quite agitated. They state quite emphatically that they do not wish, under any circumstances, to have an epidural anesthetic. What should your response to this request be?
   a. "you really have to leave it up to me to decide that"
   b. "epidural analgesia is one of many non-compulsory methods to relieve labor pain"
   c. "you better track down another doctor"
   d. "epidurals have no complications; you should really reconsider your position"
   e. none of the above

6. Which of the following statements regarding epidural analgesia is (are) true?
   a. maternal hypertension is a common side effect of epidural analgesia
   b. high spinal anesthesia is one of the most serious complications of epidural analgesia
   c. unintentional dural puncture occurs in 10% of attempted epidural analgesia
   d. prolongation of all stages of labor by epidural analgesia has been established
   e. fetal bradycardia is seen consistently with epidural analgesia

7. The couple has registered for Lamaze classes. Lamaze can best be described as which of the following?
   a. a method emphasizing the psychoprophylaxis of labor
   b. a method describing how to keep away from physicians at all costs
   c. a method concentrating on the difficulties physicians cause in obstetrics
   d. a method emphasizing the importance of "toughing things out"
   e. all of the above

8. The couple's final question concerns "routine episiotomy." They have been told that the medical profession is "cut happy" and that the vast majority of episiotomies are unnecessary. Which of the following statements regarding routine episiotomy is true?
   a. episiotomy pain may be more severe and last longer than the pain from perineal lacerations
   b. episiotomy repairs heal more rapidly than do vaginal and perineal tears

c. dyspareunia is more common after vaginal lacerations and perineal tear than after episiotomy
   d. episiotomy reduces the rate of subsequent pelvic relaxation problems
   e. episiotomy reduces the rate of third- and fourth-degree perineal lacerations

9. Which of the following is (are) an indication for the performance of an episiotomy?
   a. nonreassuring fetal heart rate in the second stage of labor
   b. significant maternal cardiac disease
   c. operative delivery using obstetric forceps
   d. delivery of the fetus with shoulder dystocia
   e. all of the above

10. Which of the following statements regarding the presence or absence of a supportive person (or coach) in labor is (are) true?
    a. the presence of a support person or coach decreases the need for analgesia in labor
    b. the presence of a support person or coach decreases the need for operative interventions such as forceps or vacuum extraction
    c. the presence of a support person or coach decreases the cesarean delivery rate
    d. all of the above are true
    e. none of the above are true

CLINICAL CASE MANAGEMENT PROBLEM

A 28-year-old primigravida presents at 16 weeks of gestation for her first prenatal visit. She is accompanied by her husband. As you begin to discuss your routine with respect to prenatal care, the couple presents you with a "list of demands." These demands include the right to decide whether an IV will be inserted, when the fetal heart can be auscultated, when the physician can "interfere" with the natural birth process, and how the infant is to be resuscitated. Describe how you would deal with this situation.

▶ ANSWERS:

1. **e.** Birth plans are an integral component of what has become known as family-centered maternity care. Family-centered maternity care allows pregnant couples the opportunity of going through labor and delivery in an informal setting, preferably with minimal medical intervention. Family-centered maternity care involves the husband or significant other as a coach in labor and allows for immediate bonding of infant to both parents.

Breastfeeding is encouraged, and rooming-in is available. A trusting doctor–patient relationship is essential to family-centered maternity care. If the couple is confident in their doctor, they feel secure that any intervention that is considered obviously will be discussed with them. If the couple is involved in the decision-making process throughout labor and delivery, any unresolved guilt related to the birth process will be avoided.

2. d. Well-controlled studies have shown that intermittent auscultation of the fetal heart rate is equivalent to EFM in assessing fetal condition when performed at specific intervals with a 1:1 nurse-to-patient ratio. EFM is associated with a small but significant increase in the incidence of cesarean delivery because of presumed "fetal distress." Perinatal outcomes as assessed by intrapartum stillbirths, low Apgar scores, need for assisted ventilation of the newborn, admission to neonatal intensive care unit, and the onset of neonatal seizures are similar with both intermittent auscultation and EFM.

3. a. Although obstetric ultrasound studies are performed routinely in many countries, the routine use of ultrasonography has not been supported from a cost–benefit standpoint. However, a 1984 consensus development conference convened by the National Institute of Child Health and Human Development proposed 27 indications for ultrasonography in pregnancy. These indications include estimation of gestational age for patients scheduled for elective cesarean delivery, identification of the cause of vaginal bleeding in pregnancy, and evaluation of significant uterine size–clinical dates discrepancy. Ultrasound exposure at intensities usually produced by diagnostic ultrasound instruments has not been found to cause any harmful biologic effects on fetuses. Infants exposed in utero have shown no significant differences in birthweight or length, childhood growth, cognitive function, acoustic or visual ability, or rates of neurologic deficits. The use of diagnostic obstetric ultrasound on an as-needed basis is supported by the American College of Obstetricians and Gynecologists.

4. a. An IV line can limit ambulation in the first stage of labor. Although it is customary in many hospitals to start IV infusions early in labor, there is seldom any real need to do so in women with uncomplicated pregnancies at least until analgesia is administered. IV hydration is indicated for the following reasons: (1) for prehydration when epidural analgesia is about to be administered; (2) to prevent dehydration and acidosis in the presence of a prolonged first stage of labor; and (3) to administer oxytocin prophylactically to prevent postpartum hemorrhage.

5. b. Epidural analgesia should be viewed as an option and only as an option. It is highly effective at significantly reducing or completely eliminating pain in the second stage of labor. There is some evidence that severe pain in labor may cause maternal vasoconstriction and subsequent decreased oxygen flow to the fetus; however, this has not been established. As with any invasive procedure, use of epidural analgesia may be associated with severe but rare complications.

6. b. One of the most serious immediate complications of epidural analgesia is a high or total spinal anesthesia. Signs and symptoms include numbness and weakness of upper extremities, dyspnea, inability to speak, and finally apnea and loss of consciousness. Maternal hypotension, not hypertension, is common and can be minimized by prophylactic intravascular volume expansion with 500-1000 ml of non–glucose-containing isotonic crystalloid solution. Unintentional dural puncture, resulting in a spinal headache, occurs in less than 2% of cases. Randomized controlled trials have shown conflicting results regarding the effect of epidurals on progress of labor. Fetal bradycardia occasionally may be seen with epidural analgesia, but it is usually easily treated by IV fluid administration and conservative management.

7. a. Patients who use the Lamaze technique have been schooled in the psychoprophylaxis of labor. Some people regard Lamaze as "anti-physician," "anti-all-intervention," and "anti-everything else." This is somewhat unfair. The Lamaze technique, if properly used, can help a select group of patients achieve the goals they have identified for their labor and delivery experience.

8. a. Episiotomy pain may be more severe and long-lasting than the pain of vaginal and perineal lacerations. Healing time for vaginal and perineal lacerations is generally shorter than the healing time for an episiotomy. Dyspareunia is more common after episiotomy than after vaginal and perineal tears, resulting in a prolongation of time before return to normal sexual activity.

Routine episiotomy neither increases nor decreases the incidence of subsequent pelvic relaxation. All randomized prospective studies have shown the rate of third- and fourth-degree perineal lacerations are increased rather than reduced by routine episiotomy.

9. e. Indications for episiotomy include nonreassuring fetal heart rate findings in the second stage of labor, significant maternal cardiac disease, prophylactic forceps, shoulder dystocia, and infants in the breech presentation when vaginal delivery is anticipated.

Contraindications to episiotomy include presence of inflammatory bowel disease, lymphogranuloma venereum, or severe perineal scarring or malformation. Complications of episiotomy include excessive blood loss and increased rates of lacerations into the anal sphincter and anal mucosa and infections.

Episiotomy rates can be reduced by following these indications and contraindications and by not performing an episiotomy routinely. Vaginal and perineal tears may be avoided by perineal massage and stretching exercises before delivery. Communication with the patient during perineal stretching will help reduce the degree and number of tears during childbirth. Also, controlling professional urgency for rapid delivery provides extra time for the fetal head to stretch the perineum, resulting in an increased possibility for an intact perineum.

Episiotomy does shorten the second stage of labor, but that in and of itself is not a reason for its performance.

10. **a.** The presence of a support person or coach decreases the need for subsequent analgesia in labor. This does not, however, apply to subsequent operative interventions including forceps delivery, vacuum extraction, or cesarean section.

SOLUTION TO THE CLINICAL CASE MANAGEMENT PROBLEM

This particular scenario, which is not uncommon, can be described in one way only: bad news. It is reasonable to attempt to talk to this couple in an effort to try and discover why they feel the way they do about the medical profession. Have they had a bad experience? Do they have any trust in you, to whom they have come seeking prenatal care? These issues in this case can be summarized as follows:

■ Is the couple prepared to accept your decisions regarding when medical intervention is necessary provided you consult and explain your position to them?
■ Is the couple prepared to allow you, as the physician, to perform your duly responsible medical functions in this case?
■ Is the couple willing to trust you, providing that you earn their trust?

If the answers to all three questions eventually can be negotiated to yes, it would be appropriate to proceed with the care of this patient's pregnancy. If, however, the answer to one or more of the questions is no, the best and safest course of action would be to inform the patient and her husband that in all good conscience you cannot look after their pregnancy. You, as a physician, have that ethical right except in the event of an emergency. In many cases it would be better for all concerned if the physician were to suggest that another care provider be sought. You must, however, continue to look after the patient until the time that a care provider is identified. The patient should be sent a registered letter to that effect.

SUMMARY OF FAMILY-CENTERED MATERNITY CARE

1. **Birth plans:** If prudently developed and open to negotiation and change, they may be of benefit in a couple's pregnancy. They have the potential to foster good doctor–patient communication.
2. Continuous EFM is no more effective than intermittent auscultation in reducing perinatal morbidity and mortality in low-risk pregnancies.
3. Current recommendations are that obstetric ultrasound should be used only for specific indications, although no adverse perinatal outcomes have been demonstrated in repetitive studies.
4. **Intravenous therapy:** Specific indications include long labor with ketones, use of epidural analgesia, and history of severe postpartum hemorrhage; it is not routinely needed in low-risk pregnancies.
5. **Anesthesia:** An epidural is the analgesic of choice and should be available should women choose it. Prepared childbirth classes may enhance the number of women seeking unmedicated childbirth.
6. **Episiotomy:** An episiotomy does not heal more quickly than a perineal tear, is more painful, has greater incidence of dyspareunia, increases the risk of third-degree and fourth-degree lacerations, and does not change the incidence of later pelvic relaxation. Although it does shorten the second stage of labor, that shortening in and of itself offers no definitive benefit to either mother or baby.

SUGGESTED READING

Banta DH, Thacker SB: Historical controversy in health technology assessment: the case of electronic fetal monitoring. *Obstet Gynecol Surv* 56(11):707-719, 2001.

Campbell DC: Parenteral opioids for labor analgesia. *Clin Obstet Gynecol* 46(3):616-622, 2003.

Hadar A, et al: Abnormal fetal heart rate tracing patterns during the first stage of labor: effect on perinatal outcome. *Am J Obstet Gynecol* 185(4):863-868, 2001.

Harman CR, Baschat AA: Comprehensive assessment of fetal wellbeing: which Doppler tests should be performed? *Curr Opin Obstet Gynecol* 15(2):147-157, 2003.

Segal S: Epidural analgesia and the progress and outcome of labor and delivery. *Int Anesthesiol Clin* 40(4):13-26, 2002.

Thallon A, Shennan A: Epidural and spinal analgesia and labour. *Curr Opin Obstet Gynecol* 13(6):583-587, 2001.

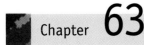

Chapter 63

Common Problems of Pregnancy

"Read my lips, Doctor. I'm never going to let this happen again."

CLINICAL CASE PROBLEM 1:

A 23-Year-Old Primigravida with Many Physical Complaints

A 23-year-old primigravida comes to your office for her second prenatal visit. You first saw her 4 weeks ago at 7 weeks of gestation. At that time you performed a complete history, a complete physical examination, and all necessary blood work. Today you note she has gained 3 lb in the last 4 weeks. She has been nauseated every day, with one episode of emesis a day. On examination, her blood pressure is 110/70 mm Hg and her general and pelvic examinations are unremarkable.

■ **SELECT THE BEST ANSWER TO THE FOLLOWING QUESTIONS:**

1. Nausea and/or vomiting in pregnancy affect approximately 80% of women at some time during pregnancy. Current theory suggests that these symptoms are the result of increased levels of which of the following hormones?
   a. estrogen
   b. progesterone
   c. human chorionic gonadotropin (hCG)
   d. human placental lactogen
   e. androstenedione

2. Which of the following should not be part of your initial advice or treatment for this patient?
   a. reassurance that this is a self-limiting condition
   b. eating small, frequent meals
   c. discontinuation of oral iron therapy
   d. avoiding contact with cooking odors
   e. prescription of an antinausea medication

3. What is the drug of choice for severe hyperemesis gravidarum in pregnancy?
   a. prochlorperazine
   b. promethazine
   c. chlorpromazine
   d. metoclopramide
   e. ondansetron

CLINICAL CASE PROBLEM 2:

A 29-Year-Old Multigravida with an Unrelenting Backache

A 29-year-old multigravida (gravida 5, para 4) comes to your office at 36 weeks of gestation with the following complaint: "For the last 10 days I've had the worst backache in my life. I've put heat on it, I've put cold on it, and I've tried rest. Nothing helps, Doctor."

On examination, the patient has no costovertebral angle (CVA) tenderness. There is moderate paralumbar tenderness. She has had no urinary tract symptoms that would suggest urinary tract infection (UTI). Flexion, extension, lateral rotation, and lateral bending all enhance the pain. She tells you that she does not recall any injury. However, the onset of the backache appeared to correspond with the baby dropping into her pelvis. She has not had any problems with her back in other pregnancies.

The patient describes the pain as dull, constant, and centered in the L2-L5 area, with no radiation to either the right leg or the left leg. It is aggravated by walking, moving, and bending. It is relieved somewhat by rest.

4. Which of the following is (are) the most likely reason(s) for her back pain?
   a. motion of the symphysis pubis
   b. motion of the lumbosacral joints
   c. general relaxation of the pelvic ligaments
   d. any of the above
   e. b or c

5. What is (are) the management(s) of choice for this patient's condition?
   a. nonpharmacologic therapy: massage, physiotherapy
   b. acetaminophen
   c. acetaminophen and codeine
   d. any of the above
   e. a and/or b only

CLINICAL CASE PROBLEM 3:

A PREGNANT 37-YEAR-OLD PROFESSIONAL WOMAN WITH VARICOSE VEINS

A 37-year-old woman (gravida 2, para 1) comes to your office at 16 weeks of gestation with severe vulvar and lower-extremity varicosities. They are bilateral and extend from her feet to her thighs. The varicosities began approximately 4 weeks ago and have been increasing gradually in severity. She is a physician and works full-time in her practice. The varicosities are unsightly and cause severe pain, especially as the day goes on. The worst varicosities are her vulvar varicosities.

6. What would you recommend at this time for the patient in Clinical Case Problem 3?
   a. discontinue work duties until after pregnancy
   b. inject sclerosing agents into the most severe veins
   c. elevate her legs and wear support hose
   d. a and c
   e. all of the above

7. Which is the most common complication of varicosities in pregnancy?
   a. deep venous thrombosis
   b. pulmonary embolism
   c. superficial thrombophlebitis
   d. ovarian vein thrombosis
   e. septic pelvic thrombophlebitis

CLINICAL CASE PROBLEM 4:

A 25-YEAR-OLD PRIMIGRAVIDA WITH SEVERE RECTAL PAIN

A 25-year-old primigravida at 36 weeks of gestation comes to your office with severe rectal discomfort of 3 weeks duration. On examination, you notice several hemorrhoids that are 1 cm in diameter.

8. Which of the following statements about hemorrhoids in pregnancy is false?
   a. hemorrhoids are varicosities of the rectal veins
   b. constipation in pregnancy aggravates the formation of hemorrhoids
   c. obstruction of venous return by the enlarged uterus worsens hemorrhoids
   d. bleeding from rectal veins may result in folate-deficiency anemia
   e. thrombosis of a rectal vein can cause significant pain

CLINICAL CASE PROBLEM 5:

A 28-YEAR-OLD MULTIGRAVIDA WITH GASTROESOPHAGEAL REFLUX DISEASE

A 28-year-old multigravida comes to your office at 30 weeks of gestation with heartburn. The symptoms are severe enough that the patient is in pain for the majority of the day.

On examination, the abdomen is soft. The patient's blood pressure is 110/70 mm Hg. There is no evidence of other conditions that may have precipitated this.

9. Which of the following statements regarding heartburn in pregnancy is false?
   a. relaxation of the lower esophageal sphincter allows reflux of stomach contents into the esophagus
   b. upward displacement and compression of the stomach by the uterus worsen symptoms
   c. usually symptoms are mild and can be relieved by small, frequent meals
   d. aluminum and magnesium hydroxide are first-line antacid choices
   e. sodium bicarbonate is an antacid that is free of side effects

10. Bizarre cravings develop during pregnancy, sometimes to the point that foods or substances considered hardly edible or nonedible are consumed in great quantities. This condition is known as and is associated with which of the following?
    a. pica associated with macrocytic anemia
    b. pica associated with iron-deficiency anemia
    c. amylophagia associated with iron-deficiency anemia
    d. geophagia associated with macrocytic anemia
    e. pica associated with none of the above

CLINICAL CASE PROBLEM 6:

A PREGNANT WOMAN WITH SWOLLEN LEGS

A patient at 32 weeks of gestation with increased swelling in both lower extremities comes to your office. The previous week she went to another physician with bilateral lower-extremity swelling from the knees down. She was prescribed both a thiazide diuretic and a loop diuretic. Now she has come to see you.

11. What should you do at this time?
    a. tell her to continue taking the thiazide diuretic but stop taking the loop diuretic
    b. tell her to continue taking the thiazide diuretic and the loop diuretic and add a potassium-sparing diuretic
    c. tell her to continue the thiazide diuretic and the loop diuretic, and add an extended release potassium capsule
    d. tell her to stop taking both the thiazide diuretic and the loop diuretic
    e. tell her to wait a few minutes, warm up the big office computer, and try to obtain the information from a data bank

CLINICAL CASE PROBLEM 7:

A 29-Year-Old Primigravida with a Copious Vaginal Discharge

A 29-year-old primigravida comes to your office complaining of increased vaginal discharge. She is 33 weeks pregnant.

On speculum examination, you confirm a copious clear vaginal discharge. There is no significant odor, a wet prep is normal, and culture results are negative. No pooling of fluid is seen in the posterior fornix.

12. Which of the following statements regarding increased vaginal discharge during pregnancy is (are) true?
    a. in most cases, the discharge is physiologic
    b. physiologic discharge arises from estrogen-mediated increased cervical mucus
    c. monilia may be identified in up to 25% of pregnant women
    d. monilia should be treated in both symptomatic women and asymptomatic women
    e. a, b, and c are true

CLINICAL CASE PROBLEM 8:

A Constipated 29-Year-Old Multigravida

A 29-year-old multigravida at 22 weeks of gestation comes to your office with a chief complaint of constipation. She states that she is having only one bowel movement every 5 or so days.

13. With regard to this complaint, which of the following statements is (are) true?
    a. constipation is uncommon in pregnancy
    b. constipation is more common in early pregnancy than in late pregnancy
    c. constipation does not need to be treated in pregnancy
    d. all of the above are true
    e. none of the above are true

14. Which of the following has (have) been implicated in the pathogenesis of constipation in pregnancy?
    a. reduced gut motility
    b. mechanical obstruction by the uterus
    c. increased water resorption
    d. increased estrogen levels
    e. a, b, and c

15. The treatment(s) of choice for constipation in pregnancy include which of the following?
    a. discontinuing iron supplements
    b. increasing the amount of fiber in her diet
    c. increasing her physical activity
    d. adding a bulk-forming agent
    e. all of the above

ANSWERS:

1. c. Nausea and vomiting in pregnancy are common complaints, especially during the first trimester. Nausea, vomiting, or other gastrointestinal symptoms may occur in up to 80% of pregnant women. The hormonal basis for the nausea and vomiting of pregnancy is not entirely clear. Severe hyperemesis is much more frequent with molar pregnancies with high levels of hCG. Empiric data supporting this include the finding that as the level of hCG declines at the end of the first trimester, the nausea and vomiting usually subside.

2. e. Nausea in pregnancy should be treated with conservative management whenever possible. Medications should be prescribed only if conservative approaches fail. Small, frequent meals; the avoidance of a high-fat foods; an intake of dry foods; and reassurance may be all that is necessary. If iron therapy has been started, it should be discontinued. Avoidance of contact with situations that may induce nausea (such as cooking odors) also is recommended.

If persistent vomiting leads to weight loss, ketonuria, or electrolyte imbalance, hospitalization and total parenteral nutrition is necessary. With persistent severe symptoms, it is imperative a workup be undertaken to rule out other serious conditions such as molar pregnancy, hyperthyroidism, pancreatitis, cholecystitis, appendicitis, hepatitis, and peptic ulcer disease.

3. d. If conservative therapy fails, antinauseant medications are indicated. Drugs that are considered safe in the treatment of nausea in pregnancy are pyridoxine, meclizine, diphenhydramine, and metoclopramide. In severe hyperemesis gravidarum, metoclopramide, a category B drug, may be used, which increases gastrointestinal motility. The category C drugs include promethazine, prochlorperazine, and chlorpromazine. These drugs are used in moderately severe hyperemesis gravidarum.

Categories B and C refer to the risk of using the drug in pregnancy. With drugs that are either category B or category C, the benefit often may outweigh the risk (see Chapter 64, Answer 3 for more details).

If treatment with prochlorperazine or promethazine is unsuccessful, other antiemetics, such as trimethobenzamide (Tigan) or ondansetron (Zofran) may be tried. Ondansetron is a serotonin antagonist used primarily in treating chemotherapy-induced nausea.

4. **d.** Backache occurs to some extent in most pregnant women in minor degrees following excessive strain or fatigue and excessive bending, lifting, or walking. A mild backache usually requires little more than elimination of the strain. In some pregnant women, as in this patient, motion of the symphysis pubis and lumbosacral joints, as well as general relaxation of pelvic ligaments, may be demonstrated. The most important disease to rule out is UTI (especially ascending).

5. **e.** Treatment of this condition involves education regarding back pain in pregnancy, rest for as much of the remaining pregnancy as possible, massage and physiotherapy, and acetaminophen. Codeine should be avoided; it has habituation potential when used chronically and can aggravate constipation.

6. **d.** Varicosities, generally resulting from congenital predisposition, are exaggerated by prolonged standing and advanced maternal age in pregnancy. They arise in up to 40% of pregnant women. Femoral venous pressure increases by twofold to threefold in pregnancy. The symptoms produced by varicosities vary from cosmetic blemishes on the lower extremities and mild pain to quite severe pain, tenderness, discomfort, and prominence. The suggested treatment is daily, frequent periods of rest and elevation of the lower extremities.

7. **c.** The most common complication of superficial varicosities is superficial thrombophlebitis. This should be treated with cold packs and rest. Superficial thrombophlebitis is not related to deep venous thrombosis, ovarian vein thrombosis, septic pelvic thrombophlebitis, or pulmonary embolism.

8. **d.** Hemorrhoids are varicosities of the rectal veins that most often are related to increased pressure on the rectal veins caused by obstruction of venous return by the large uterus and by the tendency to be constipated in pregnancy.

Pain and swelling usually can be relieved by topically applied anesthetics, warm soaks, and agents that soften the stool. Thrombosis of a rectal vein can cause considerable pain, and when this happens (usually related to an external rectal vein), the clot should be evacuated. Bleeding from the rectal veins occasionally can result in the loss of sufficient blood to cause an iron-deficiency (not folate-deficiency) anemia. The loss of only 15 ml of blood results in the loss of 6-7 mg of iron, an amount that is equal to the daily requirements during later pregnancy.

9. **e.** Heartburn, an extremely common complaint in pregnancy, is caused by the reflux of gastric contents into the lower esophagus. The increased frequency of regurgitation during pregnancy most likely results from the upward displacement and compression of the stomach by the uterus combined with decreased gastrointestinal motility. In most pregnant women the symptoms are mild and are relieved by a regimen of small, frequent meals and avoidance of bending over.

Antacid preparations may provide considerable relief, and most are completely safe. Aluminum hydroxide, magnesium hydroxide, and magnesium trisilicate, alone or in combination, should be used in preference to sodium bicarbonate. The pregnant woman who tends to retain sodium can become edematous as the result of ingestion of excessive amounts of sodium bicarbonate. Calcium carbonate also is not recommended because its use during pregnancy has been associated with hypocalcemia in the neonate.

10. **b.** Occasionally during pregnancy bizarre cravings for strange foods develop. This is called pica. These cravings may be for materials hardly considered edible. Some of those substances have included laundry starch, baking powder, baking soda, clay, baked dirt, powered bricks, and frost scraped from the refrigerator.

The desire for dry lump starch, chopped ice, or even refrigerator frost has been considered by some to be triggered by severe iron deficiency. Although women with severe iron deficiency sometimes crave these items, and although craving usually is ameliorated after correction of the iron deficiency, not all pregnant women with pica are iron deficient.

Ingestion of starch (amylophagia) or clay (geophagia) or related items is practiced more often by socioeconomically less-privileged pregnant women.

11. **d.** Lower-extremity edema, a common complication of late pregnancy, occurs because the pelvic veins and inferior vena cava are occluded as a result of the pressure from the enlarging uterus. Treatment consists of avoiding prolonged standing, elevating the lower extremities, and wearing support hose. Thiazide diuretics reduce intravascular volume as do loop diuretics. Both classes are contraindicated in pregnancy. In this patient, you should do the following: (1) discontinue the thiazide; (2) discontinue the loop diuretic; (3) suggest elevation of extremities for

1 hour three times a day; and (4) suggest that she stay off her feet as much as possible.

Warming up the big computer is never a bad idea. This would be a good second choice.

12. **e.** The most common vaginal discharge in pregnancy is a physiologic discharge. The discharge is caused by increased formation of mucus by the cervical glands under the influence of estrogen. However, it is important to rule out ruptured membranes and leaking amniotic fluid. This is accomplished by performing a speculum examination looking for pooling of fluid in the posterior fornix and identifying whether the fluid present turns Nitrazine paper blue and if ferning is seen on microscopic examination when the fluid is allowed to air dry on a glass slide.

Monilia may be identified in the vagina in up to 25% of women in late pregnancy. If the patient is symptomatic, she should be treated. If she is not symptomatic, treatment is not needed. The drugs of choice for the treatment of symptomatic monilia in pregnancy are either clotrimazole or miconazole.

13. **e.**

14. **e.** The cause of constipation in pregnancy is multifactorial. Potential causes include hormonally mediated smooth-muscle relaxation and mechanical pressure from the enlarging uterus.

15. **e.** Increasing the intake of fluids, increasing the intake of fiber, and increasing the amount of exercise (especially walking) should be encouraged. If these measures are not effective, then a bulk-forming agent such as psyllium or methylcellulose may be added. Laxatives should be used with caution because of the habituation potential.

SOLUTION TO THE CLINICAL CASE MANAGEMENT PROBLEM

Three additional common complaints of pregnancy are as follows:
1. Ptyalism is profuse salivation as a result of stimulation of the salivary glands on ingestion of starch. For treatment, the cause should be looked for and eradicated if possible.
2. In early pregnancy, most pregnant women complain of fatigue and desire excessive periods of sleep.
3. Headache is a frequent complaint in early pregnancy.

In the vast majority of cases, no cause can be demonstrated. A few cases may result from sinusitis or ocular strain caused by refractive errors. Pregnancy-induced hypertension is a potential cause in later pregnancy; at this stage any woman who presents with a headache should be assessed for preeclampsia. Treatment is largely symptomatic; by midpregnancy most of these headaches decrease in severity or disappear.

SUMMARY OF COMMON PROBLEMS IN PREGNANCY

A. Nausea and vomiting:
1. **Pathophysiology:** increased levels of circulating hCG
2. **Treatments:** reassurance; small, frequent meals and dry food; discontinuation of iron therapy (if patient is taking supplemental iron); anti-nauseants if moderately severe (Promethazine, Chlorpromazine, Prochlorperazine); if severe, metoclopramide

B. Constipation:
1. **Pathophysiology:** reduced gastrointestinal motility, mechanical obstruction of the uterus, increased water resorption

2. **Treatments:** discontinuation of iron therapy (if patient is taking iron); increasing amount of fiber in the diet; increasing the amount of total fluid intake; increasing the amount of physical activity

C. Back pain:
1. **Pathophysiology:** motion of the symphysis pubis and lumbosacral ligaments, relaxation of the pelvic ligaments and the round ligament of the uterus
2. **Treatment:** if symptomatic, heat, ice, acetaminophen, avoidance of activities that aggravate the problem

D. Hemorrhoids:
1. **Pathophysiology:** increased pressure in the rectal vein system secondary to increased intravascular volume.

Continued

SUMMARY OF COMMON PROBLEMS IN PREGNANCY—cont'd

2. **Treatments:** recumbent position; witch hazel pads (or TUCKS); hemorrhoidal cream and hydrocortisone cream, excision of external thrombosed hemorrhoid.

E. Varicosities:
1. **Pathophysiology:** congenital predisposition in weakness of vein valves, increased pressure secondary to increased intravascular volume
2. **Treatment:** rest, elevation, compression stockings
3. **Complication:** superficial thrombophlebitis most common

F. Heartburn:
1. **Pathophysiology:** displacement of uterus upward, exerting pressure on the diaphragm; and decreased pressure in lower esophageal sphincter
2. **Treatment:** antacids: magnesium hydroxide and aluminum hydroxide

G. Lower-extremity edema:
1. **Pathophysiology:** increased intravascular volume (increased by 50%), gravity
2. **Treatment:** avoid diuretics, which will further reduce the intravascular volume; rest; recumbency

H. Increased vaginal discharge:
1. **Pathophysiology:** almost always normal; results from increased hormone levels, especially estrogen
2. **Treatment:** rule out ruptured membranes and vaginitis or cervicitis; reassurance

SUGGESTED READING

Eliakim R, et al: Hyperemesis gravidarum: a current review. *Am J Perinatol* 17(4):207-218, 2000.

Jewell D: Nausea and vomiting in early pregnancy. *Am Fam Physician* 68(1):143-144, 2003.

Quinla JD, Hill DA: Nausea and vomiting of pregnancy. *Am Fam Physician* 68(1):121-128, 2003.

Chapter 64

Immunization and Consumption of Over-the-Counter Drugs During Pregnancy

"Dangers in route."

CLINICAL CASE PROBLEM 1:
A WORRIED MOTHER-TO-BE

A 22-year-old woman comes to your office asking for prenatal care. She estimates that she is about 10 weeks postconception, and her primary concern is that she will come down with an infectious disease that will harm the baby. This fear was precipitated by the fact that her sister "caught the German measles and lost her baby." In addition, she feels guilty because she has not had any immunizations for a long time. You attempt to allay her fears.

■ SELECT THE BEST ANSWER TO THE FOLLOWING QUESTIONS:

1. Which of the following immunization combinations would be acceptable for administration to a pregnant woman?
   a. tetanus and diphtheria toxoids (Td) and varicella
   b. hepatitis B and meningococcal
   c. varicella and rubella
   d. meningococcal and varicella
   e. rubella and hepatitis B

2. Which of the following statements is true about influenza in pregnancy?
   a. the immunization should not be given to high-risk patients (those with asthma, cardiovascular disease, diabetes) within the first trimester
   b. the vaccine should be administered to all pregnant women who will be in the second or third trimester of pregnancy during the influenza season
   c. pregnant women have the same severity risk level of influenza as nonpregnant women
   d. immunization of pregnant women for influenza is not safe
   e. none of the above are true

CLINICAL CASE PROBLEM 2:
A PREGNANT WOMAN CONCERNED ABOUT CONSUMING IBUPROFEN

A newly pregnant woman who comes into the office is very concerned about the fact that she took ibuprofen for a headache during the past week. She is asking whether it is safe to take in pregnancy.

3. Which of the following statements about ibuprofen in pregnancy is true?
   a. ibuprofen is considered safe during all stages of pregnancy
   b. ibuprofen is considered relatively safe during the first and second trimester but should be avoided if possible in the third trimester
   c. ibuprofen should never be taken in pregnancy; the patient should be counseled to consult a geneticist
   d. ibuprofen can be taken in the third trimester but should be avoided if at all possible in the first trimester
   e. ibuprofen can be taken in the first trimester but should be avoided if at all possible in the second trimester

4. Your patient who is newly pregnant comes in with a list of medications that she has been using during her pregnancy thus far. Which medication, several of which may be problematic, do you tell her to stop immediately?
   a. Retin A gel
   b. ibuprofen
   c. TUMS (calcium carbonate)
   d. Prozac
   e. Tylenol

CLINICAL CASE PROBLEM 3:

A PATIENT WITH PROLONGED CONSISTENT VOMITING

Your patient is vomiting on a regular basis during her 7th to 9th week of pregnancy. She comes in having lost more than 5% of her body weight in the last 2 weeks. You diagnose her with hyperemesis gravidarum.

5. Common causes of hyperemesis gravidarum include all the below *except*:
   a. gestational trophoblastic disease
   b. multiple gestation
   c. hydrops fetalis
   d. trisomy 21 (down syndrome)
   e. gestational diabetes

6. All of the following measures may be used to improve mild nausea and vomiting of early pregnancy *except*:
   a. small, frequent meals
   b. avoidance of strong smells
   c. acupressure on the Neiguan point (three finger breadths above the wrist on the volar surface).
   d. ginger
   e. nizatidine (Axid)

7. Which of the following over-the-counter (OTC) medications is not safe to take in pregnancy?
   a. kaolin and pectin (Kaopectate)
   b. bismuth subsalicylate (Pepto-Bismol)
   c. loperamide (Imodium)
   d. atropine/diphenoxylate (Lomotil)
   e. all the above are safe to take

8. Category X medications during the first trimester include:
   a. nicotine
   b. angiotensin-converting enzyme (ACE) inhibitors
   c. selective serotonin reuptake inhibitors (SSRIs)
   d. metformin (Glucophage)
   e. isotretinoin

CLINICAL CASE MANAGEMENT PROBLEM

A 20-year-old primigravida accompanied by her husband comes to your office for her first prenatal visit. As you begin to discuss routine prenatal care, the subject of alcohol consumption arises. The couple is in the habit of sharing a bottle of wine with dinner and would like to continue this routine; they find it helps them unwind after a busy day. What is your response?

ANSWERS:

1. **b.** Varicella and rubella vaccines contain live attenuated virus. Such vaccine is contraindicated in pregnancy because the effects on the fetus are unknown. Varicella and rubella immunity status should have been ascertained on a prepregnancy counseling visit and administered at least 1 and ideally 3 months prior to a woman attempting a pregnancy; however, in this case there was no pre-pregnancy care. Nonetheless, immunity can be tested during pregnancy, and there is a good chance that the patient would have been previously exposed, permitting you to inform her that she has no worry with respect to these diseases. If a susceptible pregnant woman is exposed to varicella or rubella, administration of immune globulin should be strongly considered.

In contrast to live virus, administration of inactivated virus during pregnancy is considered to be safe. Tetanus and diphtheria toxoids are recommended routinely for susceptible pregnant women. Waiting until the second trimester of pregnancy to administer Td is considered a reasonable precaution. Hepatitis B contains noninfectious hepatitis B surface antigen particles and should cause no risk to the fetus. Meningococcal vaccine contains purified polysaccharide of four serogroups of *Neisseria meningitidis*. Routine vaccination is recommended for high-risk groups, including military recruits; patients with terminal complement component deficiencies; people with anatomic or functional asplenia; and college freshmen, particularly those living in dormitories.

2. b. Influenza vaccine is a killed virus preparation and is therefore usually safe to administer. It should be administered annually between October and December to all pregnant women who will be in the second or third trimester of pregnancy during the influenza season. High-risk groups, such as women with asthma, diabetes, and cardiovascular disease, should be given the vaccine regardless of their trimester. Pregnant women in their second and third trimester of pregnancy during influenza season have higher morbidity, similar to other high-risk patients.

3. b. Ibuprofen, ketoprofen, and naproxen are associated with oligohydramnios, premature closure of the fetal ductus arteriosus with subsequent persistent pulmonary hypertension of the newborn, fetal nephrotoxicity, and periventricular hemorrhage if taken during the third trimester of pregnancy (Category D). These nonsteroid antiinflammatory drugs (NSAIDs) are considered relatively safe in the first and second trimester (Category B).

The following table outlines the U.S. Food and Drug Administration rating system:

Category	Interpretation
A	CONTROLLED STUDIES SHOW NO RISK. Adequate, well-controlled studies in pregnant women have failed to demonstrate a risk to the fetus in any trimester of pregnancy.
B	NO EVIDENCE OF RISK IN HUMANS. Adequate, well-controlled studies in pregnant women have not shown increased risk of fetal abnormalities despite adverse findings in animals, or, in the absence of adequate human studies, animal studies show no fetal risk. The chance of fetal harm is remote but remains a possibility.
C	RISK CANNOT BE RULED OUT. Adequate, well-controlled human studies are lacking, and animal studies have shown a risk to the fetus or are lacking as well. There is a chance of fetal harm if the drug is administered during pregnancy, but the potential benefits may outweigh the potential risks.
D	POSITIVE EVIDENCE OF RISK. Studies in humans, or investigational or postmarketing data, have demonstrated fetal risk. Nevertheless, potential benefits from the use of the drug may outweigh the potential risk. For example, the drug may be acceptable if needed in a life-threatening situation or serious disease for which safer drugs cannot be used or are ineffective.
X	CONTRAINDICATED IN PREGNANCY. Studies in animals or humans, or investigational or postmarketing reports, have demonstrated positive evidence of fetal abnormalities or risks that clearly outweigh any possible benefit to the patient.

4. a. Retinoids are considered Category C; the rest of the medications listed are Category B in the first trimester of pregnancy.

5. d. Hyperemesis gravidarum effects one in 200 pregnant women. Clinical features include persistent vomiting, dehydration, electrolyte disturbances, ketosis, and loss of more than 5% of body weight. All of the listed answers except fetal trisomy 21 have been associated with an increased incidence of hyperemesis gravidarum.

6. e. Nizatidine is a Category C medication that should be reserved for patients with symptoms that do not improve from the other measures.

7. b. Bismuth subsalicylate can result in the absorption of salicylate and should be avoided, especially in the third trimester. Salicylates have been associated with increased perinatal mortality, neonatal hemorrhage, decreased birthweight, prolonged gestation and labor, and possible birth defects. Bismuth subsalicylate is considered Category C in the first and second trimester and Category D in the third trimester (positive evidence of human fetal risk but the benefits from use in pregnant women may be acceptable despite the risk). Kaolin and pectin (Kaopectate) and loperamide (Imodium) are considered Category B (animal reproductive studies show no fetal risk but there are no controlled studies in pregnant women). Atropine/diphenoxylate (Lomotil) is Category C (studies in animals show adverse effects on the fetus and there are no controlled studies in women, or studies in women and animals are not available).

8. e. Of the listed medications, Accutane is the only medication considered Category X within the first trimester. SSRIs are either Category B or C throughout pregnancy. Glucophage and ACE inhibitors have increasing teratogenic potential as the pregnancy progresses and should be discontinued as soon as

possible in pregnancy. Of those drugs listed only isotretinoin (Accutane) is teratogenic in all three trimesters of pregnancy.

SOLUTION TO THE CLINICAL CASE MANAGEMENT PROBLEM

You should provide the couple with the information that will permit them to make an informed decision on their own. Point out that consumption of five or more drinks per day may lead to fetal alcohol syndrome, marked by cardiac abnormalities, low birthweight, short cracks on the eyelids (palpebral fissures), an abnormally small

midface region (midface hypoplasia), and the likelihood of mental retardation. Less severe effects are associated with consumption of smaller amounts, but nobody knows what the threshold level is. Thus you would recommend that alcohol consumption be completely curtailed throughout the whole period of pregnancy.

SUMMARY OF IMMUNIZATION AND CONSUMPTION OF OVER-THE-COUNTER DRUGS DURING PREGNANCY

1. Ideally vaccination status should be determined prior to attempting pregnancy and brought up to date at least 1 month prior to possible pregnancy.
2. If a patient has not been immunized prior to pregnancy, immunization with killed virus can be done. However, live, attenuated vaccines should not be used. Thus immunization against varicella and rubella is not recommended.
3. Patients should be counseled about the potential dangers of OTC and prescription drugs. The effects on the fetus of many common OTC drugs are unknown, and a reasonable plan is to use as

few medications as possible during pregnancy, particularly the first trimester.
4. The FDA categorizes pharmaceuticals and OTC drugs according to potential or known hazards. The categories, A, B, C, D, and X are listed and defined in Answer 3.

SUGGESTED READING

Black R, Hill D: Over-the-counter medications in pregnancy. *Am Fam Physician* 67:2517-2524, 2003.
Della-Giustina K: Medications in pregnancy and lactation. Emerg Med Clin North Am 21(3):585-613, 2003.
Quinlan J, Hill D: Nausea and vomiting of pregnancy. *Am Fam Physician* 68:121-128, 2003.
Sur D, et al: Vaccinations in pregnancy. *Am Fam Physician* 68(2):299-304, 2003.

Chapter 65

Routine Prenatal Care

"Shouldn't you see me more often, doctor?"

CLINICAL CASE PROBLEM 1:

A 24-YEAR-OLD PRIMIGRAVIDA AT 8 WEEKS OF GESTATION

A 24-year-old primigravida comes to your office at 8 weeks of gestation for her first prenatal visit. She has asked you to be her family doctor and to look after her during the entire pregnancy. You agree to provide her pregnancy care. During your first visit you

explain your general philosophy regarding prenatal care and perinatal care.

■ SELECT THE BEST ANSWER TO THE FOLLOWING QUESTIONS:

1. The Department of Health and Human Services Expert Panel on Prenatal Care (DHHSEPPC) has recommended which of the following regarding routine prenatal care?
   a. that the number of routine office visits be significantly reduced for women at low risk
   b. that focus should be on the total health and well-being of the family including medical, psychological, social, and environmental barriers affecting health

c. that provision of systematic health care start long before pregnancy because it was proved to be beneficial to the physical and emotional well-being of the prospective mother and child
d. all of the above are true
e. b and c only are true

2. The DHHSEPPC has recommended that office visits be limited to visits for specific purposes during the first how many months of pregnancy?
a. 2 months
b. 3 months
c. 4 months
d. 5 months
e. 6 months

3. A 26-year-old primigravida conceived on September 9, 2003. According to Nägele's rule, what is the patient's estimated date of delivery (assume a 28-day cycle)?
a. June 2, 2004
b. June 16, 2004
c. July 2, 2004
d. July 9, 2004
e. June 23, 2004

4. The American College of Obstetricians and Gynecologists (ACOG) has recommended intervals for routine and indicated tests in the prenatal period. Which of the intervals shown below is (are) recommended?
a. initial visit: as early as possible
b. obstetric ultrasound: 18 weeks of gestation
c. screening for gestational diabetes: 26 to 28 weeks of gestation
d. hepatitis B virus screen: as early as possible (first visit)
e. all of the above

5. What is the recommended entire weight gain recommended by the National Academy of Sciences for a pregnant woman who is 65 inches tall with a prepregnancy weight of 225 pounds?
a. 5 to 15 pounds
b. 10 to 20 pounds
c. 15 to 25 pounds
d. 25 to 35 pounds
e. 28 to 40 pounds

6. The number of calories recommended for women in pregnancy is approximately how many greater than for nonpregnant women?
a. 200
b. 300

c. 500
d. 750
e. 900

7. Which of the following statements would be regarded as reasonable nutritional advice standards in pregnancy?
a. supplementation with 30-60 mg of iron daily after the first 4 months
b. supplementation with folic acid 1 mg daily throughout pregnancy
c. a regular diet with salt added to taste
d. seek weight gain based on prepregnancy weight
e. all of the above

8. Which of the following statements regarding smoking in pregnancy is (are) true?
a. the risk of spontaneous abortion is increased significantly
b. perinatal mortality rates are increased significantly
c. abruptio placenta rates are increased significantly
d. birthweights are decreased significantly
e. all of the above are true

9. Which of the following statements regarding alcohol consumption in pregnancy and fetal alcohol syndrome is (are) true?
a. limit alcohol intake to one or two glasses of wine
b. abstain completely from alcohol during pregnancy
c. fetal alcohol syndrome is decreasing in the United States
d. a and c
e. b and c

10. Which of the following Caldwell-Moloy pelvic shape classifications is (are) both the most common and the most functional for delivery?
a. gynecoid pelvis
b. android pelvis
c. anthropoid pelvis
d. platypelloid pelvis
e. a and c are equally common and equally functional

11. Which of the following clinical examination measurements is the most critical in determining the ability of the fetus to pass through the pelvis in labor?
a. obstetric conjugate
b. diagonal conjugate

c. pelvic inlet
d. midpelvis
e. pelvic outlet

12. When is the fetal head said to be engaged?
    a. when the frontal diameter has passed through the pelvic inlet
    b. when the occipital diameter has passed through the pelvic inlet
    c. when the biparietal diameter has passed through the pelvic inlet
    d. when the biparietal diameter has passed through the midpelvis
    e. when the occipital diameter has passed through the midpelvis

13. The stage and phases of labor describe the various parts of the parturition process. Which of the following describes when effacement of the cervix primarily occurs?
    a. Stage 1, latent phase
    b. Stage 1, active phase
    c. Stage 2
    d. Stage 3

14. The active phase in a nullipara, according to the graphic labor curve of Friedman, should produce cervical dilatation of how many centimeters per hour?
    a. 0.5
    b. 1.0
    c. 1.2
    d. 1.5
    e. 2.0

15. The third stage of labor begins when the baby is delivered. What is the most frequent mistake made by physicians in this phase?
    a. allowing the third stage to progress at a very slow pace
    b. allowing the third stage to progress on its own
    c. attempting to pull or tug at the umbilical cord
    d. attempting to stop the "gush of blood" that normally accompanies the third stage of labor
    e. massaging the uterus and injecting oxytocin into the uterus

16. Which of the following statements regarding amniotomy is true?
    a. amniotomy does not change the length of labor
    b. amniotomy decreases the cesarean delivery rate
    c. amniotomy improves newborn Apgar scores
    d. amniotomy may result in prolapse of the umbilical cord
    e. none of the above

17. Which of the following has (have) been demonstrated to be of benefit in decreasing the risk of postpartum hemorrhage following the delivery of the placenta?
    a. massage of the fundus of the uterus
    b. injection of intravenous (IV) or intramuscular (IM) oxytocin
    c. injection of IV or IM ergonovine maleate
    d. traction on the umbilical cord
    e. a, and b or c
    f. all of the above

18. What are the average durations of the first stage of labor in a nullipara and the first stage of labor in a multipara?
    a. 10 hours (nullipara), 7 hours (multipara)
    b. 8 hours (nullipara), 5 hours (multipara)
    c. 12 hours (nullipara), 6 hours (multipara)
    d. 14 hours (nullipara), 8 hours (multipara)
    e. 9 hours (nullipara), 6 hours (multipara)

19. What are the average durations of the second stage of labor in a nullipara and the second stage of labor in a multipara?
    a. 1 hour 40 minutes (nullipara), 55 minutes (multipara)
    b. 1 hour 20 minutes (nullipara), 45 minutes (multipara)
    c. 50 minutes (nullipara), 20 minutes (multipara)
    d. 40 minutes (nullipara), 10 minutes (multipara)
    e. 1 hour 30 minutes (nullipara), 1 hour (multipara)

20. Which of the following options is (are) correct regarding intrapartum antibiotic prophylaxis of group B beta streptococcus (GBBS) sepsis?
    a. antibiotics are not effective in decreasing GBBS sepsis
    b. antibiotics are administered only to women with risk factors
    c. antibiotics are administered only to women with positive late pregnancy GBBS vaginal cultures
    d. antibiotics can completely prevent GBBS sepsis
    e. b and c

◢ CLINICAL CASE MANAGEMENT PROBLEM

Matching Problem:

Part A lists 10 drugs that may be useful in pregnancy. Part B lists 10 indications for treatment with those drugs. Match the numbered drug with the proper lettered condition in each case.

Continued

CLINICAL CASE MANAGEMENT PROBLEM —cont'd

Part A

1. Aspirin; 2. Zidovudine; 3. Ergonovine; 4. Aldomet; 5. Magnesium sulfate; 6. Hydralazine; 7. Penicillin; 8. Ritodrine; 9. Hydrochlorothiazide; 10. Captopril

Part B

A. Severe hypertension in pregnancy; **B**. Prophylaxis against group B streptococcus; **C**. Drug of choice: preeclampsia and eclampsia; **D**. Useful in reducing the risk of preeclampsia; **E**. Postpartum agent to enhance uterine contractions; **F**. Can prevent human immunodeficiency virus (HIV) infection in the infant of an infected mother; **G**. Teratogenic drug; **H**. No possible use in normal pregnancy; **I**. Treatment of choice in chronic hypertension; **J**. Treatment for preterm labor.

ANSWERS:

1. d. See Answer 2.

2. e. The DHHSEPPC has suggested that women at low risk can reduce the number of prenatal visits significantly. The recommendation is that office visits be limited to those necessary for indicated procedures and intervals for the first 6 months of pregnancy. This is based on the results of randomized controlled trials that found there is no difference in demonstrated quality-of-care outcomes between low-risk women who had regular "monthly" office visits and women who had prenatal visits at the time of recommended intervals for indicated tests and procedures.

Detailed recommendations also have been made regarding preconception care beginning within a year of a planned pregnancy. There should be an emphasis on prenatal care that provides an opportunity to focus on the total health and well-being of the family, including medical, psychologic, social, and environmental barriers affecting health. Systematic health care beginning long before pregnancy proves beneficial to the prospective mother and infant (e.g., folate supplementation).

The American Academy of Family Physicians suggests that the pregnant patient not only see her physician at the first indication that she is pregnant but also visit for preconception counseling during the year before she plans to get pregnant to ensure the healthiest possible outcome. Exercise, a healthy diet, and other healthy lifestyles should be encouraged many months before attempting to conceive.

3. a. Nägele's rule identifies the estimated date of delivery for women that have a 28-day menstrual cycle. The mean duration of pregnancy calculated from the first day of the last normal menstrual period (LNMP) for a large number of healthy women has been identified as to be very close to 280 days, or 40 weeks. Nägele's rule estimates the expected date of delivery by adding 7 days to the date of the first day of the LNMP and counting back 3 months. If a woman's menstrual periods are 35 days apart, add 14 days rather than 7 days. If her periods are 21 days apart, add 0 days rather than 7 days.

4. e. On the first prenatal visit, the following investigations should be performed: hemoglobin and hematocrit, urinalysis, blood group, Rh type, antibody screen, rubella antibody titer, syphilis screen, culture for gonorrhea, hepatitis B virus screen, and cervical cytology. Human immunodeficiency virus (HIV) testing should be offered for all pregnant women; Purified protein derivative (PPD) screening should be offered for women at risk of tuberculosis.

Obstetric ultrasound may be performed for dating of the pregnancy (accurate dating) at 18 weeks of gestation. Also at that time a maternal serum alpha-fetoprotein (screening for neural tube defects) or triple marker screen (screening for both neural tube defects and trisomy 18/trisomy 21) should be offered.

At 26-28 weeks of gestation the patient should have the following procedures performed: consideration for routine screen for diabetes mellitus, repeat hemoglobin or hematocrit, and repeat antibody test for unsensitized Rh-negative patients. At that time also, prophylactic administration of Rho(d) immunoglobulin can be administered to patients who are Rh negative.

At 32 to 36 weeks of gestation, testing for sexually transmitted diseases and repeat hemoglobin or hematocrit may be performed, if indicated.

Amniocentesis should be offered to high-risk women in the second trimester.

5. c. The average total pregnancy weight gain for normal healthy women eating without restrictions is 27.5 pounds (12.5 kg). However, the National Academy of Sciences summarized the published studies on weight gain during pregnancy and found that the amount of ideal weight gain varied inversely with the prepregnancy weight of the woman. Their pregnancy weight gain recommendations, based on percentage of ideal body weight (IBW), are as follows: underweight women (<90% of IBW) should gain 28 to 40 pounds (12.5 to 18 kg); normal weight women (90% to 135% of IBW) should gain 25 to 35 pounds (11.5 to 16 kg); and overweight women (>135% of IBW) should gain 15 to 25 pounds (7 to 11.5 kg). Of the recommended weight gain, approximately 9 kg comprise the normal physiologic events and features of pregnancy. These include the fetus, placenta, amniotic fluid, uterine hypertrophy, increase in maternal blood volume, breast enlargement, and dependent maternal edema as the consequence of mechanical factors. The remaining 1 to 3 kg is mostly fat.

Pregnant women should be encouraged to gain an adequate amount of weight. However, wide ranges of maternal weight gains are compatible with good clinical outcomes.

6. b. The recommended National Research Council Recommended Daily Dietary Allowances for women before, during pregnancy, and during lactation are outlined in the table.

	Nonpregnant	Pregnant	Lactating
Kilocalories	2200	2500	2600
Protein (g)	55	60	65

7. e. In general, the pregnant woman should eat what she wants to eat in amounts she desires and with salt added to taste. Care should be taken to make sure there is enough food to eat, especially in the case of the socioeconomically deprived woman.

As stated before, the pregnant woman's ideal pregnancy weight gain will be determined by her prepregnancy weight.

Periodically explore the food intake by dietary recall to uncover the ingestion of any bizarre foods. In this way, the occasional nutritionally absurd diet (pica) will be discovered.

Give tablets of simple iron salts to pregnant women that provide between 30 and 60 mg of iron per day. Supplement the pregnant patient's diet with 1 mg of folic acid per day.

Recheck the hematocrit or hemoglobin concentration at 26 to 28 weeks of gestation to detect any significant decrease.

8. e. Pregnancy outcomes are adversely affected by maternal cigarette smoking: spontaneous abortion rates are doubled; perinatal mortality rates are significantly increased; abruptio placenta is almost twice as common in smokers; and mean birthweights of infants of smokers are almost 200 g less than babies of nonsmokers. This decrease in birthweight is a combined result of preterm deliveries and growth restriction of term babies. It is estimated that 4600 infants die annually in the United States because of maternal smoking. Other conditions linked with maternal smoking include placenta previa, premature rupture of the membranes, chorioamnionitis, placental calcifications, and placental hypoxia.

The pathophysiology of maternal smoking includes (1) carbon monoxide and its functional inactivation of fetal and maternal hemoglobin; (2) vasoconstrictor action of nicotine, causing reduced placental perfusion; (3) reduced appetite and, in turn, reduced caloric intake; and (4) decreased maternal plasma volume.

9. b. The safest policy for maternal alcohol use is no use. No safe level of alcohol intake in pregnancy has been identified. Even a few drinks at a critical time in organogenesis can be teratogenic. The incidence of fetal alcohol syndrome in the United States is increasing, not decreasing. Fetal alcohol syndrome is the most common preventable cause of mental retardation.

10. a. The Caldwell-Moloy classification of four pelvis types is an attempt to predict how much difficulty there is going to be in the actual delivery of the infant. The type that is both most common and most suited for delivery is the gynecoid pelvis.

The android pelvis has convergent sidewalls, ischial spines that are prominent, and a subpubic arch that is narrow.

The anthropoid pelvis is a pelvis in which the ischial spines are narrow. This type of pelvis is much more common in African American women; the android pelvis is more common in white women.

The platypelloid pelvis has a flattened gynecoid shape. It is rare; only 3% of women have this type of pelvis.

11. b. The diagonal conjugate is the most important overall pelvic dimension. It is the distance from the sacral promontory to the lower margin of the symphysis pubis. It is the measurement that directly determines the dimensions of the pelvic inlet. The obstetric conjugate is determined by subtracting 1.5 to 2.0 cm from the diagonal conjugate. If the diagonal conjugate is greater than 11.5 cm, it is reasonable to assume that the pelvic inlet is of adequate size.

12. c. The fetal head is said to be engaged when the biparietal diameter of the fetal head has passed through the pelvic inlet. Although engagement of the fetal head usually is regarded as a phenomenon of labor, in nulliparas it commonly occurs during the last few weeks of pregnancy.

13. a. The stages and phases of labor can be described as follows:

Stage 1, latent phase: It has its onset with the onset of regular uterine contractions. It ends with acceleration of the cervical dilatation slope (usually at 3 cm or more dilatation). The purpose of the latent phase is for coordination of contractions and for cervical softening and effacement. It normally lasts less than 14 hours in a multipara or less than 20 hours in a primipara.

Stage 1, active phase: It has its onset with acceleration of the cervical dilatation slope. It ends with complete cervical dilatation at 10 cm. The purpose is threefold: active dilatation of the cervix, beginning the descent of the presenting fetal part, and beginning of the cardinal movements of labor. It normally lasts less than 4 hours in a multipara or less than 5 hours in a primipara.

Stage 2: It has its onset with complete cervical dilatation. It ends with delivery of the neonate. The purpose is to complete the descent of the presenting fetal part through the pelvis and completion of the cardinal movements of labor. It normally lasts less than 30 minutes in a multipara or less than 60 minutes in a primipara.

Stage 3: It has its onset with delivery of the neonate. It ends with delivery of the placenta. The purpose is to shear off the anchoring villi and to deliver the placenta. It normally lasts less than 30 minutes.

14. c. The graphic labor curve of Friedman is a visual representation of cervical dilatation versus time. In a primigravida the average dilatation during the first stage of labor is 1.2 cm/hour; in multiparas the average cervical dilatation is 1.5 cm/hour.

15. c. The most frequent mistake that is made in the third stage of labor is putting undue and unnecessary tension on the umbilical cord. This can cause premature separation of the placenta from the uterus and breaking or tearing of the umbilical cord. Rarely it may cause an inversion of the uterus, a life-threatening problem that is associated with severe postpartum hemorrhage.

16. d. Amniotomy describes the artificial rupture of the membranes either to induce or augment labor contractions. Other common indications for amniotomy include placement of internal electronic fetal monitoring devices when external devices do not produce a satisfactory tracing and placement of intrauterine pressure catheters for assessment of uterine contraction quality when labor progress in inadequate. The data from multiple studies show that the mean length of labor may be shortened by hours but the cesarean rates and perinatal outcomes are unchanged. Before performing amniotomy it is important to ensure that the fetal head is well applied to the cervix. Otherwise prolapse of the umbilical cord may occur, jeopardizing fetal oxygenation and requiring an emergency cesarean delivery.

17. e. The third stage of labor is best managed by massaging the uterine fundus as soon as the placenta is delivered. An IV or IM injection of either oxytocin or ergonovine maleate will contract the uterus. Traction on the umbilical cord will not speed up the contraction of the uterus, which is the primary mechanism for separating the placenta from its implantation site.

18. b. The average durations are 8 hours (nullipara) and 5 hours (multipara).

19. c. The average durations are 50 minutes (nullipara) and 20 minutes (multipara).

20. c. GBBS is a part of normal human bacterial flora with reservoirs of colonization in otherwise healthy individuals. Vaginal colonization can be as high as 35%. GBBS sepsis attacks two infants per 1000 births with a 50% mortality rate. The highest risk is found in GBBS carriers with preterm delivery, rupture of membranes greater than 12 hours, onset of labor or rupture of membranes at less than 37 weeks of gestation, or intrapartum fever. With so serious an impact on newborns, prophylactic antibiotics, often using ampicillin, have been used successfully to decrease the GBBS attack rate. Concerns have been raised, however, that widespread intrapartum prophylaxis will lead to emergence of resistant pathogens. In 1996 the Centers for Disease Control and Prevention (CDC) issued the following recommendations for the active prevention of GBBS: that antibiotic prophylaxis should be used with penicillin, that prophylaxis should be provided based on either positive late prenatal culture or a strategy based solely on clinical risk factors, and that all women with a previous GBBS-infected infant be prophylactically treated. In 2002, updated recommendations were issued by the CDC. Differences from the previous recommendations are as follows: recommendation of universal prenatal screening for vaginal and rectal GBS colonization of all pregnant women at 35-37 weeks of gestation and that prophylaxis be based on results; recommendation against routine intrapartum antibiotic prophylaxis for women who are GBS colonized and undergoing planned cesarean deliveries who have not begun labor or had rupture of membranes; a suggested algorithm for management of patients with threatened preterm delivery; and an updated algorithm for management of newborns exposed to intrapartum antibiotic prophylaxis. In short, it is hoped that this culture-based strategy will cut down on antibiotic resistance.

SOLUTION TO THE CLINICAL CASE MANAGEMENT PROBLEM

1. D   2. F   3. E   4. I   5. C   6. A   7. B   8. J   9. H   10. G

SUMMARY OF ROUTINE PRENATAL CARE

1. Routine checkups in pregnancy in low-risk patients are not indicated nearly as frequently as commonly practiced, especially in the first trimester.
2. The following are recommended as initial screening (as soon as possible after diagnosis): (a) complete blood count (CBC); (b) blood group and atypical antibody screen; (c) Rh status; (d) rubella antibody status; (e) syphilis and gonococcus screen; (f) HIV testing, (g) PPD for TB (consider); (h) hepatitis B surface antigen virus screen; and (i) urinalysis.
3. The following are recommended as initial 18-week screening: (a) obstetric ultrasound screening for fetal anomaly; (b) maternal serum alpha-fetoprotein; and (c) triple marker screen.
4. The following are recommended as initial 28-week screening:
   a. Gestational diabetes screening: 1-hour, 50-g glucose tolerance test; if results are ≥140 mg%, perform a 3-hour, 100-g glucose tolerance test
   b. Repeat atypical screen for women who are Rh negative, and administer Rh immunoglobulin, if indicated
   c. Repeat CBC
5. A GBBS vaginal culture is recommended for the initial 36-week screening.
6. Prenatal surveillance (every prenatal visit) involves the following:
   a. Fetal: (i) fetal heart rate; (ii) fundal height, actual and amount of change; (iii) presenting part and station (late in pregnancy); and (iii) fetal activity
   b. Maternal: (i) blood pressure, actual and extent of change; (ii) weight, actual and amount of change; and (iii) symptoms, including epigastric pain, headache, and altered vision.
7. Other prenatal factors:
   a. Nägele's rule estimates the date of delivery: first day of LNMP plus 7 days, then count back 3 months.
   b. Weight gain: ideal amount is based on maternal prepregnancy weight
   c. Calories: 300 additional calories in pregnancy; 400 additional calories during lactation
   d. Supplementation: iron 30-60 mg after 4 months; folic acid 1 mg/day starting before and continuing throughout the pregnancy.
   e. Smoking: stop; 4600 perinatal deaths per year in United States as a result of smoking
   d. Alcohol: none
8. Perinatal summary:
   a. Graphic labor curve of Friedman: active stage of labor (Stage 2 is 1.2 cm/hour for nullipara and 1.5 cm/hour for multipara
   b. Stage 2 of labor: 60 minutes for nullipara; 30 minutes for multipara
   c. Stage 3 of labor: 30 minutes. Use oxytocin, ergonovine, or Hemabate to enhance uterine contractility after the placenta is expelled.
   d. Engagement: when the biparietal diameter passes the pelvic inlet
9. Conjugates and pelvis:
   a. Diagonal conjugate is the measurement from the sacral promontory to the symphysis pubis. It is the most important pelvic dimension. If more than 11.5 cm, the pelvic inlet is adequate.
   b. The most favorable pelvic shape is the gynecoid (occurs in 50% of women).

SUGGESTED READING

American Academy of Family Physicians: *American Academy of Family Physicians' management of maternity care: prenatal program guide.* Available online at http://www.aafp.org/momcare.xml. Accessed February 25, 2004.

Ewigman BG, et al: Effect of prenatal ultrasound screening on perinatal outcome. *N Engl J Med* 329:821-827, 1993.

Kruszka S, Kruszka P: Does antiplatelet therapy prevent preeclampsia and its complications? *J Fam Pract* 50(5):468, 2001.

McDuffie RS, et al: Effect of frequency of prenatal care visits on perinatal outcome among low-risk women. A randomized controlled trial. *JAMA* 275:847-851, 1996.

Schrag S, et al: Prevention of perinatal group B streptococcal disease: Revised guidelines from CDC. *MMWR Recommendations and Reports* 51(RR11):1-22, August 16, 2002.

Chapter 66

Labor

There is a time to sow, a time to reap, and a time to deliver.

CLINICAL CASE PROBLEM 1:

A 28-YEAR-OLD PRIMIGRAVIDA IN LABOR

A 28-year-old primigravida at term is admitted to the delivery suite with contractions 5 minutes apart. Her cervix is found to be 3 cm dilated and 90% effaced. When examined 5 hours later she has progressed to 4 cm dilated and is 100% effaced. The station of the head is zero (0). Her contractions are mild to moderate and have become more irregular during the past 3 hours. She has been ambulating, but this has not changed the strength or the frequency of her contractions. Her membranes are intact and bulging. The baseline fetal heart rate (FHR) is 150 beats per minute (bpm). The monitor tracing shows frequent heart rate accelerations.

■ **SELECT THE BEST ANSWER TO THE FOLLOWING QUESTIONS:**

1. What is the most appropriate course of action at this time?
   a. perform an amniotomy
   b. begin oxytocin stimulation for hypotonic labor
   c. call the anesthesiologist to administer epidural analgesia
   d. reassure the patient that her contractions will pick up eventually
   e. none of the above

2. The appropriate action is taken. After 4 more hours, her contractions are still mild to moderate and irregular in frequency. The cervix is now 5 cm dilated. The electronic fetal monitor strip is reactive. What would be the most appropriate course of action at this time?
   a. perform an amniotomy
   b. begin oxytocin stimulation for hypotonic labor
   c. call the anesthesiologist to administer epidural analgesia and prepare the patient for cesarean delivery
   d. tell the patient and the nursing staff to relax; everything takes time
   e. none of the above

3. With the appropriate intervention the patient progresses to full cervical dilatation. After pushing for 2 hours, the patient is exhausted. The fetal scalp is visible at the introitus. The position of the head is occiput anterior. The FHR tracing is reactive with a baseline rate of 150 bpm. Her contractions are strong, lasting 50 seconds, and are 2-3 minutes apart. What would you do at this time?
   a. increase the oxytocin
   b. explain to the patient that she will just have to try a little harder
   c. attempt delivery with outlet forceps
   d. attempt delivery with a vacuum extractor
   e. either c or d

4. Which of the following statements concerning the use of the vacuum extractor and/or outlet forceps in the second stage of labor is true?
   a. the perinatal morbidity of infants delivered with outlet forceps is higher than if a vacuum extractor is used
   b. the perinatal morbidity of infants delivered with a vacuum extractor is higher than if outlet forceps are used
   c. intracranial compression with the vacuum extractor is higher than that with outlet forceps
   d. Apgar scores of infants delivered by the vacuum extractor are higher than those of infants delivered by outlet forceps
   e. the perinatal morbidity and Apgar scores of infants delivered by outlet forceps and vacuum extractor are similar

5. Which of the following is (are) essential for a forceps delivery to be classified as outlet forceps?
   a. the scalp is or has been visible at the introitus
   b. the skull has reached the pelvic floor
   c. the sagittal suture is in the anteroposterior diameter of the pelvis
   d. the orientation of the fetal head must be unequivocally identified
   e. all of the above

6. Which of the following is (are) maternal indication for forceps delivery?
   a. maternal exhaustion
   b. need to avoid voluntary expulsive efforts
   c. lack of maternal cooperation in pushing
   d. excessive maternal analgesia
   e. all of the above

7. Which of the following FHR patterns suggests a need for a forceps delivery if all other criteria have been met?
   a. fetal heart tones with a persistent baseline rate of >150 bpm
   b. repetitive late decelerations dropping 20 bpm lasting 20 seconds
   c. repetitive early decelerations dropping 20 bpm lasting 20 seconds

d. repetitive variable decelerations dropping 20 bpm lasting 20 seconds

e. repetitive accelerations of 20 bpm lasting 20 seconds

8. Which of the following conditions must be met before a forceps delivery is attempted?
   a. the cervix must be fully dilated
   b. the membranes must be ruptured
   c. the head must be engaged
   d. the bladder must be empty
   e. all of the above

9. Which of the following statements regarding induction of labor by stripping the membranes is (are) true?
   a. stripping of the membranes has been firmly established as a safe and efficient method to induce labor
   b. stripping of the membranes has not been associated with infection
   c. stripping of the membranes has not been associated with subsequent vaginal bleeding
   d. stripping of the membranes appears to induce labor through a prostaglandin stimulation/mediation
   e. all of the above are true

10. Which of the following is (are) a risk(s) of administering oxytocin for the induction of labor?
    a. uterine rupture
    b. fetal hypoxia
    c. uterine hypertonia
    d. all of the above
    e. none of the above

CLINICAL CASE MANAGEMENT PROBLEM

Discuss the major issues when considering the use of oxytocin for the induction of labor.

 ANSWERS:

1. a. This patient has hypotonic labor. When a patient in the active phase of labor (cervical dilatation of 4 cm or more dilation) develops hypotonic or dysfunctional uterine contractions and if the fetal head is engaged, it is appropriate to perform an amniotomy. This may augment and shorten labor. The mechanism of augmentation of contractions is thought to be release of prostaglandins from the fetal membranes when they are artificially ruptured. The patient should be kept in the Fowler's position after amniotomy to facilitate drainage of the amniotic fluid. Amniotomy should be performed under sterile con-

ditions only if the fetal head is engaged and is well applied to the cervix. There is no indication for epidural analgesia at this time.

2. b. In this patient, amniotomy has not enhanced uterine contraction regularity, intensity, and frequency. Oxytocin stimulation for hypotonic labor now should be considered. The following guidelines should be adhered to: (1) the patient must be in the active phase of labor with cervical dilatation of at least 3 cm; (2) the fetal head should be engaged or should descend through the pelvic inlet with fundal pressure; (3) the fetus should be in a cephalic presentation; (4) there should be no polyhydramnios; (5) the patient's parity should be less than 6; (6) the patient should not have a previous uterine scar; and (7) the fetal status should be reassuring.

Oxytocin infusion is turned off immediately if hyperstimulation of the uterus occurs. When infusion is restarted, it should be at half the previous dose. There should be continuous electronic monitoring of the fetal heart and uterine activity.

3. e. The mother is exhausted. Her contractions are strong and 2-3 minutes apart and are therefore not hypotonic. It would be inappropriate to increase the rate of oxytocin infusion. The head is on the perineum. Therefore delivery of the infant by either an outlet forceps or a vacuum extractor would be appropriate. When a mother has been pushing for 2 hours and is exhausted, it is inappropriate to advise her to "try harder."

4. e. The perinatal morbidity rates and Apgar scores of infants delivered by outlet forceps and by a vacuum extractor are similar. The vacuum extractor is used more commonly in Europe and Canada than in the United States. The soft silastic vacuum extractor has the advantage over older metal models of being able to be applied immediately to the fetal head. The pressure should be decreased between contractions. There is lower intracranial compression with the vacuum extractor, but there is no significant difference in perinatal morbidity or Apgar scores between infants delivered by the vacuum extractor and infants delivered by outlet forceps.

In the hands of experienced operators, both instruments are effective and safe. Proper cup placement is the most important determinant of success in vacuum extraction. The center of the cup should be over the sagittal suture and about 3 cm in front of the posterior fontanelle. Such placement prevents iatrogenic deflexion and asynclitism of the fetal head.

5. e. Forceps deliveries are classified as follows (with all criteria being present):

Outlet forceps: This refers to the application of forceps when the scalp is visible at the introitus without the need to separate the labia, the fetal skull has reached the pelvic floor, the sagittal suture is in the antero-posterior diameter of the pelvis, and rotation does not exceed 45 degrees.

Low forceps: This refers to the application of forceps when the skull has reached a station of at least +2 but is not on the pelvic floor and when the sagittal suture is in the anteroposterior or oblique diameter of the pelvis.

Midforceps: This refers to the application of forceps when the head is engaged but has not reached a station of +2.

High forceps: This refers to the application of forceps at any time before engagement of the head. There are no indications for high forceps deliveries in present-day obstetric practice.

6. **e.** Maternal indications for outlet forceps include maternal exhaustion, need to avoid voluntary expulsive effort (e.g., certain cardiac or cerebrovascular disease), lack of maternal cooperation in pushing, or excessive analgesia impairing voluntary expulsive efforts.

7. **b.** The major fetal indication for termination of the second stage of labor is a *nonreassuring fetal heart rate pattern*. This phrase has replaced the old term, *fetal distress*, because of the imprecision and inaccuracy of the latter. Nonreassuring patterns may be manifested by persistent and repetitive findings of the following: baseline FHRs of less than 100 or more than 160 bpm, late deceleration patterns of any degree, and severe variable decelerations. Severe variable decelerations can be described using the "rule of 60s": the decelerations last longer than 60 seconds, drop to lower than 60 bpm, or drop 60 beats below the baseline.

Accelerations are always reassuring. Early decelerations (head compressions) are benign and are not an indication for the termination of the second stage of labor. Variable decelerations (cord compressions) of a mild or moderate degree are not indications for intervention, but late decelerations, even 20 bpm, are nonreassuring and suggest a need for forceps delivery.

8. **e.** The use of forceps is permissible only when all of the following conditions are present, regardless of the urgency of delivery: (1) the cervix must be fully dilated; (2) the membranes must be ruptured; (3) the head must be engaged, preferably at station +2 or below, and the head must present in either vertex or face presentation with chin anterior; (4) cephalopelvic disproportion must have been ruled out; and (5) the bladder must be empty.

9. **d.** Induction of labor by stripping the membranes is a relatively common practice, although few reports documenting its efficacy and safety have been published. The potential for infection and bleeding from a previously undiagnosed placenta previa or from a low-lying placenta, as well as accidental rupture of the membranes, should be considered. Only one randomized study involving 180 pregnancies has demonstrated that membrane stripping is safe and associated with a decreased incidence of postterm gestation. If it is effective, the mechanism of action is likely to be mediated by the stimulation of prostaglandins located in the membrane itself.

10. **d.** Oxytocin is a powerful drug and has been associated with uterine rupture, hypertonic uterine contractions, and fetal hypoxia resulting from uterine hypertonia. Oxytocin must be administered on a risk–benefit basis. The risks have been discussed previously. The benefits include decreased risk of maternal exhaustion, decreased risk of intrapartum infection, and decreased risk of traumatic operative delivery. Also, failure to treat uterine dysfunction may expose the fetus to an appreciably higher risk of death.

SOLUTION TO THE CLINICAL CASE MANAGEMENT PROBLEM

Almost one-fourth of all labors are induced or augmented using oxytocin. The following protocol should be observed: (1) close observation; (2) continuous FHR monitoring; (3) continuous uterine activity monitoring; (4) parity less than 6; (5) reassuring FHR and pattern; and (6) thick meconium absent.

Numerous protocols exist for oxytocin augmentation of labor with respect to the initial dose, incremental dose increases, and intervals between dose increases. There are advantages and disadvantages to both high- and low-dose regimens. Either dosing schema is acceptable, providing the guidelines discussed earlier are adhered to before and during oxytocin administration. Low-dose regimens begin at 0.5 to 1 mU/min, increasing the dose 1 mU/min every 30-40 minutes up to a maximum dose of 20 mU/min. High-dose regimens start at 6 mU/min, advancing by 3 mU/min every 20-40 minutes up to a maximum dose of 42 mU/min. If hyperstimulation occurs, the oxytocin infusion is turned off immediately. When infusion is restarted, it should be at half the previous dose.

In 2003 a randomized controlled trial of the use of oral misoprostol for induction of labor at term reduced the use of oxytocin for women with ruptured membranes. Further trials are needed before use is widespread.

SUMMARY OF LABOR

A. Hypotonic labor:
1. Establish that the patient is in true labor.
2. If true labor is established and is not progressing, consider amniotomy.
3. If amniotomy is performed or membranes have ruptured spontaneously and labor is not progressing, consider oxytocin augmentation adhering to protocol.
4. Consider stripping of the membranes.

B. Operative vaginal delivery:
1. Forceps and vacuum are equally effective and safe if used properly.
2. Follow maternal and fetal indications for operative delivery.

3. If considering operative vaginal delivery for fetal distress or other emergency situations, weigh carefully the risks and benefits of both vaginal and abdominal delivery before making a decision.

SUGGESTED READING

Archie CL, et al: The course and conduct of normal labor and delivery. In DeCherney N: *Current Obstetric & Gynecologic Diagnosis & Treatment 2003.* The McGraw-Hill Companies, 2003, New York.

Lo JY, et al: Ruptured membranes at term: randomized, double-blind trial of oral misoprostol for labor induction. *Obstet Gynecol* 101(4): 685-689, 2003.

Stubbs TM: Oxytocin for labor induction. *Clin Obstet Gynecol* 43(3): 489-494, 2000.

Chapter 67

Spontaneous Abortion

| "Will we make it to term?"

CLINICAL CASE PROBLEM 1:
A 25-Year-Old with Vaginal Bleeding at 11 Weeks of Gestation

A 25-year-old female (gravida 2, para 0) comes to your office at 11 weeks of gestation with vaginal bleeding and mild lower abdominal cramping. She is crying and upset. Her previous pregnancy ended in a miscarriage at 9 weeks of gestation.

On examination, a bright red flow is seen coming from the cervical os. Her cervix is closed. The uterus by palpation is 8-9 weeks of gestation. Her blood pressure is 120/70 mm Hg and her pulse rate is 96. No other abnormalities are found.

▶ SELECT THE BEST ANSWER TO THE FOLLOWING QUESTIONS:

1. What is the most likely diagnosis of this patient's condition at this time?
   a. threatened abortion
   b. inevitable abortion
   c. incomplete abortion
   d. recurrent spontaneous abortion
   e. complete abortion

2. The vaginal blood flow in this patient increases slightly while in your office. She now is soaking through approximately one pad every 2 hours. What would you do at this time?
   a. observe carefully at home; order outpatient investigations
   b. admit the patient to the hospital and obtain an obstetric sonogram to assess pregnancy viability
   c. observe the patient at home; tell her not to worry about anything
   d. admit the patient to the hospital for observation only; no testing is indicated at this time
   e. it does not really matter

3. Taking into account your management, the patient goes on to spontaneously abort the fetus 3 days later. Her bleeding is minimal, and her vital signs are stable. On examination, it appears that most of the placental tissue is present. An ultrasound shows an empty uterus with a normal endometrial stripe. What would you now recommend?
   a. no further treatment
   b. ergonovine maleate to contract the uterus
   c. prophylactic antibiotics to prevent infection
   d. dilation and curettage (D&C)
   e. serial beta human chorionic gonadotropin (βhCG) titers

4. What is the spontaneous abortion rate in North American women?
   a. 10%
   b. 20%
   c. 25%
   d. 50%
   e. 75%

5. Spontaneous abortion is defined as which of the following?
   a. pregnancy loss at any gestational age
   b. pregnancy loss before 20 weeks of gestation
   c. delivery of a fetus-neonate weighing less than 250 g
   d. delivery of a fetus-neonate weighing less than 500 g
   e. none of the above

6. What is the most commonly recognized precipitating factor in spontaneous abortion?
   a. chromosomal abnormality
   b. advanced maternal age
   c. preexisting chronic maternal disease
   d. alcohol intake
   e. cigarette smoking

7. What is the most commonly recognized chromosomal anomaly associated with first-trimester spontaneous abortion?
   a. autosomal trisomy
   b. monosomy
   c. tetraploidy
   d. autosomal monosomy
   e. sex chromosome polysomy

8. Which of the following maternal conditions is (are) associated with an increased incidence of abortion?
   a. hypothyroidism
   b. controlled diabetes mellitus
   c. uncontrolled diabetes mellitus
   d. all of the above
   e. none of the above

9. Which of the following statements regarding cigarette smoking and spontaneous abortion is (are) true?
   a. smoking has been associated with an increased risk of euploidic abortion
   b. in women who smoke more than 14 cigarettes per day, the risk of spontaneous abortion is twice that of women who do not smoke
   c. smoking increases the risk of abortion by a factor of 1.2 for each 10 cigarettes smoked per day
   d. all of the above are true
   e. none of the above are true

10. Which of the following statements regarding the risk of spontaneous abortion and alcohol intake is (are) true?
    a. the risk of spontaneous euploidic abortion is increased even when alcohol is consumed "in moderation" during pregnancy
    b. the spontaneous abortion rate is doubled in women who drink twice weekly
    c. the spontaneous abortion rate is tripled in women who consume alcohol daily
    d. all of the above are true
    e. none of the above are true

11. Which of the following antibodies is associated most clearly with spontaneous abortion?
    a. anticardiolipin antibody
    b. antithyroid antibody
    c. antinuclear antibody
    d. rheumatoid factor
    e. anti–smooth-muscle antibody

CLINICAL CASE MANAGEMENT PROBLEM

Describe the currently recommended classification of spontaneous abortion.

ANSWERS:

1. **a.** The diagnosis is threatened abortion. Threatened abortion is defined as minimal vaginal bleeding, with or without mild cramping, in the first 20 weeks of pregnancy. The interval cervical os is closed. Sonographically the gestational sac appears normal, and a viable embryo or fetus is noted with cardiac motion. The incidence of threatened abortion in pregnancy is 20% to 25%; of that number, half go on to abort the fetus. Threatened abortion is associated with a higher risk of preterm labor, low birthweight, and perinatal mortality. There is, however, no increased risk of fetal malformations.

Inevitable abortion is defined as profuse vaginal bleeding and, during the first half of pregnancy, is accompanied by cervical dilatation and rupture of the gestational sac. No passage of tissue has occurred yet.

Incomplete abortion is defined when the criteria for inevitable abortion are met and some, but not all placental tissue has been passed. An ultrasound can be helpful in identifying if products of conception remain in the uterine cavity.

Completed abortion is defined when bleeding, dilation of the cervix, and complete passage of products of conception have occurred during the first half of pregnancy. This diagnosis is best confirmed with ultrasonography.

Recurrent spontaneous abortion refers to three or more consecutive abortions.

2. b. In any patient with more than slight bleeding, hospitalization is wise. With the associated cramping in this patient there is a high probability that she will go on to abort. Investigations in the hospital should include a βhCG level and an obstetric ultrasound to assess pregnancy viability and to determine intrauterine contents.

3. e. The patient appears to have undergone a completed abortion. Performing a D&C is unnecessary if the products of conception already have been removed from the uterus. The ultrasound is strongly suggestive that this is the case. However, if serial weekly βhCG levels decrease to zero, it can safely be assumed that all viable trophoblastic villi are out of the uterus.

Ergonovine maleate and prophylactic antibiotics are most useful when excessive bleeding occurs in the postpartum period and is not thought to be caused by retained products of conception.

4. b. The spontaneous abortion rate in North American women is approximately 15% to 20%.

5. b. Spontaneous abortion is defined as the termination of pregnancy before 20 weeks of gestation based on the last menstrual period.

6. a. The most commonly recognized precipitating factor in spontaneous abortion is chromosomal anomaly. Up to 50% of clinically recognized pregnancy losses have cytogenetic abnormalities. When chorionic villus sampling is performed on the placental tissue of first-trimester embryonic demises, up to 75% will be chromosomally abnormal.

7. a. The most commonly recognized chromosomal abnormality associated with first-trimester spontaneous abortion is autosomal trisomy. It can be the result of an isolated nondisjunction, maternal or paternal balanced translocation, or balanced chromosomal inversion.

8. c. Uncontrolled diabetes mellitus has been associated with an increased incidence of spontaneous abortion. Well-controlled diabetes, however, is not. There is also no association between hypothyroidism and spontaneous abortion.

9. d. Cigarette smoking is associated with an increased risk of euploidic abortion. For women who smoke more than 14 cigarettes per day, the risk of spontaneous abortion is approximately twice that of nonsmokers. This is independent of both maternal age and alcohol ingestion. The risk of spontaneous abortion increases in a linear fashion by a factor of 1.2 for each 10 cigarettes smoked per day.

10. d. The incidence of spontaneous euploidic abortion is increased even when alcohol is consumed "in moderation." Studies have indicated that the abortion rate is doubled in women who consume alcohol twice weekly and is tripled in women who consume alcohol daily when compared to nondrinkers. Increased euploidic abortion is strong evidence that both tobacco and alcohol are toxic to embryos.

11. a. Autoimmune mechanisms are those in which a cellular or humoral response is directed against a specific site within the host. Connective-tissue disorders such as systemic lupus erythematosus are associated with increased abortion and fetal death.

Antiphospholipid antibodies, including the lupus anticoagulant and anticardiolipin antibodies, are examples of autoimmune disease states that are associated with increased risk for recurrent abortion. Treatment of choice is low-dose aspirin.

SOLUTION TO THE CLINICAL CASE MANAGEMENT PROBLEM

The classification of spontaneous abortion is as follows:
Threatened abortion: any bloody vaginal discharge or vaginal bleeding that occurs before 20 weeks of gestation (based on gestational age, not on embryologic age).
Inevitable abortion: rupture of the membranes in the presence of cervical dilatation during the first 20 weeks of gestation.

Missed abortion: retention of nonviable products of conception in utero for up to 4 weeks.
Recurrent spontaneous abortion: previously known as habitual abortion. Defined by various criteria of number and sequence. The most generally accepted definition refers to three or more consecutive spontaneous abortions.

SUMMARY OF SPONTANEOUS ABORTION

1. **Classification:** See the Clinical Case Management Problem in this problem.

    Investigation of threatened abortion includes serial βhCG level determinations and ultrasound (if inconclusive, repeat in 1 to 2 weeks).
2. **Management of threatened abortion:**
    a. There is no evidence that bed rest changes the pregnancy outcome in the first trimester
    b. There is no evidence that administering any pharmacologic agent changes the outcome
    c. Conservative management if bleeding slows down or stops (document live fetus by ultrasound)
    d. D&C if heavy bleeding continues and ultrasound reveals a nonviable fetus. Expectant management or surgical D&C are options if bleeding slows or stops and ultrasound reveals a nonviable fetus or fetal demise. In most areas of the world, surgical evacuation is unnecessary

after a complete miscarriage with retained products of conception and should be indicated by clinical rather than ultrasonographic criteria.
    e. Medical management includes the addition of misoprostol (a synthetic prostaglandin E1 analogue), which induces strong uterine contractions and is recommended by some to reduce the need for surgical intervention. However, this is not a use of the drug approved by the U.S. Food and Drug Administration and improper use can cause uterine rupture in addition to gastric and other side effects. Therefore expectant management is the preferred option.

SUGGESTED READING
Ankum WM, et al: Management of spontaneous miscarriage in the first trimester: an example of putting informed shared decision making into practice. *BMJ* 322(7298):1343-1346, 2001.
Scroggins KM, et al: Spontaneous pregnancy loss: evaluation, management and follow up counseling. *Prim Care* 27(1):153-167, 2000.

Chapter 68

Postterm Pregnancy

"My baby is overdue, isn't it, Doctor?"

CLINICAL CASE PROBLEM 1:
A 24-Year-Old New Patient Who Allegedly Has Gone Past Her Due Date

A 24-year-old woman (gravida 2, para 1) comes to you as a new patient recommended by a friend. She recently has moved to your community with her 2-year-old daughter. She regrets that she lost her prenatal records when packing, but she claims to be 43 weeks pregnant by dates. When you ask her who her previous doctor was she tells you that she only went to her doctor three or four times because she did not have time and that she forgot the doctor's name.

She has not been keeping a fetal kick chart, but she says the baby has been moving. She has not had an obstetric ultrasound. On examination, her fundal height is 36 cm. Her cervix is soft, 25% effaced, and 1 cm dilated. The presentation of the fetus is cephalic, and the fetus weighs 6-7 lb. The fetal heart rate is 142 beats per minute (bpm) and regular.

SELECT THE BEST ANSWER TO THE FOLLOWING QUESTIONS:

1. At this time, what would you do?
    a. tell her to come back in a week while you think about things
    b. perform a biophysical profile and ultrasound for fetal weight
    c. schedule her for induction of labor at the maternity unit
    d. schedule her for cesarean delivery just to be on the safe side
    e. do nothing now; make an appointment to see her in 1 week

2. A pregnancy is defined as being postterm if it exceeds how many days of gestation?
    a. 280 days
    b. 287 days
    c. 294 days
    d. 273 days
    e. 301 days

3. What is the approximate prevalence of postterm pregnancy based on the last menstrual period (LMP)?
    a. 25%
    b. 15%

c. 10%
d. 5%
e. 3%

4. What is the approximate true prevalence of post-term pregnancy based on the date of conception?
   a. 25%
   b. 15%
   c. 10%
   d. 5%
   e. 3%

5. Which of the following parameters is the most sensitive test for the prediction of fetal asphyxia and resultant perinatal mortality in postterm pregnancy?
   a. a weekly nonstress test (NST)
   b. a biweekly NST
   c. lack of a 3-cm vertical pocket of amniotic fluid on ultrasound
   d. lack of a 1-cm vertical pocket of amniotic fluid on ultrasound
   e. a contraction stress test (CST)

6. What is the most common cause of a diagnosis of postterm pregnancy?
   a. lack of an obstetric ultrasound in pregnancy
   b. inaccurate dating using the LMP
   c. the postmaturity syndrome
   d. intrauterine growth restriction
   e. none of the above

7. Which of the following statements regarding post-term pregnancy is (are) true?
   a. the perinatal mortality rate is increased in patients who have, in fact, gone past 42 completed weeks of gestation
   b. the incidence of meconium staining and meconium aspiration is increased in patients who have gone beyond 42 completed weeks of gestation
   c. the true postterm fetus may continue to gain weight in utero and present a problem at birth because of fetal size
   d. the intrauterine environment in a true post-term pregnancy may predispose to the development of a dysmature or dystrophic infant
   e. all of the above are true

8. To what does the term *postmature* refer?
   a. all infants delivered by mothers diagnosed as postterm
   b. all infants verified by objective criteria to be greater than 42 weeks of gestation
   c. infants displaying specific characteristics delivered after 42 weeks of gestation

d. it is no longer a useful description
e. none of the above

9. A colleague of yours describes his approach to postterm gestation: "I deliver all my patients at 42 weeks." Without inquiring about his perinatal morbidity and mortality statistics, which of the following is (are) reason(s) not to follow his example?
   a. it is difficult to predict which fetuses will develop significant problems
   b. induction of labor is not always successful in leading to vaginal delivery
   c. delivery by cesarean birth increases the risk of serious maternal morbidity
   d. the majority of fetuses who are truly more than 42 weeks fare well
   e. all of the above are true

10. At this time, which of the following is (are) true regarding those women who have been established to be truly postterm (greater than 42 weeks of gestation)?
    a. there are two approaches to managing these pregnancies: one is conservative and the other is aggressive
    b. there appears to be no difference in perinatal outcome between aggressive management and conservative management if conservative management includes an appropriate protocol for fetal surveillance
    c. aggressive management appears to result in lower perinatal morbidity and mortality than conservative management
    d. a and b
    e. a and c

CLINICAL CASE MANAGEMENT PROBLEM

You are a family physician doing obstetrics in your local hospital. You have been asked to develop a clinical practice guideline (CPG) for the management of postterm pregnancy. Prepare this CPG based on your knowledge of the subject.

ANSWERS:

1. **b.** This patient presents a dilemma because the data you need to accurately identify her gestational age are not available. Although she appears to be in the third trimester of pregnancy by fundal height, her dates are suspect because she appears to be a poor historian. The most appropriate action at this time is to confirm fetal well-being by means of a biophysical profile and obtain an estimate of fetal weight. The ultrasound examination cannot be expected to provide a due date at this point in her pregnancy. The

normal variation in fetal size is so great in the third trimester that ultrasound estimates will vary by as much as 3 weeks. Scheduling induction or cesarean delivery is premature at this point. Doing nothing is inappropriate. Ideally assessment of gestational age is confirmed early in pregnancy using the following parameters:

Menstrual history: The LMP tends to be reliable if the patient is sure of her dates; if the pregnancy was planned; if the menstrual cycle was regular; if the menstrual cycle was usual for the patient; and if there is no recent history of oral contraceptive use, abortion, pregnancy, or lactation (all of which are associated with anovulation).

Clinical parameters include pregnancy landmarks that are identified as early as they appear: uterine size estimated by an early pelvic examination (before 12 weeks of gestation), fetal heart tones detected by Doppler stethoscope (before 12 weeks of gestation), fundal size estimated by abdominal palpation at the symphysis pubis (at 12 weeks of gestation) and the umbilicus (at 20 weeks of gestation), maternal report of feeling fetal movement (quickening) at 16-18 weeks in a multigravida and 18-20 weeks in a primigravida; and fetal heart tones heard with a fetoscope (at 18-20 weeks of gestation).

Ultrasound parameters include crown–rump length (between 8 and 12 weeks of gestation [accurate to within 5 days]) and fetal biparietal diameter (between 12 and 18 weeks of gestation [accurate to within 7 days]).

2. c. A pregnancy is postterm if it exceeds 294 days of gestation. See Answer 4.

3. c. The approximate prevalence of postterm pregnancy based on the LMP is 10%. See Answer 4.

4. e. A pregnancy is defined as being postterm if it persists beyond 294 days (or 42 weeks of gestation) from the first day of the LMP, assuming ovulation occurred on day 14 of the menstrual cycle. More precisely, however, postterm pregnancy should be defined as one that persists beyond 280 days from conception. Because only 15% of women's menstrual cycles are exactly 28 days long, many women ovulate more than 14 days after their LMP. Thus, although their pregnancies go beyond 294 days from the LMP, they have not gone beyond the 280 days from conception and are not truly postterm.

The pseudoprevalence of postterm pregnancy (the prevalence of the label of postterm pregnancy being applied or documented in the chart based on LMP) is approximately 10%. However, the true prevalence of postterm pregnancy is approximately 3%.

5. c. The most sensitive test for the prediction of fetal asphyxia and resultant perinatal mortality in postterm pregnancy is decreased amniotic fluid on ultrasound. A large study, the Canadian Postterm Pregnancy Trial, found that using the lack of a 3-cm pocket as a test for the basis for intervention was associated with a lower perinatal mortality rate than using either an NST or a CST. Thus the performance of a biophysical profile on a biweekly basis, with the demonstration of a 3-cm amniotic fluid pocket, is a sign suggesting that the fetal status is reassuring.

6. b. Postdated pregnancy is diagnosed most commonly because of incorrect or inaccurate dates based on the first day of the LMP. Although not performing an obstetric ultrasound during pregnancy will increase the probability of that diagnosis being made, it is not the true cause.

7. e. The perinatal mortality rate and the incidence of meconium staining and meconium aspiration are increased when the gestational age is 42 weeks or beyond. In true postterm pregnancy, placental function is unchanged and the fetus may continue to gain weight in utero resulting in a macrosomic fetus. This occurs in 70% of cases. In other cases the placenta may undergo aging, infarction, and calcification. In these pregnancies the intrauterine environment may predispose for loss of fetal weight, loss of subcutaneous fat and muscle, and a dystrophic or dysmature appearance. This occurs in 30% of cases.

8. c. The term *postmature* as applied to neonates refers to a specific subset of infants delivered of mothers who are truly postterm and who display the following characteristics: (1) underweight as a result of loss of subcutaneous fat; (2) long and thin in girth; (3) skin with patchy areas of desquamation; (4) skin sometimes covered with meconium; (5) wrinkled hands and feet on the ventral surfaces; and (6) long nails stained with meconium.

9. e. The following five reasons serve to discourage a policy of delivering all fetuses whose gestational age is merely suspected to be at least 42 weeks of gestation: (1) gestational age is not always known precisely, thus the fetus actually may be less mature than believed; (2) it is difficult to identify with precision those fetuses likely to develop significant morbidity if left in utero; (3) the majority of these fetuses fare rather well; (4) induction of labor is not always successful; and (5) delivery by cesarean birth appreciably increases the risk of serious maternal morbidity not only in this pregnancy but also to a degree in subsequent ones.

10. d. When a pregnancy is definitely confirmed to be 42 or more weeks in length, two management approaches appear to be equally appropriate. A randomized investigation by Hannah and colleagues compared elective induction with antepartum surveillance (NST, amniotic fluid volume, and fetal movement counting). Women were randomized to either induction of labor at 42 weeks of gestation or serial antenatal fetal testing. The findings showed that induction of labor at 42 weeks of gestation resulted in a lower rate of cesarean delivery (21%) than in the antenatal surveillance group (25%), with equivalent infant outcomes in the two study groups.

SUMMARY OF POSTTERM PREGNANCY

A good summary of this chapter is provided by the clinical practice guidelines provided in the Solution to the Clinical Case Management Problem.

SOLUTION TO THE CLINICAL CASE MANAGEMENT PROBLEM

The following are the steps that should be in the guidelines you have prepared for the management of postterm pregnancy:

1. Review the entire prenatal history. Establish whether the LMP was a normal, one and calculate an estimated date of conception (EDC) based on dates.
2. Review the early pregnancy landmarks that are documented on the prenatal chart.
3. Review any obstetric ultrasounds performed during the pregnancy, and calculate an EDC. If more than one ultrasound was performed, use the date established by the ultrasound earliest in the pregnancy.
4. Compare the EDC by dates, and compare it to the EDC from the early pregnancy landmark and the ultrasound data.
5. Determine your best estimate of the EDC from all the information available.

6. Begin antenatal monitoring at 41 weeks of gestation by best estimate EDC: charting fetal movement daily, performing NSTs twice weekly, and looking for at least one 3-cm pocket of amniotic fluid volume twice weekly.
7. Perform a pelvic examination at 42 weeks of gestation and evaluate cervical effacement and cervical dilatation. Begin induction of labor if the cervix is ripe. If not, then ripening of the cervix with a prostaglandin gel is indicated before formal induction with oxytocin.
8. Obtain a consultation from an obstetrician at this time (if one has not been done already).
9. If induction is unsuccessful or if fetal well-being cannot be assured during induction, proceed to cesarean delivery.

SUGGESTED READING

Crowley P: Interventions for preventing or improving the outcome of delivery at or beyond term. *Cochrane Database Syst Rev* (2):CD000170, 2000.

Hannah ME, et al: Canadian multicenter post-term pregnancy trial group. Induction of labor as compared with serial antenatal monitoring in post-term pregnancy. *New Engl J Med* 326:1587, 1992.

Hollis B: Prolonged pregnancy. *Curr Opin Obstet Gynecol* 14(2):203-207, 2002.

Olesen AW, et al: Perinatal and maternal complications related to postterm delivery: a national register-based study, 1978-1993. *Am J Obstet Gynecol* 189(1):222-227, 2003.

Sanchez-Ramos L, et al: Labor induction versus expectant management for postterm pregnancies: a systematic review with meta-analysis. *Obstet Gynecol* 101(6):1312-1318, 2003.

 Chapter **69**

Thyroid Diseases in Pregnancy

"You mean something in my neck makes me go to the bathroom so much?"

CLINICAL CASE PROBLEM 1:

A 28-YEAR-OLD POSTPARTUM PATIENT WITH TYPE 1 DIABETES AND FATIGUE

A 28-year-old woman with type 1 diabetes comes to your office 1 month postpartum with fatigue, weight gain, and difficulty concentrating. She is a married schoolteacher who has been breastfeeding her new baby and has been

home on family leave. Her diabetes has been well controlled during her pregnancy, her delivery was remarkably uncomplicated, and there have been no complications postpartum in either herself or her child. She initially attributed her fatigue to the stresses of caring for her new baby but states, "I have never felt this fatigued before." Her examination shows normal vital signs, is consistent with being 1 month postpartum, and is otherwise normal. A 2-hour postprandial blood sugar test is normal.

SELECT THE BEST ANSWER TO THE FOLLOWING QUESTIONS:

1. In addition to ordering a blood test for anemia, it is most appropriate to:

a. reassure her that the fatigue will pass and is consistent with her diabetes
b. suggest she discontinue breastfeeding because this is likely to be the cause of her fatigue
c. check her serum cortisol levels
d. obtain a serum thyroid stimulating hormone (TSH) level
e. none of the above

2. The appropriate test result comes back elevated. The etiology of this woman's fatigue is most likely to be which of the following:
a. pituitary infarct
b. iodine deficiency
c. hypothalamic dysfunction
d. an autoimmune disorder
e. an adrenal tumor

CLINICAL CASE PROBLEM 2:

A 27-YEAR-OLD PREGNANT WOMAN WITH UNUSUAL JITTERINESS

A 27-year-old primigravida comes to your office in her second trimester complaining of unusual jitteriness, tremors, insomnia, heat intolerance, and a racing heartbeat. In retrospect, she recalls that some of these symptoms had been present, but only rarely, prior to the pregnancy, but now they are occurring more frequently. On examination, her resting pulse is 100, her respirations are 18, her blood pressure is 110/70 mm Hg, and she is afebrile. She has not gained any weight in the last 8 weeks, and there is some evidence of a palpably enlarged thyroid. Reflexes are brisk. No other abnormalities are noted.

3. Other symptoms that frequently are associated with this condition include:
a. hyperhidrosis
b. poorly controlled hypertension
c. frequent stools
d. b and c
e. a, b, c

4. Inadequate treatment of this condition during pregnancy can lead to increased risk of which of the following:
a. preterm delivery
b. fetal loss
c. preeclampsia
d. b and c
e. a, b, and c

5. Neonatal complications of this condition include which of the following:
a. low birthweight
b. hypothyroidism
c. hyperthyroidism

d. b and c
e. a, b, and c

6. Your diagnosis is confirmed by laboratory testing, which reveals a low TSH and elevated T4 (thyroxine). Options for therapy during pregnancy include which of the following:
a. no therapy is needed after the first trimester
b. propylthiouracil (PTU)
c. methimazole
d. iodine 131
e. b or c

7. You begin a thioamide, and the patient does well. After delivery the patient wishes to breastfeed her infant. Which of the following is (are) true regarding thioamides and breastfeeding:
a. methimazole is contraindicated in lactating women
b. PTU is contraindicated in lactating women
c. women taking PTU may breastfeed
d. a and b are true
e. none of the above

CLINICAL CASE PROBLEM 3:

A 37-YEAR-OLD PREGNANT WOMAN WITH A LUMP IN HER NECK

A 37-year-old pregnant woman comes to your office at 16 weeks of gestation with difficulty swallowing. The patient is otherwise asymptomatic. On examination you discover a lump in her neck. There is a firm, noncystic nodule of approximately 2.5 cm in the left pole of the thyroid. There are no palpable surrounding lymph nodes, and the rest of the examination is normal. Thyroid function tests are normal.

8. The most appropriate course of action is to:
a. carefully watch the nodule until after delivery
b. begin thyroxine therapy
c. increase the iodine content in the patient's diet
d. send her for guided biopsy of the nodule
e. none of the above

▎ ANSWERS:

1. **d.** Thyroid disease is the second most common endocrine disorder affecting women of reproductive age. Many thyroid conditions manifest themselves during pregnancy or in the immediate postpartum period. This woman is manifesting symptoms that could be attributed to her underlying diabetes and circumstance, but the history and normal physical examination should raise the suspicion of underlying thyroid dysfunction. The TSH is the most appropriate test to rule in or out thyroid disease in this patient.

Hypocorticism, presumably resulting from a pituitary infarct, although a consideration, is unlikely given the history of normal, uncomplicated labor and delivery. Hence the serum cortisol level is not indicated as a first-line screen.

2. d. Hypothyroidism is confirmed by the elevated TSH. The most common etiology of hypothyroidism in developed countries is Hashimoto's thyroiditis, an autoimmune thyroiditis that leads to hypothyroidism. Type 1 diabetes is also an autoimmune disorder; there is an 8% incidence of hypothyroidism in women with type 1 diabetes, and these women have a 25% chance of developing the hypothyroidism in the postpartum period. Over time, Hashimoto's thyroiditis generally leads to thyroid gland enlargement and is characterized by the production of antithyroid antibodies.

Subacute thyroiditis is the second most common cause of hypothyroidism in developed countries. In developing countries, iodine deficiency is the leading cause of hypothyroidism.

3. e. This patient exhibits the classic signs of hyperthyroidism. Symptoms include unusual jitteriness or nervousness, tremors, insomnia, heat intolerance, palpitations, excessive sweating, and frequent stools. Signs include weight loss or failure to gain weight during pregnancy, hypertension that is difficult to control, hyperreflexia, enlarged or tender thyroid, a fine tremor, lid lag and retraction, and dermopathy including pretibial myxedema. Diagnosis is confirmed by a decreased TSH and T3 resin uptake levels and elevated free thyroxine (T4), total T4, total T3, and free thyroxine index levels.

4. e. Hyperthyroidism occurs in two out of 1000 pregnancies, and the vast majority (95%) of these cases result from Graves' disease. Untreated or inadequately treated maternal thyrotoxicosis is associated with increased risk of fetal loss, preterm delivery, maternal heart failure, and preeclampsia.

5. e. Fetal and neonatal complications of maternal hyperthyroidism during pregnancy include all of those listed. A large proportion of thyroid dysfunction in Graves' disease is mediated by antibodies such as thyroid-stimulating immunoglobulin and TSH-binding inhibitory immunoglobulin. These immunoglobulins act on TSH receptors to induce thyroid stimulation. The excess hormone released crosses the placenta and affects the fetus. Thus, immune mediated hypothyroidism and hyperthyroidism is possible in the fetus. Maternal hyperthyroidism also can cause intrauterine growth restriction and neonates who are small for gestational age.

6. e. Hyperthyroidism of Graves' disease in pregnancy is treated with thioamides, either PTU or methimazole. Both drugs cross the placenta and can cause transient neonatal hypothyroidism. However, the benefits of therapy are thought to outweigh the risks. Fetal growth needs careful monitoring while the woman is taking these drugs. Methimazole had been thought to be associated with a risk of fetal aplasia cutis, a skin disorder of the scalp, but recent studies have found this not to be the case.

7. c. Women taking PTU may breastfeed. Only a small amount of medication crosses into human milk, and thyroid function studies of infants whose mothers are taking PTU have been normal.

8. d. Thyroid cancer has an incidence of 1/1000 in pregnant women. Any nodule discovered during pregnancy should be diagnostically evaluated with ultrasound because up to 40% will be malignant. Fine-needle biopsy is an option to determine the presence of malignant cells. Pregnancy does not seem to alter the course of thyroid cancer, but it is unclear whether it increases the risk of a nodule becoming cancerous or the recurrence rate in women diagnosed with thyroid cancer.

SUMMARY FOR THYROID DISEASE AND PREGNANCY

Thyroid disease is the second most common endocrine disorder affecting women of reproductive age. Many thyroid conditions manifest themselves during pregnancy or in the immediate postpartum period.

A. Hypothyroidism

Autoimmune Hashimoto's thyroiditis is the most common cause, especially in women with type 1 diabetes, in whom there is a 25% incidence in the postpartum period.

1. **Symptoms:** fatigue, cold intolerance, skin dryness and thickening, and difficulty concentrating
2. **Signs:** unusual weight gain, goiter, reduced or absent reflexes
3. **Diagnostic testing:** elevated TSH confirms diagnoses
4. **Treatment:** thyroid hormone; check neonate levels after birth.

B. Hyperthyroidism

Graves' disease is the most common cause, and the incidence is 2/1000 pregnancies.

1. **Symptoms:** unusual jitteriness or nervousness, tremors, insomnia, heat intolerance, palpitations, excessive sweating, and frequent stools

Continued

SUMMARY FOR THYROID DISEASE AND PREGNANCY—cont'd

2. **Signs:** weight loss or failure to gain weight during pregnancy, hypertension that is difficult to control, hyperreflexia, enlarged or tender thyroid, a fine tremor, lid lag and retraction, dermopathy including pretibial myxedema

3. **Diagnostic testing:** decreased TSH and T3 resin uptake levels and elevated free thyroxine (T4), total T4, total T3, and free thyroxine index levels

4. **Treatment:** thioamides, either PTU or methimazole

C. Thyroid nodules discovered during pregnancy
Thyroid cancer incidence is 1/1000 pregnant women. Any nodule discovered during pregnancy should be diagnostically evaluated with ultrasound and possible biopsy; up to 40% are malignant

SUGGESTED READING

Adlersberg MA, Burrow GN: Focus on primary care. Thyroid function and dysfunction in women. *Obstet Gynecol Surv* 57(3 Suppl):S1-7, 2002.

American College of Obstetrics and Gynecology. ACOG practice bulletin. Thyroid disease in pregnancy. Number 37, August 2002. *Int J Gynaecol Obstet* 79(2):171-180, 2002.

Lazarus JH, Kokandi A: Thyroid disease in relation to pregnancy: a decade of change. *Clin Endocrinol* 53(3):265-278, 2000.

Mestman JH: Diagnosis and management of maternal and fetal thyroid disorders. *Curr Opin Obstet Gynecol* 11(2):167-175, 1999.

Chapter 70

Exercise and Pregnancy

> "My stomach may have grown big, but I am staying in good shape."

CLINICAL CASE PROBLEM 1:

A 34-Year-Old Primigravida Aerobic Dance Instructor

A 34-year-old aerobics dance instructor sees you for advice regarding her pregnancy. She is 6 weeks pregnant and wonders if she should continue her current work. Her work consists of between 4 and 5 hours of exercise daily. She currently has no problems performing this activity but wonders if all the "bouncing and stepping" will cause a miscarriage or otherwise harm the baby.

■ **SELECT THE BEST ANSWER TO THE FOLLOWING QUESTIONS:**

1. Regarding her current physical activity, you tell her which of the following:
   a. any exercise during pregnancy is not advisable
   b. aerobic and strength training exercise are likely to increase her chance of miscarriage
   c. the pregnancy-associated physiologic changes in her body make dance aerobics inadvisable
   d. continuing moderate exercise during pregnancy is desirable and not harmful
   e. none of the above

2. Which of the following is (are) an absolute contraindication(s) to exercise during pregnancy:
   a. a history of incompetent cervix or cerclage
   b. placenta previa after 26 weeks of gestation
   c. persistent second- or third-trimester bleeding
   d. a and c
   e. a, b, and c

3. Which of the following is (are) considered a relative contraindication(s) to exercise during pregnancy:
   a. severe anemia
   b. poorly controlled hypertension
   c. body mass index of less than 12
   d. b and c
   e. a, b, and c

CLINICAL CASE PROBLEM 2:

A 37-Year-Old Pregnant Woman with Severe Back Pain

A 37-year-old pregnant woman comes to your office with low back pain that has been getting worse as her pregnancy has progressed. This is her third pregnancy; the previous two were uncomplicated except for chronic back pain, and this one also has been without any other difficulty. She has tried bed rest, acetaminophen, and heat pads all without relief. She has no symptoms of dysuria or sensory/motor complaints; she says she is willing to try anything for relief. Examination is that of a normal early third-trimester pregnancy.

4. Regarding her chronic pregnancy-related back pain, you state the following:

a. step aerobics should be of therapeutic value in relieving the pain
b. water aerobics has been shown to relieve back pain in pregnant women
c. therapeutic massage is of no value in her condition
d. stationary bicycling should help her discomfort
e. none of the above

5. Your patient decides to try water aerobics, and her symptoms improve. Her mother-in-law, however, has told her swimming is harmful to the baby. She seeks your advice. You tell her:
a. water immersion late in pregnancy often is complicated by an increased rate of urinary tract infections
b. water immersion late in pregnancy often is complicated by an increase in vaginal discharges
c. water immersion late in pregnancy is dangerous because of the possibility of inducing an amnionitis
d. water immersion late in pregnancy is associated with preterm onset of labor
e. none of the above

CLINICAL CASE PROBLEM 3:

A 25-Year-Old Primigravida with Recent Onset of Lightheadedness While Exercising on the Treadmill

A 25-year-old primigravida in her second trimester returns to your office saying that she had episode of lightheadedness that occurred while exercising on her treadmill. Normally she power walks for 20 minutes each day. The episode came on suddenly, and she states she "almost passed out." Examination today is normal for her dates. Laboratory studies including hemoglobin level are normal. She asks when she can resume her exercise activity.

6. Reasons to discontinue exercise include which of the following:
a. history of preterm labor
b. dizziness or lightheadedness during exercise
c. vaginal bleeding
d. all of the above
e. none of the above

7. Which of the following forms of exercise is (are) considered safe during pregnancy:
a. scuba diving
b. gymnastics
c. basketball
d. field hockey
e. water aerobics

8. Women who engage in moderate aerobic exercise regularly during pregnancy:
a. are at greater risk for preterm labor
b. may derive significant physical and mental health benefits
c. are at risk for fetal intrauterine growth restriction (IUGR)
d. reduce their risk for preeclampsia
e. all of the above

ANSWERS:

1. **d.** Despite the importance of regular exercise in daily life, there are relatively few good studies that examine this issue. A recent Cochrane evidenced-based review concluded that regular aerobic exercise during pregnancy appears to improve (or maintain) physical fitness and body image.

2. **e.** The American College of Obstetricians and Gynecologists (ACOG) released a consensus recommendation regarding absolute and relative contraindications to exercise in pregnancy. Absolute contraindications include a history of incompetent cervix or cerclage, placenta previa after 26 weeks of gestation, persistent second- or third-trimester bleeding, hemodynamically significant heart disease, restrictive lung disease, multiple gestations at risk for premature labor, ruptured membranes, and preeclampsia/eclampsia.

3. **e.** The ACOG guidelines for relative contraindications include severe anemia, chronic bronchitis, unevaluated maternal arrhythmia, poorly controlled type 1 diabetes, morbid obesity, extreme underweight (body mass index of <12), history of sedentary lifestyle, IUGR, poorly controlled hypertension, orthopedic limitations, poorly controlled seizure disorder or hyperthyroidism, and heavy smoking.

4. **b.** Chronic back pain is a common problem in pregnancy. Conditioning the back muscles with stretching and strength training before pregnancy is a good prophylactic strategy. However, during pregnancy, water aerobics has been found in controlled trials to reduce the discomfort of low back pain in many patients. Some women feel self-conscious about exercising in pregnancy, particularly in public pools. However, many health clubs now take this into account and schedule specific times just for pregnancy water aerobics classes.

5. **e.** There are many common misconceptions regarding immersion and pregnancy. Among them are that water immersion often is complicated by urinary tract infections, vaginal discharges, leakage into the amniotic sac, and an association with preterm onset of

labor. None of these are correct. Swimming and water aerobics are perfectly safe and usually easily performed because of the buoyancy effect of water.

6. **d.** Reasons to discontinue exercise in pregnancy include vaginal bleeding, dyspnea prior to exercise, dizziness, headache, chest pain, muscle weakness, unilateral calf or leg swelling (thrombophlebitis should be ruled out), preterm labor, decreased fetal movement, and amniotic fluid leakage.

7. **e.** Although physiologic and morphologic changes of pregnancy may interfere with the ability to engage in some forms of physical activity, the patient's health status should be evaluated before prescribing an exercise program. Each sport should be reviewed individually for its potential risk, and activities with a high risk of abdominal trauma should be avoided during pregnancy. These include all contact sports and scuba diving. Scuba diving increases the fetal risk for decompression sickness during this activity.

8. **b.** Women who engage in moderate aerobic exercise regularly during pregnancy may derive significant physical and mental health benefits. To date there appears to be little or no risk for adverse outcomes such as preterm labor or fetal IUGR, and there is no effect on the risk of preeclampsia. Generally, participation in a wide range of recreational activities appears to be safe during pregnancy and should be encouraged by clinicians.

SUMMARY OF EXERCISE AND PREGNANCY

1. For most patients continuing moderate exercise during pregnancy is desirable and not harmful and should be encouraged by the physician. However, there are some limitations.
2. The ACOG consensus is that absolute contraindications for exercise during pregnancy include a history of incompetent cervix or cerclage, placenta previa after 26 weeks of gestation, persistent second- or third-trimester bleeding, hemodynamically significant heart disease, restrictive lung disease, multiple gestations at risk for premature

labor, ruptured membranes, and preeclampsia/eclampsia.

3. The AGOG consensus is that relative contraindications for exercise during pregnancy include severe anemia, chronic bronchitis, unevaluated maternal arrhythmia, poorly controlled type 1 diabetes, morbid obesity, extreme underweight (body mass index of <12), history of sedentary lifestyle, IUGR, poorly controlled hypertension, orthopedic limitations, poorly controlled seizure disorder or hyperthyroidism, and heavy smoking.
4. Controlled trials have found water aerobics reduces the discomfort of low back pain in many patients. Contrary to many "old wives' tales" immersion in water has not been shown to have any adverse affects.
5. Symptomatic reasons for discontinuing exercise in pregnancy include vaginal bleeding, dyspnea prior to exercise, dizziness, headache, chest pain, muscle weakness, unilateral calf or leg swelling (thrombophlebitis should be ruled out), preterm labor, decreased fetal movement, and amniotic fluid leakage.
6. Although, in general, participation in a wide range of recreational activities during pregnancy is safe and may provide significant physical and mental health benefits and should be encouraged by clinicians, the patient's health status and types of exercise should be evaluated before prescribing an exercise program. Participation in any sports involving abdominal contact should be discouraged as should scuba diving. Scuba diving increases the fetal risk for decompression sickness.

SUGGESTED READING

ACOG Committee Obstetric Practice: ACOG Committee opinion, No. 267, January 2002: exercise during pregnancy and the postpartum period. *Obstet Gynecol* 99:171-173, 2002.

Clapp JF: Exercise during pregnancy. A clinical update. *Clin Sports Med* 19:273-286, 2000.

De Ver Dye T, et al: Recent studies in the epidemiologic assessment of physical activity, fetal growth, and preterm delivery: a narrative review. *Clin Obstet Gynecol* 46(2):415-422, 2003.

Kramer MS: Aerobic exercise for women during pregnancy. Cochrane Pregnancy and Childbirth Group. *Cochrane Database Syst Rev* 3, 2003.

Young G, Jewell D: Interventions for preventing and treating pelvic and back pain in pregnancy. Cochrane Pregnancy and Childbirth Group *Cochrane Database Syst Rev* 3, 2003.

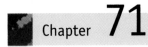

Chapter 71

Gestational Diabetes and Shoulder Dystocia

> "Twelve pounds—that is a big baby and it was vaginal."

CLINICAL CASE PROBLEM 1:

23-Year-Old Woman with Family History of Diabetes

The patient is a 23-year-old woman whose family has a history of diabetes mellitus. She is presently 28 weeks of gestation.

■ **SELECT THE BEST ANSWER TO THE FOLLOWING QUESTIONS:**

1. Which of the following statements concerning gestational diabetes screening is correct?
   a. the U.S. Preventive Task Force (USPSTF) states that there is insufficient evidence to recommend for or against routine screening for gestational diabetes (I recommendation)
   b. the USPSTF strongly recommends that clinicians routinely provide screening to eligible patients (A recommendation)
   c. the USPSTF recommends that clinicians routinely provide screening to eligible patients (B recommendation)
   d. the USPSTF makes no recommendation for or against routine provision of gestational diabetes screening (C recommendation)
   e. the USPSTF recommends against routinely providing screening to asymptomatic patients (D recommendation)

2. Which of the following is (are) NOT a major risk factor(s) for gestational diabetes mellitus (GDM)?
   a. family history of diabetes
   b. history of GDM in a previous pregnancy
   c. increased pregravid body mass index (BMI)
   d. young maternal age
   e. advanced maternal age

3. Which of the following populations is most at risk for developing GDM?
   a. Asian women
   b. Hispanic women
   c. Anglo American women
   d. Russian women
   e. Australian women

4. Which of the following statements in regard to the 50-g 1-hour glucose challenge test (GCT) done on your patient at 28 weeks is considered true?
   a. half of those with an abnormal GCT also will have a positive 100-g 3-hour oral glucose tolerance test (OGTT)
   b. a threshold of 140 mg/dL detects 90% of those with gestational diabetes when followed by a 100-g 3-hour OGTT
   c. false-negative 50-g GCT is rare (less than 2%)
   d. a venous plasma glucose cutoff of 130 mg/dL detects more than 90% of all women with a positive 100-g 3-hour OGTT
   e. all the above choices are true

5. Your patient has a positive 50-g 1-hour GCT, and her 100-g 3-hour OGTT is also positive. Which of the following are considered risk factors for macrosomia besides her GDM?
   a. primigravida status
   b. her weight gain of 30 lb
   c. her BMI of 25
   d. her gestational age of 42 weeks
   e. her height of 5 feet 2 inches

6. Which of the following statements regarding gestational diabetes is true?
   a. the 50-g GCT can only be given to a person who is fasting
   b. women with previous infants of birthweights greater than 9 lb are at decreased risk of gestational diabetes
   c. metformin therapy is approved by the U.S. Food and Drug Administration for treatment of gestational diabetes
   d. insulin therapy should begin when a woman's fasting blood sugar is greater than 105 mg/dL after medical nutrition therapy has been tried
   e. insulin therapy is indicated only when fasting blood sugar levels exceed 140 mg/dL

7. Which of the following is NOT considered a complication of fetal macrosomia?
   a. third- and fourth-degree maternal lacerations
   b. shoulder dystocia
   c. facial nerve injury
   d. increased rate of cesarean delivery
   e. postpartum hemorrhage

8. Of the following, which is the LEAST accurate predictor of macrosomia?
   a. multiparous mother's estimate of fetal weight
   b. ultrasound assessment of fetal weight
   c. clinician's Leopold maneuver
   d. choices a and c have an equivalent predictive value, which is less than that of choice b
   e. not any of the above has any predictive value

Your patient goes into labor at 40 weeks of gestation, gradually increasing to fully dilated. She then pushes for 3 hours until you elect to do a vacuum extraction because of maternal exhaustion. You notice immediate "turtling" of the infants head.

9. The following are appropriate steps in using a vacuum extractor EXCEPT:
   a. applying cup over the sagittal suture 3 cm in front of the posterior fontanelle
   b. applying continuous pressure against the vacuum until it disengages three times
   c. halting the procedure if there is no progress in three consecutive pulls
   d. releasing the vacuum when the jaw is reachable
   e. not any of the above are appropriate steps

10. Which of the following is considered an appropriate measure at this time?
    a. performing slow gradual infant nasopharyngeal suctioning
    b. requesting the nurse to do fundal pressure
    c. performing the Zavanelli procedure (replacing the infant into the uterine cavity)
    d. requesting the nurses do maternal external rotation and flexion at the hip (McRobert's maneuver)
    e. immediately going to the nurse's station to phone the ob-gyn backup

11. Elements of the Wood's screw maneuver include all except which of the following:
    a. rotating the infant's head in a counterclockwise fashion
    b. applying pressure against the posterior portion of the anterior shoulder, pressing the infant's arm closer to his chest
    c. applying pressure on the anterior portion of the posterior shoulder in an attempt to rotate the infant 180 degrees.
    d. rocking the infant's shoulder from side to side by pushing on the mother's lower abdomen
    e. pushing the posterior shoulder back up into the pelvis slightly

12. Which of the following is true regarding the incidence of shoulder dystocia?
    a. 22% of infants weighing 4000-4500 g will have shoulder dystocia
    b. more than 50% of shoulder dystocia cases occur in normal-weight infants
    c. 5% of infants weighing 2500-4000 g will have shoulder dystocia

   d. elective cesarean delivery is considered the delivery method of choice in infants who have an estimated fetal weight of more than 3800 g
   e. all of the above are true

CLINICAL CASE MANAGEMENT PROBLEM

1. Name at least four risk factors for developing gestational diabetes.
2. Name at least four abnormalities that maternal gestational diabetes puts the fetus at greater risk of developing.

ANSWERS:

1. a. The most current available literature for and against routine screening for gestational diabetes shows that there is insufficient evidence. The USPSTF gives it an I rating. The USPSTF rates their final recommendation for screening tests as A, B, C, D, or I. A recommendations mean that the USPTF found good evidence that screening improves important health outcomes and concludes that benefits substantially outweigh potential harm. B recommendation states that the USPSTF found at least fair evidence that screening improves important health outcomes and concludes that benefits outweigh potential harm. C recommendation states that the USPSTF make no recommendation for or against routine screening because the balance of benefits and harm is too close to justify a general recommendation. D recommendation states that the USPTF recommends against routinely providing the service to asymptomatic patients because there is fair evidence that the screening is ineffective or that the potential harm outweighs the benefits. An I recommendation means there is insufficient evidence to make a recommendation for or against screening.

2. d. According to the USPTF, all of the listed choices except young maternal age are major risk factors for developing GDM.

3. b. The prevalence of GDM varies in direct proportion to the prevalence of type 2 diabetes in a given population or ethnic group. GDM is more common among African American, Hispanic, and American Indian women.

4. d. There is still a great deal of confusion and debate about what is or should be considered a "positive" 1-hour GCT. Lowering the threshold of what is considered positive increases the false-positive rate. A threshold of 140 mg/dL detects only 80% of those with gestational diabetes. A threshold of 130 mg/dL detects more than 90% of those with a positive 100-g 3-hour OGTT but significantly increases the false-positive rate. The reliability of GCT is questionable for one-third of women who eventually are identified as having GDM, and even screening performed on 2 successive days often produces different results. As with all screening, the question arises as to whether screening makes a difference in outcomes, and to date the evidence in this regard is mixed.

5. **d.** Of choices provided, only her prolonged gestation and her GDM are considered risk factors for macrosomia. Other risk factors include impaired glucose tolerance, multiparity, previous macrosomic infant, maternal obesity, excessive weight gain, prolonged second stage, parental stature, male infant, and need for labor augmentation.

6. **d.** Some women with GDM may be able to control their disease by strict dietary management and glucose testing four times a day. If the woman's fasting glucose frequently is higher than 105, insulin therapy should be initiated. A 50-g GCT can be done nonfasting, and women with infants greater than 4500 g are at an increased risk of gestational diabetes. Metformin is not recommended in pregnancy.

7. **e.** Postpartum hemorrhage is not considered a common complication of fetal macrosomia, although it may occur independently as a result of a prolonged second stage. Other complications of macrosomia include brachial plexus injury and asphyxia.

8. **b.** The average weight variance for Leopold's maneuvers is 300 g (11.6 oz). The average weight variance for ultrasound is 300-550 g (11.6-19.2 oz). In a study of multiparous mothers' estimations of fetal weight, clinician's clinical estimates, and ultrasound, the ultrasound estimation was the least accurate of the three methods.

9. **b.** The traction should be halted between contractions, at which time the pressure should be released from the vacuum as well.

10. **d.** In the case of shoulder dystocia, following known protocols decrease potential morbidity and mortality of both infant and mother. Most hospitals have a set procedure for calling emergency backup. Optimally, this should involve nursing staff calling the backup physician. Because time is of the essence, gradual suctioning should be abandoned. Suprapubic, not fundal, pressure should be applied by an experienced staff person. Fundal pressure is more likely to continue jamming the obstructing shoulder into the suprapubis. The Zavanelli procedure should be avoided unless episiotomy has been done. The McRoberts' maneuver, the Wood's screw, removal of the posterior shoulder, and getting a woman onto a hands and knees position are procedures that have been successful.

11. **a.** All of the choices listed except rotating the infant's head is considered part of the Wood's screw maneuver. This maneuver allows the infants' shoulders to be delivered much like turning a threaded screw. If the shoulder is extremely impacted, it may be necessary to push either the anterior or posterior shoulder back up into the pelvis to accomplish the maneuver. Rotating the infant's head is ineffective and may increase the likelihood of brachial nerve palsy.

12. **b.** The majority of cases of shoulder dystocia occur in normal-weight infants. Elective cesarean delivery of infants with macrosomia is not considered the delivery method of choice. To prevent one case of permanent brachial plexus injury, 3700 women with infants with macrosomia would have to undergo elective cesarean delivery at a cost of $8.7 million per case prevented. Only 5% to 7% of infants weighing 4000-4500 g will have shoulder dystocia; the risk of shoulder dystocia in infants weighing 2500-4000 g is 0.3%.

SOLUTION TO THE CLINICAL CASE MANAGEMENT PROBLEM

1. Risk factors for developing gestational diabetes include obesity, a family history of type 2 diabetes, maternal age older than 35 years, and a previous history of gestational diabetes.

2. Fetal risks that are increased in gestational diabetes include fetal macrosomia, IUGR, spontaneous abortion, neural tube defects, skeletal abnormalities, gastrointestinal malformations, and cardiac malformations.

SUMMARY OF GESTATIONAL DIABETES AND SHOULDER DYSTOCIA

1. Gestational diabetes is a common condition in pregnancy with known risk factors: obesity, family history of type 2 diabetes, maternal age older than 35 years, and a previous history of gestational diabetes.
2. Presently, the USPTF states that there is insufficient evidence to screen all women for gestational hypertension in pregnancy.
3. The cutoff value for the 50-g GCT is considered controversial, with some practitioners using 130 mg/dL and others using 140 mg/dL.
4. Those with positive 3-hour GTT need to undergo strict dietary management and learn to monitor their own blood sugars four times a day. Insulin management usually is suggested for those with fasting blood sugars of more than 105 mg/dL.
5. The risk factors for shoulder dystocia include macrosomia, prolonged second stage of labor, prolonged first stage of labor, prior shoulder dystocia, high pregnancy weight and weight gain,

gestational diabetes, and an instrument-assisted delivery.
6. In a shoulder dystocia, it is wise to call for extra assistance (optimally prior to delivery), consider an episiotomy, and have your assistants help the patient with a McRobert's maneuver. Other measures to assist the delivery may include having the assistant apply suprapubic pressure, doing the Wood's screw maneuver, removing the infant's posterior arm, or having the patient roll onto a hands and knees position.

SUGGESTED READING

Baxley EG, Gobbo RW: Shoulder dystocia. *Am Fam Phys* 69(7): 1707-1714, 2004.
Gherman RB: Shoulder dystocia: an evidence-based evaluation of the obstetric nightmare. *Clin Obstet Gynecol* 45(2):345-362, 2002.
Norwitz ER, et al: Shoulder dystocia. In Gabbe SG: *Obstetrics—normal and problem pregnancies,* 4th ed. Churchill Livingstone, 2002, Philadelphia.
U.S. Preventive Services Task Force: Screening for gestational diabetes mellitus: Recommendation and rationale. *Am Fam Phys* 68(2): 331-335, 2003.
Zamorski MA, Biggs WS: Management of suspected macrosomia. *Am Fam Phys* 63:302-306, 2001.

Chapter **72**

Hypertension in Pregnancy

"Will the lid blow off?"

CLINICAL CASE PROBLEM 1:

A 35-Year-Old Primigravida with Hypertension

A 35-year-old pregnant woman (gravida 2, para 1) comes into the office for her 32-week prenatal appointment. Her blood pressure is 140/94 when taken by your nurse and is confirmed by your own measurement. She has no protein in her urine and has no headaches, blurred vision, nausea, or vomiting. The rest of the examination is consistent with dates; there is no lower-extremity edema.

■ SELECT THE BEST ANSWER TO THE FOLLOWING QUESTIONS:

1. Her diagnosis is:
   a. chronic hypertension
   b. preeclampsia/eclampsia
   c. gestational hypertension
   d. labile hypertension
   e. none of the above

2. The appropriate course of action to evaluate her elevated blood pressure includes:
   a. blood clotting studies, lactic acid dehydrogenase level
   b. starting her taking an angiotensin converting enzyme (ACE) inhibitor
   c. starting her taking Aldomet (methyldopa)
   d. inducing her labor immediately
   e. watchful waiting

On her return visit at 33 weeks, her blood pressure is now 150/94, and she has 2+ proteinuria. She had a headache yesterday, accompanied by nausea.

3. The labs that you would order include all of the following EXCEPT:
   a. serum uric acid
   b. hemoglobin and hematocrit
   c. 24-hour urine for protein
   d. serum creatinine
   e. serum magnesium level

4. Appropriate indications for induction of labor in this patient include having:
   a. preeclampsia, which is an indication by itself
   b. a "kick count" of 20
   c. a biophysical profile of 10

d. persistent severe headaches

e. a protein count of 300 mg/24 hours noted on her first urine collection last week

5. Fetal indications for delivery of this patient's baby include all the following EXCEPT:
a. signs of intrauterine growth restriction
b. suspected abruptio placentae
c. oligohydramnios
d. an amniotic fluid index of 10
e. fetus being at 40 weeks of gestation.

6. Treatment of acute severe hypertension (sustained blood pressures higher than 160 systolic and 105 diastolic) in pregnancy include the following EXCEPT:
a. labetalol (Normodyne) 20 mg
b. Nifedipine (Procardia) 10 mg orally
c. hydralazine (Apresoline) 5 mg intravenously (IV)
d. hydralazine (Apresoline) 10 mg IM (intramuscular)
e. methyldopa (Aldomet) 250 mg orally

7. The patient complains of a severe headache during labor, her blood pressure climbs to 150/100, and she now has 3+ protein on a urine sample collected by the nurse. The most appropriate treatment for your patient at this time would be:
a. labetalol (Normodyne) 20 mg IV
b. magnesium sulfate 2-g loading dose and then run at 1 g/hour
c. magnesium sulfate 4-g loading dose and then run at 2 g/hour
d. hydralazine (Apresoline) 10 mg IM
e. immediate cesarean delivery

8. Which of the following statements regarding eclampsia is true?
a. eclampsia should be treated with intravenous diazepam
b. eclampsia may occur with a diastolic blood pressure less than 90
c. eclamptic seizures frequently occur during the delivery
d. phenytoin may be administered intravenously to a patient having a preeclamptic seizure
e. none of the above are true

9. Which one of the following intrapartum conditions is associated with preeclampsia/eclampsia?
a. postpartum hemorrhage
b. postdates pregnancy with induction
c. maternal hyperglycemia
d. prolonged first stage of labor
e. venous thromboembolism

10. All of the following are criteria for hemolysis, elevated liver enzymes, low platelet count (HELLP) syndrome EXCEPT:
a. lactate dehydrogenase greater than 600 IU/L
b. aspartate aminotransferase (AST or SGOT) greater than 70 IU/L
c. abnormal peripheral blood smear
d. platelet count less than 150,000
e. increased alkaline phosphatase

11. The patient delivers vaginally. The following are considered steps to use in the active management of the third stage of labor EXCEPT:
a. administration of a uterine tonic prior to delivery of the infant
b. administration of a uterine tonic prior to delivery of the placenta
c. relatively rapid cord clamping and cutting
d. application of controlled traction to the cord
e. all of the above are steps to use in the active management of her labor

12. Risk factors for postpartum hemorrhage include:
a. prolonged first stage
b. multipara
c. large babies
d. assisted delivery (vacuum/forceps)
e. all of the above are risk factors for postpartum hemorrhage

CLINICAL CASE MANAGEMENT PROBLEM

How is pregnancy-induced hypertension distinguished from preeclampsia and preeclampsia distinguished from eclampsia?

ANSWERS:

1. **c.** Chronic hypertension is a blood pressure higher than 140/90 presenting before 20 weeks of gestation. Preeclampsia/eclampsia has associated proteinuria. Gestational hypertension is defined as elevated blood pressure without proteinuria in the second half of pregnancy.

2. **e.** The patient described has no protein in her urine and therefore does not have preeclampsia. ACE inhibitors are contraindicated in pregnancy. Most clinicians start methyldopa if the patient's blood pressures are consistently higher than 150 systolic and 100-110 diastolic and if there are signs of end-organ damage. She is not considered a candidate for immediate induction. Watchful waiting, including seeing the patient back within a week or less, is the most that is indicated at this time.

3. e. The routine labs for preeclampsia include a serum uric acid, hemoglobin, hematocrit, and platelet count; a 24-hour urine test for protein; and a serum creatinine level. Serum magnesium level is useful to monitor a patient who is taking magnesium sulfate for her preeclampsia but is not considered part of the early evaluation process.

4. d. Indications for delivery of a patient with preeclampsia include the following: favorable cervix at term, platelet count<100×10^3 per μL, progressive deterioration in liver or kidney function, suspected abruptio placentae, persistent severe headache or visual changes, and persistent severe epigastric pain with nausea and vomiting. Fetal indications for delivery include being at term, signs of intrauterine growth restriction, abruptio placentae, and oligohydramnios.

5. d. See Answer 4.

6. e. Although methyldopa is the drug of choice for chronic hypertension, its use is not recommended in the acute situation; it takes too long to become effective, is not as strong as other medications, and dosing and titration is not as flexible as other available drugs. The other agents listed in the question are considered drugs of choice for the pregnant patient with acutely severe hypertension. In addition, nitroprusside (Nipride) can be used if the other medications have failed. Nitroprusside should not be used for more than 4 hours and should be started at a dose of 0.25 mg/kg/min and titrated up to a maximum of 5 mg/kg/min.

7. c. At this point, the patient has preeclampsia. The definition of preeclampsia is as follows: blood pressure elevated higher than 140/90, proteinuria exceeding 300 mg/24 hours or a concentration of 0.1 g/L (dipstick 1+) in at least two random urine specimens collected 6 hours or more apart. Patients with blood pressures 160/110 or greater should be treated with an antiepileptic medication as well as an antihypertensive medication. The appropriate loading dose of

magnesium sulfate is 4 g, followed by a 2-4 g/hour infusion.

8. b. Of eclamptic seizures, 20% occur in patients whose diastolic blood pressure is less than 90. Diazepam and phenytoin should not be administered to a patient having a seizure. Eclampsia most frequently occurs before a delivery (79%) or within the first 24 hours after a delivery (29%) but rarely occurs during the delivery itself.

9. a. Of all the conditions listed, only postpartum hemorrhage is an associated intrapartum complication of preeclampsia.

10. e. All of the answers listed except increased alkaline phosphatase are part of the criteria of HELLP syndrome. If the platelet count is less than 50,000 per mm³, or active bleeding occurs, fibrinogen, fibrin split products, prothrombin, and partial thromboplastin times should be checked to rule out disseminated intravascular coagulation. Alkaline phosphatase is elevated in normal pregnancies.

11. a. According to studies reviewed by the Cochran Collaboration, active management of the third stage of labor decreases maternal blood loss, decreases the rate of postpartum hemorrhages more than 500 mL, and decreases the rate of a prolonged third stage of labor (Category A recommendation). Administration of a uterine tonic should be performed prior to delivery of the placenta, not prior to delivery of the infant. Delivery of the infant is the end of the second stage of labor.

12. d. Postpartum hemorrhage is classically defined as blood loss of more than 500 mL in the first 24 hours postdelivery. Clinically, it may be defined as blood loss sufficient to cause hemodynamic instability. Risk factors for postpartum hemorrhage include preeclampsia, nulliparity, multiple gestation, previous postpartum hemorrhage, previous cesarean delivery, prolonged third stage, mediolateral or midline episiotomy, arrest of descent, augmented labor, and assisted delivery. Lacerations of the cervix, vagina, or perineum also may cause a postpartum hemorrhage.

SOLUTION TO THE CLINICAL CASE MANAGEMENT PROBLEM

Hypertension, preeclampsia, and eclampsia all are marked by systolic pressure greater than 140 mm Hg and diastolic pressure greater than 90 mm Hg. Pregnancy-induced hypertension can occur anytime, but preeclampsia generally occurs after the fifth month and eclampsia occurs

near term. Moreover, proteinuria and edema accompany preeclampsia and eclampsia but are not found in pregnancy-induced hypertension. Eclampsia is distinguished from preeclampsia by the onset of seizures not attributable to other causes.

SUMMARY OF HYPERTENSION IN PREGNANCY

1. **Definitions:** Chronic hypertension = blood pressure higher than 140/90 presenting before 20 weeks of gestation. Gestational hypertension = elevated blood pressure without proteinuria in the second half of pregnancy. Preeclampsia/eclampsia = elevated blood pressure plus proteinuria. See Solution to the Clinical Case Management Problem box.

2. **Treatment of choice for chronic hypertension in pregnancy:** Methyldopa as first line; calcium channel blockers also are used.

3. **Treatment of severe acute hypertension in pregnancy:** Acceptable treatments for acute severe hypertension (sustained blood pressures higher than 160 systolic and 105 diastolic) in pregnancy include: labetalol, hydralazine IV or IM, or Procardia.

4. **Preeclampsia:** Blood pressure higher than 140/90, and proteinuria exceeding 300 mg/24 hours or a concentration of 0.1 g/L (dipstick 1+) in at least two random urine specimens collected 6 hours or more apart. Patients with blood pressure 160/110 or greater should be treated with an antiepileptic as well as an antihypertensive medication. The appropriate loading dose of magnesium sulfate is 4 g, followed by a 2-4 g/hour infusion.

5. **Indications for delivery of a patient with preeclampsia include the following:** Favorable cervix at term, platelet count of less than 100×10^3 per µL, progressive deterioration in liver or kidney function, suspected abruption placentae, persistent severe headache or visual changes, and persistent severe epigastric pain with nausea and vomiting. Fetal indications for delivery include being at term, signs of intrauterine growth restriction, abruptio placentae, and oligohydramnios.

6. **HELLP (hemolysis, elevated liver enzyme, low protelet count) syndrome:** If the platelet count is less than 50,000 per mm³, or active bleeding occurs, fibrinogen, fibrin split products, prothrombin, and partial thromboplastin times should be checked to rule out disseminated intravascular coagulation.

7. **Eclampsia:** 20% of seizures occur in patients with diastolic blood pressure of less than 90. Eclampsia most frequently occurs before a delivery (79%) or within 24 hours after a delivery (29%). It rarely occurs during the delivery itself.

SUGGESTED READING

Anderson J, et al: Postpartum hemorrhage: third stage emergency. In: *Advanced Life Saving In Obstetrics.* American Academy of Family Physicians, 2000, Leawood, KS.

Duley L, Henderson-Smart DJ: Drugs for treatment of very high blood pressure during pregnancy. *Cochrane Database Syst Rev* (4):CD001449, 2002.

Fontaine P, Sabourin ME: Medical complications of pregnancy. In *Advanced Life Saving in Obstetrics.* American Academy of Family Physicians, 2000, Leawood, KS.

Nothnagle, M, Taylor JS: Should active management of the third stage of labor be routine? *Am Fam Physician* 67:2119-2120, 2003.

Sibai BM: Diagnosis and management of gestational hypertension and preeclampsia. *Obstet Gynecol* 102(1):181-192, 2003.

Zamorski MA, Greene LA: NHBPEP report of high blood pressure in pregnancy: a summary for family physicians. *Am Fam Physician* 64:263-270, 273-274, 2001.

Chapter 73

Intrauterine Growth Restriction

"Is it too small or is it only immature?"

CLINICAL CASE PROBLEM 1:

A 36-Year-Old Multigravida with a Uterus Too Small for Dates

A 36-year-old female (gravida 4, para 2, aborta 1) is seeing you for the first time at 34 weeks of gestation. She recently moved to your area and was receiving prenatal care with another physician before her move. She brought a copy of her previous prenatal records with her.

She has noticed decreased fetal movements for the past 2 days. She states pregnancy has been complicated by chronic hypertension, and her previous prenatal visit blood pressure readings have been in the vicinity of 150/90 mm Hg.

On examination, her blood pressure is 155/95 mm Hg, and she has three+ pitting edema. Her fundal height is 29 cm. The presentation of the fetus is cephalic, and the fetal heart rate (FHR) is 125 bpm (beats per minute).

■ SELECT THE BEST ANSWER TO THE FOLLOWING QUESTIONS:

1. Which of the following would be of most help at this point in arriving at a working diagnosis with this pregnancy?
   a. take a repeat blood pressure after 5 minutes of left lateral rest
   b. confirm gestational age from a first-trimester ultrasound report

c. perform a nonstress test (NST)
d. perform a contraction stress test (CST)
e. check a spot urine sample for degree of proteinuria

2. Assume that a first-trimester ultrasound was performed that did confirm her current gestational age to be 34 weeks. What is the most appropriate next step in management?
   a. perform an amniocentesis for fetal lung maturity studies
   b. hospitalize the patient on the maternity unit for observation
   c. perform an obstetric ultrasound for fetal measurements
   d. perform an immediate cesarean delivery for fetal indications
   e. send the patient home for bed rest

3. An ultrasound shows the composite of fetal measurements is 30 weeks of gestation. Which of the following statements regarding the decreased fetal growth do you know is true for sure?
   a. the fetus is small for gestational age (SGA)
   b. the fetus has suffered brain damage
   c. the fetus has a congenital infection
   d. the fetus is constitutionally small
   e. the fetus has abnormal chromosomes

4. The fetal measurements by ultrasound showed head measurements appropriate for 33 weeks of gestation but abdominal circumference at 27 weeks of gestation. Which of the following causes for SGA would be most consistent with these findings?
   a. maternal smoking
   b. congenital rubella infection
   c. maternal lead exposure
   d. monosomy X (Turner's syndrome)
   e. maternal chronic hypertension

5. What is the leading cause of perinatal death in infants with intrauterine growth restriction (IUGR)?
   a. intrauterine asphyxia
   b. preeclampsia in the mother
   c. diabetes in the mother
   d. meconium aspiration
   e. none of the above

6. What is the single most preventable cause of IUGR in pregnancy?
   a. maternal hyperglycemia
   b. maternal malnutrition
   c. maternal cigarette smoking
   d. maternal hypertension
   e. maternal illicit drug abuse

7. What is the most common maternal disease causing IUGR?
   a. maternal hypertension
   b. maternal anemia
   c. maternal renal disease
   d. maternal inflammatory bowel disease
   e. maternal valvular heart disease

8. What is the most important screening clinical modality for a fetus with possible IUGR?
   a. inadequate maternal weight gain
   b. inadequate fundal height growth
   c. maternal hypertension
   d. maternal fetal risk status
   e. none of the above

9. IUGR is associated with which of the following neonatal conditions?
   a. hypothermia
   b. hypoglycemia
   c. hypothyroidism
   d. a and b
   e. a, b, and c

10. Which of the following statements concerning fetal alcohol syndrome is (are) false?
    a. fetal alcohol syndrome will lead to symmetric IUGR
    b. fetal alcohol syndrome is not seen when maternal intake is limited to 1 to 2 drinks a day
    c. the prevalence of fetal alcohol syndrome is extremely high in many parts of the United States
    d. all of the above are false
    e. none of the above are false

11. Which of the following statements regarding cigarette smoking in pregnancy is false?
    a. impairment of fetal growth is directly related to the number of cigarettes smoked
    b. smoking is associated with preterm birth, placenta previa, and placenta abruptio
    c. presenting the fetal hazards of cigarette smoking to a pregnant woman almost always causes her to quit
    d. cigarette smoking produces symmetric IUGR
    e. none of the above are false

12. Which of the following maternal drugs poses the greatest danger in terms of fetal growth restriction and other fetal and newborn problems?
    a. phenytoin
    b. digoxin
    c. prednisone
    d. selective serotonin reuptake inhibitors
    e. acetaminophen

13. Which of the following antepartum fetal testing methods offers the most specific evaluation of fetal jeopardy?
    a. fetal movement charts
    b. biophysical profile (BPP) testing
    c. CST
    d. NST
    e. none of the above

14. Which of the following parameters define(s) a reactive NST?
    a. the absence of late decelerations
    b. the absence of variable decelerations
    c. the absence of early decelerations
    d. all of the above
    e. none of the above

15. Which of the following parameters define(s) a positive CST?
    a. the presence of late decelerations
    b. the presence of variable decelerations
    c. the presence of early decelerations
    d. all of the above
    e. none of the above

16. Which of the following is (are) components of BPP testing?
    a. gross fetal movements
    b. fetal breathing movements
    c. fetal tone
    d. amniotic fluid volume and amniotic fluid pockets
    e. all of the above

17. Of the components of the BPP, which is the best predictor of fetal outcome with IUGR?
    a. gross fetal movements
    b. fetal breathing movements
    c. fetal tone
    d. reactive NST
    e. amniotic fluid volume

18. The presence of decelerations on an electronic fetal monitor strip during labor is variably important depending on the type of deceleration in relation to its occurrence relative to the uterine contraction. Each type of deceleration conveys a certain interpretation or a certain meaning. Which of the following pairs of deceleration type and deceleration meaning is (are) correct?
    a. early deceleration = head compression
    b. variable deceleration = cord compression
    c. late deceleration = fetal distress
    d. all of the above are correct
    e. none of the above are correct

CLINICAL CASE MANAGEMENT PROBLEM

The terminology related to decreased growth of the fetus in utero is confusing. There are two basic nomenclatures: the SGA nomenclature and the asymmetric/symmetric IUGR nomenclature. Define these two nomenclatures, and select the one considered most appropriate.

ANSWERS:

1. **b.** In this case the discrepancy in assumed gestational age and fundal height is greater than 3 cm. After 20 weeks of gestation the fundal height in centimeters and the gestational age in weeks should approximate each other. This appears to be a case of fundal height less than dates. To make that assumption, however, it is important that the dates be accurate. A first-trimester ultrasound measurement of the fetal crown–rump length is accurate to within +/– 5 days. If the patient's records reveal an early ultrasound, the results would be most helpful in identifying if this uterus is truly small for dates. Repeating the blood pressure measurement would be helpful in confirming the hypertension, but because her blood pressure is not significantly higher than it was previously, this would not give us a diagnosis. Performing an NST or a CST would assess fetal well-being but would not assess if the fundus is truly too small for dates. Assessing proteinuria would assess maternal well-being but would not confirm suspicions of being small for dates.

2. **c.** The early ultrasound provides a benchmark from which the adequacy of fetal growth can be assessed. An ultrasound at this time will allow you to assess if appropriate fetal growth has taken place since then. A fundus that appears to be smaller than dates can be the result of examiner measurement error, particularly if the patient is obese. However, if the fundus is truly too small for dates, possible causes could be decreased amniotic fluid (oligohydramnios) or decreased fetal size The acronym IUGR, formerly stood for "intrauterine growth *retardation*" but now has been replaced with "intrauterine growth *restriction*." The change in terminology came about because these small fetuses are not retarded.

3. **a.** Fetuses in the less than 10th percentile are considered to be SGA. Infants who are SGA are associated with higher rates of mortality and morbidity for their gestational ages but do better than infants with the same weight delivered at earlier gestational ages. Infants who are SGA can be divided

into two groups: those with a decreased growth potential and those with a normal potential for growth but who are prevented from reaching it because of decreased nutrition and oxygen transmission across the placenta. Although it is possible for the small fetus to have brain damage, to suffer from a congenital infection, to be constitutionally small, or to have abnormal chromosomes, the only fact we know for sure is that it is SGA.

4. **e.** Disproportionately small fetuses who are SGA (wasting of the torso while preserving the brain) are described as having *asymmetric* IUGR, whereas proportionately small fetuses who are SGA (the torso and brain are both small) are described as having *symmetric* IUGR. The fetus described in Question 4 falls into the former category. Asymmetric IUGR has been associated with fetuses that have normal growth potential that is decreased by maternal factors such as maternal hypertension, chronic renal disease, small-vessel disease, or severe malnutrition. Symmetric IUGR has been associated with fetuses that have decreased growth potential as a result of abnormal chromosomes, intrauterine infections, teratogens, anatomic anomalies, and toxins.

5. **a.** The leading cause of perinatal death in IUGR is intrauterine asphyxia. Diminished placental function resulting from factors such as cigarette smoking, diminished perfusion, placental infarction, and intrauterine infection is the most common causative factor in IUGR. The fetus with IUGR is at risk for in utero complications including hypoxia and metabolic acidosis, which may occur at any time but are particularly likely to occur during labor.

6. **c.** Cigarette smoking is the single most common preventable cause of IUGR in North America today. Cigarette smoking is more common among women of childbearing age than is alcoholism or illicit drug abuse. Birthweight is reduced by an average of 200 g in infants of mothers who smoke. The amount of reduction is related to the number of cigarettes smoked per day. Infants of mothers who smoke are also shorter in length, and there is a greater risk of perinatal death or compromise in labor.

7. **a.** Hypertension is the single most common maternal disease causing IUGR in pregnancy. Hypertension results in decreased blood flow through the spiral arteries of the placenta, resulting in decreased delivery of oxygen and nutrients to the placenta and to the fetus. Hypertension also may be associated with placental infarction. Other maternal diseases associated with IUGR include maternal anemia, severe maternal malnutrition, maternal renal disease, mater-

nal malabsorption, multiple pregnancy, extrauterine pregnancy, and maternal valvular disease. The common factor in each of these diseases is interference with uptake or delivery of nutrients or oxygen to the fetus.

8. **b.** Maternal weight gain, maternal blood pressure, maternal risk status, and especially a history of a previous fetus with IUGR are all very important with respect to fetal IUGR. However, the most important screening clinical modality is a series of carefully performed fundal height measurements throughout gestation. A tape, calibrated in centimeters, is applied over the abdominal curvature from the top of the symphysis to the top of the uterine fundus. Between 18 and 30 weeks the measurement should be within 2 to 3 cm from the gestational age in weeks.

9. **d.** Fetuses with IUGR must be observed carefully during the first few hours of life. A blood sugar level should be drawn immediately, and the infant should be wrapped in layers of blankets or placed under a warming light. These maneuvers are necessary because babies with IUGR are very prone to both hypoglycemia and hypothermia. Hypothyroidism is not increased in neonates with IUGR.

10. **b.** Fetal alcohol syndrome has a high prevalence in some areas of the United States. Prevalence rates in some populations are up to 50% of all children born. Fetal alcohol syndrome leads to symmetric IUGR. Contrary to public opinion, no amount of alcohol is a safe amount of alcohol for a pregnant woman. The prevalence of fetal alcohol syndrome in pregnant women who have an average of 1 to 2 drinks a day may be as high as 10%.

11. **c.** Cigarette smoking and its dangers increase proportionally with the number of cigarettes smoked. Cigarette smoking produces symmetric IUGR. Cigarette smoking also is associated with many other abnormal conditions in pregnancy including placenta abruptio, placenta previa, and preterm labor. It is difficult to get pregnant women to quit smoking, although success rates are greater than among nonpregnant women. If a woman does stop smoking in pregnancy, she is very likely to start again following the end of pregnancy. The most common response, when pregnant women are told of the risks to their babies, is as follows: "It won't happen to me."

12. **a.** Certain anticonvulsant medications, especially phenytoin and trimethadione, may produce specific and characteristic syndromes that include symmetric IUGR and fetal anomalies. The other medication options in this question are not associated with fetal growth problems.

13. b. The purpose of antepartum fetal assessment is to identify potential fetal compromise early enough to allow successful intervention and to avoid morbidity and mortality. The specificity of any test modality is its ability to exclude normal results. Not all antepartum fetal tests have the same specificity. The most specific fetal test is the BPP, with 70% specificity. When the BPP is low, 70% of the time the fetus truly is compromised. The other options have the following specificities: CST = 50%, NST = 20%, and fetal movement charting = 20%.

14. e. An NST is based on the assumption that FHR accelerations are associated with fetal movements after 30 weeks of gestation and indicate a normally functioning uteroplacental unit. An NST is evaluated on the presence or absence of FHR accelerations. A FHR acceleration peaks at least 15 bpm higher than the baseline and lasts at least 15 seconds from baseline to baseline. An NST is considered *reactive* (or reassuring) if there are at least two accelerations within a 20-minute period, with or without fetal movements discernible by the mother. An NST is considered *nonreactive* if there are insufficient FHR accelerations after observing for a 40-minute period. Lack of FHR accelerations can occur with any of the following: gestational age less than 30 weeks, fetal sleep cycles, fetal central nervous system anomaly, fetal sedation by maternal medications, or fetal hypoxia (in a minority of cases). If the NST is nonreactive without explanation, a vibroacoustic stimulation should be administered. A healthy fetus will move extremities and accelerate his or her heart rate in response to sound and vibratory stimulation directed through the maternal abdominal and uterine walls.

A criterion for NST evaluation is independent of uterine decelerations.

15. a. A CST is based on the assumption that uterine contractions diminish the flow of oxygenated intervillous blood to the fetus. A fetus with adequate metabolic reserve can cope satisfactorily with transient oxygen deprivation (i.e., FHR remains at stable baseline through contractions, whereas a compromised fetus will show late decelerations [FHR decelerations persisting after a contraction]). A CST is evaluated on the presence or absence of repetitive late decelerations. If they are present with three consecutive contractions in 10 minutes, the CST is positive. This is not reassuring. If late decelerations are absent, the CST is negative, which is reassuring regarding fetal status.

16. e. The BPP has five components: the NST, fetal breathing movements, fetal gross body movements, fetal tone, and amniotic fluid volume. Each of these five parameters is assigned a maximum value of two points. Thus a perfect BPP is 10/10. BPP scores of 8/10 or 10/10 are reassuring of fetal well-being. These fetuses are at low risk for chronic fetal hypoxia or asphyxia. Scores of 4/10 or 6/10 are concerning. These fetuses should be delivered if they are near term, otherwise the BPP should be repeated within 24 hours. Scores of 0/10 or 2/10 are ominous. These fetuses should be delivered expeditiously regardless of gestational age.

17. e. The best predictor of fetal outcome with IUGR is the ultrasonographic evaluation of amniotic fluid volume. The finding of a single vertical pocket of amniotic fluid measuring 3 cm or more is reassuring. If the vertical fluid pocket is less than 3 cm, the perinatal mortality increases significantly.

18. d. The definition and significance of FHR decelerations during labor are as follows:

1. **Early decelerations:**
   a. Deceleration type: early in relation to the onset of the accompanying uterine contraction. They are mirror images of the contractions and are mediated by vagal stimulation.
   b. Response to: head compression by the force of uterine contractions
   c. Significance: are not clinically significant

2. **Variable decelerations:**
   a. Deceleration type: variable in relation to the onset of the accompanying uterine contraction. They are characterized by a sudden decrease in heart rate with a sudden return to baseline.
   b. Response to: umbilical cord compression by fetal movement or uterine contractions
   c. Significance: mild to moderate variable decelerations are not clinically significant. Severe variable decelerations (prolonged, repetitive, and deep) are not reassuring. Severe variable decelerations meet the "rule of 60s": last longer than 60 seconds, drop to lower than 60 bpm, or drop 60 bpm below the baseline.

3. **Late decelerations:**
   a. Deceleration type: late in relation to the onset of the accompanying uterine contraction. They are characterized by gradual decreases in FHR with a gradual return after the end of the contraction.
   b. Response to: uteroplacental insufficiency
   c. Significance: they are never reassuring, especially if they are associated with decreased variability or tachycardia. They tend to be less dramatic on the recording paper and actually can be missed if the recording paper is not turned to a vertical position to read the strip. If persistent, late decelerations necessitate immediate intervention to correct the fetal hypoxia or asphyxia.

SOLUTION TO THE CLINICAL CASE MANAGEMENT PROBLEM

A. The SGA nomenclature

Definition: A fetus or neonate who is SGA is defined as one below the 10th percentile of the mean for a given population.

Problems with this definition: definition of the 10th percentile depends on many factors. Many reference tables use standards derived from a Denver, Colorado, population. Because Denver is at an elevation of 5000 feet, babies born in that city tend to be smaller than babies born at sea level. The birthweight considered to be in the 10th percentile at 5000 feet is less than the birthweight considered to be in the 10th percentile at sea level. Although all infants who are growth-restricted are SGA, not all infants who are SGA are growth-restricted. Of infants who are growth-restricted, 10% are small because of constitutional factors in the mother. These latter factors include maternal ethnic group, maternal parity, maternal weight, and maternal height.

B. The fetus with asymmetric IUGR versus the fetus with symmetric IUGR

Definition: The definition of asymmetric versus symmetric defines the relationship between the size of the fetal head versus the size of the rest of the fetal body.

Explanation of the definition: *Asymmetric IUGR* refers to fetuses with normal growth potential that are prevented from being actualized. Different anatomic sites respond differently to diminishing placental function. Head size is determined by brain size. As placental function diminishes, the fetal brain tends to be spared by preferential shunting of oxygen and nutrients through the foramen ovale and ductus arteriosus, allowing normal head growth. Because placental insufficiency may result in diminished glucose transfer and hepatic storage, fetal abdominal circumference (which reflects liver size) would be reduced. Muscle mass also is reduced, as are subcutaneous tissue fat stores. Asymmetric fetal IUGR is attributed to placental insufficiency resulting from a variety of hypertensive complications of pregnancy and advanced diabetes mellitus with small-vessel disease. *Symmetric IUGR* refers to fetuses with decreased growth potential resulting from a variety of causes that affected the fetus early in pregnancy (e.g., abnormal chromosomes, intrauterine infections, teratogens, anatomic anomalies, and toxins). These causative factors tend to affect all organs equally, including the brain and the liver. Thus fetal body measurements all are decreased.

The terminology of choice: previously, the terminology of choice was *SGA*. Current terminology uses asymmetric or symmetric IUGR because they tend to reflect underlying pathophysiology. However, there is considerable evidence that fetal growth patterns are more complex, and attempts to prenatally classify the cause of IUGR in fetuses is not as clear and precise as previously thought. Although all fetuses with IUGR are also fetuses who are SGA, not all fetuses who are SGA are fetuses with IUGR.

SUMMARY OF INTRAUTERINE GROWTH RESTRICTION

1. **Definitions:** See the Solution to the Clinical Case Management Problem. Current terminology uses two IUGR subtypes: symmetric and asymmetric.
2. **Prevalence:** The true prevalence of IUGR among all pregnant women is estimated at approximately 5%. Not all fetuses who are SGA are restricted in their growth potential.
3. **Differentiation:** The importance of differentiating the various types of IUGR is that it allows you to propose a management plan that is based on the pathologic condition involved. It is especially important, based on the old terminology, to separate normal from abnormal. Using the old terminology, a fetus whose mother was of a particular ethnic group, of a certain parity, of a certain weight, or of a certain height would be considered SGA and the baby probably would be labeled as IUGR when in fact this was not the case.
4. **Risk status:** True babies who are SGA are at extremely high risk for perinatal morbidity and mortality.
5. **Important connections:**
   a. Asymmetric IUGR: most commonly associated with either some form of maternal hypertensive process or collagen vascular process or maternal diabetes mellitus with small-vessel disease.
   b. Symmetric IUGR: most commonly associated with chromosomal abnormalities, cigarette smoking, fetal alcohol syndrome, or intrauterine infections.

6. **Clinical clues and investigations:**
   a. Physical examination and clinical correlates:
   b. Fundal height is less than expected by dates
   c. Failure to achieve adequate maternal weight gain

   Investigations:
   a. Establish whether gestational age is accurate.
   b. Confirm IUGR by obstetric ultrasound fetal measurements.
   c. Identify if IUGR is asymmetric or symmetric.
   d. If risk factors for IUGR are present, deal with them at each prenatal visit (e.g., smoking, drinking alcohol).
   e. An ultrasonographic search for fetal anatomic or chromosomal anomalies should be performed.
   f. Initiate fetal surveillance with a 3-cm amniotic fluid pocket being the best predictor of fetal well-being.

7. **Antepartum management:**
   a. If IUGR is diagnosed before 34 weeks of gestation and amniotic fluid volume and antepartum fetal surveillance is normal, observation usually is recommended. Assess fetal growth by ultrasound every 2-3 weeks. Consultation with a perinatologist is recommended. As long as there is continued growth and fetal evaluation remains normal, conservative management is appropriate. Unfortunately, in many cases neither a precise cause nor a specific therapy is apparent. There is no specific treatment that has been shown to improve perinatal outcome. With evidence of fetal jeopardy on antepartum surveillance, delivery is generally the best option. Again, consultation with a perinatologist is recommended.
   b. If IUGR is diagnosed near term, prompt delivery is likely to afford the best outcome for the fetus. If the diagnosis is uncertain, expectant management with regular fetal surveillance should be followed until fetal lung maturity can be assured.

8. **Intrapartum management:** A trial of vaginal delivery is appropriate in many cases. However, it is important to recognize that if the IUGR is caused by placental insufficiency, the fetus may be unable to tolerate labor. If amniotic fluid is decreased, umbilical cord compression more often is identified. This can be alleviated with amnioinfusion. Emergency cesarean delivery is necessary more frequently.

9. **Postpartum management:** Complications in neonates include hypoglycemia (caused by decreased liver glycogen reserves), hypothermia (caused by decreased subcutaneous tissue), and polycythemia (caused by relative intrauterine hypoxia). If the fetus is hypoxic at birth, meconium aspiration is more likely. Specialized neonatal care often is needed for these babies with IUGR.

SUGGESTED READING

Baschat AA, Harman CR: Antenatal assessment of the growth restricted fetus. *Curr Opin Obstet Gynecol* 13(2):161-168, 2001.

Mongelli M, Gardosi J: Fetal growth. *Curr Opin Obstet Gynecol* 12(2): 111-115, 2000.

Resnik R: Intrauterine growth restriction. *Obstet Gynecol* 99(3):490-496, 2002.

 Chapter **74**

Postpartum Blues, Depression, and Psychoses

"A bundle of joy, so why is mom so sad?"

CLINICAL CASE PROBLEM 1:

A 26-Year-Old Primigravida Who Is Tearful and Depressed 4 Days Postpartum

A 26-year-old primigravida delivers a healthy male infant at 40 weeks of gestation who she breastfeeds on demand. She is doing fairly well until the fourth day postpartum. At that time she develops insomnia, fatigue, and feelings of sadness and depression.

The patient has a history of bipolar disorder, but she has not had an episode of either hypomania or depression for the last 5 years. Despite your concern regarding her history of bipolar disorder, she begins to improve on the eighth day postpartum and returns to her normal mental state at 2 weeks postpartum. When you see her in the office in 6 weeks she is well.

■ SELECT THE BEST ANSWER TO THE FOLLOWING QUESTIONS:

1. What is the most likely diagnosis in this patient?
   a. postpartum depression
   b. postpartum blues

    c. a mild depression, definitely associated with her previous disease
    d. postpartum anxiety
    e. postpartum psychosis

2. What is the best initial choice of treatment for the patient presented in Clinical Case Problem 1?
    a. a tricyclic antidepressant
    b. lithium carbonate
    c. a monoamine oxidase inhibitor (MAOI)
    d. a selective serotonin reuptake inhibitor (SSRI)
    e. supportive psychotherapy alone

3. Considering this patient's history of bipolar disorder, which of the following statements is true?
    a. the probability of a recurrence is no greater after pregnancy than in the nonpregnant state
    b. the probability of a recurrence actually is decreased in the postpartum state
    c. the probability of a recurrence is increased in the postpartum state
    d. none of the above
    e. nobody knows for sure

CLINICAL CASE PROBLEM 2:

A 28-Year-Old Primigravida Who Is Guilt Driven, Tearful, and Depressed

A 28-year-old primigravida delivers a healthy female infant at 39 weeks of gestation. She is well until the fourth postpartum day, when she develops tearfulness, despondency, anorexia, depressed mood, insomnia, and feelings of guilt and inadequacy in coping with her infant. These feelings continue, and she is in marked distress when seen for her 3-week checkup.

4. What is the most likely diagnosis in this patient?
    a. postpartum depression
    b. postpartum blues
    c. adjustment disorder with depressed mood
    d. early bipolar disorder
    e. none of the above

5. What is (are) the treatment(s) of choice for the patient described in Clinical Case Problem 2?
    a. a tricyclic antidepressant
    b. an MAOI
    c. an SSRI
    d. supportive psychotherapy
    e. c and d

CLINICAL CASE PROBLEM 3

A 29-Year-Old Primigravida Who Is Singing

A 29-year-old primigravida is found on the fourth day after cesarean delivery loudly singing hymns at 4 AM in the hospital corridor. During the next 24 hours she causes significant turmoil on the maternity ward. She is found rushing into other patients' rooms announcing that she is about to start classes in "bioenergetics" and urges them to participate. She refuses meals and denies any need to sleep because she is "in touch with the source of superior power." She is hyperactive and talkative and invites her family physician to make love to her.

6. Which of the following statements is (are) true concerning this patient?
    a. this patient has a postpartum psychosis
    b. this patient probably has schizophrenia
    c. this patient most likely has postpartum depression
    d. a and c
    e. b and c

7. What is (are) the greatest risk(s) at this time for this patient?
    a. suicide
    b. infanticide
    c. homicide
    d. degeneration into a more or less permanent paranoid state
    e. a and b

8. Which of the following is the initial treatment of choice for this patient?
    a. intensive observation alone
    b. lithium carbonate
    c. antipsychotic medication
    d. an SSRI
    e. diazepam

9. Which of the following statements regarding the effects of maternal depression in older children is (are) true?
    a. behavioral problems are more common in children whose mothers have had a postpartum depression
    b. significant emotional problems may occur in children whose mothers have an episode of depression in the first postpartum year
    c. there is a significant correlation between reading difficulties in children and depression in their mothers
    d. all of the above are true
    e. none of the above are true

10. What is the single most important risk factor for the development of a postpartum depression?
    a. a history of depression
    b. a history of bipolar disorder
    c. a greater-than-average postpartum decrease in the serum progesterone level

d. a recent stressful life event

e. the mother's experience as a child in her family of origin

---

CLINICAL CASE MANAGEMENT PROBLEM

The relationship between the patient and her physician makes a significant difference when considering the probability that postpartum depression will develop, the early and successful recognition of mood disturbances in the postpartum period, and the successful treatment of same. This will decrease the length and severity of those mood disturbances. Provide specific suggestions to accomplish this goal.

ANSWERS:

1. b. This patient has postpartum blues, the common name for mild depressive symptoms that occur during this period. Postpartum blues occur in about 50% to 80% of puerperal women. The syndrome is transitory, resolving spontaneously within a few days to 2 weeks. Postpartum blues usually starts with a brief period of weeping on the third or fourth day after delivery and peaks between the fifth and tenth day after delivery. Symptoms include anxiety, headaches, poor concentration, and confusion.

The cause of postpartum blues is unknown, but a hormonal basis is suspected. Of the hormones involved, the most likely candidate is progesterone, and the most likely alteration is progesterone deficiency.

2. e. The treatment of choice for postpartum blues includes supportive psychotherapy; family (especially spousal) support, understanding, and reassurance; and patient education (reassuring the patient that this is completely normal). In the patient described, it is especially important to reinforce that there is no connection between the postpartum blues now experienced and her previous bipolar illness; resolution of "the blues" will occur within 2 weeks, but monitoring her condition is necessary to ensure both maternal and fetal health.

3. c. In a patient with a history of bipolar disorder there is actually an increased chance of reoccurrence in the postpartum period.

Of the 50% to 80% of women who develop postpartum blues, only 10% will go on to have a true *postpartum depression,* the common term for a major depressive disorder with postpartum onset.

4. a. This patient has a true postpartum depression because she has a major depressive episode lasting more than 2 weeks. Postpartum depression, as dis-

cussed previously, occurs in approximately 13% of women. In postpartum depression, in contradistinction to postpartum blues, the patient is disabled for a period of time greater than 2 weeks. The major symptoms are a depressed mood, a real concern about the ability to cope with the new infant, and increased guilt. Other symptoms include tearfulness, despondency, worrying about not loving the baby enough, worrying about doing something "irrational" to the baby, anxiety regarding feeding the baby, fear about the baby's sleep, fear about older siblings' jealousy, hypochondriac symptoms, irritability, impaired concentration, poor memory, and extreme fatigue.

Multiple risk factors for postpartum depression have been suggested and include the following: (1) hormonal deficiency, namely progesterone; (2) family history of depression; (3) the conduct and stress of the labor itself; (4) history of inadequate nurturing in childhood; (5) lack of an intimate confiding relationship with her partner; (6) inadequate commitment of the father to the whole process of pregnancy, labor, and delivery; and (7) concurrent presence of stressful life events including family crises, bereavement, change in housing, financial problems, and caring for her other children.

5. e. The treatment of choice for postpartum depression is a combination of supportive psychotherapy and antidepressants. SSRIs are usually the antidepressant medications of first choice because they are safer and have fewer potentially serious side effects than do tricyclic antidepressants or MAOIs. SSRIs also are started at lower doses because postpartum women are often sensitive to their side effects. In mothers who are breastfeeding, the SSRI sertraline is recommended as first-line treatment on the basis of studies that suggest that this agent may be used with little risk. The best psychotherapeutic strategy appears to involve the health care professionals (doctor, public health nurse, psychiatric nurse), the patient's immediate family (especially a supportive partner), supportive friends and relatives, and group psychotherapy (where postpartum women with this condition compare their experiences).

6. a. This patient has a postpartum psychosis. Postpartum psychoses occur in 1 to 2 per 1000 postpartum women. The presentation may be dominated by bizarre, persecutory, or grandiose delusions or thought disorganization. Manic symptoms also may be present.

Postpartum psychosis may occur as an exacerbation of preexisting bipolar disorder, major depressive disorder, or schizophrenia. When such history is absent, the diagnosis is often brief psychotic disorder with postpartum onset.

This patient is having a hypomanic episode. She is likely to have had a personal or family history of mood disorder.

7. **e.** A patient with postpartum psychosis is at risk for suicide and infanticide. In one study, 5% of patients committed suicide and 4% of patients committed infanticide.

8. **c.** Acute treatment for this patient consists of administering an antipsychotic drug to control psychosis and agitation. A high-potency antipsychotic medication such as risperidone might be a good first choice. At the same time, the patient should be observed closely by hospital staff.

Depending on the presence of an underlying psychiatric disorder or of persistent mood symptoms, antidepressant or mood-stabilizing medication may be initiated after acute control of the psychotic behavior. Additionally, supportive individual and family psychotherapy should be given. Once the psychotic episode is resolved, long-term therapy should be started. After discharge it is prudent to arrange regular visits by a mental health worker to measure general day-to-day coping skills immediately postpartum and for an extended time.

9. **d.** Enduring postpartum depression may have subtle effects on the older children of the mother. Behavioral and emotional problems and learning difficulties may develop as a result of postpartum or chronic maternal depression.

10. **d.** Of all the factors discussed previously, the single most important risk factor for the development of postpartum depression is a recent stressful life event.

 ## SOLUTION TO THE CLINICAL CASE MANAGEMENT PROBLEM

Specific suggestions to alter the course of postpartum mood disturbances in your patients should include the following:

1. Encouraging the attendance of the husband or significant other at prenatal visits.
2. Questioning the couple about prenatal education received concerning mood changes in pregnancy, during labor, and after pregnancy.
3. Providing patient education materials on specific mood disturbances.
4. Emphasizing the importance of the husband or significant other in all aspects of the pregnancy, labor and delivery, puerperium, and care of the new family member.
5. Discussing with both members of the couple the social and emotional joys and challenges of childbirth.
6. Describing all tests, all examination procedures, the reason(s) for all routine questions, and any deviation from normal protocol that may occur during pregnancy.
7. Discussing all of the uncomfortable physiologically based problems of pregnancy (edema, heartburn, ligament relaxation, hemorrhoids, and so on) that might be expected.
8. Providing clear instructions to the couple regarding when to call you and when to go to the hospital and reassuring the couple that you "would rather receive a call than not receive a call."
9. Making at least one visit to the patient during early labor.
10. Explaining every possible intervention during labor and the reason(s) for same (such as artificial rupture of the membranes, internal fetal monitoring, and augmentation of labor).
11. Encouraging the patient at every opportunity during labor and delivery.
12. Assessing the patient immediately postpartum and monitoring her condition carefully. Pay particular attention to a patient history of bipolar disorder or major depressive disorder, a family history of depression or any other significant psychiatric disease, and a patient who is going through or recently has gone through a major life stressor.

SUMMARY OF POSTPARTUM BLUES, DEPRESSION, AND PSYCHOSES

1. **Postpartum blues:**
   a. Incidence: 50% to 80%
   b. Evolution: begins on or about the third day postpartum and resolves by 2 weeks
   c. Treatment: reassurance, supportive psychotherapy; involvement of spouse or significant other is critical
2. **Postpartum depression:**
   a. Incidence: 13%
   b. Evolution: begins on the third to fifth day postpartum and lasts longer than 2 weeks
   c. Treatment: psychotherapy and pharmacologic antidepressant therapy
3. **Postpartum psychosis:**
   a. Incidence: 0.1% to 0.2%
   b. Pharmacologic treatment:
      i. Acute: antipsychotic medication, close observation to prevent self-harm and harm to the infant
      ii. Long-term: mood stabilizer if underlying bipolar disorder, manic phase is present; mood stabilizer and antidepressant if bipolar disorder, depressive phase is present; antidepressant if underlying major depressive disorder is present
   c. Psychotherapy: supportive group or individual; involvement of spouse or significant other is critical
4. **Prevention of postpartum psychopathology:**
   a. Education in the prenatal period, which must include significant attention to the psychologic consequences of pregnancy, labor and delivery, and the impact of the neonate on the family.
   b. Explanation of all procedures and interventions to allow the patient as much control as possible during labor.
   c. Significant involvement of the husband or significant other in the process.

SUGGESTED READING

Cooper PJ, et al: Controlled trial of the short- and long-term effect of psychological treatment of post-partum depression. I. Impact on maternal mood. *Br J Psychiatr* 182:412-419, 2003.

Miller LJ: Postpartum depression. *JAMA* 287(6):762-765, 2002.

Wisner KL, et al: Clinical practice. Postpartum depression. *N Engl J Med* 347(3):194-199, 2002.

PSYCHIATRY, BEHAVORIAL SCIENCE, AND COMMUNICATION

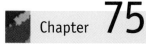 Chapter 75

Depressive Disorders

Keeping the blues from becoming black.

CLINICAL CASE PROBLEM 1:
A 34-Year-Old Female Who Is Tearful and Sad

A 34-year-old female comes to your office in a state of depression. She tells you that she has been "way down" for the past several months and has not felt much like doing anything. For the past 4 months she has been on long-term disability leave. For some 18 months before that, she had been working approximately 75 hours a week, dealing with daily difficulties and conflicts as a business executive. She found work to be increasingly stressful, ultimately compelling her to take a leave of absence.

She expresses her current situation by saying, "I have no joy left in life. I don't enjoy doing anything, even things I really liked before." She sleeps approximately 14 hours a day and constantly feels guilty and hopeless. She complains of a complete loss of energy, decreased ability to concentrate, no appetite (resulting in a 24-lb weight loss), and the inability to "move around" or get anything done.

She is married and has three children. Her marriage is described as "excellent," and her husband is very supportive. She does describe, however, a significant decrease in her sexual interest and activity. Until this time, her health had been excellent, except for a "nervous breakdown" when she was 22 years old. Both her mother and father were alcoholics, but she only drinks on occasion. She takes no drugs. Her physical examination is completely normal.

SELECT THE BEST ANSWER TO THE FOLLOWING QUESTIONS:

1. What is the most likely diagnosis in this patient?
   a. adjustment disorder with depressed mood
   b. generalized anxiety disorder
   c. major depressive disorder (MDD)
   d. mood disorder caused by a general medical condition
   e. dysthymic disorder

2. Which of the following types of psychotherapy generally is considered most effective in the illness previously described?
   a. psychoanalytic psychotherapy
   b. supportive psychotherapy
   c. psychodynamic psychotherapy
   d. cognitive behavioral psychotherapy (CBT)
   e. all of the above

3. The goals of the psychotherapy for this condition include which of the following?
   a. providing a therapeutic rationale or explanation for the patient's symptoms
   b. providing ongoing education regarding the illness, prognosis, and treatment
   c. guiding the patient with respect to interpersonal relationships, work, and major life adjustments
   d. helping to bolster the patient's morale
   e. all of the above

4. What class of drugs most often is used in the disorder described?
   a. selective serotonin reuptake inhibitors (SSRIs)
   b. tricyclic antidepressants (TCAs)
   c. monoamine oxidase inhibitors (MAOIs)
   d. benzodiazepines
   e. lithium carbonate

CLINICAL CASE PROBLEM 2:
A 41-Year-Old Male Who Is Chronically Depressed

A 41-year-old male comes to your office with a 3-year history of a "depressed mood." He states that he feels "depressed most of the time," although there are periods when he feels better. He is chronically tired, has some difficulty concentrating at work, and has found it difficult to remain productive and efficient as middle manager in a major company. He has had no other symptoms. His health is otherwise good. He is not taking any medications.

5. This 41-year-old male most likely suffers from which of the following?
   a. adjustment disorder
   b. dysthymic disorder
   c. MDD
   d. mood disorder caused by a general medical condition
   e. none of the above

6. What is the treatment of choice for the patient in Clinical Case Problem 2?
   a. relaxation therapy
   b. pharmacologic antidepressants
   c. CBT
   d. exercise
   e. b, c, and d

CLINICAL CASE PROBLEM 3:

A 35-Year-Old Female Who Is Distressed at Work

A 35-year-old female comes to your office with a 3-month history of feeling "depressed." She feels "extremely distressed at work" and tells you that she is "burned out." You discover that she moved into a managerial position at work 4 months ago and is having a great deal of difficulty (interpersonal conflict) with two of her employees.

The patient has no history of psychiatric illness. She has no other symptoms. She is not taking any medications.

7. What is the most likely diagnosis in this patient?
   a. adjustment disorder with depressed mood
   b. dysthymic disorder
   c. MDD
   d. mood disorder caused by a general medical condition
   e. burnout

8. What is the treatment of choice for the patient described in Clinical Case Problem 3?
   a. a TCA
   b. an SSRI
   c. supportive psychotherapy
   d. a and c
   e. b and c

CLINICAL CASE PROBLEM 4:

A 45-Year-Old Hard-Driving Male

A 45-year-old male who is a "hard-driving" executive comes to your office with a 4-month history of feelings of sadness, irritability, loss of appetite, inability to concentrate, and a significantly decreased ability to function in his job. He tells you that he is "completely burned out."

When you question him, he tells you that he has been "using anything and everything possible to try to relax." He has missed a number of days of work recently because he "hasn't felt up to it." He also complains of increasing stomach pains and headaches over the last 2 months.

9. From the history given, what is the most likely diagnosis in this patient?
   a. MDD
   b. dysthymic disorder
   c. mood disorder caused by a general medical condition
   d. substance-induced mood disorder
   e. adjustment disorder with depressed mood

10. What is the treatment of choice for the patient described in Clinical Case Problem 4?
    a. an SSRI
    b. a TCA
    c. an MAOI
    d. lithium carbonate
    e. none of the above

CLINICAL CASE PROBLEM 5:

A 61-Year-Old Retired Male

A 61-year-old male, a patient you have known for 20 years, comes to your office with a 4-month history of depression. He has no previous history of psychiatric illness, nor is there any evidence of psychiatric illness in his family. He also has been feeling extremely fatigued, has lost his appetite, has lost 20 lb, and has begun to experience "stomach pains" diagnosed by an Emergency Room doctor as "irritable bowel syndrome." He retired from his position as an administrative assistant with the Internal Revenue Service 6 months ago, and his symptoms began 2 months after that event.

On examination, the patient fits the criteria for MDD. However, he also has other findings that concern you. He is having many more episodes of the "irritable bowel syndrome" pain than he previously did. He also is experiencing more constipation. On physical examination you find he is mildly jaundiced.

11. On the basis of the information given, which of the following conditions is the most likely possibility in this patient?
    a. MDD
    b. substance-induced mood disorder
    c. adjustment disorder with depressed mood
    d. mood disorder caused by a general medical condition
    e. dysthymia disorder

12. What is the primary treatment for the patient described in Clinical Case Problem 5?
    a. an SSRI
    b. a TCA
    c. an MAOI
    d. lithium carbonate
    e. none of the above

13. As physicians, we need to inform our patients that depression is a disease like any other; it often affects body chemistry, just as diseases such as hypothyroidism, hyperthyroidism, and diabetes mellitus do. Which of the following hypotheses support(s) this argument?
    a. loss of the normal feedback mechanism inhibiting adrenocorticotropic hormone
    b. the lack of normal suppression of blood cortisol following the administration of dexamethasone
    c. the generalized decrease in noradrenergic function in patients who are depressed
    d. a and b
    e. all of the above

14. Which of the following neurotransmitters appears to be the most important mediator of depressive illness in humans?
    a. norepinephrine
    b. acetylcholine
    c. dopamine
    d. serotonin
    e. tryptophan

15. A thorough patient interview is most important in evaluating patients who are depressed. In a patient with depression, which of the following questions is the most important and urgent question to ask?
    a. Is there a family history of psychiatric disorders?
    b. Is there a personal history of previous episodes of depression
    c. Have you had any thoughts of suicide?
    d. Have you had hallucinations?
    e. Have you experienced any delusion?

◢ CLINICAL CASE MANAGEMENT PROBLEM

Discuss a strategy for the pharmacologic management of MDD.

 ANSWERS:

1. **c.** The diagnosis in this patient is MDD. This is based on the presence for at least 2 weeks of a distinct

change in mood (sadness or lack of pleasure) accompanied by changes in appetite and activities including decreased energy, psychomotor agitation or retardation, decreased appetite for food or sex, weight loss, changes in sleep–wake cycles, and depressive rumination or thoughts of suicide. Adjustment disorder with depressed mood is not diagnosed when symptoms are severe enough to be considered MDD.

Generalized anxiety disorder is characterized by excessive worry and nervousness about many problems. Mood disorders caused by general medical conditions are initiated and maintained by physiologic problems.

Dysthymic disorder is characterized by a depressed mood that persists for more than 2 years without the other features of MDD.

The criteria for MDD according to the *Diagnostic and Statistical Manual of Mental Disorders,* 4th ed (DSM-IV) are as follows:

1. The presence of five or more of the following symptoms during the same 2-week period. These must represent a change from previous functioning. At least one of those two symptoms must be either a or b from the following list.
   a. Depressed mood most of the day, nearly every day, as indicated by either subjective report (such as feeling sad or empty) or observation made by others (e.g., appears tearful)
   b. Markedly diminished interest or pleasure in all or almost all activities most of the day, nearly every day (as indicated by either subjective account or observation made by others)
   c. Significant weight loss when not dieting or weight gain (e.g., a change of more than 5% of body weight in a month) or a decrease or increase in appetite nearly every day
   d. Insomnia or hypersomnia nearly every day
   e. Psychomotor agitation or retardation nearly every day (observable by others and not merely subjective feelings of restlessness or being slowed down)
   f. Fatigue or loss of energy nearly every day
   g. Feelings of worthlessness or excessive or inappropriate guilt (which may be delusional) nearly every day (not merely self-reproach or guilt about being sick)
   h. Diminished ability to think or concentrate or indecisiveness nearly every day (either by subjective account or observed by others)
   i. Recurrent thoughts of death (not just fear of dying), recurrent suicidal ideation without a specific plan, a suicide attempt, or a specific plan for committing suicide
2. The symptoms do not meet the criteria for a mixed episode (manic depression).

3. The symptoms cause clinically significant distress or impairment in social, occupational, or other important areas of functioning
4. The symptoms are not caused by direct physiologic effects (such as drug abuse or a medication) or a general medical condition
5. The symptoms are not accounted for by bereavement (after the loss of a loved one); the symptoms persist for longer than 2 months or are characterized by a marked functional impairment, morbid preoccupation with worthlessness, suicidal ideation, psychotic symptoms, or psychomotor retardation

A mnemonic for MDD is SIG-**EM**-CAPS (A diagnosis is made if a patient has 5 out of the 9 following symptoms, which must include **E**nergy/fatigue or **M**ood).

S = **S**leep (hypersomnia or insomnia)
I = **I**nterest (lack of interest in life in general)
G = **G**uilt or hopelessness
E = **E**nergy/fatigue
M = **M**ood (depressed, sadness)
C = **C**oncentration (lack of)
A = **A**ppetite (increased or decreased; weight loss or weight gain)
P = **P**sychomotor (retardation or agitation)
S = **S**uicidal ideation

The other choices in this question are discussed in various other problems in this chapter.

2. d. Most studies suggest that CBT is an effective treatment for depression. CBT helps patients change the way they interpret events and encourages a greater sense of optimism and empowerment. This method of brief psychotherapy was developed over the last two decades by Aaron T. Beck. It is used primarily for the treatment of mild to moderate depression and for patients with low self-esteem. It is a form of behavioral therapy that aims to directly remove symptoms rather than resolving underlying conflicts such as is attempted in psychodynamic psychotherapies. Cognitive behavioral therapists view the patient's conscious thoughts as central to production. Both the content of thoughts and thought processes are seen as distorted in people with such symptoms. Therapy is directed at identifying and altering these cognitive distortions.

3. e. There are a wide range of psychotherapeutic interventions that may be useful in the treatment of mood disorders, particularly depressive mood disorders. The establishment of a therapeutic relationship and instilling hope are crucial in the treatment of the depressed patient. Elements of an effective psychotherapeutic relationship include the following: (1) helping the patient to understand his or her symptoms; (2) providing ongoing education regarding the condition, treatment options, and expected outcomes; (3) helping the patient improve interpersonal relationships and make lifestyle adjustments; (4) getting the patient's commitment to engage in regular exercise; (5) setting realistic goals; and (6) being available in time of crisis.

4. a. The pharmacologic treatment for patients with MDD is most often a member of the class of drugs known as SSRIs. The agents in this class include fluoxetine (Prozac), sertraline (Zoloft), paroxetine (Paxil), fluvoxamine (Luvox), and citalopram (Celexa) or escitalopram (Lexapro). These agents have significantly fewer side effects than older antidepressants. Major side effects may include gastrointestinal distress, decreased libido and inhibited orgasm, tremor, insomnia, somnolence, and dry mouth.

The SSRIs act exactly as they are named; they block the reuptake of serotonin in the brain. Mixed reuptake inhibitors (norepinephrine, 5HT, dopamine) sometimes are used instead of SSRIs and include bupropion (Wellbutrin), venlafaxine (Effexor), nefazodone (Serzone), and mirtazapine (Remeron). TCAs are used less commonly because they exhibit more anticholinergic side effects including dry mouth, urinary retention, constipation, and blurred vision. They are more sedating than most SSRIs and mixed reuptake inhibitors. Other serious significant side effects may include orthostatic hypotension (an alpha-blockade side effect), cardiac conduction abnormalities (an increased risk for patients with second-degree and third-degree heart block or right or left bundle branch block from a quinidinelike action). However, in selected cases, the sedative action of TCAs may be beneficial in the treatment of a patient who is depressed.

Antidepressants all have comparable efficacy overall, but individual patients may respond to some antidepressants but not others. It is impossible to predict with certainty which antidepressant will be effective for a particular patient, so a trial of two or more antidepressants is sometimes necessary. A patient should be switched to a different antidepressant if he or she does not respond after 6 weeks of treatment or if side effects are intolerable. If sexual side effects occur with use of an SSRI, then bupropion, an antidepressant with minimal sexual side effects (decreased libido), often is substituted.

Antidepressants exert multiple effects on central and autonomic nervous system pathways, at least partially by presynaptic blockade of norepinephrine or serotonin reuptake. MAOIs such as phenelzine or tranylcypromine may be effective in treatment of patients resistant to MDD. The most common side effects of this class of drugs are dizziness, orthostatic hypotension, sexual dysfunction, insomnia, and daytime sleepiness. The greatest risk with MAOIs is the occurrence of hypertensive crises, which may be induced by the consumption of large amounts of certain foods (i.e., aged cheese, red wine) or drugs containing sympathetic stimulant activity. MAOIs rarely are prescribed in a primary care setting because side effects and significant interactions with a multitude of other medications are common.

Pharmacologic treatment of MDD is effective in approximately 70% to 75% of cases. Electroconvulsive therapy (ECT) may be useful for individuals who do not respond to antidepressants, have contraindications to antidepressants, or are in immediate danger of committing suicide. Unlike antidepressants, which often take 4-6 weeks to have a full effect, ECT is effective almost immediately. ECT should be prescribed only by a psychiatrist; an appropriate referral is necessary.

5. b. This patient has a dysthymic disorder. Dysthymic disorder is defined as a depressive syndrome in which the patient is bothered all or most of the time by depressive symptoms. These symptoms are not of sufficient severity to warrant a diagnosis of major depressive episode.

Adjustment disorder is generally more time limited and related to a specific stressor. Mood disorders caused by general medical conditions have specific physiologic causes.

6. e. Because of the long history, this patient probably should be treated with a combination approach of exercise, psychotherapy, and pharmacotherapy.

Medications used for this disorder are as described earlier, although agents with more side effects should be avoided. Generally, if medications are used, the lowest effective dose is used, treatment is continued for 6 months, and the patient is reevaluated periodically afterward. Exercise has shown to be effective in the treatment of this disorder and should be strongly encouraged. Psychotherapy (cognitive behavioral psychotherapy as described earlier) is an important component of the treatment of this condition and has been shown to reduce recurrences.

Relaxation therapy is more appropriate for treatment of anxiety than for depression

7. a. This patient has an adjustment disorder with depressed mood, which is defined as a reaction to some identifiable psychosocial stressor(s) that occurs within 3 months of the onset of the depressed mood. The major characteristic of the disorder is an impairment in occupational or social functioning. The severity of the depression is not sufficient to warrant a diagnosis of MDD. Treatment of individuals with adjustment disorder includes counseling about stress management and brief psychotherapy.

Dysthymic disorder is characterized by 2 or more years of chronically depressed mood. Mood disorder caused by a general medical condition is caused by a known pathologic process.

Substance-induced mood disorder is directly caused by a particular substance, commonly alcohol or psychostimulants. Substance-induced mood disorder should be considered in individuals with depressive symptoms, especially those who may be under psychologic stress and using inappropriate coping mechanisms such as the use of alcohol or drugs.

8. c. The treatment of choice for adjustment disorder is brief psychotherapy consisting of counseling and stress management. If the stressful situation cannot be changed, cognitive restructuring, relaxation and other stress management techniques, and exercise are useful for improving the ability to cope with stress. The physician should suggest specific coping strategies with specific goals and objectives negotiated with the patient.

9. d. This patient most likely has a substance-induced mood disorder. The "tip-offs" to this diagnosis in this patient are as follows: (1) symptoms and signs of depression; (2) a self-described "burnout syndrome"; (3) the missing of a number of days of work recently; and (4) the clue of "I am using anything and everything to try to relax."

The sequence of events that likely took place in this patient is as follows. The drive to keep going faster and faster "to stay on the treadmill" eventually led to a depressive disorder and occupational burnout. This was followed by inappropriate "coping mechanisms" including the use of alcohol and/or drugs to keep going. Eventually he reached a point where he was unable to function because of depression, "burnout syndrome," and the number of days missed at work. Therefore his work suffered.

10. e. The steps that should be pursued in this patient's case are as follows: (1) ask the patient about alcohol intake (specific amounts, specific times, and total intake); (2) administer an alcohol abuse questionnaire; (3) involve the patient's family, if possible; (4) if a diagnosis of substance induced mood disorder is confirmed, get the patient's cooperation for initiating treatment; and (5) include an ongoing recovery program, possibly following detoxification. Individual, group, and family psychotherapy is often helpful.

Referral to a 12-step program such as Alcoholics Anonymous is extremely useful for both rehabilitation and relapse prevention.

11. d. This patient most likely has a mood disorder caused by a general medical condition. The differential diagnosis in this case includes a carcinoma of the pancreas, a likely possibility based on the associated symptoms of weight loss and stomach pains and the findings on physical examination.

The psychiatric differential diagnosis in this patient would include adjustment disorder with depressed mood associated with his retirement. The physical signs, however, point away from this.

12. e. The medical diagnosis needs to be confirmed, medical treatment should be initiated if indicated, and emotional support needs to be offered to the patient and the family.

13. e. Depression is associated with significant chemical and morphologic changes in the brain. When patients understand this, it helps to decrease the stigma of the diagnosis and decrease feelings of shame and inadequacy.

14. d. The following physiologic abnormalities have been described in MDD: (1) a "neurotransmitter imbalance" that appears to be caused by a relative deficiency of the neurotransmitter serotonin. (The new SSRIs add confirming evidence to this hypothesis);

(2) patients with MDD have hyperactivity of the hypothalamic–pituitary–adrenal axis, which results in elevated plasma cortisol levels and nonsuppression of cortisol following a dexamethasone suppression test; (3) a blunting of the normally expected increase in plasma growth hormone induced by alpha-2-adrenergic receptor agonists; and (4) a blunting of serotonin-mediated increase in plasma prolactin.

15. c. The single most important question to ask in a patient who presents with signs and symptoms of depression is whether they have contemplated suicide. The following questions are useful in exploring suicidality:

1. "You seem so terribly unhappy. Have you had any thoughts about hurting yourself?"
2. "If you have, have you thought of the means by which you would do it? Have you considered a specific plan for ending your life? Under what circumstances would you carry it out?"
3. "What would it take to stop you (from killing yourself)?"
4. "Do you feel that your situation is hopeless?"

The overall mortality from suicide in individuals with MDD is 15%. Symptoms that place a patient who is depressed at higher risk for suicide are a practical and lethal plan with feelings of hopelessness. Patients must be directly asked about suicidal ideations, and steps must be taken to protect those at high risk. Such steps include making a treatment contract, mobilizing support systems, providing close observation, ensuring immediate availability of a clinician, or placing the patient in the hospital if necessary. Suicidal risk is an acute, not a chronic, problem and has to be handled as a crisis.

SOLUTION TO THE CLINICAL CASE MANAGEMENT PROBLEM

A strategy for the pharmacologic management of MDD is as follows: (1) identify and treat causes unrelated to MDD (such as hypothyroidism or substance abuse); (2) use single-agent pharmacotherapy as the first step; (3) if there is no satisfactory response after 4 to 6 weeks and an increase of the dose does not improve the patient's condition, or if the patient cannot tolerate the first drug, switch to a different drug that minimizes the troublesome side effects or comes from a different

chemical class; and (4) if trials of two or three antidepressants are ineffective, refer to a psychiatrist for possible augmentation or other intense treatments.

A psychiatrist may elect to use ECT if several antidepressant trials in addition to nonpharmacologic treatment options have been ineffective, if there are contraindications to the use of antidepressants, or if there is a high risk of immediate suicide.

SUMMARY OF DEPRESSIVE DISORDERS

A. Prevalence:
1. Major depressive disorder (MDD):
   a. Lifetime prevalence: 3.5% to 5.8% of the population
   b. Gender difference: more common in women than in men
   c. Age: occurs in children, adolescents, adults and the elderly.
2. Dysthymia:
   a. Lifetime prevalence: 2.1% to 4.7%
   b. Gender difference: more common in women than in men
3. Prevalence for depression in medical settings has been reported to be as high as 15%.

B. Differential diagnosis of MDD as described in the DSM-IV criteria: (1) MDD; (2) dysthymia; (3) depression caused by a general medical condition; (4) adjustment disorder with depressed mood; (5) substance-induced mood disorder; (6) manic episodes with irritable mood; and (7) mixed episodes (depression, hypomania).

C. Distinguishing MDD from dysthymia: In addition to depressed mood, there are significant changes in appetite and activities, such as sleep disturbance, weight loss, severe fatigue or lack of energy, and suicidal rumination. Dysthymia is perhaps best described as "a chronic ongoing depressed mood" that lasts years rather than weeks or months.

D. Subclassifications of MDD: Once a diagnosis of depression has been made, the clinician should characterize the syndrome further if possible into the following categories:
1. Unipolar versus bipolar:
   a. MDD is unipolar
   b. Affective disorder is bipolar
2. Melancholic versus nonmelancholic: 40% to 60% of all hospitalizations are for melancholic depression. Symptoms include anhedonia, excessive or inappropriate guilt, early-morning waking, anorexia, psychomotor disturbance, and diurnal variation in mood. The patient who is depressed and melancholy may appear frantic, fearful, agitated, or withdrawn.
3. Psychotic versus nonpsychotic: Psychotic depressions are not rare. Studies suggest that approximately 10% to 25% of patients hospitalized for major depression have a psychotic depression.
4. Atypical depression: Atypical depression denotes symptoms that include hypersomnia instead of insomnia, hyperphagia (sometimes as a carbohydrate craving) rather than anorexia, reactivity (mood changes with environmental circumstances), and a longstanding pattern of interpersonal rejection sensitivity. It is much more common in women. Patients with atypical depression frequently are reported to have an anxious or irritable mood rather than dysphoria.
5. Masked depression: Masked depression is similar to atypical depression. Instead of overt depression, the depression is expressed as many psychosomatic signs and symptoms.

E. Treatment:
1. Follow the guidelines provided in the Solution to the Clinical Case Management Problem.
2. Consider the SSRIs as the drugs of first choice unless specific contraindications to their use are present.
3. Treat for at least 4 weeks before you consider the therapy you are using to be a therapeutic failure.
4. MDD should be treated with a combination of pharmacotherapy, psychotherapy, and exercise.
5. MDD is a recurrent disease: At 1 year following the start of therapy, 33% will be free of the disease, 33% will have had a relapse, and 33% still will be depressed. Using psychotherapy along with pharmacologic treatment significantly reduces the rate of relapse.

F. Three-phase approach to the treatment of depression:
1. Acute treatment phase, phase 1:
   Time = 6-12 weeks
   The goal of this phase of therapy is the remission of symptoms of depression.
2. Continuation treatment, phase 2:
   Time = 4-9 months
   The goal of this phase of therapy is to prevent a relapse of the depressive symptoms.
3. Maintenance treatment, phase 3:
   Time = patient dependent, perhaps lifetime
   The goal of this phase of therapy is to treat patients who have had three or more episodes of depression. Prevention of recurrence is the treatment goal.

Continued

SUMMARY OF DEPRESSIVE DISORDERS—cont'd

Too often medication is tapered or discontinued shortly after symptoms have been brought under control; this greatly increases the patient's risk of relapse. There is no justification for lowering the effective dose of an antidepressant drug during maintenance treatment. Once the patient is asymptomatic for at least 6 months following a depressive episode, recovery from the episode is declared.

The termination of therapy must be accompanied by patient education. The key concern is the likelihood of a recurrent episode. If this is the patient's first bout of depression that needed to be treated, the recurrence rate is approximately 50%. If there have been previous episodes of depression or a family history of depression exists, the probability of a recurrence is increased significantly. The patient must be made aware of the symptoms that indicate another episode and needs to know that subsequent attacks can be treated effectively, especially if therapy is initiated early in the disease.

SUGGESTED READING

American Psychiatric Association: *Diagnostic and statistical manual of mental disorders IV–TR*, 4th ed. American Psychiatric Association Press, 2000, Washington, DC.

Fava GA, et al: Prevention of recurrent depression with cognitive behavioral therapy: preliminary findings. *Arch Gen Psychiatry* 55(9): 816-820, 1998.

Gilbody SM, et al: Educational and organizational interventions to improve the management of depression in primary care: a systematic review. *JAMA* 289(23):3145-3151, 2003.

Gilbody SM, et al: Routinely administered questionnaires for depression and anxiety: systematic review. *BMJ* 322(7283):406-409, 2001.

Glick ID, et al: Psychopharmacologic treatment strategies for depression, bipolar disorder, and schizophrenia. *Ann Intern Med* 134(1):47-60, 2001.

Nease DE Jr, Maloin JM: Depression screening: a practical strategy. *J Fam Pract* 52(2):118-124, 2003.

Preskorn SH: Mood disorders. In Rakel R, ed: *Conn's current therapy*, WB Saunders, 2003, Philadelphia.

Remick RA: Diagnosis and management of depression in primary care: a clinical update and review. *CMAJ* 167(11):1253-1260, 2002.

Richelson E: Pharmacology of antidepressants. *Mayo Clin Proc* 76(5): 511-527, 2001.

Sutherland JE, et al: Achieving the best outcome in treatment of depression. *J Fam Pract* 52(3):201-209, 2003.

Chapter 76

Bipolar Disorder

"Anything you can do, I can do better."

CLINICAL CASE PROBLEM 1:

A 42-Year-Old Computer Science Professor Who Has Just Been Anointed By God as the New Head of the Computer Age

A 42-year-old computer science professor is brought to the Emergency Room by his wife, who complains that for the last 4 weeks her husband has become increasingly irritable, angry, and suspicious. She states: "His personality has completely changed"; "He has not slept for 6 nights and has been found by the local police using his laptop under a lamppost to work on his computer programs."

He has become preoccupied with the belief that God has anointed him as the "new leader of the computer age." Fearing that his ideas will be stolen by interpol, the CIA, the state police, and the "Red Coated Mounties" from Canada, he has constructed an elaborate mathematic code that allows only him and his appointed prophets to understand the programs. He quite proudly states that "Albert Einstein wouldn't have a chance at this. It's even too clever for him!"

His wife further states that the patient has been depressed on and off throughout his life and has been taking "all kinds of junk" for the depression, none of which helped at any time. However, she claims, the patient has never had a substance abuse problem of any kind. She describes her husband's family as "a bunch of nuts." She continues to tell you that, for instance, his mother calls him at 3 o'clock almost every morning (while he is getting his equipment and extension cords set up outside, rooting through the garage, knocking everything over, and waking up the entire neighborhood) just to tell him that she is thinking of him. His father has a history of numerous psychiatric hospitalizations for "weird behavior" and has received several courses of shock therapy.

During the interview the patient volunteers little information, is extremely agitated, and paces the floor. He makes a number of sexual advances toward the nurse who is observing him.

■ SELECT THE BEST ANSWER TO THE FOLLOWING QUESTIONS:

1. Based on the history given, what condition best describes the behavior exhibited in this patient?
   a. acute hypomania

b. acute mania
c. acute anxiety
d. dementia
e. delirium

2. Based on the patient's personal history, the condition applied in Question 1, and the family history described, this is most likely a part of a condition known as which of the following?
   a. bipolar disorder
   b. alcohol intoxication
   c. major depressive disorder (MDD)
   d. schizoid personality disorder
   e. schizophrenia

3. The DSM-IV further subclassifies this into which of the following?
   a. schizophrenia: catatonic type
   b. schizophrenia: paranoid type
   c. bipolar I disorder
   d. bipolar II disorder
   e. atypical insanity

4. At this time, what would you do?
   a. prescribe diazepam and tell his wife that you will review the situation
   b. prescribe lithium carbonate on an outpatient basis and see the patient in 3 months
   c. prescribe fluphenazine on an outpatient basis and see the patient in 1 week
   d. prescribe a tricyclic antidepressant (TCA) on an outpatient basis and see the patient in 1 week
   e. none of the above

5. Your mother has just been told that she has the illness that has just been described. You begin to wonder about the heritability of such a disorder. What is your relative risk of developing the disorder described compared with someone without a first-degree relative with the disease?
   a. half as much
   b. equal to
   c. 24 times as much
   d. twice as much
   e. 3.5 times as much

6. Which of the following statements regarding lithium carbonate in the treatment of the disorder described is (are) true?
   a. lithium carbonate is a drug of choice in the treatment of this disorder
   b. lithium prevents relapses of depressive episodes in this disorder
   c. lithium is not metabolized, and therefore problems related to active metabolites or inactive metabolites do not exist

d. regular blood level monitoring by the family physician or psychiatrist is necessary
e. all of the above

7. Patients with this disorder who are refractory to lithium carbonate could be treated with which of the following?
   a. carbamazepine
   b. L-tryptophan
   c. divalproex
   d. a and c only
   e. a, b, or c

8. Which of the following neurotransmitters is (are) implicated most clearly in the cause of the acute manic or acute hypomanic episodes in bipolar disorder?
   a. norepinephrine
   b. dopamine
   c. serotonin
   d. a and b
   e. all of the above

9. Which of the following best conceptualizes the definition of cyclothymic disorder?
   a. cyclothymic disorder is best described as a less severe form of bipolar disorder
   b. cyclothymic and dysthymic disorders are virtually identical
   c. cyclothymic disorder is a more severe, more chronic form of bipolar disorder
   d. cyclothymic disorder, by definition, has none of the elements of positive family history that characterize bipolar disorder
   e. none of the above are true

10. Which is the pharmacologic treatment of choice for cyclothymic disorder?
    a. a serotonin reuptake inhibitor (SSRI)
    b. a TCA
    c. a monoamine oxidase inhibitor (MAOI)
    d. divalproex
    e. lithium carbonate

11. What is the role of the family physician in the diagnosis and treatment of the condition described?
    a. family physicians routinely diagnose and treat this condition without the help of a psychiatrist
    b. family physicians are not involved in the diagnosis and treatment of this condition
    c. family physicians are in a unique position to diagnose this disease early because often a longitudinal relationship with the patient and the family exists

d. family physicians often are involved during the maintenance phase of treatment
e. c and d

12. Which other conditions can cause mood swings?
   a. thyroid disorders
   b. adrenal disorders
   c. neurologic disorders
   d. substance abuse disorders
   e. all of the above

CLINICAL CASE MANAGEMENT PROBLEM

Describe the basic diagnostic features of bipolar disorder: manic episode and hypomanic episode.

■ ANSWERS:

1. b. The most likely diagnosis in this patient at this time is acute mania. Mania is defined as a distinct period of abnormally and persistently elevated, expansive, or irritable mood. It may include inflated self-esteem or grandiosity, decreased need for sleep, loquaciousness, flight of ideas, distractibility, increase in goal-directed activity, activities such as unrestrained buying sprees, sexual indiscretions, and foolish business investments. These symptoms cause a marked impairment in occupational functioning.

The basic difference between mania and hypomania is that in mania there are often psychotic symptoms and a more severe impairment in normal functioning (social, occupational, etc.). In addition, the mood disturbance is more severe.

With no history of substance abuse problems, memory impairment, or general medical conditions, delirium and dementia are not likely. A diagnosis of acute anxiety does not account for many of the presenting symptoms.

2. a. This episode of acute mania is part of a bipolar disorder. For a diagnosis of bipolar disorder, at least one episode of mania or hypomania has to have occurred. This patient has a history that is very suggestive of previous episodes of major depression, which provides further evidence for a diagnosis of bipolar disorder.

His mother also may have bipolar disorder, indicated by her frequent phone calls at 3 AM. Furthermore, his father obviously had several episodes of major depression that were treated with electroconvulsive therapy.

3. c. DSM-IV subdivides bipolar disorder into two types: bipolar I and bipolar II. Bipolar I disorder identifies a patient who has had at least one true manic episode. A history of depression or hypomania also may be present in the patient with bipolar I disorder, but neither of these conditions is essential for the diagnosis. Patients with bipolar II disorder have a history of hypomania and major depressive episodes but no history of mania.

4. e. Outpatient therapy is usually not possible or safe in patients with acute mania. The treatment of choice at this time is admission to a psychiatric hospital and treatment with an antipsychotic agent such as risperidone, haloperidol, olanzapine, or clozapine until the psychotic symptoms subside. He should be started taking lithium carbonate at the same time. Lithium carbonate is the drug of choice for the treatment of bipolar disorder. It is effective treatment for acute mania and prevents relapses of both manic and depressive episodes in bipolar disorder; hence once the diagnosis has been made it should continue to be used prophylactically. In the treatment of acute mania, it may be 10-14 days before the full therapeutic effect of lithium is felt. Lithium carbonate is not metabolized and therefore does not accumulate active metabolic products. However, because the therapeutic window is very narrow, blood level monitoring is necessary to determine appropriate dosing.

Patients with bipolar disorder who do not respond to lithium carbonate or in whom lithium is contraindicated should be treated with anticonvulsants medications (carbamazepine or divalproex acid). Blood level monitoring is necessary for these agents as well. These anticonvulsants are almost as effective as lithium carbonate in the treatment of bipolar disorder. About 30% of patients with bipolar disorder will not respond to lithium and will have to be treated with other agents.

Benzodiazepines may be occasionally useful for the treatment of severe agitation during a manic episode; however, agents such as lorazepam or clonazepam are preferred.

5. c. First-degree relatives of patients with bipolar illness are reported to be at least 24 times more likely to develop bipolar illness than relatives of control subjects. The genetic evidence is very strong for bipolar disorder. The incidence of bipolar illness and MDD is much higher in first-degree relatives of patients with bipolar illness than in the general population. However, first-degree relatives of patients with MDD only have an increase in the incidence of unipolar depression.

6. **e.** Lithium is the drug of choice in the treatment of this disorder. It prevents relapses of both depressive and manic episode. It is not metabolized, so there are no active or inactive metabolites. As toxicities do occur, blood levels need to be monitored, frequently at first and later every 3 months.

7. **d.** As mentioned earlier, the anticonvulsant agents carbamazepine and divalproex are useful in the treatment of bipolar disorder if lithium is contraindicated or not helpful.

8. **d.** The most relevant pharmacologic information relating to theories of acute mania and acute hypomania is the consistent finding that direct or indirect norepinephrine and dopamine agonists (those drugs that stimulate the noradrenergic and dopaminergic receptors or increase concentrations of these neurotransmitters in the brain) can precipitate mania or hypomania in patients with underlying bipolar illness. Stimulants such as amphetamines and cocaine can induce maniclike syndromes in patients who do not appear to have an underlying vulnerability to develop a bipolar disorder. This suggests an association of mania or hypomania with hyperadrenergic or hyperdopaminergic states.

9. **a.** Cyclothymic disorder is best conceptualized as a less severe form of bipolar illness. The data indicate that approximately 30% of individuals with cyclothymia have a positive family history for bipolar illness. By definition, cyclothymic disorder is a chronic mood disturbance of at least 2 years' duration and involving numerous hypomanic and mild depressive episodes that do not meet the diagnostic criteria for mania or major depression with no periods of euthymia greater than 2 months.

10. **e.** As with bipolar disorder, the treatment of choice is lithium carbonate.

11. **e.** During the acute manic phase described earlier, patients need to be hospitalized and seen by a psychiatrist. The family physician will refer a patient with this condition until he or she is stabilized. During the maintenance phase of treatment, family physicians often resume the care of these patients, including obtaining appropriate drug levels and other blood tests. Family physicians are in a unique position to diagnose the onset of the disease because they often have longitudinal relationships with the whole family; early diagnosis and treatment of this disorder can prevent serious family and occupational disruptions. When patients have become stabilized with appropriate medication, they often are able to lead creative, productive, and satisfying lives with little impairment of social or professional functioning.

12. **e.** Many other conditions can cause mood swings. Abuse of substances such as amphetamines, cocaine and others can be diagnosed by obtaining a drug screen. Thyroid disorders can cause mood swings and are diagnosed by an appropriate physical examination and blood tests. Adrenal disorders such as Addison's disease or Cushing's syndrome; vitamin B_{12} deficiency; and certain neurologic disorders such as multiple sclerosis, brain tumors, epilepsy, or encephalitis can mimic bipolar disorder. Certain infections affecting brain function, especially acquired immune deficiency syndrome, can cause mental states resembling bipolar disorder. A number of medications, including corticosteroids and certain drugs used to treat anxiety, also can cause mood swings and need to be discontinued or their dose needs to be adjusted if these symptoms occur.

SOLUTION TO THE CLINICAL CASE MANAGEMENT PROBLEM

Key features of bipolar disorder as follows:

A. Manic episode:
1. A distinct period of abnormally and persistently elevated, expansive, or irritable mood lasting at least 1 week and of sufficient severity to cause marked impairment in social or occupational functioning.
2. During this period, at least three of the following symptoms also are present: (a) grandiosity; (b) decreased need for sleep; (c) hyperverbal or pressured speech; (d) flight of ideas or racing thoughts; (e) distractibility; (f) increase in goal-directed activity or psychomotor agitation; and (g) excessive involvement in pleasurable activities that have a high potential for painful consequences.
3. There is no evidence of a physical or substance-induced cause or the presence of another major mental disorder to account for the patient's symptoms.

Continued

SOLUTION TO THE CLINICAL CASE MANAGEMENT PROBLEM—cont'd

B. Key features of hypomanic episodes:
1. A distinctly sustained elevated, expansive, or irritable mood lasting for at least 4 days that is clearly different from the individual's nondepressed mood yet does not cause marked impairment in social or occupational functioning such as in acute mania.
2. During the mood disturbance at least three of the following symptoms also are present to a significant degree: (a) inflated self-esteem or grandiosity; (b) decreased need for sleep; (c) more talkative than usual; (d) flight of ideas or racing thoughts; (e) distractibility; (f) increase in goal-directed activity or psychomotor agitation; and (g) excessive involvement in pleasurable activities that have a high potential for painful consequences.
3. The episode is not physical or substance-induced.

SUMMARY OF BIPOLAR DISORDER

A. Prevalence:
1. The prevalence of bipolar disorders varies from 0.7% to 1.6% (lifetime).
2. The prevalence is greater in women than in men.
3. In general medical settings (settings that select for patients with emotional distress and physical illness), the lifetime prevalence rate is probably between 5% and 10%.

B. Classification of bipolar disorders:
1. Bipolar disorder I: a patient with bipolar disorder who has had at least one episode of true mania
2. Bipolar disorder II: a patient with bipolar disorder who has not had at least one episode of true mania
3. Cyclothymic disorder: a less severe form of bipolar disorder

C. Heritability of bipolar disorder:
1. First-degree relatives of patients with bipolar affective disorder are at least 24 times more likely to develop bipolar illness than relatives of control subjects.
2. The incidence of both bipolar illness and MDD is much higher in first-degree relatives of patients with bipolar illness than in the general population.

D. Diagnostic criteria:
1. See diagnostic criteria for acute mania and acute hypomania in the Clinical Case Management Problem.
2. The other mood component of bipolar disorder is depression, which is discussed in Chapter 75.

E. Cyclothymic disorder:
1. Cyclothymic disorder is defined as a less severe form of bipolar disorder. By definition, it is a chronic mood disturbance of at least 2 years' duration and involves numerous hypomanic and mild depressive episodes. These episodes do not meet the diagnostic criteria for bipolar disorder or MDD.
2. In cyclothymic disorder there are no periods of euthymia greater than 2 months' duration.

F. Treatment:
1. Acute treatment: (a) hospitalization for acute mania with psychosis; (b) antipsychotic agents (olanzapine, clozapine, risperidone, haloperidol) when psychosis is present; and (c) benzodiazepines (lorazepam, clonazepam) may be useful for severe agitation during mania.
2. Maintenance and prevention of relapse: (a) lithium carbonate is the agent of first choice (usual dosage is 900-1200 mg/day); (b) anticonvulsive agents (carbamazepine or divalproex) are useful when lithium is ineffective or contraindicated; and (c) other anticonvulsants such as lamotrigine and gabapentin may be used when the previously mentioned agents are ineffective when used alone or in combination.

SUGGESTED READING

American Psychiatric Association: *Diagnostic and statistical manual of mental disorders IV–TR,* 4th ed. American Psychiatric Association Press, 2000, Washington, DC.

Glick ID, et al: Psychopharmacologic treatment strategies for depression, bipolar disorder, and schizophrenia. *Ann Intern Med* 134(1):47-60, 2001.

Kaplan HI, Sadock BJ, eds: *Kaplan and Sadock's synopsis of psychiatry: Behavioral sciences/clinical psychiatry,* ed 8. Williams & Wilkins, 1998, Baltimore.

Thomas MR: Bipolar disorders. In: Jacobson. *Psychiatric secrets,* 2nd ed. Hanley and Belfus, 2001, Philadelphia.

Tomb DA: *Psychiatry,* 6th ed. Williams & Wilkins, 1999, Baltimore.

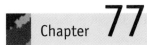

Chapter 77

Diagnosis and Management of Schizophrenia

> "You had better do what I say. I get my orders from the Great Satan himself."

CLINICAL CASE PROBLEM 1:

A 22-YEAR-OLD MALE BROUGHT TO THE EMERGENCY ROOM BY THE PARAMEDICS

A 22-year-old male is brought to the Emergency Room by the paramedics accompanied by his parents. He had begun to cut himself with a sharp knife at home and his father had called 911. The father tells you that this was the last straw. He tells you that his son has been acting very strangely for the past 15 months.

The patient stares straight ahead and refuses to answer any questions. He does, however, ask the nurse if she wants to kneel and kiss his hand. When she declines, the patient replies by saying, "You are the first woman who has refused the invitation to kiss the god of the Milky Way's hand." He points to the door entrance and remarks to the nurse, "You know, I could have you killed by my space soldiers. All it would take is one zap with the green ray gun from one of them." He tells her that he was appointed as the god of the Milky Way 14 months ago when the spaceship first landed in the back yard after having been searching for him for 400 years.

The patient's father tells you that his son essentially has locked himself in his room for the past year. He eats all his meals there. He has some carpentry skills, and he built a large "dinner decontamination center" by knocking out three of the major upstairs walls. This occurred while his father and mother were on vacation. When they do see him, he seems very sad and depressed, and his voice barely can be heard sometimes.

The patient had a job at a fast-food restaurant but was fired 9 months ago when he started to "inject all the hamburgers with a decontamination substance," which turned out to be a thick mixture of pulverized leeches. It was at that point that he locked himself in his room for good. He experienced episodes of major depression as a child. Other significant history includes enuresis, encopresis, and separation anxiety as a child. The father assures you that his son is taking no drugs, prescription or otherwise.

When you ask about family history of psychiatric disorders, alcoholism, or drug use, the father replies that "some quack of a psychiatrist labeled me as an alcoholic, which of course I am not." When you ask the patient's father what he drinks, he replies that he drinks whiskey. When you deliberately overestimate the amount—by asking whether he would have eight or more shots per

day—he replies, "No, of course not, only about four or five. The mental status examination on this patient is difficult to complete because the patient is uncooperative with testing and is mute for prolonged periods. The patient's vitals signs are normal, as is the rest of the physical examination.

■ SELECT THE BEST ANSWER TO THE FOLLOWING QUESTIONS:

1. What is the most likely diagnosis in this patient at this time?
   a. schizoaffective disorder
   b. schizophrenia
   c. schizophreniform disorder
   d. bipolar disorder
   e. delusional disorder

2. Of the following features, which one is most suggestive of the diagnosis?
   a. disorganized speech
   b. delusions
   c. hallucinations
   d. the presence of both positive and negative symptoms
   e. disorganized or catatonic behavior

3. How is the term *delusion* best defined?
   a. a false belief that is fixed and not explainable based on the cultural background of the individual
   b. a disorder of the form of thought
   c. a convincing feeling that one is being persecuted
   d. a convincing feeling that one is being controlled by a supernatural force
   e. the experiencing of stimuli in any of the senses in the absence of external stimulation

4. The differential diagnosis of this disorder described includes which of the following?
   a. bipolar disorder
   b. schizoaffective disorder
   c. delusional disorder
   d. brief psychotic disorder
   e. all of the above

5. How is the term *psychosis* best defined?
   a. behavior marked by a break from reality
   b. behavior marked by a fixed false belief not in keeping with current life situation or circumstance
   c. behavior not in keeping with the current environment in which the individual finds himself or herself

d. behavior marked by the sight of objects that are not present
e. behavior marked by the hearing of sounds that are not present

6. A patient comes to the family physician's office with almost identical symptoms to the patient described in Clinical Case Problem 1. However, the time from the beginning of the illness (the onset of the first symptom) to the termination of all symptoms is only 4 months. What is the most likely diagnosis in this patient?
   a. schizophrenia
   b. schizoaffective disorder
   c. schizophreniform disorder
   d. bipolar disorder
   e. brief psychotic disorder

7. A patient develops acute psychiatric symptoms much like those described in Clinical Case Problem 1 but in whom the symptoms of depression or mania are more prominent than the psychotic symptoms. This patient would most likely have developed which of the following conditions?
   a. schizophrenia
   b. schizoaffective disorder
   c. schizophreniform disorder
   d. bipolar disorder
   e. brief psychotic disorder

8. Disturbances in which of the following pairs of neurotransmitter systems are implicated most clearly in the pathogenesis of the condition described in Clinical Case Problem 1?
   a. serotonin/dopamine
   b. serotonin/norepinephrine
   c. serotonin/gamma-aminobutyric acid (GABA)
   d. acetylcholine/dopamine
   e. acetylcholine/GABA

9. Which of the following drugs is the best choice for the patient presented in Clinical Case Problem 1?
   a. risperidone
   b. clozapine
   c. haloperidol
   d. lithium carbonate
   e. fluoxetine

10. Which of the statements regarding the condition described in Clinical Case Problem 1 is (are) most accurate?
    a. there is a documented genetic component in the cause of the condition
    b. environmental factors affect the expression of the condition

c. lateral ventricular enlargement is common in this condition
d. increased width of the third ventricle is common in this condition
e. all of the above statements are true

11. Which test(s) is (are) indicated in the diagnostic workup of psychosis?
    a. complete blood count (CBC)
    b. a complete chemistry profile
    c. thyroid function tests
    d. a head computed tomography (CT) or magnetic resonance imaging (MRI) scan
    e. all of the above

12. Although schizophrenia is a brain disease and pharmacotherapy is the primary therapy, an approach integrating additional measures has been shown to be superior in preventing relapses. Which of the following nonpharmacologic treatment approaches is (are) appropriate?
    a. motivational interviewing
    b. community-based rehabilitation
    c. cognitive-behavioral therapy (CBT)
    d. family interventions
    e. all of the above

CLINICAL CASE MANAGEMENT PROBLEM

Describe the differential diagnosis of psychosis.

■ ANSWERS:

1. **b.** The most likely diagnosis in this patient is schizophrenia. The following features characterize schizophrenia:
   1. Psychotic symptoms, including at least two of the following symptoms, present for at least 1 month: (a) hallucinations; (b) delusions; (c) disorganized speech (incoherence, evidence of a thought disorder); or (d) disorganized or catatonic behavior
   2. Negative symptoms (flattening of affect, lack of motivation)
   3. Impairment in social or occupational functioning
   4. Duration of the illness for at least 6 months
   5. Symptoms are not primarily a result of a mood disorder or schizoaffective disorder.
   6. Symptoms are not caused by a medical, neurologic, or substance-induced disorder.

2. **d.** The most suggestive symptom of schizophrenia is the presence of both positive and negative symptoms.

Positive symptoms include the psychotic symptoms just described. The dramatic symptoms of hallucinations and delusions are the most reliably recognized symptoms of the illness.

Negative symptoms include the flattening of affect (emotional blunting), apathy, and the lack of motivation. Negative symptoms sometimes are called deficit symptoms.

3. a. A delusion is best defined as a fixed false belief that cannot be explained on the basis of the cultural background of the individual. Delusions are firmly held, pervasive personal beliefs based on incorrect interpretations of external reality despite proof or evidence to the contrary. Delusions can be bizarre, persecutory, somatic, or grandiose and may include ideas of reference.

4. e. The differential diagnosis of schizophrenia includes the following:

1. Delusional disorder: A delusional disorder is a condition in which the patient has a delusion lasting for at least 1 month in the absence of prominent hallucinations or bizarre behaviors.
2. Brief psychotic disorder: A brief psychotic disorder is a disorder characterized by a relatively sudden onset of psychosis that lasts for a few hours to a month with a quick return to normal premorbid functioning thereafter.
3. Schizoaffective disorder: A schizoaffective disorder is a psychotic disorder that is differentiated from schizophrenia by either depressive symptoms or manic symptoms that are prominent and consistent features of a patient's long-term psychotic illness (see Answer 7). In contrast, a schizophreniform disorder is a disorder displaying the signs and symptoms of schizophrenia but lasting less than 6 months (see Answer 6).
4. Bipolar disorder is distinguished from schizophrenia by a history of discreet mood disordered episodes (mania and depression). Psychosis is present only during the mood episodes. During periods of euthymia (normal mood), no psychotic symptoms are present.
5. Psychotic disorder caused by a general medical condition.
6. A substance-induced psychotic disorder: Substances commonly associated with this condition include amphetamines, cocaine, various "designer drugs," and hallucinogens.

5. a. *Psychosis* is a generic descriptive term applied to behavior marked by a break or loss of contact with reality. This often presents as disorganization of mental processes, emotional aberrations, difficulty in interpersonal relationships, and a decrease in func-

tional capacity. In a patient with psychosis, mundane daily responsibilities may become burdensome or impossible to manage.

6. c. A patient with schizophrenialike symptoms that last for a period shorter than 6 months is classified as having schizophreniform disorder. Patients with schizophreniform disorder can be classified into those with or without good prognostic features. Good prognostic features include an acute onset, good premorbid functioning, and the absence of a flat affect. Patients without good prognostic features are more likely to have a condition that persists longer than 6 months. When symptoms persist past this point, the diagnosis is changed to schizophrenia.

7. b. This patient has a schizoaffective disorder. A schizoaffective disorder usually is diagnosed when depressive or manic symptoms are a prominent and consistent feature of a patient's long-term psychotic illness. The diagnosis can be substantiated if the longitudinal course is consistent with schizophrenia and if residual schizophreniclike symptoms persist when the patient is not depressed or manic. If, however, the psychotic symptoms are present only when the patient is depressed or manic and the patient has a relatively good interim functioning between episodes, the patient should be considered to have a primary mood disorder (either a major depressive disorder with psychotic features) or a bipolar disorder.

8. a. The neurochemical basis of schizophrenia is not yet understood. However, medications that blockade some dopamine receptors (D2 and D4) and some serotonin receptors (5-HT$_2$) ameliorate symptoms of the illness. The drugs that stimulate dopamine receptors (such as amphetamines) can produce schizophrenialike symptoms. Drugs that stimulate serotonin receptors such as lysergic acid (LSD) cause hallucinations.

9. a. Risperidone and newer antipsychotic medications, including olanzapine and quetiapine, present advantages over older agents and should be used as drugs of first choice. These medications have minimal or absent extrapyramidal movement side effects and also may be more effective for treatment of negative symptoms of schizophrenia. In addition to blockading dopamine receptors, newer antipsychotic medications blockade serotonin (5-HT$_2$) receptors. Like newer antipsychotic medications, clozapine blockades both dopamine and serotonin receptors, has no movement side effects, and may be effective for negative symptoms of schizophrenia. However, it has a 5% incidence of seizures and a 1% incidence of agranulocytosis. Therefore it is not used as a first-line medication.

10. e. There is considerable evidence that schizophrenia is an illness that runs in some families, although the majority of patients do not have a first-degree relative with the disease. A first-degree relative of an individual with schizophrenia has approximately a 10% risk of developing schizophrenia. There are also unknown environmental factors that influence the expression of schizophrenia.

CT and MRI studies have demonstrated that some patients with schizophrenia have enlarged lateral ventricles, increased width of the third ventricle, and sulcal enlargement suggestive of cortical atrophy.

11. e. Blood tests such as a CBC, a serum chemistry including electrolytes, glucose, blood urea nitrogen, creatinine, calcium, phosphate and liver function tests, thyroid function tests, urinalysis, and a urine toxicology screen are obtained routinely. Sexually transmitted disease screening for syphilis and human immunodeficiency virus infection is strongly recommended. An electrocardiogram will rule out cardiac disorders. Imaging studies such as a CT or MRI of the head are useful in ruling out organic disease.

There are other imaging techniques, including single photon emission computed tomography and positron emission tomography, which can provide information on blood flow and metabolism in the brain but are not done routinely. Blood levels of therapeutic medications are obtained if appropriate.

Occasionally, additional tests, such as sleep-deprived electroencephalogram or lumbar puncture, are indicated.

12. e. Although schizophrenia is categorized as a brain disease, not a psychologic disorder, an approach integrating nonpharmacologic measures with drug therapy has shown to be superior in preventing relapses. Nonpharmacologic treatment approaches that have shown to be successful include the following: (1) motivational interviewing, which strengthens the patient's commitment to change; (2) community-based, long-term rehabilitation programs; (3) CBT, which aims to reduce the influence of delusions and hallucinations and help the patient to adapt more rationally to the demands of the environment; and (4) family interventions that present more realistic expectations for all members and improve interpersonal dynamics. These additional therapeutic modalities also improve adherence with pharmaceutical regimens. However, in the majority of cases patients with schizophrenia do not even receive routine psychiatric care with medication. Their access to primary care and preventive services is often severely curtailed, either because of the patients' social situations or their impaired social and cognitive functioning. Although care coordination services for these patients are imperative, it is rarely available.

SOLUTION TO THE CLINICAL CASE MANAGEMENT PROBLEM

A differential diagnosis of psychosis includes the following: (1) schizophrenia; (2) schizophreniform disorder; (3) schizoaffective disorder; (4) bipolar disorder (manic phase); (5) delusional disorder; (6) brief psychotic disorder; (7) psychotic disorder caused by a general medical condition; and (8) substance-induced psychotic disorder.

SUMMARY OF SCHIZOPHRENIA

1. **Prevalence:** The lifetime incidence of schizophrenia is 1% to 2%. This figure is remarkably stable across racial, cultural, and national dimensions.
2. **Characteristics of psychotic symptoms:** (a) they are nonspecific and occur in a variety of medical, psychiatric, neurologic, and substance-induced disorders; (b) the onset of schizophrenia after the age of 45 years is rare; and (c) as a consequence, first-onset psychosis after the age of 45 generally suggests a neurologic disorder, a medical condition, a substance-induced disorder, or a psychotic depression.

3. Main diagnostic clues to the diagnosis of schizophrenia are positive symptoms and negative symptoms. Positive symptoms include hallucinations, delusions, and bizarre behavior, whereas negative symptoms include emotional blunting, apathy and avolition (lack of purposeful action).

4. **Differential diagnosis of schizophrenia and clues to each one:**
   a. Delusion disorder: A disorder in which a delusion lasts at least 1 month. No other positive symptoms or negative symptoms of schizophrenia are present.
   b. Brief psychotic disorder: A disorder that is characterized by a relatively sudden onset of

psychosis that lasts for a few hours to a month with a return to premorbid functioning thereafter. No other positive or negative symptoms are present.

c. Bipolar I disorder: A disorder in which the psychotic symptoms are present only when the patient is depressed or manic; the patient has relatively good interim functioning between episodes.

d. Major depressive disorder with psychotic features: A disorder in which the psychotic symptoms are present only when the patient is depressed; the patient has relatively good interim functioning between episodes.

e. Schizophreniform disorder: Both the positive and the negative symptoms of schizophrenia are present, but the patient either recovers without residual symptoms within a 6-month period or has symptoms for less than 6 months.

f. Schizoaffective disorder: If a patient has symptoms of depression or mania with psychosis and the depressive or manic symptoms are a prominent and consistent feature of the patient's long-term psychotic illness, schizoaffective disorder is the most likely diagnosis.

g. Psychotic disorder caused by a general medical condition: A disorder that may produce psychotic symptoms include cerebral neoplasms, cerebrovascular disease, epilepsy, thyroid disorders, infections such as acquired immune deficiency syndrome, parathyroid disorders, hypoxia, hypoglycemia, hepatic disorders, renal disorders, and autoimmune disorders.

h. Substance-induced psychotic disorder: This most commonly occurs with amphetamines.

5. **Symptoms and signs of schizophrenia:**
   a. Psychotic symptoms are present for at least 1 month including two of the following: (i) delusions; (ii) disorganized speech (incoherence, evidence of a thought disorder); and (iii) disorganized or catatonic behavior.
   b. Negative symptoms are present (flattened affect, lack of motivation).
   c. There is impairment in social or occupational functioning.
   d. The illness is present for at least 6 months.
   e. Symptoms are not caused by a mood disorder or schizoaffective disorder.
   f. Symptoms are not caused by a medical, neurologic, or substance-induced disorder.

6. **Subtypes of schizophrenia:**
   a. Catatonic: dominated by motor abnormalities such as rigidity and posturing

b. Disorganized: marked by flat affect and disorganized speech and behavior
   c. Paranoid: paranoid symptoms in the absence of catatonic and disorganized features
   d. Undifferentiated: none of the previously listed symptoms predominate
   e. Residual: only negative symptoms or attenuated symptoms remain after an active phase

7. **Causation:**
   a. Schizophrenia is believed to have a pathogenesis that results from an interaction between genetic influences and environmental variables.
   b. There are gross morphologic and cytoarchitectural abnormalities in the brains of some individuals with schizophrenia, but there are no pathognomonic findings. An increased prevalence of perceptual-motor and cognitive abnormalities is described in many studies.

8. **Treatment:**
   a. Active phase includes the following: (i) hospitalization for severely disorganized or dangerous behavior; (ii) antipsychotic medications, with newer antipsychotic medications being the drugs of first choice; and (iii) reassurance and support for both patient and family members.
   b. Chronic phase includes the following: (i) continued antipsychotic medication at the lowest effective dose (often will prevent relapse for long periods) and (ii) psychosocial treatment. Underlying goals are treatment of symptoms, prevention of acute episodes through the management of stress, mobilization of social supports, and assistance with deficits in instrumental living skills caused by the illness. Comprehensive treatment aims to gradually rehabilitate the patient socially and occupationally to the most autonomous level of functioning possible for that individual.

SUGGESTED READING

American Psychiatric Association: *Diagnostic and statistical manual of mental disorders IV–TR*, 4th ed. American Psychiatric Association Press, 2000, Washington, DC.

Bustillo J, et al: The psychosocial treatment of schizophrenia: an update. *Am J Psychiatr* 158(2):163-175, 2001.

Freedman R: Schizophrenia. *N Engl J Med* 349(18):1738-1749, 2003.

Glick ID, et al: Psychopharmacologic treatment strategies for depression, bipolar disorder, and schizophrenia. *Ann Intern Med* 134(1):47-60, 2001.

Nagamoto HT: Schizophrenia and schizoaffective disorders. In: Jacobson: *Psychiatric secrets.* 2nd ed. Hanley and Belfus, 2001, Philadelphia.

Chapter 78

Alcohol Dependence and Alcohol Abuse

"Doc, I'll never be an alcoholic, I have a hollow leg."

CLINICAL CASE PROBLEM 1:

A 45-YEAR-OLD MALE WITH AN ENLARGED LIVER

A 45-year-old executive comes to your office for his periodic health assessment. He tells you that he has been feeling "weak, tired, and just not myself lately." He also tells you that he has been so tired that he "has had to stay home from work for many days at a time." He is beginning to question his ability to function effectively as the chief executive officer of a transportation company. When you inquire about other symptoms, he tells you that he also has suffered from "profound headaches" and that his sex life with his wife is "the pits." On direct questioning he tells you that the headaches "have been a problem for the past 6 months" and his "lack of interest in sex" has been a problem for about the same amount of time.

He has no serious past medical, surgical, or psychiatric illnesses. He tells you that he is taking no over-the-counter or prescription drugs.

The patient describes himself as a "social drinker," and his use of alcohol is "strictly to relax." He then states, "I hope you do not think that I'm an alcoholic, Doc!" There is no evidence of acute intoxication at this time.

He does state, on more persistent questioning, "Well, maybe I am using more alcohol than I did a few years ago. Oh sometimes, I think it might be a good idea to cut down a bit. I do get annoyed with my wife who points out that I am drinking more than I used to. Sometimes I even feel guilty and wonder if that's affecting our sex life. There are mornings that I wake up with the shakes and having an 'eye opener' really helps."

His father died of complications of "yellow jaundice" at age 61. His mother died of complications of heart failure at age 69. He has three brothers and two sisters; all are well.

On physical examination, his blood pressure is 160/104 mm Hg. His pulse is 96 and regular. Examination of the head and neck, respiratory system, and musculoskeletal system are normal. Examination of the cardiovascular system reveals a point of maximum impulse (PMI) in the fifth intercostal space on the anterior axillary line. He subsequently describes recent episodes of "waking up at night short of breath" and "shortness of breath on exertion." Examination of the gastrointestinal system reveals no tenderness or rebound tenderness. The liver edge is palpated approximately 5 cm below the right costal margin. Examination of the neurologic system reveals intermittent carpal spasms of both extremities. He has a fine tremor of his hands. He cannot perform serial 7s and has difficulty with recall of information on the mental status examination.

■ **SELECT THE BEST ANSWER TO THE FOLLOWING QUESTIONS:**

1. With the history given, what is the best description of the most likely diagnosis in this patient?
   a. somatization disorder
   b. adjustment disorder with depressed and anxious mood
   c. major depressive disorder
   d. alcohol dependence
   e. alcohol abuse

2. Which of the following signs or symptoms further substantiate your diagnosis in this patient?
   a. the location of the PMI
   b. the patient's elevated blood pressure
   c. the abdominal signs on physical examination
   d. the hand tremors
   e. all of the above

3. What are signs and symptoms of acute alcohol intoxication?
   a. facial flushing
   b. slurred speech
   c. nystagmus
   d. ataxia
   e. all of the above

4. What is the most likely cause of the patient's liver edge palpated at 5 cm below the right costal margin?
   a. tricornute liver (congenital malformation)
   b. alcoholic hepatitis or cirrhosis
   c. congestive heart failure
   d. "the deep diaphragm pushing the liver down" syndrome
   e. hepatorenal syndrome

5. There is a high correlation between the disorder diagnosed in Question 1 and which of the following syndromes?
   a. generalized anxiety disorder
   b. major depressive disorder
   c. schizophrenia
   d. opioid abuse
   e. all of the above
   f. b and d only

6. The patient's inability to perform serial 7s and information recall is most likely caused by which of the following?

a. Alzheimer's dementia
b. alcoholic dementia
c. alcoholic amnestic syndrome
d. all of the above are equally likely
e. b and c

7. At what amount of blood alcohol level is a driver determined to be "impaired" in most states?
a. 0.02% (20 mg/dl)
b. 0.05% (50 mg/dl)
c. 0.1% (100 mg/dl)
d. 0.5% (500 mg/dl)
e. 1.0% (1000 mg/dl)

8. Regarding risk factors for the condition diagnosed in Question 1, which of the following statements most accurately reflects risk factor status and identification?
a. there are no risk factors for this disease; it just happens
b. there is no single factor that accounts for increased relative and absolute risk in first-degree relatives of patients with this disorder
c. genetic, familial, environmental, occupational, socioeconomic, cultural, personality, life stress, psychiatric comorbidity, biologic, social learning, and behavioral conditioning are all risk factors or risk environments for this disorder
d. there is a clear risk factor stratification for this disorder
e. b and c

9. Which organ systems can be affected by alcohol abuse?
a. cardiovascular system
b. endocrine system
c. pulmonary system
d. hematologic system
e. all of the above

10. Which drug(s) is (are) useful in the treatment of alcohol withdrawal?
a. benzodiazepine
b. clonidine
c. barbiturates
d. anticonvulsants
e. all of the above

11. How is *alcohol withdrawal syndrome* best defined?
a. a state in which a syndrome of drug-specific withdrawal signs and symptoms follows the reduction or cessation of drug use
b. a state in which the physiologic or behavioral effects of a constant dose of a psychoactive substance decreases over time
c. a pathologic state that follows cessation or reduction in the amount of drug used

d. a and b
e. all of the above

12. How is *alcohol abuse syndrome* best defined?
a. a maladaptive state leading to clinically significant impairment
b. a maladaptive state leading to clinically significant distress
c. a maladaptive state leading to significant impairment defined by laboratory value
d. either a or c
e. either a or b

13. Considering the patient described, which of the following diagnostic imaging procedures is (are) definitely indicated?
a. chest x-ray
b. cardiac echocardiogram
c. computed tomography (CT) scan of the head
d. abdominal ultrasound
e. all of the above

14. Which of the following explanations is the most likely explanation for the tremors observed on physical examination?
a. delirium tremens (early)
b. alcohol withdrawal syndrome
c. thiamine deficiency
d. alcoholic encephalopathy (early)
e. Korsakoff's psychosis

15. A 26-year-old male comes to your office for a periodic health examination before he gets married. When you question him about his lifestyle and ask him about his alcohol intake, he replies that he is a "social drinker." Once that is established what should you do?
a. congratulate him on avoiding problems with alcohol
b. accept "social drinking" at face value and move onto the next question
c. ask him whether he ever has a drink while alone
d. ask him to very specifically define social drinking
e. request an estimate of the number of drinks per week and a specification on the kind of alcoholic beverages consumed

CLINICAL CASE PROBLEM 2:

A Patient with Short-Term Memory Deficits

A patient who you suspect of alcohol dependence demonstrates significant short-term memory deficits. He then tries to cover up those deficits by making up answers to questions.

16. Which of the following is the most likely diagnosis?
    a. Wernicke's encephalopathy
    b. alcohol-induced persisting amnestic disorder (Korsakoff's psychosis)
    c. alcohol-induced psychotic disorder with delusions
    d. alcohol-induced psychotic disorder with hallucinosis
    e. alcohol-induced persisting dementia

17. The feature described as "making up answers to questions" is known as which of the following?
    a. confabulation
    b. alcoholic lying
    c. alcoholic delirium
    d. alcoholic paranoia
    e. memory loss encephalopathy

18. What is the cause of the disorder described in Clinical Case Problem 2?
    a. riboflavin deficiency
    b. thiamine deficiency
    c. zinc deficiency
    d. cerebral atrophy caused by alcohol abuse
    e. cerebellar atrophy caused by alcohol abuse

19. The word *alcoholism* means different things to different people. Of the following, which is the best definition of alcoholism?
    a. alcohol abuse and alcohol dependency
    b. alcohol abuse but not alcohol dependency
    c. alcohol abuse or alcohol dependency
    d. alcohol abuse and/or alcohol dependency
    e. none of the above represent an adequate definition of alcoholism

20. What is the percentage of the American population who suffer from alcohol abuse or dependence?
    a. 5%
    b. 10%
    c. 23%
    d. 48%
    e. 75%

CLINICAL CASE MANAGEMENT PROBLEM

Part A: Provide a screening test for alcohol abuse that can be administered easily in the office setting.

Part B: List five objectives for short-term treatment of the patient and the patient's family in a case of alcohol dependence.

ANSWERS:

1. This patient has alcohol dependence, which is defined as at least three of the following occur-ring over a 12-month period: (1) tolerance (the need for increased amounts of a substance to achieve intoxi-cation or another desired effect or markedly diminished effect with use of the same amount of the substance); (2) characteristic withdrawal symptoms or the use of alcohol (or a closely related substitute) to relieve or avoid withdrawal; (3) substance often taken in larger amounts over a longer period than the person intended; (4) persistent desire or one or more unsuccessful attempts to cut down or quit drinking; (5) a great deal of time spent in getting the alcohol, drinking it, or recovering from its effects; (6) important social, occu-pational, or recreational activities are given up or reduced because of the alcohol; and (7) continued alcohol use despite the knowledge of having a persistent or recur-rent social, psychologic, or physical problem that is caused by, or exacerbated by, use of alcohol.

2. e. The physical signs and symptoms actually substantiate the diagnosis of alcohol dependence, not alcohol abuse. Alcohol dependence is defined as a maladaptive pattern of alcohol use with adverse clini-cal consequences. These physical symptoms include the following: (1) the location of the PMI in the fifth intercostal space suggests cardiomegaly, which either could result from alcoholic cardiomyopathy or hyper-tension (most likely also related to alcohol intake); (2) the obvious hepatomegaly suggests alcoholic hepatitis or cirrhosis of the liver; (3) the fine tremor suggests early alcoholic encephalopathy, which is substantiated by the cognitive dysfunction (lack of ability to perform serial 7s); and (4) the patient's hyper-tension suggests alcohol as a potential cause.

3. e. Acute alcohol intoxication is characterized by mood lability, poor judgment, ataxia, slurred speech, decreased concentration and memory, facial flush-ing, blood pressure elevation, enlarged pupils, and nystagmus. Increasing alcohol levels can result in depression of respiration and reflexes and a decrease in blood pressure and body temperature, potentially followed by stupor, coma, and death.

4. b. The most likely cause of the hepatomegaly is alcoholic hepatitis and possibly cirrhosis. Laboratory tests that may be abnormal in alcoholic liver disease include: γ-glutamyltransferase (GGT), alkaline phos-phatase aspartate aminotransferase (AST), and alanine aminotransferase (ALT). An ALT/AST ratio of more than 2 is especially suspicious.

Often, the mean corpuscular volume (MCV) is elevated in patients with chronic heavy alcohol con-sumption. Uric acid levels may be elevated; abnor-malities in the lipid metabolism often are present.

5. e. The National Institute of Mental Health Epidemiologic Catchment Area Program found a very high correlation rate between alcoholism and (1) suicide; (2) homicide; (3) accidents; (4) anxiety disorders; (5) major depressive disorder; (6) schizophrenia; (7) narcotic drug abuse; (8) cocaine abuse; and (9) cigarette smoking.

6. e. Chronic alcohol use is associated with the cognitive and memory deficits of alcoholic dementia and the more restrictive memory deficits of alcohol amnestic disorder. Patients with alcohol-related amnestic syndrome have the most difficulty with short-term memory (remembering recent events). However, deficits may be noted in long-term memory as well.

7. b. Drivers are determined to be "impaired" at levels of 0.05 g% (50 mg/dl) in most states. They are considered to be "under the influence" at levels of 0.1 g% (100 mg/dl). Somebody who does not exhibit signs of intoxication at alcohol levels of 100 mg/dl or higher probably is alcohol dependent because alcohol tolerance is evident.

8. e. Factors that determine an individual's susceptibility to a substance use disorder are not well understood. Studies of populations at risk for developing substance abuse have identified many factors that foster the development and continuance of substance use. Those include genetic, familial, environmental, occupational, socioeconomic, cultural, and personality factors; life stressors; psychiatric comorbidity; biologic and social learning factors; and behavioral conditioning. The concordance rate for alcoholism between fathers and sons and among identical twin pairs is very high. This suggests a strong genetic determination for this disease. Accordingly, family members of alcoholics, especially first-degree relatives, need to be screened and counseled for alcohol dependence/abuse.

9. e. Complications of the cardiovascular system include elevated blood pressures, as mentioned earlier, which usually is reversible with abstinence; alcoholic cardiomyopathy; sinus tachycardia; and arrhythmias. Endocrine complications in men include low testosterone and increased estrogen levels, decreased libido; testicular atrophy; and impotence. Women experience menstrual irregularities and sexual dysfunction. Pulmonary complications include bacterial pneumonias and aspiration pneumonias (when vomiting occurs in intoxicated patients) and increased rates of tuberculosis. Very often, pulmonary complications from smoking are present because 80% to 90% of alcoholics are cigarette smokers. Gastrointestinal complications include gastroesophageal reflux disease and peptic ulcer disease, esophagitis and esophageal varices as a late complication, alcoholic hepatitis, cirrhosis, and pancreatitis. Except for esophageal varices and cirrhosis, these conditions are often reversible with alcohol abstinence. Neurologic complications include peripheral neuropathy of the lower extremities, Wernicke-Korsakoff syndrome, hepatic encephalopathy, and alcohol dementia. Hematologic complications include iron-deficiency anemia; macrocytosis; thrombocytopenia; and neutrophil, lymphocyte and thrombocyte dysfunction.

10. e. The mainstay of therapy is long-acting benzodiazepines such as diazepam, chlordiazepoxide, and chlorazepate, given in decreasing doses. Clonidine sometimes is used to reduce noradrenergic symptoms. Antipsychotic agents such as haloperidol are useful in addition to benzodiazepines in patients with hallucinations and agitation. Barbiturates and anticonvulsants (carbamazepine and divalproex) sometimes are used as anticonvulsants.

11. a. Alcohol withdrawal syndrome is a substance-specific syndrome that develops following cessation of or reduced intake of alcohol.

12. a. Alcohol abuse describes patterns of alcohol use that do not meet the criteria for alcohol dependence. Alcohol abuse is defined as a maladaptive pattern of substance use that causes clinically significant impairment. This may include impairments in social, family, or occupational functioning; the presence of psychologic or physical problems; or the use of alcohol while or before driving a motor vehicle or operating machinery. Alcohol abuse commonly progresses to alcohol dependence.

13. e. The imaging studies indicated in this patient include a chest x-ray, a CT of the head, an abdominal ultrasound, and an echocardiogram. An echocardiogram should be done to define the thickness of the left-ventricular wall to determine whether left-ventricular hypertrophy (LVH) is present, as indicated by the position of the PMI. In addition, an electrocardiogram (EKG) will aid in the diagnosis of LVH and determine, among other things, the absence or presence of cardiac arrhythmias. A chest x-ray is justified on the basis of probable cardiac enlargement— that is, to measure the cardiac/thoracic ratio. A CT scan will rule out causes of cognitive disturbances that may be related to alcohol abuse, including intracranial bleeding. It also may detect causes of cognitive disturbances unrelated to alcohol. An abdominal ultrasound will determine the cause of the liver enlargement and help determine the spleen size.

14. d. The movement disorder that is demonstrated on physical examination suggests the early stages of liver failure and alcoholic (Wernicke's) encephalopathy. It may develop into asterixes (an arrhythmic flapping tremor of the fully extended hand), sometimes referred to as *liver flap.*

15. e. *Social drinking* is a term with little meaning. It is important to more precisely determine drinking patterns.

The first step is to determine whether a patient drinks. The second step is to determine how much alcohol a patient drinks. It helps to have the patient estimate the number of drinks per week because many drinkers have irregular patterns with heavier weekend use. Because alcoholism is a disease usually minimized, it is only when the need to drink starts to seriously interfere with social or occupational functioning or the patient is apprehended while driving under the influence of alcohol, that the alcohol abuser will become aware of having a "problem." If the family physician can express concern regarding the effect of the quantity of alcohol consumed on the patient's health, prior to there being dire consequences related to the drinking habit, treatment can be initiated at an earlier time and serious sequelae of the disease can be prevented.

A very useful instrument for screening for alcoholism in the primary care setting is the CAGE questionnaire. The CAGE questionnaire includes four questions:

1. Have you ever felt the need to **C**ut down on your drinking?
2. Have you ever felt **A**nnoyed by criticisms of your drinking?
3. Have you ever had **G**uilty feelings about drinking?
4. Have you ever taken a morning **E**ye-opener?

With the CAGE questionnaire, any more than one positive answer may suggest alcohol abuse.

Another reliable screening tool for heavy alcohol use is the Michigan Alcohol Screening Test (MAST). This 25-item scale identifies abnormal drinking through its social and behavioral consequences with a sensitivity of 90% to 98%. The Brief MAST, a shortened 10-item test, has been shown to have similar efficacy. These tests are less likely to be used in a primary care environment.

16. b. This patient has alcohol-induced persisting amnestic disorder, called *Korsakoff's psychosis.* Patients with alcohol-related amnestic disorder have the most difficulty with short-term memory (remembering recent events), although deficits in long-term memory may be noted as well.

17. a. Patients often try to conceal or compensate for their memory loss by confabulation (making up answers or talking around questions that require them to use their memory).

18. b. The cause of this particular disorder is a chronic deficiency in the vitamin thiamine. For that reason, whenever a patient is in a confused state that may be related to alcohol abuse, intravenous thiamine should be administered.

19. e. Alcoholism is defined as a repetitive but inconsistent and sometimes unpredictable loss of control of drinking that produces symptoms of serious dysfunction or disability.

20. c. In 1994 the national comorbidity study found that 23% of the population in the United States reported alcohol abuse or dependence. About 75% of the population drinks alcohol. Men are two to three times more likely than women to be problem drinkers, although women may hide their drinking more frequently. Excessive drinking causes serious digestive system disorders such as ulcers, inflammation of the pancreas, gastritis, and cirrhosis of the liver and leads to physical and nutritional neglect. Central and peripheral nervous system damage can result in blackouts, hallucinations, tremors, alcohol withdrawal syndrome, delirium tremens, and death.

When women drink even moderately during pregnancy, damage can occur to unborn children. This can include birth defects, mental retardation, learning problems, and fetal alcohol syndrome.

Heavy drinking also results in psychologic and interpersonal problems, including impaired thinking and judgment, and changes in mood and behavior. These consequences of drinking then lead to impaired social relationships, marital problems, and/or child abuse and scholastic, occupational, financial, and legal problems.

SOLUTION TO THE CLINICAL CASE MANAGEMENT PROBLEM

Part A: A good primary care screening test for alcoholism is the CAGE questionnaire. The CAGE questionnaire was described in Answer 15. Alternatives are the MAST (25 items) and the Brief MAST (10 items); however, these are not used as extensively in the family practice setting.

Part B: Five objectives for the short-term treatment of alcohol dependence in the patient and the patient's family are as follows: (1) relieving subjective symptoms of distress and discomfort caused by intoxication or withdrawal; (2) preventing or treating serious complications of intoxication, withdrawal, or dependence; (3) establishing sobriety; (4) preparing for and referral to long-term treatment or rehabilitation; and (5) engaging the family in the treatment process.

SUMMARY OF ALCOHOL DEPENDENCE AND ALCOHOL ABUSE

1. **Prevalence:** An estimated 5% to 7% of Americans have alcoholism in any given year, and 13% will have it some time during their lifetime. The prevalence of alcohol abuse is estimated at 15%, and 23% of the population has either alcohol abuse or alcohol dependency.

2. **Economic costs:** The direct economic costs of alcoholism in the United States are staggering. In 2001 total economic losses from lost productivity in the United States were $100 billion. This does not include indirect economic costs and noneconomic costs and losses.

3. **Definitions:**
   a. Alcoholism: a repetitive but inconsistent and sometimes unpredictable loss of control of drinking that produces symptoms of serious dysfunction or disability
   b. Alcohol dependence: a maladaptive pattern of alcohol use that includes any three of the following: (i) tolerance; (ii) withdrawal; (iii) increasing amounts of consumption; (iv) desire or attempts to cut down or quit; (v) substantial time spent in "hiding the habit"; (vi) important social, occupational, or recreational dysfunction; and (vii) continued use of alcohol despite knowledge of having a persistent or recurrent social, psychological, or physical problem
   c. Alcohol abuse: a residual category that describes patterns of alcohol use that do not meet the criteria for alcohol dependence
   d. Alcohol intoxication: reversible, alcohol-specific physiologic and behavioral changes caused by recent exposure to alcohol
   e. Alcohol withdrawal: an alcohol-specific syndrome that develops following cessation of or reduced intake in the amount of alcohol
   f. Alcohol-persisting disorder: an alcohol-specific syndrome that persists long after acute intoxication or withdrawal abates (such as memory impairments or dementia)

4. **Systemic disease association:** The following disease states are directly linked to the toxic effects of alcohol: (1) alcoholic cardiomyopathy; (2) systemic hypertension; (3) alcoholic hepatitis; (4) Laënnec's (alcoholic) cirrhosis; (5) esophageal varices, gastritis, ascites, and/or edema; (6) peripheral neuropathy; and (7) alcoholic encephalopathy.

5. **Neurologic syndromes include the following:** (1) alcoholic dementia; (2) alcoholic amnestic disorder; (3) Korsakoff's psychosis; (4) Wernicke's encephalopathy; (5) alcoholic hallucinosis; (6) alcoholic paranoia; and (7) alcohol delirium.

6. **Screening:** (1) the CAGE questionnaire; (2) the MAST questionnaire; and (3) the Brief MAST questionnaire

7. **Laboratory testing:** There are no diagnostic tests that are specific for alcohol dependence, but MCV, liver transaminases (ALT, AST), and GGT are the most common tests. The accuracy of a diagnosis of alcoholism increases when a number of tests are used together.

8. **Treatment:**
   a. General considerations: See the Solution to the Clinical Case Management Problem.
   b. Long-term treatment must have the following characteristics to maximize its potential: (i) active involvement with comprehensive rehabilitation and recovery program; (ii) a relapse-prevention program with peer support components and possibly pharmacologic components, including disulfiram or naltrexone; and (iii) inclusion of family and significant others in the recovery process.
   c. Goals of long-term treatment are as follows: (i) to maintain sobriety; (ii) to make significant changes in lifestyle, work, and friendships; (iii) to treat underlying psychiatric illness (dual diagnosis); and (iv) to maintain an ongoing involvement in Alcoholics Anonymous or similar groups for relapse prevention.

SUGGESTED READING

American Psychiatric Association: *Diagnostic and statistical manual of mental disorders IV–TR,* 4th ed. American Psychiatric Association Press, 2000, Washington, DC.

Brienza RS, Stein MD: Alcohol use disorders in primary care: do gender-specific differences exist? *J Gen Intern Med* 17(5):387-397, 2002.

Fiellin DA, et al: Outpatient management of patients with alcohol problems. *Ann Intern Med* 133(10):815-827, 2000.

Kennedy JA: Alcohol use disorders. In: Jacobson. *Psychiatric secrets,* 2nd ed. Hanley and Belfus, 2001, Philadelphia.

Sobell MB: Alcohol and tobacco: clinical and treatment issues. *Alcoholism: Clinical & Experimental Research* 26(12):1954-1955, 2002.

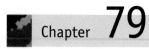

Chapter 79

Drug Abuse

One minute, euphoric.
The next, down in the dumps.

CLINICAL CASE PROBLEM 1:
A 32-Year-Old Administrator with
"Rapidly Swinging Moods"

A 32-year-old man is brought into the Emergency Room (ER) by his wife one evening. She tells you that "something is desperately wrong with my husband." She states he used to be kind, even-keeled, and fun to be with, but during the last year he has "changed drastically."

He now exhibits behavior that can best be described as "very erratic." He will go from periods of extreme depression to short intervals of "being on top of the world," "extremely elated," with "extremely fast speech and restlessness." After a few hours, he goes back into a state of depression. His wife brought him into the ER tonight because he was in a period of elation and euphoria.

She also tells you that her husband has not been performing well at work lately and that "some of his colleagues have noticed some strange behavior." In addition, she tells you that "money seems to be disappearing from our bank account at a rate far faster than I can explain."

On examination, the patient is obviously euphoric and elated. When you ask him why he agreed to come tonight, he tells you that he feels so good that he would do anything to please his wife. His speech appears extremely pressured.

On physical examination, his blood pressure is 190/110 mm Hg. His pulse is 128 and regular. His pupils are widely dilated, and he is sweating profusely. The remainder of his physical examination is normal.

■ SELECT THE BEST ANSWER TO THE FOLLOWING QUESTIONS:

1. With this history and physical examination, what is the most likely diagnosis?
   a. bipolar I disorder, rapid cycling
   b. bipolar II disorder, rapid cycling
   c. amphetamine intoxication
   d. cocaine intoxication
   e. schizophrenia: catatonic subtype

2. At this time, what would be the most appropriate course of action?
   a. arrange for a routine psychiatric consultation on an elective basis
   b. arrange for a social worker to see the patient and his wife now
   c. arrange for an immediate psychiatric consultation
   d. call the appropriate consultant and relate the history, your findings, and diagnosis and facilitate appropriate acute intervention
   e. prescribe diazepam and follow up as an outpatient in 1 week

3. The term *dual diagnosis* in psychiatry usually refers to which of the following?
   a. any two closely related psychiatric disorders in the same patient
   b. any two relatively unrelated psychiatric disorders in the same patient
   c. the manic and depressive episodes of bipolar disorder
   d. the existence of both a psychiatric disorder and a substance abuse disorder in the same patient
   e. the existence of both a chronic medical disorder and a psychiatric disorder in the same patient

4. What is the most effective interview strategy to motivate this patient to engage in treatment of his disorder?
   a. to focus on the precise details of the euphoria and the elation the patient is experiencing
   b. to focus on the precise details of the longer periods of the depression the patient is experiencing
   c. to focus on the precise details of the negative consequences that have resulted from the patient's symptoms
   d. to focus on the relationship between the patient's symptoms and the possible use or abuse of substances
   e. focusing on the relationship between the patient's symptoms and the relationship with his wife

5. Of the substances listed, which has had the most dramatic epidemic increase in the last decade in the United States?
   a. anabolic steroids
   b. crack cocaine
   c. hallucinogens
   d. marijuana
   e. alcohol

6. Following informed consent, which of the following laboratory tests will yield the most significant information concerning the confirmation of the diagnosis made in this patient?
   a. serum cotinine level
   b. urine benzoylecgonine level

c. urine opioid and serum opioid metabolite levels
d. serum gamma glutamyl transferase
e. serum barbiturate level

7. Which of the following is (are) an acute medical complication(s) of the disorder diagnosed in the patient described?
   a. sudden cardiac death
   b. cerebral hemorrhage
   c. respiratory arrest
   d. convulsions
   e. all of the above

8. Which of the following statements regarding opioid abuse in the United States is (are) true?
   a. the prevalence of human immunodeficiency virus (HIV) infection among intravenous (IV) drug abusers in the United States continues to increase
   b. opioid overdose should be suspected in any patient who is in a coma and has respiratory depression
   c. nausea, vomiting, cramps, and diarrhea are symptoms of opioid withdrawal
   d. b and c
   e. a, b, and c

9. Which of the following substances is responsible for the highest mortality rate in our society?
   a. nicotine
   b. alcohol
   c. cocaine
   d. heroin
   e. cannabis

10. Which of the following drugs most effectively ameliorates the symptoms of heroin withdrawal?
   a. naloxone
   b. naltrexone
   c. clonidine
   d. disulfiram
   e. methadone

11. Which of the following is a specific benzodiazepine antagonist?
   a. flumazenil
   b. naltrexone
   c. clonidine
   d. methadone
   e. sertraline

12. Which of the following drugs is most effective for alcohol and benzodiazepine detoxification?
   a. flumazenil
   b. naltrexone

c. carbamazepine
d. lorazepam
e. clonidine

CLINICAL CASE MANAGEMENT PROBLEM

Describe the general principles of interviewing a patient you suspect of having a substance abuse problem but who denies the problem.

ANSWERS:

1. d. This patient most likely has cocaine intoxication. Cocaine intoxication is characterized by elation, euphoria, excitement, pressured speech, restlessness, stereotyped movements, and bruxism. It causes sympathetic stimulation characterized by symptoms such as tachycardia, hypertension, mydriasis, and sweating. Paranoia, suspiciousness, and psychosis may occur with prolonged use. Overdose produces hyperpyrexia, hyperreflexia, seizures, coma, and respiratory arrest.

Amphetamines produce similar symptoms, but rapid changes in mood from elation to depression are less common because of a longer half-life. They are much less expensive than cocaine and less likely to rapidly deplete someone's savings.

2. d. Call the appropriate consultant and relate the history, your findings, and diagnosis and facilitate appropriate acute intervention, which ideally would provide detoxification and drug rehabilitation. The rehabilitation should include individual psychotherapy and group (family) psychotherapy.

3. d. The term *dual diagnosis* is used most often in psychiatry to denote the occurrence of substance abuse and another psychiatric illness. It also is used to refer to the cooccurrence of a developmental disorder (e.g., mental retardation) and another psychiatric illness.

4. c. The most effective strategy for engaging individuals in substance abuse treatment is to focus on the negative consequences resulting from drug abuse. This will produce the greatest likelihood of convincing the patient that he or she has a problem. Substance abuse treatment is rarely successful when patients do not believe that they actually have a problem. Often, the family needs to be engaged to confront the patient with the negative consequences of his or her behavior.

5. b. Of the drugs listed, the most substantial increase has been in the use of crack cocaine. In the early 1970s, about 5 million people had tried cocaine at least once, whereas in the late 1980s, about 40 million people had tried it. Cocaine is used in either powder or crystallized ("rock" or "crack") forms; it can be injected, snorted, or smoked. Crack cocaine generally is inhaled as smoke. The drug has a very rapid onset of action and thus a very high addiction potential. It is the least expensive form of cocaine.

Amphetamines are sold as prescription medications (dextroamphetamine and methamphetamine), but the majority of the drug is manufactured illicitly as powder or crystallized ("ice") methamphetamine. Amphetamines are used orally or smoked, snorted, or injected. Marijuana is the most widely used illicit drug in the United States. About two-thirds of the U.S. population has tried marijuana. According to the 1994 National Comorbidity Survey, 23% of Americans reported alcohol abuse or dependence. Men are two to three times more likely to be problem drinkers than women.

6. b. The metabolite of cocaine that can be detected in the urine is benzoylecgonine. A complete urine drug screen needs to be performed to check on possible combination drug abuse.

7. e. Complications of acute cocaine intoxication include the following: (1) sudden cardiac arrhythmias; (2) convulsions; (3) respiratory arrest; (4) cerebral hemorrhage; and (5) sudden cardiac death.

Chronic use of stimulant drugs is associated with a number of medical complications frequently encountered in the primary care setting. Any IV drug use where needles are shared can result in HIV transmission, hepatitis B or C, or endocarditis. Snorting drugs can cause chronic nosebleeds, nasal septum perforation, and sinusitis. Inhaling drugs can cause chronic cough and bronchitis. Nutritional deficiencies and weight loss frequently occur in heavy users.

8. e. Despite a number of local initiatives, the prevalence of HIV infection among IV drug abusers continues to increase because IV drug abusers frequently engage in needle sharing and unprotected sexual intercourse. Opioid overdose should be suspected in any patient who presents to the ER with coma, convulsions, and respiratory depression. Therefore naloxone, an opioid antagonist, often is indicated even before the diagnosis of opioid intoxication can be confirmed. Nausea, vomiting, cramps, and diarrhea are common signs and symptoms of opioid withdrawal. Other signs and symptoms include generalized pain, dysphoria, lacrimation, yawning, rhinorrhea, and piloerection.

9. a. Nicotine addiction and tobacco use are legally sanctioned, although restrictions on exposure of others to second-hand smoke have increased. Tobacco accounts for more than 350,000 premature deaths per year in the United States, far more than any other recreational substance. Evaluation of smoking, and, if present, counseling about tobacco cessation is an integral part of every primary care visit. Physicians' repeated questioning over time regarding the intention to quit has been shown to be an effective strategy. Using a combination of various counseling techniques, nicotine replacement products, and other medications such as bupropion may be helpful in the treatment of tobacco addiction and in managing nicotine withdrawal. Often, more than one attempt to quit is necessary before patients become permanently tobacco free.

10. e. Methadone most effectively treats the symptoms of heroin withdrawal and often is used acutely for this purpose. As a component of detoxification treatment, methadone is then gradually reduced to minimize withdrawal symptoms. Methadone maintenance programs help many addicts to lead productive lives and avoid most of the deleterious effects of heroin addiction.

The alpha$_2$-adrenergic agonist clonidine also may be used to suppress some of the signs and symptoms of opioid withdrawal. Clonidine acts at presynaptic noradrenergic nerve endings in the locus ceruleus of the brain and blocks the adrenergic discharge produced by opioid withdrawal. In most studies clonidine has been shown to suppress approximately 75% of opioid withdrawal signs and symptoms, especially autonomic hyperactivity and gastrointestinal symptoms. Withdrawal symptoms that are not significantly ameliorated by clonidine include drug craving, insomnia, arthralgias, and myalgias.

11. a. Flumazenil (Romazicon) is a benzodiazepine antagonist that binds competitively and reversibly to the gamma-aminobutyric acid (GABA)/benzodiazepine receptor complex and inhibits the effects of the benzodiazepines. The drug is approved for the treatment of benzodiazepine overdose or the reversal of benzodiazepine sedation.

12. d. Tapering doses of lorazepam or other benzodiazepines are the most effective treatment for most serious alcohol and benzodiazepine withdrawals. Carbamazepine has been demonstrated to be an effective treatment for alcohol and benzodiazepine withdrawal and has less potential than benzodiazepines for causing drug dependence. However, the adverse effects of carbamazepine, including blood dyscrasias and hepatitis, make it less useful than benzodiazepines for this indication.

SOLUTION TO THE CLINICAL CASE MANAGEMENT PROBLEM

The general principles of interviewing a patient who may be abusing drugs but who initially denies drug abuse (and that includes most patients) includes the following: (1) attempting to obtain a detailed history of any substance used (start with nicotine and alcohol); (2) asking about peer group use of these substances; (3) inquiring about physical and behavioral problems; (4) providing empathy and concern to encourage trust on the part of the patient; (5) avoiding judgmental attitudes and pejorative statements; (6) focusing on whether the patient has experienced negative consequences as a result of his or her use of psychoactive substances, has poor control of use, or has been criticized by others concerning his or her pattern of behavior or use of the substance (this can be the most effective interview strategy); (7) confronting the patient if you have solid evidence, including test results; and (8) including input from family members and significant others whenever possible.

SUMMARY OF DRUG ABUSE

Many ramifications that concern drug abuse also are outlined in Chapter 78 concerning alcoholism. Others are as follows:

1. Individuals predisposed to substance abuse often first start to abuse alcohol and marijuana and then progress to cocaine, opioids, or other dangerous drugs.
2. The most destructive recreational substance in terms of morbidity and mortality worldwide is nicotine.
3. Stimulant abuse: Crack cocaine abuse is increasingly common in the United States, and amphetamine abuse also is escalating.
4. Opioid abuse: IV heroin users are now the second largest group of patients with acquired immunodeficiency syndrome in the United States.
5. Specific drugs:
   a. Cocaine: Cocaine increases the sympathetic stimulation of the central nervous system (CNS) and produces initial euphoria as a high. Cocaine (crack) is potent and significantly less expensive than many other drugs.
   b. Caffeine: Caffeine and related methylxanthines are ubiquitous drugs in our society. These drugs produce sympathetic stimulation, diuresis, bronchodilatation, and CNS stimulation.
   c. Cannabis: Marijuana, although illegal, has been used at one time or another by 64.8% of adult Americans. Cannabis intoxication is characterized by tachycardia, muscle relaxation, euphoria, and a sense of well-being. Tachycardia, time-sense alteration, and emotional lability are common.
   d. Anabolic steroids: Some data suggest that 6.5% of adolescent American boys and 1.9% of adolescent American girls have used anabolic steroids. The medical complications of these drugs include myocardial infarction, stroke, and hepatic disease. Psychiatric symptoms associated with anabolic steroid use include severe depression, psychotic (paranoid) symptoms, aggressive behavior, homicidal impulses, euphoria, irritability, anxiety, racing thoughts, and hyperactivity. (All of these symptoms decline or are eliminated on discontinuation of the drug.)
   e. Hallucinogens: The hallucinogens include lysergic acid diethylamide, mescaline, psilocybin, dimethyltryptamine, hallucinogenic amphetamines, and methylenedioxyamphetamine. The mechanism of action of these substances includes stimulation of CNS dopamine or serotonin.
   f. Inhalants: Inhalants are volatile compounds that are inhaled for their intoxicating effects. Substances in this class include organic solvents (e.g., gasoline, toluene, and ethyl ether). Inhalants are ubiquitous and readily available in most households and can be lethal if used in overdose. These are drugs of choice for many disadvantaged youths in both urban and rural environments, along with crack cocaine.
   g. Nicotine: More than 50 million Americans smoke cigarettes daily and another 10 million use other forms of tobacco. Nicotine addiction and tobacco use are generally legally sanctioned for adults. Tobacco accounts for more than 350,000 premature deaths per year, primarily as a result of cardiovascular disease and cancer.
   h. Opioids: Opioid dependence remains a significant sociologic and medical problem in the United States. There are an estimated 500,000

Continued

SUMMARY OF DRUG ABUSE—cont'd

opioid addicts. Opioid addicts are frequent users of medical and surgical services because of multiple medical sequelae of IV drug use and associated lifestyle.

6. Treatment:
   a. The general characteristics of drug abuse treatment already have been outlined; however, the most important principles include the following: (i) detoxification and elimination of withdrawal symptoms; (ii) initial admittance of a problem and alignment of social support systems (family and others); (iii) long-term intensive individual and group therapy; and (iv) inclusion of the family members in therapy.
   b. Special treatments include the following:
      i. For opioid addiction, methadone; for short periods of opioid use, naltrexone (a long-acting orally active opioid antagonist also used for alcoholism); and for opioid withdrawal, clonidine, which blocks many symptoms.
      ii. For benzodiazepine sedation flumazenil (Romazicon) is the first benzodiazepine antagonist approved by the U.S. Food and Drug Administration. Carbamazepine (Tegretol) has been shown to be effective for ethanol and sedative detoxification. However, the adverse effects of carbamazepine, including blood dyscrasias and hepatitis, make it less useful than lorazepam or other benzodiazepines for this indication.

SUGGESTED READING

American Psychiatric Association: *Diagnostic and statistical manual of mental disorders IV–TR,* 4th ed. American Psychiatric Association Press, 2000, Washington, DC.
Kennedy J: Cocaine and amphetamine use disorders: marijuana, hallucinogens, phencyclidine, and inhalants. In: Jacobson. *Psychiatric secrets,* 2nd ed. Hanley and Belfus, 2001, Philadelphia.
Schneider RK, et al: Update in addiction medicine. *Ann Intern Med* 134(5):387-395, 2001.
Tomb DA: *Psychiatry,* 6th ed. Baltimore, 1999, Williams & Wilkins.

Chapter 80

Eating Disorders

"Mirror, mirror on the wall, why am I the fattest of all?"

CLINICAL CASE PROBLEM 1:

A 19-Year-Old Female with Rapid Weight Loss and an Intense Fear of Gaining Weight

A 19-year-old female comes to your office with a 30-lb weight loss during the last 6 months. She states that she has an intense fear of gaining weight. She has had no menstrual period during the last 4 months. When questioned about her perception of her weight, she states, "I still feel fat."

She denies episodes of binge eating and purging. She also denies the use of laxatives or diuretics.

On examination, the patient is approximately 25% below expected body weight. There is evidence of significant muscle wasting. Her blood pressure is 90/70 mm Hg, and her heart rate is 52 and regular. There appears to be significant fine hair growth over her entire body. The remainder of her physical examination is normal.

SELECT THE BEST ANSWER TO THE FOLLOWING QUESTIONS:

1. What is the most likely diagnosis in this patient?
   a. borderline personality disorder
   b. bulimia nervosa
   c. anorexia nervosa
   d. generalized anxiety disorder
   e. masked depression

2. Diagnosis of this disorder requires the maintenance of body weight at what percentage below ideal body weight?
   a. 5%
   b. 10%
   c. 15%
   d. 20%
   e. 25%

3. What percentage of individuals with the disorder described has an accompanying major depressive disorder or a coexisting anxiety disorder?
   a. 10%
   b. 20%
   c. 30%
   d. 50%
   e. 75%

4. What is the lifetime prevalence of obsessive-compulsive disorder (OCD) in patients with this disorder?
   a. 5%
   b. 15%
   c. 25%
   d. 50%
   e. 75%

5. Which complication of this disorder has the greatest potential for precipitating a life-threatening circumstance?
   a. muscle wasting
   b. generalized fatigue and weakness
   c. hypokalemia
   d. bradycardia
   e. hypotension

6. Which of the following is (are) true regarding the classification of eating disorders in the *Diagnostic and Statistical Manual of Mental Disorders,* 4th edition (DSM–IV)?
   a. there are two types of anorexia nervosa specified in DSM-IV: the restricting type and the binge-eating/purging type
   b. there are two types of bulimia nervosa specified in DSM-IV: the purging type and the nonpurging type
   c. anorexia nervosa and bulimia nervosa may be diagnosed comorbidly in a given patient
   d. a and b
   e. a, b, and c

CLINICAL CASE PROBLEM 2:

A 26-YEAR-OLD FEMALE WHO VOMITS TO PREVENT WEIGHT GAIN

A 26-year-old patient comes to your office with recurrent episodes of binge eating (approximately four times a week) after which she vomits to prevent weight gain. She says that "she has no control" over these episodes and becomes depressed because of her inability to control herself. These episodes have been occurring for the past 2 years. She also admits to using self-induced vomiting, laxatives, and diuretics to lose weight.

On examination, the patient's blood pressure is 110/70 mm Hg and her pulse is 72 and regular. She is in no apparent distress. Her physical examination is entirely normal.

7. What is the most likely diagnosis in this patient?
   a. borderline personality disorder
   b. anorexia nervosa
   c. bulimia nervosa
   d. masked depression
   e. generalized anxiety disorder

8. Examination of which of the following is most likely to be abnormal in patients with the disorder described in Clinical Case Problem 2?
   a. the mouth
   b. the cervical and axillary lymph nodes
   c. the right upper quadrant of the abdomen
   d. the sensory component of the neurologic system
   e. the motor component of the neurologic system

9. Regarding the prevalence of the disorders described in the previous two Clinical Case Problems, which of the following statements is true?
   a. the prevalence of the disorder described in Clinical Case Problem 1 is increasing, whereas the prevalence of the disorder described in Clinical Case Problem 2 is decreasing
   b. the prevalence of the disorder described in Clinical Case Problem 1 is decreasing, whereas the prevalence of the disorder described in Clinical Case Problem 2 is increasing
   c. the prevalence of both disorders is increasing
   d. the prevalence of both disorders is decreasing
   e. the prevalence of both disorders has remained unchanged over the past decade

10. The patient described in Clinical Case Problem 1 should be treated in which manner?
    a. as an outpatient: treatment focused on pharmacotherapy, psychotherapy, and behavior modification
    b. as an inpatient: treatment focused on pharmacotherapy, psychotherapy, and behavior modification
    c. as an inpatient: treatment focused on psychotherapy and behavior modification
    d. as an outpatient: treatment focused on psychotherapy and behavior modification
    e. as an outpatient: treatment focused on pharmacotherapy

11. Which of the following drugs has (have) been shown to be of benefit in the treatment of the disorder described in Clinical Case Problem 2?
    a. monoamine oxidase inhibitors (MAOIs)
    b. tricyclic antidepressants (TCAs)
    c. selective serotonin reuptake inhibitors (SSRIs)
    d. b and c
    e. a, b, and c

12. Which of the following psychotherapies is (are) generally considered most effective for the treatment of the disorder described in Clinical Case Problem 2?
    a. supportive psychotherapy
    b. psychodynamic psychotherapy
    c. psychoanalytic psychotherapy

   d. cognitive-behavioral therapy (CBT)
   e. a, b, and d

CLINICAL CASE MANAGEMENT PROBLEM

List the psychiatric disorders and associated conditions that have been shown to be related to the conditions described in this chapter.

■ **ANSWERS:**

1. c. This patient has anorexia nervosa.

2. c. Anorexia nervosa is characterized by the following: (1) a patient who refuses to maintain her minimal normal body weight for age and height leading to maintenance of body weight at least 15% below normal, or a patient who fails to gain weight as expected during growth, leading to body weight 15% below that which is expected; (2) although underweight, the patient displays an intense fear of gaining weight or becoming fat; (3) the patient experiences body weight, size, or shape in a disturbed fashion, such as claiming to feel fat even when she is clearly underweight; and (4) in female patients, at least three menstrual periods that should otherwise have been expected to occur have not occurred.

3. e. Up to 75% of patients with anorexia nervosa have a coexisting major depressive disorder or anxiety disorder.

4. c. Of patients with anorexia nervosa, 25% develop OCD some time in their life.

5. c. The medical complications of anorexia nervosa include muscle wasting, fatigue, depression of cardiovascular function leading to bradycardia and hypotension, and depression of body temperature mechanisms leading to hypothermia. Although all of these conditions can become life threatening, the abnormality of greatest medical concern is hypokalemia, caused by inadequate nutrition and sometimes exacerbated by the misuse of diuretics and laxatives. Hypokalemia can cause cardiac dysrhythmias and, if severe enough, sudden death.

6. d. There are two types of anorexia nervosa and two types of bulimia nervosa. The two types of anorexia nervosa are the restricting type and the binge-eating/purging type. Patients with restricting-type anorexia avoid weight gain primarily through limiting food intake and do not usually engage in binge eating, self-induced vomiting, or misuse of diuretics or laxatives. The binge-eating/purging type of patient regularly engages in binge eating and purging (self-induced vomiting or misuse of laxatives or diuretics).

As is the case for anorexia nervosa, two subtypes of bulimia nervosa are recognized: the purging type of patient, who regularly engages in self-induced vomiting or misuse of laxatives or diuretics and the nonpurging type of patient, who usually does not self-induce vomiting or misuse laxatives or diuretics to lose weight. Instead, the nonpurging type of patient engages in other severe compensatory behaviors such as fasting or excessive exercise.

A diagnosis of bulimia nervosa is not made if the diagnostic criteria for anorexia nervosa are present.

7. c. This patient has bulimia nervosa. Bulimia nervosa is characterized by a patient who (1) engages in repeated episodes of binge eating large amounts of food in brief periods; (2) regularly engages in severe compensatory behaviors to prevent weight gain, such as self-induced vomiting, misusing laxatives or diuretics, taking diet pills, fasting, eating very strict diets, and/or exercising very vigorously; (3) engages in at least two binge-eating and purging/severe compensatory behaviors per week for a minimum of 3 months; and (4) is relentlessly overconcerned regarding weight and body shape.

8. a. A frequently observed abnormality in bulimia nervosa is an abnormality in the examination of the oral cavity. Examination of the mouth often reveals evidence of dental caries and periodontal disease that occur because of the effects of repeated vomiting.

9. c. Studies suggest that among adolescent and young adult women in high school and college settings, the prevalence of clinically significant eating disorders is approximately 4% and, for more broadly defined syndromes, may be as high as 8%. The prevalence of these disorders seems to have increased over the past several decades. The prevalence of eating disorders may be influenced by societal attitudes regarding beauty and fashion. Over the past few years, so-called "pro-ana" Websites have appeared where anorexics claim this condition is not a disease but a lifestyle choice. These sites, usually run by young patients who are anorexic, hold a dangerous fascination for patients with an already severely disturbed body image.

10. c. A 30-lb weight loss in 6 months suggests that this patient is at immediate risk for life-threatening complications. In this circumstance, most clinicians would suggest inpatient therapy with a focus on reestablishing a reasonable weight through calorie supplementation, cognitive-behavioral treatment, and possibly other forms of psychotherapy. SSRI antidepressant medication would be indicated only for treatment of comorbid depression that commonly accompanies anorexia nervosa.

11. c. SSRI agents such as fluoxetine or sertraline have been shown to be successful in reducing binge eating and purging episodes, whether there is comorbid depression. MAOIs have no role in the treatment of bulimia.

12. d. CBT appears to be the most effective treatment for bulimia nervosa. This treatment includes several stages, each consisting of several weeks of biweekly individual or group sessions. The first stage emphasizes the patient's establishing control over eating using behavioral techniques such as self-monitoring. The second stage focuses on attempts to restructure the patient's unrealistic cognitions about eating and body image. It also instills more effective modes of problem solving. The third and final stage emphasizes maintaining the gains and preventing relapse, often by providing 6 months to a year of weekly sessions, with close follow-up during times when relapse is common. Self-help groups, especially Overeaters Anonymous, also may be useful for individuals with bulimia nervosa.

SOLUTION TO THE CLINICAL CASE MANAGEMENT PROBLEM

The psychiatric disorders that are related to the eating disorders described include the following: (1) major depressive disorder (MDD); (2) anxiety disorders (75% of patients with an eating disorder have either MDD or an anxiety disorder at the same time); (3) chemical dependency and substance abuse; and (4) personality disorders.

SUMMARY OF EATING DISORDERS

A. Prevalence: (1) the prevalence of eating disorders is 4%; (2) the prevalence of abnormal eating behaviors not classified strictly as eating disorders may be as high as 8%; (3) the prevalence of these disorders has increased significantly over the past several decades; and (4) these diseases are more common in females than in males (9:1).

B. Symptoms: the symptoms of both anorexia nervosa and bulimia nervosa have been described previously. The major diagnostic clues are as follows:
1. Anorexia nervosa: (a) failure to maintain normal weight (less than 85% of ideal weight); (b) having an intense fear of gaining weight; (c) having a distorted body image (feeling fat despite being grossly underweight); and (d) having amenorrhea.
2. Bulimia nervosa: (a) repeated episodes of rapid binge eating; (b) severe compensatory behaviors to lose weight; and (c) an unrelenting overconcern with weight and body image

C. Relationships between the two disorders: (1) both disorders involve abnormal eating behaviors and concern with body image; (2) of individuals with anorexia nervosa, 50% have binge-eating and purging behavior; and (3) a diagnosis of bulimia nervosa is not made if the criteria for diagnosis of anorexia nervosa are present.

D. Complications:
1. Anorexia nervosa: the physical complications of starvation, namely: (a) depletion of fat; (b) muscle wasting (including cardiac muscle in severe wasting); (c) bradycardia; (d) cardiac arrhythmias (sudden death may follow); (e) leucopenia; (f) amenorrhea; (g) osteoporosis; (h) cachexia; and (i) lanugo (fine body hair).
2. Bulimia nervosa: (a) dental caries and dental disease from vomiting; (b) metabolic abnormalities (hypokalemia secondary to vomiting); (c) black stools from laxative abuse; and (d) if significant weight loss occurs, physical symptoms as listed earlier for anorexia nervosa may develop.

E. Treatment:
1. Anorexia nervosa: (a) for severe cases, hospitalization to reestablish weight and correct metabolic abnormalities; (b) CBT and often family therapy focusing on dynamics related to issues of control; and (c) SSRIs for coexisting depression.
2. Bulimia nervosa: (a) CBT and (b) SSRIs to treat the binge-eating component.

SUGGESTED READING

American Psychiatric Association: *Diagnostic and statistical manual of mental disorders IV–TR,* 4th ed. American Psychiatric Association Press, 2000, Washington, DC.

Becker AE, et al: Eating disorders. *N Engl J Med* 340(14):1092-1098, 1999.

Bergh C, et al: What is the evidence basis for existing treatments of eating disorders? *Curr Opin Pediatr* 15(3):344-345, 2003.

Sandbek TJ: The deadly diet: Recovering from anorexia & bulimia, 2nd ed. New Harbinger Publications, Inc., 1993, Oakland, CA.

Tomb DA: *Psychiatry,* 6th ed. Williams & Wilkins, 1999, Baltimore.

Walsh JM, et al: Detection, evaluation, and treatment of eating disorders the role of the primary care physician. *J Gen Intern Med* 15(8):577-590, 2000.

Chapter 81

Generalized Anxiety Disorder

> "My mom won't let me play at your house.
> She is afraid a bad man will take me away."

CLINICAL CASE PROBLEM 1:

A 36-Year-Old Female with Shortness of Breath and Palpitations

A 36-year-old female comes to your office with an 8-month history of shortness of breath, palpitations, dizziness, trouble swallowing, restlessness, fatigue, and anxiety regarding her job and the health of her two children. She tells you that she constantly worries about what could happen to her children when they are playing with other children in their homes (where she cannot be constantly supervising their play activities). She also worries about them dying in a car crash. She tells you, "Well, I'm very concerned about them not only being in an automobile accident but also about the possibility of the seat belts coming loose."

When you directly question her about some of these worries she readily admits to you that "I know I'm worrying too much, Doctor, but I just can't help it."

She also complains of muscle tension, easy fatigability, difficulty concentrating, having trouble falling and staying asleep, and irritability.

At this point in the interview she becomes very tense and tells you, "You know, Doctor, this is really getting out of control; I feel I can't function anymore."

On physical examination, the patient's blood pressure is 130/70 mm Hg, and her pulse is 104 and regular. Her thyroid gland is within normal limits and nontender. Her cardiac examination reveals no abnormalities outside the tachycardia. Her neurologic examination is normal. The remainder of the physical examination is normal.

■ SELECT THE BEST ANSWER TO THE FOLLOWING QUESTIONS:

1. What is the most likely diagnosis in this patient?
   a. panic disorder
   b. major depressive disorder
   c. generalized anxiety disorder (GAD)
   d. hyperthyroidism
   e. hypochondriasis

2. Of patients with the disorder described, what percentage has at least one other similar psychiatric disorder at some time in their life?
   a. 10%
   b. 30%
   c. 50%
   d. 80%
   e. no data are available

3. What is the most common error made in the diagnosis of the disorder described?
   a. misdiagnosing this disorder when it actually is related to any one of several other general medical or mental conditions
   b. misdiagnosing this disorder as depression
   c. misdiagnosing this disorder as hyperthyroidism
   d. misdiagnosing this disorder as pheochromocytoma
   e. misdiagnosing this disorder as a multiple endocrine neoplasia syndrome

4. Which of the following symptoms is generally not characteristic of the disorder described?
   a. awakening with apprehension and unrealistic concern regarding future misfortune
   b. worry out of proportion to the likelihood or impact of feared events
   c. a 6-month or longer course of anxiety and associated symptoms
   d. association of the anxiety described with depression
   e. anxiety exclusively focused on health concerns

5. Which of the following statements regarding the disorder described is (are) true?
   a. this disorder may develop between attacks in panic disorder
   b. the symptoms of this disorder often are present in episodes of depression
   c. medical conditions that produce the major symptom associated with this disorder must be excluded
   d. the disorder is accompanied by symptoms of motor tension, autonomic hyperactivity, hypervigilance, and scanning
   e. all of the above are true

6. What is the psychotherapy of choice in this disorder?
   a. cognitive-behavioral therapy (CBT)
   b. hypnosis
   c. supportive psychotherapy
   d. psychoanalytic psychotherapy
   e. none of the above

7. What pharmacologic agents sometimes are used to treat this disorder?
   a. venlafaxine
   b. buspirone
   c. benzodiazepines
   d. selective serotonin reuptake inhibitors (SSRIs)
   e. all of the above

8. Which of the following pharmacologic agents is not recommended in the treatment of this disorder?

a. diazepam (Valium)
b. chlordiazepoxide (Librium)
c. clorazepate (Tranxene)
d. clozapine (Clozaril)
e. clonazepam (Klonopin)

9. This disorder is more common in which of the following?
a. young to middle-aged females
b. ethnic minorities
c. those currently not married
d. those of lower socioeconomic class
e. all of the above

10. Which of the following statements is (are) true regarding this disorder?
a. this disorder displays autosomal-dominant genetic transmission
b. the mechanism of symptom development in this disorder may relate to a conditioned response to a stimulus that the individual has come to associate with danger
c. a relationship between the onset of this disorder and the cumulative effects of stressful life events is possible
d. b and c
e. a, b, and c

CLINICAL CASE MANAGEMENT PROBLEM

List three substances that may precipitate the major symptoms associated with this condition.

ANSWERS:

1. c. This patient has GAD, which is defined as unrealistic or excessive worry about several life events or activities for a period of at least 6 months during which the person has been bothered more days than not by these concerns. In addition, the following six symptoms are present: muscle tension, restlessness or feeling keyed up or on edge, easy fatigability, difficulty concentrating or a sensation of the "mind going blank" because of anxiety, trouble falling or staying asleep, and irritability. Finally, the anxiety, worry, or physical symptoms significantly interfere with the person's normal routine or usual activities or cause marked distress.

2. d. Of patients with GAD, at least 80% of patients have had at least one other anxiety disorder in their lifetime.

3. a. The most common diagnostic error made is misdiagnosing GAD when another disorder is the actual cause of the anxiety. This leads to inappropriate and ineffective treatment decisions. Symptoms of anxiety are prominent in a number of conditions: (1) depressive disorders; (2) psychotic disorders; (3) substance abuse disorders including legal substances such as caffeine and diet pills; (4) somatoform disorders; (5) a number of medical conditions such as hyperthyroidism, anemia, hypoglycemia, diabetes and other endocrine disorders, and lung and heart disorders; and (6) medication side effects.

4. e. GAD is characterized by awakening with apprehension and concern regarding future misfortune, worry out of proportion to the likelihood or impact of feared events, a duration of 6 months or more of anxiety or associated symptoms, and an association with depressed moods.

GAD is usually not associated exclusively with health concerns. When health concerns become the focus of worry, a diagnosis of hypochondriasis or another somatoform disorder becomes more likely.

5. e. Generalized persistent anxiety may develop between attacks in panic disorder. GAD symptoms often are present during episodes of depression. As with panic disorder, medical conditions that may produce anxiety symptoms must be excluded (see Answer 3).

GAD is characterized by chronic anxiety about life circumstances accompanied by symptoms of motor tension, autonomic hyperactivity, hypervigilance, and scanning.

6. a. CBT is often effective in the treatment of GAD. Cognitive therapy challenges the distortions in patients' thinking that trigger and heighten their anxiety. This technique can be combined with relaxation training, including deep breathing and progressive muscle relaxation. Biofeedback and imagery are also useful to achieve systematic desensitization. Because relaxation and anxiety are mutually exclusive, these techniques help patients to achieve relief from their symptoms. Although cognitive therapy alone may alleviate GAD symptoms, the combination of cognitive and other behavioral techniques is more effective than cognitive therapy alone.

7. e. SSRIs, especially paroxetine, are agents often used in the pharmacologic treatment of GAD. Venlafaxine, a mixed serotonin–norepinephrine reuptake inhibitor can be used for short- and long-term treatment. Although commonly used, benzodiazepines have mostly short-term benefits. Although longer acting agents are preferred over short-acting benzodiazepines, their use should be limited if possible because withdrawal symptoms, dependency, and impaired performance are frequent. Buspirone, a nonbenzodiazepine anxiolytic, and other agents such as tricyclic antidepressants are used as well.

8. d. Clozapine is an antipsychotic agent used in the treatment of patients with schizophrenia. It has no role in the treatment of GAD. Benzodiazepines, including diazepam (Valium), flurazepam (Dalmane), chlordiazepoxide (Librium), clorazepate (Tranxene), and clonazepam (Klonopin), are used in the treatment of GAD; however, their usefulness is limited (see earlier comments).

9. e. GAD is slightly more common in young to middle-aged females, ethnic minorities, those not currently married, and those of lower socioeconomic class status.

10. d. Behavioral theories consider GAD, like panic disorder, to be a conditioned response to a stimulus that the individual has come to associate with danger. There is indeed some suggestion that the onset of GAD may be related to the cumulative effects of several stressful life events that have not been properly processed. There is no convincing evidence of a specific form of genetic transmission of GAD.

SOLUTION TO THE CLINICAL CASE MANAGEMENT PROBLEM

Substances that can produce significant symptoms of anxiety include the following: (1) caffeine; (2) cocaine; (3) amphetamines (methylphenidate, dextroamphetamine); (4) LSD (lysergic acid diethylamide), mescaline, psilocybin, dimethyltryptamine; (5) alcohol; and (6) appetite suppressants (herbal and pharmacologic).

SUMMARY OF GENERALIZED ANXIETY DISORDER

A. Epidemiology: the 1-month prevalence rate of GAD is 2.5%

B. Differential diagnoses includes the following: (1) panic disorder; (2) somatoform disorder; (3) hypochondriasis; (4) substance abuse including caffeine and diet pills; (5) depression (with secondary anxiety); (6) hyperthyroidism; and (7) other organic disorders (less likely).

C. Symptoms: GAD is characterized by chronic excessive anxiety concerning life circumstances accompanied by symptoms of motor tension, autonomic hyperactivity, vigilance, and scanning. These symptoms of anxiety, worry, or physical signs significantly interfere with the person's normal routine of usual activities and cause marked distress.

D. Treatment:
1. Nonpharmacologic treatment options combine behavioral interventions including: (a) CBT that challenges distortions in thinking and uses positive affirmations; (b) relaxation training, including abdominal breathing, and progressive muscle-relaxation techniques;
   (c) systematic desensitization using imagery and/or biofeedback; and (d) assertiveness training.
2. Pharmacologic treatment options include the following: (a) SSRIs; (b) tricyclic antidepressants; (c) venlafaxine; (d) benzodiazepines; and (e) buspirone.

SUGGESTED READING

American Psychiatric Association: *Diagnostic and statistical manual of mental disorders IV–TR*, 4th ed. American Psychiatric Association Press, 2000, Washington, DC.

Culpepper L: Generalized anxiety disorder in primary care: emerging issues in management and treatment. *J Clin Psychiatr* 63 Suppl 8:35-42, 2002.

Davis M, et al: *The stress and relaxation workbook*, 3rd ed. New Harbinger Publications, 1988, Oakland.

House A, Stark D: Anxiety in medical patients. *BMJ* 325(7357):207-209, 2002.

Kaplan HI, Sadock BJ: Anxiety disorders. In Kaplan HI, Sadock BJ, eds: *Kaplan and Sadock's synopsis of psychiatry: Behavioral sciences/clinical psychiatry*, 8th ed. Williams & Wilkins, 1998, Baltimore.

Nagy L, et al: Anxiety disorders. In Stoudemire A, ed: *Clinical psychiatry for medical students*, 3rd ed. JB Lippincott, 1998, Philadelphia.

Shaner R: *Psychiatry*. Williams & Wilkins, 1997, Baltimore.

Tomb DA: *Psychiatry*. 6th ed. Williams & Wilkins, 1999, Baltimore.

Tonks A: Treating generalised anxiety disorder. *BMJ* 326(7391):700-702, 2003.

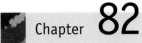

Chapter 82

Factitious Disorder

"I most certainly need another operation. You must be incompetent!"

CLINICAL CASE PROBLEM 1:

A 26-YEAR-OLD FEMALE WITH AN "ABDOMEN FULL OF SCARS"

A 26-year-old female comes to the Emergency Room (ER) with a 6-month history of "severe abdominal pain" that is relieved only by meperidine (Demerol). The patient self-reports "many, many operations" on her stomach, gallbladder, common bile duct, pancreas, large bowel, small bowel, spleen, and others that she cannot remember.

She tells you when you introduce yourself that "she has heard all about you" and is certainly glad that "you are here to solve her problems." She further tells you that she "was on the brink" until she called the Emergency Department and found out that you were the ER doctor in charge of care today.

When you try to obtain a more complete history regarding all of her abdominal problems, she tells you that she has been in 57 different hospitals in the last 37 months. She goes back to her original statement about her delight with you being on duty today.

On examination, the patient's blood pressure is 120/79 mm Hg. Her pulse is 72 and regular. Examination of the head and neck reveals "multiple scars" on her face from "gland surgery." Her abdomen has nine scars in different locations. When you press gently on her abdomen she screams very loudly. It is 3 AM and anyone in the 36-room ER who did happen to be asleep is no longer in that state.

■ SELECT THE BEST ANSWER TO THE FOLLOWING QUESTIONS:

1. On the basis of the history and physical examination, what is the most likely diagnosis in this patient?
   a. borderline personality disorder
   b. antisocial personality disorder
   c. somatization disorder
   d. factitious disorder with predominant physical signs and symptoms
   e. malingering

2. Which of the following descriptions best fits patients with this disorder?
   a. "scarface personality"
   b. "gridiron abdomen"
   c. "lost love syndrome"
   d. "deceptive fever syndrome"
   e. "multiple personality disorder"

3. In which of the following demographic groups does this disorder occur more commonly?
   a. males
   b. females
   c. health care workers
   d. b and c
   e. a and c

4. The prevalence of factitious disorders among patients admitted to general hospitals (primary and secondary care) in the United States is approximately which of the following?
   a. 0.05% of all admissions
   b. 0.1% of all admissions
   c. 0.5% of all admissions
   d. 1.0% of all admissions
   e. 5.0% of all admissions

5. Which of the following criteria is (are) important in establishing the diagnosis?
   a. intentional production or feigning of physical symptoms
   b. intentional production or feigning of psychological symptoms
   c. motivation to assume the sick role
   d. a and b only
   e. a, b, and c

6. Which of the following signs or symptoms is most predictive of this disorder?
   a. signs and symptoms of a major depressive disorder or a brief depressive disorder
   b. an obvious, recognizable goal in producing the signs and symptoms
   c. pathologic lying, lack of close relationships with others, hostile and manipulative manner, and associated substance and criminal behavior
   d. multiple admissions to different hospitals, multiple referrals to different physicians, and multiple surgical procedures
   e. the involuntary production of multiple symptoms as opposed to the voluntary production of multiple symptoms

7. When physical symptoms predominate in this disorder, what eponym sometimes is used?
   a. Briquet's syndrome
   b. Ganser syndrome
   c. Munchausen syndrome
   d. doctor abuse syndrome
   e. none of the above

8. A patient who comes to the local ER with these signs and symptoms may produce which of the following behaviors?

a. self-injection of insulin when not a diabetic
b. self-bloodletting and putting of same into urine to imitate hematuria
c. allowing the thermometer used to take temperature to be immersed in hot water
d. when producing a urine sample contaminating it with feces
e. all of the above

9. Which of the following disorders is (are) to be considered in the differential diagnosis of the condition described?
a. somatoform disorder
b. antisocial personality disorder
c. malingering
d. Ganser syndrome
e. all of the above

10. Which of the following disorders is most likely to have occurred previously in a patient who has the disorder described?
a. major depressive disorder
b. generalized anxiety disorder
c. childhood abuse or deprivation
d. childhood depression
e. autism

11. Which of the following traits often is (are) present in patients who have this disorder?
a. decreased self-worth and self-esteem
b. poor identity formation
c. masochistic personality traits
d. all of the above
e. a and b only

12. What is the most effective treatment for this disorder?
a. early diagnosis and careful documentation
b. extensive psychoanalysis type with a focus on early childhood trauma
c. cognitive psychotherapy
d. behavior-oriented psychotherapy
e. repeated confrontation about the bizarre nature of the symptoms

 CLINICAL CASE MANAGEMENT PROBLEM

Discuss the onset and development of factitious disorder.

ANSWERS:

1. d. This patient has a factitious disorder of the predominantly physical subtype.

A core feature of patients with this disorder is their intentional production of physical symptoms, often resulting in hospital admission. To support their history, the patients may feign symptoms suggestive of a disorder involving any organ system. They are often surprisingly familiar with complex medical diagnoses and may give realistic histories that deceive even experienced physicians.

The presentations that these patients manifest are myriad and include hematoma, hemoptysis, abdominal pain, fever, hypoglycemia, lupuslike syndrome, nausea, vomiting, dizziness, and seizures. As well, the urine of these patients is sometimes intentionally contaminated with blood or feces, anticoagulants are taken to simulate bleeding disorders, and insulin is used to produce hypoglycemia. (These are just a few of the symptoms produced in this disorder and the lengths gone to produce disease.)

One of the most common acts in factitious disorder patients is heating a thermometer. In this case, a patient who does not appear to be ill presents with a temperature of 104° F. This often is produced by hot water or a hot lamp.

2. b. The patients may acquire what is classically referred to as a "gridiron abdomen" from multiple surgical procedures. Complaints of pain, especially that simulating renal colic, are common. The classic description of this patient includes someone who comes in seeking meperidine (Demerol). In one of the typical scenarios, once the patient is in the hospital he or she will continue to be demanding and difficult. As each test is returned and the result is negative, the patient actually may accuse the doctor of incompetence, threaten litigation, and become abusive. Some patients may discharge themselves abruptly, especially when and if they begin to suspect that the staff is catching on or when the staff begins to confront the patient. From there the patient moves on to another hospital in the same or another city and the cycle begins again.

Some of the risk factors for this behavior and this disorder are as follows: (1) specific predisposing factors and actual physical disorders during childhood leading to extensive medical treatment; (2) anger against the medical profession or health care workers; (3) employment as a medical professional or medical paraprofessional; and (4) any type of important relationship with a physician in the past.

3. e. Factitious disorder is more common in (1) males; (2) health care workers; (3) health care professionals; and (4) individuals with a history of abuse in their family.

4. e. The prevalence of factitious disorders in admissions to primary and secondary general hospitals in the United States is thought to be about 5%. This figure may reflect an underdiagnosis of factitious disorder. Clinicians may not yet consistently recognize psychological conditions that influence interactions with health care resources.

5. e. The *Diagnostic and Statistical Manual of Mental Disorders,* 4th edition (DSM-IV) has established the following diagnostic criteria for factitious disorder: (1) the patient intentionally produces or feigns physical or psychological signs or symptoms; (2) the motivation for the patient is to assume the "sick role"; (3) external incentives for the behavior (such as economic gain, avoiding legal responsibility, or improving physical well-being) are absent or secondary.

The subtypes of factitious disorder are as follows: (1) factitious disorder with predominantly psychological signs and symptoms (if psychological signs and symptoms predominate in the case presentation); (2) factitious disorder with predominantly physical signs and symptoms (if physical signs and symptoms predominate in the case presentation); and (3) factitious disorder with combined psychological and physical signs (the classification when combined psychological and physical signs and symptoms are present but neither predominates).

6. d. The most characteristic findings in factitious disorder are visits to multiple physicians, multiple referrals, multiple ER visits and hospitalizations, and multiple surgical procedures. Although the symptoms in option **c** also may occur, they often are seen in antisocial personality disorder. The symptoms produced by patients with factitious disorder are voluntary, not involuntary.

7. c. Factitious disorder with predominantly physical signs and symptoms has been called *Munchausen syndrome.* This syndrome is named after the 18th-century German Baron von Munchausen who told exaggerated stories. Other names for the condition are hospital addiction syndrome, polysurgery addiction syndrome, and professional patient syndrome.

Briquet's syndrome, named after a 19th century French physician, is used synonymously with somatization disorder.

Ganser syndrome refers to a behavior occasionally exhibited during medical examination by inmates in correctional facilities. It is characterized by the subject using an approximate answer when questioned. For example, patients with the disorder may respond to a simple question with astonishingly incorrect answers. For instance, when an inmate is asked the color of a blue sweater, he answers, "It is red." Most patients have a comorbid personality disorder, particularly antisocial and histrionic types. Ganser syndrome is

classified as a dissociative disorder. This disorder is very rare.

8. e. A patient who comes to the local ER with signs or symptoms of a factitious disorder may self-inject insulin when not a diabetic, produce by blood-letting enough blood to simulate macroscopic or microscopic hematuria when mixed with urine, heat a thermometer either with hot water or under a lamp to produce a grossly elevated temperature reading, or mix feces with urine to simulate the possible diagnosis of an abdominal or pelvic fistula.

All of these behaviors are designed by the patient to generate among his or her physicians and other health care workers an appearance of serious organic illnesses.

9. e. Any disorder in which the physical signs and symptoms are prominent should be considered in the differential diagnosis of factitious disorder. Obviously, factitious disorder may mimic a multitude of organic diseases motivated by the patient's conscious or unconscious intention. However, many psychiatric disorders have to be distinguished from factitious disorders and are important to consider in the differential diagnosis. These include the following:

1. Somatoform disorders: various somatoform-type disorders differ from factitious disorders in the following ways:
   a. Somatization disorder: Factitious disorder is differentiated from somatization disorder by the voluntary production of factitious symptoms, the extreme course of multiple hospitalizations, and the patient's apparent willingness to undergo an extraordinary number of mutilating procedures. A patient with somatization disorder will not exhibit these signs and symptoms.
   b. Conversion disorder: Unlike patients with factitious disorder, patients with conversion disorder are not usually conversant with medical terminology and hospital routines and they have symptoms that bear a direct temporal relation or symbolic reference to specific emotional conflicts. In addition patients with conversion disorder do not voluntarily produce their symptoms.
   c. Hypochondriasis: Factitious disorder is differentiated from hypochondriasis in that patients who are hypochondriacal do not usually voluntarily initiate the production of symptoms, and patients with hypochondriasis typically have a later age of onset of the disease.
2. Personality disorders:
   a. Antisocial personality disorder.

b. Histrionic personality disorder is associated with a "dramatic flair"; this, however, sometimes also can be found in patients with factitious disorder.

c. Borderline personality disorders and schizotypal personality disorders also may need to be considered as comorbid illnesses in patients with factitious disorder.

3. Malingering disorder: Factitious disorder must be distinguished from malingering disorder. Malingerers have an obvious recognizable, external incentive for producing the signs and symptoms that they exhibit (e.g., they do not want to return to work, have legal reasons, or are looking for monetary gain.)

4. Substance abuse: Patients who are abusing substances do not exhibit symptoms of the kind described. However, substance abuse can occur in patients with factitious disorder. If a patient who has a documented factitious disorder also has a substance abuse problem, it is very important that both conditions be evaluated, diagnosed, assessed, and treated.

5. Ganser syndrome was described in Answer 7.

10. **c.** Individuals with factitious disorder often have a history of abuse and/or severe deprivation during childhood. Some clinicians believe that this has etiologic significance. In such an environment the patient learns to expect rejection and abuse and may learn to use the illusion of a genuine illness to create a closer bond with caregivers. Later in life, patients tend to repeat these interactions with health care personnel, desperately seeking their attention and angrily expecting rejection.

11. **d.** Factitious disorder is associated with (1) decreased self-worth and self-esteem; (2) inadequate identity formation; (3) masochistic personality traits; (4) learned helplessness as a child, if abuse was present; and (5) tendency to seek approval from everyone, especially caregivers.

12. **a.** The treatment of factitious disorder focuses on management of the illness rather than on its cure. Unfortunately, there is little evidence for long-term effectiveness of specific forms of psychotherapy or pharmacotherapy for this disorder. However, because patients with factitious disorder often have comorbid psychiatric disorders, selected medications and psychotherapy for these comorbid conditions may be helpful. Treatment for substance abuse if present is particularly helpful to stabilize a patient with a factitious disorder because drug-seeking behavior often complicates the situation.

The single most important factor in successful management of this condition is a physician's early recognition of the disorder with a goal of averting iatrogenic complications. As with other covert conditions such as spousal abuse, it is important to consider factitious disorder. A physician will not make this diagnosis unless it is first considered as a possibility.

SOLUTION TO THE CLINICAL CASE MANAGEMENT PROBLEM

Factitious disorder usually begins in early adulthood, although occasionally it starts in childhood or in adolescence. Characteristically, the following series of events begins the chain reaction of seeing physicians, multiple referral to more physicians, admission to hospitals, voluntary discharge from the hospital if the situation becomes uncomfortable, and quickly checking into a new hospital.

1. The onset of the disorder or of discrete episodes of treatment seeking may follow a real illness, a loss (and subsequent adjustment reaction), or an abandonment (and subsequent adjustment reaction).

2. Usually the patient or a close relative of the patient had a hospitalization in childhood or early adolescence for a genuine physical illness. Thereafter a long pattern of successive hospitalizations unfolds, beginning insidiously and progressing in a spiral that is difficult to stop.

SUMMARY OF FACTITIOUS DISORDERS

1. **Prevalence:** Approximately 5% of admissions to community hospitals are for factitious disorders.

2. **Etiology:** Etiology is associated with childhood abuse or child deprivation. In addition, there is often a history of genuine physical illness in the patient or a close relative or caregiver during childhood.

3. The cycle of illness begins in early adult life usually following discrete episodes of treatment following a real illness. After an insidious beginning, a long pattern of successive hospitalizations unfolds.
4. **Demographic characteristics:** Factitious disorder is more common in males, hospital workers, and health care workers.
5. **DSM-IV criteria for factitious disorder are as follows:**
   a. The patient intentionally produces or feigns physical or psychological signs or symptoms.
   b. The motivation for the behavior is to assume the sick role.
   c. External activities for the behavior (such as economic gain, avoiding legal responsibility, or improving physical well-being [as in malingering disorders]) are absent.
6. **DSM-IV subtypes:**
   a. Predominantly psychological signs and symptoms
   b. Predominantly physical signs and symptoms (Munchausen syndrome)
   c. Combined psychological and physical signs and symptoms
7. **Differential diagnosis of factitious disorder:**
   a. Somatoform disorders: (i) somatization disorder; (ii) conversion disorder; and (iii) hypochondriasis.
   b. Personality disorders: (i) antisocial personality disorder; (ii) borderline personality disorder; and (iii) histrionic personality disorder

c. Malingering: The most important feature distinguishing factitious disorder from malingering is that in malingering the patient has an obvious, recognizable, environmental goal for producing signs and symptoms of a particular condition.
   d. Substance abuse syndrome
8. **Course and prognosis:** (a) begins in early adult life; (b) usual history is one of severe, incapacitating emotional trauma or untoward reactions; and (c) overall prognosis for establishing a normal life is poor.
9. **Treatment:** The most important factor in any kind of successful management of factitious disorder is to make the diagnosis before iatrogenic interventions cause severe physical disability. If you do not think of the diagnosis, then you will not make the diagnosis. Successful pharmacotherapy and psychotherapeutic interventions are limited to the treatment of comorbid psychiatric conditions.

SUGGESTED READING

American Psychiatric Association: *Diagnostic and statistical manual of mental disorders IV–TR,* 4th ed. American Psychiatric Association Press, 2000 Washington, DC.

Folks D, et al: Somatoform disorders, factitious disorders, and malingering. In Stoudemire A, et al, eds: *Psychiatric care of the medical patient,* 2nd ed. Oxford University Press, 2000, New York, 458-475.

Kaplan HI, Sadock BJ: Factitious disorders. In Kaplan HI, Sadock BJ, eds: *Kaplan and Sadock's synopsis of psychiatry: Behavioral sciences/ clinical psychiatry,* 8th ed. Williams & Wilkins, 1998, Baltimore.

Tomb DA: *Psychiatry,* 6th ed. Williams & Wilkins, 1999, Baltimore.

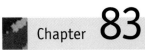

Chapter 83

Somatoform Disorders

> "Doctor, I'm sure there is not another girl in the world with a nose like mine. I need to see a plastic surgeon."

CLINICAL CASE PROBLEM 1:

A 27-Year-Old Female with 22 Different Symptoms

A 27-year-old female comes to your office for an initial consultation. She has heard from her best friend that "you are the most competent physician in the city." The symptoms described include chest pain, palpitations, "beating thyroid gland," nausea, periodic vomiting, abdominal pain, diarrhea, dizziness, gait disturbance, double vision, blurred vision, "seizures" (she falls down in the middle of crowds of people), pain on urination, back pain, abdominal pain, neck pain, headaches, vaginal paresthesias, intolerance to fatty foods, intolerance to high-fiber foods, heartburn, and "constant gas." She tells you in an authoritative and dramatic manner, "I just can't take it any more, Doctor, and I guess that is why I have come to you. I hear you are so good!"

■ SELECT THE BEST ANSWER TO THE FOLLOWING QUESTIONS:

1. What is the most likely diagnosis in this patient?
   a. somatization disorder
   b. conversion disorder
   c. thyroid cancer
   d. hypochondriasis
   e. masked depression

2. At this time, what would you do?
   a. step out of the room and ask your secretary to page you in 5 minutes
   b. tell the patient that you believe she is exaggerating her symptoms
   c. prescribe a benzodiazepine (alprazolam)
   d. make another appointment with the patient to establish a more trusting relationship and perform a thorough history and physical
   e. tell the patient that her problems are most likely emotionally based and refer her to a psychotherapist

3. What is the pharmacologic treatment of choice for the disorder described?
   a. a benzodiazepine
   b. divalproex
   c. a selective serotonin reuptake inhibitor (SSRI)
   d. a monoamine oxidase inhibitor (MAOI)
   e. none of the above

CLINICAL CASE PROBLEM 2:
A 23-YEAR-OLD FEMALE COMPLAINING OF HAVING "A PECULIARLY PROMINENT JAW"

A 23-year-old female comes to your office with a chief complaint of having "a peculiarly prominent jaw." She tells you that she has seen a number of plastic surgeons about this problem, but "every one has refused to do anything."

On examination, there is no protrusion that you can see, and it appears to you that she has a completely normal jaw and face. Although the physical examination is completely normal, she appears depressed.

4. What is the most likely diagnosis in this patient?
   a. dysthymia
   b. major depressive disorder (MDD) with somatic concerns
   c. somatization disorder
   d. body dysmorphic disorder
   e. hypochondriasis

5. Therapies that reportedly have produced successful results in this disorder include which of the following?
   a. cognitive-behavioral therapy (CBT)
   b. SSRIs
   c. tricyclic antidepressants (TCAs)
   d. individual or group psychotherapies
   e. all of the above

CLINICAL CASE PROBLEM 3:
A MOTHER OF FIVE WITH A CONSTANT HEADACHE

A 29-year-old mother of five comes to your office with a "constant headache." She states she is unable to ambu-late without assistance because of her neck, abdominal, pelvic, and rib pain. She goes on to say that she has been diagnosed as having fibromyalgia. After performing a complete history, physical examination, and laboratory and radiologic workup, you make a diagnosis of tension headache. She then tells you that she has seen a number of other physicians about the same problem and that they have come to the same conclusion (which she believes is totally incorrect). You ask her to return for a further discussion about this problem next week, shake hands, and are about to leave. However, she continues to discuss the details of her pain and the difficulties that the pain causes her.

You tell her that you will continue discussion of these problems with her when you see her next week. You again attempt to leave the office.

6. What is the most likely diagnosis in this patient?
   a. schizophrenia
   b. conversion disorder
   c. chronic pain syndrome
   d. somatization disorder
   e. none of the above

7. What is the preferred treatment for this patient?
   a. weekly (daily, if needed) visits with you
   b. group psychotherapy
   c. CBT
   d. supportive psychotherapy
   e. treatment in a multidisciplinary pain clinic

CLINICAL CASE PROBLEM 4:
A 27-YEAR-OLD WOMAN SUDDENLY BECOMING BLIND

A 27-year-old patient comes to the Emergency Room (ER) with a complaint of "having suddenly gone blind." Apparently, she was walking down the street on her way to work and, suddenly, she could not see. The visual impairment that she describes is bilateral, complete (no vision), and associated with "numbness, tingling, and weakness" in both lower extremities.

Her husband accompanies her to the ER and gruffly tells you, "Whatever it is, Doc, I want you to fix it and fix it fast."

The physical examination of the patient suggests a significant difference between the subjective symptoms and the objective complaints. Specifically, both the knee jerks and the ankle jerks are present and brisk; however, motor strength and sensation in both lower extremities appear diminished, not following anatomic pathways.

8. Based on the information provided, what is the most likely diagnosis?
   a. somatization disorder
   b. conversion disorder
   c. bilateral ophthalmic artery occlusion and spinal artery occlusion

d. histrionic personality disorder

e. none of the above

9. What is the most appropriate next step at this time?
   a. call an ophthalmologist immediately (stat)
   b. call a neurologist stat
   c. call a psychiatrist stat
   d. call a social worker stat
   e. reassure the patient and initiate discussion about stressors

CLINICAL CASE PROBLEM 5:

A 41-Year-Old Male Requesting a Cancer Checkup

A 41-year-old male comes to you for his first visit, requesting a "complete cancer checkup." You learn that this patient has had six complete cancer checkups already this year. He has had two of the six done at "executive checkup centers." He is the chief executive officer (CEO) of a large company and thus has the opportunity to take advantage of some "health perks." He provides a list of the tests he wishes to have done, including a complete history, a complete physical examination, a complete laboratory profile, a colonoscopy, an upper endoscopy, a skeletal x-ray survey, and a "head-to-toe" magnetic resonance imaging scan.

You learn that this patient is afraid that he has cancer, specifically colon cancer because a close relative was diagnosed with a colon cancer 2 years earlier and advised him to get checked as often as possible.

You are amazed that he actually has time to function as the CEO of his company. The truth is, however, that he does not. He admits that this fear is greatly interfering with his work and social life.

10. What is the most likely diagnosis in this patient?
    a. somatization disorder
    b. hypochondriasis
    c. factitious disorder
    d. obsessive-compulsive disorder (OCD)
    e. MDD

11. What is the treatment of choice for the patient described?
    a. weekly reassurance that he does not have cancer after performing all the tests he has requested
    b. weekly assurance that he does not have cancer without performing all the tests he has requested
    c. weekly assurance that he does not have cancer after refusing to perform all the tests he has requested
    d. collaboration between the primary care physician and a psychiatrist to develop a plan for regularly seeing this patient, managing his con-

dition, alleviating his anxiety, and providing coping skills training

e. all of d, lithium carbonate prophylactically, and an SSRI agent

12. The term *somatodymia*:
    a. denotes the inability to describe or be aware of emotions
    b. denotes a specific neuroendocrine syndrome
    c. communicates the inability to express physical distress in psychological language
    d. describes the use of somatically based complaints to convey emotional discomfort
    e. denotes the inability to express psychological distress in feeling terms

---

CLINICAL CASE MANAGEMENT PROBLEM

Describe the most important factors in the assessment of pain complaints.

■ **ANSWERS:**

1. **a.** This patient has somatization disorder. Somatization disorder is characterized by the following symptoms: (1) multiple physical complaints of long-standing occurrence; (2) these symptoms usually have resulted in significant medical diagnostic testing, medical interventions, and invasive procedures often causing iatrogenic sequelae; (3) the illness has resulted in significant occupational or social malfunction; (4) the patient's complaints include symptoms that are not fully explained by a known medical condition or by clinical findings; (5) pain is experienced in at least four different sites, including headache or related pain, abdominal pain, back pain, joint pain, extremity pain, chest pain, rectal pain, or dyspareunia; (6) the symptoms include two or more gastrointestinal (GI) symptoms including nausea, diarrhea, bloating, vomiting, and food intolerance; (7) also included are one or more sexual symptoms including erectile or ejaculatory dysfunction, menstrual irregularities, or decreased libido or indifference; (8) the symptoms include one or more pseudoneurologic symptoms including a conversion symptom or a dissociative symptom; and (9) these symptoms are not produced consciously.

The patient has no volitional control over these manifestations, which are believed to be expressions of underlying unacceptable emotion.

2. **d.** In this patient another visit is reasonable to establish a more trusting relationship and perform a thorough history and physical examination. Assessment and treatment of somatization disorder include the following principles: (1) the patient's illness must

be understood and addressed in a holistic fashion; (2) diagnostic procedures and therapeutic interventions must be chosen carefully to minimize adverse reactions and problems with indeterminate results fueling the disease; (3) forming an effective therapeutic alliance with the patient is essential; (4) the patient's social support system must be engaged and strengthened; (5) a regular appointment schedule with the primary care physician will help minimize crisis visits and will help to manage the condition; (6) the dialogue that occurs between the doctor and the patient must address symptoms and signs from a both a somatic and psychosocial viewpoint, including the emotional precipitants and consequences of the symptoms; (7) once the patient has gained insight into the psychological nature of the condition, a referral to a therapist may be indicated. (If this is done too early in the process, patients will be highly resistant, which will negatively affect the therapeutic alliance); (8) mood disorders and/or substance abuse problems can develop concomitantly to somatoform disorders and should be treated aggressively; (9) a possibly history of early physical, sexual, or emotional abuse should be explored; and (10) treatment of somatoform disorders needs to focus on management rather than cure.

3. **e.** Pharmacologic treatment is not helpful in the treatment of somatoform disorders. However, sometimes pharmacologic treatment of symptoms is helpful in establishing the therapeutic alliance. Concomitant psychiatric conditions may be treated with appropriate medications.

4. **d.** This patient has body dysmorphic disorder, a condition characterized by the following: (1) a preoccupation with an imagined or grossly exaggerated body defect; (2) clinically apparent distress associated with social, occupational, or functional impairment; and (3) psychiatric conditions such as OCD, anorexia nervosa, psychosis, or other psychiatric disorders cannot account for the preoccupation and the impairment.

Additionally, the differential diagnosis of body dysmorphic disorder includes the following: (1) anxiety disorders; (2) MDD; (3) hypochondriasis; (4) other somatoform disorders; (5) factitious disorders; and (6) malingering.

5. **e.** General principles for somatization disorders discussed in the previous question apply to management of body dysmorphic disorder; however, the somatic preoccupations are often persistent. Individual or group psychotherapy is sometimes useful. CBT is used increasingly for the treatment of this condition. SSRIs or TCAs have been used for some patients, especially in cases with coexisting depression. Overall,

however, pharmacologic approaches are not the mainstay of therapy for this condition.

6. **c.** The diagnosis for the patient in Clinical Case Problem 3 is chronic pain syndrome, sometimes called "pain disorder associated with psychological factors." The criteria for this diagnosis are as follows: (1) pain is the central clinical feature and is of sufficient severity to require assessment; (2) the pain results in social, occupational, or functional impairment or clinically significant distress; (3) psychological factors precipitate, exacerbate, or maintain the pain or contribute to the severity of the pain; and (4) the pain is not a component of somatization disorder or other psychiatric disorders including sexual dysfunction.

The differential diagnosis of chronic pain syndrome must take into consideration other psychiatric disorders such as a psychological factors affecting a general medical condition, somatization disorder, hypochondriasis, depressive disorders, generalized anxiety disorder, factitious disorder, and malingering.

Sometimes it is very difficult to differentiate this somatoform disorder from established medical conditions such as degenerative disc disease. Additionally, pain disorders often develop after an initial injury or illness.

Chronic pain syndrome is more common in women than men and may occur at any age. Often, patients have severe functional impairment and use pain medications extensively.

7. **e.** The treatment of choice for this patient is treatment in a multidisciplinary pain clinic. Such treatment has several objectives. Often patients first must be detoxified from analgesics and sedative hypnotics. Other nonpharmacologic treatments for pain control, including transcutaneous nerve stimulation, biofeedback, and other forms of behavioral psychotherapy, are substituted. The therapeutic emphasis must be shifted from elimination of all pain to management of pain and its consequences. Both psychological and physical therapies are used to minimize the functional limitations caused by the pain. Patients are encouraged to increase their social, occupational, and physical activities. These techniques are similar to those used in management of patients with chronic pain caused by general medical conditions. Specialized pain clinics are often the optimal treatment setting.

Depressive symptoms also must be addressed in pain management. Antidepressants are indicated when depressive disorders are present in these patients.

8. **b.** This patient has conversion disorder. Conversion disorders represent a type of somatoform disorder in which there is a loss or alteration in physical functioning during a period of psychological stress

that suggests a physical disorder but that cannot be explained on the basis of known physiologic mechanisms. Conversion disorders occasionally are seen in ambulatory care settings or emergency departments.

The *Diagnostic and Statistical Manual of Mental Disorders,* 4th edition (DSM-IV) criteria for conversion disorder are as follows: (1) the symptom(s) or deficit(s) are not consciously or intentionally produced; (2) the symptom(s) or deficit(s) are not medically explained after clinical assessment; (3) the initiation or exacerbation of the symptom(s) or deficit(s) usually is preceded by conflicts or stressors; psychological factors are prominent; (4) the symptom(s) or deficit(s) impair social or occupational functioning, create significant distress, or require medical intervention; and (5) the symptom(s) or deficit(s) are not limited to pain or sexual dysfunction and are not a component of somatization disorder or other psychiatric syndrome.

Common examples of conversion symptoms include paralysis, abnormal movements, aphonia, blindness, deafness, or pseudoseizures.

In this patient the possibility of domestic violence should be considered as a potential cause of stress leading to conversion symptoms. Although spousal abuse always should be considered, the somewhat peculiar demeanor of the husband in this Clinical Case Problem raises the index of suspicion. Diagnosis and management of spousal abuse is described in more detail in Chapter 89.

9. **e.** A wide variety of treatment techniques have been used successfully for the treatment of conversion disorder. The initial step in the management of acute symptoms is to quickly decrease the psychological stress. Brief psychotherapy focusing on stress and coping and suggestive therapy and sometimes hypnosis may be extremely effective. Pharmacologic interventions, including the acute use of benzodiazepines, also may be useful. Brief hospitalization sometimes may be indicated, particularly when symptoms are disabling or alarming. Hospitalization may serve to remove the patient from the stressful situation and to assess for possible underlying general medical conditions.

10. **b.** This patient has the disorder known as hypochondriasis, which is defined as a preoccupation with having a serious illness based on misinterpretation of physical symptoms that does not respond to physician reassurance after an appropriate evaluation. Individuals with hypochondriasis often have a profound fear of disease and an intense focus on multiple physical complaints and are hypervigilant to transient symptoms. On presentation, the medical history often is related in great detail. There is commonly a history of assessment by multiple physicians, deteriorating doctor–patient relationships, and associated feelings of frustration and anger. The clinical course is chronic, with waxing and waning of symptoms.

The DSM-IV diagnostic criteria for hypochondriasis include the following: (1) the patient is preoccupied or afraid of serious disease with misinterpretation of bodily symptoms for 6 months or longer; (2) medical evaluation and reassurance are not effective in allaying the preoccupation; (3) the preoccupation is not delusional, is not consistent with body dysmorphic disorder, and is not a component of another psychiatric disorder; and (4) significant social, occupational, and functional impairment occurs together with clinically significant distress.

The differential diagnosis of hypochondriasis includes somatization disorder, anxiety disorders, MDD, factitious disorders, malingering, and psychotic disorders manifesting hypochondriacal delusions.

Hypochondriasis may be distinguished from somatization disorder by the patient's source of concern. In hypochondriasis the concern is that the symptoms imply a serious illness. In somatization disorder, the concern is with discomfort of the symptoms themselves. The patient's anxiety regarding the experience of the symptoms is real and should not be discounted.

Factitious disorder is another important differential diagnosis. It is less likely in this Clinical Case Problem because there is no evidence of pathologic lying or recurrent, feigned, or simulated illness.

11. **d.** The primary care physician should consult with a psychiatrist about this patient and subsequently manage his condition. The patient should be seen on a regular basis to assure him that he will be followed closely and that any disease will be caught and treated in an early stage.

During these regular visits, attention must be paid to the psychosocial aspects of the patient's life. Coping skills training is useful. Psychological stress often is associated with the onset and maintenance of hypochondriasis. The general principles in caring for patients with somatization disorders should be followed, and coping skills should be taught.

Regular visits are essential to monitor symptoms, monitor anxiety or depression associated with the hypochondriacal symptoms, and help the patient come to terms with the condition. At the onset of treatment, visits should be scheduled frequently; later on, the time between visits can be increased as the patient's anxiety diminishes. Treatment of concomitant psychiatric conditions is important and may require collaboration with a mental health provider.

12. **d.** The term *somatodymia* denotes the use of physical complaints to convey emotional discomfort. Alexithymia denotes the inability or the limited capacity of some individuals to be aware of their own emotions or to articulate their feelings.

SOLUTION TO THE CLINICAL CASE MANAGEMENT PROBLEM

Pain is a prominent symptom in somatoform disorders and must be evaluated carefully. The experience of pain is real. Pain must be considered as a signal of a dysfunction in the physiologic, social, and/or psychological realms. The physician needs to determine whether the symptom of pain is caused primarily by a physical condition or is mediated predominantly by psychological factors. An assessment of the severity of impairment to the patient's functioning also must be made.

SUMMARY OF SOMATOFORM DISORDERS

1. **Somatization disorder:** Diagnostic clues include multiple physical complaints with onset before the age of 30. Tendency of these complaints is to be both chronic and longstanding. The complaints involve each of the following: pain symptoms, GI symptoms, sexual dysfunction symptoms, and pseudoneurologic symptoms. There is impairment of social or occupational functioning associated with these symptoms.
2. **Conversion disorder:** Diagnostic clues include physical symptoms primarily involving loss of motor or sensory function that are produced because of psychological conflicts or stressors. They cannot be fully explained on an anatomic basis and result in impairment of social or occupational functioning. Conversion disorder is more common among medically unsophisticated groups; it also may be a manifestation of a disturbed family or marital situation.
3. **Chronic pain syndrome:** Diagnostic clues include pain as the prominent clinical presentation, and it results in social, occupational, or functional impairment. This diagnosis is made when psychological factors are believed by the physician to have a significant role in the outset, severity, exacerbation, or perpetuation of the pain syndrome. Major depression or anxiety often are present and may be a component of the pain syndrome. The best therapeutic strategy is to limit inappropriate use of analgesics and other medical resources and to modify the patient's therapeutic expectations from cure to management of the pain while attempting to appreciate the role of psychosocial or psychological factors and stress. A multidisciplinary pain clinic is in most cases the treatment of choice.
4. **Hypochondriasis:** Hypochondriasis is characterized by a worry about having a serious disease that is based on hypervigilance and a misinterpretation of physical symptoms. It is not alleviated with appropriate physician reassurance. As with pain, the possibility of comorbid anxiety or depression should be strongly considered, and physical disease should be excluded. Treatment is most effective when there is collaboration between a primary care physician who continues regular appointments and a consulting psychiatrist. Again, the diagnosis requires significant social, occupational, or functional impairment.
5. **Body dysmorphic disorder:** The fundamental diagnostic feature is a pervasive feeling of ugliness or physical defect based on a grossly exaggerated perception of a minor (or even absent) physical anomaly. Patients frequently consult multiple primary care physicians, dermatologists, and plastic surgeons. Depressive symptoms, anxiety symptoms, social phobia, obsessive personality traits, and psychosocial distress frequently coexist. Intervention includes group or family therapy and, occasionally, the use of SSRIs or other medication to decrease obsessive concerns and depression.
6. **Malingering:** The essential feature of malingering is the intentional production of illness consciously motivated by external incentives such as avoiding military duty, obtaining financial compensation through litigation or disability, evading criminal prosecution, obtaining drugs, or securing better living conditions. Malingering is more likely when medical and legal context overshadows the presentation, marked discrepancy exists between the clinical presentation and objective findings, and a lack of cooperation is experienced with the patient. Confrontation in a confidential and empathic but firm manner that allows an opportunity for constructive dialogue and appreciation of any psychological or psychosocial problems is imperative.

SUGGESTED READING

Allen LA, et al: Psychosocial treatments for multiple unexplained physical symptoms: a review of the literature. *Psychosom Med* 64(6):939-950, 2002.

American Psychiatric Association: *Diagnostic and statistical manual of mental disorders IV–TR* 4th ed. American Psychiatric Association Press, 2000, Washington, DC.

Fischhoff B, Wessely S: Managing patients with inexplicable health problems. *BMJ* 326(7389):595-597, 2003.

Folks D, et al: Somatoform disorders, factitious disorders, and malingering. In Stoudemire A, ed: *Clinical psychiatry for medical students*, 3rd ed. JB Lippincott, 1998, Philadelphia.

Jacobson AM: Medically unexplained symptoms. In Jacobson: *Psychiatric secrets*, 2nd ed. Hanley and Belfus, 2001, Philadelphia.

Kaplan HI, Sadock BJ: Somatoform disorders. In Kaplan HI, Sadock BJ, eds: *Kaplan and Sadock's synopsis of psychiatry: Behavioral sciences/clinical psychiatry*, 8th ed. Williams & Wilkins, 1998, Baltimore.

Shaner R: *Psychiatry.* Williams & Wilkins, 1997, Baltimore.

Smith RC, et al: Treating patients with medically unexplained symptoms in primary care. *J Gen Intern Med* 18(6):478-489, 2003.

Stuart MR, Lieberman JA: The fifteen-minute hour. *Practical therapeutic interventions in primary care,* 3rd ed. WB Saunders, 2002, Philadelphia.

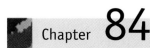

Chapter 84

Panic Disorder

> "If I try to do it, I know I'll die."

CLINICAL CASE PROBLEM 1:

A 29-YEAR-OLD FEMALE WITH A POUNDING HEART, SHORTNESS OF BREATH, CHEST PAIN, DIZZINESS, AND FEELINGS THAT SHE IS "LOSING HER MIND"

A 29-year-old female elementary school teacher comes to your office with recurrent attacks of anxiety associated with what she describes as a "pounding heart," "shortness of breath," "chest pain," "dizziness," and feelings that she is losing her mind. These attacks have been ongoing for at least 8 months and only seem to occur during school days. She tells you that these symptoms begin when she gets up in front of the class in the morning. When you question her carefully, you learn that she also develops similar symptoms when she gets into crowded stores or shopping malls.

Her history includes childhood separation anxiety. She states that her mother ran away with another man when she was 5 years old, and she was raised by her father.

Her physical examination is essentially unremarkable. Her blood pressure is 130/70 mm Hg, and the examination of the cardiovascular system and the respiratory system is normal, as is the rest of the examination.

▪ SELECT THE BEST ANSWER TO THE FOLLOWING QUESTIONS:

1. What is the most likely diagnosis in this patient?
   a. pheochromocytoma
   b. hyperthyroidism
   c. panic disorder
   d. paroxysmal atrial fibrillation
   e. generalized anxiety disorder (GAD)

2. The constellation of symptoms that this patient displays in relationship to her expressed fear of crowded stores or shopping malls is known as:
   a. social phobia
   b. specific phobia
   c. claustrophobia
   d. agoraphobia
   e. generalized phobia

3. Which of the following is (are) characteristic of this disorder?
   a. smothering sensations
   b. fear of going crazy
   c. fear of not being able to control a particular situation
   d. fear of dying
   e. all of the above

4. The "phobia" that is described in Clinical Case Problem 1 and that is specified in Question 2 is characterized by which of the following?
   a. an intense fear of being in public places
   b. acute bursts of terrifying levels of anxiety
   c. avoidance of places where help may be unavailable or escape is difficult
   d. a loss of contact with reality, including hallucinations and delusions
   e. a, b, and c

5. Which of the following is (are) true of the disorder described in Clinical Case Problem 1?
   a. it is more common in males
   b. it usually begins in middle age
   c. it is rarely confused with coronary artery disease
   d. none of the above
   e. all of the above

6. Which of the following statements regarding the pharmacologic treatment of the disorder described in this Clinical Case Problem 1 is (are) true?

a. pharmacologic therapy is effective in blocking the symptoms of the disorder described
b. pharmacologic therapy is effective in treating the "avoidance" of the specific situation
c. a combination of pharmacologic therapy, psychoeducation, and biofeedback may be most helpful in the treatment of this disorder
d. all of the above
e. a and c only

7. Which of the following is the pharmacologic treatment of choice for this disorder?
   a. alprazolam
   b. phenelzine
   c. paroxetine
   d. imipramine
   e. atenolol

8. Which of the following drugs has the greatest potential for causing dependency during treatment of this condition?
   a. alprazolam
   b. phenelzine
   c. paroxetine
   d. imipramine
   e. atenolol

CLINICAL CASE PROBLEM 2:

29-YEAR-OLD MUSICIAN WITH INTENSE FEAR BEFORE PERFORMING

A 29-year-old musician consults with you regarding what he describes as "an intense fear" before he begins his nightly performance with a civic orchestra. He tells you that it is only a matter of time before he "makes a real major mistake."

9. What is the most likely diagnosis in this patient?
   a. a specific phobia
   b. a social phobia
   c. a mixed phobia
   d. panic disorder without agoraphobia
   e. panic disorder with agoraphobia

10. Which of the following is the treatment of choice for the patient described in Clinical Case Problem 2?
    a. alprazolam before his nightly music performance
    b. phenelzine before his nightly performance
    c. atenolol before his nightly performance
    d. clomipramine before his nightly performance
    e. paroxetine before his nightly performance

CLINICAL CASE MANAGEMENT PROBLEM

List four psychiatric disorders with which the condition described in Clinical Case Problem 1 is associated.

■ ANSWERS:

1. **c.** The most likely diagnosis in this patient is panic disorder. Panic disorder is defined as recurrent episodes of panic attacks (discrete periods of intense fear or discomfort) associated with other symptoms including dyspnea, chest pain, a fear of dying, dizziness, trembling, palpitations, choking sensations, nausea, numbness, hot flushes, a fear of going crazy, a fear of not being able in control of the current situation, and feelings of depersonalization.

Although organic disease must be considered (including tachyarrhythmias and thyroid dysfunction), this constellation of symptoms is typical for panic disorder.

2. **d.** Agoraphobia is characterized by an intense fear of becoming helpless during a panic attack in a public place. This fear often leads to chronic anxiety and restriction of activities, often to the point of becoming housebound. The patient with agoraphobia avoids supermarkets, shopping malls, church services, meetings, parties, elevators, tunnels, bridges, buses, subways, and other places where help might be unavailable or where escape is difficult.

3. **e.** Symptoms of a panic attack include a discrete period of intense fear or discomfort in which at least four of the following symptoms develop abruptly and reach a peak within 10 minutes: (1) palpitations, pounding heart, or accelerated heart rate; (2) sweating; (3) trembling or shaking; (4) sensations of shortness of breath or smothering; (5) a feeling of choking; (6) chest pain or discomfort; (7) nausea or abdominal distress; (8) feeling dizzy, unsteady, lightheaded, or faint; (9) chills or hot flushes; (10) fear of losing control or going crazy; (11) fear of dying; (12) paresthesias (numbness or tingling sensations); and (13) derealization (feelings of unreality or detachment from others) or depersonalization (becoming detached from oneself).

4. **e.** As discussed in Answer 2, agoraphobia is characterized by an intense fear of being in public places, acute bursts of terrifying levels of anxiety, and avoidance of places where help may be unavailable or escape is difficult. Agoraphobia is not, however, characterized by a loss of contact with reality, although patients may complain of "being in a daze" or "being in a fog" (feelings of derealization or depersonalization). They do not experience hallucinations or delusions.

5. d. Panic disorder is a common medical illness. It usually begins in the second or third decade of life, although children and older adults also may develop the disorder. It is twice as common in women as it is in men.

Genetic and epidemiologic studies consistently have demonstrated increased rates of panic disorder among first- and second-degree relatives of patients with panic disorder. This could be a result of genetic factors, nongenetic biologic factors, or cultural factors shared by family members. Between 15% and 18% of first-degree relatives of patients with panic disorder develop the condition.

Chest pain is a common presenting complaint among patients with panic disorder. Many of these patients present to the ER and are evaluated for acute coronary syndrome. Some patients with this condition undergo coronary angiography to rule out coronary artery disease or acute myocardial infarction. Other than cardiovascular symptoms, the two most common classes of symptoms are neurologic symptoms and gastrointestinal (GI) symptoms.

6. e. Available pharmacologic treatments for panic disorder are often effective for treating the symptoms of acute panic attacks in panic disorder. Pharmacologic agents are less effective for treating the "avoidance" of the actual panic-inducing situation itself. For this component of panic disorder, cognitive behavioral treatments are useful.

The most commonly accepted therapy for panic disorder includes (1) pharmacologic treatments, (these are discussed in Answer 7) and (2) nonpharmacologic treatment:

a. First aid for acute panic attacks: patient is taught the AWARE technique:

A is for **A**nxiety: Patient labels symptom as anxiety.
W is for **W**atch it: Patient rates symptoms on a scale from 0-10.
A is for **A**ct with it: Patient does breathing to induce relaxation.
R is for **R**epeat: Patient rates symptoms again on a scale from 0-10.
E is for **E**xpect the best.

b. Graduated exposure to the phobic situation
c. Cognitive behavioral therapy to reduce irrational beliefs
d. Relaxation training and biofeedback, breathing retraining in response to exposure to somatic cues
e. Assertiveness training (can help with dependency, passivity, and suppressed anger)

f. Psychoeducation (a presentation of knowledge to the patient that includes symptoms, theories of causation, reassurance that what they believe will happen will actually not happen, and treatment strategies)
g. Group therapy (helps confirm to individuals with panic disorder that they are not alone)

7. c. Paroxetine and other selective serotonin reuptake inhibitors (SSRIs) such as fluoxetine, sertraline, and fluvoxamine are the drugs of choice for treating panic disorder. They are as efficacious as previous first-line medications such as clomipramine and imipramine and have fewer side effects and less toxicity.

Other agents that have proved effective in patients with panic disorder include the following:

1. Serotonergic tricyclic antidepressants (TCAs): Clomipramine and imipramine may be as efficacious as SSRIs but are more toxic in overdose and have more side effects.
2. High-potency benzodiazepines: The benzodiazepine of choice is alprazolam. Alprazolam often is used when SSRIs and TCAs are either contraindicated or poorly tolerated. It is highly effective for decreasing panic attacks. However, drug withdrawal symptoms are often evident several hours after the last dose and development of drug dependency is common (see later in this chapter). Clonazepam is another benzodiazepine that is used frequently for this indication because it is better tolerated by some individuals. Although the nonbenzodiazepine anxiolytic agent buspirone is effective in treating GAD, it is usually ineffective in treating panic disorder.
3. Monoamine oxidase inhibitors (MAOIs): MAOIs such as phenelzine and tranylcypromine are effective in reducing the anxiety associated with panic disorder. Necessary warnings regarding the need to maintain a low serum tyramine level sometimes may give patients with panic disorder "one more thing to worry about."
4. Beta blockers: Although the beta blockers may block symptoms such as palpitations and tremor, they are generally not as effective as SSRIs, benzodiazepines, TCAs, or MAOIs in treating panic attacks.

8. a. Alprazolam is a high-potency benzodiazepine that is very effective for treating panic attacks. Often, doses in the range of 2 mg PO qid (by mouth, four times per day) are required. The frequent daily doses are necessitated by the short half-life of the drug. Even with this dosing frequency, withdrawal symptoms may develop rapidly on discontinuation. These symptoms include anxiety and tremulousness and may be especially disturbing to patients with panic disorder. Drug dependency may develop, and it is unwise to decrease the dose without using a very gradual taper. Clonazepam causes fewer problems with dependency but is associated with more sedation. Other benzodiazepines are not as effective. Dependency issues make nonpharmacologic interventions more desirable.

9. b. This patient has what is referred to as performance anxiety, which is classified as a social phobia,

circumscribed type. This social phobia is really specific and is not at all uncommon. Most commonly, symptoms develop only in the situation of performance of the particular activity in question.

10. c. The treatment of choice in this patient is a beta-adrenergic blocking agent. The most commonly used agents include atenolol and metoprolol. Although propranolol is considered "the gold standard," a more selective beta blocker (selective in not crossing the blood–brain barrier) will produce less side effects of lightheadedness, dizziness, or fatigue.

SOLUTION TO THE CLINICAL CASE MANAGEMENT PROBLEM

A number of psychiatric disorders can be associated with panic disorder. They include (1) agoraphobia; (2) GAD; (3) MDD; and (4) substance abuse, including alcohol

Panic attacks and the anticipation of having a panic attack may cause individuals to avoid traveling and develop agoraphobia. Because of the nature of the symptoms, individuals with panic attacks and panic disorder commonly develop other associated psychiatric conditions. These include GAD and MMD. Often, patients self-medicate their anxiety with alcohol or illegal substances, leading to the association of panic attacks with alcoholism or substance abuse.

SUMMARY OF PANIC DISORDER

A. Prevalence: The lifetime prevalence is approximately 1.5%, 2.5 to 4 times greater for females than males.

B. Genetics: Risk of panic disorder in first-degree relatives of patients with panic disorder is about 15%.

C. Biochemistry: A wide range of substances are more likely to produce panic attacks in research subjects with panic disorder than in normal controls, leading to speculation as to biochemical causes. Panic-inducing substances include carbon dioxide, sodium lactate, yohimbine, and caffeine. It is likely that panic disorder may result from multiple biochemical causes.

D. Symptoms of panic disorder:
1. Recurrent panic attacks. Panic attacks are acute attacks of intense fear or discomfort associated with at least four of the following: (a) palpitations, pounding heart, tachycardia; (b) chest pain or discomfort; (c) fear of dying; (d) trem-

bling or shaking; (e) shortness of breath, smothering; (f) choking ; (g) nausea, abdominal distress; (h) sweating; (i) chills or hot flushes; (j) fear of losing control or going crazy; (k) paresthesias; (l) feeling dizzy, unsteady, lightheaded; (m) derealization; and (n) depersonalization.
2. Panic disorder is subclassified according to whether it is accompanied by agoraphobia. Agoraphobia is defined as anxiety about being in places or situations in which escape might be difficult (or embarrassing) or in which help may not be available in the event of having an unexpected or situationally predisposed panic attack. Agoraphobia may involve travel, driving, public places, or other situations such as sitting in a meeting or waiting in line.

E. Comorbid psychiatric conditions: Panic disorder is associated with alcoholism, substance abuse, GAD, major depressive disorder, and sometimes separation anxiety disorder.

F. Treatment:
1. Nonpharmacologic: Behavioral treatment, including the following:

a. First aid for acute panic attacks: Patient is taught the AWARE technique:

A is for **A**nxiety: Patient labels symptom as anxiety.
W is for **W**atch it: Patient rates symptoms on a scale from 0-10.
A is for **A**ct with it: Patient does breathing to induce relaxation.
R is for **R**epeat: Patient rates symptoms again on a scale from 0-10.
E is for **E**xpect the best.

b. Graduated exposure to the phobic situation
c. Cognitive behavioral therapy to reduce irrational beliefs
d. Relaxation training and biofeedback, breathing retraining in response to exposure to somatic cues
e. Assertiveness training (can help with dependency, passivity, and suppressed anger)
f. Psychoeducation (a presentation of knowledge to the patient that includes symptoms, theories of causation, reassurance that what they believe will happen will actually not happen, and treatment strategies)
g. Group therapy (helps confirm to individuals with panic disorder that they are not alone)

2. Pharmacologic:
   a. SSRIs, including paroxetine, fluoxetine, sertraline, and fluvoxamine, are drugs of first choice but may be associated with GI distress, increased anxiety, or sedation.
   b. High-potency benzodiazepines, especially alprazolam and clonazepam, are highly effective but may be associated with sedation and dependency.
   c. Clomipramine and imipramine are effective, but they are associated with anticholinergic effects, sedation, and toxicity in overdose.
   d. Beta blockers are useful when circumscribed social phobia (performance anxiety) is present.
   e. MAOIs sometimes are used when other medications are ineffective or contraindicated.

SUGGESTED READING

American Psychiatric Association: *Diagnostic and statistical manual of mental disorders IV–TR*, 4th ed. American Psychiatric Association Press, 2000, Washington, DC.
Beck AT, et al: *Anxiety disorders and phobias: a cognitive perspective*. Basic Books, 1990, New York.
Kaplan HI, Sadock BJ: Anxiety disorders. In Kaplan HI, Sadock BJ, eds: *Kaplan and Sadock's synopsis of psychiatry: Behavioral sciences/clinical psychiatry*, 8th ed. Williams & Wilkins, 1998, Baltimore.
Stuart MR, Lieberman JA: The fifteen-minute hour. *Practical therapeutic interventions in primary care*, 3rd ed. WB Saunders, 2002, Philadelphia.

Chapter 85

Social Phobia, Posttraumatic Stress, and Obsessive-Compulsive Disorder

"I knew it was a depraved act, but I just couldn't control myself."

CLINICAL CASE PROBLEM 1:
A 22-YEAR-OLD LAW STUDENT UNABLE TO ANSWER QUESTIONS IN CLASS

A 22-year-old law student comes to your office in a state of anxiety. He is taking a law class in which 50% of the class grade is based on class participation. Although he knows the material well, he is unable to answer the questions when posed to him by the professor. He now has gone through 2 months of the 6-month class and has not been able to answer one of the 14 questions that the professor has asked him in class.

The professor asked him to make an appointment for a "little chat" the other day. At that time, he was told that he would (in the professor's words) "fail the class" unless he began to participate.

The student describes himself as a loner. He tells you that he has always been shy, but this is the first time the shyness has really threatened to have a major impact on him. His family history is significant for what he terms "this shyness." His mother has the same characteristics, but for her it does not seem to be causing the kind of life difficulties it is causing him.

His mental status examination is essentially normal.

■ SELECT THE BEST ANSWER TO THE FOLLOWING QUESTIONS:

1. What is the most likely diagnosis in this patient?
   a. panic disorder with agoraphobia
   b. panic disorder without agoraphobia
   c. panic disorder with social phobia
   d. social phobia
   e. specific phobia

2. Which of the following is not a characteristic of the disorder described?
   a. persistent fear of humiliation
   b. exaggerated fear of humiliation
   c. embarrassment in social situations
   d. high levels of distress in particular situations
   e. fear of crowds or fear of closed-in spaces

3. Which of the following physiologic symptoms is not characteristic of the disorder described?
   a. blushing
   b. trembling
   c. bradycardia
   d. sweating
   e. elevated blood pressure

4. The neurochemical basis of the disorder described has been associated with which of the following neurotransmitters?
   a. epinephrine
   b. norepinephrine
   c. serotonin
   d. a and b only
   e. a, b, and c

5. Which of the following pharmacologic agents is used most commonly to treat this disorder?
   a. benzodiazepines
   b. monoamine oxidase inhibitors (MAOIs)
   c. tricyclic antidepressants (TCAs)
   d. newer antipsychotic medications
   e. beta blockers

6. With respect to this disorder, which of the following psychotherapies is most effective?
   a. cognitive-behavioral therapy (CBT)
   b. brief psychodynamic therapy
   c. psychoanalysis
   d. biofeedback
   e. all of the above

CLINICAL CASE PROBLEM 2:

A 27-Year-Old Woman Who Is Terrified of Flying

A 27-year-old woman is terrified of flying in airplanes and avoids all travel in them. As a result, she has lost promotional opportunities in her work and rarely sees her family, who lives in a distant city.

7. Which of the following disorders is the most likely diagnosis?
   a. panic disorder
   b. social phobia
   c. generalized anxiety disorder (GAD)

   d. specific phobia
   e. obsessive-compulsive disorder (OCD)

CLINICAL CASE PROBLEM 3:

A 73-Year-Old Male Who Is Anxious and Withdrawn

A 73-year-old male is brought to your office by his wife. His wife states that for the last 2 months her husband has been anxious and withdrawn. He was robbed at gunpoint in a shopping mall parking structure just before his symptoms began. Since that time, her husband refuses to enter parking structures or drive alone. He sleeps poorly and has complained of nightmares about the robbery. The patient himself says only that he feels unhappy but does not want to talk about the robbery. He says, "I just want to put it behind me."

8. What is the most likely diagnosis in this patient?
   a. primary insomnia
   b. adjustment disorder with anxious mood
   c. major depressive disorder (MDD)
   d. borderline personality disorder
   e. posttraumatic stress disorder (PTSD)

9. Characteristics of this disorder include which of the following?
   a. recurrent and intrusive recollections of disturbing events
   b. efforts to avoid thinking about what has happened in the past
   c. irritability or outbursts of anger
   d. a and b only
   e. a, b, and c

10. Regarding the treatment of the disorder described in Clinical Case Problem 3, which of the following statements is (are) true?
    a. treatment relies on a combination of nonpharmacologic and pharmacologic approaches
    b. nonpharmacologic treatment centers on desensitization that lowers anxiety from the conditioned stimulus
    c. TCAs have been used with some success in the treatment of this disorder
    d. MAOIs have been used with some success in the treatment of this disorder
    e. all of the above statements are true

11. Which of the following drugs has the most potential for abuse in the treatment of the disorder described in Clinical Case Problem 3?
    a. lithium carbonate
    b. phenelzine
    c. fluoxetine
    d. alprazolam
    e. desipramine

12. Which of the following medications generally would be considered the best initial choice for treatment of an acute episode of this disorder?
    a. lithium carbonate
    b. phenelzine
    c. sertraline
    d. alprazolam
    e. desipramine

CLINICAL CASE PROBLEM 4:

A COMPULSIVE 26-YEAR-OLD MALE WHO IS NEWLY MARRIED

A 26-year-old male, recently married, comes to your office with his new wife. They have been married for 3 months, and she tells you that she is very concerned about some of his behaviors. Apparently, when they go out the door in the morning and close the garage door, he goes around the block "at least eight times to make sure it is closed." Also, when he washes his hands before a meal, he often will go back and wash them at least three or four times during the meal itself "just to make sure they are clean."

The husband sits quietly and volunteers no information. He lived with his parents until he was married, and his wife tells you that apparently he was always very well protected by his mother.

When the patient finally begins to talk, he admits that everything his wife has just told you is true. He has done these things all his life, and it had never before presented a problem. His history is fairly unremarkable except for his "being a loner." Several family members, including his mother, have a history compatible with depression.

13. What is the most likely diagnosis in this patient?
    a. atypical depression
    b. schizophreniform disorder
    c. OCD
    d. GAD
    e. specific phobia

14. Which of the following medications is the best initial choice for the treatment of this disorder?
    a. clomipramine
    b. phenelzine
    c. risperidone
    d. selective serotonin reuptake inhibitors (SSRIs)
    e. peroxide

15. Which of the following psychotherapies is most useful for treatment of this disorder?
    a. psychodynamic psychotherapy
    b. humanistic psychotherapy
    c. supportive psychotherapy
    d. crisis counseling
    e. CBT

CLINICAL CASE MANAGEMENT PROBLEM

List five common obsessions and five common compulsions associated with OCD.

■ ANSWERS:

1. **d.** This patient has a social phobia, which is characterized by a marked and persistent fear of one or more social or performance situations in which the person is exposed to unfamiliar people or to possible scrutiny by others. Those patients fear that they may act in a manner that will be humiliating or embarrassing. Examples include (as in this patient) not being able to talk when asked to speak in public, choking on food when eating in front of others, being unable to urinate in a public lavatory, hand trembling when writing in the presence of others, and saying foolish things or not being able to answer questions (as in this patient) in social situations.

In addition, exposure to the feared social situation almost invariably provokes anxiety. The individual realizes that his or her behavior is abnormal and unreasonable. The feared social or performance situation either is avoided or endured with intense anxiety; and the avoidance, anxious participation, or distress in the feared social or performance situation interfere significantly with the person's normal occupational, academic, or social functioning and relationships with others.

2. **e.** Fear of crowds, in which escape may not be possible, is known as agoraphobia. Fear of closed spaces is known as claustrophobia. All the other choices correctly describe symptoms of social phobia.

3. **c.** The fear of speaking, meeting people, eating, or writing in public is related to the fear of "appearing nervous or foolish," making mistakes, being criticized, or being laughed at. This triggers elevated sympathetic arousal. Physical symptoms include blushing, trembling, sweating, elevated blood pressure, and tachycardia.

4. **e.** Symptoms reported by patients with social phobia in phobic situations suggest heightened autonomic arousal. When placed in a phobic situation, social phobics experience significant increases in heart rate that are highly correlated with self-perceived physiologic arousal (in contrast to claustrophobics, who experience less heart rate increase and negative correlations between perceived and actual physiologic arousal). Stressful public speaking situations result in twofold or threefold increases in plasma epinephrine levels. Norepinephrine increases also are seen.

Until recently, only epinephrine and norepinephrine were the neurotransmitters associated with the neurochemical basis of this disorder. However, now that the new SSRI agents have been shown to be effective in social phobic situations, serotonin is recognized as likely to be involved also. In this case, it would seem that social phobics would demonstrate a relative deficiency of serotonin-mediated activity rather than an excess, as seen with epinephrine and norepinephrine.

5. **e.** Beta blockers (such as atenolol 50-100 mg/day) commonly are used to treat circumscribed forms of social phobia such as fears of public speaking or performances.

Generalized social phobia is often less responsive to pharmacologic interventions. Although SSRIs are considered the drug class of choice, MAOIs, specifically phenelzine (45-90 mg/day), buspirone, and benzodiazepines, have all been reported to be occasionally effective.

6. **a.** CBT is particularly effective for treating social phobia. The treatment consists of desensitization through graduated exposure to social situations, modifying cognitive distortions, psychoeducation, and relaxation training.

7. **d.** The most likely diagnosis in this patient is specific phobia. Specific phobias involve intense fear and avoidance of specific objects or situations. The individual recognizes the fear and avoidance as excessive, and the symptoms result in occupational or social impairment. Common specific phobias include certain animals, heights, flying, closed spaces, crossing bridges, darkness, and blood.

8. **e.** The most likely diagnosis in this patient is PTSD. The essential features of this disorder involve the presence of intrusive recollections, emotional numbing and avoidance, difficulty sleeping and anxiety, all occurring after an event that causes feelings of danger, helplessness, and horror or after witnessing traumatic events such as the terrorist attacks of September 11, 2002.

9. **e.** There are five major criteria for the diagnosis of PTSD listed in the DSM-IV: (1) experiencing or witnessing an event that involves death, threat to life, or serious injury to himself or others that was experienced with intense fear, helplessness, or horror; (2) a traumatic event that is persistently experienced in ways such as recurrent and intrusive distressing recollections, dreams, feelings or thoughts that the event is recurring; psychological distress at exposure to symbolic events of that time, and physiologic reactivity on exposure to cues of that event; (3) persistent avoidance of stimuli associated with the trauma or numbing of general responsiveness, including efforts to avoid thoughts or feelings of the event; efforts to avoid activities, situations, or people associated with the event; inability to recall some aspect of the event (psychological amnesia); feelings of detachment or distance from others; diminished ability to have "affective feelings;" and a sense of a foreshortened future; (4) persistent symptoms of increased arousal (this is very common in war veterans) indicated by difficulty falling or staying asleep, irritability or outbursts of anger, difficulty concentrating, hypervigilance, and exaggerated startle response; and (5) marked distress or significant impairment in social or occupational functioning caused by the disturbance. Symptoms must exist for at least 1 month.

10. **e.** As is the case with other anxiety disorders, treatment for PTSD often is best accomplished with a combination of pharmacologic and nonpharmacologic therapies. SSRIs, including sertraline, often are used as medications of first choice for treating PTSD. However, many other medications have been used, and there are few controlled trials confirming the superiority of one class of drugs over another in the treatment of this disorder. Phenelzine (an MAOI) and imipramine (a TCA) have been used often. Other drugs that have shown some efficacy include clonidine, propranolol, lithium, and buspirone.

11. **d.** Alprazolam and other benzodiazepines are relatively contraindicated in this patient because of their increased potential for substance abuse and dependence in patients with PTSD. Benzodiazepines might be useful immediately after the traumatic event to help with sleep and functioning and the ability to process the event. However, their use needs to be limited to no more than 2 weeks to avoid dependence issues.

12. **d.** As discussed earlier, acute stress reactions associated with PTSD are best treated short term with a benzodiazepine such as alprazolam or clonazepam, the latter having lower incidence of dependency and a longer duration of action. This initial pharmacologic treatment should be supplemented by supportive/expressive psychotherapy (crisis counseling and/or support groups).

However, the chronic, recurrent nature of PTSD requires a more complex treatment including drugs and CBT. Drugs used to reduce anxiety symptoms of intrusion and/or avoidance behavior include tricyclics such as imipramine, desipramine, or amitriptyline; MAOIs such as phenelzine; and SSRIs such as fluoxetine or sertraline. Trazodone, a sedating antidepressant, often is used to treat insomnia.

CBTs (including relaxation training, systematic desensitization, flooding, and cognitive reframing) are most effective for decreasing symptoms of re-experiencing and hyperarousal. Hypnotherapy also has been useful.

13. **c.** This patient has OCD, which consists of either recurrent obsessions or recurrent compulsions, or both. The recurrent obsessions include persistent thoughts, impulses, or images that the patient attempts to ignore but cannot. Additionally, the obsessions are not just excessive worries about real-life problems; the patient also recognizes that these obsessions are, in fact, the product of his or her own mind.

Common obsessions include obsessions regarding contamination or illness; violent images; fear of harming others or harming oneself; perverse or forbidden sexual thoughts, images, or impulses; symmetry or exactness; somatic situations; and religious thoughts.

Compulsions are repetitive behaviors or mental acts that the individual feels driven to perform in response to an obsession or according to rigid rules. The behavior or mental act is aimed at preventing or reducing distress or preventing a dreaded event or situation. These behaviors, however, are not connected in a realistic manner with what they are designed to neutralize or prevent and are clearly excessive.

The individual realizes that the compulsions are excessive and unreasonable. They cause marked distress in the person's life or significantly interfere with the person's normal routine, occupation, or social activities.

Common compulsions include checking things (e.g., door locks, water taps, and the oven), cleaning or washing articles or parts of the body, counting objects or things, hoarding or collecting articles or things, ordering or arranging articles or things, or repeating things (such as tapping).

14. **d.** SSRIs such as fluvoxamine have become the drugs of choice for treatment of OCD and have replaced clomipramine as the first-line medications for this indication.

15. **e.** In addition to pharmacotherapy, CBT techniques are also often effective. These techniques include relaxation training, guided imagery and stimulus exposure, paradoxical intent, response prevention and thought-stopping techniques, and modeling.

SOLUTION TO THE CLINICAL CASE MANAGEMENT PROBLEM

Some common obsessions are as follows: (1) contamination and illness; (2) fear of harming others or self; (3) perverse or forbidden sexual thoughts, images, or impulses; (4) violent images; (5) symmetry or exactness; (6) exaggerated health concerns; and (7) religious thoughts.

Some common compulsions are as follows: (1) checking things (e.g., doors, locks, water taps); (2) cleaning or washing; (3) counting objects of various types; (4) hoarding or collecting objects of various types; (5) ordering or arranging articles of various types; (6) repeating things (speech, tapping); and (7) committing some unethical, immoral, or criminal acts.

SUMMARY OF SOCIAL PHOBIA, POSTTRAUMATIC STRESS DISORDER, AND OBESESSIVE-COMPULSIVE DISORDER

A. Social phobia:

1. **Epidemiology:** The estimated 6-month prevalence rate of social phobia is 1.2% to 2.2%.

2. **Definition:** Social phobia is a persistent and overwhelming fear of one or more social or performance situations in which the individual is exposed to unfamiliar people or to possible scrutiny by others. Fear of speaking in public, hand trembling, and answering questions are particular examples. The fear is one of not being able to perform the particular activity and of being humiliated in public because of

this. It produces both embarrassment and high levels of distress.

The individual either avoids the situation or endures it with intense anxiety. The individual also realizes that the fear is unreasonable but is powerless to do anything about it. Additionally, the individual experiences occupational, social, or academic impairment with normal life activities and goals.

3. **Symptoms:** Not only are intense anxiety and fear experienced, but also symptoms of autonomic hyperactivity such as blushing, trembling, tachycardia, and elevated blood pressure.

4. **Neurochemistry:** There is probable increased noradrenergic and adrenergic activity related to autonomic hyperarousal. Serotonin systems also may be involved, given the therapeutic effects of SSRIs in this disorder.

Continued

SUMMARY OF SOCIAL PHOBIA, POSTTRAUMATIC STRESS DISORDER, AND OBESESSIVE-COMPULSIVE DISORDER—cont'd

5. **Treatment:**
   a. Nonpharmacologic: CBTs (including relaxation training, systematic desensitization, flooding, and cognitive reframing) are most effective for decreasing symptoms of hyperarousal.
   b. Pharmacologic: The drug class of choice is the SSRIs. Other drug classes of benefit are MAOIs (particularly phenelzine) and beta blockers (particularly atenolol and propranolol).
6. **Concomitant disorders:** One-third of patients with social phobia report a history of MDD.

B. PTSD:

1. **Epidemiology:** It is particularly important and common in war veterans. Survivors and witnesses of terrorist attacks and other life-threatening events are at increased risk for PTSD. Lifetime prevalence rates are as high as 30% in war veterans have been reported.
2. **Definition:** PTSD is defined as a specific constellation of symptoms that present as an immediate or delayed response to a catastrophic life event. Symptoms include recurrent or intrusive distressing recollections or dreams of the event, psychological distress at exposure to events that symbolize or resemble the event, and physiologic reactivity on exposure to internal or external cues. There is also persistent avoidance of stimuli associated with the trauma or numbing of general responsiveness and persistent symptoms of increased arousal (such as being unable to fall asleep or stay asleep).
3. Examples of typical traumatic events that can generate PTSD include the following: (a) combat or war experiences; (b) terrorist attacks; (c) serious accidents (automobile, bus, plane, or train crashes); (d) natural disasters (tornado, hurricane, flood, or earthquake); (e) physical assault (rape, physical or sexual abuse, mugging, or torture); (f) other personal serious associations with danger, death, or severe injury; and (g) witnessing the mutilation, serious injury, or violent death of another person.
4. **Treatment:**
   a. Nonpharmacologic therapy includes the following: (1) CBT; (2) psychodynamic therapy; and (3) hypnotherapy.
   b. Pharmacologic therapy: Drug classes that have been shown to be effective for various symptoms include SSRIs, other antidepressants, beta blockers, mood stabilizers, and buspirone. Long-term use of benzodiazepines is contraindicated when treating this disorder because of the increased association with substance dependence.
5. **Risk factors for development of PTSD:** The risk factors for development of PTSD include separation from parents during childhood, family history of anxiety, preexisting anxiety or depression, family history of antisocial behavior, female sex, and neuroticism.

C. OCD:

1. **Epidemiology:** The measured prevalence rate has been estimated at 2% to 3%.
2. **Definition:** OCD is a mental disorder in which obsessions (recurrent distressing thoughts, ideas, or impulses) are experienced as both unwanted and senseless but at the same time irresistible. Compulsions are repetitive, purposeful, intentional behaviors, usually performed in response to an obsession, and are recognized as unrealistic and unreasonable but instrumental in temporarily relieving anxiety.

   Common obsessions and compulsions are listed in the Solution to the Clinical Case Management Problem.
3. **Treatment:**
   a. Nonpharmacologic: Prolonged exposure to ritual-eliciting stimuli together with prevention of the compulsive response resulting in desensitization.
   b. Pharmacologic: SSRIs are the drugs of choice; clomipramine is also effective, but has more untoward effects. MAOIs and alprazolam or other high-potency benzodiazepines also can be used.

D. Coexisting disorders include the following: (1) other anxiety disorders; (2) eating disorders; (3) Gilles de la Tourette's syndrome; (4) schizophrenia; and (5) separation anxiety in childhood.

SUGGESTED READING

American Psychiatric Association: *Diagnostic and statistical manual of mental disorders IV–TR*, 4th ed. American Psychiatric Association Press, 2000, Washington, DC.

Kaplan HI, Sadock BJ: Mood disorders. In Kaplan HI, Sadock BJ, eds: *Kaplan and Sadock's synopsis of psychiatry: Behavioral sciences/clinical psychiatry*, 8th ed. Williams & Wilkins, 1998, Baltimore.

Nagy LM, et al: Anxiety disorders. In Stoudemire A, ed: *Clinical psychiatry for medical students*, 3rd ed. JB Lippincott, 1998, Philadelphia.

Tomb DA: *Psychiatry*, 6th ed. Williams & Wilkins, 1999, Baltimore.

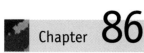

Chapter 86

Sexual Dysfunction

"Doctor, I'm not that old, but I just can't make love any more."

CLINICAL CASE PROBLEM 1:

A 65-Year-Old Male with Hypertension and Erectile Dysfunction

A 65-year-old male with hypertension, congestive heart failure, and peptic ulcer disease comes to your office for his regular blood pressure check. Although his blood pressure is now under control, he complains of an inability to maintain an erection. He currently is taking alpha-methyldopa, propranolol, verapamil, hydrochlorothiazide, and cimetidine.

On examination his blood pressure is 125/76 mm Hg. His pulse is 56 and regular. The rest of the cardiovascular examination and the rest of the physical examination are normal.

■ SELECT THE BEST ANSWER TO THE FOLLOWING QUESTIONS:

1. Which of the medications listed is the least likely to be the cause of this man's erectile dysfunction (ED)?
   a. alpha-methyldopa
   b. propranolol
   c. verapamil
   d. hydrochlorothiazide
   e. cimetidine

2. Which of the following generally is considered to be the most common cause of sexual dysfunction in both males and females?
   a. pharmacologic agents
   b. panic disorder
   c. generalized anxiety disorder (GAD)
   d. major depressive disorder (MDD)
   e. dysthymic disorder

3. Which of the following agents is not associated with sexual dysfunction?
   a. captopril
   b. labetalol
   c. hydralazine
   d. methadone
   e. all of the above have been implicated as a cause of sexual dysfunction

4. Which of the following is the most common sexual complaint in younger males?
   a. hypoactive sexual desire disorder
   b. male erectile disorder
   c. orgasmic disorder
   d. premature ejaculation
   e. none of the above

5. Which of the following is the most common sexual complaint in older males?
   a. hypoactive sexual desire disorder
   b. ED
   c. orgasmic disorder
   d. premature ejaculation
   e. none of the above

6. Which of the following statements regarding the cause of male sexual dysfunction is most accurate?
   a. male sexual dysfunction is almost always psychological in origin
   b. male sexual dysfunction is almost always organic in origin
   c. psychological factors play an important role both in primary and secondary forms of male sexual dysfunction.
   d. male sexual dysfunction in a younger patient has a greater probability of being organic in origin
   e. male sexual dysfunction in an older patient has a greater probability of being psychological in origin

7. Which of the following organic disorders is the most common cause of organic male sexual dysfunction?
   a. benign prostatic hypertrophy
   b. hyperthyroidism
   c. Parkinson's disease
   d. diabetes mellitus
   e. atherosclerosis of the abdominal aorta

8. What is the single most important aspect of the evaluation of male sexual dysfunction?
   a. the history
   b. the physical examination
   c. nocturnal penile tumescence measurement
   d. ratio of penile/brachial blood pressure
   e. serum testosterone measurement

9. Which of the following laboratory tests may be indicated in a male patient with sexual dysfunction?
   a. complete blood count (CBC)
   b. blood urea nitrogen (BUN) and serum creatinine
   c. thyroid function studies
   d. serum testosterone level
   e. all of the above

10. Which of the following is an important counseling aspect in the treatment of male sexual dysfunction?
   a. reducing performance anxiety by prohibiting intercourse
   b. reducing anxiety by identification and verbalization
   c. instructing in "sensate focus" techniques
   d. instructing in interpersonal communication skills
   e. all of the above

11. Which of the following medications are used in the treatment of male sexual dysfunction?
   a. sildenafil
   b. vardenafil
   c. testosterone
   d. tadalafil
   e. all of the above

12. Which of the following is specifically indicated as a treatment for premature ejaculation?
   a. the penile squeeze technique
   b. the injection of testosterone
   c. structured behavior-modification programs
   d. the intermittent injection of medroxyprogesterone
   e. intraarterial penile injection of local vasoconstrictors

CLINICAL CASE PROBLEM 2:

A 24-YEAR-OLD FEMALE WHO IS UNABLE TO HAVE SEXUAL INTERCOURSE

A 24-year-old female who has been married for 6 months comes to your office in tears. She and her husband have been unable to have sexual intercourse. She says that when he tries to penetrate her she "tenses up" and is "unable to go any further."

Her significant history includes being raped at the age of 12. The patient has vivid memories of this event.

Her general physical examination is normal. At this time, you do not attempt a vaginal examination.

13. Which of the following statements regarding vaginismus is false?
   a. most women with vaginismus also have difficulty with sexual arousal
   b. there is a strong association between vaginismus and an intense childhood and adolescent exposure to religious orthodoxy
   c. there is a strong association between vaginismus and a traumatic sexual experience

   d. vaginismus is a condition of involuntary spasm or constriction of the musculature surrounding the vaginal outlet
   e. vaginismus may begin with a poorly healed episiotomy following childbirth

14. Regarding the diagnosis and treatment of vaginismus, which of the following statements is false?
   a. throughout the diagnostic examination the woman must feel that she is in control and may terminate the examination at any time
   b. the diagnosis of vaginismus often can be made without inserting a speculum
   c. it is helpful if the sexual partner is involved in all aspects of the treatment process
   d. the insertion of vaginal dilators is not a recognized part of the treatment protocol
   e. "sensate focus" techniques are an important part of the treatment protocol

15. Which of the following is the most common female sexual dysfunction disorder?
   a. anorgasmy
   b. delayed orgasm
   c. hypoactive sexual desire disorder
   d. sexual aversion disorder
   e. none of the above

16. Which of the following statements regarding female sexual arousal disorder is false?
   a. it is more common in women than in men
   b. the diagnosis takes into account the focus, intensity, and duration of the sexual activity
   c. if sexual stimulation is inadequate in focus, intensity, or duration, the diagnosis cannot be made
   d. in women it is not associated with inadequate vaginal lubrication
   e. in women it often is associated with inhibited female orgasm

17. Of the following listed causes, which is the most common cause of hypoactive sexual desire disorder in women?
   a. major psychiatric illness
   b. major psychiatric illness in the woman's partner
   c. exhaustion from work and family responsibilities
   d. major physical illness in the woman
   e. alcoholism in the woman's partner

18. Which of the following statements regarding inhibited female orgasm is false?

a. it is the most common female sexual dysfunction
b. primary anorgasmia is more common among unmarried women than among married women
c. women older than age 35 years have increased orgasm potential
d. women may have more than one orgasm without a refractory period
e. fear of impregnation is a common cause

19. Which of the following statements regarding dyspareunia is (are) true?
    a. it may be caused by endometriosis
    b. it may be caused by vaginitis or cervicitis
    c. it may be caused by an episiotomy scar
    d. all of the above
    e. none of the above

20. Which of the following methods is (are) useful in the treatment of female sexual dysfunction?
    a. sexual anatomy and physiology education
    b. "sensate focus" exercises
    c. treatment of underlying anxiety and depression
    d. none of the above methods are useful
    e. all of the above methods are useful

21. Which of the following major psychiatric conditions is linked most closely to sexual dysfunction?
    a. panic attacks/panic disorder
    b. GAD
    c. MDD
    d. schizoaffective disorder
    e. schizophrenia

CLINICAL CASE MANAGEMENT PROBLEM

Describe the goal, selection, types, and duration of sexual dysfunction psychotherapies most commonly practiced today.

ANSWERS:

1. **c.** Of medications described for the patient in Clinical Case Problem 1, the only antihypertensive agent that has not been associated with sexual dysfunction is verapamil (a calcium channel blocker).

2. **a.** Recreational and medicinal drugs are the most common cause of sexual dysfunction. As described later in this chapter, arousal disorders, ED, and others have been described. This problem affects patients of both genders and all ages.

3. **e.** It is estimated that 25% of cases of ED are related to medication side effects. Many different classes of drugs have been implicated in sexual dysfunction, especially antidepressants, antihypertensive drugs, antipsychotics, and psychostimulants, but also other drugs including lithium, digoxin, indomethacin, antiparkinsonian drugs, and cimetidine.

Antihypertensive medications from a variety of classes, most recently angiotensin-converting enzyme inhibitors (particularly captopril), have been associated with sexual dysfunction. One study has confirmed that 19% of males taking captopril have worsening of their sexual function.

4. **d.** The most common sexual complaint in younger males is premature ejaculation. Estimated prevalence rates for sexual dysfunctions vary greatly, depending on the surveyed population and the survey method. Although this condition tends to lessen with age, counseling is important to avoid long-term consequences for the patient's intimate relationships.

5. **b.** The most common sexual complaint in older males is ED. This condition is associated with an increase in chronic medical problems, the concomitant increased use of medications that interfere with erection, and aging itself. The incidence of ED increases steadily with age, but it is not an inevitable consequence of aging. In one study, one-third of 70-year-old men surveyed reported no erectile difficulty. Although by the age of 80 only 8% of men still reported no difficulty, another 40% claimed only to have mild difficulty and are likely to respond favorably to treatment.

6. **c.** The cause of male sexual dysfunction may be psychological, physiologic, or a combination of both. Psychological problems often complicate male sexual dysfunction even when the original cause is physiologic. Relationship issues as a result of the sexual dysfunction often worsen the condition. In young men, most cases of male sexual dysfunction are psychological in origin. In older men, as the incidence of concurrent disease and use of medication increases, so does the prevalence of organic sexual dysfunction.

7. **d.** Diabetes mellitus is the most common organic cause of male sexual dysfunction. Patients with diabetes mellitus experience high rates of ED as a result of vascular disease and autonomic dysfunction.

Other common causes of organic male sexual dysfunction include the following: (1) atherosclerotic vascular disease; (2) congestive heart failure; (3) renal failure; (4) hepatic failure; (5) respiratory failure; (6) genetic causes (Klinefelter's syndrome); (7) hypothyroidism; (8) hyperthyroidism; (9) multiple sclerosis; (10) Parkinson's disease; (11) surgical procedures including radical prostatectomy, orchiectomy, and abdominal–perineal colon resection; and (12) radiation therapy.

8. a. The single most important aspect in the evaluation of male (and female) sexual dysfunction is the patient's history. For example, in a patient with ED, if erections are achieved under certain conditions but not others, the likelihood is high that the dysfunction is psychogenic. Normal erectile function during masturbation and extramarital sex and in response to erotic material suggests a psychological cause. Similarly, if a normal erection is lost during vaginal insertion, a psychological cause is suspected. A complete drug history is also essential.

The history should include present and previous birth control methods, a complete past medical and psychiatric history, a family history, a history of surgical procedures, a history of the marital relationship, and an assessment of present job satisfaction and other stressors. A complete physical examination including a genital examination should be performed. The physical examination will determine whether there is any evidence of organic pathology associated with the sexual dysfunction.

Measurement of nocturnal penile tumescence (most simply done using a strain gauge), the ratio of penile/brachial blood pressure, and serum testosterone levels are investigations that may have a role in the overall evaluation of sexual dysfunction but are not always indicated. Vascular impairment as a potential cause of impotence essentially can be ruled out if an injection of alprostadil (see Answer 11) induces an erection.

9. e. If the family physician suspects an organic cause, baseline screening blood work is indicated. This should include a CBC, BUN and serum creatinine, fasting blood sugar, fasting cholesterol, thyroid function studies, liver function tests, and (if indicated) a serum testosterone level.

10. e. Most cases of sexual dysfunction have, as discussed previously, a significant psychological component. The psychological treatment of male sexual dysfunction is comprised of several important steps: (1) reduction or, hopefully, elimination of performance anxiety by prohibiting intercourse during the initial treatment period; (2) anxiety reduction by identification and verbalization of the problem and relaxation and visualization techniques; (3) introduction of the process of "sensate focus" (semistructured touching that will permit focus on sensory awareness without any need to perform sexually); and (4) improvement of interpersonal communication skills.

11. e. Sildenafil (Viagra) has been used extensively for treatment of male erectile disorder and has been effective when either psychological or physiologic causes are of primary etiologic significance.

Vardenafil, marketed as Levitra, is a new drug on the market (approved by the U.S. Food and Drug Administration [FDA] in August 2003). Its mode of action is similar to that of sildenafil, although it is alleged to act a little faster.

Alprostadil (prostaglandin E1 [PGE1]) is also efficacious but must be administered through penile injection (Caverject or Edex) or intraurethral insertion via a cannula (MUSE) and is therefore not well accepted.

Yohimbine may have some effect on libido but has not been demonstrated to be efficacious in male erectile disorder.

If low testosterone levels are present, androgenic steroids may be prescribed, either by intramuscular injection or patches. These do not affect erection *per se* but may enhance desire.

Sildenafil is a relatively specific inhibitor of penile phosphodiesterase (phosphodiesterase 5 [PDE5]). Inhibition of PDE5 causes the penile smooth muscles to relax and permits more blood to flow into the cavernous spaces and thus enhances erectile function. However, the drug can work only if there is initial sexual stimulation; it cannot induce an erection itself. Although relatively specific for PDE5, sildenafil does have some affect on other PDE isozymes causing minor side effects including a mild and transient lowering of the blood pressure. Sildenafil, although a prescription drug, is widely available over the Internet and often is purchased without actually visiting a physician. Family physicians should warn their patients against this practice because serious side effects, often as a result of drug interactions, have been described, especially in patients who are taking nitrates for coronary artery disease.

Other new erection enhancers are rapidly becoming available. Tadalafil (Cialis) has been approved in Europe and by the FDA in 2004 in the U.S. Like sildenafil and vardenafil, tadalafil acts by inhibiting PDE5; however, tadalafil allegedly has a longer duration of action, which should permit greater spontaneity in sexual activity. (Because these PE5 inhibitors cannot act in the absence of sexual stimulation, there is no fear of men walking around with an erection for extended periods). A fourth oral medication, apomorphine (Uprima), presently only available in Europe, works via the central nervous system.

12. a. The initial treatment of premature ejaculation is the same as other therapies described here. In addition, an exercise known as the "penile squeeze technique" is used to raise the threshold of penile excitability. The penis is stimulated until impending ejaculation is perceived. At this time, the partner squeezes the coronal ridge of the glans penis, resulting in diminished erection and inhibited ejaculation. Eventually, with repeated practice, the threshold for ejaculation is raised. Pharmacologically, premature ejaculation may be ameliorated with SSRIs.

13. **a.** Vaginismus is defined as recurrent or persistent involuntary spasm of the musculature of the outer third of the vagina that interferes with coitus. There is an association between vaginismus and an intense childhood and adolescent exposure to strong condemnation of sexual behavior based on some religious beliefs. Vaginismus may occur when an episiotomy fails to properly heal following childbirth. Most women with vaginismus have normal sexual arousal.

In this patient, the cause of vaginismus is most likely from the traumatic sexual experience that took place during her childhood.

14. **d.** The evaluation and treatment of vaginismus begins with a carefully performed physical examination in which the patient is always in full control. She may terminate the examination at any time.

On inspection of the external genitalia, spasm and rigidity of the perineal muscles often are felt. In this case the diagnosis can be made even without inserting a speculum. From inspection, the examination may proceed to the insertion of one or more of the examiner's fingers.

The use of vaginal dilators in gradually increasing sizes has proved helpful in the treatment of vaginismus. Beginning with the smallest size, the woman inserts these herself until she becomes both comfortable and relaxed with their insertion. When the largest plastic dilator can be inserted, the couple can proceed to intercourse.

The partner should be involved in all aspects of assessment and treatment. Ideally, the partner should be present to observe the entire evaluation and treatment. Together with anatomy and physiology education, the couple learns the concept of sensate focus exercises, which plays a major part in the therapy of any sexual dysfunction.

15. **c.** The most commonly reported female sexual dysfunction disorder is hypoactive sexual desire disorder, present in up to one-third of women in some studies. Orgasmic disorder, however, is present in 5% to 10%. The prevalence of the other forms of female sexual dysfunction is less clear.

16. **d.** Female sexual arousal disorder is defined as persistent or recurrent partial or complete failure to attain or maintain the lubrication-swelling response of sexual excitement until completion of the sexual activity. The diagnosis includes the subjective sense of sexual excitement and pleasure and requires the focus, the intensity, and the duration of stimulation to be adequate. Sexual arousal disorder often is associated with inhibited female orgasm.

17. **c.** Hypoactive sexual desire disorder is defined as persistent or recurrent deficient or absent desire for sexual activity. The definition includes a lack of sexual fantasies. The major reasons for hypoactive sexual desire disorder are marital dysfunction, mismatched activity schedules, and exhaustion from work and family responsibilities.

18. **a.** Inhibited female orgasm is defined as persistent or recurrent delay in, or absence of, orgasm in a female following a normal sexual excitement phase during sexual activity. The definition takes into account the adequacy of focus, intensity, and duration of the sexual activity.

Inhibited female orgasm (as one of the orgasmic disorders) is not the most common disorder of female sexual dysfunction (5% to 10%). It is surpassed by hypoactive sexual desire disorder (33%).

Primary anorgasmia (never having had an orgasm) is more common in unmarried women than in married women. Women older than age 35 years appear to have an increased orgasmic potential.

Women may have more than one orgasm without a refractory period.

Causes for inhibited female orgasm include fear of impregnation, rejection by the woman's sexual partner, hostility, and feelings of guilt regarding sexual impulses.

19. **d.** Dyspareunia is defined as recurrent or persistent genital pain before, during, or after sexual intercourse. This dyspareunia cannot be caused exclusively by lack of lubrication or by vaginismus.

In many cases, however, vaginismus and dyspareunia are closely associated. Other causes of dyspareunia include episiotomy scars, vaginitis, cervicitis, endometriosis, postmenopausal vaginal atrophy, and anxiety regarding the sexual act itself.

20. **e.** For a woman with sexual dysfunction, it is imperative that she and her partner become knowledgeable about sexual anatomy and physiology. "Sensate focus" exercises are useful. Possible underlying anxiety and depression need to be addressed

and treated. If life and marital stressors are present, marital and stress management counseling are indicated. Because side effects of medication can cause sexual dysfunction in women as well as in men, reviewing the patient's medication is very important. As mentioned previously, antidepressants, particularly SSRIs, often cause significant sexual dysfunction, which often leads to poor acceptance of the drug. Changing the patient to a different class of antidepressant may be indicated.

21. c. The most common psychiatric condition associated with sexual dysfunction is major depressive illness in one or both mates.

In the absence of a psychiatric pathologic condition, dual sex therapy is the most accepted approach to the treatment of sexual dysfunction. One approach often used in the therapy of sexual dysfunction in couples is called the LEDO approach. The LEDO approach centers on the following:

1. **L**owering stress, tension, and anxiety levels through discussion, examination, and observation
2. **E**nsuring that both parties understand each other's desires, pleasures, and difficulties

3. **D**etermining the partner's genuine awareness and knowledge of their own and each other's sexual autonomy and the process of intercourse
4. **O**utlining, drawing, and explaining alternative approaches to arousal and excitation and intercourse techniques

The sexual problem often reflects other areas of disharmony or partner misunderstanding. The marital relationship as a whole is treated, with emphasis on sexual functioning as a part of that relationship. When a referral for sex therapy is necessary, both a female and a male therapist should be involved in the treatment of the couple's sexual problem. The therapy is short term and behaviorally oriented. The goal is to reestablish communication within the marital unit. Information regarding anatomy and physiology are given. Specific sensate focus exercises are prescribed. The couple proceeds from nongenital touching and sensory awareness to genital touching and sensory awareness, to genital touching, and finally to intercourse. The couple learns to communicate with each other through these graded exercises.

If underlying MDD, dysthymic disorder, GAD, or other anxiety disorders are present, they must be treated concurrently.

SOLUTION TO THE CLINICAL CASE MANAGEMENT PROBLEM

The description of the goal, selection, types, and duration of sexual dysfunction psychotherapies most commonly practiced today is a refinement, reinforcement, and expansion of the LEDO approach to sexual dysfunction psychotherapies, as described as follows.

1. Goal: Resolution of specific sexual dysfunctions
2. Selection: (a) All sexual dysfunction psychotherapy ideally should be performed with both partners; (b) sexual dysfunctions most suited for psychotherapy

include male erectile disorder, premature ejaculation, vaginismus, and orgasmic dysfunction.
3. Treatment: (a) make sure all medical causes are ruled out; (b) psychotherapy (types of psychotherapies used include behavior-modification techniques including systemic desensitization, homework, and education; and (c) psychodynamic approaches such as hypnotherapy, group therapy, and couples therapy as needed to deal with system dynamics.
4. Length of treatment is from weeks to months.

SUMMARY OF SEXUAL DYSFUNCTION

A. Prevalence: It is extremely difficult to estimate the prevalence of sexual dysfunction disorders. However, estimates have stated that 40% of American couples at one time or another have had a sexual dysfunction of some type. The estimated prevalence of certain disorders is as follows:

1. Males: (a) premature ejaculation, 37%; (b) hypoactive sexual desire disorder, 16%; (c) orgasmic disorder, 6%; and (d) male erectile disorder, 7%
2. Females: (a) hypoactive sexual desire disorder, 33%; (b) dyspareunia or vaginismus, not known; and (c) orgasmic disorder, 7%.
B. Most common causes are as follows: (1) pharmaceutical agents appear to be the most common cause of sexual dysfunction. (Antihypertensives and antidepressant drugs are especially important.);

(2) diabetes mellitus is the single most common organic disorder responsible for sexual dysfunction; and (3) psychological factors, even if not the predominant cause, accompany most sexual dysfunction disorders.
C. Nonpharmacologic approaches to sexual dysfunction in couples: (1) always begin by treating the relationship in reference to the couple; (2) get complete histories from both partners; (3) do complete physical examinations; (4) perform laboratory testing, which may include CBC, renal function, liver function, thyroid function, blood glucose, serum cholesterol, and hormone levels (testosterone, follicle-stimulating hormone, luteinizing hormone, estrogen, and progesterone); (5) remember there is an association between dyspareunia or vaginismus and previous sexual abuse; (6) consider the possibility of family violence in the present (such as spousal abuse leading to rape); and (7) use the LEDO approach (guidelines described in the Clinical Case Management Problem).
D. Pharmacologic treatment of male sexual dysfunction: (1) erectile dysfunction may be treated with

sildenafil, vardenafil, or tadalafil; (2) premature ejaculation may be ameliorated with SSRIs; and (3) although no reliable aphrodisiacs exist, some patients with hypoactive sexual desire disorder may respond to androgenic steroids or yohimbine. If a medication causes side effects that cannot be controlled, a change to a different medication class should be considered.
E. Pharmacologic treatment of female sexual dysfunction is under investigation.
F. Other treatments: ED also can be treated with nonprescription vacuum devices or with surgical implants.

SUGGESTED READING

American Psychiatric Association: *Diagnostic and statistical manual of mental disorders IV–TR*, 4th ed. American Psychiatric Association Press, 2000, Washington, DC.
Feldman HA, et al: Impotence and its medical and psychosocial correlates: results of the Massachusetts Male Aging Study. *J Urol* 151:54-61, 1994.
Tomb DA: *Psychiatry*, 6th ed. Williams & Wilkins, 1999, Baltimore.
Miller TA: Diagnostic evaluation of erectile dysfunction. *Am Fam Physician* 61(1):95-111, 2000.
NIH Consensus Conference on Impotence. *JAMA* 270:83-90, 1993.

 Chapter 87

Psychotherapy in Family Medicine

| "Stop the world. I want to get off!"

CLINICAL CASE PROBLEM 1:
A 29-YEAR-OLD WORKING MOTHER WITH TWO YOUNG CHILDREN WHO IS UNABLE TO COPE

A 29-year-old mother who holds a full-time out-of-the-home job has just gone back to work after the birth of her second child. The child is currently 8 weeks old. She works as an accountant in a large company. Her company is restructuring, and she worries that her job is not secure. Her husband has been laid off from his job as an assembly line worker at an automobile assembly plant.

After her maternity leave, she fears that the management was unhappy with her for "taking so much time off to have a baby." She is staying up late every night to get the housework done. She wakes up often during the night in order to feed the baby. She is too tired to spend quality time with the older child and feels guilty about that. She is crying, fatigued, and absolutely exhausted

after 10 days back on the job. She finds herself becoming "very sleepy every day at work," and the management has commented on that. She tells you, "I just can't take it any longer. I have to work to pay the mortgage and put food on the table. There are no other jobs available. What am I going to do? I just can't go on this way."

She has no history of psychiatric problems or sleep disorders. She has no family history of psychiatric disorders or personal or family history of drug or alcohol use. She is not taking any drugs at present.

■ SELECT THE BEST ANSWER TO THE FOLLOWING QUESTIONS:

1. What is the most likely diagnosis in this patient at this time?
   a. major depressive disorder (MDD)
   b. generalized anxiety disorder (GAD)
   c. adjustment disorder
   d. dysthymic disorder
   e. panic disorder

2. How is the "sleep disorder" that this patient exhibits most properly labeled?
   a. psychophysiologic insomnia
   b. adjustment sleep disorder

    c. inadequate sleep hygiene
    d. insufficient sleep syndrome
    e. idiopathic hypersomnolence

3. You decide to initiate psychotherapy. At this time, in this patient and given this diagnosis what is the single best psychotherapy to initiate in a primary care setting?
    a. cognitive psychotherapy
    b. brief psychodynamic psychotherapy
    c. behavioral psychotherapy (behavior modification)
    d. supportive psychotherapy
    e. intensive psychoanalytically oriented psychotherapy

4. What is the major goal of the psychotherapy in this patient's situation?
    a. to identify and alter cognitive distortions
    b. to understand the conflict area and the particular defense mechanisms used
    c. to maintain or reestablish the best level of functioning
    d. to eliminate involuntary disruptive behavior patterns and substitute appropriate behaviors
    e. to resolve symptoms and rework major personality structures related to childhood conflicts

5. What is the first priority at this time?
    a. foster a good working relationship with the patient.
    b. approach the patient as a "blank screen"
    c. develop a "therapeutic alliance" with the patient
    d. begin the assignment of tasks for the patient to complete
    e. develop "free association" with the patient

6. What is the therapeutic method at this time?
    a. validate and explore the patient's concerns, provide direction for problem solving, and help her deal with the situation
    b. have the patient express her anger in the "here and now"
    c. prescribe a sedative to "get things under control"
    d. have the patient "intellectualize" her concerns
    e. have the patient discuss her dreams and free associations

7. Which of the following is (are) a technique(s) of supportive psychotherapy?
    a. support problem-solving techniques and behaviors
    b. develop a short-term "mentoring" relationship
    c. develop a short-term "guiding" relationship
    d. suggest, reinforce, advise, and reality test
    e. all of the above

8. Depression is the most frequent psychiatric condition seen in the primary care setting. Which of the following psychotherapies has been shown to be most efficacious in the treatment of psychiatric conditions encountered in primary health care settings?
    a. intensive analytically oriented psychotherapy
    b. psychoanalysis
    c. cognitive-behavoral therapy (CBT)
    d. brief psychodynamic psychotherapy
    e. Gestalt psychotherapy

CLINICAL CASE PROBLEM 2:
A 39-YEAR-OLD FEMALE WITH A 4-MONTH HISTORY OF DEPRESSION

A 39-year-old female comes to your office with a 4-month history of depression. She meets the *Diagnostic and Statistical Manual,* 4th edition (DSM-IV) criteria for MDD. She was started taking an antidepressant 6 weeks ago, and it appears to be helping significantly.

9. Which of the following statements is true regarding the therapeutic approach to this patient?
    a. the best treatment for MDD combines antidepressant medications with CBT
    b. supportive psychotherapy is the ideal psychotherapy for this patient
    c. there is little evidence to support a combination of medication and psychotherapy in preference to psychotherapy alone
    d. brief psychodynamic psychotherapy has been shown to be the most effective psychotherapy when used in combination with a selective serotonin reuptake inhibitor (SSRI)
    e. none of the above statements are true

10. Which of the following statements regarding CBT is (are) true?
    a. the therapist views the interpretations that patients who are depressed make about life as different than those of patients who are not depressed
    b. CBT is best suited to patients who have depressive disorders without psychotic features
    c. formal CBT generally is conducted over a period of 15-25 weeks in weekly sessions
    d. CBT may be useful in patients who refuse to take, fail to respond to, or are unable to tolerate antidepressant medications
    e. all of the above statements are true

11. What is the major goal of CBT?
    a. to help patients "pick themselves up by the bootstraps" and change their lives
    b. to reestablish their previous best level of functioning

c. to understand the major conflict area and the particular defense mechanisms they are using
d. to identify and alter cognitive distortions
e. to clarify and resolve the focal area of conflict that interferes with current functioning

CLINICAL CASE MANAGEMENT PROBLEM

Describe the forms of psychotherapy that are useful in the family practice setting.

■ **ANSWERS:**

1. c. This patient has an adjustment disorder. Although this condition is detailed in Chapter 75, the basic characteristics of adjustment disorder are provided here again: (1) the development of a psychological reaction to identifiable stressors or events; (2) the reaction reflects a change in the individual's normal personality and is different from the person's usual style of functioning; (3) the psychological reaction is either "maladaptive" in that normal functioning (including social and occupational functioning) is impaired or greater than normally expected of others in similar circumstances; and (4) the psychological reaction does not represent an exacerbation of another psychiatric disorder.

2. d. The sleep disorder that this patient has developed secondary to her current schedule and responsibilities is known as insufficient sleep syndrome. Persons affected with this disorder voluntarily curtail their time in bed, usually in response to social and occupational demands. This results in daytime hypersomnolence and impairment.

3. d. The type of psychotherapy that best fits treatment of this patient's life situation in a primary care setting is supportive psychotherapy. Supportive psychotherapy is discussed in detail in Answers 4, 5, 6, and 7.

4. c. The major goal of supportive psychotherapy is to reestablish the best possible level of functioning given the patient's current circumstances, personality, and previous coping style. In general, this distinguishes supportive psychotherapy from the change-oriented psychotherapies that aim to modify primary disease processes, adjust thinking style, change behavior, or restructure personality.

5. a. The first priority of supportive psychotherapy is to foster a good working relationship with the patient. This will make the patient feel competent and connected, which are the two basic social needs of any human being. When people feel overwhelmed, they lose the sense of being competent and connected.

6. a. Once a working relationship is established between patient and physician, he or she encourages the patient to explore her concerns and validates her feelings. In the Clinical Case Problem in question, enlisting the husband's practical support, exploring options for temporary part-time employment, and validating the patient's need to take care of herself are important. It is extremely useful to elicit her stories about overcoming previous difficult times.

The prescription of a sedative risks compounding her problem and is contraindicated.

7. e. Some of the specific techniques used in supportive psychotherapy may include the following: (1) regular sessions in which therapy for the patient is consistently available; (2) the support by the therapist of problem solving by the patient; (3) guiding or mentoring on the part of the therapist; (4) the concomitant use of medication (especially antidepressant medication) if indicated; and (5) depending on the physician's level of expertise, specific techniques such as suggestion, reinforcement, advice, teaching, reality testing, cognitive restructuring, reassurance, the encouragement of alternate behavior, and the discussion of social and interpersonal skills.

8. c. There is an increasing amount of literature that supports the efficacy of CBT in primary care settings. Studies examining the outcome of CBT have found it to be an effective treatment in ambulatory patients with mild to moderate degrees of depression. One advantage of CBT is that the therapeutic techniques often can be learned more easily and integrated into primary care treatment than can psychodynamic techniques. Cognitive techniques include the questioning of maladaptive assumptions about problems, provision of information, and assignments for dealing with specific situations. There is a trend to combine these techniques with behavioral techniques such as relaxation training and desensitization, which are also very useful in the family practice setting.

9. a. Studies have shown that the best treatment for MDD is a combination of antidepressant medications with CBT, not supportive psychotherapy. A combination of psychotherapy and pharmacotherapy is more effective than either method alone in patients with MDD without psychotic features. If the family physician is unable to provide the psychotherapy, either because of lack of training or lack of time, a referral to a psychotherapist is indicated.

10. e. The process of CBT helps patients to reinterpret their views about their lives. It helps them to edit their stories. Although formal CBT generally is conducted over a period of 15-25 weeks in weekly sessions, family physicians can make very effective interventions during brief visits. CBT also can be used in patients who refuse to take antidepressant medication, fail to respond to antidepressant medication, or are unable to tolerate antidepressant medications.

11. CBT is a method of brief psychotherapy developed over the last 25 years primarily for the treatment of mild to moderate depression and other psychiatric conditions encountered in the primary care setting.

People who are depressed tend to have negative interpretations of the world, themselves, and the future. Also, patients who are depressed interpret events as reflecting defeat, deprivation, or disparagement and see their lives as being filled with obstacles and burdens. They also view themselves as unworthy, deficient, undesirable, or worthless and see the future as bringing a continuation of the miseries of the past.

The major goal of cognitive psychotherapy is to identify and alter cognitive distortions and thoughts. CBT helps patients to identify and alter these cognitive distortions (negative stories). The techniques that are used include behavioral assignments, reading materials, and teaching that helps these patients recognize the difference between positively and negatively biased automatic thoughts. It may seem, at first glance, completely straightforward, but it is sometimes difficult for the patient to tell the difference between the two. It also helps patients identify negative schemas, beliefs, and attitudes.

SOLUTION TO THE CLINICAL CASE MANAGEMENT PROBLEM

Family physicians can incorporate effective psychotherapeutic interventions into a brief office visit. Supportive psychotherapy and CBT are the two most appropriate psychotherapeutic approaches for use in a family physician's practice.

CBT is useful in the treatment of nonpsychotic depressive disorders and in stress management. Supportive psychotherapy is useful in the treatment of adjustment disorders, family and marital conflicts, and any condition to which importance is attached by the patient.

Family physicians should be familiar with some of the differences in goals among popular forms of psychotherapy: (1) psychoanalysis aims to resolve symptoms and perform major reworking of personality structures related to childhood conflicts; (2) psychoanalytically oriented psychotherapy aims to understand a conflict area and the particular defense mechanisms used to defend it; (3) brief psychodynamic psychotherapy is used to clarify and resolve focal areas of conflict that interfere with current functioning; (4) cognitive psychotherapy primarily identifies and alters cognitive distortions; (5) supportive psychotherapy aims to reestablish the optimal level of functioning possible for the patient; and (6) behavioral therapy (behavioral modification) aims to change disruptive behavior patterns through reinforcing positive responses and ignoring negative ones; relaxation approaches, rewards systems, and breathing techniques can be used for the patient's benefit.

Many of these psychotherapeutic modalities can be used in a group setting. This approach provides significant support to groups of patients dealing with serious general medical conditions, smoking cessation, and stress disorders.

SUMMARY OF PSYCHOTHERAPY IN FAMILY MEDICINE

1. Consider the use of supportive psychotherapy in any condition, recognizing the biopsychosocial model of illness.
2. Consider the increased efficacy of treating depressive disorders with a combination of SSRIs and cognitive psychotherapy.
3. Although formal CBT generally is conducted over a period of 15-25 weeks in weekly sessions, family physicians can make very effective interventions during brief visits.
4. Some studies point to significant cost-effectiveness of psychotherapy in relationship to other interventions.
5. Therapeutic intervention in family medicine is a skill that can be acquired with some additional training.
6. A referral to a qualified mental health professional is indicated when longstanding and complex problems are uncovered.
7. Supportive psychotherapy and CBT are the two most appropriate psychotherapeutic approaches for use in a family physician's practice.

SUGGESTED READING

American Psychiatric Association: *Diagnostic and statistical manual of mental disorders IV–TR*, 4th ed. American Psychiatric Association Press, 2000, Washington, DC.
Kaplan HI, Sadock BJ: *Psychotherapies*. In Kaplan HI, Sadock BJ, eds: Kaplan and Sadock's *Synopsis of psychiatry: Behavioral sciences/clinical psychiatry*, 8th ed. Williams & Wilkins, 1998, Baltimore.
Stuart MR, Lieberman JA: The fifteen-minute hour. *Practical therapeutic interventions in primary care*, 3rd ed. WB Saunders, 2002, Philadelphia.

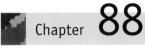

Chapter **88**

Patient Use of Alternative (Integrative) Medicine

> "Doctor, I know it is a long shot, but it seems to be my only chance."

CLINICAL CASE PROBLEM 1:
A 45-YEAR-OLD FEMALE WITH METASTATIC CANCER OF THE CERVIX

A 45-year-old female, a new patient to your practice, comes to your office to seek help in obtaining a referral to the Mexican Cancer Cure Center in a small town near Mexico City. She has metastatic carcinoma of the cervix, which has been treated with chemotherapy and radiation therapy but now has spread to her entire axial skeleton. The patient excitedly shows you the brochure that describes the brand-new facility. She tells you that she has contacted the facility and has been accepted for treatment although it is very difficult to get in. You need to formally refer her, she tells you, to the chief of staff in the center.

■ **SELECT THE BEST ANSWER TO THE FOLLOWING QUESTIONS:**

1. At this time what should you do?
   a. telephone the chief of staff at the center and make the necessary arrangements
   b. ask the patient to provide you with more information so that you can study it and make an informed decision on her behalf
   c. tell the patient that there is no way that you will have anything to do with "quack" medicine; if she wants a referral she will have to see another physician
   d. ask the patient to reconsider her request and come back to see you in 6 weeks; by that time you will have had time to discuss her case with the oncologists and will have been able to determine a more reasonable therapy for her
   e. none of the above

2. Regarding complementary and alternative/integrative medicine (CAM/IM), which one of the following statements is true?
   a. CAM/IM use is increasing in North America
   b. CAM/IM is unlikely to produce any significant adverse effects
   c. CAM/IM centers almost always provide their services at nominal cost to patients and their families
   d. CAM/IM approaches are rarely, if ever, covered by most forms of health insurance
   e. CAM/IM therapy is almost always harmful to patients

3. Regarding patients who see CAM/IM providers, which of the following is not a common characteristic?
   a. high education level
   b. high income level
   c. common coexistent psychiatric disorder
   d. previous or current conventional therapy
   e. white race

4. Regarding the total cost to patients and their families for CAM/IM therapy in North America, which of the following statements is true?
   a. the national cost may be as high as $27 billion annually
   b. the cost is likely to reflect only the cost of the products associated with CAM/IM therapies
   c. no form of CAM/IM therapy generally is funded by major health care plans
   d. CAM/IM therapy costs are easy to quantify because of the careful tracking of expenditures by government and private insurance
   e. health care costs associated with CAM/IM therapies have decreased over time

5. Regarding CAM/IM approaches, which of the following statements is true?
   a. a major advantage of CAM/IM approaches over conventional therapies is their lack of side effects
   b. all CAM/IM approaches have been shown, in randomized controlled trials, to decrease longevity in patients with cancer
   c. the U.S. Congress has decided not to fund any research trials involving CAM/IM therapies or other unconventional medical practices
   d. the simultaneous use of CAM/IM therapies and conventional therapies is extremely uncommon
   e. none of the above statements are true

6. Which of the following statements regarding alternative cancer therapy and conventional cancer therapy is true? Most patients who seek treatment with CAM/IM cancer therapies:
   a. abandon conventional cancer therapies when alternative therapy begins
   b. continue conventional cancer therapies
   c. never return to their primary physician
   d. believe that conventional cancer therapies have poisoned their organ systems irreversibly
   e. have given up all hope for conventional cures

7. What is the single most important difference between CAM/IM cancer therapies and conventional cancer therapies from the point of view of the patient?
   a. CAM/IM cancer therapies are directed at the symptoms of the cancer, whereas conventional cancer therapies are directed at the root cause of the cancer
   b. CAM/IM cancer therapies are much more likely to be successful in actual cure than conventional cancer therapies
   c. CAM/IM cancer therapies are less likely to produce fatigue than conventional cancer therapies
   d. in contrast to most conventional therapies, CAM/IM cancer therapies often focus on patients' physical, psychological, and spiritual needs and actively involve patients in their own healing
   e. CAM/IM cancer therapies are more carefully administered than conventional cancer therapies

8. Which of the following statements regarding patients seeking treatment with CAM/IM therapies is (are) true?
   a. It is always wrong for a physician to prevent a patient who wishes to use CAM/IM therapies from doing so
   b. The likelihood of a patient consulting the family physician regarding CAM/IM therapies depends on the levels of trust and the physician's cultural competence and knowledge of CAM/IM
   c. Some CAM/IM therapies appear attractive to patients because of the patient's sense that the treatment is more "natural" and "nontoxic"
   d. b and c
   e. all of the above statements are true

CLINICAL CASE MANAGEMENT PROBLEM

A 56-year-old male diagnosed with carcinoma of the pancreas comes to your office to renew his narcotic pain medications. There is no doubt that this patient has terminal cancer and needs primarily comfort care. He tells you that he has begun to take shark's cartilage to fight his cancer. He explains to you that "sharks don't get cancer and it seems that shark's cartilage works by zeroing in on the cancer cells in the pancreas." Describe how you would respond to the news that this patient of yours is taking shark's cartilage.

■ **ANSWERS:**

1. **e.** You, as the patient's family physician, should carefully discuss with the patient the following: (1) her previous therapy and her feelings about its benefit and its effect on her quality of life; (2) her relationship and feelings regarding the other physicians involved in her care; (3) her current condition including pain, other symptoms, and fears and hopes about the future; (4) her reasons for wanting to go to Mexico, her hopes and thoughts for what can be accomplished, and want she thinks will be the results of her visit; (5) her thoughts and wishes regarding further conventional therapy; and (6) the need for someone to "coordinate her care" and act as her advocate.

It would be preferable to indicate to the patient that you, as her new family physician, are willing to discuss all options and to support her in a way that you feel is in her best interest. By doing this you have the best chance of establishing good rapport with the patient and helping her evaluate her options.

2. **a.** The use of CAM/IM therapies is a growing trend. The National Institutes of Health have developed a center for the study of complementary and alternative medicine interventions and their possible benefits—the National Center for Complementary and Alternative Medicine (NCCAM).

The primary care physician should help the patient select potentially beneficial interventions and identify potentially dangerous therapies. The physician also should assure that CAM/IM therapies do not keep patients away from effective conventional therapeutic treatments. Conversely, the primary care physician should not try to prevent patients from obtaining CAM/IM treatments that might be beneficial.

3. **c.** Patients who seek CAM/IM therapies are generally well-educated patients with a relatively high income. They most commonly have had or are undergoing conventional therapy. Most are white and do not have any serious psychiatric disorder.

4. **a.** The precise total cost of CAM/IM therapies in the United States is unknown. The most recent

estimates, however, have put the approximate cost at $27 billion annually. There were 630 million documented visits to CAM/IM providers in 1997, compared with only 430 million visits to primary care allopathic physicians. Undoubtedly, many visits to CAM/IM providers are not documented.

Although more than 65% of health maintenance organizations (HMOs) cover at least one form of CAM/IM, chiropractic care is covered most commonly. However, because massage, bodywork (yoga, tai chi, etc.), acupuncture, homeopathy, naturopathy, stress management, biofeedback, specific diet programs, and herbal therapies rapidly are becoming more popular and sought after by patients, some insurers now beginning to cover these services as well. These CAM/IM therapies share a commonality of being relatively low-cost and low-tech processes that are popular with the general population, in large part because they are also high-touch.

The family physician needs to become familiar with the field of CAM approaches and begin to integrate them into the care of their patients. All therapies, complementary or mainstream, should rely on case-based evidence of their benefits, if possible. In the past 10 years, increasingly the CAM therapies are being evaluated for clinically based evidence and safety.

A recently published article about the use of CAM among patients with early-stage breast cancer found that 28% of the patients began using CAM after their diagnosis. Often, these patients were more distressed about their diagnosis and were seeking additional help.

Current CAM modalities to treat cancer include special diets; supplements; herbals, neutraceuticals, and other natural products; Eastern medical approaches such as acupuncture, and tai chi; mindfulness approaches; and spiritual or psychological support. Some of these modalities show promise in the treatment of cancers and cancer treatment–related sided effects, although further studies are needed.

Because these therapies are usually not covered by insurance and are outside of the mainstream of medicine, their costs are not effectively tracked by government or private insurance. However, undoubtedly, the cost of CAM/IM therapies will continue to increase parallel to that of conventional medicine.

5. **e.** CAM/IM therapies are not necessarily free of side effects. CAM/IM approaches are studied increasingly in randomized controlled trials. They have clearly at least provided palliative relief to a variety of conditions, and even longevity in some patients with certain cancers has been improved. Many patients undergo conventional therapy and CAM/IM therapies simultaneously, sometimes in a collaborative fashion. One major patient care and research focus is the control of side effects of aggressive chemotherapy and radiation therapies. CAM/IM approaches hold promise in this area.

The U.S. Congress in 1992 established the Office of Alternative Medicine and in 1998 established the NCCAM. The National Cancer Institute (CNI) established the Office of Cancer Complementary and Alternative Medicine (OCCAM) in 1998. These agencies are funding research in the area of CAM/IM approaches and help disseminate high-quality information about this emerging area of research and public interest.

6. **b.** Most patients with cancer who seek treatment with alternative cancer therapies continue to receive either chemotherapy or radiotherapy during or after their visits with CAM/IM providers. In 1998 the OCCAM was established to coordinate and enhance the activities of the NCI in the arena of CAM. This agency was charged with promoting and supporting research within CAM disciplines and modalities as they relate to the prevention, diagnosis, and treatment of cancer and cancer-related symptoms and side effects of conventional treatment, and with coordinating other agencies' and organizations' activities in this area.

7. **d.** One important difference between CAM/IM cancer therapies and conventional cancer therapies has nothing to do with the therapies themselves. Rather, it has much more to do with patient control and input into decision making. In contrast to treatment plans in CAM/IM therapies, many patients feel a loss of control when going through conventional cancer therapies.

8. **d.** CAM/IM therapies appear attractive to patients at least in part because of the perception that they are "natural" and "nontoxic." However, as with other interventions, they are not necessarily free of possible side effects. It is not always wrong for a physician to dissuade a patient who wishes to use CAM/IM therapies from doing so if the approach chosen has been determined to be harmful to the patient. Some therapies may be of benefit; others, as long as they are not harmful, may be a source of comfort to the patient. The probability of a patient consulting the family physician regarding CAM/IM therapies depends on the levels of trust and the physician's cultural competence and knowledge of CAM.

SOLUTION TO THE CLINICAL CASE MANAGEMENT PROBLEM

Many patients with cancer or other life-threatening illnesses will decide, at one point or another, to try a complementary treatment. You, as the family physician, should handle the situation as follows:

1. Reassure the patient and family that you will continue support throughout the course of his illness.
2. Because this patient is in a terminal stage of his disease, comfort care and support are the most important aspects of his treatment. Unless you are convinced that a particular intervention is truly harmful, you should support the patient's attempts to manage his illness and the side effects of his cancer treatment.

3. Assure that the patient's pain is controlled adequately, and ask him what kinds of interventions for pain control he would like to pursue.

There are currently a number of case-based trials looking at the effectiveness of whole shark cartilage extract, green tea, selenium, enzymes, nutritional supplements, herbals, and other regimens in the treatment of cancer. CAM approaches such as acupuncture and mind–body medicine are showing promise for use in pain control in cancer treatment.

SUMMARY OF PATIENT USE OF ALTERNATIVE (INTEGRATIVE) MEDICINE

1. Many patients with cancer seek out one or more kinds of CAM/IM therapy at some time during the course of their disease.
2. CAM/IM approaches are being examined increasingly for their effectiveness and safety in high-quality clinical trials.
3. Make every effort to become knowledgeable about the type of CAM/IM approach that your patient is considering. As with other medical approaches, do not endorse approaches that have been found to be harmful.
4. Remind the patient that no matter what, you will remain his or her advocate. Encourage the patient to maintain regular contact with you if he or she decides to pursue an alternative therapy in a distant location.
5. Patients increasingly are using CAM/IM approaches, often without informing their physicians of these therapies. If you develop cultural competence and knowledge of CAM/IM as well as a trusting relationship with your patients, they will consult you on the use of CAM therapies for their care, which likely will improve their overall care and sense of wellness.

6. In contrast to most conventional therapies, CAM/IM cancer therapies often focus on patients' physical, psychological, and spiritual needs and actively involve patients in their own healing.
7. In general, users of CAM /IM approaches are not rejecting conventional medicine; rather, they are adding CAM approaches to their biomedical treatments.
8. Treat the person, not the disease.

SUGGESTED READING

Burstein HJ, et al: Use of alternative medicine by women with early-stage breast cancer. *N Engl J Med* 340 (22):1733-1739, 1999.

Daily L: More HMOs covering alternative treatments and complementary care, *Physician's Financial News* 17(9):S1-S6, 1999.

Eisenberg DM, et al: Trends in alternative medicine use in the United States, 1990-1997: results of a follow-up national survey. *JAMA* 280(18):1569-1575, 1998.

Friedman R, et al: Behavioral medicine, complementary medicine and integrated care. *Primary Care* 24(4):949-962, 1997.

National Center for Complementary and Alternative Medicine at http://www.nccam.nih.gov.

Rakel D: *Integrative Medicine, 1st ed.* WB Saunders, 2003, Philadelphia.

Tagliaferri M, et al. Complementary and alternative medicine in early-stage breast cancer. A review. *Semin Oncol* (1):121-134, 2001.

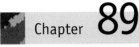

Chapter 89

Domestic Violence

"He sure does beat me, but a useless nothing like me is lucky to have any man."

CLINICAL CASE PROBLEM 1:

A 25-Year-Old Female with Pelvic Discomfort, Low Back Pain, Insomnia, and Fatigue

A 25-year-old female comes to the Emergency Room (ER) with a 6-month history of pelvic discomfort, low back pain, generalized bone pain, lethargy, and fatigue. On direct questioning, she also notes some dryness of her hair and her nails. These problems have been getting progressively worse for the past 3 months.

She tells you that she "fell down the stairs last night" when she lost her balance.

Her husband, who seems irritable and uncommunicative, accompanies her. He implies that she exaggerates her symptoms.

On examination, she has a bruise on her left eye and a number of bruises on her arms and legs that are in various stages of healing. Her blood pressure is 130/85 mm Hg. Her pulse is 108 and regular. She looks very anxious and apprehensive. Examination of the cardiovascular system and the respiratory system is normal. Examination of the abdomen reveals deep lower abdominal and pelvic tenderness.

■ SELECT THE BEST ANSWER TO THE FOLLOWING QUESTIONS:

1. Which of the following should be considered to be part of the differential diagnosis in this patient?
   a. acute leukemia
   b. hypothyroidism
   c. a bleeding disorder
   d. spousal abuse
   e. all of the above

2. Based on the constellation of findings and the relative probabilities of the various disease entities, which of the following is the most likely diagnosis?
   a. acute leukemia
   b. hypothyroidism
   c. a bleeding disorder
   d. spousal abuse
   e. none of the above

3. What is the estimated prevalence of spousal abuse in North America?
   a. 1 in 100 women
   b. 1 in 50 women
   c. 1 in 25 women
   d. 1 in 10 women
   e. 1 in 2 women

4. Which of the following is not a characteristic of the disorder described?
   a. the association of violence with alcohol intake by the batterer
   b. violent behavior in the family of origin of both victim and batterer
   c. high risk of suicide attempt or gesture in the victim
   d. high incidence of psychotropic drug use in the victim
   e. association of this disorder mainly with the lower socioeconomic classes

5. What is the psychological term or phrase that is used most commonly to describe the profile of women who are abused?
   a. intense interpersonal conflict status
   b. learned helplessness
   c. inadequate psychological functioning in general
   d. uninhibited anger focus
   e. inadequate personality disorder or thought process

6. Which of the following is the least common presenting symptom or complaint in a victim of spousal abuse?
   a. back pain
   b. headache
   c. dyspareunia
   d. spousal abuse itself
   e. abdominal pain

7. Which of the following statements about screening by primary care physicians is (are) true?
   a. only 10% of primary care providers routinely screen their patients for domestic violence
   b. more than 90% of women surveyed who were physically abused by their partners did not discuss these incidents with their physicians
   c. studies show that women would like their physicians to ask about domestic violence
   d. in specific cases, physician's recommendation of anger management training may improve the victim's situation
   e. all of the above

8. What is (are) the main fear(s) that women express about revealing spousal abuse
   a. a fear of escalation of the process
   b. a fear of being unable to function independently
   c. a fear of not being believed when they tell their story
   d. a fear of not being able to support themselves and their children
   e. all of the above

9. What is the most common site for diagnosis of the condition described?
   a. the ER
   b. the gynecologist's office
   c. the family doctor's office
   d. the internist's office
   e. all of the above are equally common

10. A woman who has been abused seeks medical help and receives it. She and her children are removed from a violent home environment and placed in a transition house where intensive counseling takes place. She leaves the transition house in 6 weeks. What is the most likely next step in this scenario?
    a. the woman and her children will establish a new life on their own
    b. the woman and her children soon will enter into another abusive relationship
    c. the woman will be unable to cope on her own and will go on to welfare; she and her children, however, will keep living independently
    d. the woman and her children will go back to their original violent home with the abuser
    e. a or c

11. It is currently estimated that what percentage of husbands or partners that abuse their wives also abuse their children?
    a. 5% to 10%
    b. 10% to 15%
    c. 15% to 20%
    d. 20% to 25%
    e. 25% to 50%

12. Following an episode of spousal abuse, the husband usually will be in what frame of mind?
    a. anger
    b. confused
    c. conciliatory
    d. silent
    e. unrepentant

13. A husband physically abuses his wife for the first time on their honeymoon. Following the episode of violence he "promises that it will never happen again." What is the most likely outcome in this situation?
    a. he is right; it will never happen again
    b. it will happen again, but the intensity of the violence will be less
    c. it will happen again, but the intensity of the violence will be greater
    d. it will happen again, and the intensity of the violence will be the same
    e. nobody really knows for sure; it depends on the situation

14. The state of learned helplessness is associated most strongly with which of the following?
    a. the upbringing of the victim
    b. the upbringing of the abuser
    c. repeated and escalating psychological abuse of the victim
    d. the economic environment (unemployment most often) that the abuser finds himself in
    e. none of the above

15. Which pharmacologic drug class is prescribed most commonly to victims of abuse when they present to physicians?
    a. antidepressants
    b. sedative-hypnotics
    c. beta blockers
    d. antipsychotic agents
    e. antimanic agents

CLINICAL CASE MANAGEMENT PROBLEM

Discuss the interventions and the order of those interventions that should take place for the victim, the victim's children, and the victim's mate in a situation similar to the one described in Clinical Case Problem 1.

ANSWERS:

1. **e.** All of the diagnostic entities listed in the question are possibilities. Although unlikely, the low back pain, generalized pain, bruising, fatigue, and lethargy could represent the signs and symptoms of an acute leukemia. The symptoms of fatigue and lethargy, along with the dry skin and dry nails,

certainly could represent hypothyroidism. Similar to the explanation for acute leukemia, the signs and symptoms could represent a bleeding disorder. Although not listed as possible responses for the question, some of the symptoms could represent a depression with somatic complaints or a somatoform disorder.

2. d. Spousal abuse is the most likely diagnostic entity. The common failure to diagnose spousal abuse may be explained by the fact that the profile presented to the clinician in cases of spousal abuse is vague. Women who are victims of spousal abuse visit physicians often, usually with somatic or conversion symptoms or psychophysiologic reactions. The most frequent complaints include fatigue, headache, insomnia, choking sensations, gastrointestinal pain, chest pain, pelvic pain, and back pain. Patients may be at risk for suicidal behavior, drug abuse, and non-adherence to medication regimens.

Unfortunately, spousal abuse often is unrecognized. If you do not think of the diagnosis, you will not make the diagnosis.

3. d. The estimated prevalence of spousal abuse in North America is 1 in 10 women. One study suggests that up to 12 million families in the United States are affected by spousal abuse. The *Diagnostic Statistical Manual of Mental Disorders,* 4th edition (DSM-IV) specifies five problems related to abuse or neglect: (1) physical abuse of a child, (2) sexual abuse of a child, (3) neglect of a child, (4) physical abuse of an adult, and (5) sexual abuse of an adult. The first three are covered in other chapters of this book, but it is important to remember that abuse is a family affair. When abuse occurs between any two members of a family, it also is very likely to occur between other members. This will be discussed in detail later.

4. e. Spousal abuse occurs in families of every racial and religious background and in all socioeconomic strata of society. Every race and religious background and all socioeconomic groups are represented. It may be true that psychosocial stressors such as unemployment, welfare status, and other financial problems increase the probability of abuse and act as precipitants. However, they are not the cause. Alcohol intake by the perpetrator also is associated with spousal abuse. The majority of men who batter their spouses have an alcohol abuse problem. Sometimes, the abuser uses alcohol as an excuse to disavow his behavior and convince others that "I was not responsible for my actions at the time."

The most important point to be made in this regard, however, is that alcohol does not cause spousal abuse. The two problems must be dealt with separately. Drug abuse, other than alcohol abuse, including the use of crack cocaine, also frequently is associated with spousal abuse.

A nuclear family of origin in which violence occurred is common in both victims and perpetrators.

5. b. The psychological term that is used most often to describe women who are abused is *learned helplessness,* a situation in which a woman who has been abused and continually told that she is worthless eventually comes to believe just that. Not only do the victims often see themselves as worthless, but they also believe that everything that has happened and is happening is, indeed, their fault. As the emotional and/or physical abuse continues, this pattern becomes more and more deeply ingrained into the psyche of abuse victims.

6. d. Spousal abuse is almost never the presenting problem. Women who are abused visit physicians frequently. Those visits, however, consist mainly of complaints or concerns regarding various somatic symptoms (back pain, headache, abdominal pain, pelvic pain, and dyspareunia) and anxiety and depression. Victims rarely volunteer information about the abuse. Usually this information has to be carefully sought, initially through the asking of general, open-ended questions and later by a more close-ended, direct approach. If you suspect spousal abuse as the cause of the patient's presenting complaints, you could begin with an open-ended question such as the following:

> "We know that domestic violence is a very common problem. About 30% of women in this country are abused by their partners at some time in their lives. Has this ever happened to you?

or

> "I don't know if this is a problem for you, but many of the women I see are dealing with abuse in their relationships. Some are too afraid or uncomfortable to bring it up themselves, so I've started to ask about it routinely."

After this opening, you could explore the situation further with more direct questions such as: "When you and your husband argue, does this ever lead to shoving or hitting?"

To open up, patients must feel understood, supported, and respected by the physician. Active listening skills and the spirit of collaboration can build a trusting relationship.

7. e. Although domestic violence is a frequent occurrence, only 10% of primary care providers routinely screen their patients for domestic violence. Studies have shown that more than 90% of women who were physically abused by their partners did not volunteer this information to their physicians but would have liked their physicians to ask them about domestic violence. In specific cases, physicians' recommendation of anger management training for the perpetrator may be effective.

8. e. All of the fears listed are reasons for victims choosing to stay in abusive relationships. Fear of escalation of violence and even of murder is a common reason for staying in the relationship. A significant percentage of the total homicides in the United States are committed by husbands who kill their wives. In fact, this is the single most common type of homicide in this country.

Fear of being unable to function independently and support both herself and her children is an almost universal fear.

Perhaps the greatest fear, and the fear that is linked to nondisclosure of spousal abuse, is the fear on the part of the victim that they will not be believed.

9. a. The most common site for the diagnosis of spousal abuse is the ER. The reason for this is the cycle of violence in which there are three distinct phases: (1) escalating tension, (2) violence erupting, and (3) reconciliation.

The victim almost always seeks help immediately after the eruption of violence. At this time the individual is most vulnerable to suggestions for therapy. Because the abuse often involves significant physical injuries, the ER is the most likely place that the initial contact with health care professionals will take place. This does not mean, however, that the other medical facilities listed are not important; it simply puts the ER at the top of the list. As well, it illustrates the point that the most cost-effective screening with the highest rate of pickup will occur in the ER.

10. d. Leaving an abusive relationship is difficult for many reasons, including fears of the victim that already have been discussed. On average, a woman will return four times to her residence of origin (i.e., go back to the abuser) before she permanently separates.

Many women who are abused seek financial assistance because inadequate child care resources make full-time work almost impossible. The availability of child care is an essential component of any plan to move single-parent families off of welfare rolls.

Choice b occurs all too often. Victims of spousal abuse who leave the original abusive relationship commonly enter into new abusive relationships.

Reasons for this probably are related to both environmental and psychological factors.

Another outcome of an abusive relationship may be rehabilitation of the abuser. Current estimates suggest that approximately 25% of abusers can and do seek help to correct their behavior. Treatment often involves substance rehabilitation; individual, marital, and group counseling; and anger management training. Court mandates for treatment also may play a role.

11. e. It is important to recognize that 25% to 50% of husbands and mates who physically abuse their wives also physically abuse their children. Thus domestic violence is indeed often a family affair. From this, the obvious follows: whenever one form of family violence exists, all other potential types must be considered and evaluated. Just as abusers often witnessed or were victims of abuse in their childhood, they are likely to abuse their children.

Family violence is a learned behavior and can take many forms, within and between generations and genders, including same-sex relationships.

12. c. Going back to the cycle of violence described in Answer 9, the husband is often in a very conciliatory mood after the episode of violence. He will seek the forgiveness of his wife with apparently heartfelt words such as, "It will never happen again, Honey. It was just a mistake and a misunderstanding. I'm sorry." This is called the "honeymoon phase." Along with this apology often will come gifts and tokens of affection. The wife, wanting desperately to believe this, often will go back at that time or shortly thereafter. Although in medicine we say "never say never and never say always," spousal abuse has a serious prognosis: without counseling and help, the abuse almost surely will recur.

13. c. As stated previously, the violence will recur in increasingly severe episodes. It may culminate in murder. As mentioned earlier, spousal abuse is the single most important and prevalent category of homicide in the United States. In some of these cases an abuser also kills his children and then himself. This is obviously a tragic end to a situation that might have been averted with proper diagnosis, assistance for both victim and abuser, and the provision of an ongoing safe environment for the children.

14. c. Learned helplessness is characterized by a deep belief on the part of the victim that she can do nothing to change her environment. Growing up in an abusive household may predispose the victim to accept this situation. Additionally, a victim may believe that it is she who is ultimately responsible for all the violence that has occurred in the relationship. The abuser almost always encourages this belief. Part of the psychological abuse consists of isolating and controlling the victim and limiting her ability to obtain social support elsewhere.

15. a. Frequently, physicians misidentify the anxiety and depression associated with abuse as resulting from an underlying psychiatric disorder. Victims commonly are given prescriptions for antidepressants or anxiolytics without having been assessed adequately.

SOLUTION TO THE CLINICAL CASE MANAGEMENT PROBLEM

The interventions that should take place include the following:

A. Victim and children: (1) establish the diagnosis by asking open-ended questions followed by more direct, closed-ended questions; (2) explain the importance of the removal of both the spouse and her children to a safe environment (preferably a transition house where peer counseling and other specific therapy is available); (3) facilitate the placement of the victim and the children in this safe environment; (4) use supportive psychotherapy in the safe environment to reestablish the victim's self-esteem and to reverse the ingrained feeling in the victim of learned helplessness; (5) after a period of approximately 6 weeks, facilitate the victim's and the children's assumption of new roles and relationships; and (6) continue contact and supportive psychotherapy for the victim and assist the children with any difficulties that they are having (such as school problems).

B. Abuser (husband or mate): (1) group psychotherapy, especially focusing on anger management, appears to work best for perpetrators because it facilitates the sharing of experiences with other individuals who have had the same experience; (2) treatment of concurrent psychiatric problems (especially alcoholism and drug abuse) is essential; and (3) reuniting families should be done gradually and with caution.

SUMMARY OF DOMESTIC VIOLENCE

1. **Definition of spousal abuse:** the physical or psychological abuse usually directed by a man against his female partner in an attempt to control her behavior or intimidate her
2. **Prevalence:** current prevalence estimated as 10% of American women
3. **Presenting symptoms:** usually vague somatic or psychophysiologic symptoms
4. **Diagnosis:** First, think of the diagnosis. Proceed from open-ended questions to more direct closed-ended questions. Primary care physicians need to screen patients for intimate partner abuse in a variety of clinical situations.
5. **Treatment:**
   a. Victim or children: removal to a safe environment and supportive psychotherapy for the victim to reestablish self-esteem and reverse learned helplessness. It is important to remember, however, that it may take several attempts before the victim is ready to permanently separately from her abuser.
   b. Abuser: group psychotherapy to help the abuser accept responsibility for his actions, to help him learn to express anger and frustration in other ways, and to treat concomitant psychiatric problems (especially alcoholism and drug abuse)
   c. Remember, one form of abuse begets another: where spousal abuse is present, consider the very high probability of child abuse and elder abuse

SUGGESTED READING

American Psychiatric Association: *Diagnostic and statistical manual of mental disorders IV–TR*, 4th ed. American Psychiatric Association Press, 2000, Washington, DC.

Punukollu M: Domestic violence: screening made practical. *J Fam Pract* 52(7):537-543, 2003.

Ramsay J, et al: Should health professionals screen women for domestic violence? *BMJ* 325(7359):314, 2002.

Rodriguez MA, et al: Screening and intervention for intimate partner abuse: practices and attitudes of primary care physicians. *JAMA* 282(5):468-474, 1999.

Tomb DA: *Psychiatry*, 6th ed. Williams & Wilkins, 1999, Baltimore.

Chapter 90

Ethics and Responsibilities Associated with Referrals and Consultations

| "I need a second opinion!"

CLINICAL CASE PROBLEM 1:

A 35-YEAR-OLD FEMALE WITH A 4-YEAR HISTORY OF CHRONIC ABDOMINAL PAIN

A 35-year-old female comes to your office for a periodic health examination. She is a well-known patient of yours who has a 4-year history of chronic abdominal pain (diagnosed by you as irritable bowel syndrome). During this encounter she mentions that she would like to see a specialist about her condition; although you have completely investigated her symptoms, she continues to be concerned about intermittently occurring abdominal pain. She states that she really is not sure that her complaints have been investigated sufficiently and asks you to make a referral to a gastroenterologist who has been recommended to her.

■ **SELECT THE BEST ANSWER TO THE FOLLOWING QUESTIONS:**

1. Considering the situation, what should you do now?
   a. explain to the patient that you have investigated the condition completely and that there is no need for a referral
   b. tell the patient that if that is the way she feels she probably should find another family physician
   c. empathize with the patient regarding her symptoms and refer her to a gastroenterologist of your choice
   d. empathize with the patient regarding her symptoms and refer her to the gastroenterologist she mentions unless there is a specific reason not to
   e. tell the patient that you are deeply offended by her request; she has no right to question your competence

2. Considering a patient's request for a second opinion, which of the following statements is true?
   a. a patient does not have the right to ask for a second opinion
   b. a patient who asks for a second opinion is demonstrating lack of trust in you as a family physician

   c. a patient has the right to ask for a second opinion
   d. the request for a second opinion should be granted only if you have some uncertainty about either diagnosis or therapy
   e. obtaining a second opinion is required for all chronic conditions

3. Regarding access to specialist care, which of the following statements is true?
   a. patients should have an identifiable family physician who coordinates access to consultants
   b. access to specialist consultants needs to occur in a timely manner
   c. family physicians need to be able to obtain brief, timely, informal advice from specialists
   d. the referral process needs to be streamlined and user-friendly
   e. all of the above

4. What is the primary purpose of consultation or referral to a specialist?
   a. to validate the findings of the family physician
   b. to make sure that the family physician hasn't missed anything
   c. to provide reassurance to the patient that the family physician is concerned about his or her welfare
   d. to improve the quality of health care by making available to patients and referring physicians the knowledge and skills of specialist or consultant at appropriate times
   e. to provide protection for the family physician against a malpractice suit

5. It generally is agreed that family physicians, given the proper training, can adequately care for what percentage of the patients they see in their practices without the aid of consultation or referral?
   a. 50%
   b. 60%
   c. 75%
   d. 85%
   e. 95%

6. Which of the following responsibilities is (are) of the physician making the referral to a specialist?
   a. ensure that patients understand the need for and purpose of referral for consultation.
   b. clearly specify whether the patient is being sent for consultation, is being sent for joint management, or is being transferred to the specialist's care.

c. communicate clearly to the specialist the purpose and problems for which help is needed

d. send specialists (when necessary and possible) the results of findings and investigations so that they will be available at the time of the consultation

e. all of the above

7. In which of the five following situations is a referral made in an inappropriate manner:

a. A family physician has carefully worked up a patient with multiple joint pains by careful history, physical examination, and laboratory testing. He is unable to find any abnormalities and refers his patient to a rheumatologist. His referral letter contains the essence of the patient's history, his physical examination, copies of the laboratory investigations, and his differential diagnosis and opinion.

b. A family physician sees an elderly woman with multiple medical problems who is taking multiple medications. The physician decides to refer the patient to a general internist and writes her a brief note stating: "Elderly patient with congestive heart failure, hypertension, diabetes, and osteoarthritis on multiple medications. PLEASE ASSESS. Thank you."

c. A family physician sees a middle-aged man with what appears to be chronic fatigue syndrome. She takes a complete history; does a complete physical examination; and does laboratory work to exclude anemia, other blood abnormalities, and hypothyroidism. She also rules out major depression. She refers the patient to an infectious disease specialist for a second opinion.

d. A family physician sees a patient who has the signs and symptoms of a major depressive illness. The patient, however, does not accept this diagnosis and asks to be referred to a general internist for a second opinion. The family physician agrees to this referral.

e. A family physician sees a new patient who has been to four other physicians with complaints of chronic lumbar pain. She requests a referral to a pain clinic. The family physician takes a complete history, does a complete physical examination, and agrees to the patient's request for referral to a pain clinic.

8. Regarding the responsibilities of patients in referral to a consultant or specialist, which of the following statements is (are) true?

a. the patient should explain to the specialist why he or she been referred

b. the family physician's office should make the appointment for the patient

c. patients have the choice to have the specialist take care of all their subsequent medical needs

d. it is the responsibility of the patient to report the specialist's findings

e. none of the above

9. Regarding the responsibilities of specialists or consultants in the referral process, which of the following statements is false?

a. the consultant has the responsibility to provide his or her services in a timely manner depending on the urgency of the condition

b. the consultant has the responsibility to communicate his or her findings in a timely manner to the referring physician

c. the consultant has the responsibility of deciding whether the patient should continue to be seen on an ongoing basis or should return to the family physician for ongoing care

d. the consultant has the responsibility to advise referring physicians promptly of their patients' admission to the hospital

e. the consultant has the responsibility to participate in peer and system review of the consultation and referral process

CLINICAL CASE PROBLEM 2:
A 28-Year-Old Female Seeking Referral to a Neurologist

A 28-year-old female with chronic headaches comes to your office for the specific purpose of seeking referral to a neurologist. She has seen five neurologists already but is not satisfied with what any of them have told her.

10. What is the most appropriate action for you to take at this time?

a. agree to refer her to another neurologist and get out of the room as quickly as possible

b. refuse to refer the patient to another neurologist

c. ask the patient to come back in a few weeks; you have to think carefully about this request

d. tell the patient that although you will refer her to another neurologist, this is a complete waste of everyone's time and money; there is obviously nothing wrong with her

e. none of the above

11. Which of the following statements is true regarding the future number of family physicians in the United States relative to specialists or consultants?

a. the relative proportion of family physicians to specialists is likely to remain the same
b. the relative proportion of family physicians to specialists is likely to decrease
c. the relative proportion of family physicians to specialists is likely to increase
d. it is difficult to predict which way the trend will develop over the next several years
e. there are likely to be decreases in both the number of family physicians and the number of specialists relative to other health care professionals

12. Regarding the definition of lateral referrals and the ethical implications of the same, which of the following statements is true?
a. lateral referrals are referrals in which a family physician refers a patient from one specialist to another; such lateral referrals are completely ethical
b. lateral referrals are referrals in which a specialist who has been consulted refers the patient to another specialist without the knowledge or consent of the family physician; such lateral referrals are completely ethical
c. lateral referrals are referrals in which a specialist who has been consulted refers the patient to another specialist without knowledge of the family physician; lateral referrals without the knowledge of the referring family physician may not be in the patient's best interest and should be discouraged
d. lateral referrals are referrals in which a family physician refers a patient to another family physician with expertise in the particular area; such lateral referrals may not be in the best interest of the patient
e. lateral referrals are referrals in which a family physician refers a patient to another family physician with expertise in the particular area; such lateral referrals are always ethical and in the best interest of the patient

13. Regarding referrals from one family physician to another, which of the following statements is true?
a. family physicians rarely develop expertise in a specific area; thus referrals from one family physician to another are rarely appropriate
b. family physicians may develop significant expertise in a specific area; referrals from one family physician to another may be in the best interest of the patient
c. family physicians who develop specific areas

of interest are really straying away from the foundations of their specialty
d. family physicians should always consider referral to a specialist or consultant rather than to another family physician
e. family physicians are not in a position to identify each other's areas of expertise with any degree of knowledge

CLINICAL CASE PROBLEM 3:
A 35-Year-Old Female Patient of Yours Who Is Admitted to a Hospital by a Surgeon

A 35-year-old female with colon cancer is admitted for surgery to her local hospital by the surgeon who is going to perform her hemicolectomy.

14. How should the patient's family physician be notified regarding the admission?
a. via an admitting slip from the hospital once the patient is admitted
b. through the ward clerk in charge of the ward to which the patient is admitted
c. through the charge nurse who is looking after the patient on the day of the admission
d. through the resident on the surgery service
e. none of the above

CLINICAL CASE PROBLEM 4:
A 40-Year-Old Woman Who Is Pregnant and Has Diabetes

A 40-year-old pregnant woman who has diabetes who originally was seen by an obstetrician for care during pregnancy subsequently is referred to an internist, a neurologist, a dermatologist, and a gastroenterologist for multiple other problems. No family physician is involved in the patient's care.

15. Regarding this type of referral pattern, which of the following statements is true?
a. this pattern of referral is likely to lead to optimal patient care
b. this pattern of referral is likely to be followed by close communication among the various specialists
c. this pattern of referral, without the coordinating role of a family physician, may create significant problems in the care of this patient and her family
d. this pattern of referral is extremely uncommon
e. none of the above statements are true

CLINICAL CASE MANAGEMENT PROBLEM

Your 28-year-old female patient is hospitalized for repair and reconstruction of a left anterior collateral knee ligament, removal of a left lateral meniscus, and partially torn left medial meniscus. After the surgery the patient is in severe pain, but the surgeon tells her that the pain is not severe enough to warrant a strong analgesic. As her family physician, you do not have admitting or order-writing privileges on the surgical floor. You are called by a close friend and informed of the patient's condition. Discuss your approach to help solve this problem.

■ ANSWERS:

1. d. Unless there is a specific reason not to, you should refer the patient to the gastroenterologist of her choice. Patients with chronic symptoms are difficult to manage. You may find that a second opinion not only validates your findings but also improves the relationship between you and the patient. She may in fact find the chronic abdominal pain to be less of a problem. In this case, it would prove to be less of a problem for both you and her.

2. c. A patient has the right to ask for a second opinion. In this case, you should look at her request as an opportunity to confirm your findings and as an opportunity for the patient to receive the reassurance she needs to manage the abdominal pain more effectively. In the long term, this may turn out to be beneficial for the doctor–patient relationship.

3. e. All patients should have an identifiable family physician who coordinates their care and, when necessary, refers them to specialist consultants who should see the patient in a timely manner. For this process to be efficient family physicians need to be able to obtain brief, timely, informal advice from the specialists they use; communications between family physicians and specialists should be two-way and user-friendly.

4. d. The primary purpose of consultation or referral is to improve the quality of health care by making available to patients and referring physicians the knowledge and skills of specialists or consultants at appropriate times.

There may be situations in complicated cases in which you wish to validate your findings or make sure that nothing has been overlooked. There also may be times when patients need additional reassurance.

To refer to specialists for the sole purpose of protecting yourself against malpractice (especially on a regular basis) is inappropriate.

5. e. A recent study funded by the Agency for Healthcare Research and Quality confirmed the long-held belief that family physicians can look after the vast majority of patient problems that they encounter. The researchers examined more than 5000 visits to family physicians throughout the United States and found that 95% of patient visits were handled by the family physician.

The type of medical problem involved is a powerful determinant of whether a patient is referred, and obtaining advice is by far the most common reason for referral. In the majority of cases, family physicians recommended a specific specialist to the patients because of their personal knowledge of the specialist.

6. e. In addition to the responsibilities listed in the choices, the referring physician should participate in peer and system review of the consultation and referral process.

7. b. This is a common occurrence and is really a situation of a family physician "dumping" a complicated patient on a consultant or specialist with little significant information given to the consultant. This type of referral is a time-consuming waste of resources because the specialist will have to start from the beginning.

All of the other situations describe appropriate referrals.

8. e. The important point in this question is that patients, as well as their physicians, have a responsibility to make the consultation process work in an efficient, timely, and cost-effective manner. Although patients should understand the reasons and purpose for the referral and make and keep their own appointments, it is not their role to communicate medical findings between physicians. Patients should return to the referring physician after the presenting problem has been addressed. In some cases, specialists will continue to comanage a patient's problems along with the family physician.

9. c. The consultant or specialist should return the patient to the referring physician once the consultation is complete. A consultation is just that: a consultation. It is inappropriate for consultants to take over the care of patient. However, it may take a consultant or specialist a number of visits to feel that he or she has dealt with the problem adequately. Also, it may be totally appropriate for the consultant (with the family physician's permission) to see the patient on a periodic basis to maximize quality of care.

In general, specialists should provide their services in a timely manner depending on the urgency of the condition; communicate clearly and promptly the results of the consultation, including all test results and findings; and notify the referring physician at once when his or her patient has been admitted to the hospital. To improve the consultation process, specialists and family physicians should participate in peer and system review of the consultation process.

10. **e.** This situation is more common than initially may be thought. There are many situations in which patients request to see a number of doctors of the same specialty for second, third, and fourth opinions. One should start by determining why the patient has been unsatisfied with the advice she has obtained previously. This should be followed by a complete history, a complete physical examination, and an exploration of the psychosocial aspects related to the patient's problem. Using the acronym BATHE (Background, Affect, Trouble, Handling, and Empathy) you would find out the following:

1. **B**ackground: what is happening in the patient's life (i.e., what stressors is she dealing with?)
2. **A**ffect: how it makes her feel
3. **T**rouble: what about the situation troubles her the most
4. **H**andling: how she is handling the situation
5. **E**mpathy: finish by making an empathic statement to the effect that you can understand that the situation is difficult and might be a factor in triggering her headaches

This technique not only helps the patient connect her emotional and physical responses but also establishes rapport with a physician who has just demonstrated an interest in her as a person. It may be that what this patient needs is someone to listen to her and to help her manage her chronic headaches. Although it is possible that there is something else causing the headaches, it would appear that this patient needs a relationship with a good family physician much more than a referral to another neurologist.

11. **d.** Although there is a need in the United States at this time for well-trained family physicians to balance the number of specialists, many factors affect the proportion, including medical student choice, availability of residency programs, demographic trends of the physician population, and immigration, to name just a few. Additionally, the increasing availability of mid-level providers (advanced practice nurses and physicians' assistants) complicates the picture.

12. **c.** Lateral referrals are referrals that take place from one specialist or consultant to another. If the original referring family physician is not notified, the ethics of such process is questionable. If a consultant feels that a patient requires another specialist or consultant, the referral should be made with the knowledge and involvement of the initial referring family physician.

13. **b.** Family physicians often develop areas of expertise and certificates of additional qualifications in various areas such as sport medicine, adolescent medicine, geriatrics, women's health, and complementary and alternative medicine. This additional training and expertise makes these practitioners ideal referral sources for patients with specific problems or preferences.

14. **e.** The surgeon who is going to perform the operation should inform the patient's family physician and seek input and help from him or her. At the time when a patient is about to undergo a major cancer operation, the patient's family physician can make a significant contribution to the patient's care. One of the most frequent errors is that the family physician of record is not notified at all or is notified in a way in which a significant delay occurs. The patient, meanwhile, is often left wondering where his or her family physician is and who to turn to for the answers to the many questions that may arise during a significant medical or surgical procedure.

As a principle, miscommunication often is avoided if the contact and communication is direct from attending physician to attending physician. In most cases, this route of communication will optimize patient care.

15. **c.** Unfortunately, this particular scenario is all too common and in many cases leads not only to a breakdown in communication among the various specialists but also to a lower overall quality of patient care. The role of the family physician in treating patients with multiple medical problems is even more critical than in a patient without such problems. The family physician understands the patient and the patient's family and is likely to be able to significantly improve the overall care delivered because of this knowledge.

SOLUTION TO THE CLINICAL CASE MANAGEMENT PROBLEM

One of the family physician's roles is to be a patient advocate. In the Clinical Case Management Problem, presented, it is reasonable to believe that your patient is in severe pain. Therefore the family physician should express his or her concerns directly to the surgeon and offer to undertake the responsibility of managing the patient's pain. Should the issue of hospital privileges create difficulties, it may be possible to transfer the patient's care to the family physician. Because the referral to the surgeon most likely was made via the family physician, it seems probable that the surgeon would permit the family physician to participate in the patient's care.

SUMMARY OF THE ETHICS AND RESPONSIBILITIES ASSOCIATED WITH REFERRALS AND CONSULTATIONS

1. The referral or consultation process requires the participation and commitment of the family physician, the specialist or consultant, and the patient. All three have responsibilities.
2. Patients are ethically entitled to a second opinion; a physician should not feel offended when one is requested.
3. Family physicians need to be able to obtain brief, timely, informal advice from the specialists they use; communications between family physicians and specialists should be two-way and user-friendly.
4. The primary purpose of referral or consultation is to improve the quality of care delivered to patients by making available the knowledge, skills, and experience of someone skilled in the management of a particular problem.
5. Family physicians can manage the vast majority of patient care problems without the need for consultation with specialist colleagues.
6. Family physicians that refer a patient to a specialist have the responsibility of providing a detailed summary of the patient's history, physical findings, and laboratory investigations. To refer a patient to a specialist with a brief one- or two-sentence note is inappropriate.
7. Specialists or consultants have the responsibility of seeing patients in a timely fashion; in an urgent situation if they are unable to see the patient, they should make arrangements for someone else to do so.
8. Specialists or consultants who admit a patient to a hospital should inform the patient's family physician personally and invite the family physician to participate in the care of the patient when indicated.
9. Lateral referrals from specialist to specialist without the involvement of the original referring family physician compromise patient care.
10. Patients who go from one consultant to another looking for answers should be listened to and cared for by a compassionate family physician.
11. Patient advocacy is a major responsibility of the family physician.

SUGGESTED READING

Primary care and family medicine in Canada—a prescription for renewal. College of Family Physicians in Canada. http://www.cfpc.ca/prescription-oct00.htm, October 2000.

Report of a Joint Task Force of The College of Family Physicians of Canada and The Royal College of Physicians and Surgeons of Canada: Relationship between family physicians and specialists/consultants in the provision of patient care, *Can Fam Physician* 39:1309-1312, 1993.

Starfield B, et al: Variability in physician referral decisions. *J Am Board Fam Pract* 15:473-480, 2002.

Stuart MR, Lieberman JA: The fifteen-minute hour. Practical therapeutic interventions in primary care, 3rd ed. WB Saunders, 2002, Philadelphia.

Chapter 91

How to Break Bad News

> "Well, Doc, how did the tests come out?"

CLINICAL CASE PROBLEM 1:
A 34-Year-Old Female Just Diagnosed with Metastatic Malignant Melanoma

You have just received the computed tomography (CT) scan report on a 34-year-old mother of three who had a malignant melanoma removed 3 years ago. Originally, it was a Clark's level I and the prognosis was excellent. The patient came to your office 1 week ago complaining of chest pain and abdominal pain. A CT scan of the chest and abdomen revealed metastatic lesions throughout the lungs and the abdomen. She is in your office, and you have to deliver the bad news of the significant spread of the cancer.

■ SELECT THE BEST ANSWER TO THE FOLLOWING QUESTIONS:

1. Regarding the delivery of bad news to patients who are unaccompanied when they come to the office, which of the following statements is true?
   a. the fact that the patient is alone is irrelevant.
   b. you have no right to interfere with her decision to come alone to the office
   c. you should go into the consultation room and explain that the situation is complex and it would be better if her husband or significant other were present when the test results were explained and treatment options were discussed
   d. patients do not remember much of anything after bad news is delivered, so it does not really matter whether someone else is present
   e. having a significant other present only will complicate an already difficult situation

2. Which of the following settings is not acceptable for the delivery of bad news?
   a. a physician's office
   b. a quiet room in a hospital setting
   c. the patient's home
   d. a private hospital room
   e. a multibed hospital room

3. The first step in breaking bad news is to:
   a. deliver the news all in one blow and get it over with as quickly as is humanly possible
   b. fire a "warning shot" that some bad news is coming

   c. find out how much the patient knows
   d. find out how much the patient wants to know
   e. tell the patient not to worry

4. Which of the following would be an appropriate statement to use in breaking bad news?
   a. "I'm sorry, I have bad news to tell you."
   b. "I can't talk to you without your family here."
   c. "The test results show that you have a very aggressive malignancy. Fortunately, that means we may be able to kill more cells with the chemotherapy."
   d. "I've asked Dr. Smith, the oncologist, to join us so that he can explain the cancer treatment to you."
   e. "Unfortunately, the cancer has spread all over your body. I think it's time you called your lawyer and started to get things wrapped up."

5. The next step is to find out how much the patient knows. Which of the following questions is not helpful in this regard?
   a. What's your understanding of what the tests were designed to tell us?
   b. Do you want me to tell you what is wrong with you?
   c. What did the previous doctors tell you about the illness or operation?
   d. What have you been most concerned about?
   e. When you first had symptom X, what did you think it might be?

6. Which of the following statements regarding finding out how much the patient wants to know is not true?
   a. every patient should be told everything about their condition
   b. some patients would rather not know all of the details of their disease
   c. most patients initially don't know how much they want to be told
   d. some patients want to know the whole truth right away
   e. in some instances patients should not be told the full extent of their condition

7. There are two languages that physicians use in talking to patients: English and "medispeak." Unfortunately, patients usually only understand English. Which of the following is an example of "medispeak"?
   a. lesion
   b. malignancy
   c. tumor
   d. cancer
   e. leukemia

8. Which of the following statements is false regarding the involvement of family physicians in the care of a patient with cancer?
   a. ideally, the family physician should be present when the patient is told of a bad diagnosis or prognosis
   b. the family physician and the primary consultant should be in contact and should be certain that the same message is delivered
   c. family physicians have a limited role to play once the patient is enrolled in a tertiary care cancer treatment center
   d. the family physician has a responsibility to follow up on the care of his or her patients regardless of whether he or she is actively involved in all aspects of care
   e. as cancer becomes a more chronic rather than fatal condition, much of the long-term care can be managed by the family physician

9. Which of the following is (are) true regarding the delivery of bad news to patients with a serious disease?
   a. check the patient's reaction to the situation frequently
   b. reinforce and clarify the information you are giving
   c. check the patient's understanding of the facts
   d. elicit the patient's concerns
   e. all of the above are true

10. In an interview in which news of a serious disease is presented, which of the following is the thing to do before the patient leaves the office?
    a. make sure the patient understands every word
    b. make sure the patient understands that you are doing everything you can
    c. make sure you leave the patient with a follow-up plan and provide the patient with some hope
    d. make sure the patient understands the dismal prognosis
    e. make sure that you have left no question unanswered

CLINICAL CASE PROBLEM 2:
LIFE AFTER THE BAD NEWS

A physician diagnosed with a terminal illness returns to his home university to continue the pursuit of his academic career to the best of his ability after having received bad news about his medical condition. He purposefully does not tell his colleagues the truth about his disease and continues to teach, write, receive grants, publish, and practice medicine. His condition deteriorates and he becomes more and more physically disabled.

11. Which of the following scenarios is (are) most likely to occur?
    a. he is apt to receive more phone calls from concerned colleagues and more inquiries as to whether they can be of assistance to him
    b. when his colleagues see him in the hall, they will go out of their way to talk to him and offer any assistance they can
    c. once his colleagues are aware of the full extent of his illness, they will offer not only moral support but support in terms of assistance in teaching, assistance in looking after his patients, and assistance in keeping his research programs viable
    d. all of the above are likely to occur
    e. none of the above are likely to occur

CLINICAL CASE MANAGEMENT PROBLEM

You are the physician caring for an 85-year-old woman who you have just diagnosed as having breast cancer. Before you have an opportunity to talk to the patient, her son and daughter come to your office to advise you that they do not wish you to tell their mother anything about her diagnosis. Describe how you would respond to the request.

ANSWERS:

1. c. You should go into the patient's room and explain that the situation is complex; it would be better if her husband or significant other were present when the test results were explained and treatment options were discussed. To have devastating news delivered to a patient in an unsupported environment is less than optimal. If a spouse, son, daughter, brother, sister, or other significant other cannot be present during the delivery of the news, it is useful to invite a social worker, psychologist, or member of the clergy to be present for patient support.

2. e. A multibed hospital room or an exposed area of an ER is not an acceptable location for the delivery of bad news. Patients in beds next to your patient obviously will be able to hear all or most of the conversation. Being in an exposed area would add to patients' feelings of vulnerability. Just pulling a hospital curtain is not an acceptable option.

When breaking bad news, attention to privacy, the physical environment, and the presence of a support person are important. Obviously, the other alternatives in the question are acceptable.

3. b. A "warning shot" prepares the patient psychologically to hear something negative.

4. a. The most appropriate warning shot in a situation like this is simply to state that you have bad news to deliver. It is important to pause before going on. Then it is useful to find out the patient's understanding of the condition.

5. b. To find out how much the patient knows, useful questions include finding out the patient's understanding of what the tests were designed to clarify, their previous discussions with other providers, their concerns, and their personal interpretation of their symptoms.

6. a. Most patients will want to be told the whole truth, but there are some exceptions. Every patient is different. The "whole truth" also does not have to be told all at once. Most patients initially are not even aware how much they want to be told. In some cultures it may be inappropriate to convey medical facts directly to the patient. It is useful to encourage patients to ask questions and tailor your responses to meet their needs. Open-ended questions—such as, "How much technical detail about your condition would you like me to share with you right now?"—would be helpful.

7. a. Most health care professionals unconsciously use their own professional jargon. Using "medispeak" to explain something to a patient makes it less likely that the patient will be able to ask relevant questions. It also tends to isolate and alienate patients who find it unfamiliar. A comparison of English and "medispeak" is shown in the table (Buckman R, 1992).

English	Medispeak
Leukemia	Blast cells
Multiple sclerosis	Demyelination
Cancer	Space-occupying lesion
The situation is serious	The prognosis is guarded

8. c. Family physicians assume and maintain a coordinating role in the care of patients with cancer. Although at a certain time a patient may be receiving treatment in a tertiary care treatment center, the family physician must be seen as coordinating that care. Communication between the family physician, the family, and the specialist(s) involved should be maintained.

Much of the long-term care can be managed by the family physician as cancer becomes a more chronic rather than fatal condition. The family physician's role can best be described in terms of the 5 Cs: **c**ontinuous, **c**omprehensive, **c**ompassionate, **c**oordinated, and **c**ompetent care.

9. e. While providing information to the patient, it is imperative that the physician keep the following principles in mind: (1) provide the information in small chunks—after firing the "warning shot"; (2) use English, not "medispeak"; (3) check patients' reactions both in terms of information processing and emotional state; (4) reinforce and clarify information you are giving; (5) elicit and address the patient's concerns; and (6) adjust your agenda to the patient's agenda.

10. c. Make sure before the patient leaves your office that you provide him or her with a follow-up plan. This will reinforce the belief that you are indeed in charge of his or her care and will ensure that the care plan is implemented. In addition, be sure to leave the patient with some hope for the future. That hope must be realistic hope, but hope nevertheless.

11. e. This case is a true story and was told eloquently by a physician named Rabin in the *New England Journal of Medicine* in 1982. The observations made of both the consultation with the neurologist and the reaction and treatment that the physician patient received when he returned to his home university have been summarized.

"My first reaction to the neurologist was one of deep disappointment from his impersonal manner. The neurologist exhibited no interest in me as a person and did not make even a perfunctory inquiry about my work. He gave me no guidelines about what I should do, either concretely—in terms of daily activities—or, what was more important, psychologically, to muster the emotional strength to cope with a progressive degenerative disease. The only thing my doctor did offer me was a pamphlet setting out in grim detail the future that I already knew about too well."

The reaction of colleagues to another problem is illustrated very well in the following description:

"By early 1980, however, the limp was worse, and I now held a cane in my right hand. The inquiries ceased and were replaced by a very obvious desire to avoid me. When I arrived at work in the morning I could see, from the corner of my eye, colleagues changing their pace or stopping in their tracks to spare themselves the embarrassment of bumping into me. As the cane became inadequate and was replaced by a walker, so my isolation from my colleagues intensified."

One has to ask why this happened. The author (Rabin D, 1982) suggests the following:

"Perhaps it is because we, as physicians, are the healers. We dispense treatment, counsel, and support; and we represent strength. The dichotomy of being both doctor and patient threatens the integrity of the club. To this guild of healers, becoming ill is tantamount to treachery. Furthermore, the sick physician makes us uncomfortable. He reminds us of our own vulnerability and mortality, and this is frightening for those of us who deal with disease every day while arming ourselves with an imaginary cloak of immunity against personal illness. This account is meant to draw attention to our frequent inability as physicians to deal with members of our profession who no longer fit the mold of complete healer."

The author also suggests some very simple steps that we can take to support our colleagues in time of illness, stress, trouble, or other difficulty. First, do not ignore ill colleagues. Greet them, inquire about their health, and visit them. Offer them support if they are physically handicapped. Second, be conscious of the physician patient's family and extend support to them. The spouse and children are suffering at least as much as the physician and need support, encouragement, and acknowledgment of their difficulties. Third, remember that the absence of a magic potion against the disease does not render you impotent. No one can assume the burden, but the patient knowing that he or she has not forgotten does ease the pain.

This special type of communication and caring among physicians (or any other professional group) is essential as we enter an era of change unlike any other era health care has ever seen. Remember that the word *doctor* is translated from the Latin "doktor," meaning teacher. As physicians we are all teachers, some in more diverse ways than others. Medical students, residents, patients, other health care professionals, and most of all students play the role at one time or another.

Confucius: *When the student is ready, the teacher will appear.*

SOLUTION TO THE CLINICAL CASE MANAGEMENT PROBLEM

This is not an infrequent occurrence. In this situation, it is extremely important to remember who the patient is and what rights the patient has and does not have. Proceed in the following manner:

1. First, remember who the patient is: the mother, not the son or the daughter.
2. Invite the son and daughter to come in for a discussion with you. Start off by acknowledging that you understand how much they love their mother and obviously have her best interest in mind. Then, explain that as their mother's physician you have an ethical responsibility to talk to her about her disease.

Offer to do it in such a way that allows their mother an opportunity to communicate how much information about the disease she wants. Ask the mother (in the presence of her son and daughter) how much detail she would like to hear about her condition and whether she wants to make her own decision or rather delegate this responsibility to her children.

3. In the unusual event that the son and daughter remain in disagreement about the process of information sharing and insist that their mother not be told about her condition, you might have to resort to including other parties such as a hospital ethics committee.

SUMMARY OF HOW TO BREAK BAD NEWS

A. **The seven-step protocol to breaking bad news is as follows:**
   1. Getting started: (a) get the physical setting right; (b) ensure family support at the time of breaking the news; and (3) fire a warning shot.
   2. Find out how much the patient already knows.
   3. Find out how much the patient wants to know.
   4. Decide on your objectives.

5. Share the information: (a) give the information in small chunks—start with the "warning shot"; (b) use English, not "medispeak"; (c) reinforce and clarify the information frequently; (d) listen for the patient's concerns; (e) blend your agenda with the patient's agenda; and (f) offer hope.
6. Respond to the patient's feelings.
7. Follow through with your planned objectives.

B. **Remember your colleagues:** physicians as patients are just as vulnerable if not more

Continued

SUMMARY OF HOW TO BREAK BAD NEWS—cont'd

B. Remember your colleagues—cont'd
vulnerable than patients who are not physicians and need our friendship, encouragement, help, and hope.

C. Guidelines and suggestions:
1. Always leave the patient with realistic hope.
2. Realize that the patient will not absorb all the information on the first visit; schedule follow-up visits frequently.
3. Facilitate and coordinate the patient's care from this point on.
4. Remember the 5 Cs of the family physician: **c**ontinuous, **c**omprehensive, **c**ompassionate, **c**oordinated, and **c**ompetent care.
5. Try to unlearn "medispeak."

SUGGESTED READING

American Psychiatric Association: *Diagnostic and statistical manual of mental disorders IV–TR,* 4th ed. American Psychiatric Association Press, 2000, Washington, DC.

Buckman R: *How to break bad news: A guide for health care professionals.* University of Toronto Press, 1992, Toronto.

Ptacek JT, Eberhardt TL: Breaking bad news: A review of the literature. *JAMA* 276(6):496-502, 1996.

Rabin D: Compounding the ordeal of ALS: Isolation from my fellow physicians. *N Engl J Med* 307(8):506-509, 1982.

CHILDREN AND ADOLESCENTS

 Chapter 92

Attention Deficit–Hyperactivity Disorder, Conduct Disorder, and Oppositional Defiant Disorder

The riddle of Ritalin.

CLINICAL CASE PROBLEM 1:

A 6-Year-Old Child Who Is "Always On the Go," "Into Everything," and "Easily Distractible"

A mother brings her 6-year-old son to the office for a complete assessment. She states that "there is something very wrong with him." He just sprinkled baby powder all over the house, and last night he opened a bottle of ink and threw it on the floor. He is unable to sit still at school, is easily distracted, has difficulty waiting his turn in games, has difficulty in sustaining attention in play situations, talks all the time, always interrupts others, does not listen when talked to, and is constantly shifting from one activity to another.

As you enter the examining room, the child is in the process of destroying it. On examination (what examination you can manage), you discover that there are no physical abnormalities demonstrated.

■ SELECT THE BEST ANSWER TO THE FOLLOWING QUESTIONS:

1. What is the most likely diagnosis in this patient?
   a. mental retardation
   b. childhood depression
   c. attention deficit–hyperactivity disorder (ADHD)
   d. maternal deprivation
   e. childhood schizophrenia

2. Which of the following is (are) associated with the disorder described?
   a. feelings of low self-esteem
   b. feelings of depression
   c. feelings of demoralization
   d. propensity to sustain severe injuries
   e. all of the above

3. Who is the person who usually makes this diagnosis?

   a. the child psychiatrist
   b. the family physician
   c. the mother or father
   d. the schoolteacher
   e. the grandparents

4. The differential diagnosis of this disorder includes which of the following?
   a. adjustment disorder
   b. bipolar disorder
   c. anxiety disorder
   d. childhood schizophrenia
   e. a, b, and c
   f. a, b, c, and d

5. Which of the following is (are) true regarding the prevalence of the disorder?
   a. prevalence rates are higher in preschool children than in school-age children
   b. affected boys outnumber girls in surveys of school-age children
   c. prevalence rates fall as a cohort of children ages into adulthood
   d. a, b, and c
   e. none of the above

6. This disorder is linked most closely to which of the following disorders?
   a. childhood depression
   b. childhood anxiety
   c. conduct disorder
   d. oppositional defiant disorder (ODD)
   e. c and d

7. The diagnosis of conduct disorder is made when which of the following criteria is (are) fulfilled?
   a. repetitive and persistent patterns of behavior that violate the rights of others
   b. stealing
   c. lying
   d. vandalism
   e. a and any two of b, c, and d

8. What is the best definition of the term *oppositional defiant disorder*?
   a. chronic behavior patterns in children and adolescents that are more severe than those in conduct disorder

449

b. chronic behavior patterns in children and adolescents that result in serious violation of the law and incarceration
c. chronic behavior patterns in children and adolescents that are less severe than those seen in conduct disorder
d. a and b
e. none of the above

9. Which of the following disorders often appear together in the same individual at various life stages?
a. mental retardation, ADHD, and learning disability
b. childhood depression, ADHD, and early-onset adult schizophrenia
c. ADHD, conduct disorder, and antisocial personality disorder
d. adjustment disorder, ADHD, and major depression
e. ADHD, bipolar disorder, and conduct disorder

10. Conduct disorder appears to result from an interaction of which of the following factors?
a. temperament
b. attention to problem behavior and ignoring good behavior
c. association with a delinquent peer group
d. a and c only
e. a, b, and c

11. Which of the following are pharmacologic treatment options in ADHD?
a. methylphenidate or its derivatives
b. dextroamphetamine or amphetamine derivatives
c. magnesium pemoline
d. modafinil
e. a or b only

12. What are the pharmacologic treatment alternatives for ADHD in patients who do not respond to stimulants?
a. desipramine
b. fluoxetine
c. guanfacine
d. clonidine
e. a, c, or d

13. Which of the following statements regarding the comparison between the effects of stimulants on children, adolescents, and adults is (are) correct?
a. in children and adolescents the use of stimulants has a paradoxic effect: they are "slowed down," as opposed to adults, in whom stimulants increase activity and awareness

b. normal and hyperactive children, adolescents, and adults have similar cognitive responses to comparable doses of stimulants
c. normal and hyperactive children, adolescents, and adults have similar behavioral responses to comparable doses of stimulants
d. b and c
e. nobody really knows for sure; it depends on the patient

14. A given child who is being treated with methylphenidate does not respond well to the medication; there is essentially no change in this behavior after 3 months of therapy. At this time, what would you do?
a. continue methylphenidate at one and one-half times the dose (for another 3 months)
b. switch the child to dextroamphetamine
c. discontinue stimulants altogether and prescribe desipramine
d. continue methylphenidate and add desipramine
e. b or c

15. What is the most common reason for referral to either a child psychiatry service or an adolescent psychiatry service?
a. conduct disorder
b. ADHD
c. ODD
d. childhood–adolescent depression
e. childhood–adolescent schizophrenia

CLINICAL CASE MANAGEMENT PROBLEM

Part A: List four psychiatric disorders that are associated with ADHD.

Part B: List five parental behaviors, disorders, or situations that may be associated with ADHD.

Part C: Comment on the association between ADHD and the schoolteachers.

ANSWERS:

1. **c.** This child has ADHD. Diagnostic criteria from the American Psychiatric Association's *Diagnostic and Statistical Manual of Mental Disorders,* 4th edition (DSM IV) for ADHD require a pattern of behavior that appears no later than the age of 7 years, has been present for at least 6 months, and is excessive for age and intelligence. The symptoms of the disorder are divided into inattention and hyperactivity/impulsivity; either must be present often, although not necessarily all of the time or in every situation. Either six inattention symptoms or six hyperactivity symptoms are required for the diagnosis.

For a diagnosis of inattention, six or more of the following symptoms must be present: (1) does not pay attention to details or makes careless mistakes; (2) has difficulty sustaining attention; (3) does not seem to listen when spoken to; (4) does not follow through on instructions and fails to finish; (5) has difficulty organizing tasks or activities; (6) avoids, dislikes, or is reluctant to engage in tasks that require sustained mental effort; (7) loses things; (8) is easily distracted by stimuli; and (9) is forgetful.

For a diagnosis of hyperactivity–impulsivity: six or more of the following symptoms must be present: (1) fidgets or squirms; (2) leaves seat when staying put is expected; (3) inappropriately runs about or climbs; (4) has difficultly in quietly engaging in leisure activities; (5) seems "on the go" or "driven by a motor"; (6) talks excessively; (7) bursts out answers before questions are asked; (8) has difficulty waiting for his or her turn; and (9) interrupts or intrudes.

2. **e.** Commonly associated features of ADHD are low self-esteem, feelings of depression, feelings of demoralization, and lack of ability to take responsibility for one's actions. In social situations these young children are immature, bossy, intrusive, loud, uncooperative, out of synchrony with situational expectations, and irritating to both adults and peers. Children with ADHD are more likely to sustain severe injuries than those without ADHD.

3. **d.** The most common person to make the diagnosis of ADHD is the schoolteacher. There is considerable controversy concerning the fact that many children who are hyperactive take medication because of the remarks or diagnosis of the schoolteacher. There may be some truth to this statement. Inexperienced or overly critical teachers may in fact confuse normal age-appropriate overactivity with ADHD.

4. **e.** The differential diagnosis of ADHD includes the following: (1) adjustment disorder (an identifiable stressor is identified at home and the duration of symptoms is less than 6 months); (2) an anxiety disorder (instead of or in addition to the diagnosis of ADHD); (3) bipolar disorder (bipolar disorder in children may manifest as a chronic mixed affective state marked by irritability, overactivity, and difficulty concentrating; (4) mental retardation; (5) a specific developmental disorder; (6) drugs (phenobarbital prescribed for children as an anticonvulsant, and theophylline prescribed for asthma); (7) systemic disorders (hyperthyroidism); and (8) other disruptive behavioral disorders including ODD and conduct disorder but does not include childhood schizophrenia.

5. **d.** Some studies suggest between 14% and 20% of preschool and kindergarten boys and approximately one-third as many girls have ADHD. In elementary-school studies, 3% to 10% of students have ADHD symptoms. Affected boys outnumber girls until young adulthood, where women predominate.

6. **e.** In clinical settings, at least two-thirds of patients with ADHD also have either ODD or conduct disorder. The characteristics of these two disorders are discussed in Answers 7, 8, and 10.

7. **e.** The diagnosis of conduct disorder requires a repetitive and persistent pattern of behavior that violates the basic rights of others or age-appropriate rules of society, manifested by at least three of the following behaviors: (1) stealing; (2) running away from home; (3) staying out after dark without permission; (4) lying so as to "con" people; (5) deliberately setting fires; (6) repeatedly being truant (beginning before the age of 13); (7) vandalizing; (8) being cruel to animals; (9) bullying; (10) being physically aggressive; and (11) forcing someone else into sexual activity.

Conduct disorder is a purely descriptive label for a heterogenous group of children and adolescents. Many of these individuals also lack appropriate feelings of guilt or remorse, empathy for others, and a feeling of responsibility for their own behavior.

8. **c.** ODD is best described as a milder form of conduct disorder. Children who are diagnosed as having ODD are certainly at risk for developing conduct disorder.

9. **c.** ADHD commonly leads to conduct disorder. Adolescents who develop conduct disorder are predisposed to develop antisocial personality disorder or alcoholism as adults.

10. **e.** Conduct disorder appears to result from an interaction among the following factors: (1) temperament; (2) parents who provide attention to problem behavior and ignore good behavior; (3) association with a delinquent peer group; (4) a parent "role model" of impulsivity and rule-breaking behavior; (5) genetic predisposition; (6) marital disharmony in the family; (7) placement outside of the home as an infant or toddler; (8) poverty; and (9) low intelligence quotient or brain damage.

11. **e.** The pharmacologic agents of choice for the management of ADHD are the stimulant medications (1) methylphenidate or derivatives or (2) dextroamphetamine or amphetamine derivatives.

As many as 96% of children with ADHD have at least some positive behavioral response to stimulants, of which methylphenidate or dextroamphetamine are the two tried and true medications. Both are available in various formulations including longer-acting derivatives. Methylphenidate is available in short (Ritalin), intermediate (Ritalin-SR), and long-acting (Concerta) preparations. Dextroamphetamine also is available as short (6-8 hours; Dexedrine, Adderall) or longer acting (Dexedrine spansules, Adderall XR) formulations. Unfortunately, side effects may limit efficacy or require discontinuation of medication in some children. Both preschool children and adolescents may require lower weight-adjusted doses than school-aged children and manifest a greater likelihood of side effects and somewhat lower therapeutic efficacy. Pemoline was removed from the market because of liver toxicity and should not be used. Modafinil (Provigil) is a stimulant medication used in narcolepsy under study for use in ADHD; preliminary studies are promising. Atomoxetine, an inhibitor of presynaptic norepinephrine, is also under study and may be a therapeutic option in the future.

12. e. Desipramine is an alternative drug in patients who do not respond to stimulants, who develop significant depression while taking stimulants, who have a personal or family history of tics, or who develop tics when taking a stimulant. Because several deaths have been linked to this drug, it has fallen into disfavor in some circles. Use requires careful monitoring by electrocardiogram for signs of prolonged QT intervals, necessitating discontinuation.

The other choices are clonidine or guanfacine. These alpha-adrenergic agents (clonidine, given either in pill form or transdermal form) are useful for a subgroup of children with ADHD, including those with tics or a family history of Tourette's syndrome or those in whom a stimulant is only partially effective.

13. d. Contrary to previous belief, normal and hyperactive children, adolescents, and adults have similar cognitive and behavioral responses to comparable doses of stimulants. Stimulants do not have a paradoxic sedative action; they do not lead to drug abuse or addiction, and many adolescents with ADHD continue to require and benefit from their use.

14. b. As many as 25% of children who respond poorly to one stimulant have a positive response to another stimulant. Stimulants reliably decrease physical activity, especially during times when children are expected to be less active (such as during school). They also decrease vocalization, noise, and disruption in the classroom to the level of normal peers and improve handwriting. Stimulants consistently improve compliance to adult commands.

Stimulants also produce improvement on cognitive laboratory tasks measuring sustained attention, distractibility, impulsivity, and short-term memory. Stimulants increase productivity and decrease errors in tests of arithmetic, reading comprehension, sight vocabulary, and spelling and increase the percentage of assigned work completed.

Because of these benefits, it is strongly suggested that if one of the stimulants is not effective, try another one before switching to a drug of another class.

15. a. The single most common reason for referral to a child or adolescent psychiatry clinic or hospital is conduct disorder.

SOLUTION TO THE CLINICAL CASE MANAGEMENT PROBLEM

Part A: Four psychiatric disorders associated with ADHD are as follows: (1) childhood depression; (2) conduct disorder; (3) ODD; and (4) alcoholism.

Part B: Five parental behaviors, disorders, or situations that may be associated with ADHD are as follows: (1) providing attention to problem behavior and ignoring good behavior; (2) parental modeling (impulsivity and rule-breaking); (3) parental marital conflict; (4) family poverty; and (5) inheritance (genetic predisposition).

Part C: The relationship between ADHD and schoolteacher input in many cases is that the diagnosis of ADHD is made by the teacher, not by the physician. Instead of carefully considering the diagnostic criteria elaborated in the DSM-IV, the physician may simply accept the word of the schoolteacher and begin treatment with stimulant medication. The basic problem is the inability, in some cases on the part of the schoolteacher and ultimately on the part of the physician, to distinguish between ADHD and normal appropriate-for-age overactivity. Most school systems in the U.S. now by law provide for a comprehensive developmenal assessment by a child study team of professionals. These evaluations provide important information for the physician, and nicely complement the medical assessment. Physicians and other clinicians must learn to work in tandem with school systems and parents to provide optimal diagnosis and care to patients with ADHD. High levels of communication among all parties are essential.

SUMMARY OF ATTENTION DEFICIT–HYPERACTIVITY DISORDER, CONDUCT DISORDER, AND OPPOSITIONAL DEFIANT DISORDER

A. ADHD:
1. **Prevalence:** highest in preschoolers, 7% of school-age children; decreases with age; males predominate; between 18% and 35% of affected children have an additional psychiatric disorder
2. **Signs and symptoms:** See the diagnostic criteria described in Answer 1.
3. **Treatment:**
   a. Nonpharmacologic: Behavior modification can improve both academic achievement and behavioral compliance if they are targeted specifically.
   b. Pharmacologic:
      i. First choice: stimulants, such as methylphenidate, dextroamphetamine, or derivatives
      ii. Second choice: desipramine, clonidine or guanfacine
   c. Stepwise therapy:
      i. Begin first stimulant (usually methylphenidate).
      ii. Increase dose gradually.
      iii. End of dose failure: Consider another one of the two recommended stimulants.
      iv. Failure: Switch to nonstimulant
   d. Length of time and dosing:
      i. Consider early morning and noon dosing.
      ii. Consider "drug holidays" on weekends and vacations.
      iii. Use for as long as is needed.

B. Conduct disorder:
1. **Prevalence:** estimated at 3% to 7%; males predominate
2. **Signs and symptoms:** See the criteria listed in Answer 7. Conduct disorder is the most common reason for referral to a child or adolescent psychiatry service.
3. **Treatment:**
   a. Nonpharmacologic: Cognitive-behavior modification (when used together) is the single most effective nonpharmacologic therapy.
   b. Pharmacologic: Lithium is used for severe impulse aggression. Carbamazepine is used for severe impulse aggression accompanied by emotional lability and irritability. Propranolol is used for uncontrollable rage reactions, especially when associated with impulse aggression. Neuroleptics (e.g., haloperidol) may reduce aggression, hostility, negativism, and explosiveness in severely aggressive children, and antidepressants may help if the conduct disorder is secondary to major depression.

C. ODD:
1. **Prevalence:** 6% to 10%; males predominate
2. **Differential diagnosis:** "stubbornness"
3. **Signs and symptoms:** Best described simply as a less severe form of conduct disorder.
4. **Treatment:**
   a. Nonpharmacologic: An operant approach using environmental positive and negative contingencies to increase or decrease the frequency of behaviors is most useful.
   b. Pharmacologic: If ADHD and ODD coexist, treat with stimulant medication.

D. Possible progression: ADHD to conduct disorder or ODD to antisocial personality disorder to alcoholism

E. Major differential diagnosis of disruptive behavior disorders include the following: (1) major depressive illness; (2) bipolar affective disorder; (3) anxiety disorder; (4) mental retardation; (5) specific developmental disorder; (6) adjustment disorder; (7) pharmacotherapy (phenobarbital, theophylline); and (8) systemic disorders (hyperthyroidism).

SUGGESTED READING

American Psychiatric Association: *Diagnostic and statistical manual of mental disorders-CM*, 4th ed. American Psychiatric Association Press, 2000, Washington, DC.

Anonymous: Clinical practice guideline: diagnosis and evaluation of the child with attention-deficit/hyperactivity disorder. American Academy of Pediatrics. *Pediatrics* 105(5):1158-1170, 2000.

Collett BR, et al: Ten-year review of rating scales. V: scales assessing attention-deficit/hyperactivity disorder. *J Am Acad Child Adolesc Psychiatry* 42(9):1015-1037, 2003.

Guevara JP, Stein MT: Evidence-based management of attention deficit hyperactivity disorder. *BMJ* 323(7323):1232-1235, 2001.

Kirby K, et al: Attention-deficit/hyperactivity disorder: a therapeutic update. *Curr Opin Pediatr* 14(2):236-246, 2002.

Weiss M, Murray C: Assessment and management of attention-deficit hyperactivity disorder in adults. *CMAJ* 168(6):715-722, 2003.

Chapter 93

Child Abuse

"All I wanted to do is to shut that brat up!"

CLINICAL CASE PROBLEM 1:

A 2-Month-Old Infant Who Fell Off a Sofa and Fractured His Humerus

A 2-month-old infant is brought to the hospital emergency room (ER) by his mother. She says that he rolled off the sofa the previous night and injured his right arm.

On examination, the infant is crying inconsolably and has a swollen, bruised right arm. An x-ray reveals a spiral fracture of the right humerus. There are also a number of old abrasions and old bruises that appear to be in various stages of healing. The remainder of the physical examination is normal. The mother says that the child has been well since birth. He has not had any significant medical illnesses.

■ SELECT THE BEST ANSWER TO THE FOLLOWING QUESTIONS:

1. Given the history, the physical examination, and the x-ray report, what should you do now?
    a. obtain an orthopedic consultation
    b. prescribe a sling for the child's arm
    c. investigate the child for possible coagulopathy
    d. suggest that the mother purchase a walker instead of laying her child on a sofa
    e. discuss the details of the incident more fully with the mother and contact the hospital social worker

2. After your initial intervention or recommendation, what is the next step you should take?
    a. ask the mother to return with the child for follow-up in 3 weeks
    b. ask the mother to return with the child for follow-up in 1 week
    c. arrange for the family physician to see the child at home the following day
    d. hospitalize the child
    e. none of the above

3. Which of the following has the lowest priority as part of this child's initial workup?
    a. obtaining a skeletal survey
    b. performing a funduscopic examination
    c. contacting the state child protection services

    d. testing for osteogenesis imperfecta
    e. obtaining a computed tomography (CT) scan of head

4. A physician should report suspected child abuse to the state agency for child protection:
    a. only if the physician is certain that the child is being abused
    b. only if the perpetrator confesses
    c. any time the physician has a reasonable suspicion of abuse
    d. only if the child is being abused physically
    e. only if the abuse is witnessed

CLINICAL CASE PROBLEM 2:

A 1-Year-Old Male Whose Weight Is Below the 5th Percentile for His Age

A 1-year-old male child is admitted to the hospital for investigation of failure to thrive. The child's weight is below the 5th percentile for his age. He appears withdrawn and avoids eye contact. His mother states that there is something wrong with him and says she cannot understand "why she had to get a kid like this."

Apart from the child being below the 5th percentile for weight, no other abnormalities are found on physical examination.

A complete blood count, a complete urinalysis, and serum electrolytes are within normal limits.

5. What is the most likely diagnosis for this child's behavior?
    a. the "white-coat" syndrome
    b. psychotic depression
    c. child abuse or neglect
    d. childhood schizophrenia
    e. acute paranoia of childhood

6. Which of the following statements regarding the parent(s) of a child with the disorder described in Clinical Case Problem 2 is (are) true?
    a. the parent(s) may be overwhelmed
    b. the parent(s) may be depressed
    c. the parent(s) may be isolated
    d. the parent(s) may be impoverished
    e. all of the above statements may be true

7. You make the proper diagnosis for the child described in Clinical Case Problem 2 and hospitalize him. You would expect that the child will:
    a. not gain significant weight during the initial hospitalization period

b. gain weight during the initial hospitalization period only if put on a significant antipsychotic agent
c. gain weight quickly during the initial hospitalization period
d. lose weight during the initial hospitalization period
e. none of the above

8. Which one of the following statements most accurately reflects the situation in a family in which there has been documented child abuse?
   a. in most cases the child has to be permanently removed from the family and placed in a foster home
   b. rehabilitation of parents that have been involved in child abuse is almost always unsuccessful
   c. with comprehensive and intensive treatment of the entire family, 80% to 90% of families involved in child abuse or neglect can be successfully rehabilitated
   d. in most cases child abuse will leave a permanent scar on the child's personality
   e. in a situation in which one child in a family has been abused, there is usually no increased risk to other children in the same family

9. Which of the following statements concerning child abuse in relation to spousal abuse is true?
   a. women who are abused are unlikely to abuse their children
   b. men who abuse their wives or partners are unlikely to abuse their children
   c. men who abuse their wives are much more likely to abuse their children than are men who do not abuse their wives
   d. there is no correlation between the various forms of family violence
   e. parents who abuse their children are unlikely to have come from families in which they themselves were abused or their mother was abused

10. Regarding the epidemiology of child abuse, which of the following statements is (are) true?
    a. in 1997 the National Committee for the Prevention of Child Abuse estimated that more than 3 million cases of child abuse and neglect were reported to public social service agencies in the United States
    b. approximately 1000 deaths are caused by child abuse and neglect each year in the United States
    c. each year more than 200,000 new cases of child sexual abuse are reported in the United States
    d. it is estimated that by the age of 18 years one out of every three or four girls will be sexually assaulted and one out of every six to eight boys will be sexually assaulted
    e. all of the above are true

CLINICAL CASE PROBLEM 3:
A Blistered 8-Month-Old Baby

An 8-month-old child is brought to the hospital ER with a large blistering burn covering both feet and ankles. There are also burns on the child's buttocks. The father states that the patient's 5-year-old brother must have turned on the hot water while they were bathing together.

11. As the ER doctor in charge, what is your next step?
    a. treat the burn and move on to the next patient: time is money!
    b. call the police and have the hospital security guards detain and restrain the father
    c. obtain a more detailed history of the child's present injury and his previous health; at the same time immerse the child's buttocks in cold water in an attempt to minimize damage from the burn
    d. obtain a more detailed history of the child's present injury and his previous health, try to make the child comfortable with analgesics, and apply a burn dressing as soon as possible
    e. use a confrontational approach and accuse the father of concealing information and abusing the child; have your resident deal with the immediate burn injury

12. Sexual abuse of children includes:
    a. penetrating vaginal, anal, or oral intercourse
    b. inappropriate touching
    c. visual exposure to masturbation
    d. sexually explicit, suggestive talk or threats
    e. all of the above

ANSWERS:

1. **e.** Such a child is almost always a victim of child abuse. Child abuse is defined as any maltreatment of children or adolescents by their parents, guardians, or other caretakers. The definition includes physical abuse, sexual abuse, physical neglect, medical neglect, emotional abuse, and emotional neglect.

The physician must be able to distinguish accidental from nonaccidental injury. Clues to nonaccidental injury in this case include the following:

A discrepant history: The explanation given by the parents or significant other does not fit the pattern and severity of the medical findings. Thus the "baby rolling off the sofa" is a totally inadequate explanation for a fractured humerus.

A delay in seeking care: The injury had occurred the previous night, but the mother had waited until the next day to bring the baby into the ER.

Story inappropriate for developmental level: 2-month-old babies should not be able to coordinate rolling activity. Although all parents still should be counseled against leaving any baby unattended on a table, adult bed, or sofa, the story does not fit the developmental level of the baby.

The treatment of the fracture itself, although it must be treated, should not be the focus of attention. An orthopedic consultation may be appropriate depending on the severity of the fracture.

It would be inappropriate to suggest the purchase of a walker at the best of times because this is associated with an increased incidence of falls and injuries, and the American Academy of Pediatrics has counseled against their use.

A coagulopathy could explain excessive bleeding with mild trauma; it could not explain the fractures in this child's case.

2. d. The most appropriate action at this time is to hospitalize the child. This removes the child to a safe environment and permits time for a complete evaluation. Trusting a family to follow up, especially when abuse is suspected, would be inappropriate.

3. d. Any infant with a suspicious injury needs a skeletal survey. This should be done in parts with multiple views instead of one anterior-posterior (AP) x-ray view (the so-called "babygram"). Suspicious lesions include multiple fractures, fractures at different stages of healing, spiral fractures, metaphyseal chip fractures (so-called "bucket handle fractures"), and posterior rib fractures. A funduscopic examination is needed to rule out retinal hemorrhages. Children with evidence of "shaken baby syndrome" (i.e., multiple fractures, retinal hemorrhages, and posterior rib fractures) require a head CT scan to rule out subdural hemorrhages. Infants have very large heads in relation to the rest of their bodies and are very susceptible to shearing and impact injuries with shaking.

Physicians are mandated reporters and are required by law to report suspected abuse to the state agency. A complete evaluation of family dynamics and a detailed history of family members (including psychiatric, substance abuse, and domestic violence history) also should be obtained. Although osteogenesis imperfecta is in the differential diagnosis of multiple fractures, it is a rare disorder and is much less likely in this case. Nonetheless, this possibility should be considered and ruled out before any other action is taken.

4. c. Physicians are mandated reporters of child abuse. This includes any type of child abuse. The physician is obligated by law to report any suspicion of abuse to child protection authorities. It is not the physician's duty to "prove" the abuse, although the physician must document all history and statements carefully (and sometimes take photographs) because they may be used as evidence. The physician is not liable if the investigation finds the claim of abuse to be false. Reporting is made in good faith and with good intentions whenever there is suspicion. The physician may be liable if there was clear evidence of abuse and the abuse was not reported.

5. c. The most likely diagnosis in this child is failure to thrive as a result of child abuse or neglect. A maltreated child often demonstrates no obvious evidence of being battered but has multiple signs of minor deprivation, neglect, and abuse. Such a child often is taken to a hospital or a private physician and has a history of failure to thrive, malnutrition, poor skin hygiene, irritability, withdrawal, and other signs of psychologic and physical neglect.

Children who have been neglected may show overt failure to thrive at younger than 1 year of age, and their physical and emotional development is impaired drastically. The child may be physically small and not able to show appropriate social interaction. Hunger, chronic infection, poor hygiene, and inappropriate dress may be present. Malnutrition is common.

These chronically neglected children may be socially unresponsive and withdrawn, or indiscriminately affectionate, even with strangers. Child abuse or neglect is one of the most common causes of failure to thrive, even in familiar social situations. Older neglected children may present either as runaways or as children with a conduct disorder.

6. e. Parents who neglect their children often are overwhelmed, depressed, isolated, or impoverished. Unemployment, lack of a two-parent family, and substance abuse may exacerbate the situation.

There are several prototypes of neglectful mothers that have been suggested. Again, the term *neglect* seems to be somewhat disparaging and some may object to it. Some mothers are young, some are inexperienced, some are socially isolated, and some cannot comprehend what is going on around them. Others have been portrayed as chronically passive and withdrawn; these women often have been raised in chaotic, abusive, and neglectful homes.

7. c. Once the neglected child is hospitalized and in a safe environment, the child should gain weight rapidly if given unlimited feedings. This is almost diagnostic of a nonorganic etiology for failure to thrive.

8. c. With comprehensive and intensive treatment of the entire family, 80% to 90% of families involved in child abuse or neglect (excluding incest) can be rehabilitated to provide adequate and appropriate care for their children. Approximately 10% to 15% of such families can only be stabilized and will require an indefinite continuation of support services until the children in the family become independent. In only 2% to 3% of cases is termination of parental rights or continued foster care necessary (again excluding incest).

9. c. Men who abuse their wives are more likely to abuse their children than men who do not abuse their wives. In fact, the abuse of a spouse is an absolute red flag to inquire about child abuse. It is estimated that approximately 25% to 50% of men who abuse their wives also abuse their children.

Women who currently are abuse (as spouses or partners) or who have been abused in the past (as children) are also more likely to abuse their children than women who are not abused or who have not been abused (either as a spouse or as a child).

Parents who abuse their children are much more likely than not to have come from nuclear families in which abuse occurred. Most commonly they were abused as children, although the witnessing of abuse as a child is also a common characteristic.

Thus abuse is very much a family affair and moves not only from generation to generation at different times but also occurs among different generations at the same time. That is, it may well be that child abuse, spousal abuse, and elder abuse are occurring at the same time in the same family.

10. e. According to the National Committee to Prevent Child Abuse and The National Clearinghouse on Child Abuse Information, in 1997 almost 3.2 million cases of child abuse and neglect were reported to public social service agencies; 33% of that number were substantiated. Neglect accounts for some 52% of the reports, physical abuse for some 24% to 26%, sexual abuse for some 7% to 13%, emotional mal-treatment for about 6%, and medical neglect for about

3%. Each year in America about 1000 children die as the result of fatal physical injuries from beatings or other physical trauma. It is estimated that one in every three or four girls will be sexually assaulted by the age of 18 years, and one out of every six to eight boys will be sexually assaulted. It should be remembered that the actual occurrence rates are likely to be higher than those estimates because many maltreated children go unrecognized and many are reluctant to report the abuse, particularly sexual abuse.

11. d. The most appropriate next steps at this time are as follows:
1. Treat the child's burn injury: use analgesics and apply an appropriate sterile dressing. Cold-water immersion is inappropriate and actually may extend the injury and trauma. Because of the extent of the burns and the fact that they cross joint lines (over the toes and ankles), the child should be admitted (preferably to a burn center) for observation, burn care, and possible intravenous fluids.
2. Obtain a more detailed history of the child's present injury and his previous health. This is the classic "stocking" distribution of an immer-sion burn. The child is held over hot water and the feet are forced into the water. When the child tries to pull up the feet, the buttocks are now the lowest point and are immersed. If the child had indeed been sitting in the bath when the hot water was turned on, the burn would be more diffuse. Regardless, an 8-month-old and a 5-year-old never should be bathing alone together.

Although it seems obvious what actually has happened here, it is important that as complete a history as possible be taken and documented for legal purposes.

12. e. Sexual abuse does not only include penetra-tion and sexual intercourse. Forcing a child to watch masturbation or copulatory activity, fondling and touching a child's private areas, and using sexually explicit language with or without threats also can be sexual abuse. Internet chat rooms are a more recent area where parents need to make sure that their children are safe. Although some children inadver-tently find sexually explicit chat rooms, there are also people targeting children and young adolescents under the supposed safety and anonymity of the Internet.

A few generalities follow:
1. Mothers abuse their children more often than fathers do. Roughly two-thirds of the perpetra-tors are women who are responsible for some

75% of neglect and medical neglect cases. However, men are responsible for about 75% of the sexual abuse cases.

2. Girls are abused more often than boys. The overall ratio is about 53%:46%. However, girls are subjected to sexual abuse at almost twice the rate as boys. For both sexes some 22% to 23% of the incidents of sexual abuse occurred before the age of 8 years.

3. Strangers are seldom the perpetrators of the child abuse. Of the abusers, 77% are a parent and another 11% are a close relative.

4. One parent is usually the active perpetrator, and the other parent passively accepts the abuse.

SUMMARY OF CHILD ABUSE

1. **Prevalence:** Some 3 million cases are reported each year in the United States; more than 1000 children die every year of injuries incurred from child abuse in the United States.

2. **Definition:** Child abuse can be defined as any short-term, intermediate-term, or long-term situation in a family in which a child is physically abused, sexually abused, emotionally or psychologically abused, physically neglected, emotionally neglected, or medically neglected by any other member of that family.

3. **Characteristics:** Child abuse occurs across all races and socioeconomic levels. Most commonly child abuse is perpetrated by a close relative, usually the parent. Mothers abuse their children more often than fathers; girls are abused more often than boys; one parent is usually the "active perpetrator" and the other parent is the "passive perpetrator." Strangers rarely are involved in child abuse. Risk factors for abuse include parents brought up in a harsh family environment, increasing home stressors, a decreased ability to cope with frustration or stress in a parent, a parental history of being abused, unplanned or unwanted pregnancy, socially isolated single parents, unemployment, alcohol or drug abuse, depression in a parent, a mentally impaired or physically impaired child, poverty, and unrealistic parental expectations.

4. **"Red lights" for child abuse:** Suspect child abuse if (a) there is a discrepant history (what is said to have happened does not match the injury pattern); (b) there is a delay in seeking care; (c) there was a recent family crisis; (d) there are unrealistic expectations put on the child by the parents; (e) there is a pattern of increasing severity of so-called accidents; (f) families are living under stressful living conditions including overcrowding and poverty; (g) there is a real lack of a support system for the family and the family members, (h) aggressive behavior is displayed by the child; (i) you are aware of underlying psychiatric disease in either the father or the mother; or (j) there is either alcohol abuse or drug abuse in the father or the mother.

5. **Acute treatment:** The acute treatment (no matter what type of child abuse is being dealt with) is hospitalization of the child. This allows time to subcategorize the type of child abuse that has occurred (often more than one type); observe the child and the child's behavior in a safe environment; investigate the child from a physical, psychologic, and social perspective; obtain all details necessary to clearly understand this episode of abuse and any others that have taken place before this; and interview the parents, grandparents, and other family members.

6. **Immediate and long-term treatment:** The ultimate goal in a situation in which child abuse has occurred is to eventually return the child to the home. However, first it is necessary to (a) restore the child to a healthy state; (b) identify and understand the reason for the abuse; (c) provide individual and family counseling to the parents and the family; (d) treat coexisting psychiatric conditions in both parents (alcoholism, drug abuse, depression); and (e) set up an ongoing counseling program for the individuals in the family.

7. Establish a contract with the abusing parents ("I will call if I get to a stage where I think I can no longer handle it"). Remember that family violence begets family violence. Where you find one type you will likely find another type (child abuse, spousal abuse, or elder abuse).

SUGGESTED READING

Holmes WC, Slap GB: Sexual abuse of boys: definition, prevalence, correlates, sequelae, and management, *JAMA* 280(21):1855-1862, 1998.

Lahoti SL, et al: Evaluating a child for sexual abuse. *Am Fam Physician* 63:883-892, 2001.

Nagler J: Child abuse and neglect. *Curr Opin Pediatr* 14(2):251-254, 2002 Apr.

National Clearinghouse on Child Abuse Information: 330 C Street, SW, Washington, DC, 20447, *http://www.nccanchcalib.com.*

Santucci KA, Hsiao AL: Advances in clinical forensic medicine. *Curr Opin Pediatr* 15(3):304-308, 2003 Jun.

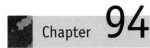

Chapter 94

Neonatal Jaundice

"Oh, is my baby very sick? See how yellow her skin appears to be."

CLINICAL CASE PROBLEM 1:

A Breastfed Baby that Became Jaundiced 48 Hours after Birth

A 3750-g male infant was delivered at 40 weeks of gestation. The prenatal course was unremarkable. The mother's blood type is Group A, and she is Rh positive. The neonate's blood type is the same. At approximately 48 hours of life, the neonate begins to develop jaundice. The baby is being breastfed and is feeding vigorously every 2 hours. There have been approximately 10 wet diapers noted per day. The baby's hemoglobin is 175 g/L. His total bilirubin is 10 mg/dL, and his indirect bilirubin is 9 mg/dL. His direct and indirect Coombs' tests are negative. On physical examination, he appears healthy and happy. There is no lethargy, no feeding difficulties, and no other abnormalities. He is jaundiced on his face, sclera, and upper chest. There is no organomegaly.

■ SELECT THE BEST ANSWER TO THE FOLLOWING QUESTIONS:

1. What is the most likely diagnosis in this infant?
   a. neonatal sepsis
   b. breast milk jaundice
   c. physiologic jaundice
   d. jaundice caused by minor antigen blood group incompatibility
   e. ABO blood group incompatibility

2. Which of the following characteristics would make you question your diagnosis in the previous question?
   a. jaundice beginning in the first 24 hours of life
   b. an increase in serum bilirubin greater than 5 mg/dl during the first 24 hours
   c. the total serum bilirubin exceeds 17 mg/dl at any time
   d. the neonate has a large cephalohematoma
   e. any of the above would cause you to question the diagnosis made in response to Question 1

3. Which of the following causes of jaundice is the least common in the newborn?
   a. ABO blood group incompatibility
   b. neonatal sepsis
   c. physiologic jaundice
   d. breast milk jaundice
   e. biliary atresia

4. What is the treatment of choice for the infant described in Clinical Case Problem 1?
   a. immediate transfer to the nearest neonatal intensive care unit for exchange transfusion
   b. intensive phototherapy
   c. tell the mother to stop breastfeeding and start bottle feeding
   d. start intravenous fluids at 1.5 times maintenance per 24 hours
   e. none of the above

CLINICAL CASE PROBLEM 2:

A Breastfed Baby that Became Jaundiced 5 Days after Birth

A full-term infant weighing 3650 g develops jaundice on the fifth day of life. He is breastfeeding well, every 2 hours, and having normal urine and stool output. On examination, the infant is not lethargic or irritable, feeds well, and has no signs or symptoms of systemic disease. The mother is blood group A and Rh positive. The baby has the same blood type. The infant's hemoglobin is 165 g/L. The direct and indirect Coombs' tests are negative. The total serum bilirubin is 14 mg/dL, and the indirect bilirubin is 13.5 mg/dL.

5. What is the most likely diagnosis to explain this infant's jaundice?
   a. breast milk jaundice
   b. physiologic jaundice
   c. neonatal sepsis
   d. minor blood group incompatibility
   e. dehydration

6. The treatment of choice for the infant described in Clinical Case Problem 2 is:
   a. exchange transfusion
   b. phototherapy
   c. change from breastfeeding to bottle feeding
   d. intravenous fluids
   e. none of the above

CLINICAL CASE PROBLEM 3:

A Breastfed Baby that Became Jaundiced 18 Hours after Birth

A 2900-g infant born at term develops jaundice at approximately 18 hours of life. The infant appears well, is not lethargic, and is breastfeeding well. Vital signs and physical examination reveal no abnormalities. The infant's serum bilirubin at 24 hours is 12.9 mg/dL, with the indirect bilirubin at 12 mg/dL. The neonate is blood group B and Rh positive. The mother is blood group O and Rh positive. The neonate's hemoglobin is 135 g/L, and the reticulocyte count is 10%.

7. What is the most likely cause of jaundice in this infant?
   a. neonatal sepsis
   b. breast milk jaundice
   c. physiologic jaundice
   d. jaundice caused by minor blood group antigen incompatibility
   e. ABO blood group incompatibility

8. What is the treatment for choice for the infant described in Clinical Case Problem 3?
   a. phototherapy
   b. exchange transfusion
   c. cessation of breastfeeding and change to bottle feeding
   d. intravenous fluids
   e. none of the above

9. What is the most dreaded complication of neonatal hyperbilirubinemia?
   a. profound hemolytic anemia
   b. seizures
   c. hepatic failure
   d. encephalopathy
   e. bronze baby syndrome

10. In which of the following situations would ABO blood group incompatibility be the most likely?
   a. the mother is blood group O and the infant is blood group O
   b. the mother is blood group O and the infant is blood group A or B
   c. the mother is blood group A and the infant is blood group A
   d. the mother is blood group A and the infant is blood group B
   e. ABO blood group incompatibility can occur with any of the above situations

11. Jaundice develops in approximately what percentage of full term neonates?
   a. 10%
   b. 30%
   c. 60%
   d. 80%
   e. 95%

12. What is the mechanism of action for phototherapy in the treatment of neonatal jaundice?
   a. hemolysis of the fetal hemoglobin f blood cells remaining in the circulation
   b. increase in the activity of the liver enzyme glucuronyl transferase
   c. increase of enterohepatic circulation
   d. increase in the activity of the liver enzyme gamma glutamyl transferase
   e. none of the above

ANSWERS:

1. c. The most likely cause of jaundice in the neonate described in Clinical Case Problem 1 is normal physiologic jaundice. Physiologic jaundice usually begins on the second or third day of life. It is caused by the breakdown of fetal red blood cells into bilirubin and the transient limitation in the neonate's ability to conjugate bilirubin.

Physiologic jaundice always is caused by unconjugated (indirect) bilirubinemia. The primary pathophysiology behind the hyperbilirubinemia is a relative deficiency or inactivity of the enzyme bilirubin glucuronyl transferase. Neonates are more prone to this as a result of relative polycythemia and increased red blood cell turnover.

Physiologic jaundice usually peaks on days 3 or 4 of life and gradually recedes over about 1 week. The bilirubin level usually peaks at about 5-6 mg/dL but does reach higher levels in some neonates, especially those with risk factors.

Risk factors for exaggerated physiologic jaundice include previous siblings with jaundice, gestational age of 35-38 weeks, exclusive breastfeeding, Asian race, maternal age greater than 25 years, and male gender.

2. e. Jaundice appearing in a neonate within the first 24 hours of birth, increasing more than 5 mg/dL during 24 hours, and bilirubin exceeding 17 mg/dL at any time are all characteristics that would support a diagnosis of a pathologic cause for neonatal jaundice, not physiologic jaundice. Large cephalohematomas and other causes of bleeding cause rapid red blood cell breakdown and pathologic jaundice. Other causes for concern would be a large fraction of conjugated bilirubin, poor feeding, lethargy, high or low body temperature, and rashes such as petechiae and purpura.

3. e. Among the choices listed, biliary atresia would be the least common diagnosis of an infant with neonatal jaundice. Biliary atresia would cause a conjugated hyperbilirubinemia. It is a good diagnosis to entertain as a part of a differential but will show itself rarely. Physiologic jaundice would be the most common etiology, followed by breast milk jaundice, which is also quite common. Jaundice caused by ABO blood group incompatibility, minor blood group antigen incompatibility, Rh incompatibility, and neonatal sepsis are all less common.

4. e. At this time, no therapy is required. Close observation will be critical to ensure that the serum bilirubin level is not rising. The levels at which phototherapy is started are controversial and differ from institution to institution. The level of 10 mg/dL at

48 hours of age should place this infant in a low-risk group for complications of hyperbilirubinemia such as kernicterus. The mother should be encouraged to continue breastfeeding. Feeding helps to stimulate conjugation of bilirubin. Breast milk has many proven advantages for the infant and should continue to be encouraged. Intravenous fluids can help if a neonate is clinically dehydrated, but it will not help in decreasing the level of serum bilirubin.

5. a. Breast milk jaundice is the most likely diagnosis in this case. Breast milk jaundice usually presents between the fourth and fourteenth days of life. The serum bilirubin usually is elevated to between 12 and 20 mg/dL. The etiology for breast milk jaundice is not completely understood; it is postulated that breast milk may contain varying amounts of a substance that inhibits bilirubin metabolism. Hyperbilirubinemia caused by breast milk jaundice is always unconjugated hyperbilirubinemia.

Breast milk jaundice must be clearly distinguished from breastfeeding jaundice. The term breastfeeding jaundice is used to describe jaundice that usually occurs on about day 3 of life and is primarily the result of low volume of feeding. Maternal breast milk has not fully come in, and the volume of feeds is smaller. The infant therefore has less ability to conjugate and excrete bilirubin.

6. e. Treatment for breast milk jaundice is controversial. In the past, practitioners would recommend that the mother stop breastfeeding for a period of time. In fact, if breastfeeding is discontinued, the serum bilirubin will decrease quickly. However, current recommendations are to continue breastfeeding as long as possible but to increase the frequency of feeds. Increasing the frequency of feeds will aid in processing and conjugating the bilirubin. Studies also have shown that after discontinuing breastfeeding, many mothers will not resume, even after the threat of hyperbilirubinemia has passed. An important danger of stopping breastfeeding is implying that there is something "wrong" with the breast milk that is making the infant ill, which may send a mixed message to the mother. Encouraging breastfeeding and maintaining breastfeeding throughout the first year of life is one of the strongest recommendations of the American Academy of Pediatrics.

Phototherapy can be added as therapy if the bilirubin continues to increase. If this is not effective, then breastfeeding may have to be discontinued. If there is uncertainty about the diagnosis, discontinuation of breastfeeding can be diagnostic. Practitioners must be very careful about discontinuing breastfeeding and about the messages that they send.

7. e. In this case ABO blood group incompatibility is the most likely diagnosis. The early onset of jaundice (less than 24 hours) and high bilirubin level for 24 hours of life are red flags for a pathologic basis for the jaundice. The infant's and mother's blood types are a set-up for hemolytic disease.

8. a. The treatment of choice in Clinical Case Problem 3 would be phototherapy. The serum bilirubin level is high after only 24 hours of life and probably is increasing rapidly. If phototherapy failed to prevent a dramatic increase in serum bilirubin, then exchange transfusion would be indicated. ABO blood group incompatibility is one of the pathologic causes of neonatal jaundice that can cause kernicterus.

9. d. The most dreaded complication of neonatal hyperbilirubinemia is kernicterus (bilirubin encephalopathy). Elevated levels of serum bilirubin are toxic to the basal ganglia and the brainstem nuclei. Infants with kernicterus in the acute stage will be lethargic and hypotonic. The chronic stage is characterized by hypertonicity, athetoid cerebral palsy, mental retardation, and other severe handicaps. The risk of kernicterus is related to the highest serum bilirubin level, the duration of time in which the serum bilirubin was elevated, and the gestational age of the neonate.

10. b. The most likely scenario would be that the mother is blood group O and therefore would make antibodies against blood group antigens A or B if she were exposed. These antibodies are immunoglobulin G (IgG) and can cross the placenta. An infant with blood group A or B would be a set-up for ABO incompatibility and therefore hemolytic disease. Depending on the patient population, ABO incompatibility can occur in about 20% of pregnancies. However, only about 10% of these cases actually develop hemolytic disease.

11. c. Jaundice develops in approximately 60% of normal-term neonates during the first week of life. This increases to 80% for preterm infants.

12. e. Years ago, it was noted that infants placed near the window in the sunlight were less likely to be jaundiced than their neighbors in the shade. Clinical jaundice and indirect hyperbilirubinemia are reduced on exposure to a high intensity of light in the visible spectrum. Bilirubin absorbs light maximally in the blue spectrum. Bilirubin in the skin absorbs light energy, which changes bilirubin into a photoisomer that can be excreted in the bile without conjugation. Phototherapy also changes bilirubin to another isomer, which can be excreted in the urine without conjugation. These isomers are also less toxic and less permeable through the blood–brain barrier and thus are less likely to cause kernicterus. Infants are placed in a bassinet under single or double phototherapy lights, naked except for eye shields. Complications include loose stool, skin rash, and dehydration, so the infant should continue to feed as much as possible (which also helps to excrete the bilirubin), and all output should be quantified and followed.

Phototherapy is contraindicated with conjugated hyperbilirubinemia, which can cause a permanent discoloration of the skin known as bronze baby syndrome.

SUMMARY OF NEONATAL JAUNDICE

1. **Prevalence** of neonatal jaundice is about 60% in full term infants and about 80% in preterm infants.
2. **Differential diagnosis:** (a) physiologic jaundice; (b) breast milk jaundice; (c) ABO blood group incompatibility with hemolysis; (d) trauma (severe bruising, cephalohematoma) with blood degradation; (e) neonatal sepsis; (f) Rh incompatibility; (g) minor blood group antigen incompatibility; (h) toxoplasmosis; (i) rubella, cytomegalovirus, and herpes simplex virus (torch) infections; and (j) conjugated hyperbilirubinemia—biliary atresia, intrinsic liver disease.
3. **Pathophysiology:**
   a. Physiologic jaundice: caused by normal breakdown of fetal red blood cells coupled with a transient inability to conjugate all of the bilirubin. Onset on day numbers 2 and 3, usually disappears by the end of the first week of life. Risk factors for more severe physiologic jaundice include Asian race, male sex, prematurity, and breastfeeding.
   b. Breast milk jaundice: caused by inhibitors of bilirubin conjugation found in breast milk. Onset between days 4 and 14, usually persists about 3 weeks.
   c. ABO blood group incompatibility: usually arises when mother is blood type O and infant is blood type A or B; may appear within 24 hours with elevated bilirubin and low hemoglobin for age.
   d. Minor blood group incompatibility and Rh incompatibility: keep in mind, minor blood group incompatibility is usually not as severe as Rh incompatibility, which is rare now with prenatal testing and use of Rhogam.
   e. Neonatal sepsis: always important differential for any newborn with any abnormality. Jaundice and poor feeding are important signs, along with high or low temperature, rash, or lethargy.
4. **Treatment**
   a. Physiologic jaundice: careful observation and serial measurements of serial bilirubin. Most textbooks carry guides for serum bilirubin by age in hours, classifying different bilirubin levels as low, medium, and high risk for complications such as kernicterus. Phototherapy also is used, especially for more severe physiologic jaundice.
   b. Breast milk jaundice: increase frequency of feedings, may consider phototherapy. Try not to discontinue breastfeeding unless jaundice is very severe.
   c. ABO and other blood group incompatibilities: increased feeding frequency, phototherapy, serial measurements of hemoglobin and serum bilirubin.
   d. Exchange transfusion for very severe hyperbilirubinemia
5. **General points**
   a. Jaundice within the first 24 hours of life is a red flag for pathology.
   b. Hyperbilirubinemia is treated aggressively to prevent kernicterus, or bilirubin encephalopathy.
   c. Infants discharged early from the hospital (48 hours or less) must follow up within 2-3 days for examination and evaluation.

SUGGESTED READING

Atkinson RL, et al: Phototherapy use in a large managed care organization. Do clinicians adhere to the guidelines? *Pediatrics* 111(5), 555-561, 2003.

Carbonell X, et al: Prediction of hyperbilirubinaemia in the healthy term newborn. *Acta Paediatr* 90(2):166-170, 2001.

Dennery PA, et al: Neonatal hyperbilirubinemia. *N Engl J Med* 344(8): 581-590, 2001.

Maisels MJ, Newman TB: Predicting hyperbilirubinemia in the newborn: the importance of timing. *Pediatrics* 103(2):493-495, 1999.

Newman TB, Maisels MJ: Less aggressive treatment of neonatal jaundice and reports of kernicterus. Lessons about practice guidelines. *Pediatrics* 105(1suppl):242-245, 2000.

Porter ML, Dennis BL: Hyperbilirubinemia in the term newborn. *Am Fam Physician* 65(4):599-606, 2002.

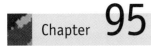

Chapter 95

Colic

"My baby cries constantly.
Can't you do something to help her?"

CLINICAL CASE PROBLEM 1:

An 8-Week-Old Infant with Inconsolable Crying for Many Hours and Days

A 28-year-old mother of two comes to your office with her 8-week-old infant. Her baby has been "crying constantly" for the last 4 weeks, and she is at her "wit's end." She is bottle feeding her baby and is having no significant feeding problems apart from what may be "excessive" gas and burping following feeding. No other symptoms have been identified. The mother also states that her first child had "some crying" spells but it was "nothing like this." The baby has had no other problems, specifically no constipation or diarrhea.

On examination, the infant is afebrile and has no abnormalities of the ears, throat, and lungs. The abdomen is soft, and there are no palpable masses.

■ SELECT THE BEST ANSWER TO THE FOLLOWING QUESTIONS:

1. What is the most likely diagnosis in this infant?
   a. infantile colic
   b. excessive spasm syndrome of infancy
   c. early Crohn's disease
   d. psychosocial stress syndrome of infancy
   e. urinary tract infection

2. Investigations that should be undertaken in the infant described include which of the following?
   a. complete blood count (CBC)
   b. CBC with white cell count differential, and erythrocyte sedimentation rate (ESR)
   c. CBC with white cell count differential, ESR, and urinalysis
   d. urinalysis
   e. none of the above; no investigations need be done

3. What is the most likely underlying cause of the infant's symptom of excessive crying?
   a. bottle feeding
   b. hormone abnormalities produced by the newly diagnosed psychiatric condition labeled "baby stress"
   c. gastrointestinal hyperperistalsis
   d. maternal stress
   e. none of the above; the cause of these symptoms is unknown

4. Which of the following definitions correctly identifies infants with the syndrome described?
   a. unexplained fussiness or crying lasting longer than 3 hours/day, 3 days/week, and continuing for more than 3 weeks in infants younger than 3 months old
   b. unexplained fussiness or crying lasting longer than 6 hours/day, 3 days/week, and continuing for more than 2 weeks in an infant younger than 4 months old
   c. unexplained fussiness or crying lasting longer than 4 hours/day, 3 days/week, and continuing for longer than 2 weeks in an infant younger than 6 months old
   d. unexplained fussiness or crying lasting longer than 6 hours/day, 5 days/week, and continuing for more than 3 weeks in an infant younger than 8 months old
   e. unexplained fussiness or crying lasting longer than 7 hours/day, 6 days/wk, and continuing for more than 7 weeks in an infant younger than 6 months old

5. At this time, what should you do?
   a. tell the mother to relax and to call you in 4 weeks if the crying has not improved
   b. set up an appointment for the baby with the infant psychiatrist
   c. do nothing
   d. discontinue cow's milk and begin soy formula
   e. none of the above

6. Which of the following statements regarding treatment of the condition described is true?
   a. treatment should begin and should be continued until the condition improves
   b. treatment is ineffective; it is not worth the bother
   c. the most effective treatment is reassuring the mother about the benign nature of the condition
   d. treatment with oral analgesics appears to be the most effective therapy that can be offered
   e. treatment with antibiotics should be started

7. Which of the following statements regarding drug therapy for the condition described is true?
   a. antispasmodic medications are safe and effective
   b. antihistamines given to the infant may be beneficial in sedating the baby and settling everybody down
   c. antispasmodics and antihistamines together offer the best form of drug therapy
   d. aspirin should be considered as a first-line option
   e. none of the above statements are true

ANSWERS:

1. a. This infant most likely has infantile colic, which is defined as spells of unexplained fussiness or crying lasting longer than 3 hours/day, 3 days/week, and continuing for more than 3 weeks in infants younger than 3 months old. "Unexplained fussiness or crying" implies that other causes (particularly infection) have been ruled out.

Excessive spasm syndrome of infancy and psychosocial stress syndrome of infancy do not exist. Early Crohn's disease is not possible.

Urinary tract infection, along with otitis media, pharyngitis, pneumonitis, and other infections, should be considered carefully before labeling the child as having infantile colic.

2. d. A urinary tract infection is the first infection that should be ruled out by performing a urinalysis. In addition, a complete physical examination should be performed to rule out any other causes. At this age otitis media, pharyngitis, pneumonia, meningitis, pyelonephritis, intussusception, or volvulus may present initially only with excessive crying. If your index of suspicion is raised following a physical examination, particularly in the presence of a fever, a more complete laboratory workup and hospitalization is indicated.

3. e. The cause of excessive crying in infancy is unknown. Although gastrointestinal hyperperistalsis, cow's milk protein allergy, lactose intolerance, disturbances in the parent–infant relationship, and a neurophysiologic response of the immature newborn to external and internal stimuli have all been proposed as potential underlying causes of infantile colic, nobody really knows for sure. The cause is likely multifactorial.

The newly diagnosed psychiatric condition known as "baby stress" does not exist.

4. a. Although you may argue correctly that the only type of person who would ask a question like this is one who was really strapped for good questions in the first place, it does reinforce the Wessel criteria for the diagnosis of infantile colic: unexplained fussiness or crying lasting longer than 3 hours/day, 3 days/week, and continuing for longer than 3 weeks in an infant younger than 3 months old.

5. e. The most reasonable course of action in this case (after you have ruled out other causes) is to (1) describe the condition to the mother; (2) explain that the cause is unknown; (3) reassure the mother that the colic will pass by the age of 3 months, or shortly thereafter, and if it does continue longer it certainly will continue to improve; (4) discuss maternal coping strategies with the mother; and (5) ask the mother to call you in 2 weeks if the symptoms have not improved or sooner if any other symptoms develop.

6. c. The most effective and important treatment is reassurance, stressing the benign nature of the condition and the assurance of resolution of the condition.

Reassure the mother that there is nothing that she is doing wrong and that there is no reason to switch to a soy-based formula. The prevalence, pattern, and amount of crying associated with infantile colic are reportedly similar in both human milk and formula-fed infants. Colic is not less common in soy-based feeding compared with ordinary infant formula.

To simply tell the mother to relax is not particularly helpful to anyone and indicates your lack of sensitivity to a very difficult problem.

7. e. Many different pharmacologic treatments frequently have been used to treat infantile colic, including dicyclomine (Bentyl), Phenergan (an antihistamine), aspirin, acetaminophen, and codeine. Dicyclomine has been associated with apnea and respiratory difficulties, and antihistamines may cause significant central nervous system difficulties.

Although you may consider using simple acetaminophen, even with this drug there are no good data to indicate its safety in very young infants.

SUMMARY OF COLIC

1. Infantile colic is extremely common; it occurs in up to 25% of infants.
2. Although there are a number of theories as to its cause, the cause at this time is idiopathic.
3. The most important differential diagnosis is infection: if the ears, throat, and lungs are clear and if no abnormalities are detected on abdominal examination, a urinalysis is the only investigation that is necessary.
4. Diagnosis of infantile colic is based on Wessel criteria: 3,3,3, and 3 (see Answer 4).
5. During episodes infants may have a tense abdomen, lift the head, clench the fists, flex the

legs to the abdomen, and appear flushed. The episodes tend to peak at age 6 weeks and are most common in the late afternoon and evening.

6. Reassurance of the parent is as effective as any other therapy and is the treatment of choice.

7. Medications including dicyclomine (Bentyl), antihistamines, and aspirin should not be used.

SUGGESTED READING

Balon AJ: Management of infantile colic. *Am Fam Physician* 55(1):235-242, 245-246, 1997.

Curran JS, Barness LA: The feeding of infants and children. Chapter 41. In: Behrman RE, et al, eds: *Nelson textbook of pediatrics*. Philadelphia, 2000, WB Saunders.

Gupta SK: Is colic a gastrointestinal disorder? *Curr Opin Pediatr* 14(5): 588-592, 2002.

Wade S, Kilgour T: Infantile colic (Clinical review: Extracts from "Clinical Evidence"). *BMJ*. 323(7310):437-440, 2001.

Chapter 96

Immunizations

> "That shot made my baby ill."

CLINICAL CASE PROBLEM 1:

A 2-Month-Old Infant with a High Fever 8 Hours after Receiving Her First Set of Immunizations

A 2-month-old infant is brought to your office by his mother following his first set of immunizations. His mother states that approximately 8 hours after being immunized, the infant developed a temperature of 39.9° C. The child is screaming and irritable. On physical examination, no localizing signs of infection are found. Examination of the ears shows hyperemia of both tympanic membranes. You realize, of course, that this probably is caused by the crying itself. The throat is normal. The lungs are clear. The cardiovascular system and abdomen are normal. Skin is without rash.

■ SELECT THE BEST ANSWER TO THE FOLLOWING QUESTIONS:

1. Which immunization(s) is (are) the most likely cause of the fever and the irritability in this child?
   a. poliomyelitis
   b. pertussis
   c. diphtheria
   d. tetanus
   e. any of the above

2. Considering this is an adverse reaction that appears to be related to the immunization, what would you do?
   a. hospitalize the child
   b. advise the mother to give the child aspirin to bring down the fever
   c. advise the mother to give the child acetaminophen to bring down the fever
   d. obtain immediate blood cultures, complete blood count, and urine for analysis and culture and perform a lumbar puncture
   e. none of the above

3. Which of the following statements regarding future immunizations for the child in Clinical Case Problem 1 is true?
   a. all future diphtheria–tetanus–pertussis (DTaP) and polio immunizations should be canceled
   b. irritability seen in this child is a contraindication to future immunization
   c. future immunizations should omit tetanus toxoid
   d. future immunizations should not be affected; DTaP and polio immunizations should be given as before
   e. none of the above statements are true

4. Which of the following statements regarding vaccination against poliomyelitis is true?
   a. at this time, although two forms of vaccination against poliomyelitis exist, only one is licensed for use in the United States
   b. oral polio vaccine (OPV) is a live, attenuated, trivalent vaccine known as the Salk vaccine
   c. inactivated poliomyelitis vaccine (IPV) is an inactivated (killed), trivalent vaccine known as Sabin vaccine
   d. the most recent recommendation calls for an all-IPV dosing regimen
   e. OPV and IPV both are associated with a small risk of vaccine-associated paralytic poliomyelitis (VAPP)

5. Which of the following statements is true regarding hepatitis B vaccine in children?
   a. it is not recommended as a routine immunization
   b. it is recommended as a routine immunization, and the first dose should not be given before the age of 2 months
   c. it is recommended as a routine immunization, and the first dose should be given at 6 months
   d. it is recommended as a routine immunization, and the first dose should be given at birth
   e. none of the above statements is true

6. Which of the following statements is (are) true regarding reactions that follow the immunization of infants and children with whole-cell DTP?
   a. there are three different types of adverse reactions that may occur
   b. the fever that may develop from one type of reaction often reaches 40.5° C
   c. this vaccine is no longer recommended
   d. a, b, and c
   e. none of the above statements are true

7. Which of the following is a true contraindication to immunization?
   a. prematurity
   b. recent exposure to an infectious disease
   c. current antimicrobial therapy
   d. moderate or severe illness with or without a fever
   e. history of penicillin or other allergies

8. Which of the following statements regarding immunization against *Haemophilus influenzae* Type b is (are) true?
   a. the vaccine is known as the Hib vaccine and is available in combination with the hepatitis B vaccine
   b. the first dose of *H. influenzae* Type b vaccine should be given at age 2 months
   c. the *H. influenzae* Type b vaccine is given to protect the infant only from *H. influenzae* Type b infections that lead to meningitis
   d. all of the above statements are true
   e. a and b only

9. Which of the following vaccines is recommended for first administration at age 12-15 months?
   a. hepatitis B
   b. *H. influenzae* Type b vaccine
   c. measles–mumps–rubella (MMR) vaccine
   d. hepatitis A
   e. pneumococcal

10. By the time a child reaches 7 years old, how many doses of DTaP should have been administered?
    a. 2 doses
    b. 3 doses
    c. 4 doses
    d. 5 doses
    e. none of the above

11. Which of the following statements about tetanus toxoid (Td or DT) is false?
    a. routine boosters are recommended every 10 years
    b. it is contraindicated during pregnancy
    c. it is given to children age 7 and older
    d. it should be given to patients presenting to the emergency department with dirty wounds if they have not had the last booster within the past 5 years
    e. Td should be given to children younger than age 7 years who have a contraindication to pertussis vaccine

12. All of the following are true about pneumococcal infection and the pneumococcal conjugate vaccine (PCV) except:
    a. it is indicated for all children younger than 24 months and for high-risk children up to their fifth birthday (includes splenic, other immunologic, and cardiopulmonary disorders)
    b. PCV is highly effective at preventing pneumococcal meningitis, pneumonia, sepsis, and nasal carriage (including resistant strains)
    c. the minimum interval between doses in the primary series is 8 weeks
    d. it is a heptavalent vaccine
    e. pneumococci cause more cases of otitis media than any other single pathogen

13. Which of the following is false in regards to the varicella vaccine?
    a. it should not be given before 12 months of age
    b. two doses are needed at least 4 weeks apart in those age 13 and older
    c. it is not effective in preventing or modifying disease if given after exposure
    d. a mild varicellalike syndrome can develop in 1% to 4% of those vaccinated
    e. the vaccine is 71% to 91% effective in preventing all symptoms of this disease

14. Which statement about vaccines is true?
    a. there is evidence that the MMR vaccine induces autism
    b. most vaccine-preventable diseases have been reduced by more than 99% since the introduction of vaccines

c. vaccines can cause autoimmune disorders and allergic disease

d. less than 100,000 of the nation's children are not fully immunized

e. 85% of children nationally have received all recommended vaccinations

CLINICAL CASE MANAGEMENT PROBLEM

Discuss some of the important causes for the reduction in neonatal, infant, and childhood mortality that have occurred during the past century. Indicate whether these causes are still a concern in certain parts of the world.

ANSWERS:

1. **e.** Although in the past pertussis most frequently was associated with fever, the new recommendations for use of acellular in place of whole-cell pertussis makes any of these vaccines equally culpable. Non-immunization causes should be considered.

2. **c.** Hospitalization or an intensive septic workup is unnecessary. Acetaminophen is the analgesic of choice for the treatment of fever in children. Aspirin should not be given because of its possible link with Reye's syndrome. This child should be reassessed within 24 hours if the symptoms (especially the fever) do not improve with the administration of the antipyretic acetaminophen or if any other symptoms or signs develop.

3. **d.** Much progress has been made in reducing the incidence of adverse reactions to vaccines. Although all vaccines may produce minor reactions— particularly local soreness, redness, and swelling following the administration of an injectable antigen— these are not absolute contraindications to further immunizations.

4. **d.** Two types of vaccine are licensed in the United States for prevention of polio: OPV, a live, attenuated, trivalent poliovirus vaccine known as Sabin; and an IPV, an inactivated (killed) trivalent vaccine known as Salk. Since 2000 the Advisory Committee for Immunization Practices (ACIP) has recommended an all-IPV vaccine regimen scheduled at 2 months, 4 months, 6-18 months, and 4-6 years. The reason for the change was to eliminate any VAPP, which occurs in 1 case in 2.4 million doses with OPV. IPV is not known to cause VAPP.

5. **d.** Vaccination against hepatitis B is routinely recommended for all children born in the United States. The easiest schedule for hepatitis B immunization is birth, 2 months, and 6 months. Thimerosal-free vaccines are recommended. It is acceptable to give the first dose of hepatitis B at 2 months if the infant's mother is known to be hepatitis B surface antigen (HBsAg) negative.

6. **d.** There are three types of adverse reactions that can occur with whole-cell DTP: local reactions, mild systemic reactions, and serious systemic reactions.

Whole-cell pertussis vaccines commonly are associated with local adverse events such as erythema, swelling, and pain at the injection site. Mild systemic events include fever, fretfulness, drowsiness, and anorexia. More serious systemic reactions are seizures and hypotonic hyporesponsive episodes, which occur in approximately 1 in 1750 doses administered. Acute encephalopathy occurs even more rarely (0-10.5 cases in 1 million doses administered). Concerns about the safety of DTP vaccine prompted the development of purified (acellular) pertussis vaccines (DTaP), which is now the recommended vaccine.

7. **d.** There are three true contraindications to the administration of childhood immunizations: (1) an anaphylactic reaction to a vaccine; (2) an anaphylactic reaction to a vaccine constituent contraindicates the use of vaccines containing that substance; and (3) moderate or severe illness with or without a fever. Mild acute illness with or without a fever is not a contraindication. Convulsions, encephalopathy, collapse, or shocklike state within 48 hours of receipt of any vaccine is a cause for concern and may be considered a contraindication to further vaccination. Such episodes, which had been related to the whole-cell DTP vaccine, are extremely rare with the acellular DTaP vaccine. For live attenuated vaccines, known immunodeficiency and pregnancy are also contraindications.

8. **e.** Vaccination against *H. influenzae* Type b is recommended at 2, 4, 6, and 12-15 months of age. *H. influenzae* vaccine is given at these times because of the age at which *H. influenzae* meningitis affects infants and children. Meningitis caused by this organism usually occurs between the ages of 1 month and 4 years. Major neurologic sequelae of *H. influenzae* Type b meningitis include behavior problems, language disorders, delayed development of language, impaired vision, mental retardation, motor abnormalities, ataxia, seizures, and hydrocephalus.

About 6% of patients with *H. influenzae* type b meningitis are left with some hearing impairment. Other significant infections caused by *H. influenzae* are acute epiglottis; pneumonia; septic arthritis;

cellulitis; osteomyelitis; pericarditis; bacteremia without an associated focus; neonatal disease; and miscellaneous infections such as urinary tract infection, cervical adenitis, uvulitis, endocarditis, primary peritonitis, periappendiceal abscess, and otitis media. The Hib immunization should, theoretically, be effective against all of these infections.

The early scheduling of the Hib vaccine and the hepatitis B (Hep B) vaccine is similar and they are available in combination.

9. c. Only two vaccinations are given for the first time at 12-15 months of age: MMR and varicella. They can be administered at the same time, but if not, at least a 4-week interval needs to separate the two.

10. d. By the time a child reaches 7 years of age, five doses of DTaP should have been administered. DTaP is given at 2, 4, 6, and 12-18 months of age and at 4-6 years of age.

11. b. Td is not contraindicated during pregnancy. It is not teratogenic and is not a live vaccine so it can be administered during pregnancy. The first dose of dT should be between 11-12 years of age if at least 5 years elapsed since the last dose of tetanus and diphtheria. The subsequent booster should be every 10 years unless a major or dirty wound is sustained, then the dose should be given if it has not received in the previous 5 years. Children older than age 6 years receive dT and not DTaP.

12. c. The minimal interval between doses in the primary series for the heptavalent PCV is 4 weeks. PCV is given to children younger than age 2 years, whereas the PPV (pneumococcal polysaccharide vaccine) is given to those older than age 2 who are high risk such as those with asplenia, sickle cell disease, diabetes, chronic cardiac and pulmonary disease, human immunodeficiency virus, and congenital immune deficiency. PPV is not effectively immunogenic in patients younger than 2 years of age.

13. c. The varicella vaccine is effective in preventing or modifying disease if given within 72 hours of exposure and possibly up to 120 hours of exposure. It should not be given prior to 12 months because of passive immunity transferred maternally. The vaccine has a 96% seroconversion rate. It is 95% to 100% effective in preventing severe disease and 71% to 91% efficacious in preventing all symptoms of this disease.

14. b. Nationwide, immunization levels are high, and there has been a 99% reduction in vaccine-preventable disease in this country. Yet, more than 900,000 of children in the United States are not fully immunized. The rate of immunization varies, with approximately 71% of African Americans, 76% of Hispanics, and 79% of whites being fully immunized. Although many hypotheses exist linking vaccines with chronic diseases such as autism, multiple sclerosis, allergies, and other autoimmune diseases, there is no good evidence to support these claims.

SOLUTION TO THE CLINICAL CASE MANAGEMENT PROBLEM

The reductions in neonatal, infant, and childhood mortality in the developed world during the last century are truly remarkable. These reductions are a result of better prenatal care and prenatal assessment of high-risk status; improved perinatal care; immunizations; antibiotics; other diagnostic and therapeutic tools; and public health measures including filtration and chlorination of water, hygienic food handling (especially of milk), mosquito control, and isolation of individuals infected with a communicable disease.

In addition, the health of children has been directly affected by improvements in social conditions, economic conditions, and educational advances in the developed world. Little more can be done to further reduce mortality rates apart from a paradigm shift from acute episodic care of children to primary preventive care on visits that occur for a different reason. For example, if a 6-month-old child is brought to your office by his mother for assessment of fever and irritability, it is a perfect opportunity to discuss the inadvisability of walkers near stairs, the use of child safety seats in automobiles, and locations of potential toxic substances and medicines in the home.

There is, however, a startling contrast between neonatal, infant, and childhood health in the developed world and the health of the same-aged population in the developing world, especially in areas of continual war and strife. In some areas of the developing world neonatal, infant, and childhood mortality is significantly higher today than it was in the United States in the eighteenth century.

RECOMMENDED CHILDHOOD AND ADOLESCENT IMMUNIZATION SCHEDULE—UNITED STATES, JANUARY–JUNE 2004

Vaccine ▼ / Age ►	0 Birth	1 mo	2 mos	4 mos	6 mos	12 mos	15 mos	18 mos	24 mos	4-6 yrs	11-12 yrs	13-18 yrs
Hepatitis B[1]	HepB #1	only if mother HBsAg(−)									HepB series	
		HepB #2				HepB #3						
Diphtheria, Tetanus, Pertussis[2]			DTaP	DTaP	DTaP		DTaP			DTaP		Td
Haemophilus influenzae Type b[2]			Hib	Hib	Hib	Hib						
Inactivated Polio			IPV	IPV		IPV				IPV		
Measles, Mumps, Rubella[4]						MMR #1				MMR #2		MMR #2
Varicella[5]						Varicella				Varicella		
Pneumococcal[6]			PCV	PCV	PCV	PCV				PCV	ppV	
Hepatitis A[7]										Hepatitis A series		
Influenza[8]						Influenza (yearly)						

Legend: range of recommended ages; catch-up vaccination; preadolescent assessment

Vaccines below this line are for selected populations

Figure 96-1

SUMMARY OF IMMUNIZATIONS

Figure 96-1 indicates the recommended ages for routine administration of currently licensed childhood vaccines, as of June 2004, for children through age 18 years. Any dose not given at the recommended age should be given at any subsequent visit when indicated and feasible. Tables 96-1 and 96-2 indicate age groups that warrant special effort to administer those vaccines not previously given. Additional vaccines may be licensed and recommended during subsequent years. Licensed combination vaccines may be used whenever any components of the combination are indicated and the vaccine's other components are not contraindicated. Providers should consult the manufacturers' package inserts for detailed recommendations.

1. Hepatitis B vaccine (Hep B)

All infants should receive the first dose of hepatitis B vaccine soon after birth and before hospital discharge; the first dose also may be given by age 2 months if the infant's mother is HBsAg-negative. Only monovalent Hep B can be used for the birth dose. Monovalent or combination vaccine containing Hep B may be used to complete the series. Four doses of vaccine may be administered when a birth dose is given. The second dose should be given at least 4 weeks after the first dose, except for combination vaccines, which cannot be administered before age 6 weeks. The third dose should be given at least 16 weeks after the first dose and at least 8 weeks after the second dose. The last dose in the vaccination series (third or fourth dose) should not be administered before age 6 months.

Infants born to mothers who are HBsAg-positive should receive Hep B and 0.5 mL hepatitis B immune globulin (HBIG) within 12 hours of birth at separate sites. The second dose is recommended at age 1-2 months. The last dose in the vaccination series should not be administered before age 6 months. These infants should be tested for HBsAg and anti-HBs at 9-15 months of age.

Continued

SUMMARY OF IMMUNIZATIONS —cont'd

Infants born to mothers whose HBsAg status is unknown should receive the first dose of the Hep B series within 12 hours of birth. Maternal blood should be drawn as soon as possible to determine the mother's HBsAg status; if the HBsAg test is positive, the infant should receive HBIG as soon as possible (no later than age 1 week). The second dose is recommended at age 1-2 months. The last dose in the vaccination series should not be administered before age 24 weeks.

2. Diphtheria and tetanus toxoids and acellular pertussis vaccine (DTaP)

The fourth dose of DTaP may be administered as early as age 12 months, provided 6 months have elapsed since the third dose and the child is unlikely to return at age 15-18 months. Tetanus and diphtheria toxoids (Td) is recommended at age 11-12 years if at least 5 years have elapsed since the last dose of tetanus and diphtheria toxoid-containing vaccine. Subsequent routine Td boosters are recommended every 10 years.

3. Haemophilus influenzae type b (Hib) conjugate vaccine

Three Hib conjugate vaccines are licensed for infant use. If PRP-OMP (PedvaxHIB® or ComVax® [Merck]) is administered at ages 2 and 4 months, a dose at age 6 months is not required. DTaP/Hib combination products should not be used for primary immunization in infants at ages 2, 4, or 6 months but can be used as boosters following any Hib vaccine.

4. Measles–mumps–rubella vaccine (MMR)

The second dose of MMR is recommended routinely at age 4-6 years but may be administered during any visit, provided at least 4 weeks have elapsed since the first dose and that both doses are administered beginning at or after age 12 months. Those who have not previously received the second dose should complete the schedule by the 11-12-year-old visit.

5. Varicella vaccine

Varicella vaccine is recommended at any visit at or after age 12 months for susceptible children (i.e., those who lack a reliable history of chickenpox). Susceptible persons aged 13 years or older should receive two doses given at least 4 weeks apart.

6. Pneumococcal vaccine

The heptavalent pneumococcal conjugate vaccine (PCV) is recommended for all children age 2-23 months. It also is recommended for certain children age 24-59 months. Pneumococcal polysaccharide vaccine (PPV) is recommended in addition to PCV for certain high-risk groups. (See *MMWR* 49(RR-9):1-38, 2000.)

7. Hepatitis A vaccine

Hepatitis A vaccine is recommended for children and adolescents in selected states and regions and for certain high-risk groups; consult your local public health authority. Children and adolescents in these states, regions, and high-risk groups who have not been immunized against hepatitis A can begin the hepatitis A vaccination series during any visit. The two doses in the series should be administered at least 6 months apart. See *MMWR* 48(RR-12):1-37, 1999.

8. Influenza vaccine

Influenza vaccine is recommended annually for children age 6 months or older with certain risk factors (including but not limited to asthma, cardiac disease, sickle cell disease, HIV, diabetes, and household members of persons in groups at high risk (see *MMWR* 51(RR-3):1-31, 2002) and can be administered to all others wishing to obtain immunity. In addition, healthy children age 6-23 months are encouraged to receive influenza vaccine if feasible because children in this age group are at substantially increased risk for influenza-related hospitalizations. Children aged 12 years or older should receive vaccine in a dosage appropriate for their age (0.25 mL if age 6-35 months or 0.5 mL if aged 3 years or older). Children aged 8 years or older who are receiving influenza vaccine for the first time should receive two doses separated by at least 4 weeks.

The ACIP has indicated that beginning in fall 2004, children 6 to 23 months should receive annual influenza vaccine. For additional information about vaccines, including precautions and contraindications for immunization and vaccine shortages, please visit the National Immunization Program Website at www.cdc.gov/nip or call the National Immunization Information Hotline at 800-232-2522 (English) or 800-232-0233 (Spanish).

Approved by the Advisory Committee on Immunization Practices (www.cdc.gov/nip/acip), the American Academy of Pediatrics (www.aap.org), and the American Academy of Family Physicians (www.aafp.org).

Table 96-1 Catch-up schedule for children age 4 months through 6 years

	MINIMUM INTERVAL BETWEEN DOSES			
Dose One (Minimum Age)	Dose One to Dose Two	Dose Two to Dose Three	Dose Three to Dose Four	Dose Four to Dose Five
DTaP (6 wks)	4 weeks	4 weeks	6 months	6 months[1]
IPV (6 wks)	4 weeks	4 weeks	4 weeks[2]	
HepB[3] (birth)	4 weeks	8 weeks (and 16 weeks after first dose)		
MMR (12 mos)	4 weeks[4]			
Varicella (12 mos)				
Hib[5] (6 wks)	4 weeks: if 1st dose given at age 12–14 mos, 2nd dose given at age >15	4 weeks[6]: if current age <12 mos 8 weeks (as final dose)[6]: if current age >12 mos and 2nd dose given at age <15 mos No further doses needed: if previous dose given at age >15 mos	8 weeks (as final dose): this dose only necessary for children age 12 mos to 5 yrs who received 3 doses before age 12 mos	
PCV[7]	4 weeks: if 1st dose given at age <12 mos and current age <24 mos 8 weeks (as final dose): if 1st dose given at age >12 mos or current age 24–59 mos No further doses needed: for healthy children if 1st dose given at age >24 mos	4 weeks: if current age <12 mos 8 weeks (as final dose): if current age >12 mos No further doses needed: for healthy children if previous dose given at age >24 mos	8 weeks (as final dose): this dose only for children age 12 mos to 5 yrs who received 3 doses before age 12 mos	

[1]DTaP: The fifth dose is not necessary if the fourth dose was given after the fourth birthday.

[2]IPV: For children who received an all-IPV or all-OPV series, a fourth dose is not necessary if a third dose was given at age >4 years. If both OPV and IPV were given as part of a series, a total of four doses should be given, regardless of the child's current age.

[3]HepB: All children and adolescents who have not been immunized against hepatitis B should begin the hepatitis B vaccination series during any visit. Providers should make special efforts to immunize children who were born in, or whose parents were born in, areas of the world where hepatitis B virus infection is moderately or highly endemic.

[4]MMR: The second dose of MMR is recommended routinely at age 4-6 years but may be given earlier if desired.

[5]Hib: Vaccine is not generally recommended for children age >5 years.

[6]Hib: If current age is <12 months and the first two doses were PRP-OMP (PedvaxHIB or ComVax), the third (and final) dose should be given at age 12-15 months and at least 8 weeks after the second dose.

[7]PCV: Vaccine is not generally recommended for children age >5 years.

Table 96-2 Catch-up schedule for children age 7 through 18 years

MINIMUM INTERVAL BETWEEN DOSES		
Dose One to Dose Two	Dose Two to Dose Three	Dose Three to Booster Dose
Td: 4 weeks	Td: 4 weeks	Td[1]: 6 months: if 1st dose given at age <12 mos and current age <11 yrs
IPV[2]: 4 weeks	IPV[2]: 4 weeks	IPV[2]

Continued

Table 96-2 Catch-up schedule for children age 7 through 18 years—cont'd

MINIMUM INTERVAL BETWEEN DOSES		
Dose One to Dose Two	Dose Two to Dose Three	Dose Three to Booster Dose
HepB: 4 weeks MMR: 4 weeks Varicella[3]: 4 weeks	HepB: 8 weeks (and 16 weeks after 1st dose)	

[1]**Td:** For children age 7-10 years, the interval between the third and booster dose is determined by the age when the first dose was given. For adolescents age 11-18 years, the interval is determined by the age when the third dose was given.
[2]**IPV:** Vaccine is not generally recommended for persons age >18 years.
[3]**Varicella:** Give a two-dose series to all susceptible adolescents age >13 years.
Report adverse reactions to vaccines through the federal Vaccine Adverse Event Reporting System. For information on reporting reactions following vaccines, please visit www.vaers.org or call the 24-hour national toll-free information line at 800-822-7967.
Report suspected cases of vaccine-preventable diseases to your state or the local health department.
For additional information about vaccines, including precautions and contraindications for immunization and vaccine shortages, please visit the National Immunization Program Website at www.cdc.gov/nip or call the National Immunization Information Hotline at 800-232-2522 (English) or 800-232-0233 (Spanish).
Adapted from: http://www.aafp.org/x7666.xml?printxml

SUGGESTED READING

American Academy of Pediatrics: *2000 Red Book: report of the Committee on Infectious Diseases,* 25th ed. American Academy of Pediatrics Press, 2000, Oakbrook Terrace, IL.

Atkinson WL: General recommendations on immunization. Recommendations of the Advisory Committee on Immunization Practices (ACIP) and the American Academy of Family Physicians (AAFP). *MMWR Recomm Rep* 51(RR-2):1-35, 8-Feb. 2002.

Centers for Disease Control and Prevention National Immunization Program: http://www.cdc.gov/nip/home-hcp.htm.

Fombonne E: No evidence for a new variant of measles-mumps-rubella-induced autism. *Pediatrics* 108(4):E58, 2001.

Offit PA: Addressing parents' concerns: Do vaccines cause allergic or autoimmune diseases? *Pediatrics* 111(3):654-659, 2003.

Peter G: Immunization practices. In: Behrman RE, et al, eds: *Nelson textbook of pediatrics,* 16th ed. WB Saunders Company, 2000, Philadelphia.

Prince A: Infectious disease: prevention. In: Behrman RE, Klegman RM, eds. *Nelson essentials of pediatrics,* 4th ed. WB Saunders, 2002, Philadelphia, 359-365.

Swain G, Bower D: Office based immunization practice. In: Rakel RE, Bope ET, eds. *Conn's Current Therapy 2003,* 55th ed. Elsevier, 2002, Philadelphia.

Chapter 97

Infant Feeding

"Breast is best."

CLINICAL CASE PROBLEM 1:

AN ANXIOUS MOTHER WITH A 3-WEEK-OLD INFANT AND MANY QUESTIONS CONCERNING FEEDING

A mother who just delivered her first baby 3 weeks ago comes to your office for her first neonatal visit. She has many questions concerning breastfeeding and has been getting much advice from her friends and especially her mother-in-law. The infant appears to be growing well and, according to her mother, is happy and content. The mother-in-law has suggested that her daughter-in-law change from breastfeeding to cow's milk because she feels the infant's crying is waking up her son (the baby's father) and preventing him from getting "the rest that the poor boy needs." The mother appears somewhat tired herself. The child is at the 50th percentile for weight and the 50th percentile for length. More importantly, the child has gained an average of 50 g/day since discharge from the hospital. The child is feeding every 2 hours at this time.

SELECT THE BEST ANSWER TO THE FOLLOWING QUESTIONS:

1. What is the minimal appropriate weight gain (and a sign of both infant health and maternal–infant bonding with breastfeeding) following discharge from hospital?
   a. 15 g/day
   b. 20 g/day
   c. 30 g/day
   d. 50 g/day
   e. 75 g/day

2. What would be your suggestion to the mother in terms of feeding her infant?

a. ask her mother-in-law; she seems to know all the answers
b. decrease the feeds of the infant to every 3 hours
c. feed the infant on demand
d. switch from breastfeeding to bottle feeding
e. a and c

3. Regarding the feeding of infants when they cry, which of the following offers the best advice to the mother?
a. feed the baby; no ifs, and, or buts
b. let the infant cry for at least 30 minutes; if the infant is still crying it's likely to be either a diaper problem or a food problem
c. supplement breastfeeding; crying may indicate inadequate milk supply
d. crying may or may not indicate hunger; assume that the baby needs to be fed until proved otherwise; if the baby refuses the breast, check for other causes of crying
e. crying is usually the first sign of hunger in a baby

4. Which of the following statements regarding milk production and maternal anxiety is (are) true?
a. there is little correlation between milk production and maternal anxiety
b. maternal anxiety may significantly increase milk let-down
c. maternal anxiety may significantly decrease milk let-down
d. the main determinant of a good milk supply is frequent, effective milk removal
e. c and d

5. Human colostrum is the precursor to human milk. What is (are) the major components found in colostrum that offer(s) a significant advantage to breastfed infants?
a. macrophages that synthesize complement, lysozyme, and lactoferrin
b. bacterial antibodies that protect the infant against bacterial organisms entering through the gastrointestinal (GI) tract
c. antibodies that protect the infant against viral organisms entering through the GI tract
d. b and c
e. a, b, and c

6. Which of the following antibodies is of particular importance and is found in abundance in human colostrum?
a. immunoglobulin A (IgA)
b. IgG

c. IgM
d. IgE
e. none of the above

CLINICAL CASE PROBLEM 2:
A 28-Year-Old Primigravida with Mastitis

A 28-year-old primigravida develops an erythematous skin discoloration in the upper outer quadrant of the left breast. You suspect bacterial mastitis.

7. At this time, what would you do?
a. stop breastfeeding and have the mother express her breast milk until the infection is cleared up
b. continue breastfeeding and treat the mother with hot compresses and antibiotics
c. continue breastfeeding and treat both the mother and the infant with antibiotics
d. discontinue breastfeeding for now and provide antibiotics to the mother
e. discontinue any further breastfeeding and perform an incision and drainage immediately

8. What is (are) the organism(s) most likely responsible for the condition described in Clinical Case Problem 2?
a. Streptococcus pneumoniae
b. Staphylococcus aureus
c. Escherichia coli: subtype H-57
d. Bacteroides fragilis
e. b and d

9. Which of the following statements comparing human milk with cow's milk is false?
a. cow's milk may be responsible for diarrhea, intestinal bleeding, and occult melena
b. spitting up, infantile colic, and atopic dermatitis are more common in infants fed with cow's milk (or infant formula)
c. human milk contains bacterial and viral antibodies, antibodies mainly of the IgA class
d. breastfed babies do not require iron supplementation until the age of 1 year
e. human milk has an adequate amount of vitamin C

10. The mother described in Clinical Case Problem 1 has been told that she should be "giving the baby lots of every vitamin under the sun." Her mother-in-law even offers to purchase the 37 different vitamins for the baby. The mother-in-law actually may be right with respect to which of the following vitamins?

a. vitamin A
b. vitamin C
c. vitamin D
d. b and c
e. a, b, and c

11. Fluoride supplementation for both breastfed babies and bottle-fed babies should not be required if the fluoride concentration in the water supply of the community exceeds which of the following?
a. 1.0 ppm
b. 2.0 ppm
c. 5.0 ppm
d. 10.0 ppm
e. 100.0 ppm

12. Human milk, in comparison to cow's milk, has which of the following?
a. a higher fat content
b. a lower carbohydrate content
c. a lower protein content
d. a greater concentration of the protein casein
e. a greater number of kilocalories per gram of milk

13. Which of the following statements is false regarding infant feeding?
a. infants establish their own feeding pattern; there is considerable variation from one infant to another
b. for the first 1-2 months of life, frequent feedings occur throughout the 24-hour period
c. breastfed babies should be fed on an established schedule
d. during the first month of life, feedings average 8 to 12 every 24 hours
e. as age-appropriate solid foods are added after 6 months of age, the frequency of breastfeeding tends to decrease

14. The mother-in-law in Clinical Case Problem 1 recommends that solids be introduced on day 8 and that one new solid food be introduced every 4 days until a total of 28 different solids are being consumed regularly. You have a different recommendation. Your recommendation is that solid foods do not have to be introduced into the infant's diet until what age?
a. 1 month of age
b. 2 to 3 months of age
c. 6 months of age
d. 9 months of age
e. 12 months of age

15. Six weeks later, you see the same mother presented in Clinical Case Problem 1. She has switched from breastfeeding to infant formula feeding because she had to go back to her full-time job as an accountant. She tells you that her infant is now constipated. On careful questioning, you determine that the infant is having one hard bowel movement every 4 days. The physical examination is completely normal, including anal sphincter tone. What should you do now?
a. advise the mother to go home and relax
b. suggest supplementation with extra fluids, addition of corn syrup to the formula, or change to a less-constipating formula if appropriate
c. suggest the use of milk of magnesia at bedtime
d. suggest the addition of two teaspoons of bran to the formula every 3 hours
e. advise the use of glycerine suppositories twice a day for 6 weeks

CLINICAL CASE PROBLEM 3:
A MOTHER WITH A BABY WHO SPITS UP HER FORMULA

A mother comes to your office with her infant. Her baby is 6 weeks of age and has been "spitting up" all of her formula for the last 3 weeks. She believes the infant is malnourished and has been told so by another very helpful mother-in-law. You weigh the baby; she is 11 pounds, 3 ounces. Her birth weight was 7 pounds, 6 ounces.

16. At this time, you should advise the mother to do which of the following:
a. return home and relax; the child will grow out of it
b. increase the time spent burping the infant and keep the infant semi-upright after feedings
c. investigate the child for pyloric stenosis
d. suggest the use of a GI tract motility modifier such as metoclopramide
e. immediately refer the child to a pediatric gastroenterologist

CLINICAL CASE PROBLEM 4:
A MOTHER WITH BREASTFEEDING PROBLEMS

A mother comes to your office with her 8-week-old infant girl. The mother is tearful and depressed. She has been trying to breastfeed, but she tells you that "I'm obviously inadequate. I'm not producing enough milk, and the baby is fussy all of the time." On examination, the infant looks thin. Since her last checkup 3 weeks ago, she has gained only 90 g. The rest of the physical examination is normal.

17. At this time, what should you do?
    a. ask some very direct questions about the mother's feeding technique
    b. refer the mother to a lactation consultant
    c. encourage the mother to start pumping and include the baby's father or other family member in feeding her milk to the baby, adding formula if necessary until her milk supply is adequate for the baby's catchup growth
    d. schedule a reassessment within 3 days after interventions have been undertaken
    e. all of the above

18. Which of the following statements regarding breastfeeding is (are) true?
    a. early postpartum hospital routines can adversely affect breastfeeding
    b. most breastfeeding problems can be prevented by frequent, unscheduled feedings and ensuring good positioning and latch
    c. maternal fatigue may impair breastfeeding
    d. the rate of milk production increases with a more thoroughly drained breast and decreases when a breast is not as completely drained
    e. all of the above statements are true

CLINICAL CASE MANAGEMENT PROBLEM

Compare the composition of human milk with infant formula or cow's milk.

 ANSWERS:

1. **b.** The minimal acceptable weight gain in the neonatal period and infancy is 20 g/day. If weight gain equals or exceeds that, you can be reasonably confident that the infant is thriving.

In an excellent review article, Dr. Nancy Powers (see Suggested Readings) states: "*There are few normative data regarding weight gain for fully breastfed infants in the first 1-4 weeks of life....data confirm clinical guidelines that thriving, breastfed infants lose less than 10% of their birth weight and return to birth weight by 2 weeks of age. ....data also show that between 2 and 6 weeks of age, average daily weight gain is 34 g for girls and 40 g for boys....The fifth percentile for boys and girls is approximately 20 g per day... Several studies in the United States have shown that healthy, breastfed infants do not necessarily follow the National Center for Health Statistics (NCHS) growth curves....Infants who fail to return to birth weight by age 2 weeks or are not gaining a minimum of 20 g per day thereafter should be evaluated thoroughly.*"

2. **c.** During the first few weeks and months of life the ideal feeding schedule is feeding on demand. This will vary from infant to infant but eventually will settle into a reasonable schedule averaging 8-12 feedings per day.

3. **d.** Infants cry for a variety of reasons, and crying may not always be a sign of hunger. Some infants are placid, some are unusually active, and some are irritable. Sick infants are often uninterested in food. We should encourage mothers to put the baby to breast whenever it is exhibiting any signs of distress. If the baby refuses the breast, they should check for other things. Breastfeeding is more than just a feeding method. It is a way of nurturing a baby. If we perpetuate the bottle-feeding model by stressing the feeding role of nursing and neglecting the nurturing dimensions, we are sending the wrong message. Bottle-fed babies can only take the bottle when they are hungry; in fact, they often overfeed because they get more milk because of their inability to regulate the flow, and that may be one reason they are more likely to regurgitate. When a bottle-fed baby needs to suck for comfort, a bottle is not the answer because the baby does not want milk. A pacifier may be more appropriate. However, breastfed babies can regulate their intake of milk at the breast by altering their suckling patterns. That way, a breastfed baby can nurse actively and vigorously for hunger, less actively for thirst, and even do very light "flutter" sucking with minimal milk intake when they just want to suck for comfort. A mother's milk supply depends on frequent and effective breast milk removal.

It is best for the mother to try feeding whenever the baby demonstrates feeding cues. If the baby does not wish to nurse, he or she will refuse. Then the mother can check other possible causes of crying. Infants who awaken and cry consistently at short intervals simply may need nurturing. Some infants cry to gain sufficient attention, whereas other infants deprived of adequate mothering become indifferent. Some infants simply need to be held. Those who stop crying when they are picked up or held do not usually need food, but those who continue to cry when held and when food is offered should be carefully evaluated for other causes of distress.

4. **e.** Maternal anxiety, fatigue, postpartum depression, and stress from other causes are causal candidates for decreased milk production and let-down. The main determinant of a good milk supply is frequent, effective milk removal.

5. **e.** Colostrum provides macrophages that synthesize complement, lysozyme, and lactoferrin and

antibodies against bacteria and viruses that protect the infant against infection through the GI tract.

6. a. Human colostrum contains antibodies of the IgA class that protect the infant from bacterial species such as *E. coli* and certain viruses. In addition, human colostrum contains macrophages that are able to synthesize complement, lysozyme, lactoferrin, and the iron-binding whey protein that is normally about one-third saturated with iron.

7. b. See Answer 8.

8. b. Unless exceptional circumstances dictate otherwise, the recommended course of action with maternal mastitis is to continue breastfeeding and treat the mother with both symptomatic treatments such as hot compresses and antibiotics effective against *S. aureus* (including coagulase-positive *Staphylococcus*). The antibiotic of choice in this case is either cloxacillin or methicillin.

9. d. Advantages of human milk include convenience, digestibility, transfer of antiviral and antibacterial antibodies, lack of allergic phenomena, low incidence of regurgitation, lower incidence of colic, and no constipation or GI bleeding. Breastfeeding may facilitate maternal–infant bonding. Additionally, breastfeeding delays or reduces the incidence of atopic diseases such as eczema, allergies, and asthma and helps prevent obesity and type 1 diabetes. Breastfeeding has increased in frequency from a low of 52% in the late 1980s to two-thirds of postpartum women at discharge today. Human milk usually contains adequate supplies of all vitamins, with the possible exception of vitamin D. Vitamin C is not required for supplementation. Although human milk contains small amounts of highly bioavailable iron, iron-fortified foods are recommended to be introduced at 6 months of age to prevent iron-deficiency anemia.

10. c. Vitamin D is the only vitamin that may be required for supplementation in a breastfed baby. If a baby is not exposed to adequate sunlight or has dark skin, the quantity of vitamin D in breast milk may not be sufficient. The daily recommended vitamin D intake is 400 IU/day.

11. a. Fluoride supplementation for infants (both breastfed and bottle-fed) is not required if the fluoride concentration of the water supply exceeds 1.0 ppm, and it should not be started before 6 months of age. Additional fluoride given to formula-fed babies in a community with a fluoridated water supply could result in fluorosis.

12. c. In comparison to cow's milk, human milk has a higher carbohydrate concentration, a lower protein concentration, different protein composition (lactalbumin and lactoglobulin rather than casein), a higher percentage of polyunsaturated fat (qualitative difference), and the same caloric content (20 kcal/oz).

13. c. As stated previously (in Answer 2) neonates and infants should be fed on demand, not on a strictly imposed schedule. However, the following statements concerning infant feeding are true: (1) there is considerable variation in feeding patterns from infant to infant; (2) during the first month or 2 of life, feedings are taken frequently throughout the 24-hour period; (3) during the first few months of life, feedings average 8-12 per 24-hour period; and (4) as age-appropriate solid foods are added after 6 months of age, the frequency of breastfeeding tends to decrease.

14. c. Solid foods should not be introduced into an infant's diet until approximately 6 months of age. New foods should not be introduced more often than one every 1-2 weeks. The order of food introduction appears relatively unimportant. The introduction of one food at a time will help determine if there is an allergic or atopic reaction to any particular newly introduced food. Iron-containing foods are desirable. The wording in the American Academy of Pediatrics recommendations does say "approximately." After all, there is nothing magical that happens on the 6-month birthday. Some babies are truly ready for solids a couple of weeks earlier, and some are really not at all ready for another few weeks. We should teach parents the signs of readiness for solids (e.g., ability to sit unsupported, loss of the tongue-protrusion reflex, ability to grasp the food and bring it to the mouth).

15. b. Constipation is a common problem in formula-fed infants. It is extremely rare in a breastfed baby. Constipation in a formula-fed baby may be caused by an insufficient amount of food or fluid, a diet too high in fat or protein, or a diet deficient in bulk. The addition of extra fluids or the addition of corn syrup to the formula may be appropriate. Certainly, soy formulas are the most constipating, so if the baby is on soy but can tolerate a cow's milk–based formula, that might be worth a try. If the infant is drinking a conventional cow's milk formula, consider a switch to a partially hydrolyzed formula. In older infants, but certainly not at 6 weeks of age, constipation may be alleviated by adding or increasing the amounts of cereal, vegetables, or fruit or offering prune juice (0.5 to 1 ounce). The use of milk of magnesia and glycerine suppositories as anything but a temporary measure is inappropriate. The addition of 2 teaspoons of bran to pablum, although theoretically sound as a measure of increasing the bulk in the infant's diet, would be inappropriate in a 6 week old. Telling the mother to go home and relax is not appropriate.

16. **b.** Regurgitation, or spitting up, is a common problem in infants. The mechanism appears to be an incompetent gastroesophageal sphincter. Regurgitation can be reduced by adequate eructation of swallowed air during and after eating, by gentle handling, by avoidance of emotional conflicts, and by holding the infant against the shoulder or placing in a semi-upright position (e.g., infant car seat) after eating. The head should not be lower than the rest of the body during rest periods. Unless the child (especially a male) demonstrates projectile vomiting and has a palpable mass in the pylorus, pyloric stenosis is not likely.

17. **e.** This is a very common scenario in family practice. The mother should be questioned carefully and, ideally, observed regarding feeding technique. Before assuming that the mother has insufficient milk, other possibilities should be excluded: errors in feeding technique responsible for the infant's inadequate progress; remediable maternal factors related to diet, rest, or emotional distress; or physical disturbances in the infant that interfere with eating or with weight gain. Occasionally infants who seem to be nursing well may not thrive because of milk insufficiency; in this case increased frequency of feedings and increased maternal nutrition and hydration may be indicated. Usually once there has been this slow of a weight gain, however, insufficient maternal milk supply is a strong possibility (most often because of infrequent or inadequate milk removal), and she needs to pump every 2-3 hours with a heavy-duty double-pumping hospital grade electric pump to bring it back. In the meantime, there may not be enough of her milk to get this baby back from the brink. This is one of the few situations in which formula really is needed.

Referral to the La Leche League or a certified lactation consultant is an alternative that can be recommended to this mother. The La Leche League is a volunteer organization composed of successfully nursing mothers willing to assist other mothers desiring to nurse. If the mother is exhausted but able to successfully express sufficient milk, the husband or significant other may be able to assist the mother in feeding. This alternative is attractive because it gives the mother time to rest and recover her strength. This infant should be reassessed soon after the previously mentioned interventions are undertaken to monitor nutritional progress. Infant formulas provide adequate nutrition for the infant and may be the last alternative. Although "breast is best," a dogmatic approach to breastfeeding should be avoided. Yet, remember that most breastfeeding problems can be solved without having to give up the multiple benefits of breast milk.

18. **e.** All of the statements are true.

SOLUTION TO THE CLINICAL CASE MANAGEMENT PROBLEM

A succinct comparison between human milk and formula or cow's milk follows: (1) human milk has higher carbohydrate content than formula or cow's milk; (2) human milk has lower protein content than cow's milk; (3) human milk has lactalbumin and lactoglobulin, whereas formula or cow's milk has casein as the major protein; (4) human milk has a higher percentage of polyunsaturated fat; (5) human milk, cow's milk and formula have equivalent caloric content (20 kcal/oz); (6) only breastfeeding has been demonstrated to protect the child against obesity, atopic disease, and type 1 diabetes, and (7) breastfeeding protects the nursing child against a variety of acute and chronic illnesses, and because they do not get equivalent protection, formula-fed infants have more illnesses and incur a higher cost to the health care system.

Breastfeeding also promotes maternal health. It provides short-term benefits such as a reduced risk of postpartum hemorrhage and iron deficiency and long-term benefits including decreased risk of breast, ovarian, and uterine cancers.

SUMMARY OF INFANT FEEDING

1. **Breastfeeding:** Breastfeeding is best. Advantages of breastfeeding include convenience, digestibility, transfer of antiviral and antibacterial antibodies, decreased risk of allergic phenomena, maternal–infant bonding, low incidence of regurgitation, and no constipation. In addition, breastfeeding delays or reduces the incidence of infectious diseases and atopic diseases such as eczema, allergies, and asthma, and it may help prevent

Continued

SUMMARY OF INFANT FEEDING —cont'd

1. **Breastfeeding—cont'd**

   obesity and type 1 diabetes. Breastfeeding has increased in frequency from a low of 52% in the late 1980s to two-thirds of postpartum women at discharge today.

   Breastfeeding needs to be encouraged: Education and planning should begin optimally during the early part of pregnancy. Lactation assistance by breastfeeding-knowledgeable health care professionals after birth is important for first-time mothers. After delivery, before assuming that milk production is insufficient for the infant, you should consider errors in feeding techniques, remediable maternal factors such as lack of confidence and/or lack of support, anatomic anomalies in the mother or infant, and physical disturbances in the infant.

   Feeding should be on demand: although erratic in the first few months, infants tend to regulate themselves after a short time.

2. **Vitamin, fluoride, and iron supplements:** Vitamins are unnecessary in most babies, particularly if maternal supplies during pregnancy were adequate. If the baby is not exposed to sufficient sunlight or is darkly pigmented, supplemental vitamin D is recommended. Fluoride supplementation is unnecessary if the community water supply contains 1.0 ppm or more fluoride. Iron supplements (in the form of iron-fortified food) may be begun at the age of 6 months to reduce the possibility of anemia.

3. **Solid foods:** Breast milk is an excellent food through at least the first year of life, and may be continued as long as mother and child like. Solid foods should be introduced at approximately 6 months of age; introduce one new food every 1-2 weeks.

4. Do not assume that nutrition information received from other sources (including well-meaning family members) is valid information.

5. Advantages of human colostrum include the following: It provides macrophages, viral and bacterial antibodies of the secretory IgA class. Colostrum also supplies immunomodulating agents such as complement, lysozyme, lactoferrin, cytokines, and interleukins.

6. **Growth and development:** The minimum standard for the neonate is a weight gain of 20 g/day.

7. As a general rule, any drug that can be given safely to a neonate is probably safe to use during breast-feeding. The American Academy of Pediatrics publishes a review of drugs and chemicals that can be safely used during lactation. Although the "jury is still out" in terms of studies, the prime contraindication to breastfeeding is maternal human immunodeficiency virus infection.

SUGGESTED READING

Bottcher MF, Jenmalm MC: Breastfeeding and the development of atopic disease during childhood. *Clin Exper Allergy* 32(2):159-161, 2002.

Briggs GG: Drug effects on the fetus and breast-fed infant. *Clin Obstet Gynecol* 45(1):6-21, 2002.

Fulhan J, et al: Update on pediatric nutrition: breastfeeding, infant nutrition, and growth. *Curr Opin Pediatrics* 15(3):323-332, 2003.

Lawrence RA: Breastfeeding: benefits, risks and alternatives. *Curr Opin Obstet Gynecol* 12(6):519-524, 2000.

Li L, et al: Breast feeding and obesity in childhood: cross sectional study. *BMJ* 327(7420):904-905, 2003.

Powers N: How to assess slow growth in the breastfed infant. *Pediatr Clin N Am* 48(2):345-363, 2001.

Chapter 98

Failure to Thrive and Short Stature

"How come he seems so skinny and small?"

CLINICAL CASE PROBLEM 1:

AN 8-MONTH-OLD INFANT WHO APPEARS MALNOURISHED

An 8-month-old infant is brought to the emergency department by his mother for an assessment of an upper-respiratory tract infection. He has been coughing for the past 3 days and has had a runny nose.

On examination, his temperature is 37.5° C. His weight is below the 3rd percentile for his age, his length is at the 25th percentile, and his head circumference at the 50th percentile. He appears malnourished and has thin extremities, a narrow face, prominent ribs, and wasted buttocks. He has a prominent diaper rash, unwashed skin, a skin rash that resembles the skin infection impetigo contagiosum on his face, uncut fingernails, and dirty clothing.

▐ SELECT THE BEST ANSWER TO THE FOLLOWING QUESTIONS:

1. What is the most likely diagnosis in the infant described?

a. nonorganic failure to thrive (FTT)
b. organic FTT
c. child neglect
d. a and c
e. b and c

2. What is the most likely cause of this child's condition?
   a. maternal deprivation
   b. cystic fibrosis
   c. constitutionally small for age
   d. infantile autism
   e. congenital bilateral sensorineural hearing loss

3. What is (are) the procedure(s) of choice for this infant at this time?
   a. provision of a high-calorie formula; reassessment of the infant in 1 week
   b. initiation of outpatient investigations in the child to exclude serious organic disease
   c. treatment of the respiratory tract infection and instruction to the mother in correct feeding practices
   d. all of the above
   e. none of the above

4. Where is follow-up of this child best performed?
   a. in the hospital outpatient department
   b. in the hospital emergency room
   c. in the family physician's office
   d. in the home by the public health nurse
   e. in the social worker's office

5. The initial follow-up plan suggests the frequency of visits for the child to be which of the following?
   a. every month
   b. every 3 months
   c. every week
   d. every 6 weeks
   e. every 6 months

6. The environment that exists for this child should be thoroughly assessed for which of the following?
   a. child abuse or potential for child abuse
   b. spousal abuse or potential for spousal abuse
   c. level of family income
   d. inappropriate parental coping mechanisms: alcohol and drug use
   e. all of the above

CLINICAL CASE PROBLEM 2:

A 13-YEAR-OLD FEMALE WHO IS SHORT WITH A WEBBED NECK

A 13-year-old female is brought to your office for assessment of her short stature. On examination the child has a height and weight below the 5th percentile, a webbed neck, lack of breast bud development, a high-arched palate, and a low-set posterior hairline.

7. What is the most likely diagnosis in this child?
   a. Noonan's syndrome
   b. trisomy 21
   c. Turner's syndrome
   d. fragile X syndrome
   e. constitutional delay of growth

8. What is the most common cause of short stature in children?
   a. familial short stature
   b. chromosomal abnormality
   c. constitutional delay of growth
   d. hypothyroidism
   e. psychosocial dwarfism

9. Bone age sometimes can be used to differentiate certain causes of short stature in children. With respect to bone age, which of the following statements is true?
   a. bone age is normal in both familial short stature and in constitutional delay of growth
   b. bone age is normal in familial short stature and delayed in constitutional delay of growth
   c. bone age is normal in constitutional delay of growth and delayed in growth hormone deficiency
   d. bone age is delayed in both familial short stature and in short stature caused by hypothyroidism
   e. bone age is variable and cannot be used to differentiate familial short stature and constitutional delay

10. Psychosocial dwarfism is a situation in which poor physical growth may be associated with an unfavorable psychosocial situation. With respect to psychosocial dwarfism, which of the following statements is (are) true?
    a. sleep and eating aberrations occur in these children
    b. growth usually returns to normal when the stress is removed
    c. behavioral problems are common in these children
    d. a, b, and c are true
    e. a, b, and c are false

11. Which of the following investigations should be performed in a child with FTT or a child in which short stature is unlikely to be familial in nature?
    a. complete blood count (CBC)
    b. complete urinalysis
    c. serum blood urea nitrogen (BUN) and creatinine

   d. T4 and thyroid-stimulating hormone (TSH)
   e. all of the above

CLINICAL CASE MANAGEMENT PROBLEM

List at least 10 disorders that may manifest
themselves as FTT in infants and children.

ANSWERS:

1. d. This child most likely has nonorganic FTT,
secondary to child neglect.

2. a. FTT may be a result of organic causes, nonorganic causes, or both. Nonorganic causes predominate. Nonorganic FTT includes psychologic FTT
(maternal deprivation), child neglect, lack of education
regarding feeding, and errors in feeding. Nonorganic
FTT is most often attributable to maternal deprivation
(as in this case) or lack of a nurturing environment at
home. Organic FTT is caused most commonly by a
medical condition impairing the child's ability to take
in, absorb, or metabolize adequate calories.

3. e. The treatment of choice at this time is to
hospitalize the child and to give unlimited feedings
for a minimum period of 1 week. At the same time, a
careful physical examination and laboratory investigations including CBC, complete urinalysis, renal
function testing, and serum TSH level can be completed. If the child lives in an inner-city neighborhood
with older housing stock, a serum lead level test also
should be done. The family physician should involve
social services and also should initiate a detailed
assessment of the child's home environment. Before
the child is discharged home, the home environment
must be assessed and the parents of the child must be
given explicit instructions in feeding practices.

4. d. If the child begins to gain weight rapidly and
reestablish his health in the hospital (which is very
likely), reassessment ideally should be done in the
environment that allowed the development of the
problem in the first place (at least on some occasions).
This is obviously the home, and the health care professional in the best position to do this is probably the
public health nurse or the community health nurse.

5. c. The initial follow-up supervision should be
close and frequent—every week for the first 6 weeks
following discharge from the hospital is reasonable.

6. e. Maternal neglect resulting in nonorganic FTT
should not be just left at that; the reasons need to

be investigated. A mother who neglects her child (a
form of child abuse) is also at risk for committing
other forms of child abuse. In addition, she herself is
at greater-than-average risk of being abused by her
husband or partner. Remember that family violence
begets family violence, and in this case we already
have established that a form of family violence (child
abuse [neglect]) exists.

7. c. The most likely cause of this child's short
stature is Turner's syndrome. Noonan's syndrome
(an autosomal dominant trait with widely variable
expressivity) also has short stature and neck webbing
as its most common presentation. It can be distinguished from Turner's syndrome easily, however, by its
normal chromosome complement and characteristic
facies including hypertelorism and ptosis. Patients
with Turner's syndrome will have either a 45 XO
chromosome complement or a mosaic involving loss
of sex chromosomal material. Trisomy 21 usually will
be recognized long before the age of 13 years. The
fragile X syndrome is a syndrome associated with
mental retardation and macroorchidism in males.

8. a. The most common cause of short stature in
children is short parents. When a short child who is
growing at a normal rate and has a normal bone age
is found to have a strong family history of short
stature, familial short stature is the most likely cause.
Other causes of short stature include constitutional
delay of growth, chromosomal abnormalities, intrauterine growth restriction, chronic diseases such as
renal disease or inflammatory bowel disease, hypothyroidism, adrenal hyperplasia, growth hormone
deficiency or resistance, psychosocial dwarfism, and
idiopathic short stature.

9. b. Bone age determination can distinguish
between the two most common causes of short
stature: familial short stature and constitutional delay
of growth. Children with familial short stature have
normal bone ages. Constitutional delay of growth,
which is really a delay in reaching ultimate height and
sexual maturation, presents with delayed bone age
and delayed sexual maturation. Hypothyroidism and
growth hormone deficiency usually present with a
delayed bone age.

10. d. Inadequate growth in children may be associated with an unfavorable psychologic environment.
In this situation the child may show transiently low
human growth hormone levels during periods of
stress. He or she also may have behavioral, sleep, and
eating disturbances. Both growth and growth hormone
levels return to normal when the psychologic stressors
are removed.

11. **e.** Recommended investigations in a child with FTT or a child in which short stature is unlikely to be familial in nature should include CBC, complete urinalysis, serum BUN and creatinine, erythrocyte sedimentation rate (ESR), serum thyroxine, TSH, and bone age hand x-ray. Serum lead level, stool for ova and parasites, and liver enzymes (serum bilirubin, alanine aminotransferase, and aspartate aminotransferase) may be considered when the clinical history is suggestive.

SOLUTION TO THE CLINICAL CASE MANAGEMENT PROBLEM

Disorders that may manifest themselves as FTT in infants and children include the following: (1) emotional/psychologic factors; (2) ventral nervous system (central nervous system [CNS]) abnormality; (3) gastrointestinal (GI) malformation (pyloric stenosis, tracheoesophageal fistula, cleft palate) or disease (Hirschsprung's disease, gastroesophageal reflux, chronic diarrheal syndromes and malabsorption diseases, inflammatory bowel disease, liver disease, or parasites); (4) congenital or acquired heart disease (cardiac failure); (5) chronic renal disease (anomalies, renal failure); (6) chromosomal disorders (Down syndrome, Turner's syndrome); (7) chronic infection (GI system, kidney, pulmonary system, CNS, tuberculosis, human immunodeficiency virus, hepatitis); (8) inborn error of metabolism (hypothyroidism/hyperthyroidism/hyperaldosteronism); (9) malignancies (neuroblastoma, nephroblastoma, glioma); (10) anemias; (11) congenital low birthweight syndrome (fetal alcohol or drug exposure); (12) cystic fibrosis, (13) bronchopulmonary dysplasia; and (14) drug reactions.

SUMMARY OF FAILURE TO THRIVE AND SHORT STATURE

A. FTT:

1. Nonorganic: psychologic FTT; maternal deprivation; child neglect; lack of education regarding feeding; errors in feeding. Suspect family dysfunction and monitor carefully in these cases.
2. Organic FTT: See the Solution to the Clinical Case Management Problem.
3. Treatment:
   a. An initial period of hospitalization is indicated in most cases. Unlimited feedings (especially to any infant) should be given in these cases, and a complete investigation should be performed to attempt to elucidate the cause.
   b. When the child goes home, careful and frequent observation is indicated especially in the initial period. Some of these observations should take place in the environment (the home) in which the problems began (for nonorganic FTT). Weekly observation is indicated initially.

B. Short stature:

1. Familial short stature is the most common cause.
2. Familial short stature can be differentiated from constitutional delay of growth (the second most common cause) by bone age.
3. Other causes of short stature include chromosomal abnormalities, intrauterine growth restriction, hypothyroidism, psychosocial dwarfism, Turner's syndrome, and growth hormone deficiency.
4. Investigations of a child with short stature should include CBC, complete urinalysis, serum BUN/creatinine, liver enzymes and bilirubin, ESR, serum thyroxine, TSH, and x-ray of the hands and wrist for bone age.

SUGGESTED READING

Jolley CD: Failure to thrive. *Curr Prob Pediatr Adolesc Health Care* 33(6):183-206, 2003.
Shah MD: Failure to thrive in children. *J Clin Gastroenterol* 35(5):371-374, 2002.
Vance ML, Mauras N: Growth hormone therapy in adults and children. *N Engl J Med* 341(16):1206-1216, 1999.
Wright CM: Identification and management of failure to thrive: a community perspective. *Arch Dis Childhood* 82(1):5-9, 2000.

Chapter 99

Respiratory Syndromes

> "Do something!
> My baby can't breathe."

CLINICAL CASE PROBLEM 1:
AN 18-MONTH-OLD INFANT WITH AN UPPER-RESPIRATORY TRACT INFECTION

An 18-month-old is brought to the emergency department by his mother. He developed an upper-respiratory tract infection 2 days ago and suddenly this evening developed a harsh, barky cough and difficulty breathing.

On examination, the child is coughing and his temperature is 38.5° C. His respiratory rate is 40 per minute, and he is in some respiratory distress. The breath sounds that are heard appear to be transmitted from the upper airway. There are nasal flaring and suprasternal, infrasternal, and intercostal retractions.

■ **SELECT THE BEST ANSWER TO THE FOLLOWING QUESTIONS:**

1. What is the most likely diagnosis in this child?
   a. viral pneumonia
   b. acute epiglottis
   c. bronchiolitis
   d. croup
   e. bacterial pneumonia

2. The causative agent responsible for this child's condition is most likely which of the following?
   a. adenovirus
   b. *Pneumococcus*
   c. parainfluenza virus
   d. *Haemophilus influenzae*
   e. respiratory syncytial virus (RSV)

3. What is the treatment of choice for moderate cases of the disorder described?
   a. racemic epinephrine
   b. aerosolized budesonide
   c. humidification
   d. dexamethasone intravenously
   e. a, b, and c

CLINICAL CASE PROBLEM 2:
A 19-MONTH-OLD BOY WITH A COUGH, WHEEZING, DYSPNEA, AND IRRITABILITY

A 19-month-old boy with an acute onset of rhinorrhea and cough, which has progressed to wheezing, dyspnea, and irritability, is brought to the emergency department by his mother. On examination, the child's temperature is 38° C. His respiratory rate is 50 per minute, and he

exhibits flaring of the alae nasi and use of the accessory muscles of respiration resulting in intercostal and subcostal retractions. There are rhonchi heard in all lobes, and widespread fine rales are heard at the end of inspiration and in early expiration. The expiratory phase is prolonged, and wheezing is audible throughout the lung fields.

4. What is the most likely diagnosis in this patient?
   a. viral pneumonia
   b. acute epiglottis
   c. bronchiolitis
   d. croup
   e. bacterial pneumonia

5. What is the causative agent most likely responsible for this child's condition?
   a. adenovirus
   b. *Pneumococcus*
   c. rhinovirus
   d. *H. influenzae*
   e. RSV

6. The treatment of this child at this time may include which of the following?
   a. humidified oxygen
   b. nebulized bronchodilators
   c. ribavirin
   d. all of the above
   e. none of the above

CLINICAL CASE PROBLEM 3:
A 5-YEAR-OLD CHILD WHO HAS BEEN TALKING STRANGELY AND IS ANOREXIC

A 5-year-old child is brought to the emergency department by his mother. The mother tells you that for the past 24 hours the child has been "talking strangely" and drooling. He has had no appetite and has not been drinking.

7. Based on this history, what is the diagnosis of major concern?
   a. viral pneumonia
   b. acute epiglottitis
   c. bronchiolitis
   d. croup
   e. bacterial pneumonia

8. What is the diagnostic procedure that can substantiate the diagnosis you made in response to Question 7 for the patient described in Clinical Case Problem 3?
   a. a white blood cell count (WBC)
   b. an erythrocyte sedimentation rate
   c. a chest x-ray

d. a lateral x-ray of the neck

e. a computed tomography scan of the head and neck

9. What is the treatment of choice for the patient described in Clinical Case Problem 3?
   a. intubation and full respiratory support
   b. PO (oral) ampicillin and careful observation
   c. Intravenous (IV) ceftriaxone
   d. supplemental oxygen by mask
   e. a and c

CLINICAL CASE PROBLEM 4:
A 6-YEAR-OLD IN SEVERE RESPIRATORY DISTRESS

A 6-year-old male is brought to the emergency department with an acute asthmatic attack. His mom says he developed a respiratory tract infection 3 days ago and began wheezing 24 hours ago. He had his first asthma attack 2 years ago and usually has one attack per month. He is not taking medications. On examination, the child is in severe respiratory distress. His respiratory rate is 48 per minute. He has marked indrawing of the accessory muscles of respiration. Generalized wheezes are heard throughout the lung fields.

10. Which of the following statement(s) concerning wheezing in childhood is (are) true?
    a. most wheezing in childhood is related to asthma
    b. there appears to be a relationship between bronchiolitis and ongoing airway hyperreactivity
    c. many children with bronchiolitis go on to develop asthma
    d. none of the above statements are true
    e. all of the above statements are true

11. What is the treatment of choice in this patient at this time?
    a. IV sodium cromoglycate
    b. IV fluids and corticosteroids
    c. nebulized beta-agonist
    d. humidified oxygen
    e. b, c, and d

12. After stabilization and treatment, pulmonary function tests are performed on the patient described in Clinical Case Problem 4. Which of the following parameters of pulmonary function would be expected to increase after administration of a bronchodilator?
    a. forced vital capacity (FVC)
    b. forced expiratory volume in 1 second (FEV_1)
    c. maximum expiratory flow between 25% and 75% of the vital capacity (MEF 25-75)

d. total lung capacity (TLC)

e. b and c

13. The patient described in Clinical Case Problem 4 is treated and eventually discharged. You learn his attacks occur at least weekly and are interfering with normal daily activities such as play. Which of the following is the pharmacotherapeutic agent of choice?
    a. an inhaled beta-agonist
    b. PO theophylline
    c. an inhaled corticosteroid
    d. sodium cromoglycate
    e. a PO corticosteroid

CLINICAL CASE PROBLEM 5:
A 12-YEAR-OLD BOY WITH EXERCISE-INDUCED ASTHMA

A 12-year-old boy comes to your office for assessment of exercise-induced asthma. The child is fine when at rest but develops shortness of breath and wheezing at the end of or during a vigorous exercise session.

14. What is the treatment of first choice in this child?
    a. daily inhaled sodium cromoglycate
    b. an inhaled beta-agonist prior to exercise
    c. PO theophylline the day of exercise
    d. an inhaled corticosteroid prior to exercise
    e. a PO corticosteroid an hour before exercise

CLINICAL CASE MANAGEMENT PROBLEM

Defend the statement, "All that wheezes is not asthma."

ANSWERS:

1. **d.** This child has croup. A child with croup (the most common form being acute laryngotracheobronchitis) usually has a typical upper-respiratory tract infection for several days before the brassy, barking cough, inspiratory stridor, and respiratory distress become apparent. As the infection extends downward involving the bronchi and the bronchioles, respiratory difficulty increases and the expiratory phase of respiration becomes labored and prolonged.

The child often appears restless, agitated, and frightened. The child's temperature may be only slightly elevated, or it may be as high as 39° C to 40° C (102° F to 104° F).

Croup can be characterized based on the severity of symptoms. In mild croup, stridor is present with excitement only or is present at rest without signs of respiratory distress. In moderate croup, stridor occurs at rest and there is intercostal, suprasternal, or subcostal retractions. In severe croup, there is severe respiratory distress, decreased air entry, and an altered level of consciousness. Children with severe croup should be hospitalized and intubated under controlled conditions.

2. c. Most cases of croup (the most common form being acute laryngotracheobronchitis) are caused by the parainfluenza group of viruses. RSV, influenza, and adenoviruses may be implicated in some cases.

3. e. Until recently, the treatment of choice for mild to moderate cases of croup was simple humidification. However, it has been clearly established that nebulized budesonide (an inhaled glucosteroid) or PO (not IV) dexamethasone are of significant benefit in young children with mild to moderate croup. In moderate or severe cases, nebulized racemic epinephrine has been proven to be of value.

4. c. This child has bronchiolitis. The signs and symptoms of bronchiolitis have been well described in the clinical history just noted. Roentgenographic examination reveals hyperinflation of the lungs and an increased anteroposterior diameter of the chest on lateral view. Scattered areas of consolidation are found in about one-third of patients and are caused by either atelectasis secondary to obstruction or to inflammation of the alveoli. The WBC and the differential are usually within normal limits.

5. e. The agent responsible for most cases of bronchiolitis is RSV. Other causes include the parainfluenza 3 virus, mycoplasma, some adenoviruses, and occasionally other viruses. Adenovirus-caused bronchiolitis may be responsible for long-term complications including bronchiolitis obliterans and unilateral hyperlucent lung syndrome.

6. d. Humidified oxygen is of benefit in the treatment of infants and children with bronchiolitis. Ribavirin (Virazole), an antiviral agent, is effective in reducing the severity of bronchiolitis caused by RSV infection when administered early in the course of the illness. Its use is indicated in children younger than 2 years of age who have severe infection documented by fluorescent antibodies or culture or strongly suspected on epidemiologic grounds and whose hospitalization is likely to exceed 3 days. It also should be administered to patients with milder bronchiolitis caused by RSV infection who have underlying severe chronic illness as a result of cardiac disease.

Bronchodilating aerosolized drugs frequently are used empirically, and a subset of infants demonstrate response to bronchodilator therapy. However, corticosteroids, epinephrine, or alpha-adrenergic agents have not been shown to improve outcomes in recent randomized controlled trials. Antibiotics have no therapeutic value unless there is a secondary bacterial infection.

7. b. This child must be suspected of having acute epiglottitis until proved otherwise. Acute epiglottitis, a potentially lethal condition, occurs in children ages 2-7 years old and peaks at the age of 3.5 years. The incidence of this disease has dropped 10-fold thanks to routine immunization against *H. influenzae*. Acute epiglottitis is characterized by a fulminating course of fever, sore throat, dyspnea, rapidly progressive respiratory obstruction, and prostration. In minutes or hours, epiglottitis can lead to complete obstruction of the airway and death unless adequate treatment is administered.

Respiratory distress is the first symptom. The child may be well at bedtime but awakens later in the evening with a high fever, aphonia, drooling, and moderate to severe respiratory distress with stridor. An older child or adult often will complain of a "sore throat". Severe respiratory distress may ensue within minutes or hours of the onset.

8. d. On physical examination, the child is noted as having moderate to severe respiratory distress with inspiratory and, at times, expiratory stridor. There is drooling and an abundance of mucus and saliva, which also may result in rhonchi. With progression, stridor and breath sounds may become diminished as the patient tires. If this diagnosis is suspected, necessary equipment should be obtained and someone qualified to intubate the child should be summoned immediately; both the equipment and person should accompany the patient for any diagnostic studies. The diagnosis can be made by a lateral x-ray of the neck, which will clearly show the swollen epiglottis (thumb sign).

9. e. The child's pharynx should not be examined with a tongue depressor. The diagnosis requires direct visualization by laryngoscopy with the ability to intubate immediately. The treatment of choice for a child with acute epiglottis is as follows:
1. An artificial airway must be established immediately. Untreated patients have a substantial mortality even when observed in the hospital with appropriate intubation equipment nearby. Oxygen is administered.
2. IV ceftriaxone or ampicillin and chloramphenicol should be given pending culture and susceptibility reports because of the multiple possible agents being the cause of the condition.

10. e. All of the statements are true. Most wheezing in childhood is related to asthma. There is a fear among many physicians in labeling a child as having asthma. Much of this has to do with fear of the consequences of having to explain to the parent what this means or mislabeling a child with a chronic illness when one does not exist. The reality is that asthma is a protean disease having many degrees of severity from mild to severe. There appears to be a relationship between bronchiolitis and ongoing airway hyper-reactivity. There also appears to be a relationship between bronchiolitis and asthma, with many young infants with bronchiolitis at an increased risk of developing asthma later in childhood. By taking the time to talk with parents, much of the fear and misunderstanding about asthma can be allayed.

11. e. This child is in severe respiratory distress from the current asthmatic attack and should be treated with a combination of an IV corticosteroid (determined on a milligram-per-kilogram basis) and a nebulized beta-agonist. Oxygen and fluids also should be administered. Early and aggressive treatment will prevent deterioration and possibly even death.

12. e. Pulmonary function testing before and after administration of an aerosol bronchodilator will assess the degree of reversibility of airway obstruction. Normally the administration of a bronchodilator will result in an increase in FEV_1 and MEF 25-75. FVC and TLC, which already may be increased in patients with bronchial asthma, will not increase further after administration of a bronchodilator.

13. c. Asthma is classified into four categories: (1) intermittent, (2) mild, (3) moderate, or (4) severe persistent. Asthma is the most common chronic illness in children. It is a chronic inflammatory condition. Therefore, in persistent asthma, inhaled steroids are the drugs of choice. Sodium cromolyn is an effective prophylaxis agent but is not a primary agent in treatment of persistent asthma. In addition to inhaled steroids, leukotriene modifiers, long-acting beta-2 agonists, and theophylline can be used in chronic asthma. However, an inhaled beta-agonist remains the drug of choice in acute exacerbation.

14. b. Exercise-induced asthma may be manifested by both an early (in terms of time following exercise) and late bronchoconstriction. Early bronchoconstriction begins 3-8 minutes following exercise, and late bronchoconstriction occurs 4-6 hours after exercise. This boy has early bronchoconstriction. Inhaled sodium cromoglycate will block both early and late bronchoconstriction but is less effective than inhaled beta-agonists. Inhaled beta-agonists only will block early bronchoconstriction but are extremely effective. Corticosteroids will block only late bronchoconstriction. Prophylactic daily leukotriene modifiers and long-acting beta-agonists also have been found to be effective in athletes with exercise-induced asthma.

SOLUTION TO THE CLINICAL CASE MANAGEMENT PROBLEM

It is important to realize that there are causes for wheezing in infancy and childhood other than asthma. Although asthma remains the most common cause of wheezing, it is by no means the only cause. The second most common cause is bronchiolitis. As described earlier, there is an association between bronchiolitis and the subsequent development of asthma. It may very well be that RSV alters lung structural elements in ways that predisposes a child to develop asthma at a later date.

In addition to asthma and bronchiolitis as causes of wheezing, remember airway obstruction. This most commonly would be caused by the lodging of a foreign body in the trachea or in one of its branches.

As a corollary to "all that wheezes is not asthma" we can add "all asthma does not wheeze." This is particularly true in children in which the principal manifestation at onset is often nighttime cough.

SUMMARY OF RESPIRATORY SYNDROMES

1. Major worrisome symptoms:
   a. Harsh, barky cough
   b. Stridor and respiratory distress

   c. Drooling
   d. Wheezing
2. Croup: Most common form is acute laryngotracheobronchitis. A harsh, barky cough in a young infant is almost pathognomonic of croup. Respiratory distress can be pronounced.

Continued

SUMMARY OF RESPIRATORY SYNDROMES—cont'd

   a. Causative agent: parainfluenza virus
   b. Treatment: humidified oxygen; plus PO or nebulized corticosteroids; racemic epinephrine in moderate to severe cases
3. Bronchiolitis: may produce very significant respiratory distress and stridor, rales, and wheezing—expiratory phase prolonged
   a. Causative agent: multiple viruses, RSV most common
   b. Treatment: humidified oxygen and ribavirin; corticosteroids and racemic epinephrine not effective; antibiotics for secondary infections only
4. Acute epiglottitis: drooling, very sore throat, and difficulty swallowing liquids (this can be used as a diagnostic test)
   a. Do not attempt visualization of the epiglottis unless prepared to intubate
   b. Lateral x-ray of the neck for diagnosis (thumb sign swollen epiglottis)
   c. Causative agent was *H. influenzae* (before immunization), now strep and others
   d. Treatment: intubation, respiratory support, and IV ceftriaxone
5. Asthma: most common chronic illness in children; nighttime cough, wheezing, dyspnea; chronic inflammatory condition of lower airways with episodic, reversible airway obstruction via bronchoconstriction, mucous plug formation, and edema.
   a. Causative agent: hyperresponsiveness to allergens; outdoor and indoor air pollution (including ozone and cigarette smoke); atopic history, often familial

   b. Classification: four levels (intermittent and mild, moderate, and severe persistent)
   c. Treatment: based on classification level; environmental control in all cases
      i. For acute attack rescue, beta-2 agonist via metered-dose inhaler or nebulizer; in severe cases, use IV fluids, steroids, nebulized beta-agonists, and oxygen
      ii. For all forms of persistent: inhaled corticosteroids are drugs of first choice; add leukotriene modifier, consider cromolyns, long-acting beta-2 agonists, oral theophyllines; steroid effect on growth (minimal, <1 cm/year) must be balanced against prospect of achieving normal daily functioning
      iii. Exercise-induced: Beta-agonists prior; consider prophylactic daily leukotriene modifiers or long acting β-2 agonists in athletes
   d. Other information:
      i. Asthma kills; treat aggressively
      ii. Not all that wheezes is asthma; think airway foreign body
      iii. Not all asthma wheezes

SUGGESTED READING

Ewig JM: Croup. *Pediatr Ann* 31(2):125-130, 2002.
Malhotra A, Krilov LR: Viral croup. *Pediatr Rev* 22(1):5-12, 2001.
Panitch HB: Bronchiolitis in infants. *Curr Opin Pediatr* 13(3):256-260, 2001.
Stroud RH, Friedman NR: An update on inflammatory disorders of the pediatric airway: epiglottitis, croup, and tracheitis. *Am J Otolaryngol* 22(4):268-275, 2001.
Wainwright C, et al: A multicenter, randomized, double-blind, controlled trial of nebulized epinephrine in infants with acute bronchiolitis. *N Engl J Med* 349(1):27-35, 2003.
Wright RB, et al: New approaches to respiratory infections in children. Bronchiolitis and croup. *Emerg Med Clin N Am* 20(1):93-114, 2002.

Chapter **100**

Otitis Media

"My child won't become deaf, will he?"

CLINICAL CASE PROBLEM 1:

A 24-Month-Old Child Who Is Constantly Crying and Who Complains of a Right-Sided Earache

A mother comes to your office with her 24-month-old daughter. The child developed an upper-respiratory tract infection approximately 1 week ago. The infection started with cough, congestion, and rhinorrhea. Two days ago the child began complaining of pain in the right ear.

On examination, the child has nasal congestion and a hyperemic throat. The left tympanic membrane is normal, and the right tympanic membrane is bulging and red. There appears to be fluid behind it. The lungs are clear. The child's temperature is 39.5° C.

SELECT THE BEST ANSWER TO THE FOLLOWING QUESTIONS:

1. What is the most likely diagnosis in this child?
   a. acute otitis media (AOM)
   b. otitis media without effusion

c. chronic otitis media (COM)
d. otitis media with effusion (OME)
e. none of the above

CLINICAL CASE PROBLEM 2:
An 8-Month-Old Male with an Upper-Respiratory Tract Infection but No External Signs of Acute Ear Infection

An 8-month-old male is brought to your office the same day as the child in Clinical Case Problem 1. He, too, has had an upper-respiratory tract infection but has no signs of acute ear infection such as irritability, poor sleeping, pulling at his ears, or fever.

On examination, there is a middle-ear effusion, confirmed by pneumatic otoscopy, and the tympanic membrane is dull but not red. The rest of the examination is benign besides a mild clear rhinorrhea.

2. What is the most likely diagnosis in this child?
   a. AOM
   b. otitis media without effusion
   c. COM
   d. OME
   e. none of the above

CLINICAL CASE PROBLEM 3:
A 7-Month-Old Child with an Upper-Respiratory Infection and Erythema of the Tympanic Membrane

A 7-month-old child is brought to your office by his mother the same day as you saw the children in Clinical Case Problems 1 and 2. He has had an upper-respiratory tract infection for the past 3 days.

On examination, there is erythema of the left tympanic membrane with opacification. There are no other signs or symptoms.

3. What is the most likely diagnosis in this patient?
   a. AOM
   b. otitis media without effusion
   c. COM
   d. OME
   e. none of the above

CLINICAL CASE PROBLEM 4:
A 9-Month-Old Child with a Discharge from His Ear

This is obviously "ear day" in your practice. A fourth child, 9 months of age, is brought to your office with a discharge from the left ear that has been present for the last 6 weeks. The child has a history of frequent ear infections, all of which have been treated with antibiotics.

4. What is the most likely diagnosis in this patient?
   a. AOM
   b. otitis media without effusion
   c. COM with perforation
   d. OME
   e. none of the above

5. Referring again to the patient you saw in Clinical Case Problem 1, which of the following statements regarding her condition described is false?
   a. this condition usually begins a few days after the onset of an upper-respiratory tract infection
   b. this condition usually is associated with eustachian tube dysfunction
   c. environmental factors such as pollen, dusts, molds, and cigarette smoke are unlikely to be associated with an increase in the incidence of this condition
   d. many cases of this condition are considered to be bacterial in origin
   e. none of the above statements are false

6. What are the three most common bacterial organisms in order of frequency that are responsible for the condition described in Clinical Case Problem 1?
   a. *Streptococcus pneumoniae*, group A streptococci, *Haemophilus influenzae*
   b. *S. pneumoniae, H. influenzae, Staphylococcus aureus*
   c. *S. pneumoniae, H. influenzae, Moraxella catarrhalis*
   d. *H. influenzae, S. pneumoniae*, group A streptococci
   e. *H. influenzae, S. pneumoniae, M. catarrhalis*

7. What is the drug of choice for the condition described in Clinical Case Problem 1?
   a. penicillin
   b. amoxicillin
   c. erythromycin–sulfamethoxazole
   d. cefaclor
   e. amoxicillin–clavulanic acid

8. A family practice resident who is working with you describes the condition of a child he has just seen. He describes a normal tympanic membrane behind which is significant fluid. He tells you, however, that there are no other symptoms associated with this effusion. He asks you what he should do. You should tell him to do which of the following:
   a. forget about it; it is not bothering him
   b. perform a myringotomy and suck out all the fluid that is present
   c. perform a pneumatic otoscopy to assess the movement of the tympanic membrane
   d. refer the child to an ear, nose, and throat (ENT) surgeon for myringotomy, tubes, and an adenoidectomy (you might as well suggest a

tonsillectomy at the same time and get everything over at once)

e. none of the above

9. Which of the following statements regarding treatment of the condition described in Clinical Case Problem 1 is (are) true?

a. earache and fever should be treated with aspirin

b. topical decongestants are useful in improving eustachian tube dysfunction

c. eardrops do not provide significant relief in children with the condition described in Clinical Case Problem 1

d. systemic antihistamine–decongestants have been shown to improve the symptoms and shorten the course of the condition described in Clinical Case Problem 1

e. all of the above statements are true

10. How is *recurrent otitis media* defined?

a. three or more episodes of AOM that occur within 6 months, or four episodes that occur within a year

b. four or more episodes of AOM that occur within 6 months, or five episodes that occur within a year

c. five or more episodes of AOM that occur within 6 months, or six episodes that occur within a year

d. six or more episodes of AOM that occur within 6 months, or eight episodes within a year

e. two or more episodes of AOM that occur within 6 months, or three or more episodes that occur within a year

11. Which of the following statements regarding recurrent otitis media is true?

a. recurrent bouts of AOM usually occur in the winter or early spring

b. recurrent bouts of AOM should be managed by myringotomy and the insertion of ventilation tubes

c. medical management appears to be less effective and is not as safe as myringotomy and tubes in children with recurrent AOM

d. amoxicillin does not have a major role to play in the management of recurrent AOM

e. antibiotic prophylaxis should be given for at least 6 months to a year

12. Which of the following intracranial complications may occur with otitis media?

a. meningitis

b. subdural empyema

c. brain abscess

d. all of the above

e. a and c only

13. Which of the following is not a possible extra-cranial complication of otitis media?

a. mastoiditis

b. cholesteatoma

c. labyrinthitis

d. facial paralysis

e. otic hydrocephalus

14. Which of the following is true in regards to the patient in Clinical Case Problem 2?

a. steroids should be prescribed because they have been shown to decrease the duration of this condition

b. in most cases this condition resolves spontaneously within 3 months

c. topical or systemic decongestants should be prescribed to improve eustachian tube function

d. eustachian tube–middle ear inflation should be performed as soon as possible to decrease the likelihood of developing hearing loss and language delay

e. if present for more than 3 months, bilateral myringotomy with ventilation tube placement is necessary

15. All of the following about the management of OME is true except:

a. environmental risk factor control should be part of parent counseling

b. a course of antibiotics is an acceptable treatment

c. a hearing evaluation should be done if the effusion persists for more than 3 months

d. myringotomy and ventilation tube placement along with tonsillectomy and adenoidectomy are indicated in those with chronic effusion and hearing loss

e. for children with chronic effusions, evaluation for anatomic abnormalities such as nasopharyngeal tumors or submucous cleft palate should be considered

16. All of the following are true about AOM except:

a. infants and young children are at highest risk

b. 40% of children will have an effusion that persists for 4 weeks

c. boys tend to have a higher incidence of AOM than girls do

d. nearly 90% of children will have an episode of AOM by age 3 years

e. incidence of AOM peaks between 6 to 13 months of age

17. Tympanocentesis with aspiration of middle ear fluid should be considered in all of the following patients except:

a. a child who presents with AOM and complains of tinnitus, vertigo, and hearing loss

b. a child who develops a suppurative intra-cranial complication of OM

c. an patient who is immunologically impaired and has AOM who does not improve with antibiotic treatment

d. a child who has extreme ear pain and appears toxic

e. a child who is already taking antibiotics who develops an AOM

CLINICAL CASE MANAGEMENT PROBLEM

A mother comes to your office with her 18-month-old child following the treatment of an episode of AOM. She states that the child was in considerable pain despite analgesics and antibiotics and asks you to refer her child to an ENT surgeon. She wishes to have "tubes" inserted in her child's ears. She has a number of friends who have had this done to their children following the first episode of AOM and it has been extremely successful. Discuss how you would approach this problem.

ANSWERS:

1. a. AOM also is known as acute suppurative, acute purulent, or acute bacterial otitis media. The pathophysiology is basically an effusion of the middle ear that becomes infected with viruses and/or bacteria. There is often a rapid onset of signs and symptoms such as fever; ear pain; a red, bulging, tympanic membrane; and fluid behind the middle ear.

2. d. OME also is known as nonsuppurative, serous, or mucoid otitis media. This is manifested as otitis media without signs or symptoms of acute disease but with a middle-ear effusion. OME may be subdivided into acute, subacute, and chronic based on the duration of the effusion. OME with effusions present for less than 3 weeks are acute; subacute effusions are present 3 weeks to 3 months; lastly, chronic effusions are those present for longer than 3 months.

3. b. Otitis media without effusion also is known as myringitis. It indicates the presence of erythema (redness) and opacification of the tympanic membranes without the presence of an effusion. This may be seen in the early stages of AOM or as otitis media resolves.

4. c. COM is synonymous with chronic suppurative, purulent, or intractable otitis media. There is a pronounced, intractable middle-ear pathologic condition with or without suppurative otorrhea.

Suppurative refers to an active infection, and *otorrhea* refers to a discharge through a perforated tympanic membrane.

5. c. AOM usually begins a few days after the onset of an upper-respiratory tract infection. The upper-respiratory tract infection usually produces eustachian tube dysfunction and obstruction. This subsequently leads to the accumulation of fluid in the middle ear. This fluid then becomes infected with a virus, a bacteria, or a virus followed by bacteria.

Environmental factors such as exposure to respiratory tract irritants (cigarette smoke, pollen, dust, molds) may increase the incidence of upper-respiratory tract infection and AOM. Supine nursing (habitually putting the infant to bed with a bottle) also may contribute to the incidence of otitis media.

6. c. The bacteriology of AOM suggests that the following bacterial organisms (in this order of incidence) are responsible for most cases of AOM: (1) *S. pneumoniae* (30% to 50%); (2) *H. influenzae* (20% to 30%); (3) *M. catarrhalis* (1% to 5%); (4) group A streptococci; and (5) *Staphylococcus aureus*.

As mentioned previously, viruses also have been implicated as primary causative agents. Also, if a virus produces the primary infection, many of these cases will become secondarily infected with a bacterium.

7. b. The drug of choice for AOM in primary care practice is still amoxicillin. The duration of treatment depends on the patient's age and other patient factors. In children older than 2 years of age without underlying medical conditions, 5-7 days of antibiotics is usually sufficient treatment. Younger children and those with craniofacial abnormalities, chronic or recurrent otitis media, or perforation of the tympanic membrane should be treated for 10 days.

A patient who does not improve while taking amoxicillin most likely has an infection with a beta-lactamase–producing organism. In this case, second-line agents including cefuroxime axetil, amoxicillin–clavulanate, and intramuscular ceftriaxone would be appropriate choices.

8. c. The most reasonable maneuver to perform at this time is pneumatic otoscopy to assess the movement of the tympanic membrane. This will provide an accurate indication of whether there is fluid present in the middle-ear cavity. This easily performed maneuver often is omitted in primary care. Tympanometry is an acceptable alternative.

Referral to an ENT surgeon for myringotomy, tubes, adenoidectomy, and tonsillectomy is not indicated at this time. Similarly, the performance of a myringotomy in the office is an invasive and painful procedure. Observation or antibiotic treatments are options for therapy. See the Agency for Healthcare Research and Quality (see Answer 15).

9. c. Ear drops do not provide any symptomatic relief in otitis media and interfere with otoscopic examination and follow-up. Symptoms of earache or fever should be treated with acetaminophen. Aspirin should be avoided because of the possible link to Reye's syndrome.

Topical decongestants (sympathomimetic nose drops and sprays), used to relieve obstruction in the eustachian tube, and systemic antihistamine–decongestant combinations have not been shown to be effective in the treatment of otitis media. They affect neither the duration nor the severity of symptoms.

10. a. Recurrent otitis media is defined as three or more episodes of AOM that occur within 6 months or four episodes within a year.

11. a. Recurrent bouts of acute otitis usually occur in the winter or early spring. Such recurrent episodes can be managed to some extent with prophylactic antibiotics. Prophylaxis should not be given for more than 6 months to decrease the likelihood of colonization by resistant bacteria. Although a myringotomy and the insertion of ventilation tubes ultimately may have to be performed, it is not the first-line option. Medical management with antibiotics has been shown, in most studies, to be just as effective. Half-strength amoxicillin or sulfisoxazole is reasonable prophylactic therapy.

12. d. Otitis media is not always an innocuous diagnosis. Intracranial complications associated with otitis media include meningitis, subdural empyema, brain abscess, lateral sinus thrombosis, and focal otitis encephalitis.

13. e. Extracranial complications and sequelae associated with otitis media include hearing loss, tympanic membrane perforation, chronic suppurative otitis media, mastoiditis, cholesteatoma, facial paralysis, tympanosclerosis, and labyrinthitis. Otic hydrocephalus is an intracranial complication consisting of increased intracranial pressure without other abnormalities of the cerebral spinal fluid that occurs with either AOM or chronic otitis media.

14. b. OME is a middle ear effusion without signs or symptoms of acute infection. Most often the effusion clears spontaneously by 3 months in 90% of children. Neither oral or nasal steroids nor decongestants have proved to be effective for this condition. Using the method of Politzer or the Valsalva maneuver to open the eustachian tubes has not been shown to be effective in the treatment of OME. Even if the effusion is present for more than 3 months, myringotomy and ventilation tubes are not indicated unless there is a 20-decibel or worse bilateral hearing level.

15. d. According to the U.S. Agency for Healthcare Research and Quality, tonsillectomy alone or with adenoidectomy has not been proven to be effective in the treatment of OME. Adenoidectomy is indicated only if there is adenoid pathology or obstruction. Environmental risk factor control counseling should be done. Parents should be advised of the increased incidence of OME in children attending group day-care facilities, those exposed to passive tobacco smoking, and children who are bottle-fed rather than breastfed. A 10-day course of antibiotics is an acceptable treatment option that has shown a 14% increase in the resolution rate of effusions. Hearing evaluations are warranted in children with effusions persisting more than 3 months and may be considered in those with effusions more than 6 weeks. Evaluation for anatomic abnormalities causing OME should be considered in patients with chronic effusions.

16. d. By age 3 years, nearly 70% (not 90%) of children have at least one case of AOM. Half of children actually will have two or more episodes by age 3. Incidence does peak at 6-13 months, and risk decreases with age, with a sharp decline of AOM after age 6 years. Boys do have a higher incidence. After AOM about 40% of children will have an effusion present for 4 weeks and 10% will have an effusion that persists at 3 months.

17. a. The diagnosis of AOM is made clinically based on symptoms and appearance of the tympanic membrane; however, in certain circumstances, tympanocentesis with aspiration of the middle ear fluid may be considered to aid in diagnosis (by culture) but also in alleviating severe pain. Patients who appear toxic or who develop either suppurative intratemporal or intracranial complications should have tympanocentesis. A newborn or otherwise immunologically deficient patient who does not improve with empiric therapy may warrant tympanocentesis because unusual organisms may be involved. Similarly, a child who is taking antibiotics already who develops a new AOM also may be considered for tympanocentesis to culture for resistant organisms.

Complaints of tinnitus, hearing loss, and vertigo are not that uncommon, especially in older children, and do not implicate a need for tympanocentesis.

SOLUTION TO THE CLINICAL CASE MANAGEMENT PROBLEM

This is a difficult issue because the mother has come to your office expecting and wanting a referral to an ENT surgeon. You should do the following:

1. Discuss the incidence of AOM and point out to the mother that more children have had it than have not had it.
2. Emphasize that in most cases the symptoms resolve with simple antibiotic therapy.
3. Describe briefly the anatomy of the eustachian tube and point out that as her child grows, the probability of infections will continue to decrease.
4. Try to establish why she is so concerned and wants a

referral at this time. Often (referring back to the biopsychosocial model) there are other issues that need to be addressed with the mother.
5. If the mother, despite all of your reassurance, insists on a referral, give her one. However, point out to the mother that the ENT surgeon is unlikely to want to put in tubes at this time.
6. Offer to discuss the issue of her child's otitis media or any other issues at any time. Provide for the mother a framework in which she can begin to view you, the family physician, as her advocate in health care. She probably needs this more than anything else.

SUMMARY OF OTITIS MEDIA

1. AOM is common in childhood. By 12 months of age, 62% of children have had at least one infection.
2. When discussing otitis media, use the correct terminology:
   a. Acute otitis media: middle-ear effusion with acute signs of infection such as otalgia, fever, and irritability
   b. Otitis media with effusion: middle-ear effusion with no signs of acute infection
   c. Chronic otitis media: middle-ear effusion present for more than 3 months
   d. Chronic suppurative otitis media: nonintact tympanic membrane with 6 weeks or more of drainage
3. Most common bacterial causative agents in order of frequency are *Pneumococci, H. influenzae, M. catarrhalis*, and group A streptococci.
4. Treatment of choice for AOM in the primary care setting is still amoxicillin.
5. The definition of acute otitis is otalgia, fever, and irritability associated with a full or bulging tympanic membrane with effusion.

6. Decongestants–antihistamines and ear drops have not been shown to influence either the severity or duration of the symptoms.
7. Consider prophylactic antibiotics before considering myringotomy and tubes for the treatment of recurrent otitis media.
8. Remember that otitis media can produce complications. Treat otitis media with an antibiotic. Treatment duration depends on the patient characteristic. See Answer 7.

SUGGESTED READING

Glaszious PP, et al: Antibiotics for acute otitis media in children. Cochrane database of systematic reviews. Hamilton, Canada: 2002, BC Decker.

Hendley JO: Otitis media. *N Engl J Med* 347:1169-1174, 2002.

Jacobs MR: Prevention of acute otitis media: Role of pneumococcal conjugate vaccines in reducing incidence and antibiotic resistance, *Journal of Pediatrics* 141:287-293, 2002.

Pensak M: Otitis Media. In: Rakel RE, Bope ET, eds: *Conn's current therapy 2003.* Elsevier 2002, Philadelphia.

Pichichero ME: Acute otitis media (pt I). Improving diagnostic accuracy. *Am Fam Physician* 61:2051-2056, 2000.

Pichichero ME: Acute otitis media (pt II). Treatment in an era of increasing antibiotic resistance. *Am Fam Physician* 61:2410-2416, 2000.

Rothman R, et al: Does this child have acute otitis media? *JAMA* 290(12):1633-1640, 2003 Sep 24.

Semchenko A, et al: Management of acute sinusitis and otitis media. *Am Fam Physician Monograph No.1,* 4, 2001.

Chapter 101

The Common Cold

"Since my youngest started nursery school, all I do is wipe his runny nose."

CLINICAL CASE PROBLEM 1:
A 4-Year-Old Child with a Runny Nose, a Sore Throat, and a Nonproductive Cough

A 4-year-old child with a runny nose, a sore throat, a feeling of "fullness" in his ears, and a nonproductive cough comes to your office with his mother. He has had these symptoms for the last 4 days and is not improving. He has had no fever, no chills, or any other symptoms.

On examination, the child's temperature is 37.6° C. His ears are clear, his throat is slightly hyperemic, and both sides of his nose look congested and red. His lung fields are clear, there is no significant cervical lymphadenopathy, and no other localizing signs are present.

The child's history is unremarkable, and he has had no significant medical illnesses.

■ SELECT THE BEST ANSWER TO THE FOLLOWING QUESTIONS:

1. What is the most likely diagnosis in this child?
   a. early streptococcal pharyngitis
   b. early mycoplasma pneumonia
   c. early acute otitis media
   d. early viral pneumonia
   e. viral upper-respiratory infection (URI)

2. What is the most likely pathogen responsible for this condition?
   a. *Streptococcus pneumoniae*
   b. rhinovirus
   c. parainfluenza A
   d. adenovirus
   e. respiratory syncytial virus (RSV)

3. Investigations at this time should include which of the following?
   a. complete blood count (CBC)
   b. throat swab
   c. rapid strep test
   d. chest radiograph
   e. nothing at this time

4. Which of the following statements regarding the common cold is true?
   a. adults are affected less than children
   b. the highest incidence of the common cold is among children of kindergarten age
   c. adults with young children at home have an increased number of colds
   d. infants with older siblings in school or daycare have an increased incidence of colds
   e. all of the above are true

5. Which of the following statements regarding treatment of the condition described is true?
   a. the use of antibiotics in the condition described in Clinical Case Problem 1 has shown to decrease the probability of complications; their routine use is reasonable
   b. vitamin C has definitely shown to decrease the frequency of occurrences of the condition described in Clinical Case Problem 1
   c. zinc lozenges have been shown to be ineffective therapy in children
   d. rhinoviruses associated with the condition described in Clinical Case Problem 1 have not been shown to be temperature sensitive
   e. antihistamines have not been shown to be effective in reducing symptoms in the condition described in Clinical Case Problem 1

6. Children of kindergarten age are subject to how many colds on an average yearly basis?
   a. 12
   b. 7
   c. 3
   d. 6
   e. 5

7. What is the most effective preventive measure against the common cold?
   a. megadoses of vitamin C
   b. meticulous hand washing
   c. extra sleep
   d. avoiding all contact with children and adults who have a cold
   e. pleconaril

CLINICAL CASE PROBLEM 2:
A 6-Month-Old with Nasal Congestion and Difficulty Feeding

A 6-month-old infant is brought to your office by her mother who states the child has been having nasal congestion for 5 days. The mother states the child's had a clear runny nose at first but now the drainage is thick and yellow and she seems to be having difficulty with taking the bottle because, "she just starts to snort and then spits it out." She also reports the baby has had only low-grade temperatures of less than 100.4° F. The mother tells you the baby seems cranky but is consolable and has had difficulty sleeping because of the breathing. She is concerned because her 5-year-old child's birthday party is in 2 days and she does not want to get everyone infected. She asks you for an antibiotic.

On examination, the infant is afebrile. There is no tachypnea. The conjunctivae are slightly hyperemic but without purulent exudates. The nose is congested with erythematous mucosa and thick yellow drainage bilaterally. The ears are clear. The throat is pink, but postnasal drip is noted. The chest is without retractions and is clear to auscultation.

8. What is the diagnosis?
   a. bronchiolitis
   b. bacterial rhinosinusitis
   c. viral rhinosinusitis
   d. bacterial conjunctivitis
   e. allergic rhinitis

9. Which of the following agents is the least likely cause of the condition described in Clinical Case Problem 2?
   a. RSV
   b. rhinovirus
   c. parainfluenza virus
   d. adenovirus
   e. *Chlamydia psittaci*

10. Which of the following questions about the treatment of this condition in infants is false?
    a. aspirin should be avoided
    b. medications other than acetaminophen and ibuprofen should be avoided
    c. nasal saline drops are helpful
    d. decongestants and antihistamines are helpful
    e. expectorants have not been proven to be effective

11. Which of the following is the most common bacterial complication of this condition?
    a. sinusitis
    b. pneumonia
    c. meningitis
    d. otitis media
    e. pharyngitis

12. Which of the statements below is true and is the best answer to the mother's concern in Clinical Case Problem 2?
    a. the infant is no longer infectious so there is no need to worry about spread of infection
    b. evidence does not support the use of antibiotics in URIs, and in fact there is an increased risk of adverse effect with their use
    c. viral shedding lasts up to 14 days so the infant most likely will spread the infection to all those that come to her sibling's party
    d. the color of the baby's nasal discharge suggests a bacterial infection and antibiotics will be prescribed, so there should be no concern for transmission to others
    e. none of the above is true

13. Which of the following statements about echinacea is false?
    a. prophylactic use has a significant impact on the frequency, severity, or duration of URIs
    b. when used as a treatment of URI, it shows a modest positive effect
    c. use for more than 8 weeks can cause hepatotoxicity
    d. use for more than 8 weeks potentially can cause immunosuppression
    e. it is one of the top 3 selling herbs in the United States

---

CLINICAL CASE MANAGEMENT PROBLEM

An 8-year-old male is brought to your office with "a cold." He has had the cold for approximately 10 days, and his rhinorrhea, cough, and congestion continue. His mother tells you that she has just seen her family doctor for the same symptoms and an antibiotic was prescribed. She asks you to prescribe the same for her son. On examination, the boy has nasal congestion and a hyperemic throat. No other abnormalities are found. Discuss your approach to this patient's request.

■ **ANSWERS:**

1. **e.** This child most likely has the common cold or URI. Although the fullness in his ears may be associated with fluid in the middle-ear cavity, the absence of fever, pain, and hyperemia on the tympanic membranes makes acute otitis media unlikely. Movement of the tympanic membranes would further clarify the likelihood of fluid collection in the middle ear.

The presence of a runny nose and a cough significantly diminishes the probability of streptococcal pharyngitis.

Although viral pneumonia or mycoplasma pneumonia may develop, there is no evidence of either of these now.

2. b. The most common cause of the common cold is a rhinovirus. Rhinoviruses are responsible for approximately 30% to 40% of all cases of the common cold. Influenza virus; parainfluenzae types A, B, and C; RSV, and mumps and measles viruses are responsible for many others. Other viruses that cause coldlike symptoms include coronaviruses, adenoviruses, certain enteric cytopathic human orphan (echo) viruses, and coxsackievirus. More than 100 serospecific rhinovirus types have been established, and many viruses remain untyped.

The absence of significant fever, cervical lymphadenopathy, and exudates along with the presence of rhinorrhea and cough significantly decrease the probability of *S. pneumoniae* as a cause of this patient's symptoms.

3. e. No investigations should be initiated yet. Because the pretest probability of a streptococcal pharyngitis is very low, it is inappropriate to order a CBC, a throat swab, a rapid antigen test for streptococcus, or any other investigations at the present time.

4. e. In general, the common cold affects children significantly more frequently than adults. The highest incidence is among children of kindergarten age. Adults with young children in the home have an increased number of colds, as do infants with older siblings. At times parents often notice the latter (the "second sibling syndrome") and sometimes need reassurance that their children do not have some other constitutional weakness.

5. c. The use of zinc lozenges for treating the common cold in children has been demonstrated to be ineffective; however, evidence of the effects of zinc lozenges for the common cold in adults has been inconclusive.

Antibiotics have not been shown to reduce the incidence of complications and thus should not be used in a prophylactic fashion.

Vitamin C has not been shown to be effective in reducing the frequency or severity of symptoms. This is, however, a difficult area to study objectively because of problems associated with measuring improvement in symptoms.

Rhinoviruses are temperature sensitive. A controlled study testing warm (30° C) humidified air against hot (45° C) humidified air to provide nasal hyperthermia for 20-30 minutes has demonstrated a significant reduction in the severity and duration of common cold symptoms. Thus it may be that this "old-fashioned" remedy has some basis in fact.

Antihistamines have been found to be helpful in reducing symptoms of the common cold. Antihistamines act through nonspecific sedating or anticholinergic mechanisms rather than through any histamine-releasing action of the virus. Also, pseudoephedrine, alone or in combination with antihistamines, is also effective in reducing symptoms. Analgesics, such as acetylsalicylic acid (ASA) or acetaminophen, have not been shown to have any significant effect on the duration or the severity of the common cold; however, they are useful for symptomatic relief as antipyretics and analgesics. ASA should not be used because of the possibility of Reye's syndrome.

6. a. Children of kindergarten/nursery school age are subject to 8-12 colds annually, whereas school-aged children are subject to an average of 6-8 colds annually. Adolescents and adults are subject to an average of 2-4 colds annually.

7. b. The most effective preventive measure against the common cold is meticulous hand washing and avoidance of contact with the face or nose. There is increasing evidence that aerosol spread of the cold viruses is less important than indirect spread. Experiments suggest that cold-causing viruses can be spread by self-inoculation from deposits of virus on such surfaces as plastics to the surface of the finger and then transferred to mucous membranes of the nose and eye. This is particularly true if the inoculum is still moist.

Extra sleep and megadoses of vitamin C have not been shown to be at all effective.

It is unrealistic to suggest avoiding all contact with children and adults who have colds. Cold viruses are everywhere and will continue to be everywhere.

Placinoral is a rhinovirus capsid-function inhibitor that exhibits antiviral activity; however, the U.S. Food and Drug Administration did not approve use of the drug based on questions of its safety.

8. c. The infant has a common cold, in this case causing mostly a rhinosinusitis. In infants, bacterial and viral rhinosinusitis are difficult to distinguish from one another. Bacterial rhinosinusitis is a possible complication of viral rhinosinusitis and should be expected if the patient has symptoms over 14 days with purulent rhinorrhea and fever higher than 39° C.

The patient does not have bacterial conjunctivitis because there is no drainage from the eyes. Bronchiolitis most often is caused by RSV, which is the most common viral pathogen causing lower-respiratory tract illness in infants. Tachypnea and respiratory distress including wheezing are common presentations. Other manifestations of RSV in infants can be lethargy, irritability, apneic episodes, and poor feeding.

Allergic rhinitis does not present with fever and usually is associated with pale, edematous, or violaceous turbinates.

9. e. *Chlamydia psittaci, Coccidiodes immitis, Histoplasma capsulatum, Bordetella pertussis,* and *Coxiella brunetti* are all bacteria that are very rare causes of cold symptoms. All the other choices include the viruses that most frequently cause the common cold.

10. d. Decongestant and antihistamine use in infants has the potential for unusual central nervous system or cardiovascular side effects such as extreme lethargy or irritability that far outweigh the small potential benefits. For most URIs the best treatment is no pharmacologic treatment; however, in those with fever antipyretics should be used. Aspirin (ASA) should be avoided because of the risk of Reye's syndrome. Expectorants have not been proven to be effective for cough. Cough suppressants also are contraindicated for infants and, in fact can cause paradoxical bronchoconstriction in some. Nasal saline drops followed by gentle bulb syringe suction can help to loosen secretions and relieve obstruction temporarily and can be particularly helpful just prior to feeding.

11. d. Otitis media is the most common bacterial complication of the common cold, occurring in approximately 2% of patients with colds. Sinusitis, pneumonia, and pharyngitis are less common complications. Meningitis is not a typical complication of viral URIs but rarely can be caused by adenovirus in infants or patients who are immunocompromised.

12. b. There is not enough evidence of important benefits of antibiotics for the treatment of URIs. Indeed, studies have shown significant increases of adverse effects with their use.

The infant is likely still infectious. Viral shedding during a URI usually lasts 7-14 days and occasionally longer. Even so, most transmission is thought to be by self-inoculation by contaminated hands and somewhat by droplet spread through sneezing; it is unlikely that the infant will spread the infection to all the guests unless parents and sibling neglect to wash their hands and inoculate most household surfaces just before the guests arrive (because viruses can live up to a few hours on plastic surfaces).

The color and thickness of nasal secretions do not help to differentiate between bacterial, viral, or allergic cause.

13. a. Echinacea for prophylaxis of URIs does not significantly decrease the frequency, severity, or duration of URIs; however, when used as treatment very early in the disease, a modest positive effect has been shown in multiple studies with a decrease in severity of symptoms and decrease in duration by 1 or 2 days.

Although short-term use is thought to cause immunostimulation, extended use for more than 8 weeks has the potential to cause immunosuppression and hepatotoxicity.

There is great difficulty in interpreting the research on echinacea because of the heterogeneity of the product (i.e., there is no standardization of any particular component). Regardless, it is one of the top-three herbs sold in the United States.

SOLUTION TO THE CLINICAL CASE MANAGEMENT PROBLEM

The prescription of antibiotics for an obvious viral infection (the common cold is probably the best example) is likely the most frequent "mistake" made by family physicians. It is obviously a lot easier to prescribe an antibiotic for the child than to explain to the parent why one is not needed. Considering that URIs are a frequent presenting complaint to a family physician's office, this "mistake" actually may happen several times a day in an average practice. A reasonable approach to take to this patient's request may be as follows:
1. Explain the viral nature of the symptoms and your certainty in coming to that conclusion in the patient.
2. Explain the side effects of antibiotics including drug intolerance, drug allergy, and the possibility of creating an environment in the patient's body that promotes the growth of resistant organisms.

Continued

SOLUTION TO THE CLINICAL CASE MANAGEMENT PROBLEM—cont'd

3. Carefully go over some alternatives to antibiotic therapy that the patient may pursue for symptom relief. For children older than age 5 years, these include the use of steam, antihistamines, decongestants, and cough suppressants. Also suggest increased rest and fluid hydration.

4. Take the opportunity to discuss how meticulous hand washing and related hygienic measures can significantly decrease spread of the common cold among family members.

5. Repeat the following age-old edict to the parent: "The symptoms will abate in a week with antibiotics and in 7 days without." (Having said that, remember that 30% of patients with common cold symptoms who

had visited a physician still had a cough and a runny nose by the eighth day.)

6. Do not compromise your principles and prescribe an antibiotic when you know it is, at best, not indicated and possibly harmful. If the parent insists on an antibiotic, consider this an opportunity to discuss your philosophy of care with the patient: have the parent consider whether he is comfortable with the advice you are giving. If not, you should ask the parent if she really wishes to continue care in your practice.

This actually can be done in a very pleasant manner. There is rarely a problem in reaching a mutually agreeable position. It really comes down to a question of trust between the parent, the patient, and the physician.

SUMMARY OF THE COMMON COLD

1. As the most common presentation of an URI, it is the most common problem presenting to the family physician.

2. Viral infections are the major, if not the only, cause of common colds.

3. Rhinovirus is the most common pathogen (30% to 40%); influenza; parainfluenza A, B, and C; and RSV make up another 15%.

4. No laboratory investigations are necessary: the combination of rhinorrhea, cough, congestion, sneezing, and a sore throat (or some reasonable combination) in the absence of significant fever, cervical nodes, or an exudate virtually rules out streptococcal pharyngitis.

5. Prevention of spread to family members is best accomplished by meticulous hygiene. Self-inoculation is more important than aerosol spread.

6. Treatment is symptomatic: steam, nasal saline, decongestants and antihistamines.

7. Resist the temptation to prescribe antibiotics. Remember, "a week with antibiotics, 7 days without."

SUGGESTED READING

American Academy of Pediatrics: *AAP 2000 Red Book: Report of the Committee on Infectious Diseases,* 25th ed.

Arroll B, Kenealy T: Antibiotics for the common cold (Cochrane Review). In: *The Cochrane Library,* 3, 2001.

Chua D: Chronic use of Echinacea should be discouraged. *Am Fam Physician* 68(4):617; author reply 617:15, 2003.

Hayden F: Introduction: emerging importance of the rhinovirus. *Am J Med* 112 6A:1S, 2002.

Herendeen N, Szilagy P: Infections of the upper respiratory tract. In: Behrman RE, et al, eds.: *Nelson Textbook of Pediatrics,* 16th ed. WB Saunders, 2000, Philadelphia.

Kligler B: Echinacea. *Am Fam Physician* 67(1):77-80, 2003.

Macknin ML, et al: Zinc gluconate lozenges for treating the common cold in children. A randomized controlled trial. *JAMA* 279: 1962-1967, 1998.

Senior K: FDA panel rejects common cold treatment. *Lancet Infect Dis* 2(5):264, 2002.

Simoes E: Viral upper respiratory tract infections In: Rakel RE, Bope ET, eds.: *Conn's Current Therapy, 2003.* Elsevier, 2002, Philadelphia.

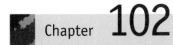

Chapter 102

Streptococcal Infections

"You mean by not treating my boy's sore throat earlier he may develop heart trouble?"

CLINICAL CASE PROBLEM 1:

A 6-YEAR-OLD WITH A SORE THROAT

A 6-year-old is brought to the family health center by her mother. The child today had sudden onset of a painful sore throat, difficulty swallowing, headache, and abdominal pain. The child has had no recent cough or coryza and was exposed to someone at school that recently was diagnosed with a "strep throat."

On examination the child has a temperature of 40° C. She has tender anterior cervical nodes and exudative tonsils. The lungs, heart, and abdominal examinations are benign.

■ **SELECT THE BEST ANSWER TO THE FOLLOWING QUESTIONS:**

1. What is the most likely diagnosis in this child?
   a. adenovirus
   b. corona virus
   c. group A beta-hemolytic streptococcus
   d. influenza a
   e. influenza b

2. What is the most practical way to confirm the diagnosis for this child?
   a. throat culture
   b. rapid streptococcal test
   c. antistreptolysin-O (ASO) titers
   d. a and b
   e. none of the above

3. What treatment would you offer for this child?
   a. Zithromax
   b. amoxicillin
   c. ciprofloxacin
   d. no antibiotics, rest, fluid, acetaminophen, and saline gargles
   e. none of the above

4. In the pediatric population what is the incidence of group A streptococcus causing pharyngitis
   a. 5% to 15%
   b. 15% to 30%
   c. 10% to 20%
   d. 20% to 30%
   e. nobody really knows for sure

5. The entire reason for treating group A beta-hemolytic streptococcus is to prevent which of the following sequelae.
   a. pyelonephritis
   b. rheumatic fever
   c. glomerulonephritis
   d. a and c
   e. all of the above

6. Which specific infections are associated with group A beta-hemolytic streptococcus?
   a. erysipelas
   b. scarlet fever
   c. impetigo
   d. all of the above
   e. none of the above

7. Recent practice guidelines recommend which of the following regarding diagnosis of group A beta-hemolytic streptococcus in children?
   a. clinical presentation alone should enable a physician to diagnose a streptococcal throat
   b. a negative rapid strep test rules out streptococcal throat
   c. a negative rapid strep test must be confirmed by a throat culture to rule out streptococcal throat
   d. a positive rapid strep test alone is 100% proof of a streptococcal infection
   e. none of the above

8. An appropriate throat swab involves sampling of which of the following regions?
   a. tonsils
   b. pharyngeal wall
   c. uvula
   d. a and b
   e. all of the above

9. What percentage of patients seen for a sore throat in a primary care setting receive antimicrobials?
   a. 40%
   b. 50%
   c. 60%
   d. 70%
   e. 80%

10. What percentage of children are colonized (asymptomatic carriers) of group A beta-hemolytic streptococcus?
    a. 5% to 10%
    b. 10% to 15%
    c. 15% to 20%
    d. 20% to 25%
    e. 25% to 30%

11. Recurrent tonsillitis usually is caused by which of the following?
    a. group A beta-hemolytic streptococcus
    b. parainfluenzae virus
    c. rhinovirus
    d. adenovirus
    e. Epstein-Barr virus

12. Which of the following statements regarding tonsillitis and recurrent sore throat is (are) correct?
    a. the frequency of recurrent sore throats in young children often decreases after tonsillectomy
    b. in many cases children who have not undergone a tonsillectomy experience a decreased frequency of recurrent sore throats similar to that observer after tonsillectomy
    c. tonsillectomy often decreases the frequency of recurrent upper-respiratory tract infections (colds) in young children
    d. a and b
    e. all of the above statements are true
    f. none of the above statements are true

13. Regarding tonsillar size and the frequency of tonsillitis, which of the following statements is (are) true?
    a. most hypertrophic tonsils are actually normal in size
    b. tonsils are relatively larger in younger children than in older children
    c. hypertrophic tonsils are more likely to become infected than nonhypertrophic tonsils
    d. a and b
    e. all of the above

14. Which of the following is (are) a complication(s) of tonsillectomy?
    a. hemorrhage
    b. postoperative throat infection
    c. pulmonary edema
    d. a and b
    e. a, b, and c

15. Which of the following is (are) a manifestation(s) of adenoidal hypertrophy?
    a. mouth breathing
    b. persistent rhinitis
    c. snoring
    d. a and c
    e. a, b, and c

CLINICAL CASE MANAGEMENT PROBLEM

List the indications for performance of a tonsillectomy.

ANSWERS:

1. **c.** This child has signs and symptoms of group A beta-hemolytic streptococcal pharyngitis, namely fever, sore throat, difficulty in swallowing, headache, and tender anterior cervical lymph nodes. Also, the absence of cough and coryza also favors a bacterial rather than a viral etiology.

2. **b.** The newer rapid streptococcus tests are 75% to 87% sensitive and greater than 90% specific. A positive result should confirm your clinical suspicion. However, even if the rapid streptococcus test is negative, a throat culture should be sent out to confirm the diagnosis and the patient should be started taking antibiotics until the results are confirmed.

   The rapid streptococcal test is an enzyme-linked immunosorbent assay (ELISA) test designed to detect antibodies against multiple streptococcal extracellular antigens. It has a very high specificity and a very low false-positive rate. The sensitivity of the test ranges from 75% to 87%, and the specificity ranges from 90% to 96%. The sensitivity of the test is lower, and therefore the false-negative rate can be somewhat high. Therefore in practical clinical terms, if a test is positive it can be assumed that the patient has the disease; however, if it is negative it cannot be assumed that the patient does not have a streptococcus infection, particularly if signs and symptoms are suggestive. The "gold standard" for the diagnosis of streptococcal pharyngitis remains culture with a throat swab. It should be performed in most patients suspected of having streptococcal pharyngitis and who have a negative rapid streptococcal test.

3. **b.** Penicillin and amoxicillin are first line in the treatment of streptococcal pharyngitis. Patients who are allergic to penicillin can be treated with erythromycin.

4. **b.** Group A streptococcus causes 15% to 30% of cases of acute pharyngitis in children but only 5% to 10% in the adult population.

5. **b.** Group A streptococcus pharyngitis is usually a self-limited disease; fever and constitutional symptoms disappear spontaneously within 3-4 days of onset, even without antimicrobial treatment. Therapy can be safely postponed for up to 9 days after the onset of symptoms and still prevent the occurrence of acute rheumatic fever. Therapy does not reduce the incidence of poststreptococcal glomerulonephritis.

6. **d.** All of the above.

7. **c.** The diagnosis of acute group A streptococcus infection should be suspected on clinical grounds and then supported by performance of laboratory testing.

A positive result either of a throat culture or a rapid streptococcal test provides adequate confirmation of the presence of group A beta-hemolytic streptococcus in the pharynx. However, for children and adolescents a negative rapid streptococcus test should be confirmed by a throat culture because of the higher prevalence (15% to 30%) of this infection and the higher number of false-positive results using the rapid streptococcal test.

Although false-positive results are obtained in fewer than 10% of the analyses, they do occur. Thus the statement that a positive rapid strep test alone is 100% proof of a streptococcal infection is false.

8. **d.** Throat swab specimens should be obtained from the surface of both tonsils or tonsillar fossae and the posterior pharyngeal wall. Other areas of the oral pharynx and the mouth are not acceptable sites and should not be touched with the swab before or after the appropriate areas have been sampled. In children this can be difficult at times, and a cooperative effort is sometimes needed involving the family, physician, and nursing staff.

9. **d.** Recent national data have shown that antibiotics, frequently more expensive and broader spectrum ones, are prescribed for approximately 70% of individuals who consult a community primary care physician for a sore throat.

10. **c.** Of children, 15% to 20% have nonvirulent group A beta-hemolytic streptococcus colonization in the nasopharynx. This makes the interpretation of the throat swab difficult because of the false-positive results produced. This is a diagnostic dilemma. These organisms lack the M-protein virulence factor.

11. **a.** Recurrent tonsillitis almost always is caused by group A beta-hemolytic streptococcus. We must, however, differentiate between cases of clinically suspected streptococcal tonsillitis and culture-proven streptococcal tonsillitis. Often, a parent will come to your office with a child, complaining that the child has "continual tonsillitis" or "recurrent tonsillitis." It is very important to document whether these cases of tonsillitis are laboratory group A streptococcal tonsillitis or simply recurrent pharyngitis assumed to be streptococcal. This is especially important when the issue of tonsillectomy for recurrent tonsillitis is raised.

12. **d.** The frequency of recurrent sore throats in young children often decreases after tonsillectomy. However, a similar rate of decrease in the frequency of recurrent sore throats occurs in children as they grow older despite not having had a tonsillectomy. It is difficult, therefore, to suggest a "relative value" of tonsillectomy in this age group.

Tonsillectomy does not decrease the incidence of recurrent upper-respiratory tract infections (colds) in young children. Thus an important distinction exists between recurrent sore throats and recurrent upper-respiratory tract infections in relationship to the efficacy (or lack of efficacy) of tonsillectomy.

13. **d.** Most hypertrophic tonsils are actually normal in size; the misinterpretation results from failure to appreciate that "normal" tonsils are relatively larger in young children than in older children. There is no evidence that hypertrophic (or larger) tonsils become infected any more frequently than nonhypertrophic (or smaller) tonsils.

14. **e.** Complications of tonsillectomy include minor hemorrhage, postoperative throat infection, severe postoperative hemorrhage, and pulmonary edema. Pulmonary edema is not uncommon after the relief of upper-airway obstruction with tonsillectomy or adenoidectomy. The possibility of severe postoperative hemorrhage also makes this operation a risky procedure. The indications for the procedure (discussed in the Solution to the Clinical Case Management Problem) should be followed closely.

15. **e.** Reasons for adenoidectomy include persistent mouth breathing, persistent rhinitis, chronic otitis, and persistent snoring.

 ## SOLUTION TO THE CLINICAL CASE MANAGEMENT PROBLEM

The indications for the performance of a tonsillectomy include the following: (1) one episode of peritonsillar abscess; (2) airway obstruction (as a result of markedly hypertrophied tonsils); (3) seven episodes of throat-culture–proven streptococcal tonsillitis in 1 year; or (4) five episodes of throat-culture–proven streptococcal tonsillitis per year in 2 successive years.

SUMMARY OF STREPTOCOCCAL INFECTIONS

1. **Neonates:** Group B streptococcus is now the most frequent cause of neonatal septicemia and meningitis.
2. **Streptococcal pharyngitis:**
   a. Only 15% of pharyngitis cases in children have group A beta-hemolytic streptococcus as the cause.
   b. Streptococcal pharyngitis is suggested by (i) age older than 5 years; (ii) high fever; (iii) tonsillar exudates; (iv) tender anterior cervical lymphadenopathy; (v) scarlatiform rash; (vi) history of exposure; (vii) absence of cough; and (viii) absence of rhinitis.
   c. Only 25% of patients with exudates have streptococcal pharyngitis. The presence of either cough or rhinitis makes the probability of streptococcal pharyngitis very low. Some authorities believe that the predictive value of physicians in distinguishing streptococcal pharyngitis from viral pharyngitis is at best 50%.
   d. Of children, 15% to 20% carry group A beta-hemolytic streptococcus as a normal commensal organism.
3. **Erysipelas:** acute, well-demarcated infection of the skin caused by group A beta-hemolytic streptococcus (a.k.a. *streptococcus pyogenes*)
4. **Impetigo:** caused primarily by group A beta-hemolytic streptococcus; may lead to more serious conditions such as cellulitis; also many cases caused by *S. aureus*
5. **Scarlet fever:** Fine, diffuse, erythematous rash in the setting of pharyngeal streptococcal infection. It is not as common or as virulent as in past decades but has a cyclic incidence.
6. **Bacterial endocarditis:** in children, typically caused by *S. viridans*
7. **Tonsillitis and tonsillectomy:** tonsillectomy should be performed only if there is one episode of peritonsillar abscess, a history of airway obstruction, or seven documented episodes of group A beta-hemolytic streptococcal infections in a 12-month period or five documented episodes in each of 2 successive years. Remember the following: (i) most hypertrophied tonsils are normal tonsils; (ii) tonsils grow smaller as the child grows older; (iii) large tonsils are no more prone to

tonsillitis than small tonsils; and (iv) not all tonsillitis is caused by beta-hemolytic streptococcus (approximately 25%; the other 75% of causes are viral in origin).
8. **Adenoids and adenoidectomy:** the only indication that is similar for both tonsillectomy and adenoidectomy is airway obstruction. The other indications for adenoidectomy are chronic otitis media and chronic rhinitis.
9. **Other streptococcal infections:** human infection with streptococci of groups C, D, E, F, G, H, K, L, M, N, and O has been reported in normal infants and children. Penicillin G provides effective therapy for non–group-A streptococcus except for group D (enterococci). This organism is generally susceptible to ampicillin.
10. **Treatment for streptococcal infections:**
    a. Group A beta-hemolytic streptococcal pharyngitis: laboratory diagnosis and begin treatment with penicillin V for 10 days (in unreliable patients use benzathine penicillin G); amoxicillin may be a reasonable alternative.
    b. *S. viridans*: bacterial endocarditis: use ampicillin and an aminoglycoside
    c. Infection with Lancefield group G streptococcus has been recognized as an increasingly serious and frequent cause of human disease. This group can cause endovascular infection, endocarditis, and septic arthritis.
    d. Early treatment of group A beta-hemolytic streptococcal pharyngitis (i) decreases the virulence and severity of the infection; (ii) decreases the length of symptoms of the infection; (iii) protects against rheumatic fever, once again an increasing problem in the United States; and (iv) it does not, however, protect against poststreptococcal glomerulonephritis.

SUGGESTED READING

Bisno AL: Acute pharyngitis. *N Engl J Med* 344(3):205-211, 2001 Jan 18.

Cunningham MW: Pathogenesis of group A streptococcal infections. *Clin Microbiol Rev* 13(3):470-511, 2000.

Curtin-Wirt C, et al: Efficacy of penicillin vs. amoxicillin in children with group A beta hemolytic streptococcal tonsillopharyngitis. *Clin Pediatr* 42(3):219-225, 2003 Apr.

Gerber MA: Group A streptococcus. In: Behrman RE, et al, eds.: *Nelson textbook of pediatrics*, ed 17. Elsevier, 2004, Philadelphia.

Musher DM: How contagious are common respiratory tract infections? *N Engl J Med* 348(13):1256-1266, 2003 Mar 27.

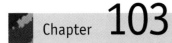

Chapter 103

Viral Exanthems

| "Don't judge a rash too rashly." |

CLINICAL CASE PROBLEM 1:

A 3-Year-Old with a Rash and Fever

A 3-year-old comes to your office with fatigue and irritability and a low-grade fever that he has had for 3 days. The father relates to you that the child attends daycare where a virus is "going around." The father used Tylenol, which has helped to decrease irritability; although the child's appetite is suppressed, he is still taking in a good amount of fluids.

On physical examination the child does not look ill. His temperature is 38° C. His skin examination shows scattered small vesicles on an erythematous base. The rash was seen first on the face and seems to be spreading to the trunk.

■ SELECT THE BEST ANSWER TO THE FOLLOWING QUESTIONS:

1. What is the most likely diagnosis in this child at this time?
   a. rubella (German measles)
   b. adenoviral exanthem
   c. varicella zoster
   d. mumps
   e. rubeola

2. What is the most outstanding feature of this illness?
   a. constitutional symptoms
   b. the appearance of a rash at the same time as the temperature falls
   c. the description of the lesion as a "dew drop on a rose petal"
   d. recurrence of the rash in adulthood
   e. benign nature of this infection

3. What is the causative agent of this infection?
   a. human parvovirus
   b. adenovirus
   c. rhinovirus
   d. herpesvirus
   e. Epstein-Barr virus

4. This infection can occur in adulthood. Which of the following is a unique feature in this recurrence?
   a. incidence varies with gender and race
   b. there is no long-term sequelae with the recurrence
   c. there is dermatomal distribution of the lesions

   d. diagnosis usually is made on clinical findings
   e. these lesions are not seen in immunocompromised patients

5. The American Academy of Family Physicians recommends which of the following for the treatment and prevention of this condition?
   a. no antibiotics, no vaccinations
   b. no antibiotics, an antiviral agent to prevent complications
   c. no antibiotics, one vaccination in childhood
   d. antibiotics, no vaccinations in childhood
   e. no antivirals, two vaccinations in childhood

CLINICAL CASE PROBLEM 2:

A 5-Year-Old with Cough, Coryza, and Conjunctivitis

A 5-year-old whose family believes that immunizations can cause autism is brought into the office with a 3-day history of fever, nonproductive cough, coryza, and conjunctivitis. This morning a rash appeared on his forehead and behind the ears and appears to be spreading to his upper arms and chest.

On physical examination you note a fine maculopapular rash over the face that appears to be spreading to the back and thighs.

6. What is the most likely diagnosis in this patient?
   a. erythema infectiosum
   b. streptococcal infection
   c. cytomegalovirus
   d. rubeola
   e. rubella

7. What are the hallmark signs and symptoms of this infection?
   a. Koplik spots
   b. coalescing erythematous maculopapular rash
   c. suboccipital and postauricular lymph node enlargement
   d. conjunctivitis
   e. all of the above

8. Which of the following is a relatively common complication of this infection?
   a. encephalitis
   b. myocarditis
   c. pneumonia
   d. thrombocytopenic purpura
   e. keratoconjunctivitis

9. What treatment recommendations will you make to the father?
   a. amoxicillin
   b. erythromycin

c. symptomatic treatment
d. vitamin A
e. ribavirin

10. What is the recommended immunization schedule for the prevention of this infection?
   a. four doses at 2, 4, 6 months with a booster at 15 months
   b. three doses at 2, 4, and 6 months.
   c. two doses at 12-15 months and 4-6 years
   d. three doses at 0, 1, and, 6 months
   e. two doses at 1 year and 15 months

CLINICAL CASE PROBLEM 3:
A 4-YEAR-OLD WITH A BRIGHT RED RASH ON BOTH CHEEKS

A 4-year-old is brought to the office by his mother. The child has had a low-grade fever, headache, and a sore throat for the past 1 week. Four days ago he suddenly developed a bright red rash on his cheeks, which now over the last 2 days has spread to the trunk, arms, and legs.

On physical examination, the child has erythema of the cheeks and a maculopapular rash on the trunk spreading to the extremities. There are no other significant findings.

11. What is the most likely diagnosis in this child?
   a. rubella
   b. adenoviral exanthem
   c. human herpesvirus 6
   d. erythema infectiosum
   e. rhinovirus

12. What is the causative agent of this infection?
   a. herpes virus 6
   b. human papillomavirus
   c. rhinovirus
   d. human parvovirus B19
   e. adenovirus

13. What are the morphologic features of this infection?
   a. circumoral pallor and sandpaperlike appearance of the trunk
   b. fine pustular appearance and a bright red macular–papular rash with central clearing
   c. erythematous cheeks with a lacy reticular pattern
   d. coalesced lesions in various stages (vesicles, bullae, and papules)
   e. none of the above

14. The mother asks you what can she do about the slap-cheeked appearance. People are staring at her as though she has been abusing her child.

   a. tell her to tell them to stop staring; it's none of their business
   b. tell her to give the child Tylenol every 4-6 hours
   c. tell her to wash the face repeatedly with cold water
   d. advise her to keep the child out of the sun
   e. reassure her that this will resolve on its own

15. The mother then tells you that she is 4 months pregnant and asks whether she should she be worried about anything. What do you tell her?
   a. there is no cause for concern; this is a self-limiting illness
   b. there is a small chance for fetal demise or congenital defects
   c. tell her you are too busy and ask her why doesn't she just look it up on the Internet like everyone else
   d. all of the above
   e. none of the above

Questions 16 to 26 are matching questions. Eleven disease-producing pathogens or disease entities are listed in the left-hand column, and 11 disease-defining characteristics are listed in the right-hand column. Beside each disease-producing pathogen or disease entity, put the letter of the disease-defining characteristic to which it corresponds.

16. Herpes varicella
17. Herpes simplex
18. Coxsackievirus A16
19. Kawasaki disease
20. Adenovirus
21. Lyme disease
22. Parainfluenza virus
23. Tinea versicolor
24. Tinea corporis
25. Pityriasis rosea
26. Molluscum contagiosum

a. discrete, dome-shaped papules
b. herald patch
c. erythema chronicum migrans
d. hand-foot-and-mouth disease
e. acute gingivostomatitis
f. ringworm
g. primary cause of conjunctivitis
h. primary cause of infectious croup
i. hyperpigmented or hypopigmented lesions
j. coronary vasculitis
k. "crops of lesions": vesicles

CLINICAL CASE MANAGEMENT PROBLEM

Define the following primary skin lesions seen in children: macule, bullae, papule, pustule, nodule, wheal, vesicle, and cyst.

ANSWERS:

1. c. This is a classic presentation of chickenpox (varicella zoster). A prodrome of low-grade fever and general malaise usually precedes the defining rash 1-2 days. The classic rash begins as scattered small vesicles with erythematous bases, seen first on the trunk and face. The lesions spread centrifugally to involve all skin surfaces and possibly mucous membranes (lips, vulva). The lesions are pruritic, and many patients will scratch. Intact and ruptured vesicles will be present simultaneously; scratching may yield excoriations and superficial skin infections. Treatment is symptomatic.

2. c. The classic description of the lesion is a "dew drop on a rose petal," corresponding to a clear vesicle on an erythematous base.

3. d. The herpesviruses are a large group of double-stranded DNA viruses that includes oral and genital herpes (herpes simplex virus [HSV] Types 1 and 2), Epstein-Barr virus, cytomegalovirus, and varicella zoster virus.

4. c. Herpes zoster (shingles) is caused by the varicella zoster virus, the same virus that causes chickenpox. Shingles is seen primarily in the elderly or in the immunocompromised, especially those with human immunodeficiency virus or lymphoreticular malignancies. Herpes zoster occurs when the virus is reactivated from its latent state in the dorsal root ganglia. Inflammatory changes occur in the sensory root ganglia and in the skin of the associated dermatome. The clinical presentation is that of an erythematous vesicular rash associated with pain before, during, and after the rash in a dermatomal distribution.

5. c. All relevant professional organizations recommend no antibiotics and one vaccination in childhood.

6. d. Rubeola (measles) has an incubation period of 8-12 days. The prodromal phase includes fever, nonspecific upper-respiratory inflammation (i.e., cough, coryza, conjunctivitis, and a low- to moderate-grade fever). Koplik's spots (1-mm, bluish white lesions on an erythematous base) can be seen only in the first couple of days of symptoms. They usually appear on the buccal mucosa opposite the lower molars and quickly coalesce into larger lesions. The temperature in rubeola increases as the rash appears. The maculopapular rash usually begins on the face and neck and spreads to the entire body from the neck down. The rash begins to disappear in about 3 days in the same manner (from head down). Fine desquamation may occur during healing. The total duration of the rash is about 7 days.

The major complications of rubeola are otitis media, bronchopneumonia, and gastrointestinal symptoms including nausea, vomiting, and diarrhea. Patients with rubeola are ill appearing. Prevention can be achieved with active immunization at 12-15 months and a booster at ages 4-6.

7. e. In brief the major symptoms of measles are Koplik spots, a coalescing erythematous maculopapular rash, suboccipital and postauricular lymph-node enlargement, and conjunctivitis.

8. c. The more common complications, as mentioned in Answer 6, are bronchopneumonia and otitis media. The remainder (encephalitis, myocarditis, thrombocytopenic purpura, and keratoconjunctivitis) are much less common; however, all of them are possible.

9. c. As with most viral infections, treatment is primarily symptomatic.

10. c. The recommended immunization schedule for measles is two doses at 12-15 months and 4-6 years (also see Chapter 96).

11. d. See Answer 14.

12. d. See Answer 14.

13. c. see Answer 14.

14. d. Erythema infectiosum is caused by human parvovirus B19. It occurs mostly during spring months; localized outbreaks among children and adolescents are common. The infection begins as a low-grade fever and produces a "slapped-cheek" rash appearance on the face associated with a lacy, reticularlike maculopapular rash pattern on the trunk and extremities. Constitutional symptoms include headache, pharyngitis, myalgias, arthritis, gastrointestinal upset, and coryza. The illness usually lasts 5-10 days. The rash may last from a few days to several weeks. It is frequently pruritic. Recurrences after exercise, after application of heat, or after emotional distress are not uncommon. Treatment is symptomatic.

15. b. There is a small chance for fetal demise or congenital defects as a result of infection with human parvovirus B19 during pregnancy. Therefore the mother should try to avoid contagion.

16. k. The viral agent is herpes varicella (chicken pox). Disease-defining characteristics are crops of small, red papules that develop into oval vesicles on an erythematous base.

17. **e.** The viral agent is herpes simplex virus. Disease-defining characteristic is acute herpetic gingivostomatitis, which is the most common cause of stomatitis in children ages 1-3 years old.

18. **d.** The viral agent is coxsackievirus A16. Disease-defining characteristics are hand, foot, and mouth disease and an enteroviral exanthem–enanthem with the distribution portrayed by the name.

19. **j.** The disease entity is Kawasaki disease. The disease-defining characteristic is coronary vasculitis, also known as mucocutaneous lymph-node syndrome or infantile polyarteritis. Cardiac involvement is the most important manifestation of Kawasaki disease (10% to 40% of children within the first 2 weeks of illness). The causal agent is unknown.

20. **g.** The viral agent is adenovirus. The disease-defining characteristic is adenovirus, the single most common cause of conjunctivitis.

21. **c.** The disease entity is Lyme disease. The disease-defining characteristic is erythema chronicum migrans, which begins as an erythematous macule or papule at the site of a tick bite. The causative organism is *Borrelia burgdorferi,* which develops into an expanding erythematous annular lesion with central clearing and often reaches a diameter of 16 cm.

22. **h.** The viral agent is parainfluenza virus. The disease-defining characteristic is that it is the most common cause of infectious croup.

23. **i.** The disease entity is tinea versicolor. The disease-defining characteristic is hypopigmented or hyperpigmented macules covered with a fine scale. Lesions begin in a perifollicular location, enlarge, and form confluent patches, most commonly on the neck, upper chest, back, and upper arms. The causative organism is dimorphic yeast (*Pityrosporon orbiculare [Malassezia furfur]*).

24. **f.** The disease entity is tinea corporis. The disease-defining characteristic is ringworm, the common name for a group of disorders known as dermatophytoses. The three principal genera responsible for dermatophyte infections are Trichophyton, Microsporum, and Epidermophyton. A classical lesion begins as a dry, mildly erythematous, elevated, scaly papule or plaque and spreads centrifugally as it clears centrally to form the characteristic annular lesion responsible for the designation ringworm.

25. **b.** The disease entity is pityriasis rosea. The disease-defining characteristic is the herald patch, a solitary, round, or oval lesion that may occur anywhere on the body and is often but not always identifiable by its large size. The herald patch usually precedes the generalized maculopapular eruption of oval or round lesions that crop. The rash can assume a characteristic Christmas-tree appearance on the back.

26. **a.** The disease entity is molluscum contagiosum. The disease-defining characteristic describes a disorder characterized by discrete, dome-shaped papules varying in size from 1 to 5 mm. Typically these lesions have a central umbilication from which a cheesy material can be expressed. The papules may occur anywhere on the body, but the face, eyelids, neck, axillae, and thighs are sites of predilection. The causative agent is a DNA virus, the largest member of the poxvirus group.

SOLUTION TO THE CLINICAL CASE MANAGEMENT PROBLEM

Macule: An alteration in skin color that cannot be felt

Papule: Palpable solid lesions smaller than 1.0 cm

Nodule: Palpable solid lesions larger than 1.0 cm

Vesicle: Raised, fluid-filled lesions less than 0.5 cm in diameter

Bullae: Raised, fluid-filled lesions larger than 0.5 cm in diameter

Pustules: Raised lesions that contain pustular material

Wheals: Flat-topped, palpable lesions of variable size and configuration that represent dermal collections of edema fluid

Cyst: Circumscribed, thick-walled lesions that are located deep in the skin; are covered by a normal epidermis; and contain fluid or semisolid material

SUMMARY OF VIRAL EXANTHEMS

Because so many conditions were described in this chapter, the summary will be limited to a discussion of what are termed the "big five" viral exanthems in children. (Note that erythema infectiosum also is known as fifth disease.)

1. **Exanthem subitum (roseola infantum):** high fever followed by defervescence with the appearance of an erythematous maculopapular rash at the same time
2. **Erythema infectiosum:** low-grade fever followed by the appearance of a rash: "slapped-cheek" appearance followed by a generalized lacy-reticular pattern rash
3. **Rubella:** mild fever; significant tender retroauricular, posterior, and postoccipital lymphadenopathy
4. **Rubeola:** prodromal symptoms include the 3 Cs: cough, coryza, and conjunctivitis. Koplik's spots are pathognomonic. Photophobia is common. The temperature increases abruptly as the rash

appears. The severity of the disease is directly related to the extent and confluence of the rash. The mnemonic is cc-CPK: cough, coryza, conjunctivitis, photophobia, Koplik's spots.

5. **Scarlet fever:** group A beta-hemolytic streptococcal infection that presents as fever, chills, headache, vomiting, and pharyngitis. Exanthem has the texture of coarse sandpaper. Circumoral pallor is common. Penicillin V is the drug of choice.

SUGGESTED READING

Gerber MA: Group A streptococcus. In: Behrman R, et al, eds.: *Nelson's textbook of pediatrics*, ed 17. Elsevier, 2004, Philadelphia.

Koch WC: Parvovirus B19. In: Behrman R, et al, eds.: *Nelson's textbook of pediatrics*, ed 17. Elsevier, 2004, Philadelphia.

Leach CT: Human herpesviruses 6 and 7. In: Behrman R, et al, eds.: *Nelson's textbook of pediatrics*, ed 17. Elsevier, 2004, Philadelphia.

Maldonado Y: Measles. In: Behrman R, et al, eds.: *Nelson's textbook of pediatrics*, ed 17. Elsevier, 2004, Philadelphia.

Maldonado Y. Rubella. In: Behrman R, et al, eds.: *Nelson's textbook of pediatrics*, ed 17. Elsevier, 2004, Philadelphia.

Scott LA, Stone MS: Viral exanthems. *Dermatology Online Journal* 9(3):4, 2003 Aug.

Chapter 104

Childhood Pneumonia

"How did my baby get water in her lungs? I always was so careful when I gave her a bath."

CLINICAL CASE PROBLEM 1:

A 2-Day-Old Infant with Pneumonia

A 4000-g infant born at 39½ weeks gestation appeared healthy at birth. His Apgar scores were 7 and 9. On the second day of life he begins to have difficulty feeding, his temperature increases to 40.5° C, his breathing becomes labored, and he appears ill.

His chest x-ray shows a reticulogranular pattern, a pattern that appears exactly like hyaline membrane disease. On physical examination, you also note apnea, tachypnea, grunting, flaring of the nares, and subcostal retractions. There are adventitious breath sounds heard in all lobes of the lungs.

■ SELECT THE BEST ANSWER TO THE FOLLOWING QUESTIONS:

1. Based on the information provided to this point, what is the most likely diagnosis?
   a. group A streptococcal pneumonia
   b. *Klebsiella* pneumonia
   c. adenoviral pneumonia
   d. group B streptococcal pneumonia
   e. staphylococcal pneumonia

2. What is the most likely source of this infant's infection?
   a. airborne droplets
   b. oral–fecal transmission
   c. direct spread from the mother
   d. intrauterine colonization
   e. none of the above

3. What is the treatment of choice in this child at this time?
   a. ampicillin plus cefotaxime
   b. amoxicillin
   c. trimethoprim–sulfamethoxazole
   d. clavulanic acid
   e. penicillin G and metronidazole

CLINICAL CASE PROBLEM 2:

A 3-Year-Old Female with Fever, Chills, Nasal Flaring, Subcostal Indrawing, and a Harsh Cough

A 3-year-old female is brought to your office with a 4-day history of fever, chills, nasal flaring, subcostal indrawing, and a harsh cough. The child is in respiratory distress.

Before the onset of the present symptoms, the child had a recent respiratory tract infection. The child's symptoms were bilateral conjunctivitis, rhinorrhea, nonproductive cough, and sore throat.

On physical examination, the child's temperature is 39° C. Her respiratory rate is 32 per minute. There are rales and rhonchi in all lobes. The child is using her accessory muscles of respiration, especially her intercostal muscles and sternocleidomastoid muscles.

4. What is the most likely diagnosis in this case?
   a. *Mycoplasma pneumoniae*
   b. adenoviral pneumonia
   c. *Streptococcus pneumoniae*
   d. *Haemophilus influenzae* pneumonia
   e. group B streptococcal pneumonia

5. What is the most common causative agent responsible for pneumonia in children age 5 years and younger?
   a. respiratory syncytial virus (RSV)
   b. *Mycoplasma pneumoniae*
   c. adenovirus
   d. *S. pneumoniae*
   e. *H. influenzae*

6. What is the most common bacterial causative agent responsible for pneumonia in children under the age of 5 years?
   a. *S. pneumoniae*
   b. *Staphylococcus aureus*
   c. group A beta-hemolytic *Streptococcus*
   d. *H. influenzae*
   e. *Klebsiella pneumoniae*

7. A child who is considered low risk for complications and who develops the clinical picture described in Clinical Case Problem 2 should be treated with which of the following?
   a. ribavirin
   b. ampicillin
   c. erythromycin
   d. penicillin
   e. supportive/symptomatic treatment

8. A child who is considered high risk for complications and who develops the clinical picture described in Clinical Case Problem 2 should be treated with which of the following?
   a. ribavirin
   b. ampicillin
   c. erythromycin
   d. hospitalization
   e. a and d

9. A high-risk child who develops a secondary pneumonia infection caused by the causative agent most likely responsible for bacterial pneumonia in children younger than age 5 years should be treated with which of the following?
   a. ribavirin
   b. ampicillin
   c. penicillin G
   d. hospitalization
   e. b and d

10. What is the most common nonviral pneumonia in children older than age 5 years?
    a. *M. pneumonia*
    b. *S. pneumoniae*
    c. *Listeria monocytogenes* pneumonia
    d. *H. influenzae* pneumonia
    e. group B *S. pneumoniae*

11. What is the second most common bacterial agent responsible for pneumonia in children older than age 5 years?
    a. *S. pneumoniae*
    b. *H. influenzae*
    c. *Staphylococcus aureus*
    d. *K. pneumoniae*
    e. group B *S. pneumoniae*

12. Which of the following causative agents usually evolves into a pneumonia that often includes an empyema or a pleural effusion?
    a. *S. pneumoniae*
    b. *Staphylococcus aureus*
    c. group B *S. pneumoniae*
    d. *H. influenzae*
    e. *K. pneumoniae*

13. What is the most sensitive sign of pneumonia in infants younger than 6 months of age?
    a. fever
    b. cough
    c. tachypnea
    d. crackles
    e. wheezing

14. Which of the following statements about viral pneumonia is false?
    a. radiographs show diffuse interstitial infiltrates
    b. the rate of hospitalization decreases with increasing age
    c. antibiotics play no role in treatment
    d. rapid antigen detection tests are available for RSV and influenza
    e. RSV is the most common pathogen

15. Which of the following is the least common complication of pneumonia?
    a. abscess
    b. empyema
    c. effusion
    d. pericarditis
    e. dehydration

CLINICAL CASE MANAGEMENT PROBLEM

With respect to viral, mycoplasmal, and bacterial pneumonias in neonates, infants, and children, list the following: (1) the most common causative agent in the age group in question; (2) the most common bacterial causative agent in the age group in question; and (3) the recommended treatment for each of the pneumonias in question.

■ ANSWERS:

1. **d.** This neonate most likely has group B streptococcal pneumonia. Other potential pathogens that are much less likely include *Escherichia coli*, *Listeria*, and group D *streptococci*. These former pathogens usually occur in preterm infants of mothers with chorioamnionitis and cause earlier onset of respiratory distress.

2. **c.** In newborns this is primarily a disease in which the organism is colonized by passage through the birth canal, thus a direct spread from the mother.

3. **a.** The empiric treatment of choice for neonatal pneumonia is ampicillin 100 mg/kg/day plus cefotaxime 100 mg/kg/day. The treatment should be continued for at least 10 days.

4. **b.** The initial presentation of conjunctivitis, nonproductive cough, rhinorrhea, and sore throat is most compatible with adenoviral infection. The real clue in this case is the conjunctivitis, a symptom much more common with adenovirus infection than with any other viral infection.

The probable sequence of events is minor adenoviral upper-respiratory tract infection proceeding to adenoviral pneumonia.

5. **a.** The most common cause of pneumonia in children younger than age 5 years is RSV pneumonia.

The typical signs and symptoms of viral pneumonia in children include a dry, tight, and nonproductive cough; fever or chills absent as frequently as present; and auscultatory findings including rhonchi, fine rales, and audible wheezing.

In general, the younger the infant the more severe the disease symptoms, these may include significant respiratory distress, listlessness, and apnea.

Radiographic findings are more likely to include air trapping, bilateral fine/fluffy infiltrates, and atelectasis. Secondary bacterial invasion must be considered when consolidation is present.

The five most common viral agents causing pneumonia in infants and children are as follow: (1) RSV; (2) parainfluenza virus; (3) influenza virus (in children mostly influenza B); (4) adenovirus; and (5) enterovirus.

6. **a.** The most common bacterial cause of pneumonia in a child younger than age 5 years is *S. pneumoniae*.

Bacterial pneumonias usually present with a clinical picture that is quite different from viral pneumonias. Signs and symptoms of bacterial pneumonias include fever, chills, cough productive of purulent sputum, pleuritic chest pain, and dyspnea and tachypnea. Also, the use of the accessory muscles of respiration is very common, especially in children.

The chest x-ray frequently will show lobar consolidation. The complete blood count often will reveal an extremely high white blood cell count with a shift to the left.

7. **e.** The treatment of an infant or child with probable adenoviral pneumonia is symptomatic. No antibiotics or antiviral agents have been shown to be effective for the treatment of this infection. The major decision regarding this child will be whether hospitalization is necessary. This will depend on the child's clinical condition and, most importantly, on the degree of respiratory distress that the child demonstrates.

If you even think about hospitalizing a child with pneumonia, do it. You will not have made a mistake.

8. **e.** A child with possible adenoviral pneumonia who is at high risk for complications (congenital heart disease, cystic fibrosis, malignancy, chronic immunosuppression, or any primary immune deficiency) should be hospitalized and given supplementary oxygen (with or without a mist tent). It also is reasonable to treat such high-risk children with ribavirin to reduce potential coinfection with RSV, the most common cause of viral pneumonia in this age group.

9. **e.** The treatment of choice for a high-risk child who has a secondary streptococcal pneumonia includes antibiotic therapy (IV ampicillin is the drug of first choice) and ribavirin and hospitalization with supplementary oxygen and close monitoring as described in Answer 8.

As the child improves, it is not uncommon for the chest x-ray changes to lag significantly behind the clinical improvement. In a child with this picture, arterial blood gases or pulse oximetry are also a very good way of measuring response to treatment and improvement.

10. **a.** The most common cause of nonviral pneumonia in children older than age 5 years is *M. pneumoniae.* In a child with mycoplasma pneumonia there is often a significant discrepancy between the clinical findings and the radiologic findings. The most important clinical symptom is a persistent, hacking, nonproductive cough that is difficult to treat. Often auscultation of the lungs will be normal. The chest x-ray, however, may very well be quite revealing (with a significant bilateral infiltrate being the most common picture).

The treatment of choice for *M. pneumoniae* in a child is erythromycin.

11. **a.** In children older than age 5 years, streptococcal pneumonia is the most common cause of bacterial pneumonia after mycoplasma.

12. **b.** The answer is staphylococcal pneumonia. Most patients with staphylococcal pneumonia have roentgenographic evidence of nonspecific bronchopneumonia early in the course of the illness.

However, the infiltrate may soon become patchy and limited in extent or, alternatively, dense and homogenous and involve an entire lobe or hemithorax. The right lung is involved in approximately 65% of cases; bilateral involvement occurs in fewer than 20% of cases. A pleural effusion or empyema is noted during the course of illness in most patients; pyopneumothorax occurs in approximately 25% of patients. Pneumatocele occur frequently and vary considerably in size.

Although no x-ray change can be considered diagnostic, progression over a few hours from broncho-

pneumonia to effusion or pyopneumothorax with or without pneumatocele is highly suggestive of staphylococcal pneumonia.

The treatment of choice for staphylococcal pneumonia is a semisynthetic, penicillinase-resistant penicillin (such as methicillin) given intravenously.

13. **c.** Although tachypnea is not specific for bacterial pneumonia, it is the most sensitive sign of pneumonia in infants. Tachypnea is classified as a respiratory rate of >50 breaths/minute in infants younger than 1 year of age.

14. **c.** Antibiotics are not indicated if the pneumonia is certain to be viral and the patient is not toxic or in any respiratory distress. However, one must remember that bacterial coinfection is not rare and many would consider treating with antibiotics appropriate, especially in children who appear more ill.

15. **d.** Dehydration is the most common systemic complication occurring as a result of decreased intake and increased losses from fever, tachypnea, and vomiting. Local complications such as effusion, empyema, and abscess are more common than systemic complication from hematologic spread by bacteremia such as pericarditis, meningitis, and septic arthritis.

SUMMARY OF CHILDHOOD PNEUMONIA

This topic is well summarized in the Solution to the Clinical Case Management Problem.

SOLUTION TO THE CLINICAL CASE MANAGEMENT PROBLEM

A reasonable approach to diagnosis includes an understanding of prevalence of different types of pneumonia based on age:

1. Age <2 weeks:
   a. Most common organism: group B streptococcus
   b. Treatment: Ampicillin plus gentamicin
2. Age 2 weeks to 4 months:
   a. Most common organism: *Chlamydia trachomatis*
   b. Treatment: erythromycin plus cefotaxime
3. Age 4 months to 4 years:
   a. Most common organism: viral
   b. Most common viruses causing pneumonia are as follows: (i) RSV; (ii) parainfluenza viruses; (iii) influenza; (iv) adenovirus; and (v) enterovirus.

   c. Treatment: symptomatic or also ribavirin for severe RSV
   d. Most common type of bacterial pneumonia: *S. pneumoniae*
   e. Treatment: amoxicillin, outpatient; ampicillin (nonlobar) or cefotaxime (lobar), inpatient via IV
4. Age >4 years:
   a. Most common cause: viral
   b. Most common bacterial cause: *M. pneumoniae*
   c. Treatment: erythromycin
   d. Second most common type of bacterial pneumonia: *S. pneumoniae*
   e. Treatment: penicillin or macrolide, outpatient; cefotaxime, inpatient

SUGGESTED READING

Bradley JS: Management of community-acquired pediatric pneumonia in an era of increasing antibiotic resistance and conjugate vaccines. *Pediatr Infect Dis J* 21(6):592-598; discussion 613-614, 2002 Jun.

Darr C, et al: Reactive airway disease and pneumonia. In: Marx J, ed. *Rosen's emergency medicine: concepts and clinical practice.* Mosby, Inc., 2002, Philadelphia.

Gaston B: Pneumonia. *Pediatr Rev* 23(4):132-140, 2002.

Kercsmar CM: Chapter 12. The respiratory system. In: Behrman RE, Kliegman RM: *Nelson essentials of pediatrics, 4th ed.* WB Saunders, 2002, Philadelphia, 515-554.

Lichenstein R: Pediatric pneumonia. *Emerg Med Clin North Am* 21(2):437-451, 2003.

McIntosh K: Community-acquired pneumonia in children. *N Engl J Med* 346(6):429-437, 2002 Feb 7.

Prober C: Pneumonia. In: Behrman RE, et al, eds.: *Nelson essentials of pediatrics, 4th ed.* WB Saunders, 2002, Philadelphia, 383, 714.

 ## Chapter 105

Fever

> "My child seems OK except he has had a fever for the last month."

CLINICAL CASE PROBLEM 1:

A 15-MONTH-OLD CHILD WITH PERSISTENT FEVER

A 15-month-old is seen in your office for the fourth time this month with unexplained intermittent episodes of fever of 39° C. The mother has used children's Advil to treat the fever and has been able to bring the temperature down to 38° C. However, the mother now is frustrated because this is her fourth visit to the office and nobody knows why her child is continuing to have these fevers. The child is not in daycare and has no history of any serious illnesses, travel, or sick contacts. The child has had no symptoms of an upper-respiratory infection.

On examination the child is actively playing with his toys. He does not look ill or toxic. His rectal temperature is 39° C. The head, neck, lungs, cardiovascular, abdominal, neurologic, and musculoskeletal examination are all normal.

Your clinical judgment is that the child looks well and has no serious illness.

■ SELECT THE BEST ANSWER TO THE FOLLOWING QUESTIONS:

1. What is your diagnosis at this time?
   a. recurrent viral infection
   b. fever without a focus
   c. infantile febrile response
   d. fever of unknown origin
   e. periodic fever, aphthous ulcers, pharyngitis and adenopathy (PFAFA) syndrome

2. What is the most appropriate next step in the workup of this patient?
   a. obtain an immediate consultation with an infectious disease specialist
   b. start the child empirically taking antibiotics
   c. order a complete blood count (CBC) and urinalysis
   d. obtain a more detailed history
   e. obtain a chest x-ray

3. Which of the following represents the strict definition of fever of unknown origin (FUO)?
   a. fever in a child that persists for more than 1 month
   b. fever for more than 3 weeks with no diagnosis after three outpatient visits or 3 days in the hospital
   c. no diagnosis after 1 week of intelligent and intensive evaluation in the hospital
   d. b and c
   e. all of the above

4. Which of the following is the one preliminary diagnosis in this case that you always should consider?
   a. drug fever
   b. factitious fever
   c. occult bacteremia
   d. malignancy
   e. collagen vascular disease

5. The mother is very frustrated and wants to know what initial test you are going to do to figure out what is going on with her son. Which of the following will you tell her?
   a. chest x-ray
   b. lumbar puncture
   c. white blood cell (WBC) count
   d. urine culture
   e. blood culture

6. What is the most common organism causing occult bacteremia in children?
   a. *Haemophilus influenza*
   b. *Mycoplasma pneumoniae*
   c. *Streptococcus pneumoniae*
   d. *Salmonella*
   e. *Neisseria meningitidis*

7. The most common cause(s) of a child with recurrent fever occurring at regular intervals is (are).

a. PFAPA
b. Epstein-Barr virus
c. parvovirus B19
d. cytomegalovirus
e. all of the above

8. What is the most common condition seen in infants with occult bacteremia?
    a. cellulitis
    b. pneumoniae
    c. otitis media
    d. pharyngitis
    e. osteomyelitis

9. Which of the following statements regarding the presumptive use of antibiotics in infants with and FUO is (are) false?
    a. presumptive use of antibiotics in infants with an FUO decreases morbidity and mortality
    b. the later the use of antibiotics the greater the risk of morbidity and mortality
    c. presumptive use of oral antibiotics reliably prevents the risk of meningitis
    d. all of the statements are false
    e. b and c

10. In a child between the ages of 3-36 months the probability of occult bacteremia is decreased if:
    a. temperature is less than 39° C
    b. WBC range is between 5000-15,000 cells/mm^3
    c. there is a negative exposure history
    d. all of the above decreases probability
    e. none of the above decreases probability

CLINICAL CASE PROBLEM 2:

A 3-YEAR-OLD WITH A RASH AND FEVER

A 3-year-old girl presents to the Family Health Center with a fever for the last 36 hours. Maximum temperature was 104° F at 2 AM, which came down to 101.6° F with children's Advil. Her appetite and fluid intake has decreased over the last 24 hours.

Physical examination shows an ill-appearing child. Her temperature is 99° F. The skin has a macular–papular petechial rash on the chest and back. The remainder of the physical examination is normal.

11. Which of the following best describes your clinical impression at this time?
    a. viral syndrome
    b. meningitis

c. sepsis
d. b and c
e. any of the above

12. Which laboratory testing would you order at this time?
    a. CBC
    b. blood culture
    c. urine culture
    d. lumbar puncture
    e. all of the above

13. Which of the following is the most likely organism that you need to consider in this situation?
    a. *S. pneumoniae*
    b. *H. influenzae*
    c. *Neisseria meningitidis*
    d. *M. pneumoniae*
    e. *Listeria monocytogenes*

14. Which one of the following antibiotics would you consider in the treatment of this condition?
    a. Fortaz
    b. Rocephin
    c. Unasyn
    d. Zithromax
    e. Tequinol

15. What would you do next concerning this patient?
    a. immediate hospitalization
    b. outpatient antibiotics
    c. symptomatic treatment with analgesics and antipyretics only
    d. blood and urine cultures with outpatient follow-up in 24 hours
    e. all of the above

■ CLINICAL CASE MANAGEMENT PROBLEM

Describe a reasonable approach to the diagnosis and management of a fever without a focus in a 1-year-old infant.

■ **ANSWERS:**

1. **d.** This child has a fever of unknown origin. Most FUOs are the result of atypical presentation of common illnesses. A thorough evaluation, including history, physical examination, and selected tests, will reveal the etiology in most cases. Fever without localizing signs and symptoms is a common diagnostic dilemma

for physicians caring for children younger than age 2 years. The classic definition of FUO is a fever of 38° C or higher for more than 3 weeks with no diagnosis after three outpatient visits or 3 days in the hospital.

In contrast, fever without focus is usually of acute onset and presents for less than 1 week.

PFAFA syndrome is characterized by periodic episodes of high fever (39° C) lasting 3-6 days and recurring every 21 days, accompanied by aphthous stomatitis, pharyngitis, and cervical adenopathy. The cause of PFAFA is unknown, although viral and autoimmune mechanisms have been postulated. This is by far the most common cause of predictable recurrent fevers with regular intervals.

2. d. The next step is to obtain a more detailed history, including the fever itself (remittent, intermittent, hectic, or sustained) and a history of exposure to infective agents such as siblings, pets, or chemicals.

3. d. See Answer 1.

4. c. Fever without focus is caused by occult bacteremia until proved otherwise.

5. c. The diagnosis of FUO rarely is made with screening laboratory tests. Screening labs may direct further investigations. The suspicion of a presence of occult bacteremia depends in part on the value of the WBC. This is the most appropriate next step in the workup for infants who are 3-24 months of age.

6. c. The most common organism causing occult bacteremia in children is *S. pneumoniae*. This organism is responsible for approximately 65% of cases of occult bacteremia. *H. influenzae* is the second-leading cause with approximately 25%. *N. meningitides*, *Listeria monocytogenes*, and group B streptococcus account for the remaining 10%.

7. a. The other choices cause recurrent fevers at irregular intervals. PFAFA is the only one that causes recurrent fevers at regular intervals.

8. c. The most common condition in infants and children associated with occult bacteremia is otitis media. This most commonly is caused by *S. pneumoniae*, followed by *H. influenzae* type b.

S. pneumoniae also causes pneumonia and meningitis in infants and children.

9. d. The use of presumptive or prophylactic antibiotics in the prevention of morbidity or mortality associated with bacteremia is controversial. Although oral antibiotics may retard the emergence of some less serious focal bacterial disease (strep throat, otitis media, and pneumonia), they do not reliably prevent meningitis. There is no evidence that the sooner a presumptive antibiotic is used, the greater it will affect morbidity and mortality from any disease.

10. d. The probability of occult bacteremia is decreased if any of the following criteria are met: (1) temperature of less than 39° C; (2) WBC 5000-15,000 cells/mm^3; and (3) negative exposure history.

11. b. A prodromal respiratory illness or sore throat often precedes the fever, headache, stiff neck, and vomiting that characterizes acute meningitis. In infants between the ages of 3-24 months symptoms and signs are less predictable. There are some red flags in this presentation that should alarm the physician. There are no localizing signs for an infection. The rash is suspect because it could be secondary to septicemia.

12. e. All the above.

13. a. Although all of these organisms can cause meningitis. *S. pneumoniae* is still the leading cause in this age group.

14. b. A third generation cephalosporin usually is added because it is highly effective against common meningeal pathogens in patients of all ages. However, in areas of high pneumococcal resistance, vancomycin with or without rifampin should be added. In newborns ampicillin usually is added to cover *Listeria* and gentamicin may be added to expand the gram-negative coverage. These patterns of treatment are changing continually based on resistance in the community and availability of newer antibiotics. For example, Levaquin is a newer antibiotic that has a very broad range of coverage including gram-positive/negative anaerobic and atypical organisms. The dilemma is that inappropriate or overuse of these antibiotics also has led to increased resistance within the community.

15. a. This child requires immediate hospitalization for a septic workup including a lumbar puncture and intravenous antibiotics. Meningitis is a very insidious disease and can be rapidly fatal if treatment is not instituted immediately.

SOLUTION TO THE CLINICAL CASE MANAGEMENT PROBLEM

A reasonable approach to the diagnosis and management of fever without a focus in a 1-year-old child is as follows:

1. A proper history and physical examination are both sensitive and specific in determining the prevalence of occult bacteremia. Does the child appear ill? If no, then reassure the parent. If yes, then consider this a serious sign and continue investigation. Consider the following in an infant: quality of cry, reaction to parent stimulation, color hydration, and response (talk, smile) to social overtones

2. Remember the risks for occult bacteremia: fever higher than 40° C; WBC <5000 cells/mm^3; WBC >15,000 cells/mm^3; and positive exposure history.

3. Remember the importance of repeated examinations and continuing contact with parents if fever without a focus is diagnosed and the child is allowed to go home.

4. Remember the most common organisms associated with occult bacteremia: *S. pneumoniae, H. influenzae,* group A beta-hemolytic *Streptococcus, N. meningitidis.*

5. Remember the most common conditions associated with occult bacteremia: otitis media, bacterial pneumonia, streptococcal pharyngitis, and meningitis. Consider the possibility of febrile convulsions if the temperature is >40.0° C.

6. Remember that not all infants with fever have to be treated with antipyretics. Antipyretics do not speed the resolution of the condition. They may, in fact, hide certain symptoms.

7. Remember that symptomatic treatment (tepid sponge baths) may be just as effective as antipyretics.

8. Remember the importance of repeated reassessment of a child with fever without a focus until either the fever abates or the condition becomes overt.

9. Remember that if you are going to use an antipyretic to treat a child with a fever without a focus, the preferred agent is acetaminophen or ibuprofen.

10. Remember that blood cultures should be obtained before the increase in temperature.

SUMMARY OF FEVER

The Solution to the Clinical Case Management Problem adequately summarizes this chapter.

SUGGESTED READING

Mourad O, et al: A comprehensive evidence-based approach to fever of unknown origin. *Arch Intern Med* 165(5):545-551, 2003.

Titus MO, Wright SW: Prevalence of serious bacterial infections in febrile infants with respiratory syncytial virus infection. *Pediatrics* 112(2):282-284, 2003.

Chapter 106

Gastroenteritis

"Why don't you want to use an antibiotic for my child's tummy ache?"

CLINICAL CASE PROBLEM 1:

An 18-Month-Old Infant with Diarrhea

A mother comes to your office with her 18-month-old infant son who has had diarrhea for the past 5 days. When asked about the diarrhea, the mother states that the infant has "six to eight loose bowel movements every day." There has been no blood in the stools. The infant has a mild fever (38.5° C) and appears to have some abdominal discomfort. The child vomited several times in the first 3 days of the illness, but this has subsided. The infant has two siblings; neither one of them has any abnormal symptoms.

On physical examination, the child is active and does not appear to be significantly dehydrated. Examination results of the ears, throat, lungs, and abdomen are normal. There are no abdominal masses and no tenderness.

SELECT THE BEST ANSWER TO THE FOLLOWING QUESTIONS:

1. What is the most likely cause of this infant's diarrhea?
   a. Norwalk agent
   b. rotavirus
   c. coxsackievirus
   d. echovirus
   e. *Shigella*

2. What is the treatment of choice in this infant at this time?
   a. admission to the hospital for intravenous (IV) therapy
   b. observation in the hospital and oral rehydration therapy
   c. treatment at home with fluids including fruit juices and noncarbonated beverages
   d. treatment at home with an oral rehydrating solution
   e. none of the above

3. Which of the following statement(s) regarding the infection caused by the agent identified in response to Question 1 is (are) true?
   a. upper-respiratory tract symptoms frequently precede the gastrointestinal symptoms
   b. it is the cause for hospitalization in up to 60% of children with diarrhea worldwide
   c. it is seen most commonly in summer months
   d. a and b
   e. frequent complications include meningitis and osteomyelitis

4. Which of the following represents the composition of an ideal rehydrating solution for moderate dehydration (all numbers are represented in mEq/L except CHO, which is given in g/dL)?
   a. Na^+, 23; K^+, 53; Cl^-, 15; CHO, 3.0
   b. Na^+, 40; K^+, 10; Cl^-, 20; CHO, 3.0
   c. Na^+, 90; K^+, 20; Cl^-, 80; CHO, 2.0
   d. Na^+, 140; K^+, 50; Cl^-, 80; CHO, 5.0
   e. Na^+, 100; K^+, 40; Cl^-, 100; CHO, 7.5

5. What is the most common bacterial cause of diarrhea in children?
   a. *Salmonella*
   b. *Shigella*
   c. *Campylobacter*
   d. *Escherichia coli*
   e. *Enterococcus*

6. Which of the following infectious agents may produce bloody diarrhea in infants and children?
   a. *Shigella*
   b. *Salmonella*
   c. enteroinvasive *E. coli*
   d. *Enterococcus*
   e. a, b, and c
   f. all of the above

7. Which of the following statements about enterohemorrhagic *E. coli* O157:H7 is false?
   a. infection is transmitted by undercooked ground beef, unpasteurized milk, and other vehicles contaminated with bovine feces
   b. outbreaks have been linked to contaminated apple cider, raw vegetables, and drinking water
   c. person-to-person transmission is uncommon in outbreaks
   d. the dose necessary to cause infection is low
   e. hemolytic uremic syndrome is a serious complication of infection

8. What is the most common cause of antibiotic-associated diarrhea in infants and children?
   a. ampicillin
   b. clindamycin
   c. erythromycin
   d. penicillin
   e. none of the above

CLINICAL CASE PROBLEM 2:
A 23-MONTH-OLD INFANT WITH SUNKEN EYEBALLS AND DOUGHY SKIN

An infant, age 23 months, is brought to the emergency department by his mother. He has had diarrhea and vomiting for the past 3 days and appears to be at least 15% dehydrated. His eyeballs are sunken, and his skin is doughy. The child has no satisfactory veins in which to place an IV line.

9. What should you do now?
   a. attempt oral rehydration therapy
   b. perform a venous cutdown in the ankle
   c. begin an interosseous infusion
   d. begin a subcutaneous infusion
   e. any one of the above

10. Which of the following investigations should not be performed on any child who has ongoing diarrhea and severe dehydration?
    a. urine-specific gravity
    b. stool evaluation for blood
    c. stool evaluation for fecal leukocytes
    d. stool cultures
    e. serum electrolytes

CLINICAL CASE PROBLEM 3:
A 3-YEAR-OLD MALE WITH DIARRHEA WHO HAD BEEN CAMPING

A mother comes to your office with her 3-year-old boy who has developed severe crampy diarrhea and mild fever. The family has just returned from a camping trip in the Rocky Mountains; the child became sick on the third day. He was apparently drinking water from the local stream.

11. What is the most likely diagnosis in this patient?
   a. viral gastroenteritis
   b. *Shigella* gastroenteritis
   c. *Salmonella* gastroenteritis
   d. giardiasis
   e. amebiasis

12. Which of the following pediatric infections often present(s) with diarrhea as the initial symptoms?
   a. acute appendicitis
   b. otitis media
   c. urinary tract infections
   d. pneumonia
   e. all of the above

13. Which of the following is the most common cause of acute abdominal pain in children?
   a. constipation
   b. intussusception
   c. volvulus
   d. gastroenteritis
   e. mesenteric lymphadenitis

14. All of the following factors are associated with an increased risk of gastroenteritis except:
   a. daycare attendance
   b. recent antibiotic use
   c. winter and summer months
   d. age older than 5 years
   e. poor sanitation

CLINICAL CASE MANAGEMENT PROBLEM

Discuss the most common cause of childhood death from gastroenteritis (worldwide). Comment on community health aspects of this condition.

ANSWERS:

1. **b.** The most common cause of childhood gastroenteritis is rotavirus. Symptoms of rotavirus infection include low-grade fever, anorexia, nausea, vomiting, diarrhea, and abdominal cramps. Dehydration may occur. The disease typically runs its course in a 4- to 10-day time frame.

Other causes of viral diarrhea in children include the following: (1) parvoviruses such as the Norwalk agent; (2) coxsackievirus; (3) echovirus; (4) adenovirus; and (5) calicivirus.

2. d. Because this child does not appear to be significantly dehydrated, hospitalization is not required. The treatment of choice is home oral rehydration therapy. Fruit juices (undiluted) and commercial beverages are not recommended because of high osmolarity and the danger of hypernatremia or exacerbation of stool losses.

Details of oral rehydrating solutions are discussed in Answer 4.

3. d. Viruses are the most common cause of wintertime diarrhea in infants. Rotavirus, as mentioned previously, is the most common agent. It is responsible for more than 50% of cases of acute diarrhea in children and accounts for 20% to 60% of hospitalization for children with diarrhea worldwide. The other viral causes are listed in Answer 1. The majority of infants and children who develop rotavirus develop an upper-respiratory tract infection preceding the gastrointestinal symptoms. The respiratory tract symptoms include rhinorrhea, cough, pharyngeal erythema, and otitis media. Dehydration is the most common complication. Meningitis and osteomyelitis are infrequent complications that can occur with bacterial causes of gastroenteritis such as shigella, salmonella, and *E. coli*.

4. c. Oral rehydration therapy effectively resolves most cases of pediatric gastroenteritis.

The World Health Organization-recommended standard for oral rehydration therapy is Na^+ 90 mEq/L, K^+ 20 mEq/L, Cl^- 80 mEq/L, HCO_3^- 30 mEq/L, and CHO 2 g/dL.

Among the common oral rehydration solutions used, Rehydralyte has the closest composition to the World Health Organization's formula. Pedialyte is less ideal because it contains only 45 mEq/L of sodium instead of 90 mEq/L. Although these solutions are best suited as maintenance solutions, they can satisfactorily rehydrate children who are mildly or moderately dehydrated.

Clear liquids should not be given to infants with diarrhea because they have a low sodium content, a low potassium content, and a high carbohydrate content. Examples of clear liquids include apple juice, carbonated beverages, and sports beverages.

5. c. The most common cause of bacterial gastroenteritis in both children and adults is *Campylobacter jejuni*.

Campylobacter gastroenteritis typically begins with fever and malaise, followed by nausea, vomiting, diarrhea, and abdominal pain. The diarrhea is often profuse and may contain blood. The illness is self-limited, lasting less than 1 week in 60% of cases. Recurrences and chronic symptoms can occur, especially in infants.

Symptoms caused by *C. jejuni* usually occur as a result of endotoxin production. Invasive strains also occur and produce disease. *Campylobacter* is treated effectively with erythromycin, although the infection is usually self-limiting and clears up when left untreated.

6. e. *Salmonella* gastroenteritis begins with watery diarrhea and is accompanied by fever and nausea. As with *Campylobacter*, *Salmonella* produces disease both by mucosal invasion and endotoxin production, and the diarrhea may be bloody. Most cases of *Salmonella* gastroenteritis do not require antibiotic therapy.

Shigella gastroenteritis begins with watery diarrhea, high fever, and malaise; this usually is followed in 24 hours by tenesmus and frank dysentery. Mucosal invasion with frank ulceration and hemorrhage often occur. Dehydration is common. *Shigella* gastroenteritis should be treated with trimethoprim–sulfamethoxazole.

E. coli gastroenteritis may occur as an enteropathic infection, an enterohemorrhagic infection, an enterotoxigenic infection, or an enteroinvasive infection. Enteropathic *E. coli* usually produces a mild self-limited illness. Enterohemorrhagic *E. coli* produces diarrhea that is initially watery and later becomes bloody. Enterotoxigenic *E. coli* is the most common cause of traveler's diarrhea. Enteroinvasive *E. coli* invades the mucosa and produces a dysenterylike illness with bloody stool.

In infants and children, *Yersinia enterocolitica* may produce acute and chronic gastroenteritis and mesenteric lymphadenitis. Mesenteric lymphadenitis is, at times, extremely difficult to distinguish from acute appendicitis. Diarrhea, fever, and crampy abdominal pain are the most common presenting symptoms. Treatment is symptomatic only; antibiotic therapy is unnecessary.

Enterococcus is not a cause of bacterial gastroenteritis in children.

7. c. *E. coli* O157:H7 infections in the United States have become more common. Outbreaks have been linked to contaminated water, apple cider, salami, yogurt, undercooked beef, and raw vegetables. Person-to-person transmission is high during outbreaks, and the infectious dose is low (about 100 organisms). Enterohemorrhagic *E. coli* infection can progress to hemolytic uremic syndrome (especially O157:H7).

Enteropathic *E. coli* infection is seen primarily in infants. Enterotoxigenic *E. coli* infection is usually brief and self-limited. This is the most common cause of traveler's diarrhea.

8. a. The most common cause of antibiotic-associated diarrhea is ampicillin. Ampicillin and other antibiotic-associated diarrheas are common and generally self-limiting. Most cases resolve on discontinuation of the drug. However, on occasion a pseudomembranous colitis may develop because of an overgrowth of *Clostridium difficile* or release of its toxin. The prognosis of severe *C. difficile*–induced pseudomembranous colitis cases is poor with a 20% to 30% fatality rate and a 10% to 20% relapse rate. Treatment of severe cases consists of oral vancomycin or metronidazole.

9. c. In a young infant or child who presents with severe dehydration, it is often very difficult to establish good IV access. A skull vein is a possibility, but even that is difficult. An excellent alternative is an interosseous infusion (usually placed in the tibia). A large bore needle is used after local anesthesia has been infiltrated around the bone. This allows easy access and affords an excellent alternative to venous access.

10. d. The investigations that should be performed on all children who have ongoing diarrhea include urine-specific gravity, stool analysis for blood, and stool analysis for fecal leukocytes. A urine-specific gravity of less than 1.015 suggests adequate hydration.

If a patient presents with bloody diarrhea, high fever, persistent symptoms, tenesmus, or a history of foreign travel, a stool culture and examination of the stool for ova and parasites should be performed. Routine stool culture, however, is not cost-effective.

Other investigations that should be considered in a toxic child include complete blood count, serum electrolytes, and serum osmolality.

11. d. Gastroenteritis that begins while camping in the Rocky Mountains most likely is caused by giardiasis. Giardiasis needs a very low "organism load" to produce a very painful gastroenteritis. Giardiasis is the most common parasitic cause of gastroenteritis; however, parasitic infections in total only account for less than 10% of all cases of gastroenteritis. The recommended treatment is metronidazole and rehydration.

12. e. Many nonenteric infections may produce diarrhea as the first and most prominent symptom. These include otitis media, urinary tract infection, acute appendicitis (from inflammation extending to involve the ureter on the right side of the body), lower lobe pneumonia, and mesenteric lymphadenitis (*Y. enterocolitica*).

13. d. The most common medical cause of abdominal pain in children is gastroenteritis. The most common surgical cause is appendicitis. Intussusception and volvulus are not common; however, intussusception is the most common cause of bowel obstruction in childhood. Patients often will have emesis and bloody stool, but only about 50% will have the characteristic "currant-jelly" stool. Although constipation is common, it does not most commonly present as acute abdominal pain. Mesenteric lymphadenitis often presents similar to appendicitis and can be caused by *Yersinia enterocolitica* and pseudotuberculosis and *Giardia lamblia*.

14. d. Gastroenteritis risk is increased with travel to underdeveloped countries, exposure to untreated drinking water, daycare center attendance, recent antibiotic treatment, and contact with animals. There is no predominate age in gastroenteritis because it occurs in all ages. Disease manifestation, however, may differ across ages depending on etiologic agent.

SOLUTION TO THE CLINICAL CASE MANAGEMENT PROBLEM

The most common cause of gastroenteritis-produced death in infants and children is cholera. Cholera is both endemic and epidemic, and both have a seasonal pattern. Contaminated water is the major source of infectivity and transmission, and cholera becomes an epidemic when crowded conditions such as refugee camps are established.

The responsible organism is *Vibrio cholerae*. The resulting illness is sudden in onset and produces severe rice-water diarrhea and severe dehydration that can lead to death quickly. Most cases can be treated effectively by oral rehydration with a balanced electrolyte solution.

SUMMARY OF GASTROENTERITIS

1. **Prevalence:** During the first 3 years of life a child experiences an estimated one to three acute, severe episodes of diarrhea.
2. Most common causes are as follows:
   a. Rotavirus is the most common cause (50%). Rotavirus gastroenteritis usually is preceded by upper-respiratory tract symptoms.
   b. *C. jejuni* is the most common bacterial cause.
   c. Other viral agents producing gastroenteritis include the following: (i) Norwalk agent (parvovirus); (ii) coxsackievirus; (iii) echovirus; (iv) adenovirus; (v) calicivirus; and (vi) astrovirus.
   d. Other bacterial agents include the following: (i) *Salmonella;* (ii) *Shigella;* (iii) *Yersinia;* and (iv) *E. coli*.
   e. Parasites include the following: (i) giardiasis ("beaver fever") most common and (ii) amebiasis
3. **Diagnosis:** Routine laboratory testing is not necessary in most children. All children who are severely dehydrated or who have failed oral replacement therapy should be evaluated by having a complete urinalysis performed, including urine-specific gravity and a stool examination for blood and fecal leukocytes. Specific gravity of 1.015 or less suggests adequate hydration.

If bloody diarrhea, persistent symptoms, fever, tenesmus, or recent foreign travel are present, a stool culture for ova and parasites should be done. In mild and self-limiting diarrhea, a stool culture is not cost-effective.
4. **Treatment:** Most children can be managed by oral rehydration therapy using a solution containing Na^+ 90 mEq/L; K^+ 20 mEq/L; Cl^- 80 mEq/L; HCO_3^- 30 mEq/L; and carbohydrate 2.0 g/dL.

Antibiotic therapy should be initiated for *Shigella* (trimethoprim–sulfamethoxazole) and *C. jejuni* (erythromycin).

SUGGESTED READING

Burkhart D: Management of acute gastroenteritis in children. *Am Fam Physician* 60:2555-2561, 1999.

Guarino A, et al: Working Group on Acute Gastroenteritis. Oral rehydration: toward a real solution. *J Pediatr Gastroenterol Nutr* 33 Suppl 2:S2-12, 2001 Oct.

Jiang X, Pickering LK: Update on caliciviruses and human acute gastroenteritis. *Pediatr Infect Dis J* 21(11):1069-1070, 2002 Nov.

Leung A, Sigalet D: Acute abdominal pain in children. *Am Fam Physician* 67:2321-2331, 2003.

Mitchell DK: Astrovirus gastroenteritis. *Infect Dis J* 21(11):1067-1069, 2002 Nov.

Pickering L, Snyder J: Gastroenteritis. In: Behrman RE, et al, eds. *Nelson textbook of pediatrics* 16th ed. WB Saunders, 2000. Philadelphia.

Report of the Committee on Infectious Diseases. *AAP 2000 Red Book*, 25th ed. www.cdc.gov/

Walter JE, Mitchell DK: Astrovirus infection in children. *Curr Opin Infect Dis* 16(3):247-253, 2003 Jun.

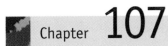

Chapter 107

Recurrent Abdominal Pain

> "I just can't go to school.
> My tummy aches again."

CLINICAL CASE PROBLEM 1:
A 12-Year-Old Female with Recurrent Abdominal Pain

A 12-year-old female is brought to your office with a history of recurring abdominal pain. She is having episodes of abdominal pain once or twice a week. These episodes last approximately 8 hours. She has been seen on many occasions for the same problem and has been investigated completely. The investigations have included a complete blood count (CBC); urinalysis; stool for ova and parasites; an ultrasound of the kidneys, ureter, and bladder; and an abdominal plain film. All investigations were normal. The pain is described as umbilical in location with a quality described as a "dull ache." She rates the pain at a baseline quantity of 6/10, with increases to 8/10 and decreases to 4/10. It is not associated with any food intake, and it is not associated with any diarrhea or constipation.

On physical examination, the young girl is in no apparent distress. Her vital signs, height, and weight are normal for her age. On examination of the abdomen, there is slight tenderness in the area of the periumbilical region. There is no hepatosplenomegaly and no other masses.

SELECT THE BEST ANSWER TO THE FOLLOWING QUESTIONS:

1. What is the most likely diagnosis in this patient?
   a. recurrent abdominal pain (RAP) syndrome
   b. lactose intolerance
   c. Crohn's disease
   d. mesenteric lymphadenitis
   e. chronic appendicitis

2. What is the prevalence of this condition in children?
   a. 1%
   b. 5%
   c. 10%
   d. 20%
   e. 25%

3. Regarding the physiologic basis for the pain that occurs in the condition described in Clinical Case Problem 1, which of the following statements is (are) true?
   a. the pain can be conceptualized as a disorder that provokes pain pathways
   b. the pain can be conceptualized as an alteration in the patient's threshold to pain
   c. there is evidence that an abnormality in the autonomic nervous system is involved in this condition
   d. there is evidence that intestinal motility can be affected along with the occurrence of hyperalgesia
   e. all of the above statements are true

4. Which of the following statements regarding school attendance and the condition described in Clinical Case Problem 1 is true?
   a. there is no association between school attendance and the condition described
   b. school phobia (reluctance to attend school) may be an important contributing factor in many cases of this condition
   c. children with this condition usually achieve higher marks than their counterparts without this condition
   d. there is no association between stressful events at school and this condition
   e. none of the above statements are true

5. Which of the following investigations should be reordered in the patient described in Clinical Case Problem 1 at this time?
   a. urinalysis
   b. CBC
   c. kidneys, ureter, and bladder (KUB) x-ray
   d. abdominal ultrasound
   e. none of the above

6. Which of the following organisms has been commonly associated with organic recurring abdominal pain in children?
   a. enterotoxigenic *Escherichia coli*
   b. enteropathogenic *E. coli*
   c. *Giardia lamblia*
   d. *Entamoeba histolytica*
   e. *Salmonella*

7. Which of the following is the treatment of choice for the condition described?
   a. muscle relaxants
   b. tricyclic antidepressants
   c. narcotic analgesics
   d. nonsteroidal antiinflammatory drugs
   e. none of the above

CLINICAL CASE MANAGEMENT PROBLEM

List nine frequent causes of acute abdominal pain for each of the following: (1) infancy (<2 years); (2) preschool (age 2-5 years); (3) school age (5-10 years); and (4) adolescence (11-15 years).

ANSWERS:

1. a. The most likely diagnosis in this patient is RAP syndrome. The signs and symptoms of RAP syndrome are marked by their lack of specificity. The crucial separation of organic from nonorganic pain can be based on a few important findings, including the specificity and consistency of the pain and the relationship of the pain to meals and movement. The patient with nonspecific RAP tends to look well, to have pain that is inconsistent in relationship to meals and to movement, and to be free of the occurrence of additional symptoms such as nausea, vomiting, or dysuria. In some 10% to 15% of cases of RAP, there lurks an underlying organic etiology; most cases are said to be "functional."

Lactose intolerance often is confused with RAP syndrome in childhood and with irritable bowel syndrome in adults. In fact, these two syndromes can coexist. Lactose intolerance usually is associated with flatus and diarrhea. Crohn's disease and mesenteric lymphadenitis usually are associated with systemic symptoms. The lack of systemic symptoms in this patient is strong evidence against these diagnoses. Chronic appendicitis, if it exists, is more likely to be associated with pain in the right lower quadrant and with nausea and vomiting.

2. c. The prevalence of RAP syndrome in childhood is 10%. RAP affects males and females equally until age 9 years, after which time females have a slightly higher incidence. The overall incidence of RAP peaks between the ages 10 to 12. RAP is virtually nonexistent in those younger than age 5, and an organic cause should be considered likely in this age group.

3. e. There are many theories related to RAP syndrome in children. Pain in children is conceptualized as a disorder that provokes pain pathways or an alteration in the patient's threshold to pain. A widely held plausible explanation in these cases is some abnormality in the functioning of the autonomic nervous system. This is thought to result in altered intestinal motility and the occurrence of hyperalgesia and altered secretory pathways.

There are some clear warning signs and symptoms that should raise the likelihood of underlying organic disease. Complaint of localizing pain, pain associated with change in bowel habits, repeated vomiting, altered vital signs, anorexia or weakness, and RAP syndrome occurring in a child younger than age 4 years should be investigated vigorously. Constitutional signs of weight loss, growth restriction or cessation, organomegaly and localized tenderness, hernias, or swelling similarly should be pursued.

4. b. School phobia (reluctance to attend school) may be an important contributing factor in many cases of RAP syndrome in childhood. There is a significant association between stressful events at school and RAP syndrome. Children with this condition, on average, achieve lower grades than their cohorts without this condition. This actually may be more associated with diminished school attendance than anything else. There is a significant association between stressful events at school and exacerbations of this condition.

5. e. Because this child already has had numerous investigations, including all of the investigations described in Question 5, it is pointless to repeat them unless her condition is markedly different from previous episodes. Because the possible mechanisms associated with abdominal pain are so numerous and not completely understood, the investigation and treatment of these cases of RAP in childhood test not only the physician's scientific acumen but also their skill in the practice of the art of medicine. There is a great temptation to "overdo" the testing and treatment when reliance on a careful clinical evaluation is the most important first step toward resolving the problem. Recall that in only 10% of cases of RAP syndrome is an organic cause found. Therefore, in most cases, investigations can be limited to a CBC, urinalysis, stool specimen for occult blood, white cells, culture, and ova and parasite examination. A flat plate of the abdomen can define significant constipation if this is suspected by history or examination, and abdominal ultrasonography may be of use for diagnosing renal, gynecologic, or cystic etiologies.

6. c. *Giardia lamblia* is sometimes the cause of a recurrent pain syndrome in children. Thus every child with recurrent pain should have an examination of the stool for ova and parasites.

7. e. Treatment for RAP syndrome in childhood should not be based on pharmacotherapy, especially pharmacotherapy that may do more harm than good. Therapy should emphasize the patient's response to the pain. In most cases, these efforts should involve the parents.

First, the patient and parents need to be reassured that the problem is not life threatening. Second, the physician should be realistic and frank and warn the patient and family that the problem may persist for an extended period. As mentioned, the physician should avoid prescribing medications and other therapies that may be harmful. Sedatives, antispasmodics, and analgesics are not only not beneficial but actually also harmful. These agents, in addition to having potentially deleterious effects on the intestinal motility and appetite, also may create dependency.

Laxatives and, at times, enemas may be beneficial when there is some evidence of retained stool or, in difficult cases, even a suspicion of constipation. General measures such as the promotion of full activity and a sense of normal health are extremely important. A well-balanced diet that is not excessive in fiber content and adequate fluid intake are recommended. A systematic review of evidence of efficacy found usefulness in therapies that use famotidine, pizotifen, cognitive–behavioral therapy, biofeedback, and peppermint oil enteric-coated capsules. Improvement is greater when therapy targets specific functional gastrointestinal disorders (e.g., dyspepsia, irritable bowel syndrome). Behavioral interventions also have a positive effect in RAP. Although many of these therapies have not been widely used, and in many cases the mechanism of action is not understood, each is believed to be safe.

Every attempt should be made to maintain school attendance. In some otherwise physically well patients, a cycle of emotional turmoil, school absenteeism, and pain evolve. Identifying the stressors and breaking the cycle by ongoing counseling is the most important first step. The prognosis for children with RAP is unclear. There is certainly no increased risk of intra-abdominal disease, and in most cases symptoms improve before the age of 20 years. Some children with RAP syndrome do, however, go on to develop an irritable bowel syndrome as adults.

SOLUTION TO THE CLINICAL CASE MANAGEMENT PROBLEM

Nine frequent causes of acute abdominal pain in infancy, preschool, school age, and adolescence are listed in the table.

Additional causes for all ages include mesenteric lymphadenitis, tumor, pneumonia, constipation, sickling syndrome, cystic fibrosis, diabetes mellitus, and celiac disease.

Infancy	Preschool	School Age	Adolescence
Colic	Gastroenteritis	Gastroenteritis	Gastroenteritis
Gastroenteritis	Urinary tract infection	Urinary tract infection	Urinary tract infection
Milk intolerance	Trauma	Appendicitis	Appendicitis
Intussusception	Intussusception/constipation	Recurrent abdominal pain syndrome	Pelvic inflammatory disease/dysmenorrhea
Urinary tract infection	Henoch-Schönlein purpura/Sickle-cell disease	Inflammatory bowel disease	Inflammatory bowel disease
Trauma/abuse	Appendicitis	Ingestions	Peptic ulcer disease
Volvulus/intestinal anomaly (Meckel's)	Hemolytic uremic syndrome	Gonadal torsion	Ingestion
Incarcerated hernia	Lead and other ingestions	Lactose intolerance	Gonadal torsion
Other	Ketoacidosis	Wilms' tumor	Pregnancy

SUMMARY OF RECURRENT ABDOMINAL PAIN

1. The diagnosis of RAP syndrome in childhood usually can be made from the history and physical examination, supplemented with a few investigations including CBC, urinalysis, erythrocyte sedimentation rate, stool for ova and parasites, occult blood, KUB x-ray, and abdominal ultrasound.

2. RAP in childhood is common; the prevalence is estimated at 10%, both sexes are equally affected, and peak incidence is at ages 10-12 years.

Continued

SUMMARY OF RECURRENT ABDOMINAL PAIN—cont'd

3. Do not overinvestigate or overtreat patients with RAP in childhood. The vast majority of cases (85% to 90%) are nonorganic in origin.
4. Treatment should be supportive and should consist of reestablishing a healthy lifestyle, eating a well-balanced diet, exercising daily, and avoiding stress (especially at school).
5. There is a strong association between school phobia (school avoidance) and RAP syndrome. Take a careful history of school performance, school fears, and general feelings about attending school.

SUGGESTED READING

Leung AK: Acute abdominal pain in children. *Am Fam Phys* 67(11): 2321-2323, 2003.
Thiessen PN: Recurrent abdominal pain. *Pediatr Rev* 23(2):39-46, 2002.
Weydert JA: Systematic review of treatments for recurrent abdominal pain. *Pediatrics* 11(1):e1-11, 2003.
Zeiter DK: Recurrent abdominal pain in children. *Pediatr Clin North Am* 49(1):53-71, 2002.

 Chapter **108**

The Limping Child

> "Mom! Can you rub my legs? They hurt so much."

CLINICAL CASE PROBLEM 1:
A 9-Year-Old Male with Leg Pain

A 9-year-old boy comes to your office with his mother. He complains of a recurrent (nightly) pain in both legs. The pain is so severe that it wakes him from sleep. It is described as a "deep pain." The pain is bilateral and usually is gone by morning. There is no associated fever, chills, limp, or other symptoms. There is no pain during the day.

His history has been excellent. He has had no significant medical illnesses. On examination, the child has no limp and no leg-length discrepancy.

SELECT THE BEST ANSWER TO THE FOLLOWING QUESTIONS:

1. What is the most likely diagnosis in this child?
   a. slipped capital femoral epiphysis (SCFE)
   b. Legg-Calve-Perthes disease
   c. osteogenic sarcoma
   d. Ewing's sarcoma
   e. "growing pains"

2. What is the preferred treatment for this condition?
   a. surgical fixation
   b. bracing or traction
   c. amputation
   d. radiotherapy followed by chemotherapy
   e. none of the above

3. Regarding limb pain in children, which of the following statements is (are) true?
   a. limb pain is a common presenting complaint in children
   b. there is significant association between limb pain, headache, and abdominal pain
   c. there is frequently an association between limb pain in children and pain of other types in family members
   d. there is frequently an emotional component to limb pain in children
   e. all of the above statements are true

4. The following criteria describe which of the following childhood orthopedic conditions listed: (1) The condition occurs as a result of acute trauma or in a more subtle fashion over time; (2) The typical patient is a somewhat overweight and sedentary teenage boy; (3) Pain is located either in the groin or on the medial side of the knee; (4) The hip is held in abduction and external rotation, and there is marked limitation of internal rotation; and (5) Diagnosis is made by x-ray.
   The possible conditions are:
   a. SCFE
   b. Legg-Calve-Perthes disease
   c. osteogenic sarcoma
   d. Ewing's sarcoma
   e. "growing pains"

5. What is the preferred treatment for the condition chosen in response to Question 4?

a. surgical fixation
b. bracing or traction
c. amputation
d. radiotherapy followed by chemotherapy
e. none of the above

6. The following criteria describe which of the orthopedic conditions listed?
   Criteria: (1) It is also known as *avascular necrosis* of the femoral head; (2) it is found mainly in children younger than age 10 years; (3) it is suggested by pain in the area of the hip or knee; (4) demonstration of a limp and a decreased range of motion on physical examination is most likely.
   Possible Conditions:
   a. SCFE
   b. Legg-Calve-Perthes disease
   c. femoral head abnormality
   d. hypermobile femur
   e. none of the above

7. What is the preferred treatment for the condition described in Question 6?
   a. surgical fixation
   b. bracing or traction
   c. casting
   d. any of the above may be indicated, depending on the case
   e. none of the above are indicated

8. The following criteria describe which of the following orthopedic conditions listed?
   Criteria: (1) There is localized tenderness and swelling present over the tibial tubercle, (2) the pain is aggravated by running, jumping, going up and down stairs, and kneeling; (3) the condition is an overuse syndrome that occurs commonly in physically active males around puberty, and (4) Significant athletic activity and a recent growth spurt may result in detachment of cartilage fragments from the tibial tuberosity.
   Possible Conditions:
   a. chondromalacia
   b. osteochondritis dissecans
   c. Osgood-Schlatter disease
   d. patellofemoral syndrome
   e. lateral diskitis

9. What is the preferred treatment for the condition described in Question 8?
   a. surgical removal
   b. casting
   c. bracing or traction
   d. splinting
   e. none of the above

10. The following criteria describe which of the following orthopedic conditions?
    Criteria: (1) The condition is characterized by subchondral bone necrosis and complete or partial separation of articular fragments; (2) the condition usually is caused by repeated trauma to a segment of the bone with tenuous vascularity; (3) The clinical manifestations may include episodic knee pain, aching after exercise, stiffness, clicking, muscle atrophy, mild joint swelling, and occasional locking; and (4) the demarcated fragments of subchondral bone are best demonstrated radiographically by a "notch view" of the knee.
    Conditions:
    a. chondromalacia
    b. osteochondritis dissecans
    c. Osgood-Schlatter disease
    d. patellofemoral syndrome
    e. lateral diskitis

11. What is the usual preferred treatment for the condition described in Question 10?
    a. surgical removal
    b. casting
    c. bracing and/or traction
    d. splinting
    e. none of the above

CLINICAL CASE PROBLEM 2:

A 13-Year-Old Female with Pain and a Grating Sensation in Her Knee

A 13-year-old female, a star on the junior high school basketball team, comes to your office with left anterior knee pain and a grating sensation aggravated by activities involving knee flexion such as climbing stairs and running.

On physical examination, you ask the patient to extend her knee while you compress the patella against the femoral condyle. The patient refuses to extend the femoral condyle because of pain.

12. What is the most likely diagnosis?
    a. patellofemoral syndrome
    b. osteochondritis dissecans
    c. Osgood-Schlatter disease
    d. soft patella syndrome
    e. none of the above

13. What is the preferred treatment for most cases of this condition?
    a. surgical removal
    b. casting
    c. bracing or traction
    d. splinting
    e. none of the above

14. The following criteria describe which of the following orthopedic conditions?
Criteria: (1) It is the most common cause of non-traumatic limb and hip pain in the 3- to 6-year-old age group; (2) it is characterized as an idiopathic, nonspecific, common, unilateral, inflammatory arthritis involving the hip joint; (3) symptoms of upper-respiratory tract infection often precede hip symptoms in this condition, and (4) this condition is more common in boys than in girls.
Conditions:
a. toxic synovitis
b. Legg-Calve-Perthes disease
c. SCFE
d. septic arthritis
e. osteomyelitis

15. What is the preferred treatment for the condition described in Question 14?
a. surgical decompression
b. casting
c. bracing or traction
d. splinting
e. none of the above

ANSWERS:

1. e. This child has typical "growing pains" or idiopathic limb pain.

Growing pains occur in 15% to 30% of otherwise normal children. It consists of deep pain often in the lower limbs that can be severe enough to wake the child from sleep. The pains occur intermittently, are always bilateral, are poorly localized, and are usually completely gone in the morning. The pains sometimes can be aggravated by heavy exercise during the day, but day pain is never a regular characteristic of growing pains. They can be improved by nonpharmacologic therapies such as heat, massage, and physiotherapy. There is no limp or apparent disability and the cause is unknown.

There is often a psychologic component to growing pains. There seems to be a relationship between limb pain, abdominal pain, and headaches in children and an inherited or environmentally determined link between siblings with pain and parents with pain.

2. e. Treatment consists of reassuring the family about the benign, self-limited course of the condition. Systematic treatment such as heat and an analgesic can be provided. Although avoidance of activities that aggravate the condition should be advised, this must be balanced against the positive benefits of maintaining some type of exercise program. Inform the family that if clinical features change, the child should be brought back to the office for reevaluation.

3. e. Limb pain is a common presenting complaint in primary care practice. It is estimated to account for 5% to 10% of pediatric visits.

With limb pain in childhood, there is frequently an emotional component. There is a relationship between growing pains and headache and abdominal pain in children with these symptoms, who often come from "pain-prone" families. The parents often have had pain as children that sometimes persisted into adulthood. In up to 33% of cases, this "childhood pain syndrome" persists.

4. a. This child has SCFE, the characteristics of which are listed as criteria in Question 4. Physiologically, SCFE occurs before the epiphyseal plate closes and usually at a time before and during the maximal pubertal growth spurt (13-15 years old in males; 11-13 years old in females). This condition is the most common adolescent hip disorder. Obesity is present in 80% of children with this disorder. It is more common in males. In nearly 50% of cases, both hips ultimately will be affected.

5. a. An SCFE is an orthopedic emergency. Immediate hospitalization and operative fixation is indicated. Stabilization of the SCFE is essential if acute or gradual slipping is to be prevented. In severe chronic (and poorly aligned) SCFE, osteotomies are required to realign and stabilize the capital femoral epiphysis. Prompt intervention also is required to minimize avascular necrosis of the femoral head as a result of slippage.

6. b. These criteria describe Legg-Calve-Perthes disease. The major criteria have been listed in Question 6. Legg-Calve-Perthes disease, in pathologic terms, is a juvenile idiopathic avascular necrosis of the femoral head. The cause is unknown, although repeated trauma, variation in the vascularity of the proximal femur, coagulation abnormalities, and other mechanisms have been suggested. An association also has been found between avascular necrosis of the femoral head and multiple courses of systemic steroids.

Legg-Calve-Perthes disease occurs in about 1 of every 750 children. It primarily occurs between the ages of 4 and 10 years and primarily affects boys.

7. d. Legg-Calve-Perthes disease is difficult to treat because of the necessity for long-term treatment and the need to limit activities. The psychologic status of the child during treatment must be monitored. A biopsychosocial approach is often necessary to treat both the psychologic and orthopedic aspects of the problem. Braces and casting may be required for 1-2 years. Surgery, the other option, will allow the child to return to normal activity in 4-6 months.

The prognosis for Legg-Calve-Perthes disease is, at best, fair. In the middle years, approximately 50% of patients go on to develop severe degenerative hip disease and require hip replacement.

8. c. Osgood-Schlatter disease results from overuse of the lower extremity. It is a traction apophysitis of the tibial tubercle resulting from repetitive micro-trauma. Athletic activity with or without a recent growth spurt may lead to cartilage detachment. The diagnosis is made by localizing the point of maximal tenderness over the tibial tuberosity and can be confirmed by x-ray. Very rarely, the patella tendon can pull off of the tibial tubercle, creating a small avulsion fracture of the tibial tubercle.

9. e. The preferred treatment for Osgood-Schlatter disease is a reduction in physical activity as dictated by symptoms. The disease process itself is usually self-limited with complete remission when there is fusion of the tibial tubercle to the diaphysis. Resolution occurs over a period of months.

Local corticosteroid injections should not be used; injections of this nature may weaken the quadriceps tendon and produce local cutaneous thinning and depigmentation.

10. b. Osteochondritis dissecans is a condition characterized by subchondral bone necrosis and, on occasion, by complete or partial separation of the articular fragments.

The most common site for osteochondritis dissecans is the lateral aspect of the medial femoral condyle. It also may occur in the patella and the lateral condyle of the femur.

Males are affected more often than females (3:1), and there appear to be two peaks of incidence: children younger than 12 years of age and young adults.

11. e. In most cases of osteochondritis dissecans the treatment (in the patient with open growth plates) is conservative. Isometric quadriceps exercises, limitation of activities, and time lead to resolution of most lesions. Open arthrotomy or arthroscopic surgery is indicated when the fragments are displaced or greater than 1 cm in diameter or if conservative treatment fails.

12. a. Patellofemoral syndrome is a common cause of anterior knee pain in teenagers. It is an overuse syndrome. Most affected individuals show some degree of patellofemoral malalignment.

The principal symptoms (anterior knee pain and a grating sensation aggravated by activities involving knee flexion, such as climbing stairs or running) are reflected by a tender undersurface on the medial side of the patella and some crepitus.

13. e. The treatment for patellofemoral syndrome includes an active isometric progressive resistance exercise program to strengthen the quadriceps. The goal is to optimize the tracking of the patella in the intercondylar groove of the femur. Concentrating on strengthening of the medial portion of the quadriceps muscles, or the vastus medialis, will help to keep the patella aligned properly. During the acute phase, non-steroidal antiinflammatory drugs may be of benefit. Avoiding squats, excessive stairs, and prolonged sitting will help with symptoms. Braces have not been shown to effectively maintain proper tracking of the patella. In very few cases arthroscopy may be needed to remove bone or cartilaginous fragments, to shave the under-surface of the patella, or to release the lateral reti-nacular tethering structures.

14. a. Toxic, or transient, synovitis is an idiopathic, transient, nonspecific, common, unilateral (5% bilat-eral) inflammatory arthritis involving the hip joint. It principally occurs in children between the ages of 3 and 6 years and is the most common cause of limp with hip pain in this age group.

Toxic synovitis usually follows a viral upper-respiratory infection and begins 3 to 6 days after the respiratory symptoms abate. In addition to guarded hip rotation, there is pain in the hip and pain in the anteromedial aspect of the thigh and knee. There also may be constitutional symptoms. These include a low-grade fever (less than or equal to 38° C [101° F]) and slight elevation of the erythrocyte sedimentation rate (ESR).

Aspirated fluid from the hip joint is clear, and x-ray demonstrates normal hips with an increased space between the medial acetabulum and the ossified femoral head. Because the bones are normal, the prob-ability of aseptic necrosis, osteomyelitis, and other serious conditions is greatly diminished. Ultrasound of the hips usually demonstrates a joint effusion.

Note that it is extremely important to differentiate toxic synovitis from septic arthritis. Unlike toxic synovitis, septic arthritis demonstrates higher fever, malaise, more pronounced spasm, guarding and fixed positioning, and a higher white blood cell count and ESR. Aspirated fluid from the hip joint helps to differentiate, with fluid from septic arthritis usually demonstrating a more turbid color, white blood cell count of greater than 50,000/hpf, and a positive culture in about 33% of cases.

15. e. The preferred treatment for toxic synovitis is conservative, including non–weightbearing on the affected leg, nonsteroidal antiinflammatory medica-tions, and symptomatic treatment. Close follow-up is necessary to continue to distinguish this benign entity from more serious conditions.

SUMMARY OF LIMPING CHILD

1. A child with a limp is a common presentation in family medicine. History and physical examination are critical. A careful observation of gait and preferred position of the affected leg will aid in diagnosis. Frequent follow-up is often critical to reassure that a condition is benign. The most important distinction to make is the difference between urgent and nonurgent conditions. Urgent conditions often require consultation with a specialist and/or hospitalization for treatment. Nonurgent conditions can be reassured, treated with conservative measures, and followed closely.
2. Common causes of childhood limp are as follows:
   a. Urgent: (i) toxic or transient synovitis; (ii) septic arthritis; (iii) osteomyelitis; (iv) Legg-Calve-Perthes disease; (v) slipped capital femoral epiphysis; and (vi) malignancies (uncommon).
   b. Nonurgent: (i) growing pains; (ii) school phobias; (iii) Osgood-Schlatter disease; (iv) osteo-

chondritis dissecans (consultation strongly suggested); (v) chondromalacia patellae; and (vi) other patellofemoral disorders or syndromes.
3. The most common cause of organic hip pain for each age group follows:
   a. Toxic synovitis at age 3-6 years
   b. Legg-Calve-Perthes disease at 4-10 years
   c. SCFE at 11-15 years

SUGGESTED READING

Eilert R, Georgopoulos G: Orthopedics. In: Hathaway WE, et al, eds.: *Current pediatric diagnosis and treatment,* ed 11. Appleton & Lange, 1993, Norwalk, CT.

Kim M, Karpas A: The limping child. *Clin Pediatr Emerg Med* 3(2):129-137, 2002.

Leet AI, Skaggs D: Evaluation of the acutely limping child. *Am Fam Physician* 61(4):1011-1018, 2000.

Thompson GH: Common orthopedic problems of children. In: Behrman RE, Kliegman RM, eds.: *Nelson essential of pediatrics,* 4th ed. WB Saunders Co., 2002, Philadelphia, 821-857.

Chapter 109

Foot and Leg Deformities

"I would just die if I had a daughter with crooked legs."

CLINICAL CASE PROBLEM 1:

AN ANXIOUS MOTHER WITH A 3-MONTH-OLD INFANT WITH CROOKED FEET

A 3-month-old infant is brought to your office by his mother. She states that he has "crooked feet." She has been told by her friend that he will "need a number of casts to correct this."

On examination, the infant's feet are everted. The heel position as viewed from behind with his feet dorsiflexed is valgus. No other abnormalities are found on examination.

The mother's pregnancy was unremarkable. The birthweight of the infant was 10 pounds, 8 ounces.

SELECT THE BEST ANSWER TO THE FOLLOWING QUESTIONS:

1. What is the most likely diagnosis in this infant?
   a. congenital calcaneovalgus
   b. metatarsus valgus
   c. metatarsus varus
   d. talipes equinovarus
   e. clubfoot

2. What is the treatment of choice in this child?
   a. serial casts
   b. bilateral osteotomies
   c. Denis-Browne splints
   d. immediate referral to an orthopedic surgeon
   e. reassurance and foot exercises

CLINICAL CASE PROBLEM 2:

A 4-WEEK-OLD INFANT WITH "TOEING IN"

A mother brings her 4-week-old infant to the office for assessment of her child's "toeing in." She states that another physician has told her that this probably will require "serial casts" to correct.

On physical examination, both feet deviate medially. The feet dorsiflex easily, and the heels are in a neutral position. The lateral borders of the feet are convex.

3. What is the most likely diagnosis in this patient?
   a. calcaneovalgus
   b. metatarsus varus
   c. metatarsus valgus
   d. talipes equinovarus
   e. clubfoot

4. What is the most likely predisposing factor to the diagnosis described in Clinical Case Problem 2?
   a. abnormality at the embryo stage of development
   b. hereditary susceptibility to the condition
   c. position of the fetus in utero
   d. abnormality in the shape of the maternal uterus
   e. abnormality in the formation of the fetal legs and feet

5. What is the treatment of choice for the majority of patients with the condition described in Clinical Case Problem 2?
   a. serial casts
   b. bilateral osteotomies
   c. Denis-Browne splints
   d. immediate referral to an orthopedic surgeon
   e. reassurance and foot exercises

CLINICAL CASE PROBLEM 3:

A 15-MONTH-OLD WITH "BOWLEGS"

A mother brings her 15-month-old infant into your office for an assessment of "his bowlegs." She states that he has been "bowlegged" since he began to walk 3 months ago.

On examination, the toddler's feet point inward and his knees point straight ahead.

6. On the basis of the information provided, what is the most likely diagnosis?
   a. internal tibial torsion
   b. internal femoral torsion
   c. metatarsus varus
   d. fixed tibia varum
   e. calcaneovalgus

7. What is the treatment of choice for the child described in Clinical Case Problem 3?
   a. serial casts
   b. bilateral osteotomies
   c. Denis-Browne splints
   d. immediate referral to an orthopedic surgeon
   e. reassurance and leg exercises

CLINICAL CASE PROBLEM 4:

AN 18-MONTH-OLD WITH TWISTED LEGS

A mother comes to your office with her 18-month-old infant. She tells you that her child appears to have "both legs twisted inward from the hips." You examine the child and confirm that the mother's impression appears to be correct. The anterior aspect of the patellae is directed medially, and hip internal rotation is greater than external rotation.

8. What is the most likely diagnosis in this patient?
   a. internal tibial torsion
   b. excessive femoral anteversion
   c. flexible flat feet
   d. metatarsus adductus
   e. metatarsus varus

9. What is the most common cause of intoeing in children older than age 3?
   a. internal tibial torsion
   b. excessive femoral anteversion
   c. metatarsus adductus
   d. metatarsus varus
   e. none of the above

10. What is the initial treatment of choice for the condition described in Clinical Case Problem 4?
    a. serial casts
    b. bilateral osteotomies
    c. Denis-Browne splints
    d. immediate referral to an orthopedic surgeon
    e. watchful expectation

11. What is the most common method of measuring the degree of the condition described in Clinical Case Problem 4?
    a. computed tomography scan of the lower leg
    b. ultrasonography of the lower leg
    c. biplanar radiography of the lower leg
    d. magnetic resonance imaging scan of the lower leg
    e. none of the above

CLINICAL CASE PROBLEM 5:

A 6-MONTH-OLD WITH CROOKED FEET

A mother brings her 6-month-old infant to your office for assessment. She tells you that her child's feet are "completely crooked" and that there is no way she can correct it.

On examination, you are unable to dorsiflex either foot. You notice that the heels are in the varus position (medial deviation) and the sole is kidney-shaped when viewed from the bottom.

12. What is the most likely diagnosis in this infant?
    a. talipes equinovarus
    b. metatarsus adductus
    c. internal tibial torsion
    d. excessive femoral anteversion
    e. none of the above

13. Which of the following treatments may be indicated for correction of the condition described in Clinical Case Problem 5?

a. posterior medial release of the heel cords
b. serial casts
c. reassurance and foot exercises
d. a and b
e. a, b, and c

14. Which of the following may be associated with the condition described in Clinical Case Problem 5?
    a. congenital dislocation of the hip
    b. spina bifida
    c. myotonic dystrophy
    d. a and b
    e. a, b, and c

CLINICAL CASE PROBLEM 6:
A 21-MONTH-OLD CHILD WITH FLAT FEET

A mother comes to your office with her 21-month-old infant. She tells you that he "slaps his feet when he walks." Her mother-in-law has informed her that he has "flat feet" and instructed her to "make darn sure the doctor does something about it." On examination, you observe the child walking. There certainly does seem to be a difference between the contour of the foot when weightbearing as compared to when not weightbearing.

15. Assuming that the abnormalities in this child's feet involve arch support and ligamentous laxity, what is the most likely diagnosis?
    a. muscular dystrophy
    b. cerebral palsy
    c. flexible flatfeet
    d. osteochondrosis
    e. obesity

16. What is the most likely difference between weightbearing and non–weightbearing?
    a. a difference in "heel lift"
    b. a difference in "toe lift"
    c. a difference in foot varus
    d. a difference in foot valgus
    e. a difference in sag versus nonsag weightbearing

17. Which of the following coexisting conditions is (are) associated with this condition?
    a. muscular dystrophy
    b. cerebral palsy
    c. congenital heel cord tightness
    d. a and c
    e. a, b, and c

18. What is the treatment of choice for the primary condition described in Clinical Case Problem 6?
    a. corrective orthopedic shoes
    b. orthotic inserts

c. flexible, well-fitted soft shoes
d. specially designed shoes
e. none of the above; watchful waiting is more appropriate

■ ANSWERS:

1. **a.** The most likely diagnosis is congenital calcaneovalgus.

2. **e.** The calcaneovalgus foot is a common neonatal foot deformity. It is the result of positional confinement in utero. The foot has a banana-shaped sole (lateral deviation); dorsiflexes quite easily because of a stretched, abnormally long heel cord; and has a heel that deviates laterally.

Prognosis is excellent; most cases improve spontaneously and rapidly. Parents who are uncomfortable with the prescription of observation alone should be encouraged to exercise the child's foot at each diaper change by stretching the ligaments and stretching the dorsal tendons.

Only in the rare instance that the foot remains severely deformed should corrective casts be applied. If the calcaneovalgus foot can be only partially corrected, a flexible flatfoot results.

This calcaneovalgus foot must be differentiated from a congenital vertical talus (congenital convex pes valgus), which is associated with neurologic disorders such as spina bifida or arthrogryposis in about 50% of cases. The vertical talus foot has a "rocker-bottom" appearance with a tight heel cord.

3. **b.** This child has metatarsus adductus and metatarsus varus. They are used synonymously in practice, although they describe slightly different variations in the forefoot. In both cases, the sole is kidney bean–shaped (medial deviation), and the foot is easily dorsiflexed.

4. **c.** Metatarsus adductus (varus) may be either bilateral or unilateral; it is probably secondary to in utero confinement. Two conditions associated with metatarsus adductus are muscular torticollis and congenital hip dysplasia.

5. **e.** Metatarsus adductus usually improves spontaneously; this applies to at least 85% of cases. The severity of the metatarsus adductus, determined from the examination, should be documented. Severity is classified as follows: Category A is mild/flexible, Category B is moderate/fixed, and Category C is severe/rigid.

The vast majority of cases fall into the mild/flexible group (Category A).

The parents can be taught to stretch the child's foot by firmly holding and stabilizing the heel and stretching the forefoot laterally, holding it to a count of five. The exercise can be performed five times at each diaper change.

Category B metatarsus adductus may need to be treated by serial casting. Category C metatarsus adductus may need corrective surgery.

6. a. Internal tibial torsion is a normal finding in the newborn. The mean tibial torsion at maturity is 15 degrees to 20 degrees. At birth, the mean tibial torsion is 5 degrees—that is, 10-15 degrees inward compared with adults. Internal tibial torsion usually presents at walking age, and affected children have an inward foot progression angle. When the child walks, it can be observed that the kneecaps point forward but the foot points inward.

Internal tibial torsion is thus a physiologic bowing of the lower extremities produced by the external rotation of the femur and internal rotation of the tibia.

7. e. The natural history of internal tibial torsion is spontaneous resolution in more than 95% of children. Internal tibial torsion usually resolves by 7 or 8 years of age, at which time the rotatory conformation of the bones is largely established. Reassurance and leg exercises are the treatment of choice for the management of internal tibial torsion.

8. b. The most likely diagnosis is excessive femoral anteversion.

9. b. The most common cause of intoeing in children older than age 3 years is excessive femoral anteversion. The femoral neck is normally anteverted 10 degrees to 15 degrees with respect to the axis of the femoral condyles in the knee of adults. The femoral neck is more anteverted in children. In one large study the average degree of anteversion of the femur in children between the ages of 3 months and 12 months was 39 degrees and 31 degrees in 1- to 2-year-old children.

10. e. The treatment of choice in children with excessive femoral anteversion is "watchful waiting." In 90% to 95% of children, the degree of anteversion will decrease progressively to a level that is both within the normal range and completely acceptable.

11. c. A number of techniques have been devised to accurately measure the degree of femoral anteversion. The most commonly used techniques involve biplanar radiography.

In children who have excessive femoral anteversion as the cause of their intoeing, the typical clinical finding is that the child is observed to walk with his or her patellae and feet pointing inward. The clinical diagnosis is made by having the child lie prone or supine with the hips extended and externally rotating the hip. In children with excess femoral anteversion, most of the arc of rotation of the hip will be inward.

12. a. This child has talipes equinovarus (clubfoot). When a child develops clubfoot, you notice the following: (1) the inability to dorsiflex the clubfoot (heel equinus); (2) the presence of heel varus (medial deviation); and (3) a sole that is kidney-shaped (forefoot and midfoot adductus).

Mild cases of clubfoot can be attributed to deformation caused by intrauterine compression, whereas more severe, fixed cases are usually secondary to underlying anatomic abnormalities such as an abnormal talus.

13. d. Treatment options for talipes equinovarus include corrective serial casts and posterior medial release of the heel cords.

The proportion of children requiring corrective surgery varies from 75% if full anatomic, radiographic, and clinical correction is attempted to less than 50% if mild radiographic and clinical deformity is accepted.

14. e. Accompanying deformities with talipes equinovarus include congenital dislocation of the hip, spina bifida, myotonic dystrophy, and arthrogryposis.

15. c. This child has flexible flatfeet. The flexible flatfoot is extremely common, with an incidence ranging from 7% to 22%.

16. e. The condition often is hidden by normal adipose tissue and usually becomes noticeable after a child begins to stand. The most common cause of the flexible flatfoot is ligamentous laxity, which allows the foot to sag with weightbearing. Children often present with accompanying hyperextension of fingers, elbows, and knees and a family history of flatfeet and ligamentous laxity.

A child with flexible flatfeet secondary to ligamentous laxity can form a good arch when asked to stand on tiptoe. The heel rolls into a varus position (medial deviation) on tiptoe, and good strength of the ankle and foot muscles is assured.

When the child walks, the difference that can be seen immediately is that when the child is not bearing weight there is an arch. When the child is bearing weight, there is no arch.

17. e. Although flexible flatfeet are usually not associated with any secondary conditions (i.e., primary flexible flatfeet), it must be recognized that flexible flatfeet can be secondary to muscular dystrophy, mild cerebral palsy, or congenital tightness of the heel cords.

18. **e.** Although many treatments have been advocated for flatfeet (corrective shoes, custom orthotics, corrective inserts, and flexible flatfoot wear), none of them have been shown to be better than "no treatment" or "watchful expectation."

SUMMARY OF FOOT AND LEG DEFORMITIES

1. Prevalence of foot and leg deformities: common (up to 10% of infants)
2. Foot deformities in infants and children:
   a. Congenital calcaneovalgus foot: very common neonatal foot deformity. It results from the fetal position in utero. The foot has a banana-shaped sole (lateral deviation) and dorsiflexes quite easily because of a stretched, abnormally long heel cord and a heel that deviates laterally. Treatment consists of watchful waiting.
   b. Metatarsus adductus (metatarsus varus): most common congenital foot deformity. The sole is kidney bean–shaped (medial deviation), and the foot is easily dorsiflexed. Treatment consists of foot exercises and watchful waiting.
   c. Talipes equinovarus (clubfoot): this disorder is characterized by the inability to dorsiflex the foot, the presence of a heel varus (medial deviation), and a sole that is kidney bean–shaped when viewed from the bottom. The tarsal navicular position is abnormal. A tight heel cord is exceedingly common. Many cases are caused by intrauterine position. Treatment consists of serial casts or surgical posterior medial heel cord release.
3. Other causes of intoeing in young children:
   a. Internal tibial torsion: In internal tibial torsion, the entire foot points inward and the patella points straight ahead (medial tibial torsion). Treatment consists of watchful waiting.
   b. Excessive femoral anteversion: The entire leg turns in so that both the patella and the foot are facing medially (medial femoral torsion or increased anteversion of the hips). Treatment consists of watchful waiting.
4. Flexible flatfeet: In a child with flexible flatfeet, when the foot is not bearing weight, the arch of the foot is preserved. When the child is bearing weight, the arch of the foot is not preserved. Treatment consists of watchful waiting.
5. Establish a therapeutic alliance with parents:
   a. Begin with a complete history of the pregnancy and birth (pay particular attention to any complications).
   b. Carry out a complete physical examination in which the following are especially noted: (i) foot varus versus foot valgus and (ii) flexibility of varus or valgus deformity.
   c. Explain to the mother the various causes of intoeing and the very high frequency with which they self-correct (90% to 95%).
   d. Have the patient return regularly for follow-up.
   e. Refer to a specialist when indicated.

SUGGESTED READING

Churgay C: Diagnosis and treatment of pediatric foot deformities. *Am Fam Physician* 47(4):883-889, 1993.
Dietz F: Intoeing—fact, fiction, and opinion. *Am Fam Physician* 50(6): 1249-1259, 1994.
Sass P, Hassan G: Lower extremity abnormalities in children. *Am Fam Physician* 68:461-468, 2003.
Thompson GH: Common orthopedic problems in children: The foot. In: Behrman RE, Kliegman RM, eds.: *Nelson essentials of pediatrics*, 4th ed. WB Saunders Co, 2002, Philadelphia, 837-843.
Tolo VT, Wood B: *Pediatric orthopaedics in primary care*. Williams & Wilkins, 1993, Baltimore.

 Chapter **110**

Adolescent Development

> "I'm doing good. My mom just gets uptight easily."

CLINICAL CASE PROBLEM 1:
14-YEAR-OLD COMES FOR A SPORTS PHYSICAL

A 14-year-old comes to the office for a sports physical. According to his mom he used to see a pediatrician, but he feels too old for that now. This is his initial visit to the family health center.

On taking the history you notice that he seldom makes eye contact and appears anxious, more than usual for a child his age. The physical examination is benign, including a complete musculoskeletal and neurological examination.

▎ **SELECT THE BEST ANSWER TO THE FOLLOWING QUESTIONS:**

1. Regarding the patient described, you should do which of the following?

a ask the parent if she has any concerns about his growth and development

b. refer the patient to a psychologist

c. attempt to identify an underlying agenda

d. consult a school counselor

e. all of the above

2. To facilitate further discussion with this patient at this time you should say?

a. you are in good health so I'll see you next year

b. we need to schedule you for some routine blood work

c. why don't you ask your mom if she has any questions?

d. I get the feeling that there is something on your mind that you would like to talk about....I'm listening

e. I am too busy, but why don't you make a follow-up appointment with your guidance counselor.

3. During this first visit, which of the following issues should be addressed?

a. body image

b. home environment

c. education

d. sex, drugs, and alcohol

e. all of the above

4. In the United States the leading cause of death among people ages 15-24 years is:

a. homicide

b. suicide

c. accidents

d. human immunodeficiency virus infection

e. cancer

5. Which psychiatric disorder is least common in adolescents?

a. depression

b. anxiety

c. schizophrenia

d. adjustment disorder

e. antisocial personality disorder

6. Children in mid-adolescence primarily are concerned with which of the following?

a. strong emphasis on the new peer group

b. struggle with sense of identity

c. realization that parents are not perfect and identification of their faults

d. movement toward independence

e. a and d

7. What major factor(s) is (are) most important to ensure healthy development of the adolescent?

a. encouragement toward independence

b. the establishment of boundaries

c. teaching of discipline

d. a prolonged supportive environment

e. a and d

8. Risk factors for alcohol and drug use in the adolescent include all of the following except:

a. divorce or separation of parents

b. poor school performance

c. sexual promiscuity

d. peer group

e. socioeconomic status

9. Regarding visits to family physicians by adolescents, which of the following are true?

a. adolescents make regular visits to the doctor

b. 25% of adolescents have chronic conditions necessitating a visit to the doctor

c. adolescents are open about asking questions regarding sexual issues

d. a and c

e. none of the above

10. What is the second leading cause of death among people age 15-24 years of age in the United States?

a. motor vehicle accidents

b. suicide

c. homicide

d. cancer

e. acquired immune deficiency syndrome

CLINICAL CASE PROBLEM 2:
MY SON'S GRADES ARE SLIPPING

A mother brings her 15-year-old to the office stating that she is suspicious that her son may be using drugs. According to the mom, her son has always been an A student until recently, when his grades have slipped. The mother relates to you that she is separated from her husband and is in the midst of a bitter divorce. She also has an older son who is away at college.

On evaluation the patient complains of fatigue, hypersomnolence, and increased appetite. This has resulted in a 40-pound weight gain over the past year. The patient's physical examination is normal except for a body mass index (BMI) of 40.

11. What is your initial approach to this patient?

a. tell the mom you are going to order a drug screen

b. tell the mom that he has a poor self-image secondary to the weight gain and exercise and diet will resolve this issue

c. tell the mom to leave the room so you can spend some time obtaining a more thorough history
d. evaluate the adolescent for hypothyroidism
e. a and c

12. Given this presentation, what type of things should you screen this adolescent for?
a. body image
b. depression
c. substance abuse
d. hypothyroidism
e. all of the above

13. Which medical problem is on the rise in the United States in adolescents with an elevated BMI?
a. sleep apnea
b. osteoarthritis
c. hypertension
d. diabetes mellitus
e. none of the above

14. The boy in Clinical Case Problem 2 would be classified as being:
a. underweight
b. overweight
c. obese
d. morbidly obese
e. toxically obese

15. What advice would you give to the mother in dealing with her son described in Question 14?
a. to have her child speak to a guidance counselor at school
b. to have her child admitted to a rehabilitation program
c. to obtain a family therapist to work on a myriad of psychosocial issues
d. a and c
e. none of the above

16. What is the third leading cause of death in the United States among people ages 15-24 years old?
a. substance abuse
b. cancer
c. suicide
d. homicide
e. motor vehicle accidents

CLINICAL CASE MANAGEMENT PROBLEM

Describe the preventive medicine strategies that should be incorporated into an office visit in which an adolescent comes to see his or her physician for acute episodic care.

ANSWERS:

1. **c.** This adolescent is obviously very anxious about something. The physical examination may be the perfect opportunity to have the parent leave so that you can have a discussion in private and attempt to identify why he is so anxious. There is a high probability that the patient may have some issues that he may disclose to you.

2. **d.** At this time you should attempt, if possible, to identify exactly what the patient's agenda may be. An appropriate opener would be "I get the feeling that there is something you would like to talk about....I'm listening." More direct questions would be about school, friends, peers, sexual orientation, drugs, alcohol, and the like. A good way to approach these issues would be "I know that a lot of people your age are starting to have sex or use drugs and alcohol. Are you aware of anyone in your school that may be doing this?" This is a nonthreatening way of approaching a sensitive topic.

3. **e.** Body image; home environment; education; and sex, drugs, and alcohol are all topics that may be important to find out about the adolescent.

4. **c.** The leading cause of death among people ages 15-24 is accidents.

5. **c.** Schizophrenia is the least likely mental illness that adolescents have. The peak incidence is usually ages 18-25. The other conditions are much more prevalent in the adolescent population.

6. **e.** Although there is a continuum of development, there are three identified phases of adolescent development. In early adolescence there is a preoccupation with bodily changes. Early adolescents often feel uncertain about their appearance, and their interests are directed toward themselves. This is a period marked by high levels of physical activity and mood swings.

In mid-adolescence the major concern is independence. The peer group dominates social life, and risk behaviors become more prevalent. This is a time of heightened sexual curiosity and exploration.

In late adolescence there is greater emotional stability with the establishment of a firmer self-identity. There is goal-directed behavior and more adult-type thinking, with an acceptance of social and cultural institutions. The adolescent begins to act like an adult, thinking about the future and weighing risks, benefits, and consequences of life decisions.

7. **e.** Experts tell us that the key ingredient to ensure healthy adolescent development is a prolonged supportive environment with graded steps toward autonomy. Healthy development is encouraged by a

process of mutual positive engagement between the adolescent, various adults, and peers. Youth groups and other social organizations (e.g., Boy Scouts) can have a very positive impact toward the development of an independent mature adolescent

8. e. Divorce or separation of parents, poor school performance, sexual promiscuity, and peer group pressure are all risk factors for alcohol and substance abuse. Socioeconomic status is not.

9. e. Acute episodic care is the most frequent reason why adolescents visit physician's offices. These visits most frequently involve respiratory tract infections, skin conditions, genitourinary concerns, musculoskeletal injuries, or psychological disorders.

Among adolescents 10% have chronic medical conditions (e.g., diabetes, asthma, epilepsy, irritable bowel disorder, juvenile rheumatoid arthritis, malignancies) necessitating regular visits.

School and sports physicals are the only other times when adolescents will make a regular visit to the physician's office. Therefore it is incumbent for physicians to attempt to discuss a healthy lifestyle in any of these visits.

10. c. It is a poor commentary on our social conditions, but homicide is the second leading cause of death among young people aged 15-24 years old in the United States.

11. c. This obviously is a complicated case with a variety of issues that need to be explored. As always, a good history and thorough psychosocial evaluation including assessment of anxiety, depression, and risk for suicide needs to be done. This adolescent has multiple risk factors, personal and social, that may require the need for a psychiatrist, psychologist, or both.

12. e. Questions relating to body image, depression, substance abuse, and hypothyroidism all need to be addressed.

13. d. There is an epidemic of type 2 diabetes in the adolescent population in the United States. This is a direct result of physical inactivity, computer video games, and a diet that is high in calories and rich in carbohydrates. For the first time in its history, the American Academy of Pediatrics has advocated an hour of vigorous physical activity for all children and adolescents on a daily basis.

14. d. This adolescent has a BMI that corresponds to morbid obesity. This is an independent risk factor for hypertension, diabetes, sleep apnea, heart disease, and osteoarthritis. A BMI of 27 corresponds to overweight. A BMI of 30 is obese, and a BMI of 16 is anorexic.

15. d. Professional counseling appears to be the best approach to work on the variety of psychosocial issues both at home and at school.

16. c. Once again it is a sorry commentary, but suicide is the third leading cause of death among people 15-24 years of age.

 # SOLUTION TO THE CLINICAL CASE MANAGEMENT PROBLEM

1. Universal: Adolescence is a period when at least one health maintenance examination should be carried out. Episodic care visits are an ideal time to carry out these health screenings and assessments. Two mnemonics useful in screening adolescents are "safe times" and "heads":

SAFE TIMES
S = Sexuality issues
A = Affect (depression) and abuse (drugs)
F = Family (function and medical history)
E = Examination (sensitive and appropriate)
T = Timing of development (body image)
I = Immunizations
M = Minerals (nutritional issues)
E = Education, employment (school and work issues)
S = Safety (vehicle)

HEADS
H = Home
E = Education, employment (school/work)
A = Activities, affect, anxieties, ambitions
D = Drugs
S = Sex, stress, suicide, self-esteem

2. Phases of adolescent development:
   a. Early adolescence: Preoccupation with body changes. Early adolescents often feel uncertain about their appearance, and their interests are directed toward themselves. This is a period marked by high levels of physical activity and mood swings.
   b. Mid-adolescence: In mid-adolescence the major concern is independence. The peer group dominates social life, and risk behaviors become more prevalent. This is the time when sexual matters receive much interest.

Continued

SOLUTION TO THE CLINICAL CASE MANAGEMENT PROBLEM—cont'd

c. Late adolescence: In many ways, youths in the late-adolescence phase appear to be adults. They are more capable of future orientation, mutual caring, and internal control. However, most late adoles-

cents also have uncertainties about sexuality, future relationships, and future work possibilities. Allowing them to be adolescents is very important.

SUMMARY OF ADOLESCENT DEVELOPMENT

The Solution to the Clinical Case Management Problem is an excellent summary of adolescent development.

SUGGESTED READING

Culbertson JL: Childhood and adolescent psychologic development. Pediatr Clin North Am 50(4):741-764, vii, 2003.

DiClemente RJ: The psychological basis of health promotion for adolescents. *Adolesc Med* 10(1):13-22, 1999.

Goran MI: Obesity and risk of type 2 diabetes and cardiovascular disease in children and adolescents. *J Clin Endocrinol Metab* 88(4): 1417-1427, 2003.

Juszczak L, Sadler L: Adolescent development: Setting the stage for influencing health behaviors. *Adolesc Med* 10(1):1-11, v, 1999.

Lammers C, et al: Influences on adolescents' decision to postpone onset of sexual intercourse: a survival analysis of virginity among youths age 13 to 18 years. *J Adolesc Health* 26(1):42-48, 2000.

Story M, Neumark-Sztainer D: Promoting healthy eating and physical activity in adolescents. *Adolesc Med* 10(1):109-123, vi, 1999.

Windle M, Windle RC: Adolescent tobacco, alcohol, and drug use: current findings. *Adolesc Med* 10(1):153-163, 1999.

Chapter 111

Enuresis

> "Doctor, I still need to use rubber sheets. Will it never end?"

CLINICAL CASE PROBLEM 1:

A 6-YEAR-OLD MALE WHO STILL WETS THE BED

A mother brings her 6-year-old son to your office for a periodic health assessment. The child continues to wet his bed at night (an average of two to three times per week). He is dry during the day. The child has no history of significant medical problems. Specifically, he has had no urinary tract infections. Labor and delivery were normal, as was the neonatal period. His growth (both weight and height) always has been in the 10th percentile. He started school last year but did not do well. He had to repeat the first grade. His blood pressure measured today is 85/60 mm Hg. The examination of all other body systems is normal.

SELECT THE BEST ANSWER TO THE FOLLOWING QUESTIONS:

1. What is the most likely diagnosis in this child?
   a. school phobia
   b. nocturnal enuresis
   c. small bladder syndrome (SBS)
   d. masked childhood depression
   e. none of the above

2. With respect to this condition, which of the following statements is false?
   a. at age 5, 15% to 25% of children have this condition
   b. the condition is more common when one or both parents had the condition
   c. the condition is three times more common in boys
   d. the condition usually implies significant psychopathology in the child
   e. bladder capacity is normal in children with enuresis, but functional bladder capacity is less

3. A child is defined as enuretic if he or she has not attained full bladder control by what age?

a. 3 years
b. 4 years
c. 5 years
d. 6 years
e. 8 years

4. Which of the following factors regarding bed-wetting is (are) true?
   a. families with low socioeconomic status have higher incidence of bedwetting
   b. nocturnal enuresis is a psychologic condition
   c. stressful events associated with toilet training have minimal effect on the achievement of continence
   d. bedwetting may be a sign of rebellion on the part of the child
   e. b and d

5. Which of the following investigations is the most important to be performed in a child with enuresis?
   a. urinalysis
   b. urine culture
   c. complete blood count (CBC)
   d. complete cystometric evaluation
   e. intravenous pyelography (IVP)

6. Which of the following is not a consideration in the differential diagnosis of enuresis?
   a. diabetes mellitus
   b. diabetes insipidus
   c. petit mal seizures
   d. separation anxiety disorder
   e. posterior urethral valve syndrome

7. Which of the following is the drug of choice in the pharmacologic treatment of this disorder?
   a. oxybutynin chloride
   b. imipramine
   c. chlorpromazine
   d. diazepam
   e. desmopressin

8. Which of the following statements most accurately reflect(s) the treatment of this condition?
   a. most nonpharmacologic therapies have been shown to be no more effective than placebo in the treatment of this condition
   b. behavior modification has been shown to be superior to pharmacologic therapies
   c. pharmacologic therapy is recommended in children with enuresis who do not respond to nonpharmacologic therapies
   d. b and c
   e. all of the above

9. What is the most effective form of behavior modification in the treatment of the disorder described?
   a. biofeedback
   b. electric shock treatment (spontaneously triggered when the child wets the bed)
   c. a bell or buzzer system
   d. the behavior-modification theory of logical consequences
   e. all of the above are equally effective

10. True statement(s) regarding the use of bedwetting alarms is (are):
    a. for resolution of bedwetting, the alarm may need to be used for 15 weeks
    b. the treatment dropout rate is up to 30%
    c. the alarm should not be used in children younger than 5 years old
    d. a and c
    e. a, b, and c

11. Which of the following is (are) important in the treatment of this condition?
    a. using a reward system for dry nights achieved
    b. establishing a rule that older children should be expected to launder their own soiled bed-clothes and pajamas
    c. elimination of liquids before bedtime
    d. voiding just before bedtime
    e. all of the above

12. Which of the following should not be used in the treatment of this condition?
    a. punishing the child
    b. postponing bedtime in an effort to decrease the frequency of the problem
    c. providing the child with a feeling of inferiority for having the problem
    d. all of the above
    e. a and c

■ **ANSWERS:**

1. **b.** Nocturnal enuresis is urinary leakage that occurs at night during sleep. Enuresis can be primary (if the individual has never been dry at night for any substantial time) or secondary (i.e., returning after having one or fewer wetting episodes per month for at least 1 month).

The *Diagnostic Statistical Manual of Mental Disorders*, 4th edition (DSM-IV) classification of enuresis (which this child has) is based on the following criteria: (1) repeated voiding of urine into bed or clothes (whether involuntary or intentional); (2) the behavior is clinically significant as manifested by either frequency of twice a week for at least 3 consecutive weeks or the presence of clinically significant distress or impairment in social, academic (occupational), or other important areas of functioning; (3) age of at least 5 years; and (4) not caused by the direct physiologic effect of a substance (such as a diuretic) or a general medical condition (such as diabetes, spina bifida, or a seizure disorder).

DSM-IV further subclassifies enuresis into the following categories: (1) nocturnal only; (2) diurnal only; and (3) nocturnal and diurnal.

This child does not meet the criteria for school phobia, and there is no information that suggests a diagnosis of masked depression.

There is no such condition as SBS.

2. **d.** Nocturnal enuresis once was thought to be a psychologic condition. It now appears that the psychologic problems are the result of enuresis and not the cause. Children with nocturnal enuresis have not been found to have an increased incidence of emotional problems. It has been found that although real bladder capacity is identical in children with and without enuresis, functional bladder capacity may be less in those with enuresis.

3. **c.** Enuresis usually is defined as the involuntary discharge of urine after the age at which bladder control usually should have been established (age 5). As just classified, this child has nocturnal enuresis (only at night).

The prevalence of enuresis decreases with increasing age. Thus 82% of 2-year-old children, 49% of 3-year-old children, 26% of 4-year-old children, and 15% to 25% of 5-year-old children still wet beds or clothes on a regular basis. Enuresis is definitely more common in children when one or both parents were enuretic as children.

4. **c.** There appears to be a developmental immaturity leading to a decreased functional bladder capacity in children with enuresis. Uropathies may be associated with enuresis. Urethral valves, neurogenic bladder, and ectopic ureter occasionally may be the cause of primary enuresis. Urinary tract infections are a common organic cause of enuresis, especially secondary enuresis, in girls.

Familial factors that have been found to have no relationship to the achievement of continence include social background, stressful life events, and the number of changes in family constellation or residences. Bedwetting is not a sign of rebellion in most children. The key points to consider in discussing the relationship between enuresis and psychologic or psychiatric problems in children are as follows: (1) the vast majority of children with enuresis have no associated psychologic or psychiatric pathologic condition, and

(2) chronic psychologic stress (unrelated to toilet training experiences) can impair the child's ability to achieve bladder control.

5. **a.** The only mandatory laboratory evaluation for children with enuresis is a urinalysis. The presence of white blood cells in the urine as a result of a urinary tract infection; low urinary specific gravity as a result of diabetes insipidus; proteinuria; or hematuria as a result of renal disease; and glucosuria as a result of diabetes mellitus are all important abnormalities that may be associated with enuresis.

Urine culture, CBC, IVP, and cystometric evaluation should be performed only if specific indications suggest the need. Posterior urethral valves (especially in boys) may be associated with enuresis.

6. **d.** The only disorder listed in Question 5 that is not part of the differential diagnosis of enuresis is separation anxiety disorder.

7. **e.** At one time the pharmacologic therapy of choice for enuresis was imipramine. However, because its administration is generally effective only briefly and drug tolerance, exacerbation of symptoms after the discontinuation of the drug, and medication side effects are common, recommendations presently discourage its use in children with enuresis. Use of the antidiuretic hormone analogue 1-(3-mercaptoproprionic acid)–8-D-arginine vasopressin (or desmopressin acetate nasal spray [DDAVP]) for treatment of nocturnal enuresis has been increasing. Although DDAVP can reduce the number of wet nights in many children, it is not curative. Relapses occur commonly on cessation of the drug.

8. **d.** Behavior modification has been shown to be superior to pharmacologic therapies. However, pharmacologic therapy is recommended in children with enuresis who do not respond to nonpharmacologic therapies.

9. **c.** The most effective form of behavior modification in the treatment of enuresis is a bell or buzzer system.

10. **e.** For resolution of bedwetting, the alarm may need to be used for 15 weeks. The treatment dropout rate is up to 30%, and the alarm should not be used in children younger than 5 years old.

11. **e.** See Answer 12.

12. **e.** Because there is usually no identifiable cause of enuresis and the disorder tends to remit spontaneously even if not treated, treatment should be

conservative. The methods approved for the treatment of enuresis include the following:

1. Appropriate toilet training (scheduled voiding times especially in the evening; wake up to urinate in the middle of the night)
2. Behavior modification (bell or buzzer) and pad: These treatments are the most successful in achieving cure. The alarm should not be used in children younger than age 5 and may be needed for up to 15 weeks to establish continence. There is a 10% to 30% dropout rate. Possible predictors of a poor response include an unstable or chaotic family situation, behavioral deviance in the child, high parental anxiety level, and low parental education level.
3. Positive reinforcement system that charts the child's progress: Although all of the approved methods are effective and should be used together, it appears that the most effective behavior-modification method is the buzzer or bell and pad system.

Here are some general recommendations that may prove helpful in the treatment of enuresis:

1. Enlist the support and cooperation of the child in treating the condition.
2. Have older children launder their own soiled bedclothes and pajamas (not as a punishment but rather as participation in their own illness).
3. Prohibit liquids after dinner.
4. Make sure the child voids before retiring.

Here are some general recommendations to avoid in the treatment of enuresis:

1. Waking the child repeatedly during the night to take him or her to the bathroom; this has negative consequences in most children because it disturbs sleep and may further engender or aggravate anger in the child or the parent
2. Punishing the child for wetting the bed
3. Intimidating the child or lowering his self-esteem
4. Postponing the child's bedtime in an effort to decrease the frequency of bedwetting

SUMMARY OF ENURESIS

1. **Prevalence:** 7% at the age when bladder control should have been fully achieved (i.e., after 5 years of age)
2. Classification of subtypes of enuresis is based on whether the child ever has achieved bladder control:
   a. Primary enuresis: child never has been dry.
   b. Secondary enuresis: child has been dry for a period but becomes enuretic later.
3. Classification based on period when child does not have bladder control:
   a. Nocturnal enuresis: enuresis at night only
   b. Diurnal enuresis: enuresis during the day only
   c. Nocturnal and diurnal enuresis: enuresis during both day and night
4. **Pathophysiology**: immaturity of the part of the autonomic nervous system that controls the bladder in the vast majority of cases. Infrequently, enuresis is associated with organic problems such as congenital urinary tract system abnormality or urinary tract infection.
   a. Only 20% of children with enuresis have a psychodevelopmental disorder (lower intelligence quotient or behavioral disorder).
   b. Regressive enuresis usually is associated with some stressful environmental event.
5. **Investigations:** urinalysis is the only mandatory investigation for nocturnal enuresis. If enuresis occurs also in the daytime or if urinary flow is small or interrupted, a renal ultrasound and a careful neurologic examination (including inspection of the sacral area for structural abnormalities) are indicated.
6. **Treatment:**
   a. Pharmacologic: Imipramine is no longer recommended for the treatment of enuresis in most children. Desmopressin nasal spray or tablets are useful in achieving dry nights but is not curative.
   b. Nonpharmacologic: A behavior-modification program is the treatment of choice: (i) buzzer or bell system and a pad; (ii) positive reinforcement; (iii) charting progress to increase confidence and self-esteem of the child; (iv) urinating before bed; (v) avoiding liquids after supper; and (vi) relationship to psychopathology.

SUGGESTED READING

American Psychiatric Association: *Diagnostic and statistical manual of mental disorders*, ed 4, American Psychiatric Association Press, 1994, Washington, DC.

Cendron M: Primary nocturnal enuresis: current concepts. *Am Fam Physician* 59:1205-1218, 1219-1220, 1999.

Sulkes SB, Dosa NP: Chapter 1. Developmental and behavioral pediatrics: Enuresis. In: Behrman RE, Kliegman RM, eds.: *Nelson essentials of pediatrics*, 4th ed. WB Saunders, 2002, Philadelphia, 32-31.

Thiedke CC: Nocturnal enuresis. *Am Fam Physician* 67:1499-1506, 1509-1510, 2003.

Chapter **112**

Allergic Rhinitis

*"My little girl has had this
cold for the past year!"*

CLINICAL CASE PROBLEM 1:
A 5-YEAR-OLD GIRL WITH A PERSISTENT STUFFY, RUNNY NOSE

A 5-year-old girl is brought into your office by her father who states she has had a "stuffy, runny nose for what seems forever." The father states his daughter started to have a runny nose 9 months ago with associated congestion and at times "fits of sneezing." She has not had any fever, cough, wheezing, headache, or ear pain. Over-the-counter oral "cold medicines" have helped somewhat.

When asked about changes around the home, the father states they had wall-to-wall carpeting installed almost a year ago. The only significant past medical history is some mild eczema.

On examination, there is bilateral clear rhinorrhea and obvious turbinate swelling with a violaceous mucosa. The child is obviously mouth breathing and several times during the examination is noted to rub her nose upward with the palm of her hand. The pharynx is pink, but you do notice cobblestoning posteriorly. The chest examination is totally negative.

■ **SELECT THE BEST ANSWER TO THE FOLLOWING QUESTIONS:**

1. What is the most likely diagnosis in this child?
   a. infectious rhinitis
   b. vasomotor rhinitis
   c. seasonal allergic rhinitis
   d. perennial allergic rhinitis
   e. rhinitis medicamentosa

2. The condition described above is a risk factor for all of the following except:
   a. epistaxis
   b. sinusitis
   c. otitis media
   d. nasal polyps
   e. nasopharyngeal tumors

3. Which of the following immunoglobulins is associated with the condition described in case 1?
   a. immunoglobulin A (IgA)
   b. IgE
   c. IgG
   d. IgM
   e. no immunoglobulin is associated with the condition

4. What is the single most important factor that predisposes a child to develop the condition described in Clinical Case Problem 1?
   a. eczema
   b. chronic aspirin use
   c. family history
   d. smoke exposure
   e. asthma

5. Which of the following physical signs associated with the condition described in Clinical Case Problem 1 is found most commonly in children and not adults?
   a. "shiners"
   b. nasal crease
   c. mouth breathing
   d. the "salute sign"
   e. posterior pharyngeal wall lymphoid hyperplasia

6. Which of the following is the most common cause of the condition described in Clinical Case Problem 1?
   a. mold spores
   b. cockroaches
   c. feathers
   d. dust mite
   e. eggs

7. What is the most common cause of seasonal allergic rhinitis?
   a. mold spores
   b. insects
   c. pollens
   d. animal dander
   e. flowers

8. What is the first principle of therapy in treating the condition in Clinical Case Problem 1?
   a. immunotherapy
   b. use of intranasal cromolyn sodium
   c. use of intranasal corticosteroids
   d. use of antihistamines
   e. avoidance of the inciting cause

9. Which of the following therapies for the condition described in Clinical Case Problem 1 has the least side effects?
   a. immunotherapy
   b. intranasal cromolyn sodium
   c. intranasal corticosteroids
   d. antihistamines
   e. leukotriene receptor antagonists

10. What is the single most effective pharmacologic treatment for the condition described in Clinical Case Problem 1?

a. intranasal cromolyn sodium
b. intranasal corticosteroids
c. antihistamines
d. oral or topical decongestants
e. leukotriene receptor antagonists

11. Which of the following statements about diagnostic tests for the condition described in Clinical Case Problem 1 is false?
    a. laboratory testing is not essential for diagnosis or initiation of treatment
    b. more than half of patients have normal serum levels of associated immunoglobulin
    c. a nasal smear that is negative for eosinophils rules out the disease
    d. skin testing is slightly more sensitive than radioallergosorbent test (RAST) testing
    e. skin testing should be avoided in patients with significant dermatographism or diffuse skin disease

12. Which of the following statements about vasomotor rhinitis is false?
    a. nasal smears lack eosinophils
    b. predominant feature is congestion and rhinorrhea, not sneezing and itching
    c. symptoms are associated with changes in temperature or humidity
    d. it is common in children
    e. hot or spicy foods can elicit symptoms

13. Which of the following is not a physiologically based treatment for allergic rhinitis?
    a. leukotriene receptor antagonist
    b. oral corticosteroids
    c. anticholinergics
    d. guaifenesin
    e. antihistamines

14. Which of the following systemic diseases is not associated with rhinitis?
    a. hypertension
    b. sarcoidosis
    c. Wegener's granulomatosis
    d. hypothyroidism
    e. amyloidosis

15. All of the following statements about immunotherapy are true except:
    a. about 80% to 85% of patients will have significant long lasting relief with continued therapy
    b. it should not be initiated during pregnancy
    c. anaphylaxis is rare
    d. skin testing must be done prior to initiation
    e. it is more effective for allergens of perennial rhinitis than seasonal rhinitis

CLINICAL CASE MANAGEMENT PROBLEM

Define and describe rhinitis medicamentosa.

■ **ANSWERS:**

1. d. The child has allergic rhinitis with no seasonal pattern and seems to have perennial symptoms. There is no fever, purulent rhinorrhea, fetid breath, headache, or ear pain to suggest an infection. Allergic rhinitis is the sixth leading type of chronic disease in the United States and the most common nasal problem.

Symptoms of allergic rhinitis include nasal congestion; rhinorrhea; sneezing; watery eyes; and pruritus of the nose, palate, pharynx, ears, and eyes. Systemic symptoms also may occur including weakness, malaise, irritability, fatigue, and difficulty concentrating.

Physical signs include bilateral nasal obstruction with boggy, often bluish mucous membranes; clear mucoid nasal discharge; mouth breathing; a horizontal nasal crease from chronic rubbing of the nose upward; allergic shiners, which are dark and puffy lower lids from venous stasis; and the allergic salute sign, which is an upward nasal rubbing.

2. e. Sinusitis and otitis media are common complications of untreated allergic rhinitis caused by inflammation and obstruction of the sinus ostia and eustachian tube. Nasal polyps are a rare complication of allergic rhinitis and occur less in children than adults. Nasal polyps, however, are a feature of cystic fibrosis. Epistaxis can occur with severe acute allergic rhinitis. Allergic rhinitis is not a risk factor for nasopharyngeal tumors, but tumor should be in the differential diagnosis of chronic nasal congestion.

3. b. The response in allergic rhinitis is initiated by IgE. After sensitization of the nasal mucosa by a formerly encountered allergen, subsequent exposure results in cross-linking specific IgE receptors on mast cells. The activation of mast cells leads to release of multiple inflammatory mediators including histamine that result in vasodilation, edema, and pruritus. Subsequent recruitment of lymphocytes, eosinophils, basophils, and neutrophils also adds to the early and late-phase allergic response.

4. c. Family history is the single most important factor that predisposes a child to develop allergies. Smoke exposure can precipitate symptoms in someone who already has the disease. Aspirin intolerance along with nasal polyposis and asthma constitute the triad asthma syndrome. Eczema or atopic dermatitis is associated with allergic rhinitis. About 50% to 80% of children with atopic dermatitis develop allergic rhinitis, asthma, or both. However, only 10% of patients with allergic rhinitis go on to develop asthma.

5. **d.** All of the listed physical findings are found in patients with allergies; however, one is most likely to actually visualize the upward motion of nose rubbing (the salute) in children and not adults. Chronic nose rubbing and wrinkling of the nose is theorized to cause the horizontal nasal crease that is commonly seen at the junction of the bridge of the nose with the bulbous tip of the nose. Posterior pharyngeal wall lymphoid hyperplasia is also commonly known as "cobblestoning."

6. **d.** Perennial allergic rhinitis is most often the result of sensitivity to indoor inhalant allergens. House dust mites and cat dander are the most common causes. Cockroaches, feathers, and mold are all possible indoor inhalant allergens. Foods in general are not considered important causes of allergic rhinitis.

7. **c.** Seasonal allergic rhinitis (also known as hay fever or pollinosis) is caused by outdoor inhaled allergens including tree, grass, and weed pollens. Allergic rhinitis is not caused by insect-pollinated flowers and plants. Typically, animal dander/roaches do not cause "seasonal" symptoms. Mold can be an outdoor allergen as well, but it is not nearly as common a cause as the pollens.

8. **e.** The first principle of treatment with allergic rhinitis is to avoid exposure to the inciting allergen as much as possible. Avoiding outdoor allergens is difficult, although minimizing outdoor time when allergen levels are high and minimizing the indoor flux of these allergens can be done to some extent. Avoiding opening windows (using air conditioning instead) and avoiding fans that draw air into the home are some methods. Showering and changing clothes after outdoor activities on windy, high pollen days also is helpful.

Indoor allergens are also challenging. Most patients with pets are not willing to remove the pet from the household; however, not allowing the pet in the bedroom helps considerably. Dust mite control especially in the bedroom is also important. Removing carpets whenever feasible is one method (a suggestion that should be made to the patient's father in Clinical Case Problem 1). Mattresses and pillows should be encased in impermeable covers; humidity should be reduced because dust mites need it to survive; upholstered furniture should be avoided whenever possible; and bedding should be washed in hot water.

9. **b.** Intranasal cromolyn sodium has almost no side effects other than possible local irritation and sneezing. The problems with this therapy are that it is not very efficacious and it is prophylactic, so it should be started prior to onset of symptoms and needs to be used four to six times daily; therefore compliance is an issue. Antihistamines can cause sedation and interfere with school or work function. Immunotherapy can cause local reactions and more importantly anaphylaxis. Intranasal steroids can cause local irritation and bleeding and rarely septal perforation. Topical steroids do have some systemic absorption; however, in recommended doses they do not cause hypothalamic–pituitary axis suppression. Some studies do show minor effects on growth, so for children the lowest effective dose for the shortest amount of time necessary is recommended. Leukotriene receptor antagonists can cause influenzalike symptoms.

10. **b.** Intranasal corticosteroids are by far the most efficacious agents for allergic rhinitis. For children, intranasal cromolyn should be first-line therapy, with nasal steroids being second-line therapy if cromolyn is not enough. Antihistamines are useful for rhinorrhea and pruritus; however, they do not relieve congestion. Newer nonsedating forms such as loratadine, ceterizine, and fexofenadine are better choices because studies have shown that older antihistamines can cause psychomotor or cognitive impairment even without sedation. Topical decongestants can be used only for 3-5 days; if used longer they can cause rebound congestion. Oral decongestants can be used with antihistamines but can cause hyperactivity and insomnia. They should be used with caution in patients with hypertension, thyroid disease, diabetes, and enlarged prostates. Leukotriene antagonists have similar efficacy to antihistamines but work better in combination with them.

11. **c.** Nasal smears are helpful in ruling out infectious causes of rhinitis; however, lack of eosinophils does not rule out allergic rhinitis. Smears that are positive also do not rule out NARES, which is the not-well-understood syndrome of nonallergic rhinitis with eosinophilia. Laboratory studies are not always necessary, especially in patients with a clearcut seasonal pattern and classic history. Serum IgE is not an appropriate screening test for allergies because more than half of patients with allergies have normal levels.

12. **d.** Vasomotor rhinitis is seen rarely in children. This disorder is poorly understood and is theoretically

the result of an imbalance of the autonomic nervous system control of mucosal vasculature and mucous glands in which symptoms mimic allergic rhinitis but no allergic cause is found on testing.

13. **d.** Guaifenesin is an expectorant and is not indicated for the treatment of allergic rhinitis. Leukotriene antagonists inhibit the immune cascade that potentially can cause allergic symptoms and have been discussed prior. Oral corticosteroids are not routinely recommended but can be used for severe, acute disease for a short term as potent antiinflammatory agents. Anticholinergics and topical ipratropium bromide are effective in treating the watery rhinorrhea of allergies. Antihistamines also help with pruritus.

14. **a.** Although antihypertensive agents such as reserpine can cause rhinorrhea, hypertension itself is not associated with allergic rhinitis. The other systemic diseases can be associated with rhinitis.

15. **e.** Immunotherapy is indicated in patients who do not have adequate relief from pharmacologic treatment, who cannot tolerate the medications, or in whom the pharmacologic treatments are contraindicated for other medical reasons. Immunotherapy has been proved to be effective for seasonal-type allergens such as grass, ragweed, and trees. Its efficacy in controlling dust and mold-related symptoms is still not clear. There is no absolute recommendation for duration of therapy, but most believe that with 3-5 years of adequate symptom control, immunotherapy then can be stopped and that 65% of those patients will have continued longlasting relief. If a patient does not show any improvement after 1 year of immunotherapy, it should be discontinued. All of the other statements about immunotherapy are true.

SOLUTION TO THE CLINICAL CASE MANAGEMENT PROBLEM

Rhinitis medicamentosa is the term used to describe the chronic nasal congestion that results as a rebound effect of prolonged or excessive use of topical nasal decongestant nose drops that work by vasoconstriction. The rebound swelling is caused by interstitial edema, not vasodilation. Topical decongestants therefore should not be used for more than 5 days. Similar consequences can be produced by chronic topical use of other vasoconstrictors, such as cocaine. On examination the nasal mucosa appears beefy red and swollen and may show areas of punctate bleeding.

SUMMARY OF ALLERGIC RHINITIS

A. **Classification:** Seasonal allergic rhinitis (also known as hay fever or seasonal pollinosis) causes include tree, weed, and grass pollen; mold spores are a less likely cause; temporally related to seasons with high pollen counts, variable on geographic location

 Perennial allergic rhinitis: symptoms present at least 9 months out of the year; causes include dust mite, animal dander, feathers, mold, and cockroaches

B. **Symptoms:** nasal congestion; rhinorrhea; pruritus; sneezing; nasal discharge; and eye redness, itching, and tearing

C. **Signs:**
 1. Allergic shiners: dark, puffy lower eyelids from venous stasis caused by impaired blood flow through inflamed, edematous nasal mucous membranes
 2. Allergic salute: rubbing nose with palm of hand in an upward motion, usually only seen in children
 3. Horizontal allergic nasal crease: results from chronic nose rubbing, wrinkling, scrunching
 4. Pale, blue, boggy nasal turbinates and mucosa
 5. Lymphoid hyperplasia of posterior pharyngeal wall
 6. Mouth breathing and snoring

D. **Diagnosis:** clinical history and physical, nasal smear with eosinophils, RAST testing, and skin allergy testing

E. **Associated disorders:** otitis media (acute and chronic), sinusitis, adenoid and tonsillar hypertrophy, asthma, and atopic dermatitis

Continued

SUMMARY OF ALLERGIC RHINITIS —cont'd

F. **Differential diagnosis:** eosinophilic nonallergic rhinitis, infectious rhinitis, vasomotor rhinitis, and rhinitis medicamentosa

   Systemic diseases (Sarcoidosis, Wegener's granulomatosis, amyloidosis, hypothyroidism)

G. **Treatment:** avoidance of allergen as much as is feasible; inhaled corticosteroids are most efficacious and first-line therapy; nonsedating antihistamine; leukotriene receptor antagonists (not any more efficacious than antihistamines alone, but better when added to antihistamines); use decongestants sparingly; immunotherapy

SUGGESTED READING

Eggleston PA: Environmental allergen avoidance: an overview. *J Allergy Clin Immunol* 107(3 Suppl):S403-405, 2001.

Naclerio RM, Wood R: Allergic rhinitis: a practical review. *Resident & Staff Physician* 49(8):10-17, 2003.

Scadding GK: Corticosteroids in the treatment of pediatric allergic rhinitis. *J Allergy Clin Immunol* 108(1 Suppl):S59-64, 2001.

Skoner DP: Allergic rhinitis: definition, epidemiology, pathophysiology, detection, and diagnosis. *J Allergy Clin Immunol* 108(1 Suppl):S2-8, 2001.

Stone KD: Atopic diseases of childhood. *Curr Opin Pediatr* 14(5):634-646, 2002 Oct.

Chapter 113

Diaper and Other Infant Dermatitis

> "Doctor, can't you do something? He is so uncomfortable."

CLINICAL CASE PROBLEM 1:

A 2-MONTH-OLD INFANT WITH A RASH ON HIS CHEEKS

A 2-month-old infant is brought to your office by his mother. He developed an erythematous, dry skin rash on both cheeks approximately 1 week ago. Although the rash is always present, the mother states that it seems to be worse after she feeds him.

The mother breastfed for the first 4 weeks of life but returned to work 4 weeks ago and switched the baby from breastfeeding to bottle feeding. The mother has a history of asthma, and the father has seasonal allergies.

On examination, the child appears healthy. He has an erythematous maculopapular eruption that covers his cheeks, and he appears to be developing an erythematous rash on his neck, both wrists, and both hands. The rest of the physical examination is within normal limits.

■ SELECT THE BEST ANSWER TO THE FOLLOWING QUESTIONS:

1. What is the most likely cause of this infant's skin rash?
   a. atopic dermatitis
   b. allergic contact dermatitis
   c. seborrheic dermatitis
   d. infectious eczematoid dermatitis
   e. none of the above

2. What is (are) the recommended treatment(s) of the skin rash in the infant presented?
   a. skin hydration
   b. local corticosteroid therapy
   c. systemic antihistamines
   d. minimizing the use of soap
   e. all of the above

3. What other conditions are associated with this condition?
   a. asthma
   b. allergic rhinitis
   c. wool sensitivity
   d. keratosis pilaris
   e. all of the above

4. Which statement is false regarding the prognosis and treatment of this condition?
   a. topical steroids achieve good control in 90% of patients
   b. smallpox vaccine is contraindicated in these patients because of the risk of eczema herpeticum.
   c. up to 30% of patients have spontaneous resolution by puberty
   d. some adults continue to have localized rash
   e. atopic dermatitis is relatively rare in geriatric patients

5. Which statement is true regarding this condition?
   a. a cotton diaper is preferred over a disposable diaper in this condition

b. breastfeeding offers no advantage over formula feeding in this condition
c. sun exposure may be helpful in this condition
d. patients do better in a dry climate
e. antihistamines can be curative in this condition

CLINICAL CASE PROBLEM 2:

*A 1-MONTH-OLD INFANT WITH
A 2-WEEK-OLD DIAPER RASH*

A 1-month-old infant is brought to your office by his mother. She states that the infant has had a diaper rash for the past 2 weeks that has not cleared up with the use of zinc oxide three times a day. She tells you that she must be doing something wrong, and she is extremely upset.

On examination, the infant has a mildly erythematous, greasy, scaly rash in the diaper area. He also has a scaly rash on the scalp, the ear, the sides of the nose, and the eyebrows and eyelids. The rest of the physical examination is normal.

6. What is the most likely diagnosis in this infant?
   a. atopic dermatitis
   b. allergic contact dermatitis
   c. seborrheic dermatitis
   d. infectious eczematoid dermatitis
   e. none of the above

7. What is (are) the treatment(s) of choice for the condition described in Clinical Case Problem 2?
   a. wet compresses
   b. topical corticosteroids
   c. topical ketoconazole
   d. a and b
   e. a, b, and c

CLINICAL CASE PROBLEM 3:

*AN 8-MONTH-OLD INFANT WITH A
LONG-TERM PERSISTENT DIAPER RASH*

An 8-month-old infant is brought to your office by his mother for assessment of a diaper rash. His mother has tried cornstarch, talcum powder, vitamin E cream, zinc oxide, and three different prescribed corticosteroid creams from three different physicians as remedies. She tells you that she went to three doctors because the first two said, "Oh, don't worry, dear. It's just a little diaper rash. It will go away. Don't worry your pretty little head about it."

On examination, the infant has an intensely erythematous diaper dermatitis that has a scalloped border and a sharply demarcated edge. There are numerous "satellite lesions" present on the lower abdomen and thighs.

8. What is the most likely diagnosis in this infant?
   a. atopic dermatitis
   b. allergic contact dermatitis
   c. seborrheic dermatitis
   d. infectious eczematoid dermatitis
   e. candidal diaper dermatitis

9. What is the treatment of choice for the diaper rash of the infant described in Clinical Case Problem 3?
   a. a topical corticosteroid
   b. a topical antibiotic
   c. a systemic antibiotic
   d. a topical antifungal agent
   e. none of the above

CLINICAL CASE PROBLEM 4:

*A 4-MONTH-OLD INFANT WITH A DIAPER
RASH CAUSED BY DIRTY DIAPERS*

A 4-month-old infant is brought to your office by her mother. Her mother complains that the child has a diaper rash that is probably related to her "lack of changing by the babysitter." Apparently, the infant went for long periods wearing a dirty diaper while the babysitter sat on the couch watching television. Needless to say, the babysitter is no longer in the employment of the mother.

On examination, the infant has erythematous, scaly, papulovesicular diaper dermatitis with numerous bullous lesions, fissures, and erosions.

10. What is the most likely diagnosis in this infant?
    a. atopic dermatitis
    b. primary irritant contact dermatitis
    c. seborrheic dermatitis
    d. fungal dermatitis
    e. allergic contact dermatitis

11. What is (are) the treatment(s) of choice for the infant described in Clinical Case Problem 4?
    a. zinc oxide paste
    b. topical hydrocortisone
    c. systemic antibiotics
    d. a and b
    e. a, b, and c

12. What differentiates a candidal diaper rash from irritant diaper dermatitis?
    a. irritant diaper dermatitis spares the crural folds
    b. candidal diaper rash spares the crural folds
    c. irritant diaper dermatitis involves the crural folds
    d. none of the above
    e. a, b, and c

ANSWERS:

1. a. This child has atopic dermatitis. Atopic dermatitis is an inflammatory skin disease characterized by erythema, edema, pruritus, exudation, crusting, and scaling.

Atopic dermatitis usually begins in infancy. The areas most commonly affected include the cheeks, neck, wrists, hands, and extensor aspects of the extremities. Spread often occurs from extensor to flexor. Pruritus may lead to intense scratching and secondary infection.

Atopic dermatitis usually is precipitated by or exacerbated by the introduction of certain foods to the infant's diet, particularly cow's milk, wheat, or eggs. Environmental factors such as dust mites, mold, and cat dander also may trigger the condition.

2. e. The treatment of atopic dermatitis begins with the avoidance of any environmental factors that precipitate the condition.

Smooth-textured cotton garments help reduce added irritation in this disorder. The use of soaps and detergents abstracts lipids from the skin and should be minimized. Bathing without bath oil should be avoided when possible. Ideally, the child should be in the tub for at least 15 minutes before the bath oil is added to the water.

Atopic dermatitis is best managed with local therapy. Flareups of the condition are treated with topical corticosteroid creams or lotions. To further prevent scratching, the fingernails should be cut short. Percutaneous absorption of corticosteroid does occur, and atrophy of the skin should be watched for. This can be avoided by using a moderate potency topical corticosteroid for 7 days followed by a low-potency topical hydrocortisone preparation (0.5% hydrocortisone) for 2-3 weeks until the lesions have resolved.

Systemic antihistamines such as diphenhydramine, promethazine, and hydroxyzine may have to be used to control pruritus (use with caution). Nonsedating antihistamines such as loratadine or cetirizine also can provide relief from itching and scratching, but they are not curative.

Infected atopic dermatitis is best managed by antibiotic therapy. Systemic antibiotics are the mainstays of treatment for infected atopic dermatitis. However, the newer, nonsensitizing local antibiotic preparations such as mupirocin may be used for local infections.

3. e. Atopic dermatitis often is associated with a family history of allergies, asthma, hay fever, or atopic dermatitis. Individuals are more sensitive to certain fibers, particularly wool. Rough fibers tend to be more irritating than smooth fibers in clothing textiles.

Keratosis pilaris, which is characterized by asymptomatic horny follicular papules on the upper arms, buttocks, and thighs, is another manifestation of atopic dermatitis.

4. c. Atopic dermatitis is largely a condition of children. It typically manifests in infants in the first 6 months of life, and 90% of patients will have disease presentation by age 5 years. Close to 90% of patients have resolution of symptoms by puberty. Topical steroids are well-proven in achieving good rash control, but care must be used to prevent steroid overuse and the development of skin atrophy and striae. Some adults continue to have atopic dermatitis, but these patients often manifest with hand and foot dermatitis. Atopic dermatitis is rare in geriatric patients.

5. c. A randomized controlled study found no difference in eczema scores with cotton diaper versus cellulose core/absorbent gel disposable diapers. Breastfeeding is clearly advantageous over formula feeding in atopic dermatitis. Sun exposure may be helpful in atopic dermatitis. Patients do better in humid environments. Antihistamines can be symptom controlling but not curative in this condition.

6. c. This infant has seborrheic dermatitis, an inflammatory disorder that often begins in the first month of life. The initial manifestation of seborrheic dermatitis is often a diffuse or focal scaling and crusting of the scalp, a condition known as *cradle cap.* A dry scaly, erythematous, papular dermatitis, which is usually nonpruritic, may develop, involving the face, neck, retroauricular areas, axillae, and diaper area. The dermatitis may be patchy or focal or may spread to involve the entire body.

7. e. Wet compresses (saline) are an effective first treatment for seborrheic dermatitis. A soft brush can be used to remove some of the scales associated with cradle cap. Scalp lesions also may be controlled with an antiseborrheic shampoo such as selenium sulfide.

Topical corticosteroids (hydrocortisone 0.5% to 1%) may be applied to inflammatory lesions. The use of topical ketoconazole (2%) has been found to be of benefit in the treatment of seborrheic dermatitis.

8. e. This infant has candidal diaper dermatitis, which presents as an erythematous confluent plaque formed by papules and vesiculopustules, with a scalloped border and a sharply demarcated edge.

Candidal diaper dermatitis usually can be distinguished from other childhood diaper dermatoses by the presence of "satellite lesions" produced at some distance from the primary eruption.

9. d. The treatment of choice in candidal diaper dermatitis is a topical antifungal agent. Topical miconazole, clotrimazole, or ketoconazole can be used after soaking the inflamed area with wet aluminum acetate compresses. In an infant with a severe inflammatory reaction, a topical corticosteroid may be mixed 50/50 with a topical antifungal agent and applied on a regular basis for a few days to a week.

The attitude displayed by the first two physicians (condescending and arrogant) is not as uncommon as we think. Doctor–patient communication in something as simple as diaper dermatitis can significantly affect not only the efficacy of treatment but also compliance and postdiagnostic attitudes.

10. b. This child has a primary irritant contact dermatitis. Irritant contact dermatitis is a reaction to friction, maceration, and prolonged contact with urine and feces. It usually presents as an erythematous, scaly dermatitis with papulovesicular or bullous lesions, fissures, and erosions. The eruption can be either patchy or confluent. The genitocrural folds often are spared.

Secondary infection with either bacteria or yeast can occur. The infant can be in considerable discomfort because of the marked inflammation that sometimes is associated with this type of diaper rash.

Primary irritant diaper dermatitis should be managed by frequent changing of diapers and thorough washing of the genitalia with warm water and a mild soap. Occlusive plastic pants that promote maceration should be avoided. Highly absorbent disposable diapers should be used instead of cloth diapers. Drying out the skin by allowing the infant to go without diapers can be helpful but can be logistically challenging.

11. d. An occlusive topical agent such as zinc oxide can be applied until healing occurs. Topical 1% hydrocortisone ointment is also very useful in the management of diaper dermatitis in its more severe form. Systemic antibiotics are not indicated in the treatment of primary irritant diaper dermatitis.

12. a. A useful diagnostic pearl for differentiating candidal diaper rash from irritant diaper dermatitis is that candidal diaper rash tends to involve the warm, moist folds of the skin, whereas irritant diaper dermatitis tends to spare the folds, chiefly occurring in the areas of greatest skin contact with urine and feces. Candidal diaper rash also tends to present with satellite lesions.

SUMMARY OF DIAPER AND OTHER INFANT DERMATITIS

A. Atopic dermatitis:
1. **Diagnostic clue:** usually begins and is more prominent on the cheeks of infants
2. **Treatment:** moisturization, mild topical corticosteroids, systemic antihistamines (with caution), systemic or topical antibiotics for secondary infection

B. Seborrheic dermatitis:
1. **Diagnostic clue:** cradle cap often associated with this type of diaper dermatitis
2. **Treatment:** wet compresses (saline), mild topical corticosteroids, topical ketoconazole

C. Candidal dermatitis:
1. **Diagnostic clue:** satellite lesions around the peripheral area of the main area of dermatitis
2. **Treatment:** topical miconazole, topical ketoconazole, mild topical hydrocortisone mixed 50/50 with a topical antifungal agent when severe inflammation is present

D. Primary irritant dermatitis:
1. **Diagnostic clue:** maceration, often a history of the use of cloth diapers or plastic pants
2. **Treatment:** occlusive topical agent such as zinc oxide or petroleum jelly or zinc oxide applied over hydrocortisone base when severe inflammation is present

SUGGESTED READING

Allen DM, Drolet BA: Chapter 20. Pediatric dermatology. In: Behrman RE, Kliegman RM, eds.: *Nelson essentials of pediatrics,* 4th ed. WB Saunders, 2002, Philadelphia, 875-877.

Ghidorzi A: Atopic dermatitis. *emedicine.com.* June 28, 2001.

Johnson BA, Nunley JR: Treatment of seborrheic dermatitis. *Am Fam Physician* 61:2703-2710, 2713-2714, 2000.

Smethurst D, Macfarlane S: Atopic eczema. Clinical evidence concise. *BMJ* Publishing Group. June 2003.

TePas EC, Umetsu DT: Chapter 8. Immunology and allergy: atopic dermatitis. In: Behrman RE, Kliegman RM, eds.: *Nelson essentials of pediatrics,* 4th ed. WB Saunders, 2002, Philadelphia, 330-333.

Chapter 114

Cardiac Murmurs

> "My baby has heart problems? Does that mean he is going to die young?"

CLINICAL CASE PROBLEM 1:

A 3-Year-Old Child with a Cardiac Murmur

A 3-year-old child is brought to your office by his mother for a periodic health examination. The child has been well and has no history of significant medical illness. He has reached all of his developmental milestones.

On physical examination, the child is in the 50th percentile for weight and height. His blood pressure is 90/70 mm Hg. He has a grade II/VI short ejection systolic murmur heard maximally along the left sternal edge from the midsternum to the lower end of the sternum. There is no radiation of the murmur to either the neck or back. There is no associated thrill with this murmur. The child's pulse is 84 per minute and regular. The femoral artery pulses are normal and are not delayed. The rest of the physical examination is normal.

■ **SELECT THE BEST ANSWER TO THE FOLLOWING QUESTIONS:**

1. Which of the following statement(s) best reflect(s) the character of this heart murmur?
   a. the location of the heart murmur (mid to low sternum) increases the probability of this murmur being pathologic
   b. systolic timing of the heart murmur increases the probability of this murmur being pathologic
   c. grade of the murmur (II/VI rather than I/VI) increases the probability of this murmur being pathologic
   d. none of the above
   e. a, b, and c

2. This murmur is best referred to as which of the following?
   a. Mustard's murmur
   b. Fallot's murmur
   c. Still's murmur
   d. De Bakey's murmur
   e. Framingham's murmur

3. Which of the following signs or symptoms is not associated with "innocent" cardiac murmurs?
   a. low frequency
   b. an associated thrill
   c. short ejection systolic in timing
   d. grade I or grade II in audibility
   e. a and b

4. The murmur described is intensified by which of the following?
   a. sitting the patient up
   b. increasing the heart rate
   c. fever
   d. anxiety
   e. all of the above

5. At this time, which of the following investigations should be performed on the child?
   a. a chest x-ray
   b. an electrocardiogram (ECG)
   c. an echocardiogram
   d. none of the above
   e. a, b, and c

6. At this time, what should you do?
   a. call the pediatric cardiologist immediately
   b. tell the child's mother that the child has a heart murmur but "not to worry...It probably isn't anything important"
   c. tell the mother that all heart murmurs need to be taken very seriously; therefore, it is probably best to have the pediatric cardiologist do "every test he can"
   d. tell the mother that the heart sound you hear (a very soft murmur) is very common and occurs in at least half of all children
   e. tell the mother nothing; there is no need to cause her unnecessary worry

CLINICAL CASE PROBLEM 2:

A 6-Month-Old Infant with a Harsh Grade III/VI Pansystolic Heart Murmur

A 6-month-old infant is brought to your office by his mother. She came in for a periodic health assessment. You have not seen the child before. The mother states that the child has been well and has had no medical problems.

On examination, the child has a grade III/VI harsh pansystolic heart murmur heard along the lower left sternal edge. There is no radiation of the murmur. The heart rate is 72 beats per minute and regular. There is no thrill. The blood pressure is 80/60 mm Hg.

No other abnormalities are found on examination. Most importantly, the child is in the 50th percentile for weight and length.

7. What is the most likely cardiac diagnosis in this infant?
   a. innocent cardiac murmur
   b. tetralogy of Fallot
   c. pulmonary atresia
   d. ventricular septal defect (VSD)
   e. coarctation of the aorta

8. At this time, the child described in Clinical Case Problem 2 should:
   a. have immediate surgery
   b. be managed with digoxin and diuretics
   c. be managed with digoxin, diuretics, and an angiotensin-converting enzyme inhibitor
   d. have an immediate cardiac catheterization performed followed by surgical closure within 3 months
   e. none of the above

9. What preventive health practices should be followed for the child described in Clinical Case Problem 2?
   a. prophylaxis against bacterial endocarditis if dental work is to be done
   b. cardiac catheterizations every 3 months until resolution
   c. echocardiograms every 3 months until resolution
   d. a and c
   e. none of the above

10. What is the prevalence of cardiac murmurs in childhood?
    a. 5%
    b. 10%
    c. 20%
    d. 50%
    e. 90%

11. What is the most common pathologic cardiac murmur in childhood?
    a. atrial septal defect (ASD)
    b. tetralogy of Fallot
    c. VSD
    d. transposition of the great arteries
    e. aortic stenosis

12. Which of the following is (are) a common innocent cardiac murmur(s) in childhood?
    a. neonatal pulmonary artery branch murmur
    b. "venous hum" of late infancy
    c. "Still's aortic vibratory" murmur
    d. pulmonary valve area "flow" murmur
    e. all of the above

CLINICAL CASE PROBLEM 3:

A BABY WITH ABNORMAL FACIES AND A MURMUR

A mother brings her child in for a 2-month visit. She gives a history of no prenatal care and a normal vaginal delivery. The baby has received no medical care since discharge. The infant has a large, protruding tongue; short palpebral fissures; and epicanthal folds. He has a simian palmar crease and a large space between the first and second toes. On cardiac examination, you note a harsh 3/6 systolic murmur on the left sternal border.

13. Your leading cardiac diagnosis is:
    a. Still's murmur
    b. venous hum
    c. teratology of Fallot
    d. atrioventricular canal
    e. hypoplastic left heart

■ ANSWERS:

1. **e.** This murmur has all the characteristics of an innocent murmur: it is located at the mid to low sternal border, it is systolic in timing, and it has no associated thrill. Most importantly, the child appears healthy and is growing and developing normally. The grading of murmurs is from I to VI. Grade I is very faintly auscultated with the stethoscope. Grade II can be heard more clearly. Grade III is a loud murmur with no associated thrill. Grade IV is also loud, with a palpable thrill. Grade V can be heard with the stethoscope tilted off of the patient's chest, and Grade VI can be heard without a stethoscope. Location, quality, and timing (systole or diastole) are critical characteristics of a murmur.

2. **c.** This murmur, which is described as "vibratory" or "musical" in nature, is known as Still's murmur. Still's murmur is safely diagnosed clinically, and laboratory studies add nothing to its assessment. However, any murmur associated with failure to thrive, no matter how innocent sounding, should prompt further investigation.

3. **b.** There is no such thing as an innocent thrill. A palpable thrill demands a further workup.

4. **e.** Other characteristics of an innocent cardiac murmur (such as a Still's murmur) include the following: it is low in frequency and localized; it is seldom greater than grade II/VI in intensity; and it is accentuated by the sitting position, anxiety, fever, anemia, and increasing heart rate. Once again note that an innocent cardiac murmur in a child is never associated with a thrill.

5. **d.** This Still's murmur is safely diagnosed clinically, and laboratory and diagnostic imaging studies add nothing to its assessment.

6. **d.** In explaining heart murmurs to parents, not just what you say but how you say it is very important. It is important to be reassuring in your tone and to point out that 50% of children have cardiac murmurs.

Make sure that you provide an opportunity for the mother to ask any questions that she may have.

It is extremely unwise not to tell the parents when you detect a heart murmur in a young child. Sooner or later someone is going to hear it and mention it. At that time it will come back to haunt you. It is far better to tell the parent(s) that a heart murmur exists but that you are confident that it is innocent. If you are not positive, an elective referral to a pediatric cardiologist would be reasonable.

7. d. The most likely cardiac diagnosis in this infant is VSD. The typical heart murmur associated with a VSD is harsh, pansystolic, and best heard at the lower left sternal edge. Even as the VSD becomes smaller, it maintains its regurgitant characteristic of starting off with the first heart sound (holosystolic timing). As a VSD closes and becomes smaller, the murmur actually can become louder until the VSD is closed.

8. e. The treatment recommended at this time is none of the above. Watchful expectation should be pursued. The prognosis is excellent, and the defect likely will close spontaneously. As the VSD becomes smaller, the murmur becomes shorter and (as mentioned) maintains its regurgitant characteristics (i.e., it starts off with the first heart sound). At least 50% of VSDs will close by the end of the first year or shortly thereafter. Pediatric cardiology referral is appropriate for serial examinations and echocardiograms.

9. a. The only prophylaxis that needs to be followed in this child is protection with antibiotic therapy (penicillin, amoxicillin, or erythromycin for patients allergic to penicillin) before any dental procedure or any other procedure that would increase the probability of bacterial endocarditis. This obviously can be discontinued when the defect closes. Serial echocardiograms are indicated. Different cardiologists have different recommendations for the frequency of examination, but every 6-12 months is the range, not every 3 months. Cardiac catheterization is not indicated for this lesion.

10. d. The prevalence of cardiac murmurs in childhood is at least 50%, probably considerably higher to the sensitive ear. The vast majority of these murmurs are innocent in nature and do not reflect any cardiac pathologic condition.

11. c. The most common pathologic cardiac murmur in childhood is VSD. With a VSD, the cardiac murmur is often not present at birth but is first heard at the 2- to 4-week well-baby checkup. As discussed previously, the most common outcome of this congenital heart defect is spontaneous closure. In some cases, however, surgical closure is indicated. The most uncommon scenario is the development of congestive cardiac failure secondary to VSD.

The relative frequency of pathologic cardiac murmurs in childhood are as follows: VSD, 38%; ASD, 18%; pulmonary valve stenosis, 13%; pulmonary artery stenosis, 7%; aortic valve stenosis, 4%; patent ductus arteriosis, 4%; mitral valve prolapse, 4%; and all others, 11%.

12. e. The common functional or common innocent murmurs of infancy and childhood include the following: (1) neonatal pulmonary artery branch murmur; (2) venous hum of late infancy and early childhood; (3) Still's aortic vibratory systolic murmur; and (4) pulmonary valve area "flow" murmur of late adolescence and childhood.

13. d. This infant has the characteristic stigmata of Down syndrome, or trisomy 21. At least 50% of infants with Down syndrome have some type of congenital heart disease. Atrioventricular canal, or an endocardial cushion defect, is one of the most common lesions in this population. Congestive heart failure can develop in these infants. Most infants with congenital heart disease and trisomy 21 should be identified on prenatal screening. Care must be taken in patients with no prenatal care and little medical follow-up. Any newborn identified with the stigmata of trisomy 21 should have a screening echocardiogram.

SUMMARY OF CARDIAC MURMURS

1. Prevalence of murmurs:
   a. Overall prevalence: at least 50% of all children
   b. Innocent/pathologic: 10/1
2. Epidemiology: Experienced clinical assessment is just as sensitive and specific as echocardiography and more sensitive and specific than electrocardiography. Any concern or doubt on the part of the primary care physician should warrant referral to a pediatric cardiologist. Evaluation should include a complete history and physical examination, including careful palpation of pulses and cardiac impulses, assessment of skin color, and complete cardiac examination.
3. Innocent murmurs:
   a. Still's murmur (most common)
   b. Venous hum (second most common)

c. Pulmonary flow murmur

d. Neonatal pulmonary artery branch murmur

4. Pathologic murmurs:

a. VSD (most common)

b. ASD (second most common)

c. Pulmonary valve stenosis

5. Clinical signs and symptoms that are reassuring for the family physician as he or she evaluates a childhood cardiac murmur include the following:

a. Is there any evidence of failure to thrive in the child? If no, this suggests an innocent murmur.

b. Are there any symptoms (shortness of breath, blue lips, lethargy) or signs (cyanosis, diastolic murmur, parasternal heave, thrill, loud murmur greater than II/VI, holosystolic murmur) to suggest pathologic murmur? If no, this suggests an innocent murmur.

c. Is the murmur accentuated by sitting forward? If yes, this suggests an innocent murmur.

d. Is the murmur accentuated by exercise or increased heart rate resulting from another cause? If yes, this suggests an innocent murmur.

e. Is the murmur accentuated by fever? If yes, this suggests an innocent murmur.

f. Is the murmur accentuated by anxiety, restlessness, or crying? If yes, this suggests an innocent murmur.

g. Is the murmur a murmur without any radiation (i.e., to the neck or to the back)? If yes, this suggests an innocent murmur.

h. Is the murmur present lower (rather than higher) along the left sternal edge? If yes, this suggests an innocent murmur.

i. Did the mother bring the child in for a specific reason that may be associated with cardiac disease (such as having to stop and rest while playing)? If no, this suggests an innocent murmur.

j. Are there any other characteristics of abnormal murmurs including: sweating while eating, clubbing, associated anomalies or abnormal facies, edema, and arrhythmias? If not, this suggests an innocent murmur.

SUGGESTED READING

Allen H, et al: Heart murmurs in children: When is a work-up needed? *Contemp Pediatr* 11:28-52, 1994.

Ando M, et al: Infective endocarditis affecting both pulmonary and systemic circulations predisposed by a ventricular septal defect. *Japan J Thoracic Cardiovasc Surg* 48(7):451-454, 2000.

Brook MM: Chapter 13. The cardiovascular system. In: Behrman RE, Kliegman RM, eds.: *Nelson essentials of pediatrics*, 4th ed. WB Saunders, 2002, Philadelphia, 555-604.

Clark EB: Etiology of congenital cardiovascular malformations: epidemiology and genetics. In: Allen H, et al, eds.: *Moss and Adam's heart diseases in infants, children and adolescents including fetus' and young adults*. Volume 1. 6th ed. Williams and Wilkins, 2000, Philadelphia.

Park MK: *Pediatric cardiology for practitioners*, 3rd ed. Mosby, 1996, St. Louis.

Symthe J, et al: Initial evaluation of heart murmurs: Are laboratory tests necessary? *Pediatrics* 86(4):497-500, 1990.

Chapter 115

Over-The-Counter Drugs

"You mean that medicine from the drug store can be bad for my baby?"

CLINICAL CASE PROBLEM 1:

A 6-MONTH-OLD INFANT WITH AN UPPER-RESPIRATORY TRACT INFECTION

A 6-month-old infant is brought to your office by his mother. He has had an upper-respiratory tract infection (URI) consisting of a runny nose, cough, and a mild fever for the last 4 days. The infant's mother is concerned because his temperature reached 39° C last evening.

On physical examination, the child looks well. He has nasal congestion and a hyperemic pharynx. His lungs are clear; no adventitious breath sounds are heard.

■ SELECT THE BEST ANSWER TO THE FOLLOWING QUESTIONS:

1. Regarding the child's fever, what should you tell the mother?

a. treat the fever with baby aspirin if it reaches 39° C again

b. treat the fever with elixir of acetaminophen if it reaches 39° C again

c. treat the fever with a combination of baby aspirin and elixir of acetaminophen if it reaches 39° C again

d. use only symptomatic treatment (cool clothes, fan in the room)

e. tell the mother that everyone has a different opinion; as far as you are concerned, she can do whatever she wants

2. What is the analgesic agent of choice in the treatment of childhood fever and mild childhood pain?

a. elixir of naproxen
b. elixir of hydromorphone
c. elixir of acetaminophen
d. children's aspirin: 75 mg
e. elixir of acetaminophen and codeine

3. Regarding the use of aspirin and acetaminophen in childhood analgesia, which of the following statements most accurately reflects current recommended practice?
   a. aspirin is still the analgesic of choice in the treatment of infant and childhood pain
   b. aspirin is not contraindicated in the treatment of infant and childhood pain associated with URIs
   c. aspirin is a more potent analgesic than acetaminophen
   d. acetaminophen is the drug of choice for the treatment of infant and childhood pain
   e. acetaminophen should be used in all infants and children

4. Regarding the use of antihistamines in children, which of the following statements is true?
   a. antihistamines shorten the duration of respiratory tract illness in children
   b. antihistamines reduce the incidence of otitis media following the beginning of a URI in a young child
   c. the prescription of an antihistamine in a child with a viral URI is considered good practice
   d. antihistamines may produce seizures in young children who are given antihistamine doses (tablets or suppositories) that are meant for older children (on a milligram-per-kilogram basis)
   e. none of the above statements are true

5. Regarding the relief of nasal congestion in infants and children, which of the following statements is true?
   a. antihistamines produce excellent relief of pediatric nasal congestion
   b. antihistamines, when compared to cool or warm steam, produce superior relief of nasal congestion in pediatric patients
   c. cool or warm steam, when compared to antihistamines, produce superior relief of nasal congestion in pediatric patients
   d. antihistamines and cool or warm steam are equally efficacious in providing relief of nasal congestion
   e. nobody really knows for sure

The child described in Clinical Case Problem 1 returns in 3 days with his mother. She states that despite your treatment the child has not improved. He now has significantly greater nasal congestion and is having a difficult time breathing at night.

On examination, the ears and throat remain clear. You do not notice any change in the state of the nasal congestion.

6. With respect to treatment of this infant at this time, which of the following statements is true?
   a. a decongestant to relieve nasal congestion is a reasonable therapeutic maneuver now
   b. decongestants have been shown to reduce the duration of viral URI symptoms
   c. topical sympathomimetic agents are unlikely to be systemically absorbed
   d. overstimulation is a common side effect when decongestant preparations are given to children
   e. none of the above statements are true

CLINICAL CASE PROBLEM 2:
A 6-MONTH-OLD INFANT WITH A PERSISTENT COUGH

A mother brings her 6-month-old daughter to your office for assessment of a persistent cough. The cough has been present for the past 10 days. It is nonproductive, and the mother believes it is interfering significantly with the child's sleep. You are considering prescribing an antitussive or an expectorant.

7. Which of the following statements regarding the use of antitussives or expectorants in infants and children is true?
   a. dextromethorphan suppresses cough and is unlikely to produce any significant adverse reactions in infants and children
   b. the combination of a cough suppressant and an expectorant is a logical combination to try in a child with a persistent cough
   c. dextromethorphan has been shown to significantly decrease the duration of respiratory tract infection symptoms in children
   d. respiratory depression in children has been reported with dextromethorphan
   e. none of the above are true

CLINICAL CASE PROBLEM 3:
A 13-MONTH-OLD INFANT WITH NAUSEA AND VOMITING

A mother brings her 13-month-old infant to the office for assessment of nausea and vomiting. She stopped in at the local emergency department 24 hours previously and was told to purchase childhood dimenhydrinate suppositories for the nausea. Apparently, the emergency department physician did a complete workup and there were no other significant findings.

However, the nausea and vomiting continued. At this time the child appears to be approximately 5% dehydrated. On physical examination, there are no other abnormalities found. The child appears somewhat sedated and lethargic.

You decide to admit the child for observation, reevaluation, and rehydration.

8. Which of the following statements regarding the use of antiemetics in children is (are) true?
   a. dimenhydrinate is effective for the treatment of nausea and vomiting associated with gastrointestinal infection and is devoid of significant side effects
   b. the sedation that is seen in this infant may be secondary to the dimenhydrinate
   c. dimenhydrinate toxicity may be difficult to distinguish from worsening of the illness
   d. b and c
   e. a, b, and c

CLINICAL CASE PROBLEM 4:

AN 8-MONTH-OLD INFANT WITH FEVER, DIARRHEA, AND RED CHEEKS

A mother brings her 8-month-old infant to your office for assessment of fever, diarrhea, and red cheeks that she attributes to teething. She was advised by her neighbor to purchase a preparation of topical benzocaine. This has not helped.

On examination, the infant has a temperature of 39° C. There are no other abnormalities on physical examination.

9. Which of the following statements regarding this infant is (are) true?
   a. the symptoms described probably are caused by teething
   b. acetaminophen is a reasonable treatment for a child that is teething
   c. teething often begins at 4-6 months of age and carries on intermittently up to the age of 2 years
   d. b and c
   e. a, b, and c

10. In addition to the side effects of the various ingredients in over-the-counter (OTC) cough and cold preparations, which of the following are also potential hazards when these medications are given?

a. dosing errors
b. not intending to do any harm, parents sometimes intentionally give higher than recommended doses
c. parents are often unaware of the possible side effects
d. parents sometimes give the medications for one of the side effects: sedation
e. all of the above

ANSWERS:

1. **d.** The basic axiom relevant to this question is that "not all fever has to be treated with drugs." In fact, there are good reasons for suggesting that fever only be treated when it reaches a level of 39.5° C. Fever is a normal body response mechanism. In children, the major concern with very high fever is the possibility of a febrile convulsion.

2. **c.** The analgesic agent of choice in the treatment of childhood fever and mild to moderate childhood pain is acetaminophen. Hydromorphone is a strong narcotic. Naproxen is a nonsteroidal antiinflammatory agent, and aspirin is contraindicated (see Answer 3).

Acetaminophen with codeine elixir is available and may be indicated in more severe pain syndromes in childhood.

3. **d.** Acetaminophen is the analgesic of choice for the treatment of infant and childhood pain. Aspirin use basically should be discouraged; this is by far the safest policy. Aspirin use has been linked to Reye's syndrome, and it seems wise to avoid this drug in children. Not all childhood pain needs to be treated with drugs. Many children will do just as well and feel just as well without drug use.

4. **d.** Most cough and cold remedies contain antihistamines. Antihistamines, however, never have been shown to be of value in the treatment of viral URIs. In fact, OTC cold and cough preparations have no demonstrated benefit in children younger than age 5 years. Antihistamines do not shorten the duration of respiratory tract illness in children and do not reduce the subsequent incidence of otitis media following the onset of a viral upper-respiratory illness. They may, however, produce seizures in children if given in toxic amounts. The younger the child, the easier it is to inadvertently produce antihistamine toxicity.

Treatment of a viral URI in an infant or young child should consist of reassurance and cool steam or saline nasal drops (if nasal congestion is present).

5. **c.** Cool or warm steam is actually superior to antihistamines in producing relief of nasal congestion

in infants and young children. If steam is being used in a humidifier in the child's room, it is safer to use a humidifier that emits cool steam to avoid the risk of burns. However, the use of warm steam (as from turning on the shower in the bathroom) also does produce significant symptomatic relief of nasal congestion.

6. **d.** Decongestants have not been shown to shorten the duration of viral URI symptoms. Topical sympathomimetic agents are absorbed systemically and may result in elevation of blood pressure, tachycardia, and overstimulation of the central nervous system, leading to irritability, insomnia, and sometimes even frank psychosis. Overstimulation is a particularly common side effect in children. Thus, as with antihistamines, the risks of using decongestants in children outweigh any potential benefits.

It may be reasonable to use a very dilute nasal sympathomimetic for a short period (2 days) in this child if all else fails; however, it is still preferable to stick to steam if possible.

7. **d.** Dextromethorphan is the most common ingredient in OTC cough medicines. As well as producing drowsiness, it has been reported to produce respiratory depression, abnormal limb movements, and coma in infants and children. As with antihistamines and decongestants, dextromethorphan has not been shown to shorten the duration of respiratory tract illness in children or adults.

Many cough preparations also contain an expectorant. The combination of a cough suppressant and an expectorant is not recommended.

Time remains the best cure for the viral URI symptoms. The use of a nasal aspirator (bulb syringe) will help to clear a young infant's nasal secretions and make feeding easier. Saline nasal drops also may be used. In infants who are irritable and feverish from viral symptoms, the use of acetaminophen is the safest OTC drug to use.

8. **d.** Dimenhydrinate should not be used for the treatment of nausea and vomiting secondary to gastroenteritis in children (especially very young children). Even in adults the use of this agent is questionable; it has been demonstrated to be of value only in the treatment of motion sickness in adults. Dimenhydrinate may produce significant sedation (and even a semicomatose state) in children. It may be difficult for the physician to differentiate dimenhydrinate toxicity from a worsening of the illness itself. This makes the use of this agent in children dangerous.

9. **d.** Teething usually begins at 4-6 months and continues until the age of 2 years. Although often blamed on teething, there is no good evidence that rash, fever, diarrhea, vomiting, nasal congestion, irritability, or sleeplessness are related to teething.

Although topical benzocaine usually does not produce any side effects, cases of methemoglobinemia have been reported in children who have been treated with this agent.

Teething is best treated with reassurance and appropriate doses of acetaminophen.

10. **e.** All are potential hazards when OTC cold and cough medications are given to infants and children. It is very important for physicians to inquire about and educate parents about the use of all OTC medications.

 ## SUMMARY OF OVER-THE-COUNTER DRUGS

1. **URIs:** There is no evidence to suggest that antihistamines, decongestants, cough suppressants, or expectorants are of any value in the treatment of viral URI symptoms in infants and young children. Potential toxicity is present with all of these agents.
2. **Nausea and vomiting:** Dimenhydrinate is not useful and is potentially toxic.
3. **Teething:** There is no evidence to suggest that rash, diarrhea, vomiting, nasal congestion, irritability, and sleeplessness are associated with teething.

Benzocaine preparations should be avoided. Reassurance and judicious use of acetaminophen may be indicated.
4. Physicians need to inquire about the use of all OTC medications and need to educate parents about their effectiveness and safety.

SUGGESTED READING

Gal P, Reed MD: Medications. In: Behrman RE, et al, eds.: *Nelson textbook of pediatrics*, 16th ed. Philadelphia: WB Saunders Company, 2000.
Gunn VL, et al: Toxicity of over-the-counter cough and cold medications. *Pediatrics* 108(3):E52, 2001.
Simoes EAF: Viral upper respiratory tract infections. In: Rakel RE, Bope ET, eds.: *Conn's current therapy*. WB Saunders, 2003, Philadelphia.

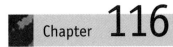

Chapter 116

Sickle Cell Disease

> "It's not fair. Why should our family have this disease? We have lived in the United States for generations and will never be exposed to malaria."

CLINICAL CASE PROBLEM 1:

A 10-YEAR-OLD MALE WITH DIFFUSE MUSCULOSKELETAL PAIN

A recently immigrated family from the Middle East comes to the office with their 10-year-old son. The child has been experiencing acute abdominal and diffuse musculoskeletal pain for the last 24 hours. The family states that he has had previous attacks with similar symptoms, usually treated with hospitalization.

On physical examination the child is in acute distress and complaining of neck, back, and chest pain. A thorough physical examination is positive for acute tenderness in the musculoskeletal areas. The remainder of the examination is normal.

▪ SELECT THE BEST ANSWER TO THE FOLLOWING QUESTIONS:

1. Given the case presentation what is the most likely diagnosis in this patient?
   a. viral syndrome (flu)
   b. acute chest syndrome
   c. sickle cell disease
   d. gastroenteritis
   e. thalassemia

2. What is the pathophysiology of this condition?
   a. replacement of normal hemoglobin A by hemoglobin C
   b. replacement of normal hemoglobin A by hemoglobin F
   c. substitution of glutamic acid by valine in the 6th position of the beta chain of hemoglobin A
   d. substitution of glutamic acid by lysine in the 6th position of the beta chain of hemoglobin A
   e. a and c

3. What is the most likely type of acute crisis that this patient is experiencing?
   a. aplastic crisis
   b. hemolytic crisis
   c. neutropenic crisis
   d. sequestration crisis
   e. vasoocclusive crisis

4. In children which of the following are the possible acute complications of this condition?
   a. cerebrovascular accident
   b. splenic sequestration
   c. priapism
   d. acute chest syndrome
   e. all of the above

5. In this situation what treatment would you recommend to the family?
   a. immediate hospitalization
   b. outpatient hydration with pain management and observation
   c. transfer to a tertiary care center that specializes in this condition
   d. narcotic analgesics
   e. none of the above

6. Given this patient's history, which laboratory test(s) would be most helpful?
   a. reticulocyte count
   b. complete blood count (CBC)
   c. a and b
   d. hemoglobin electrophoresis
   e. chest x-ray

7. In which of the following ethnic groups does sickle cell disease not occur?
   a. African Americans
   b. Italians
   c. Saudi Arabians
   d. Northwestern whites
   e. Greeks

8. Which of the following vaccinations is this patient going to need in the future?
   a. pneumovax
   b. influenza
   c. meningococcal
   d. a and c
   e. a, b, and c

9. Which of the following statements regarding this disease and priapism is true?
   a. attacks of priapism in boys and men are uncommon
   b. hospitalization often is indicated
   c. beta blockers are first line in the treatment of priapism
   d. the incidence of priapism is significantly higher in older men
   e. priapism when it occurs is generally self-limiting

10. Chronic manifestations of this condition include all of the following except:
    a. proliferative retinopathy
    b. pulmonary hypertension

c. avascular necrosis
d. cholelithiasis
e. dactylitis

CLINICAL CASE MANAGEMENT PROBLEM

List the major complications of the disorder described.

■ **ANSWERS:**

1. c. This child has sickle cell disease. The acute pain that this child is experiencing at this time is caused by a vasoocclusive phenomenon. Throughout their lives, patients with sickle cell disease are plagued by recurrent painful crises. These episodes may occur with explosive suddenness and may attack various parts of the body, particularly the abdomen, back, chest, and joints. Approximately 25% of these patients' crises are preceded by a viral or bacterial infection. A given patient may have months or even years without a crisis and then have a cluster of frequent, severe attacks. In some patients these crisis occur more frequently in the cold weather; this may be a result of reflex vasospasm. In others the attacks occur in warm weather and presumably are caused by dehydration.

2. c. Sickle cell disease is an inherited hemolytic anemia that results when both copies of normal hemoglobin A (HbA) are replaced by the mutant hemoglobin (HbS) (genotype HbS/HbS). This major variation is caused by one amino acid substitution (valine for glutamic) at the 6th position of the beta chain of HbA. Heterozygotes (HbS) have "sickle cell trait" and are almost free of clinical symptoms.

Sickle cell disease as a result of inheritance of a defective genes is present in about 1 out of 375 African Americans. There is also a higher incidence in Mediterranean, Middle Eastern, Indian, Caribbean, and Central and South American ancestry.

The one thing in common among these various regions and ethnic groups is that malaria *(Plasmodium falciparum)* is endemic. It is believed that this mutation is an evolutionary event that prevents and curtails malaria's infectivity in the red blood cells of heterozygous individuals. Such people are said to have the sickle cell trait and only have minimal symptoms.

3. e. This patient is experiencing an acute vasoocclusive crisis resulting from ischemia to various regions of the body, especially the osseous structures, and a variety of organs.

A sequestration crisis is an acute increase in splenic trapping of red blood cells resulting in worsening anemia, which can be rapidly fatal; this is an emergency requiring admission to the hospital and rapid blood transfusion.

Aplastic crisis is a failure of red blood synthesis. Pain is associated with a dropping hematocrit and a reticulocyte count less than 10%.

Hemolytic crisis is anemia associated with increasing hemolysis, the bilirubin is increased and the patient is jaundiced.

Neutropenic crisis would result from a marked decrease in production of white blood cells with an absolute neutrophil count less than or equal to 500. Sickle cell disease does not affect leukocyte synthesis.

4. e. All of the above are possible complications of an acute crisis of sickle cell disease. A cerebrovascular event maybe prevented by transfusion if the patient is assessed to be high risk by ultrasound evaluation of the Circle of Willis.

As mentioned before, splenic sequestration is a life-threatening event that can be rapidly fatal if not treated immediately.

Priapism is a common recurrent condition that can occur in children and is usually self-limiting. However, prolonged priapism of more than 2-4 hours requires immediate surgical intervention.

Acute chest syndrome presents with fever, cough, dyspnea, and pulmonary infiltrates. These patients need to be monitored very closely because they can progress rapidly to respiratory failure. It is difficult to differentiate between this and pneumonia, so it is necessary to start antibiotics early.

5. b. This appears to be a straightforward recurrent vasoocclusive crisis, given that the patient is clinically stable and the overall examination is negative except for musculoskeletal. It would be appropriate to manage this patient on an outpatient basis with hydration and analgesics along with some basic laboratory testing and close follow-up.

6. c. A CBC would be useful to assess the severity of the anemia or any other evidence of infection. A reticulocyte count would give you an assessment of bone marrow functioning and thus the ability of the body to cope with the crisis.

7. d. The disease is virtually nonexistent in white people whose ancestors evolved in malaria-free zones.

8. **e.** Children with sickle cell disease should receive the usual recommended immunizations. Children need to be monitored closely postvaccination for fever because it may be sepsis. Additional immunizations that are recommended include influenza vaccine annually and a single quadrivalent meningococcal vaccine after age 2 years.

9. **e.** As mentioned before, priapism is usually a self-limiting condition in children. It often occurs in the early morning hours, and episodes usually last fewer than 2 hours. A prolonged episode that lasts more than 2-4 hours eventually may result in impotence and requires immediate treatment including hydration, analgesics, aspiration, and irrigation by an urologist.

10. **b.** Pulmonary hypertension is not a consequence of chronic sickle cell disease. However, adults can develop cardiomegaly from chronic anemia.

Proliferative retinopathy is seen secondary to microvascular occlusion and ischemia.

Avascular necrosis of the femoral head is very common in patients with sickle cell disease and can lead to significant disability.

Cholelithiasis results from high bilirubin levels from constant hemolysis.

Dactylitis presents as a painful swelling of either the hand or foot and is caused by infarction of bone marrow in metacarpal or metatarsal bones and phalanges. This is a self-limiting condition that usually resolves within 1 week.

 SOLUTION TO THE CLINICAL CASE MANAGEMENT PROBLEM

Sickle cell disease is characterized by the following complications:

1. Hemolytic anemia: Sickle cell disease (genotype HbS/HbS) is associated with a severe hemolytic anemia with hematocrit values varying between 18% and 30%. The mean red blood cell survival is between 10 and 15 days.

2. Acute pain crises and chronic organ damage: The morbidity and mortality of sickle cell disease are primarily a result of recurrent vasoocclusive phenomena. This vasoocclusive damage can be divided into microinfarcts that produce the painful crisis and macroinfarcts that produce organ damage. Although almost any organ can be involved, the most common organs involved are the lungs, kidneys, liver, skeleton, and skin.

3. Pulmonary function restriction: Impairment of pulmonary function is a common complication of sickle cell disease. Resting arterial PO_2 is reduced in part because of the intrapulmonary arterial-venous shunting. Because HbS/Hbs red blood cells have decreased oxygen affinity, arterial blood is significantly undersaturated. This creates an increased tendency for red blood cells to sickle when they reach the peripheral circulation.

4. Congestive cardiac failure: HbS/Hbs homozygotes frequently develop overt congestive heart failure (CHF). The pathophysiology of this CHF is associated with the severe chronic anemia and hypoxemia (high-output cardiac failure).

5. Cerebrovascular accidents (CVAs): The primary cause of a CVA in patients with sickle cell disease is cerebral thrombosis. The other cause, however, is subarachnoid hemorrhage. A patient with sickle cell disease has approximately a 25% lifetime chance of developing some type of neurologic complication. Hemiplegia is encountered more frequently than coma, convulsions, or visual disturbances. Patients generally make a full recovery, particularly after only one CVA.

6. Ophthalmologic complications: A variety of ocular abnormalities are encountered in patients with HbS/Hbs disease. These include retinal infarcts, peripheral vessel disease, arteriovenous anomalies, vitreous hemorrhage, proliferative retinopathy, and retinal detachment.

7. Genitourinary complications: Patients with sickle cell disease develop significant and prolonged painless hematuria as a result of papillary infarcts. The amount of blood loss can be so significant that iron deficiency develops.

   Longer surviving patients with HbS/Hbs disease (patients living into their fourth or fifth decade) develop progressive renal failure. Boys and young men with sickle cell disease occasionally develop priapism. The treatment of this condition was discussed in Answer 9.

8. Hepatobiliary complications: Patients with sickle cell disease are icteric because of the hemolytic anemia discussed previously. The hyperbilirubinemia that is associated with sickle cell disease is nonconjugated hyperbilirubinemia. Patients with sickle cell disease are also at increased risk of gallstone formation.

Continued

SOLUTION TO THE CLINICAL CASE MANAGEMENT PROBLEM—cont'd

9. Skeletal complications: The skeletal complications associated with HbS/Hbs disease develop as a result of expansion of the red marrow, bony infarcts, and avascular necrosis of joints in hip and shoulder. The biconcave, or "fishmouth," vertebrae are virtually pathognomonic for sickle cell disease. The previously mentioned hand–foot syndrome is a painful swelling of the hand or foot caused by infarction of the bone marrow in metacarpal or metatarsal bones and phalanges.

10. Skin disease: Chronic skin ulcers often occur in the lower extremities. These skin ulcers appear to be associated with patients with HbS/Hbs disease that have more severe hemolytic anemia.

Splenic sequestration: The spleen becomes enlarged as a result of the rapid sequestration of sickled blood. The acute anemia that results may be rapidly fatal and should be treated with emergency blood transfusions.

11. Aplastic crises: The previously mentioned aplastic crises, which usually occur when a child is recovering from an infection, are caused by human parvovirus B19. Profound anemia occurs, and blood transfusions are necessary to treat it.

SUMMARY OF SICKLE CELL DISEASE

1. Population at greatest risk: African Americans, 1 in 12 (8%) carry the sickle cell trait HbA/HbS (are heterozygous for sickle cell trait); homozygous genotype HbS/HbS have the disease.

2. Diagnosis:
   a. Blood smear: red blood cells sickle and hemolyze
   b. Hemoglobin electrophoresis

3. Clinical manifestations are discussed in the Clinical Case Management Problem.

4. Treatment:
   a. Treatment and, whenever possible, prevention of complications (recurrent cerebrovascular accidents [CVAs] may be prevented by starting the child on a chronic transfusion program)
   b. Nutritional supplements: Folic acid, 1 mg/day
   c. Immunizations or vaccines: *H. influenzae B*, *pneumococcal vaccine*, and all other routine vaccinations recommended for other children, as summarized in Chapter 96.
   d. Prophylactic antibiotics: penicillin V 125 mg bid up to age 3 years; then 250 mg bid up to age 5 years.
   e. Pain control for acute pain crises and other painful events: intravenous fluids and analgesics as needed; do not be afraid to use narcotic analgesics
   f. Painless hematuria: aminocaproic acid
   g. Transfusion: indicated for symptomatic episodes of acute anemia, severe symptomatic episodes of acute anemia, severe symptomatic chronic anemia, prevention of recurrent strokes in children, acute chest syndromes with hypoxia, and surgery with general anesthesia
   h. Hydroxyurea: indicated for adolescents or adults with frequent episodes of pain, a history of the acute chest syndrome, or other severe vasoocclusive complications, or severe symptomatic anemia
   i. Transplantation: bone marrow (stem-cell) transplantation has been successful; a consideration in children and adolescents under 16 years old who have severe complications and an HLA-matched donor available

SUGGESTED READING

Fixler J: Sickle cell disease. *Pediatr Clin North Am* 49(6):1193-1210, vi, 2002.

Scott JP: Chapter 17. Hematology: sickle cell disease. In: Behrman RE, Kliegman RM, eds.: *Nelson essentials of pediatrics*, 4th ed. WB Saunders, 2002, Philadelphia, 623-625.

Steinberg MH: Drug therapy: Management of sickle cell disease. *N Engl J Med* 340(13):1021-1030, 1999.

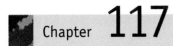

Chapter 117

Physical Activity and Nutrition

> "Boy, Mom, the food in the school cafeteria sure has improved. Now we can get french fries, cokes, doughnuts, and all sorts of yummy food like that."

CLINICAL CASE PROBLEM 1:

A 12-Year-Old Boy Who Is Overweight

A mother comes into your clinic with her 12-year-old son. She is concerned that he might be overweight and wants some advice on weight-loss programs. The patient has been healthy with no medical problems. On examination, he is in the 90th percentile for height and more than 97th percentile for weight.

■ SELECT THE BEST ANSWER TO THE FOLLOWING QUESTIONS:

1. Questions that you want to ask this mother include:
   a. how much time does the patient spend watching television and playing video games?
   b. how much physical activity does the patient receive at home and how much physical education at school?
   c. what type of snacks does he eat and how frequently?
   d. how much juice and soda does he consume?
   e. all of the above

2. Barriers to effective interventions designed to encourage a healthy diet include all of the following except:
   a. parental food shopping
   b. cognitive developmental stage of the child and ability to understand cause and long-term effects
   c. perceived lack of time
   d. expense of supplemental nutritional shakes
   e. plenitude and availability of inexpensive fast food, junk food, and soda

3. Perceived barriers to physical activity include:
   a. lack of time
   b. weather conditions
   c. access to facilities or equipment
   d. perceived lack of safety
   e. all of the above

4. Strength training in children:
   a. has been shown to be beneficial when provided in a supervised environment
   b. has no proven benefit in increasing fitness or helping with weight loss
   c. actually can cause children to gain significant amounts of weight
   d. endangers growth plates and increases risk of injuries
   e. should focus on heavy weights and few repetitions

5. Effective nutritional interventions for obese children include:
   a. allowing the child/adolescent to choose food at the market
   b. very low-carbohydrate/high-fat diets
   c. increasing consumption of fruit drinks
   d. eating while watching television
   e. none of the above

6. Which of the following statements is false?
   a. peak bone mass is achieved in childhood and adolescence
   b. smoking cigarettes can decrease calcium absorption and decrease bone mineral density
   c. increased calcium intake in childhood and adolescence is associated with increased bone mineral density and decreased fractures later in life
   d. soft drinks have an adverse effect on bone mineralization
   e. weightbearing physical activity and strength training puts extra stress on bones and increases risk for decreased bone mineral density and stress fractures

CLINICAL CASE PROBLEM 2:

An Overweight Fourth-Grade Class

You are hired as a school physician at a school-based health center located in an elementary school. You are reviewing the charts of all of the students in the fourth-grade class. To your dismay, you find that 25% of the children are over the 97th percentile for weight. You decide to investigate some of the reasons behind these findings, with the hope of developing an effective intervention.

7. The overall prevalence of being overweight in United States children is closest to:
   a. 1%
   b. 5%
   c. 10%
   d. 20%
   e. 40%

8. Which of the following statements is false:
   a. health behaviors established in childhood/adolescence have little correlation with adult health behaviors

b. increased physical activity in adults is associated with a decreased risk of coronary artery disease, myocardial infarction, cerebral vascular attacks, cancer, and diabetes mellitus

c. the prevalence of obesity in adults has increased by approximately 60% since 1990

d. physical activity declines as children pass into adolescence

e. television viewing is strongly associated with obesity

9. As you research the physical education programs in your school and others across the nation, you find that the following is a true statement:
a. all of the physical education period is dedicated to physical activity
b. physical education classes have decreased dramatically in frequency and duration across the nation
c. daily physical education classes in school have no association with physical activity as adults
d. recess periods are equivalent to structured physical education periods
e. school physical education programs meet the current recommendations for physical activity in children

10. The results of increasing physical activity in children include all of the following except:
a. increased fitness levels
b. decreased risk of obesity and some chronic diseases such as diabetes mellitus
c. increased skills in teamwork, leadership, and socialization
d. decreased anxiety and stress
e. worsening academic performance as a result of time spent exercising

11. Which one of the following statements is true?
a. television commercials have no influence on food choices made by children/adolescents
b. schools generally provide attractive and tasty healthy food choices in cafeterias
c. soft drink companies often sponsor schools to allow their products to be features prominently in the schools
d. when faced with a choice, children generally will choose a healthier meal with a greater percentage of fruits and vegetables over a high-fat meal
e. school-age children should have four to five servings of fruit drinks per day

ANSWERS:

1. e. Obesity is increasing at epidemic proportions in the United States and other industrialized countries, especially among children and adolescents. All of the choices listed are important in evaluating an obese child. Television and video games have been associated with childhood and adolescent obesity. The amount of physical activity and physical education at school are important factors in weight maintenance and general health. High-fat snacks and juice and soda consumption are important culprits in childhood and adolescent obesity. Sometimes, a food diary requested from the mother or patient will help in getting an accurate picture of true intake.

2. d. Parents are generally responsible for food shopping. If the parents want their children to eat healthy food, then they cannot buy junk food and not expect the children to want it. The cognitive developmental stage of children is also important to institute changes in behavior. Children and early adolescents have more difficulty understanding the importance of long-term effects on health. Perceived lack of time is a major barrier to behavioral changes. In this modern age, children's schedules are packed like never before. Fast food seems a convenient option for many families without time or resources to cook healthier meals. Soda and junk food are usually cheaper and more available than fruits and vegetables. Nutritional shakes should not be a regular part of a normal child's diet. Nutritional recommendations should be met with the basic food groups. Parents who need further help in constructing healthy diets for themselves and their children can benefit by the knowledge of a trained nutritionist.

3. e. All of the above are barriers to physical activity. As in Answer 2, lack of time is an issue for busy children and adolescents. Setting aside daily time for exercise can be difficult for anyone. Weather conditions also can affect choices to participate in physical activity. Depending on the climate, there can be rain, snow, smog, and hot and cold temperatures that make exercise less appealing. Access to facilities and equipment is another barrier, especially in urban areas where such facilities are limited. Neighborhood playgrounds are often not felt to be safe, creating another barrier. Busy traffic makes bicycling and walking more dangerous as well. Sedentary lifestyle in a child's parents is a critical barrier in encouraging physical activity. Children often model their parents' behaviors. A household that watches television and does not encourage physical activity will raise children with the same values and expectations.

4. a. Strength training in children has been shown to be beneficial in increasing fitness and in helping to lose weight. Muscle burns more calories at baseline than fat, so building muscles actually can help burn calories. Muscle weighs more than fat, so as muscle mass grows body weight can actually increase slightly, but when this occurs it is negligible and is offset by the health benefits. When children learn strength training in a supervised environment with good technique, there is very low risk for injury and no risk to growth plates. Strength training in children should emphasize low weights and more repetitions.

5. **e.** None of the above answers are correct. Children can participate in shopping at the market for healthy food, but left to their own devices generally will choose high-fat snacks over fruits and vegetables. Fad diets popular with adults, such as very low-carbohydrate/high-fat and very low-fat diets have not been studied in children and are therefore not recommended. General nutritional guidelines from the U.S. Department of Agriculture recommend that fat intake be approximately 30% of total calories for the day. An obese child or adolescent should have less fat in the diet than this recommendation but should continue to eat a well-balanced diet. Fruit drinks are a hidden source of calories. Many parents feel that fruit drinks must be healthy for their children. They also taste good, and children enjoy drinking them. However, many fruit drinks only contain about 5% to 10% of actual fruit juice. Even 100% fruit juice is high in calories and low in fiber and other nutrients essential to a healthy diet. School-age children and adolescents should not drink much more than 10-12 ounces of juice per day. Eating while watching television has been shown to increase food intake. Television commercials also feature high-fat foods that make children want fast food and junk food instead of healthier choices.

6. **e.** Peak bone mass is achieved in childhood/ adolescence and is improved by increased calcium intake at that time. Soft drinks and smoking cigarettes both have adverse effects on bone mineralization. Weightbearing physical activity and strength training increases bone density and decreases the risk of osteoporosis and stress fractures.

7. **d.** The overall prevalence of overweight children in the United States is closest to 20%. Among African Americans, the prevalence is about 21.5%, among Hispanics it is 21.8%, and among non-Hispanic whites it is about 12.3%. In 2000 the Centers for Disease Control and Prevention (CDC) found that the prevalence of obesity for United States adults was 19.8%.

8. **a.** Health behaviors established in childhood and adolescence (healthy diet, physical activity, not smoking) have been shown to be strongly associated with health behaviors as adults. Physical activity has been shown to decrease from childhood into adolescence, especially among girls. Therefore childhood is the ideal time to encourage healthy behaviors. Physical activity has been associated with a decreased prevalence of many major diseases, including coronary artery disease, myocardial infarctions, cerebral vascular events, different types of cancers, and diabetes mellitus. According to the CDC, the prevalence of obesity among adults in the United States has increased approximately 60% since 1990. Multiple studies have shown television viewing to be strongly correlated with obesity.

9. **b.** School physical education programs do not even come close to meeting the current recommendations for physical activity in children. Current recommendations advocate 30-60 minutes of moderate to vigorous physical activity a day at least 5 days per week. Physical education in schools is shaped by state law. Over recent years, with increasing demand for students' time and decreasing availability of qualified teachers, physical education programs have suffered. Many schools have physical education classes one to three times per week. Very few schools have daily classes. Some schools try to use open recess periods to meet requirements. Some children are active during free recess periods, but many are not, choosing to stand and socialize or read. Even in dedicated physical education classes, more than half of the allotted time can be wasted with changing and showering. Physical education programs need to be supported in schools to help children meet current recommendations for physical activity.

10. **e.** Physical activity in children has many benefits. Children can achieve increased fitness levels, increased strength, and decreased risk of obesity and related health problems such as insulin resistance. Children who participate in physical activity and team sports are found to have improved skills in teamwork, leadership, confidence, and socialization. Anxiety and stress are decreased, and depression is improved. In one study, adolescents who engaged in regular physical activity were statistically less likely to have thoughts of suicide. Academic performance actually has been found to be improved by participation in regular physical activity. Some researchers feel that students who play sports have to budget their time more efficiently and are more disciplined and organized. Some also feel that participating in regular physical activity provides increased energy and a sense of well-being that allows greater concentration.

11. **c.** School budgets are being cut now more than ever. One of the places that often suffers is the school

cafeteria. Unfortunately, fast foods and junk food are almost always cheaper and more plentiful than good fresh fruits and vegetables. The few low-fat choices are often not very attractive choices, especially not to a child or adolescent, who when faced with a choice almost always will choose something that tastes better and is high in fat. Television commercials constantly advertise fast food, and soft drink companies some-times do pay schools much needed money for the privilege of featuring their products. When children are overwhelmed by so many messages combined with convenience and cheapness, they generally will choose fast food and soda. Children should have five servings of fruits and vegetables per day, and only up to 10-12 ounces of fruit drink per day, as described earlier.

SUMMARY OF PHYSICAL ACTIVITY AND NUTRITION

Obesity is a public health problem of epidemic proportions, with more than 20% of the U.S. population, including children, being overweight.

Obesity is related to many chronic health problems, including cancer and heart disease, the most important causes of adult morbidity and mortality.

The CDC and Healthy People 2010 recommend 30-60 minutes of moderate to vigorous physical activity per day at least 5 days per week in all children.

Physical activity has been associated with decreased risk of many chronic diseases. In adolescents, participation in regular physical activity has been associated with decreased smoking; decreased drug use; increased fruit and vegetable consumption; decreased risk of pregnancy and sexually transmitted disease; decreased anxiety, stress, and depression; decreased illicit drug use; increased seatbelt use; and increased academic performance. Therefore physical activity is strongly associated with other positive health-related behaviors.

Health behaviors, including physical activity and nutrition, that are started as children/adolescents carry over into adulthood. Therefore, to prevent adult chronic disease, practitioners should concentrate especially on these behaviors in children and adolescents.

There are many perceived and real barriers to adequate physical activity. These include lack of time, bad weather, access to facilities or equipment, lack of safety, and lack of energy. Attempts must be made to further characterize and eliminate these barriers. Physical education classes are currently inadequate to meet the physical activity recommendations for children and adolescents. Strength training in a well-supervised environment is beneficial for children in terms of overall fitness and strength.

Adequate nutrition and a healthy diet are also critical in childhood and adolescence. Parents must be the ones to model good eating behavior and to make good food purchases. Despite the convenience and inexpensive price tag on many fast food meals, parents must make the added effort to find and prepare well-balanced and healthy meals, providing plenty of fresh fruits and vegetables and less than 30% of total calories as fat. Fruit juice is an often unrecognized culprit in childhood obesity and is not a substitute for fresh fruits.

Peak bone mass is achieved in adolescence. Calcium intake and physical activity during this time can help to determine later bone mineral density and the risk of future osteoporosis and stress fractures.

SUGGESTED READING

American Academy of Pediatrics: Policy statement on strength training by children and adolescents. *Pediatrics* 107(6):1470-1472, 2001.

Centers for Disease Control and Prevention: *Healthy People 2010.* www.cdc.gov.

Flegal KM, et al: Prevalence of overweight in US children: comparison of US growth charts from The Centers for Disease Control and prevention with other reference values for body mass index. *Am J Clin Nutr* 76(6):1086-1093, 2001.

Goran MI, et al: Obesity and risk of type 2 diabetes and cardiovascular disease in children and adolescents. *J Clin Endocrinol Metab* 88(4):1417-1427, 2003 Apr.

Hill JC, et al: What are the most effective interventions to reduce childhood obesity? *J Fam Pract* 51(10):891, 2002 Oct.

Kohl HW, Hobbs KE: Development of physical activity behaviors among children and adolescents. *Pediatrics* 101(3); suppl, Part2/2: 549-554, 1998.

Mascarenhas MM, et al: Nutritional interventions in childhood for the prevention of chronic diseases in adulthood. *Curr Opin Pediatr* 11(6):598-604, 1999.

Sothern MS, Gordon ST: Prevention of obesity in young children: a critical challenge for medical professionals. *Clin Pediatr* 42(2):101-111, 2003 Mar.

Strauss RS, Pollack HA: Epidemic increase in childhood overweight, 1986-98. *JAMA* 286(22):2845-2848, 2001.

Trudeau F, et al: Daily primary school physical education: effects on physical activity during adult life. *Med Sci Sports Exerc* 31:111-117, 1999.

Trudeau F, et al: A follow up on the Trois-Rivières growth and development studies for health fitness and risk factors. *Am J Human Biol* 12:207-213, 2000.

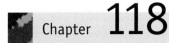

Chapter **118**

Lymphomas and Leukemias

"Doc, it is hard to believe that not too
many years ago this would have been
a death sentence for my little boy."

CLINICAL CASE PROBLEM 1:

*A 10-YEAR-OLD BOY WITH
A MEDIASTINAL MASS*

A 10-year-old male is brought into the office by his
parents. For the past 2 weeks he has been very tired and
has felt short of breath. The mother tells you that she
thinks he has been losing weight. On physical examination the child is alert and in no distress; vital signs are
normal, but he has lost 3 pounds since his last visit
6 months ago. The lungs are clear bilaterally, and the
heart examination is normal. You palpate an enlarged
supraclavicular node. Chest radiography reveals a large
mediastinal mass.

■ **SELECT THE BEST ANSWER TO THE
FOLLOWING QUESTIONS:**

1. What is the most likely diagnosis?
   a. acute streptococcal pneumonia
   b. mycoplasma pneumonia
   c. mononucleosis
   d. Hodgkin's disease
   e. tuberculosis

2. Which of the following is commonly associated
   with non-Hodgkin's lymphoma?
   a. intussusception in a child older than 5 years
      of age
   b. intraabdominal mass
   c. superior vena cava obstruction
   d. airway obstruction
   e. all of the above

3. The presence of Reed-Sternberg cells in tissue is
   diagnostic of which disease?
   a. Hodgkin's disease
   b. lymphoblastic lymphoma
   c. Burkitt lymphoma
   d. large cell lymphoma
   e. non-Hodgkin's disease

4. The most common malignancy in childhood is:
   a. acute lymphoblastic leukemia (ALL)
   b. acute myeloid leukemia (AML)
   c. chronic myelogenous leukemia
   d. Hodgkin's disease
   e. non-Hodgkin's lymphoma

CLINICAL CASE PROBLEM 2:

*A 4-YEAR-OLD BOY WITH
FEVER AND PAINS*

A mother brings her 4-year-old son into the office. He
has had intermittent fevers to 101.2° F over the past
3 weeks and has been complaining of pain in his legs
and back. On physical examination, the vital signs are
normal and there is a generalized lymphadenopathy. The
liver and spleen both feel enlarged. A complete blood
count (CBC) reveals a white blood cell (WBC) count of
33,000/mm³ and a platelet count of 81,000/mm³. The
peripheral blood smear shows blasts, and the lactate
dehydrogenase (LDH) activity is elevated.

5. The most likely diagnosis is:
   a. juvenile rheumatoid arthritis
   b. infectious mononucleosis
   c. ALL
   d. Hodgkin's disease
   e. none of the above

6. Which of the statements regarding the disease
   described in Clinical Case Problem 2 is true?
   a. the peak age of onset is 12 years
   b. at the time of diagnosis most patients have a
      thrombocytosis
   c. a CBC with differential is the most useful
      initial test
   d. a chest x-ray is the most useful initial test
   e. none of the above

7. Which of the following increases the risk of a child
   developing AML?
   a. previous exposure to benzene
   b. previous exposure to ionizing radiation
   c. neurofibromatosis
   d. a and c
   e. a, b, and c

■ **ANSWERS:**

1. **d.** The correct answer is Hodgkin's disease. There
are two types of lymphomas: Hodgkin's disease and
non-Hodgkin's lymphoma. Hodgkin's disease is the
more common type of lymphoma.

Nonspecific signs and symptoms observed in children with lymphoma include malaise, fever, painless
adenopathy, headache, nausea, vomiting, weight loss,
abdominal pain, intussusception, intermittent obstruction, diarrhea, pruritus, swelling of the face and neck,
cough, and shortness of breath with no history of
reactive airway disease.

Hodgkin's disease commonly presents with painless cervical adenopathy. Early lymph-node biopsy
should be considered if there is no identifiable

infection in the region drained by an enlarged node, a node is greater than 2 cm, there is supraclavicular adenopathy or an abnormal chest x-ray, or a lymph node is increasing in size after 2 weeks or does not resolve after 4-8 weeks.

When Hodgkin's disease is suspected, a chest x-ray should be ordered. Half of all patients will have either mediastinal adenopathy or an anterior mediastinal mass. The blood count is usually normal, and acute phase reactants such as the erythrocyte sedimentation rate often are elevated.

2. e. All of the above. The onset of symptoms is more rapid in non-Hodgkin's lymphoma than Hodgkin's disease. Shortness of breath and abdominal symptoms such as intussusception, obstruction, and abdominal mass are more common in non-Hodgkin's lymphoma.

Non-Hodgkin's lymphoma is divided into three groups: lymphoblastic, small noncleaved cell, and large cell. The presentation of non-Hodgkin's lymphoma depends on the cell type. Lymphoblastic lymphoma commonly presents with symptoms of airway obstruction or superior vena cava obstruction. This is the result of mediastinal disease. Small noncleaved cell lymphomas and large cell lymphomas often present with signs or symptoms related to abdominal disease.

3. a. The presence of Reed-Sternberg cells in tissue is diagnostic of Hodgkin's disease. These cells are large and multinucleated and have abundant cytoplasm.

4. a. ALL is the most common malignancy of childhood. It accounts for approximately 25% of all cancer diagnosis in children under age 15 years.

5. c. Most patients with ALL are between the ages of 2 and 10 years with the peak age of onset at 4 years. Intermittent fevers and bone pain, especially in the pelvis, femurs, and lower spine, are common presenting complaints. Fevers may be the result of an infection secondary to the leukopenia or from cytokines induced by the leukemia. Other presenting signs and symptoms may include cutaneous or mucosal bleeding, easy bruising, petechiae, purpura, pallor, lymphadenopathy, hepatosplenomegaly, swelling of the face, testicular enlargement, and subcutaneous nodules known as leukemia cutis.

The most useful initial test to perform in patients suspected of having ALL is a CBC with differential. In most cases, there will be an increase or decrease in at least one or two cell types. The WBC count may be decreased, normal, or elevated and the differential will show a neutropenia. Blasts may be seen on the peripheral smear. Most patients with ALL will have a decreased hemoglobin and platelet count at the time of diagnosis. The diagnosis of ALL is confirmed by a bone marrow examination showing more than 25% lymphoblasts.

A chest radiograph should be obtained to look for a possible mediastinal mass.

With combination chemotherapy, the prognosis of ALL is very good.

6. c. As discussed in Answer 5, a CBC with differential is the most useful initial test to obtain when the diagnosis of ALL is suspected.

7. e. A less common type of leukemia seen in children is AML. Risk factors for AML include exposure to ionizing radiation or benzene, previous treatment with cytotoxic chemotherapeutic agents, and certain congenital syndromes such as neurofibromatosis. Most patients will have no identifiable risk factor. The incidence of AML is bimodal and peaks at the ages of 2 years and 16 years, and leukemia during the first 4 weeks of life is most often AML.

Children with AML may present with fever, pallor, weight loss, or fatigue. In some cases, sepsis or bleeding may be the initial presentation of AML. A CBC will show anemia, thrombocytopenia, and an elevated or low WBC count. Bone marrow aspirate will show more than 30% myeloblasts.

SUMMARY OF LYMPHOMAS AND LEUKEMIAS

I. Lymphoma
A. Hodgkin's disease
1. Most common type of lymphoma (incidence about 5.5 to 12.1 cases per 100,000)
2. Commonly presents with painless cervical adenopathy
3. If diagnosis is suspected, a chest radiograph should be obtained to look for mediastinal adenopathy or anterior mediastinal mass
4. Reed-Sternberg cells are diagnostic of Hodgkin's disease. Viral DNA has been found in Reed-Sternberg cells. Epstein-Barr virus has been implicated in about 50% of all cases Hodgkin's lymphoma in the United States.
5. Treatment involves multiagent chemotherapy and in some cases radiation therapy. Patients with lower-stage disease have more than a 90% survival rate; those with a higher-stage disease have more than a 70% survival rate.

B. **Non-Hodgkin's lymphoma** (somewhat less common than pediatric Hodgkin's)
1. Groups
   a. Lymphoblastic
   b. Small noncleaved cell
   c. Large cell
2. More rapid onset of symptoms than in Hodgkin's disease
3. Shortness of breath, intussusception, bowel obstruction, and abdominal mass are more common in non-Hodgkin's lymphoma than Hodgkin's disease
4. Presentation of non-Hodgkin's lymphoma depends on cell type
   a. Lymphoblastic lymphoma commonly presents with airway obstruction of superior vena cava obstruction
   b. Small noncleaved cell and large cell lymphomas commonly present with signs and symptoms related to abdominal disease.
5. Treatment is based on multiagent chemotherapy based on the histologic subtype. Since the late 1960s, treatment has progressed rapidly. Rather than an inevitable death sentence, the present cure rate is around 65% to 90%.

II. Leukemias
A. ALL
1. Most common malignancy of childhood, accounting for about 33% of all childhood malignancies. There are about 2,000-2,500 new cases per year.
2. Peak age of onset is 4 years, usual range 2-5 years of age
3. Common presentation: (a) intermittent fevers, (b) bone pain; (c) cutaneous or mucosal bleeding; (d) petechiae, purpura; (e) pallor; (f) lymphadenopathy; (g) hepatosplenomegaly; (h) swelling of the face; (i) testicular enlargement; and (j) subcutaneous nodules (leukemia cutis)
4. CBC with differential: (a) WBCs increased, decreased, or normal; (b) neutropenia; (c) anemia and (d) thrombocytopenia
5. Bone marrow shows large number of leukemic blasts.

6. Obtain chest radiograph to look for mediastinal widening or mass.
7. Treatment is chemotherapy based. Although a death sentence a few decades ago the present cure rate is more than 70%. The more resistant cases have leukemic blood cells with a BCR-ABL fusion.

B. AML
1. Less common than ALL. Overall accounts for about 20% of childhood leukemias.
2. Peak incidence at 2 and 16 years of age. Because the incidence of ALL starts later and falls more rapidly, AML accounts for a larger fraction of cases in children younger than 2 years and older than 5 years.
3. Leukemia during the first 4 weeks of life is most often AML and accounts for some 50% by adolescence.
4. Risk factors: (a) previous exposure to benzene, ionizing radiation, or cytotoxic chemotherapeutic agents and (b) certain congenital syndromes such as neurofibromatosis and chromosomal aberrations
5. Common presentation: (a) fever; (b) pallor; (c) weight loss; (d) fatigue; (e) cutaneous or mucosal bleeding; and (f) menorrhagia
6. CBC with differential: (a) anemia; (b) thrombocytopenia; and (c) elevated or low WBCs
7. Bone marrow aspirate shows more than 30% myeloblasts
8. Treatment is intensive chemotherapy. Overall cure rate is about 50%. (Children with Down's syndrome do best with less intensive treatment.)

SUGGESTED READING

Albano EA, et al: Neoplastic disease. In: Hay WW, et al, eds.: *Current pediatric diagnosis & treatment*. Lange Medical Books/McGraw-Hill, 2003, New York.

Brown VI: Acute lymphoblastic leukemia. In: Schwartz MW, ed.: *The 5-minute pediatric consult*: Lippincott-William & Wilkins, 2003, Philadelphia.

Kang T, Shankar SM: Acute myeloid leukemia. In: Schwartz MW, ed.: *The 5-minute pediatric consult*: Lippincott-William & Wilkins, 2003, Philadelphia.

Reaman GH: Pediatric oncology: current views and outcomes. *Pediatr Clin N Am* 49(6):1305-1318, 2002.

Velez MC: Lymphomas. *Pediatr Rev* 24(11):380-386, 2003.

GENERAL SURGERY AND SURGICAL SUBSPECIALTIES

 Chapter **119**

Acute Appendicitis

The great imitator.

CLINICAL CASE PROBLEM 1:
A 29-YEAR-OLD FEMALE WITH NAUSEA, VOMITING, AND CENTRAL ABDOMINAL PAIN

A 29-year-old female comes to your office with a 1-day history of nausea, some vomiting, and vague central abdominal pain. The pain has begun to move down and to the right. She also describes mild dysuria. Anorexia began 24 hours ago, and the patient also has "felt warm." Her last menstrual period was 2 weeks ago.

Her past health has been excellent. She has no drug allergies and is not taking any medication. On physical examination, the patient looks ill. Her temperature is 38.1° C. She has tenderness in both the right lower quadrant and the left lower quadrant, but tenderness is greatest in the right lower quadrant. Rebound tenderness is present. The rectal examination discloses tenderness on the right side. There is no costovertebral angle tenderness.

▶ **SELECT THE BEST ANSWER TO THE FOLLOWING QUESTIONS:**

1. What is the most likely diagnosis in this patient?
   a. pelvic inflammatory disease (PID)
   b. twisted ovarian cyst
   c. acute appendicitis
   d. acute cholecystitis
   e. acute pyelonephritis

2. At this time, what would be the most reasonable course of action?
   a. advise the patient to go home and return for follow-up in 24 hours
   b. hospitalize the patient for observation, evaluation, and possible operation.
   c. begin outpatient oral antibiotic therapy and see the patient in 48 hours
   d. advise the patient to go home and call you if no improvement occurs within the next 72 hours
   e. none of the above

3. The investigations you perform heighten your suspicion of the primary diagnosis. The white blood cell (WBC) count is elevated, and there is a definite abnormality seen on the abdominal x-ray. At this time, you, the family physician, should do which of the following?
   a. continue to observe the patient for improvement or deterioration
   b. arrange for a computed tomography (CT) scan to definitely establish the diagnosis
   c. a and b
   d. arrange for an ultrasound to definitely establish the diagnosis
   e. none of the above

4. A consultant sees your patient and makes an appropriate suggestion. Which of the following is the suggestion likely to be?
   a. perform an abdominal laparoscopy or laparotomy
   b. begin intensive triple-drug intravenous antibiotics
   c. continue the period of observation
   d. perform further diagnostic tests
   e. order another consult

5. Which of the following is not a clear complication of the original condition and definitive therapy?
   a. wound infection
   b. subphrenic abscess
   c. pelvic abscess
   d. appendiceal abscess
   e. infertility

6. In which of the following groups are the signs and symptoms of the condition described likely not to be classic?
   a. infants
   b. young adult males
   c. the elderly
   d. a and c
   e. b and c

7. In which of the following age groups is the diagnosis of the condition described in Clinical Case Problem 1 most likely to be confused with another serious intraabdominal inflammatory condition?

a. infants
b. young children
c. young adult males
d. young adult females
e. elderly males and females

8. The condition described has been called which of the following?
    a. the "great imitator"
    b. the "typical condition"
    c. a diagnosis "unable to miss"
    d. a diagnosis "unable to make under the best of conditions"
    e. none of the above

9. Regarding the pathophysiology of the described condition, which of the following is not a usual component of the pathologic process?
    a. obstruction of the organ accounting for early symptoms and signs
    b. hypoperistalsis leading to abdominal cramping
    c. rapid invasion of the wall of the organ by bacteria leading to inflammation
    d. spreading of the inflammation to involve the whole wall of the organ
    e. gangrene and perforation of the organ

10. Mortality the highest in which of the following groups?
    a. infants
    b. young adults with rupture of the organ
    c. children with rupture of the organ
    d. elderly with rupture of the organ
    e. pregnant women

11. Which of the following statements about the condition described in Clinical Case Problem 1 is false?
    a. it is the most common acute surgical condition of the abdomen
    b. vague, dull abdominal pain is usually the first clinical symptom
    c. Rovsing's sign can be present on physical examination
    d. the chandelier sign can be associated with this condition
    e. it is the most common extrauterine surgical emergency in pregnancy

12. All of the following statements about the management of this condition when rupture occurs are true except:
    a. more aggressive fluid resuscitation is usually necessary
    b. intravenous antibiotics should be given for 7-10 days or until the patient is afebrile

c. insertion of a percutaneous drain prior to surgery is recommended
d. open laparotomy or laparoscopy can be performed
e. expect a prolonged recovery with longer duration of fever and elevated WBC count

13. The radiographic test with the highest sensitivity in diagnosing this condition is:
    a. ultrasonography
    b. barium enema
    c. abdominal x-ray
    d. CT with intravenous and oral contrast
    e. nuclear medicine WBC-labeled scan

CLINICAL CASE MANAGEMENT PROBLEM

Discuss the management of the condition described in Clinical Case Problem 1 when it presents with abscess formation.

■ ANSWERS:

1. **c.** The most likely diagnosis in this patient is acute appendicitis.

The typical history of acute appendicitis is vague central abdominal discomfort followed by anorexia, nausea, and some vomiting. The pain, which is continuous but often not severe, usually moves into the right lower quadrant. The pain is aggravated by movement, walking, or coughing.

In patients with retrocecal appendicitis (which this description fits) there may be dysuria and hematuria with rectal tenderness because of the proximity of the appendix to the ureter and bladder. With perforation (as in this patient) there is generalized abdominal tenderness and rebound tenderness. Retrocecal appendicitis often produces poorly localized epigastric pain and only mild nausea and vomiting. Thus retrocecal appendicitis can be significantly more difficult to diagnose than classic appendicitis. Peritonitis can develop very rapidly. Temperature elevation is usually mild in appendicitis.

The most important differential diagnosis in this case is acute PID. The constellation of signs and symptoms, however, favors appendicitis. Acute cholecystitis, acute pyelonephritis, and acute PID will be discussed in separate problems.

2. **b.** This patient has an acute abdomen and therefore should be hospitalized for further evaluation and possible operation. A WBC count, a urine analysis, a serum pregnancy test, and three views of the abdomen are all investigations that should be performed in this patient.

In acute appendicitis the average leukocyte count is 15,000/mm^3, and 90% of patients have a leukocyte count greater than 10,000/mm^3. In 75% of patients, the differential count will show greater than 75% neutrophils.

Three views of the abdomen may show localized air-fluid levels, localized ileus, and an increased soft-tissue density in the right lower quadrant. In addition, an altered right psoas shadow or an abnormal right flank stripe may be seen. However, they may show nothing specific.

With an acute abdomen, definitive treatment, as described in Answer 3, should not be delayed. This will be discussed in a subsequent question.

Antibiotics should not be given to this patient because they may mask the signs of peritonitis by reducing the inflammation of the peritoneum without treating the underlying pathology.

3. e. At this time the probability of the diagnosis of acute appendicitis with perforation and peritonitis is very high, and the most important intervention is a surgical consult as soon as possible.

4. a. The most appropriate action at this time would be an abdominal laparoscopy or laparotomy to confirm the diagnosis and treat the condition. The laparoscope now is being used for the removal of appendices by some surgeons. Advantages to laparoscopy include the ability to examine the entire abdomen without the need for extending the operative incision. In addition, there are significantly fewer infectious wound complications. However, there is controversy over whether patients with perforation should have laparoscopy because there is suggestion of higher incidence of postoperative intra-abdominal abscess seen when compared to open laparotomy. Once the decision to operate has been made, it is appropriate to start the patient taking broad-spectrum antibiotics that are effective against both aerobic and anaerobic organisms. The probability of an anaerobic organism as part of the bacterial process is extremely high, and the polymicrobial nature of perforated appendicitis has been clearly established.

5. e. The risk of infertility in women who have had appendicitis is not clear. One large study found no increased risk of infertility in women with nonperforated disease but a several-fold increase in infertility in women with perforated appendicitis. Another study showed no increased risk.

Clear complications of appendectomy include the following:
1. Wound infection: This complication occurs in less than 1% of patients with unperforated appendicitis but increases to 20% with perfora-tion. With perforation, delayed primary closure of the wound may be a good strategy. Treatment is directed at drainage of the infection followed by the administration of appropriate antibiotics.
2. Subphrenic abscess: The persistence of spiking fevers beginning on day 4 or day 5 without obvious cause should raise the suspicion of an intraabdominal collection of pus. The diagnosis is established by physical examination demonstrating an elevated diaphragm and a pleural effusion. There is often tenderness over the seventh and eighth ribs laterally and edema or erythema of the lower chest wall.
3. Pelvic abscess: A patient with recurrent fever and diarrhea after appendectomy suggests the formation of a pelvic abscess. Diagnosis is made by rectal examination and is confirmed by ultrasonography or a CT scan.
4. Appendiceal abscess: Although uncommon, a small percentage of patients seek treatment after the acute infection has become walled off. Under these conditions, it may be preferable to delay appendectomy until the inflammation has settled down.

6. d. Infants, young children, and elderly patients may all present with unclassic symptoms, making the diagnosis of appendicitis difficult. In infants and young children, the presenting symptoms may be nonspecific and include only lethargy and irritability, especially in the early stages. In elderly patients, the same situation applies. Moreover, in elderly patients, the probability of rupture increases from 20% to 70%.

7. d. This question is meant to reiterate both the difficult issue raised previously and the importance of distinguishing acute appendicitis from acute PID and its complications such as tuboovarian abscess. Laparoscopy is definitely indicated in this circumstance.

8. a. Acute appendicitis often is called the "great imitator." This name arises from the different presentations of the disease that are possible, especially at the extremes of life. Elderly patients, infants, and children often will have signs and symptoms that may not be "classic textbook." Thus appendicitis is one of those conditions in which you often will not make the diagnosis unless you think about the diagnosis and have a high level of suspicion.

9. e. The small size of the appendix accounts for its ability to produce symptoms quickly. The pathologic process can be divided into stages:

Stage 1 involves the obstruction of the appendix by a fecalith, a mucous plug, a foreign body, a parasite, lymphoid hyperplasia, or a tumor. This obstruction and hyperperistalsis (not hypoperistalsis) is associated with the early signs of periumbilical cramping and vomiting as a result of distention of the appendix.

Stage 2 involves the rapid invasion of the wall of the organ by bacteria, with secondary inflammation. Gradual onset of systemic signs such as anorexia and malaise, low-grade fever, and leukocytosis then occur.

Stage 3 involves spreading of the infection/inflammation to involve the entire wall of the organ and neighboring peritoneum, leading to a change in character of the pain to constant and localized. At this stage the differential diagnosis may include pyelonephritis, cholecystitis, or tuboovarian abscess.

Young women with right-sided ovarian disease are particularly difficult to differentiate from young women with acute appendicitis. One clue may lie in the point of maximal tenderness. In appendicitis, the point of maximal tenderness is McBurney's point (two-thirds of the distance from the umbilicus to the anterior superior iliac spine). In right-sided ovarian disease the point of maximal tenderness is 2-3 cm below this point.

Stage 4 is the last stage and involves perforation of the appendix. All four stages may develop within a very short period (24-48 hours).

10. d. Elderly patients with rupture have the highest mortality rates. Overall mortality from appendicitis is less than 1% since the era of antibiotics; however, mortality rates increase to 3% in the general population with rupture. Although rupture in infants and the elderly is common, elderly patients have a much higher mortality rate (up to 15%). Pregnant women do not have high rates of mortality but are much more likely (2-3 times more) to perforate, in which case maternal death is rare but fetal abortion reaches a rate of 20%.

11. d. The chandelier sign is associated with PID and is described elsewhere. The rest of the statements are all true regarding appendicitis. Rovsing's sign can be elicited when pressure over the left lower quadrant refers pain to the right lower quadrant. Other signs that can be found in appendicitis include the psoas sign, which is elicited while the patient lies on their left sign and the right hip is extended, producing increased pain as the psoas muscle is stretched under an inflamed appendix. The obturator sign is elicited with the patient lying supine and passively rotating the flexed right hip. When positive the patient reports increased pain with the maneuver.

12. c. Percutaneous drainage is indicated only with late perforated appendix that has resulted in abscess formation at time of diagnosis. Morbidity increases from 0.1% to almost 4% with perforation (and much higher in the elderly), and perforation always results in a prolonged recovery compared to unperforated appendicitis. Although laparoscopy can be performed, as mentioned earlier it can be associated with higher rates of postoperative abscess formation than open laparotomy once the appendix has ruptured. Once appendicitis has been diagnosed, antibiotics are indicated. For uncomplicated appendicitis, one preoperative prophylactic dose of broad-spectrum antibiotic such as cefotetan or cefoxitin should be administered. For ruptured appendicitis, a broad-spectrum antibiotic should be continued for 7-10 days or until the patient is afebrile and has a normal WBC count. Before surgery fluid resuscitation is always necessary, but with perforation the patient usually will be even more volume depleted and will need much more aggressive fluid replacement.

13. d. The sensitivity of CT with intravenous and oral contrast is 96%. The sensitivity of ultrasonography is 75% to 90% and is very operator-dependent. Barium enema is 80% to 90% sensitive but is no longer recommended because up to 40% of studies can be equivocal secondary to only partial filling of the appendix. Abdominal radiographs are not routinely recommended because of very low sensitivity and specificity. Nuclear magnetic scans are 87% to 93% sensitive. Remember, the diagnosis of appendicitis primarily is made by history and physical and imaging should be reserved for cases that are equivocal.

SOLUTION TO THE CLINICAL CASE MANAGEMENT PROBLEM

Of patients with appendicitis, 2% present with a right lower quadrant mass, which can be an abscess or phlegmon. Currently the preferred management of these patients includes ultrasound or CT-guided percutaneous drainage and intravenous antibiotics. Elective appendectomy then can be pursued after 6 weeks. This approach now is favored over immediate surgery for appendiceal abscess, which can lead to disseminate a local infection and result in fistulas and the need for more extensive surgeries such as cecectomy or right hemicolectomy with subsequent longer hospitalization.

SUMMARY OF ACUTE APPENDICITIS

Acute appendicitis is the "great imitator." If you do not think of appendicitis, you will not make the diagnosis. Maintain a high index of suspicion, especially in the young and in the elderly.

1. Classic symptoms of appendicitis: periumbilical abdominal pain, initially vague, but later localizes to the right lower quadrant; anorexia; low-grade fever; and leukocytosis
2. Retrocecal or retroileal appendicitis: poorly localized abdominal pain, mild nausea and vomiting, mild diarrhea, urinary frequency, and hematuria
3. Diagnostic tests: WBC, urinalysis, three views of the abdomen, ultrasonography, and CT scanning if needed
4. Definitive therapy: laparoscopic appendectomy or laparotomy and open removal (laparoscopic appendectomy is being performed more and more commonly. The procedure itself is associated with fewer postoperative complications)
5. Complications: wound infection, subphrenic abscess, pelvic abscess, and appendiceal abscess

SUGGESTED READING

Brown CV: Appendiceal abscess: immediate operation or percutaneous drainage? *Am Surg* 69(10):829-832, 2003.

Lally KP, et al: Appendix. In: Townsend CM, ed.: *Sabiston's textbook of surgery*. WB Saunders Company, 2001, Philadelphia.

Lasson A: Appendiceal abscesses: primary percutaneous drainage and selective interval appendicectomy. *Eur J Surg* 168(5):264-269, 2002.

Mourad J, et al: Appendicitis in pregnancy: new information that contradicts long-held clinical beliefs. *Am J Obstet Gynecol* 182:1027-1029, 2000.

Wilcox CM: Miscellaneous inflammatory diseases of the intestine. In: Goldman, ed: *Cecil's textbook of medicine*, WB Saunders Company, 2000, Philadelphia.

Wolfe JM, Henneman PL: Acute appendicitis. In: Marx J, ed. *Rosen's emergency medicine: concepts and clinical practice*. Mosby, 2002, St. Louis.

Chapter 120

Biliary Tract Disease

"Stones and groans but not bones."

CLINICAL CASE PROBLEM 1:
A 43-Year-Old Female with Recurrent Right Upper Quadrant Pain

A 43-year-old female comes to your office with a 3-hour history of right upper quadrant (RUQ) pain. The pain is described as spasmodic and sharp. It radiates through to the back. The patient describes several episodes of this pain within the past 6 months. Nausea and vomiting accompany most of these episodes. Fever and chills are usually absent. The pain usually comes on after a meal.

On examination, there are no abdominal masses or tenderness. The chest is clear, and the cardiovascular system is normal. The patient's blood pressure is 140/70 mm Hg. The patient has no drug allergies and is not taking any medications at the present time.

■ SELECT THE BEST ANSWER TO THE FOLLOWING QUESTIONS:

1. What is the most likely diagnosis in this patient?
   a. acute cholecystitis
   b. biliary colic
   c. acute pancreatitis
   d. ileocecal appendicitis
   e. Crohn's disease

The patient's symptoms subside before your consultation is complete. You elect a wait-and-see policy. In 3 weeks the patient returns. On this occasion the patient's symptoms have been present for the last 24 hours. The patient is nauseated and has vomited three times since this pain began. The pain, as well as radiating to the back, also is radiating to the right shoulder.

On examination, there is tenderness in the RUQ. On deep inspiration and palpation the patient's pain is accentuated and actually interrupts inspiration. The patient also has a mild fever.

2. What is the most likely diagnosis at this time?
   a. acute cholecystitis
   b. biliary colic
   c. acute pancreatitis
   d. ileocecal appendicitis
   e. Crohn's disease

3. Given this patient's signs and symptoms, which of the following investigative procedure is likely to yield the best information?
   a. a white blood cell count
   b. an oral cholecystogram
   c. an abdominal ultrasound
   d. an electrocardiogram
   e. three views of the abdomen

4. What is (are) the treatment(s) of choice for the patient at this time?
   a. intravenous fluids
   b. parenteral antibiotics
   c. nasogastric suction
   d. all of the above
   e. none of the above

5. Regarding the definite procedure to correct this condition, which of the following statements is true?
   a. a definite procedure should not be contemplated at this time; if required it should be performed several months later
   b. a definitive procedure should not be contemplated at this time; if symptoms continue to recur, you can reconsider
   c. a definitive surgical procedure should be performed at this time
   d. a definitive procedure is contraindicated given the signs and symptoms with which this patient presents
   e. a definitive procedure should not be considered until all other methods of treatment have failed

6. Which of the following statements about gallbladder disease in the United States is (are) true?
   a. more than 20 million Americans have gallstones
   b. in the United States more than 300,000 cholecystectomies are performed annually
   c. most gallstones are composed predominantly of cholesterol
   d. all of the above statements are true
   e. none of the above statements are true

7. Regarding the use of oral dissolution therapy in gallstone disease, which of the following statements is true?
   a. oral dissolution therapy is an excellent option for most patients
   b. few, if any, gallstones that are dissolved with oral dissolution therapy recur
   c. the preferred agent for oral dissolution therapy is ursodiol
   d. oral dissolution therapy should not be combined with extracorporeal shock wave lithotripsy (ESWL)
   e. oral dissolution therapy works best in patients with large gallstones

8. Which of the following statements regarding the treatment of asymptomatic gallstones is most accurate?
   a. asymptomatic gallstones should be treated with cholecystectomy
   b. asymptomatic gallstones should not be treated
   c. whether asymptomatic gallstones should be treated depends on the presence or absence of comorbid conditions
   d. asymptomatic gallstones should or should not be treated; it all depends on who you talk to
   e. asymptomatic gallstone treatment has changed radically since the introduction of laparoscopic cholecystectomy

9. What is the most common complication during laparoscopic cholecystectomy?
   a. excessive bleeding
   b. small bowel perforation
   c. injury to the biliary tract system
   d. inability to remove the gallbladder through the laparoscope
   e. liver laceration

10. Which of the following statements is (are) true of laparoscopic cholecystectomy?
    a. laparoscopic cholecystectomy provides a safe and effective treatment for most patients with symptomatic gallstones; it is the treatment of choice
    b. laparoscopic cholecystectomy provides distinct advantages over open cholecystectomy
    c. laparoscopic cholecystectomy can be performed at a treatment cost equal to or slightly less than that for open cholecystectomy
    d. during laparoscopic cholecystectomy, when the anatomy is obscured because of excessive bleeding or other problems, the operation should be converted promptly to open cholecystectomy
    e. all of the above statements are true

CLINICAL CASE MANAGEMENT PROBLEM

The two most common diagnostic conditions associated with gallbladder disease are biliary colic and acute cholecystitis. Describe the differences in presentation and pathophysiology between biliary colic and acute cholecystitis.

ANSWERS:

1. **b.** This patient exhibits a typical presentation of biliary colic, which is characterized by transient obstruction of the cystic duct. The pain, located in the RUQ, lasts from minutes to several hours. The pain is best described as spasmodic and constant. Postprandial presentation is common. Nausea and vomiting usually accompany the pain.

2. **a.** The persistent nature of the pain in acute cholecystitis is major clinical symptom that differentiates it from bilary colic. In addition, there is RUQ

abdominal tenderness, voluntary guarding, and continuation of the other signs.

The pain sometimes is referred to the right scapula, and the gallbladder may be palpable. Moreover, mild jaundice may occur.

Acute cholecystitis is manifested pathologically by gallbladder distention (hydrops), serosal edema, and infection secondary to obstruction of the cystic duct. Although the other choices presented sometimes can present atypically with RUQ pain only, the probability is low.

3. **c.** The diagnostic procedure of choice in this patient is an abdominal ultrasound. Gallstones will be demonstrated in approximately 95% of cases, and the specificity of the procedure is very high.

4. **d.** In a patient with acute cholecystitis, intravenous fluids should be given to correct dehydration and possible electrolyte imbalance, and a nasogastric tube should be inserted if the patient has protracted vomiting. For acute cholecystitis, appropriate parenteral antibiotics should be given.

5. **c.** In years past, acute cholecystitis was managed either aggressively or conservatively. Because the disease resolves spontaneously in approximately 60% of cases, the conservative approach was to manage the patient expectantly, with a plan to perform elective cholecystectomy after recovery, reserving early surgery for those patients with severe or worsening disease.

The preferred treatment plan at this time, however, is to perform cholecystectomy in all patients following an episode of acute cholecystitis unless there are specific contraindications to performing the operation. The most common contraindication is severe concomitant disease. The reasoning for this approach is as follows: (1) the incidence of technical complications is no greater with early surgery; (2) early surgery reduces the total duration of illness by approximately 30 days, the length of hospitalization by 5-7 days, and direct medical costs by several thousand dollars; and (3) in the absence of surgery, recurrent episodes are not uncommon, which may increase morbidity.

In addition, the following factors affect the decision as to when to operate: (1) the diagnostic certainty; (2) the general health of the patient; and (3) signs of local complications of acute cholecystitis such as gangrene or empyema.

6. **d.** More than 20 million Americans have cholelithiasis; approximately 300,000 operations are performed annually for the disease. The incidence of cholelithiasis increases with age.

Most gallstones (70% to 95%) are comprised predominantly of cholesterol. The remainder are pigment stones. The composition of the gallstone affects neither the symptoms associated with biliary colic nor the symptoms associated with acute cholecystitis.

7. **c.** Oral dissolution therapy with bile acids first was introduced in the early 1970s. The first agent available was chenodiol, which has been replaced by ursodiol. Oral dissolution therapy is indicated only in a small minority of patients. The most effective use of bile acids occurs with small gallstones (50 mm in diameter or less), which are floating, cholesterol in nature, and within a functioning gallbladder. This represents approximately 15% of patients. Patients must be treated within between 6 and 12 months, and monitoring is necessary until dissolution is achieved. In such patients 60% to 90% of gallstones will dissolve. Unfortunately, at least 50% of these stones reoccur within 5 years.

Dissolution rates are higher and recurrence rates are lower in patients with single stones, in nonobese individuals, and in young patients. Unfortunately, many patients suffer distressing side effects such as nausea from this treatment. Indications for bile acid therapy are limited to patients with a comorbid condition that precludes safe operation and patients who choose to avoid operation.

ESWL is not commonly used by itself; it is used along with oral dissolution therapy. This technique may be successful in up to 95% of patients with a functioning gallbladder and solitary noncalcified stones 20 mm in diameter or less. Recurrence is infrequent following therapy with ESWL for a single small stone, but it is more common in patients with multiple stones. Again, the gallbladder remains and the probability of further stone formation is high.

8. **b.** Current opinion suggests that asymptomatic gallstones should not be treated. The vast majority of gallstones remain silent throughout life. Only 1% to 4% per year of asymptomatic patients will develop symptoms or complications of gallstone disease. Existing data suggest that 10% of patients will develop symptoms within the first 5 years following diagnosis and approximately 20% within 10 years. Almost all patients will experience symptoms for a time period before they develop a complication. Therefore, with few exceptions, prophylactic treatment of asymptomatic patients cannot be justified.

9. **c.** All of the complications listed are possible, but the most common complication of laparoscopic cholecystectomy is bile duct injury. The frequency of bile duct injury is dependent on the skills of the surgeon and has been decreasing consistently as more experience with this procedure has been gained.

10. e. Laparoscopic cholecystectomy provides a safe and effective treatment for most patients with symptomatic gallstones. It is the treatment of choice for most patients at this time, providing distinct advantages over open cholecystectomy. It decreases pain and disability without increasing mortality or overall morbidity. Although the rate of common bile duct injury is slightly increased, this rate is still sufficiently low to justify the use of this procedure.

Laparoscopic cholecystectomy can be performed at a treatment cost that is equal to or slightly less than that of open cholecystectomy and will result in substantial cost savings to the patient and society because of reduced loss of time from work.

The outcome of laparoscopic cholecystectomy is influenced greatly by the training, experience, skill, and judgment of the surgeon performing the procedure. Multiple studies have found that improved outcome is directly related to volume of procedures performed. Therefore, choosing a surgeon is often the critical decision a family physician can make that influences a patient's outcome. During laparoscopic cholecystectomy, when anatomy is obscured, excessive bleeding occurs, or other problems arise, the operation should be converted promptly to open cholecystectomy. Conversion under these circumstances reflects sound surgical judgment and should not be considered a complication of laparoscopic cholecystectomy.

SOLUTION TO THE CLINICAL CASE MANAGEMENT PROBLEM

Biliary colic results from transient obstruction of the cystic duct with a gallstone. The pain associated with biliary colic usually begins abruptly after a meal and subsides gradually, lasting from a few minutes to several hours. It is located in the upper right quadrant and may or may not be associated with abdominal tenderness. There is no associated inflammation of the gallbladder with biliary colic because of the transient nature of the condition.

Acute cholecystitis, however, is associated pathophysiologically with inflammation of the gallbladder wall, with secondary infection in the gallbladder caused by blockage of the cystic duct. The first symptom is abdominal pain in the RUQ, with referral of the pain to right scapula. The pain persists and becomes associated with abdominal tenderness. There is nausea, vomiting, and a positive Murphy's sign (arrest of inspiration with palpation in the RUQ). The pain does not resolve spontaneously. There may be fever.

SUMMARY OF BILIARY TRACT DISEASE

A. **Acute cholecystitis:**
   1. Symptoms and signs: (a) acute RUQ pain and tenderness; (b) mild fever and leukocytosis; (c) nausea and vomiting; (d) palpable gallbladder; and (e) gallstones on ultrasound scan
   2. Treatment: (a) nasogastric suction; (b) parenteral fluids; (c) analgesics; (d) intravenous antibiotics; and (e) laparoscopic cholecystectomy as soon as possible

B. **Biliary colic:**
   1. Symptoms and signs: (a) recurrent abdominal pain (usually RUQ); (b) dyspepsia; and (c) gallstones on ultrasound
   2. Treatment: laparoscopic cholecystectomy when recurrent episodes occur

C. **Choledocholithiasis/cholangitis:** choledocholithiasis occurs in 15% of patients with gallstones. Preoperative endoscopic retrograde cholangiography with sphincterotomy or intraoperative common duct exploration are options in concert with cholecystectomy.

Choledocholithiasis is the major cause of cholangitis. Symptoms of cholangitis include biliary colic, jaundice, fever, and chills. Treatment of cholangitis includes intravenous antibiotics, cholecystectomy, and intervention to the common duct.

D. **Laparoscopic cholecystectomy:** Laparoscopic cholecystectomy is the treatment of choice for the vast majority of patients with biliary tract disease. It is a much more conservative operation, causes much less postoperative pain, and is associated with a much earlier return to work. Choice of surgeon is key, with higher quality outcomes tied to higher volume of cases performed.

E. **Asymptomatic gallstones:** Asymptomatic gallstones should be left where they are; do not create a problem where one does not exist.

SUGGESTED READING

Indar AA, Beckingham IJ: Acute cholecystitis. *BMJ* 325(7365):639-643, 2002 Sep 21.
Trowbridge RL, et al: Does this patient have acute cholecystitis? *JAMA* 289(1):80-86, 2003.

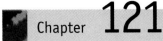

Chapter 121

Common Procedures in Office Surgery

> "Are you sure you can cut it out, right here in your office?"

CLINICAL CASE PROBLEM 1:

A 37-Year-Old Female with a Skin Lesion on Her Back

A 37-year-old female comes to your office for assessment of a skin lesion on her back that has been present for the last 3 years. It recently has increased in size, and the patient is concerned about it. The lesion is pigmented, raised, and dark brown. It is approximately 1.5 cm in greatest diameter. There are other, smaller lesions that have a similar appearance on the patient's back, but they have neither increased in size nor changed color.

You decide to remove the skin lesion in your office.

■ SELECT THE BEST ANSWER TO THE FOLLOWING QUESTIONS:

1. In removing the skin lesion from your patient's back, what should you do?
   a. follow Langer's lines
   b. use silk sutures for skin closure
   c. use catgut sutures for subcutaneous tissue closure
   d. all of the above
   e. none of the above

2. In considering the deep subcutaneous tissue on your patient's back and your selection of suture material, you should be aware that it takes approximately how many days for fibroblasts to grow across the wound line and develop enough strength to hold together the deep portion of the wound?
   a. 10 days
   b. 15 days
   c. 21 days
   d. 28 days
   e. 35 days

3. In deciding on the use of needles for suture placement on skin surfaces in deep layers, which of the following statements is true?
   a. a cutting needle should be used for skin closure; a taper needle should be used for deeper tissues
   b. a taper needle should be used for skin closure; a cutting needle should be used for deep tissue
   c. a cutting needle should be used for both skin closure and deep-tissue closure

   d. a taper needle should be used for both skin closure and deep-tissue closure
   e. both cutting and taper needles may be used for either skin or deep-tissue closure

4. What is the local anesthetic of choice for the patient described?
   a. lidocaine with epinephrine
   b. lidocaine plain
   c. bupivacaine plain
   d. bupivacaine with epinephrine
   e. none of the above

5. Which of the following is (are) useful in controlling bleeding from a skin lesion base?
   a. application of pressure
   b. electrocautery
   c. a pressure dressing
   d. hemostatic sutures
   e. all of the above

6. Which of the following techniques is (are) recommended for the removal of pigmented skin lesions?
   a. punch biopsy
   b. shave biopsy
   c. electrocautery
   d. a or b
   e. any of the above

7. What is (are) the treatment(s) of choice for the removal of plantar warts?
   a. cryosurgery
   b. electrocautery
   c. salicylic acid plaster
   d. podophyllin application
   e. any of the above

8. The treatment(s) of choice for the removal of venereal warts include which of the following?
   a. electrocautery
   b. cryosurgery
   c. surgical excision
   d. podophyllin application
   e. all of the above

CLINICAL CASE PROBLEM 2:

A 5-Year-Old Child with a Second-Degree Burn on Her Right Hand

A 5-year-old child is brought to your office with a small second-degree burn on her right hand. The burn was sustained when she put her hand on a kettle of boiling water. On examination, there is an area of 3 cm × 5 cm on the left hand that has undergone blister formation. Her mother wrapped the burn in a gauze dressing.

9. At this time, what would be the most appropriate first course of action?
   a. debride the wound
   b. cool the burn site by immediately immersing the hand in cold water
   c. aspirate the fluid underneath the blister
   d. clean the area and redress it with gauze
   e. debride the wound, aspirate the fluid, and apply an antibiotic cream

10. Following the initial step described in Question 9, what should be the next step(s)?
    a. arrange for a revisit in 48 hours
    b. debride the burn site
    c. provide tetanus prophylaxis
    d. a and c
    e. a, b, and c

CLINICAL CASE PROBLEM 3:

A 4-Year-Old Male Who Banged His Thumb

A 4-year-old boy is brought to your office by his mother after having banged his thumb in a door. He is crying and irritated. His left thumb has a purplish discoloration under the nail.

11. At this time, what should you do?
    a. reassure the mother and send the child home with a pat on the head
    b. reassure the mother and give the child some plain acetaminophen
    c. under local anesthetic remove the nail
    d. under local anesthetic perform a wedge resection
    e. none of the above

CLINICAL CASE PROBLEM 4:

A 25-Year-Old Female with a Sore Big Toe

A 25-year-old female has had a sore left great toe for the past 4 weeks. On examination, the lateral aspect of the left toe is erythematous and puffy, with pus oozing from the corner between the nail and the skin tissue surrounding the nail. This is the first occurrence of this condition in this patient.

12. At this time, what should you do?
    a. nothing
    b. have the patient soak her toe in hydrogen peroxide three times daily
    c. have the patient apply a local antibiotic cream, and prescribe systemic antibiotics to be taken for 7-10 days

d. under local anesthesia, remove the whole toenail
e. b and c

13. If the treatment advocated in Question 12 is unsuccessful, what should you do then?
    a. still do nothing; these things have a habit of going away if you wait long enough; tell the patient she will be in pain only for another 3 or 4 months at the most
    b. have the patient continue to soak her toe in hydrogen peroxide; tell the pharmacist to mix up a double-strength mixture for her
    c. change both the local and the systemic antibiotics to the big, all-inclusive, all-pervasive, kill-everything-in-sight guns
    d. under local anesthesia, remove the whole toenail
    e. none of the above

CLINICAL CASE PROBLEM 5:

A 45-Year-Old Male with Rectal Pain

A 45-year-old male comes to your office with a 4-day history of rectal pain. The pain is dull, constant, and made worse by defecation. On examination, there is a 3 cm × 2 cm thrombosed mass present at the 3 o'clock position in the anal area.

14. At this time, what should you do?
    a. advise the patient to take five sitz baths per day
    b. advise the patient to apply a local antiinflammatory cream three times a day
    c. under local anesthesia, remove the contents of the mass with a straight incision
    d. under local anesthesia, remove the contents of the mass with an elliptical incision
    e. apply a band to this mass and wait for it to fall off

CLINICAL CASE PROBLEM 6:

A 28-Year-Old Male with Rectal Bleeding

A 28-year-old male comes to your office with rectal bleeding and local burning and searing pain in the rectal area. The patient describes a small amount of bright red blood on the toilet paper. The pain is maximal at defecation and following defecation. The burning and searing pain that occurs at defecation is replaced by a spasmodic pain after defecation that lasts approximately 30 minutes.

15. What is the most likely diagnosis in this patient?
    a. adenocarcinoma of the rectum
    b. squamous cell carcinoma of the rectum

c. internal hemorrhoids
d. anal fissure
e. an external thrombosed hemorrhoid

16. What is (are) the treatment(s) of choice for large prolapsing internal hemorrhoids?
    a. excision and drainage
    b. sclerotherapy
    c. internal banding
    d. all of the above are equally effective
    e. none of the above

 CLINICAL CASE MANAGEMENT PROBLEM

Discuss the classification of burns and how that classification affects office or hospital treatment.

■ **ANSWERS:**

1. a. For skin incision, it is extremely important that the skin lines of tension be followed (Langer's lines). This is especially important on areas such as the face, where Langer's lines tend to run horizontally on the upper face and vertically on the lower face.

2. c. It takes approximately 21 days for fibroblasts to grow across a wound line and for the wound to develop enough strength to hold deep portions of a wound together. If deep portions of a wound pull apart, a depression on the skin surface may develop, which represents a poor cosmetic outcome.

3. a. Cutting needles always should be used on the skin. Almost all cutting needles now have a reverse cutting design (flat surface is on the inside of the curve). For deeper layers, taper needles are less likely to cut through a blood vessel and start bleeding that is difficult to control.

4. a. The anesthetic agent of choice for this patient is lidocaine with epinephrine. The epinephrine will decrease the amount of bleeding from the incision site. The prepackaged solution of lidocaine with epinephrine has a very low pH (pH 4.05) and produces much more pain on injection than lidocaine plain. The pain reaction can be avoided by buffering the lidocaine with sodium bicarbonate in a combination of 10 parts of lidocaine to 1 part of sodium bicarbonate. When this combination is used, the pH is near neutral and the stinging sensation is eliminated.

Other measures that reduce the pain of injection include warming the solution to body temperature, injecting the solution extremely slowly, and cooling the injection site with ice or ethyl chloride before injection. In addition, very small caliber needles can be used for the initial injection (such as a 30 gauge, ½-inch needle), or a local anesthetic such as tetracaine, epinephrine, and cocaine (TAC) or 20% benzocaine liquid or gel can be used.

5. e. Common methods for controlling bleeding after incision include (1) application of pressure with a sponge held firmly against the bleeding areas; (2) electrocautery; (3) use of local anesthesia containing epinephrine; (4) topical epinephrine; (5) Drysol solution (aluminum chloride, 20% in alcohol); (6) hemostatic sutures; (7) elevation; (8) pressure dressings; and (9) various methods of cooling.

6. d. A pigmented skin lesion should be removed intact to ensure an "unharmed" specimen for pathologic evaluation. If electrocautery is used to remove the lesion, the lesion obviously will be destroyed in the process.

7. a. Multiple different ablative methods have been used to treat plantar warts.

The first step is to pare down the excess callus in the area of the wart. This is best done by shaving off thin layers of the callus with a straightedge razor blade held by hand or a scalpel with a #10 blade. This process should be continued until most of the callus is gone and normal-appearing pliable skin is seen.

The shaving is kept superficial to any bleeding or sensation of pain. The circular plantar wart then becomes much clearer and more evident. Some of the keratin plug then can be excised with the corner of the razor blade or the tip of the scalpel blade. Following callus removal, the ablative method chosen will be more effective, although no treatment is 100% successful and many warts resolve on their own.

8. d. The treatment of choice for venereal warts is 25% podophyllum in tincture of benzoin. Care must be taken to apply the agent only to the wart to avoid damaging the surrounding normal skin. This can be accomplished with the application of petroleum jelly to the surrounding tissue. The patient should be instructed to wash off the podophyllin in 2-4 hours to avoid a chemical burn. Pregnant patients should not be treated with podophyllin.

9. d. The burn should be cleaned and dressed with a nonadherent dressing. Cooling runs the risk of compromising circulation to marginally surviving areas of the burn and should not be done for serious burns. If the blister is intact, the burn should not be débrided. Oral analgesia should be provided.

However, the pain associated with minor first-degree burns will be alleviated to some degree by cooling. Moreover, because tissue damage is minimal it will do no harm.

10. d. Cleaning the burn site with a surgical soap to remove dirt, oil, or other foreign matter is the first step. The use of 4×4 gauze sponges or cotton balls can facilitate cleansing. If cleansing is done gently and the burn site is properly cooled, minimal pain should result.

Tetanus prophylaxis is important in all patients with serious burns. If this child's tetanus is not up to date, it must be brought up-to-date.

For a second-degree burn, as in this child, expert opinion is divided on whether débridement should take place. Most experts elect to leave the blister intact for several days. The skin of a natural blister may act as a natural dressing, protecting the wound against infection and reducing the amount of pain.

After the initial cleansing, the blistered area may be covered with a layer of silver sulfadiazine ointment (Silvadene) or, in patients who are allergic to sulfa, Polysporin. A nonadherent dressing then should be applied. Following that, a conforming protective material, such as Kling or Kerlix, should be applied. The wound should be rechecked within 48 hours.

11. e. This patient has a subungual hematoma that needs to be released. The best method of release is to heat a wire (a paper clip), reassure the patient that this is not going to hurt, and gently press the hot metal tip directly over the central portion of the hematoma. As soon as penetration is complete, blood flows through the opening and relief of pain is immediate. An antibiotic ointment will help protect against infection.

12. e. See Answer 13.

13. e. This patient has an ingrown toenail. It is perfectly reasonable to try a conservative approach first. The conservative approach consists of prescribing topical and oral antibiotics for infection, having hot soaks or hydrogen peroxide soaks, practicing good nail care (make sure that the nail is cut straight across), and wearing wider shoes. The corner of the nail that is causing the problem (i.e., the corner of the nail that is infected) often can be encouraged to grow out over the skin at the end of the toe by elevation. The corner may be held up by some articles such as a wisp of cotton, a folded piece of Telfa, or petroleum jelly gauze or other dressing.

This first attempt at conservative treatment has the additional advantage of decreasing the swelling and inflammation and facilitating injections of the local anesthetic if wedge resection does, in the end, have to be performed. Wedge resection of the nail (the next step) is a procedure whereby the offending curve is cut off at an angle of approximately 30 degrees. Only in recurrent cases is it necessary to completely remove the nail.

14. d. This patient has a thrombosed external hemorrhoid. This condition is painful and causes the patient a great deal of discomfort. Treatment consists of removal of the contents (a clot) using an elliptic

SOLUTION TO THE CLINICAL CASE MANAGEMENT PROBLEM

Burns are classified as follows:

1. *First-degree:* Symptoms and signs include pain and redness but no blistering. Dressing is unnecessary. Pain from small burn areas can be relieved by cooling or application of topical creams, ointments, and lotions containing a "caine" medication.

    In areas of clothing, the burn can be covered, and a medicated ointment followed by the application of a nonadherent dressing is recommended.

    Pain can be treated with acetaminophen, aspirin, or another nonsteroidal antiinflammatory drug.

2. *Second-degree:* The hallmark of a second-degree burn is blister formation. Second-degree burns may be either superficial or deep. Treatment options include cleaning and application of a topical antibiotic and dressing. In most cases, leave the blister intact.

3. *Third-degree:* These are full-thickness skin burns. Referral to a plastic surgeon as soon as possible is mandatory. Third-degree burns are much more likely to be more serious, be more extensive, have a much greater chance of developing sepsis, and often require an intensive care unit situation if the burn covers a significant portion of the body.

incision with a #15 scalpel under local anesthetic. The area should be cleansed and, once bleeding is controlled, an antibiotic ointment and 4×4 gauze pads should be applied.

15. d. This patient has an anal fissure, which is a common cause of rectal bleeding. A crack or a fissure in the skin of the anal canal results from the passage of large, hard boluses of stool. A small amount of bright red blood is noted on the toilet paper. The bleeding most often occurs after defecation. Pain is an important symptom; it is usually a local burning or searing pain and is often very severe.

Examination reveals a semi-elliptical defect or crack in the anal skin running in a radial direction.

Initially, treatment of anal fissures involves the application of a local steroid cream applied twice daily for 2 or 3 weeks. The use of stool softeners and daily hot sitz baths are recommended. In most cases this treatment will promote complete healing.

16. c. The treatment of choice for internal hemorrhoids is banding. This office procedure should be performed with no more than two hemorrhoids at once. If there are three or more hemorrhoids, wait 3 or 4 weeks before repeating the procedure.

SUMMARY OF OFFICE SURGERY

1. **Remember the ABCs:** Always have an emergency cart available if you are planning on doing office surgery.
2. **Skin lesion removal:** (a) follow Langer's lines; (b) use an elliptic incision (long enough to avoid puckering at the ends); (c) for local anesthesia use lidocaine with epinephrine, except on the fingers and toes; (d) suture skin with monofilament nylon 3-0, 4-0, 5-0, 6-0, using a cutting needle; (e) for suturing deep wounds use a tapered Dexon needle; (f) do not use electrocautery on anything that should rightly go for biopsy; and (g) for small skin lesion removal use punch biopsy. If you are not absolutely, 100%, sure of what a skin lesion is, then biopsy it.
3. **Sebaceous cysts:** These are most frequent on the scalp and back and can be a cause of significant irritation. Try wherever possible to shell out the whole cyst. If you are unable to remove the entire cyst, there is a significant chance of recurrence.
4. **Incision and drainage of abscesses:** Make sure you know exactly what you are incising and draining and why you are doing it. Be very careful of both the vascular supply and the nerve supply if you go deep.
5. **Common warts:** Cryosurgery with liquid nitrogen is a common treatment. Be careful on the digits so as not to disturb blood flow.
6. **Plantar warts:** (a) pare down excess callus to the bleeding point; (b) remove keratin plug if possible; and (c) use ablative method of your and patient's choice.
7. **Burns:** Described in the Solution to the Clinical Case Management Problem
8. **Paronychia:** (a) try conservative management first and (b) remove the proximal segment of fingernail and then dress it.
9. **Subungual hematoma:** Remove with the old, wise, worn, and true heated paper clip.
10. **Thrombosed external hemorrhoids:** (a) use local anesthesia and (b) use an elliptic incision and remove the clot.
11. **Lacerations:** Use rules as stated for skin lesion removal.
12. **Anal fissures:** (a) it is mandatory that further episodes be prevented, which is best achieved by preventing constipation; and b) use conservative treatment using sitz baths and local steroid cream.
13. **Internal hemorrhoids:** (a) make sure you know what you are banding before you band it; and (b) once sure, banding is the preferred method of treatment.

SUGGESTED READING

Achar S, Kundu S: Principles of office anesthesia: part I. Infiltrative anesthesia. *Am Fam Physician* 66(1):91-94, 2002.
Kundu S, Achar S: Principles of office anesthesia: part II. Topical anesthesia. *Am Fam Physician* 66(1):99-102, 2002.
Zuber TJ: Fusiform excision. *Am Fam Physician* 67(7):1539-1544, 1547-1548, 1550, 2003.
Zuber TJ: The mattress sutures: vertical, horizontal, and corner stitch. *Am Fam Physician* 66(12):2231-2236, 2002.
Zuber TJ: Ingrown toenail removal. *Am Fam Physician* 65(12):2547-2552, 2554, 2002.
Zuber TJ: Dermal electrosurgical shave excision. *Am Fam Physician* 65(9):1883-1886, 1889-1890, 1895, 2002.
Zuber TJ: Minimal excision technique for epidermoid (sebaceous) cysts. *Am Fam Physician* 65(7):1409-1412, 1417-1418, 1420, 2002.
Zuber TJ: Punch biopsy of the skin. *Am Fam Physician* 65(6):1155-1158, 1161-1162, 1164, 2002.

Chapter **122**

Pancreatitis

> "All I need is another drink
> to settle my stomach."

CLINICAL CASE PROBLEM 1:
A 44-YEAR-OLD MALE WITH A HISTORY OF VERY HEAVY ALCOHOL INTAKE

A 44-year-old male with a 20-year history of heavy drinking comes to your office with his wife. His wife is very concerned about her husband's condition and, specifically, about an abdominal pain that began 4 days ago. The pain has been so severe that her husband has been crying at night. Despite this severe pain, the patient managed to make it to his local bar last evening and straggled home at 3 AM.

On examination, you observe a stoic, overweight male who looks much older than his stated years. When you ask him what is wrong, he says, "Nothing, just a little indigestion." As you examine him you clearly smell alcohol on his breath. The patient's blood pressure is 90/70 mm Hg. He has a marked tenderness in the epigastric region along with "bruising" in the epigastric area. There is also a sensation of a mass present in the epigastric area. When questioned about the bruising, the patient states that he fell down the stairs yesterday. No other abnormalities are present.

■ SELECT THE BEST ANSWER TO THE FOLLOWING QUESTIONS:

1. Following the history and physical examination, which of the following is the next step?
   a. send the patient for blood work
   b. send the patient for x-rays
   c. send the patient for both blood work and x-rays
   d. consult a psychiatrist to assess his alcohol intake and subsequent family problems
   e. none of the above

2. Following the step taken in Question 1, what would you do now?
   a. order additional blood tests and x-rays if any abnormalities were found
   b. order an ultrasound of the abdomen
   c. call a colleague who specializes in the gastrointestinal system and ask him to see the patient within a few days
   d. do a complete mental status examination to determine suicidal ideation
   e. none of the above

3. What is the most likely diagnosis in this patient?
   a. alcoholic esophagitis
   b. severe alcoholic gastritis
   c. acute pancreatitis
   d. perforated duodenal ulcer
   e. early alcoholic encephalopathy with underlying alcoholic gastritis

4. The "bruising" present in the epigastrium is most likely the result of which of the following?
   a. the patient's wife's floor wax
   b. trauma secondary to a barroom brawl
   c. retroperitoneal bleeding
   d. superior mesenteric artery erosion
   e. disseminated intravascular coagulation

5. What is the most likely disease complication associated with the "bruising?"
   a. a defect in the intrinsic coagulation pathway
   b. a defect in the extrinsic coagulation pathway
   c. diffuse intravascular coagulation as a result of the alcohol intake
   d. pseudocyst formation
   e. hemorrhagic abscess formation

6. What is (are) the essential diagnostic feature(s) of the condition of the patient described in Clinical Case Problem 1?
   a. abrupt onset of epigastric pain with radiation to the back
   b. nausea and vomiting
   c. elevated serum amylase
   d. all of the above
   e. none of the above

7. The treatment of this condition must include all of the following except:
   a. gastric suction
   b. fluid replacement
   c. calcium replacement
   d. oxygen
   e. an H_2 receptor blocker

8. Which of the following statements about the disease discussed is (are) true?
   a. many cases of this disease are associated with a pathologic condition of the biliary tract
   b. strong evidence suggests a link between this disease and alcohol
   c. the chronic condition of this disease is more likely to be associated with alcohol abuse rather than biliary tract disease
   d. all of the above statements are true
   e. none of the above statements are true

9. In approximately two-thirds of cases of this disease, a plain film of the abdomen is abnormal. Which of the following abnormalities is this plain film most likely to show?
   a. a "sentinel loop"
   b. the "colon cutoff sign"
   c. air under the diaphragm
   d. distention in both the small bowel and the large bowel
   e. feces throughout the colon

10. Complications of the condition described in Clinical Case Problem 1 include which of the following?
   a. ascites
   b. pleural effusion
   c. abscess formation
   d. all of the above
   e. none of the above

CLINICAL CASE MANAGEMENT PROBLEM

Describe the four essential features of the diagnosis of chronic pancreatitis.

ANSWERS:

1. **e.** This patient is extremely ill and should be hospitalized now.

2. **e.** The combination of low blood pressure, abdominal pain, and a history of heavy alcohol intake strongly suggest the diagnosis of an acute abdomen. No time should be taken for doing laboratory investigations or x-rays at this time; that can wait until the patient has been assessed and is hemodynamically stabilized.

3. **c.** This patient has acute pancreatitis. His admission to an intensive care unit would be the best course of action. His blood pressure should be stabilized and input and output measurements should be started immediately.

4. **c.** This patient has Cullen's sign, an ecchymosis in the periumbilical area caused by the dissection of blood retroperitoneally. This also confirms the diagnosis of hemorrhagic pancreatitis. Another sign that sometimes can be found in patients with acute pancreatitis is called Grey-Turner's sign. In Grey-Turner's sign there is the same ecchymosis, only the location is the flank area rather than the periumbilical area.

5. **d.** The most likely complication is bleeding into a pancreatic pseudocyst that has formed as a com-

plication of acute pancreatitis. Such bleeding must be stopped. This may be accomplished by embolization of the artery. If the bleeding cannot be stopped by embolization, emergency surgery should be performed. In this patient it may be necessary to open the pseudocyst, ligate the bleeding vessel in the cyst wall, and drain the cyst.

6. **d.** The essential diagnostic features of acute pancreatitis include abrupt onset of epigastric pain with radiation to the lower lumbar spine, nausea and vomiting, and elevated serum or urinary amylase. Acute pancreatitis usually is caused by cholecystitis or alcoholism.

The essential diagnostic features of pancreatic pseudocyst include an epigastric mass and pain, mild fever and leukocytosis, persistent serum amylase or serum lipase elevation, and demonstration of pseudocyst by computed tomography (CT) scan.

7. **e.** The essentials of treatment of acute pancreatitis include (1) gastric suction to eliminate gastric secretions and decompression; (2) fluid replacement to replace sequestered fluid in the retroperitoneal space; (3) replacement of calcium and magnesium (in severe attacks of pancreatitis both hypocalcemia and hypomagnesemia may occur and need to be treated); (4) oxygen therapy (severe hypoxemia develops in 30% of patients; the onset is often insidious and can result in adult respiratory distress syndrome); (5) peritoneal lavage in severe cases to remove toxins; (6) nutrition: nothing by mouth (NPO) and total parenteral nutrition (TPN); and (7) when hemorrhage into either the pancreas or a pancreatic pseudocyst occurs, a blood transfusion.

Although the use of H_2 receptor blockers, anticholinergic drugs, glucagon, and antibiotics is reasonably common, their efficacy has not been demonstrated.

8. **d.** Gallstone disease and alcohol abuse each are responsible for approximately 40% of cases of acute pancreatitis. Other causes include hyperparathyroidism, hyperlipidemia, familial pancreatitis, postoperative (iatrogenic) pancreatitis, protein deficiency, use of certain drugs, obstruction of the pancreatic duct, and trauma.

Chronic pancreatitis is much more likely to be associated with alcoholism than with biliary tract disease. In fact, a patient with alcoholism who presents with one attack of acute pancreatitis is very likely to go on to subsequent attacks and to chronic disease.

9. **a.** In approximately two-thirds of cases, a plain film of the abdomen is abnormal. The most frequent

finding is isolated dilatation of a segment of gut (the sentinel loop) consisting of jejunum, transverse colon, or duodenum adjacent to the pancreas.

Gas distending the right colon that abruptly stops in the mid or left transverse colon is called the colon cutoff sign. This is caused by colonic spasm adjacent to the pancreatic inflammation.

Air under the diaphragm is suggestive of a perforated peptic ulcer.

A completely distended small and large bowel suggests a distal bowel obstruction.

Constipation is not associated with acute pancreatitis.

10. **d.** In addition to chronic pancreatitis and pancreatic pseudocyst formation, acute pancreatitis also may be associated with pancreatic abscess (fatal if not treated surgically), pancreatic ascites, and pancreatic pleural effusion.

SOLUTION TO THE CLINICAL CASE MANAGEMENT PROBLEM

The four essential features of chronic pancreatitis are as follows: (1) persistent or recurrent abdominal pain in almost all cases; (2) pancreatic calcification on x-ray in 50% of cases, (3) pancreatic insufficiency in 30% of cases, which may lead to either steatorrhea or diabetes mellitus; and (4) most often caused by alcoholism.

SUMMARY OF PANCREATITIS

1. Acute pancreatitis usually is caused by either alcohol abuse or biliary tract disease (40% biliary tract–gallstone associated; 40% alcohol intake).
2. Essential features of diagnosis: abrupt onset of epigastric pain radiating through to the back; nausea and vomiting; and elevated serum amylase, serum lipase, or urinary amylase
3. Laboratory investigations: complete blood count; serum amylase and urine amylase; serum lipase; serum glucose; serum lactate dehydrogenase (LDH), serum bilirubin, serum aspartate aminotransferase (AST)/alanine aminotransferase (ALT); serum calcium, serum magnesium, electrolytes, cholesterol and triglycerides, blood gases, plain film of abdomen, abdominal ultrasound, CT scan
4. Ranson's criteria of severity of acute pancreatitis:
   a. Criteria initially present: (i) age >55 years; (ii) white blood cell count >16,000/mm^3; (iii) blood glucose >200 mg%; (iv) serum lactate dehydrogenase >350 IU/L; and (v) aspartate aminotransferase (serum glutamate oxaloacetate transaminase) >250 IU/L
   b. Criteria developing within 48 hours of admission: (i) hematocrit decreases more than 10%; (ii) blood urea nitrogen increases more than 5 mg/dL; (iii) serum Ca: 8 mg/dl or less; (iv) arterial PO$_2$ <60 mm Hg; (v) base deficit >4 mEq/L; and (vi) estimated fluid sequestration ≥600 ml (volume requirement)
   c. Morbidity and mortality rates correlate with number of criteria present: (i) 0 to 2 criteria 1% mortality; (ii) 3 or 4 criteria 15% mortality; (iii) 5 or 6 criteria 40% mortality; and (iv) 7 or 8 criteria 50% or greater mortality
5. Essentials of management: NPO; nasogastric suction; urine output (a measure of fluid sequestration); fluid replacement of sequestered fluid; replacement of calcium and magnesium if low; oxygen; peritoneal lavage; and TPN
6. Resolution within a week in most cases.
7. Complications: pseudocyst formation, abscess formation, hemorrhage, ascites, pleural effusion, chronic pancreatitis
8. Chronic pancreatitis almost always is associated with alcohol-induced problems; complications of chronic pancreatitis include malabsorption (steatorrhea), diabetes mellitus, and chronic pain.

SUGGESTED READING

Beckingham IJ, Bornman PC: ABC of diseases of liver, pancreas, and biliary system. Acute pancreatitis. *BMJ* 322(7286):595-598, 2001.

Munoz A, Katerndahl DA: Diagnosis and management of acute pancreatitis. *Am Fam Physician* 62:164-174, 2000.

Vlodov J, Tenner SM: Acute and chronic pancreatis. *Prim Care* (3):607-628, 2001.

Yousaf M, et al: Management of severe acute pancreatitis. *Br J Surg* 90(4):407-420, 2003.

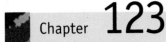

Pancreatic Carcinoma

| A little organ; big problems.

CLINICAL CASE PROBLEM 1:
A 62-YEAR-OLD MALE WITH ABDOMINAL PAIN

A 62-year-old male comes to your office for a third opinion. He has seen two other physicians during the last 3 months regarding an abdominal pain that is, according to the patient, "getting worse and worse." It is unrelated in any way to food intake except that the patient has become significantly anorexic since developing the pain. The first physician told him that he had irritable bowel syndrome; the second physician told him that the pain was a psychoneurotic pain: "Basically, sir, that means it is all in your head." The patient tells you that he was very disappointed with the two physicians, especially because the first one had been his family doctor for more than 15 years.

You decide to spend your time today on a very focused history. The most important information you gather is (1) the patient has lost 20 lb in 3 months; (2) the pain is constant; (3) the patient has never had abdominal pain before; (4) the patient's mood has definitely changed over this period (in fact, the first symptom was depression, even before the pain started); and (5) the pain is central abdominal, radiating through to the back, dull and aching in character, and described as a 10/10 in terms of severity.

On examination, the patient looks "unwell." You cannot describe it any more clearly than that. He just looks unwell. There is no clinical evidence of anemia, jaundice, or cyanosis. Examination of the abdomen reveals some tenderness in the midabdominal region. The liver edge is felt 2 cm below the left costal margin.

■ **SELECT THE BEST ANSWER TO THE FOLLOWING QUESTIONS:**

1. The differential diagnosis in this patient would include all except which of the following?
   a. inflammatory bowel disease
   b. carcinoma of the stomach
   c. carcinoma of the pancreas
   d. irritable bowel syndrome
   e. none of the above can be excluded

2. If you could order only one investigation at this time, which one of the following would you order?

   a. a magnetic resonance imaging (MRI) scan of the abdomen
   b. gastroscopy
   c. a computed tomography (CT) scan of the abdomen
   d. a colonoscopy
   e. serum amylase or serum lipase

3. Which of the following statements regarding the relationship between this patient's depressive symptoms and his abdominal symptoms is correct?
   a. the abdominal symptoms are unrelated to the depression
   b. the abdominal symptoms are indirectly related to the depression
   c. the abdominal symptoms are directly related to the depression
   d. the abdominal symptoms and the depressive symptoms usually do not coexist in this disorder
   e. nobody really knows for sure

4. The appropriate investigation is ordered. What is the sensitivity of this investigation in the disorder described?
   a. 70%
   b. 80%
   c. 90%
   d. 95%
   e. 100%

5. The patient had planned a vacation for the week after the investigation was performed. You persuaded him to return to your office when he gets back from his vacation in 6 weeks for further evaluation. You encourage him to take his vacation because of your suspicions regarding his disease. Before he leaves for his vacation, however, you must provide the patient with one other treatment. What is the single most important treatment to be undertaken at this time?
   a. begin the patient taking an antiinflammatory medication
   b. begin the patient taking an oral corticosteroid
   c. begin the patient taking an antidepressant
   d. begin the patient taking an oral chemotherapeutic agent
   e. none of the above

6. Cancer pain is an extremely important medical problem. Which of the following statements regarding the management of cancer pain in the United States is true?
   a. cancer pain is extremely well managed by most American physicians

b. the overtreatment of cancer pain is much more of a problem than the undertreatment of cancer pain in the United States

c. the undertreatment of cancer pain is much more of a problem than the overtreatment of cancer pain in the United States

d. most Americans with cancer pain die in very good control; few have cancer pain that is not well controlled

e. none of the above statements are true

7. The patient returns to your office in 6 weeks following an overseas tour. Because of your therapy, he was able to enjoy most of his holiday. Three days ago, his pain began to become acutely worse. The patient now appears jaundiced. He has lost another 15 lb, and there is a palpable mass in the periumbilical region. The investigation performed earlier is repeated, and a mass measuring 6 cm × 5 cm now is seen in the appropriate region. At this time, what should you do?

a. explore with a surgeon the possibility of a Whipple's procedure

b. begin aggressive radiotherapy and chemotherapy

c. begin high-dose prednisone to increase his weight

d. explore with a surgeon the possibility of the total removal of the organ in question

e. none of the above

8. What is the most clearly established risk factor for the disease described?

a. alcohol consumption

b. cigarette smoking

c. high fat intake

d. environmental toxins

e. previous exposure to radiation

9. With respect to the molecular biology of this disease, which of the following statements is true?

a. no genetic mutations have been established for this disease

b. the CK-Ras gene mutates to become the CK-Ras oncogene in 25% of patients with this disease

c. the CK-Ras oncogene is present in 50% of patients with this disease

d. the CK-Ras oncogene is present in 75% of patients with this disease

e. the CK-Ras oncogene is present in 90% of patients with this disease

10. A patient with this disease will demonstrate which of the following physical findings?

a. decreased pain when assuming the supine position

b. increased pain when assuming the supine position

c. decreased pain with flexion of the spine

d. increase pain with flexion of the spine

e. b and c

f. a and d

◢ CLINICAL CASE MANAGEMENT PROBLEM

Discuss the impact of this disease on the American population under the following headings: (1) disease prevalence over the last 30 years (increase or decrease); (2) place as a killer of Americans (among all cancers); (3) risk factors; (4) symptoms and signs; (5) treatment; and (6) prognosis.

■ ANSWERS:

1. **d.** From the history and the physical examination, you determine that the patient has a serious disease. In forming a differential diagnosis, you should consider diagnostic possibilities in the following categories: (1) infectious/inflammatory; (2) neoplastic or not; (3) circulatory; or (4) traumatic.

From the history alone, the following are diagnostic possibilities:

A. Infectious/inflammatory: (1) inflammatory bowel disease, Crohn's disease, or ulcerative colitis; (2) pancreatitis; or (3) cholecystitis

B. Neoplastic: (1) carcinoma of the stomach (linitis plastica); (2) carcinoma of the head of the pancreas; or (3) carcinoma of the colon

C. Circulatory: (1) aortic aneurysm (leaking) or (2) mesenteric ischemia

D. Traumatic: pancreatic pseudocyst

2. **c.** Obviously, before you decide on which investigation to order, you have to make a commitment to your primary diagnosis. The most likely diagnosis is adenocarcinoma of the pancreas. The reasons are as follows: (1) the abdominal pain is constant and unrelated to food; (2) the patient has experienced a 20-lb weight loss; and (3) the patient is depressed.

Therefore the investigation of choice is a CT scan of the abdomen.

3. **c.** There is a significant correlation between carcinoma of the pancreas and depression. In many cases, as in this Clinical Case Problem, the depression actually precedes the abdominal pain.

4. d. The sensitivity of the CT scan in the diagnosis of adenocarcinoma of the pancreas is 95%—that is, only one out of every 20 patients with adenocarcinoma will have false-negative CT scan results.

5. e. Although it is reasonable to start the patient taking an antidepressant, it is the second most important treatment. The most important treatment is to start the patient on an adequate pain relief program. It would seem that, because of the severity of the pain, an oral narcotic analgesic would be the drug of first choice. You suggest that while he is on vacation he telephone on a regular basis so you can advise medication changes.

6. c. Cancer pain is an enormous medical problem in the United States and Canada. It is likely to become even more of a problem in the future because the population is aging. It is estimated that close to 50% of patients in North America with cancer die in moderately severe to severe pain. The reason appears to be multifactorial and related to inadequate education in medical school, in residency, and in continuing medical education; reluctance to use narcotic analgesics when they need to be used; and fear of licensure difficulties if "too many narcotics" are prescribed.

7. e. You should (1) break the news to the patient with his spouse or significant other be present, if possible; (2) discuss with the patient his treatment options, including palliative radiotherapy, palliative chemotherapy, and palliative radiotherapy and chemotherapy; (3) suggest an aggressive pain control program, consider a celiac plexus block, changing narcotic analgesics, and continuing to increase his dosage of narcotics; and (4) in terms of symptoms, maintain control of nausea or vomiting, maintain control of constipation, and consider an appetite stimulant (Megace).

8. b. The most likely established risk factor for adenocarcinoma of the pancreas is cigarette smoking. There is some controversy regarding alcohol intake, but most authorities consider it a significant risk factor as well.

9. e. There is insufficient evidence to suggest a particular genetic predisposition for adenocarcinoma of the pancreas. However, more than 90% of patients who develop adenocarcinoma of the pancreas have a mutation of the Ki-ras gene on chromosome 12. This is simply an example of the powerful influence of genetics on cancer and the explosion of new knowledge that eventually will result in more effective, more precise, and more targeted treatments for most or all cancers in the future.

10. e. One of the most important tests in the physical examination of a patient suspected of having a malignancy is known as a provocative maneuver. A provocative maneuver attempts to reproduce the pain (gently). An example of a provocative maneuver for somatic pain caused by bony metastatic disease is to put pressure on the bone in question. The provocative maneuver for a patient with a tumor that is retroperitoneal is to have the patient lie flat or lie with a pillow or other object underneath the small of his or her back. This will reproduce the pain. The same patient will obtain relief from their pain when leaning forward.

SOLUTION TO THE CLINICAL CASE MANAGEMENT PROBLEM

Adenocarcinoma of the pancreas:
1. Prevalence over last 30 years: The prevalence of adenocarcinoma of the pancreas among Americans has been increasing rapidly. Until recently, the incidence of the disease was increasing in the United States at an annual rate of 15%. It now appears to have leveled off.
2. Mortality from adenocarcinoma: Approximately 28,000 new cases of adenocarcinoma of the pancreas occur each year. After squamous cell carcinoma of the lung and adenocarcinoma of the colon, adenocarcinoma of the pancreas is the third leading cause of death caused by cancer in men between the ages of 35 and 54 years old.
3. Risk factors for adenocarcinoma of the pancreas: Some 10% of the cases have a strong familial relationship, and cigarette smoking in all cases clearly remains the number one risk factor. Other implicated factors include history of gastrectomy (more than 20 years ago); alcohol intake; African American or white race; high consumption of meat and fat; and presence of diabetes mellitus, although recent work has

Continued

SOLUTION TO THE CLINICAL CASE MANAGEMENT PROBLEM—cont'd

disputed the latter two. Obviously more controlled studies are required.

High intake of fruits and vegetables appears to have a protective effect.

4. Symptoms and signs:
   a. Abdominal symptoms and signs: (i) central abdominal pain radiating through to the back; dull, aching and steady in character; most commonly described as a "deep" pain; (ii) weight loss; (iii) hepatomegaly (50% of patients); (iv) palpable abdominal mass (indicates inoperability); (v) a palpable nontender gallbladder in a jaundiced patient suggests neoplastic obstruction of the common bile duct (Courvoisier's law).
   b. Nonabdominal symptoms and signs: depression as a result of the patient's general medical condition (*Diagnostic and Statistical Manual*, 4th edition) is often the initial symptom appearing before any of the abdominal symptoms or painless jaundice.

5. Treatments:
   a. Surgical: Carcinoma of the pancreas is resectable in only 20% of patients (Whipple's procedure).
   b. Chemotherapy/radiotherapy: Palliative chemotherapy or radiotherapy can be offered; at this time there a several clinical trials having some promise of reducing mortality.
   c. Pain control: Pain control appears to be the single most important part of therapy (celiac plexus block and/or narcotic analgesics).
   d. Symptom control: control nausea and vomiting with combination antiemetics, and control constipation with lactulose or stool softener and a peristaltic stimulant.

6. Prognosis: The prognosis for adenocarcinoma of the pancreas is dismal. A 5-year survival rate is approximately 5%. However, encouraging early results have been obtained with the use of gemcitabine and other adjuvant, x-ray, and molecular biologic therapies.

SUMMARY OF PANCREATIC CARCINOMA

See the Solution to the Clinical Case Management Problem.

SUGGESTED READING

Abrams RA: Adjuvant therapy for pancreatic adenocarcinoma: what have we learned since 1985? *Int J Rad Oncol Biol Phys* 56 (supplement 4):3-9, 2003.

Bornman PC, Beckingham IJ: ABC of diseases of liver, pancreas, and biliary system. Pancreatic tumours. *BMJ* 322(7288):721-723, 2001.

Michaud DS, et al: Dietary meat, diary products, fat and cholesterol and pancreatic cancer risk in a prospective study. *Am J Epidemiol* 157(12):1115-1125, 2003.

Rocha Lima CM, Centeno B: Update on pancreatic cancer. *Curr Opin Oncol* 14(4):424-430, 2002 Jul.

Rulyak SL, et al: Risk factors for the development of pancreatic cancer in familial pancreatic cancer kindreds. *Gastroenterology* 124(5): 1292-1299, 2003.

Chapter 124

Colorectal Cancer and Other Colonic Disorders

"Doctor, the idea of that snakelike instrument stuck up my rear is disgusting."

CLINICAL CASE PROBLEM 1:

A 48-Year-Old Male with Weakness, Fatigue, and Lower Right-Sided Abdominal Fullness

A 48-year-old male comes to your office with a vague lower right-sided abdominal fullness (not pain). He describes to you a general feeling of "not feeling well," fatigue, and a somewhat tender area "down near my appendix." He states, "I have no energy. I'm tired all the time." He also suspects that his skin changed color, first to a pale color and then to a slightly yellow color.

On direct questioning he admits to anorexia, weight loss of 30 lb in 6 months, nausea most of the time, vomiting twice, some diarrhea that seems to be mucus, and blood in the stool almost every day for the past 3 months. When you ask him what he makes of all this he tells you, "Maybe a very bad flu."

On examination, the patient looks very pale. Examination of the abdomen reveals abdominal distention. You record the abdominal girth as a baseline. There is a sensation of "fullness" in the right lower quadrant of the abdomen. This area also is dull to percussion and is slightly tender. There is definite percussion of tympany on both sides of the area of dullness. The liver span is approximately 20 cm. The sclerae are yellow.

SELECT THE BEST ANSWER TO THE FOLLOWING QUESTIONS:

1. At this time, what would you do?
   a. tell the patient to relax and recheck with your office in 6 months
   b. diagnose the irritable bowel syndrome and start the patient on dietary therapy
   c. tell that patient that he probably is going through a viral illness; relax and come back in 2 months if the symptoms have not improved
   d. order a complete workup on the patient—the good old shotgun approach (every test known to man and then some)
   e. none of the above

2. What is the definitive diagnostic procedure of choice in this patient?
   a. complete blood count (CBC)
   b. fecal occult blood samples
   c. air-contrast barium enema
   d. colonoscopy
   e. three views of the abdomen

3. What is the most likely diagnosis in this patient?
   a. irritable bowel syndrome
   b. lactose intolerance
   c. adenocarcinoma of the pancreas
   d. adenocarcinoma of the colon
   e. ruptured appendix

4. Having made a correct diagnosis from Question 3, what is the definitive treatment of choice?
   a. colonic segmental resection
   b. total colectomy
   c. removal of the appendix
   d. abdominoperineal resection of the rectum
   e. neodymium:yttrium-aluminum garnet (Nd:YAG) laser photocoagulation of the identified lesion

5. Carcinoma of the colon most commonly originates in which of the following?
   a. an adenomatous polyp
   b. an inflammatory polyp
   c. a hyperplastic polyp
   d. a benign lymphoid polyp
   e. a leiomyoma

6. Adenomatous polyps are found in approximately what percentage of asymptomatic patients who undergo screening?
   a. 5%
   b. 10%
   c. 15%
   d. 20%
   e. 25%

7. A barium enema is performed on a patient with a suspected carcinoma of the descending colon following an unsuccessful colonoscopy. What is the best radiologic description that fits the probable diagnosis in this patient?
   a. a "strawberry cutout" lesion
   b. an "orange dimpled" lesion
   c. an "apple core" lesion
   d. a "cabbage fulgurating" lesion
   e. a "banana peel" lesion

8. Colorectal polyps are thought to be the origin of most colorectal cancers. Which of the following statements regarding colorectal polyps is false?
   a. the larger the colorectal polyps, the greater the chance of malignancy
   b. hyperplastic polyps have the highest malignant potential of all colorectal polyps
   c. adenomatous polyps increase in incidence with each decade after the age of 30 years
   d. routine removal of adenomas from the colon reduces the incidence of subsequent adenocarcinoma
   e. villous adenomas carry the highest malignant potential of all adenomas

9. Which of the following statements best describes the current evidence for fecal occult blood screening as a measure to reduce the morbidity and mortality from colorectal cancer?
   a. there is excellent evidence to include fecal occult blood testing in screening asymptomatic patients older than age 50 years for colorectal carcinoma
   b. there is fair evidence to include fecal occult blood testing in screening asymptomatic patients older than age 50 years for colorectal carcinoma
   c. there is insufficient evidence to include or exclude fecal occult blood testing as an effective screening test for colorectal cancer in asymptomatic patients older than age 50 years
   d. none of the above

10. Which of the following statements regarding carcinoembryonic antigen (CEA) and colorectal cancer is true?
    a. CEA is a cost-effective screening test for colorectal cancer
    b. elevated preoperative CEA levels correlate well with postoperative recurrence rate in colorectal cancer
    c. CEA is a sensitive test for colorectal cancer
    d. CEA is a specific test for colorectal cancer
    e. CEA has no value in predicting recurrence in colorectal cancer

CLINICAL CASE PROBLEM 2:
A 78-Year-Old Male with Acute and Severe Abdominal Pain

A 78-year-old male comes to your office with acute and severe abdominal pain, left lower-quadrant tenderness, a left lower-quadrant mass, and a temperature of 39° C. The patient has had no significant illnesses in the past. He is very healthy. He sees his physician once a year and has had a normal heart, normal blood pressure, and normal "everything else," as he says, for many years.

On examination, the patient's temperature is 39.5° C. His pulse is 96 and regular. His blood pressure is 210/105 mm Hg. There is significant tenderness in the left lower quadrant. Rebound tenderness is not present. There is a definite sensation of a mass present.

11. What is the most likely diagnosis in this patient?
    a. adenocarcinoma of the colon
    b. diverticulitis
    c. diverticulosis
    d. colorectal carcinoma
    e. atypical appendicitis

12. What is the treatment of choice for the patient described in Clinical Case Problem 2?
    a. primary resection of the diseased segment with anastomosis
    b. primary resection of the diseased segment without anastomosis
    c. colectomy
    d. abdominal perineal resection
    e. none of the above

13. Which of the following is (are) a component(s) of the acute treatment of this patient's condition?
    a. intravenous (IV) fluids
    b. IV (broad-spectrum) antibiotics
    c. nasogastric (NG) suction, if abdominal distention or vomiting are present
    d. all of the above
    e. a and c only

14. Which of the following investigations is contraindicated at this time in the patient described in Clinical Case Problem 2?
    a. computed tomography (CT) scan of the abdomen and pelvis
    b. magnetic resonance imaging scan of the abdomen and pelvis
    c. three views of the abdomen
    d. air-contrast barium enema
    e. none of the above are contraindicated

15. Which of the following statements regarding this patient's blood pressure elevation is true?

    a. this patient most likely has essential hypertension
    b. this patient's abdominal pain is most likely related to his hypertension
    c. this elevation of blood pressure could be caused by the pain he is experiencing
    d. this patient's physician (the one he has been seeing every year) obviously has made a very serious mistake in labeling this patient as normotensive
    e. none of the above statements are true

16. What is the analgesic of choice for control of pain in this patient?
    a. morphine
    b. hydromorphone
    c. methadone
    d. pentazocine
    e. codeine

17. Which of the following organism(s) is (are) the most likely cause(s) of the condition described?
    a. *Escherichia coli*
    b. *Bacteroides fragilis*
    c. *Streptococcus pneumoniae*
    d. a and b only
    e. all of the above

CLINICAL CASE PROBLEM 3:
A 35-Year-Old Male with Rectal Bleeding and Mucoid Discharge from the Rectum

A 35-year-old male comes to your office with rectal bleeding, mucoid discharge from the rectum, and protrusion of certain structures through the anal canal. On proctoscopic examination, large internal hemorrhoids are seen.

18. What is the best next step in the management of this patient?
    a. proceed with definitive treatment
    b. proceed with further investigations
    c. prescribe a hemorrhoidal cream
    d. do nothing; ask the patient to return in 6 months for review
    e. none of the above

19. What is the treatment of choice for the patient described in Clinical Case Problem 3?
    a. a hemorrhoidal cream
    b. a hemorrhoidal ointment
    c. hemorrhoidectomy
    d. injection of phenol into the hemorrhoidal tissue
    e. rubber band ligation of the internal hemorrhoids

20. Which of the following statements regarding angiodysplasia is (are) true?

a. angiodysplasia is an acquired condition most often affecting individuals older than age 60 years

b. angiodysplasia is a focal submucosal vascular ectasis that has the propensity to bleed profusely

c. most angiodysplastic lesions are located in the cecum and proximal ascending colon

d. multiple lesions occur in 25% of cases

e. all of the above statements are true

CLINICAL CASE MANAGEMENT PROBLEM

In the fourth edition of this book it was possible to write: "Regarding colorectal cancer, there appears to be almost universal support for the following: (1) decreasing the amount of fat in the diet, especially saturated fat (this also will lead to decreased body mass index or total body weight); (2) increasing the amount of fiber in the diet; (3) increasing the intake of cruciferous vegetables and fiber; (4) decreasing alcohol intake; and (5) decreasing the intake of salted, smoked, and nitrate-based foods." In which way has this belief been altered in the new millennium by evidence-based randomized clinical trials?

ANSWERS:

1. e. None of the answers are appropriate or sufficiently focused.

2. d. The colonoscopy will allow for a tissue biopsy and diagnosis as well.

3. d. In this patient the problem list at this point is as follows: (1) a middle-aged male with nonspecific feelings of "ill health"; (2) there is a right lower-quadrant mass on physical examination, raising the question of carcinoma; (3) the liver is enlarged, possibly indicating metastases; (4) the pale appearance suggests anemia; (5) icterus suggests elevated conjugated hyperbilirubinemia; and (6) the clinically apparent abdominal distention indicates possible ascites.

With this constellation of symptoms and signs, the working diagnosis is adenocarcinoma of the cecum with liver metastases.

The investigations that must be performed at this time include the following:

1. Laboratory: (a) CBC; (b) serum bilirubin; (c) liver enzymes (aspartate aminotransferase, alanine aminotransferase, and γ-glucuronosyltransferase); (d) alkaline phosphatase; (e) serum calcium; (f) serum electrolytes; and (g) carcinoembryonic antigen (CEA).

2. Radiology: (a) chest x-ray; (b) three views of the abdomen; and (c) abdominal ultrasound

3. The diagnostic procedure of choice in this patient is a total colonoscopy to confirm a mass lesion, to determine the location of that lesion, and to obtain a biopsy of the lesion if possible.

4. For colon carcinoma the essentials of diagnosis are as follows:

a. Right colon: (i) an unexplained weakness or anemia; (ii) occult blood in the feces and diarrhea with mucus; (iii) dyspeptic symptoms; (iv) persistent right abdominal discomfort; (v) palpable abdominal mass; (vi) characteristic x-ray findings; and (vii) characteristic colonoscopic findings.

b. Left colon: (i) change in bowel habits with thin stools; (ii) gross blood in the stool; (iii) obstructive symptoms; (iv) characteristic x-ray findings; and (v) characteristic colonoscopic or sigmoidoscopic findings

c. Rectum: (i) rectal bleeding; (ii) alteration in bowel habits; (iii) sensation of incomplete evacuation; (iv) intrarectal palpable tumor; and (v) sigmoidoscopic findings

4. a. The definitive surgical treatment of choice in this patient (if feasible) is colonic resection. The preliminary location of the lesion based on physical examination is in the area of the cecum. If this proves to be correct, the colonic resection will involve the removal of the area from the vermiform appendix to the junction of the ascending and transverse colons. With the presence of liver metastasis, this procedure is palliative.

5. a. The vast majority of colonic adenocarcinomas evolve from adenomas. Adenomas are a premalignant lesion, and in the large bowel the sequence is adenoma, dysplasia in the adenomas, and adenocarcinoma.

6. e. Both adenomas and the subsequent evolved adenocarcinomas increase in incidence with age, and the distribution of adenomas and cancer in the bowel is similar. Overall, adenomatous polyps are found in approximately 25% of asymptomatic patients who undergo screening colonoscopy. The age-related prevalence of adenomatous polyps is 30% at age 50 years, 40% at age 60 years, 50% at age 70 years, and 55% at age 80 years. The mean age of patients with adenomas is 55 years, which is approximately 5-10 years earlier than the mean age for patients with adenocarcinoma of the colon. Approximately 50% of polyps occur in the sigmoid colon or in the rectum and thus can be revealed by sigmoidoscopy. About 50% of patients with adenomas have more than one adenoma, and 15% have more than two adenomas. There is an interesting correlation between patients with breast cancer and adenomatous polyps in the colon and rectum. Those patients with breast cancer have an increased risk of adenomatous polyps. Studies suggest that taken beta-carotene supplements, as in lung cancer, increased the risk of cancer in smokers and in individuals consuming one or more drinks of alcohol per day. Conversely, calcium supplements and vitamin supplements have been reported to decrease the risk.

The malignant potential of the adenoma depends on the growth pattern, the size of the polyp, and the degree of atypia or dysplasia. Adenocarcinoma of the colon is found in approximately 1% of adenomas less than 1.0 cm in diameter, in approximately 10% of adenomas between 1.0 cm and 2.0 cm in diameter, and in approximately 45% of adenomas with a diameter greater than 2.0 cm.

The potential for cancerous transformations increases with increasing degrees of dysplasia.

Sessile lesions are more apt to be malignant than pedunculated ones. The time it takes an adenoma to proceed through the process to frank adenocarcinoma is between 10 and 15 years.

The following is a summary of the types of adenomas and their malignant potential: (1) villous adenoma, 40% become malignant; (2) tubulovillous adenoma, 22% become malignant; and (3) tubular adenoma, 5% become malignant.

7. c. This patient most likely suffers from a constricting carcinoma of the descending colon. A barium enema (preferably an air-contrast barium enema) of a constricting carcinoma of the descending colon presents what is best described as an "apple core" lesion. On the barium enema you will note the loss of mucosal patterns, the "hooks" at the margins of the lesion, the relatively short length of the lesion, and the abrupt ending of the lesion.

8. b. Hyperplastic polyps are polyps that are designated as "unclassified" but are totally benign. The highest malignant potential is carried by villous adenomas.

9. a. The current United States Preventive Services Task Force (USPSTF) recommendation for screening colorectal cancer is for all people aged 50 or older to be screened at least by annual fecal occult blood testing. Screening reduces mortality (USPSTF level 3ai). Colonoscopy provides an alternative method that will find abnormalities throughout the track and allows removal of polyps at the same time; however, the major complication rate of 1 in 1000 procedures makes some patients afraid of the process. Flexible sigmoidoscopy also provides a clear picture but only of the distal third of the colon. So-called virtual colonoscopy done via a CT scan at this time cannot replace colonoscopy.

10. b. CEA is a glycoprotein found in the cell membranes of a number of tissues, a number of body fluids, and a number of secretions including urine and feces. It also is found in malignancies of the colon and rectum. Because some of the CEA antigen enters the bloodstream, it can be detected by the use of a radioimmunoassay technique of serum.

Elevated CEA is not specifically associated with colorectal cancer; abnormally high levels of CEA also are found in patients with other gastrointestinal (GI) malignancies and non-GI malignancies. CEA levels are elevated in 70% of patients with an adenocarcinoma of the large bowel, but less than 50% of patients with localized disease are CEA-positive. Thus because of these difficulties with sensitivity and specificity, CEA does not serve as a useful screening procedure, nor is it an accurate diagnostic test for colorectal cancer at a curable stage. However, elevated preoperative CEA levels correlate with postoperative recurrence rate, and failure of CEA to fall to normal levels after resection implies a poor prognosis. CEA is helpful in detecting recurrence after curative surgical resection; if high CEA levels return to normal after operation and then increase progressively during the follow-up period, recurrence of cancer is likely.

11. b. This patient has diverticulitis, an infection and inflammation of one or more diverticula that, in its noninflammatory state, is known as *diverticulosis*. In the United States and Canada approximately 50% of patients have diverticula, 10% by age 40 and 65% by age 80. The prevalence of diverticula varies tremendously around the world.

Cultural factors, especially diet, play an important causative role. Among dietary factors, the most important one is the fiber content of ingested food.

The essentials of diagnosis of diverticulitis are as follows: (1) acute abdominal pain (usually left lower); (2) left lower-quadrant tenderness with or without a mass in the same area; and (3) fever with leukocytosis.

The imaging findings are as follows:
1. Plain films: if inflammation is localized: ileus, partial colonic obstruction, small bowel obstruction, or left lower-quadrant mass
2. CT scans: no perforation: effacement of pericolic fat with or without abscess or fistulas
3. Barium enema: contraindicated during an acute attack of diverticulitis; the risk of perforation and barium escape into the peritoneal cavity is high

12. e. The treatment of choice for diverticulitis is expectant unless surgical treatment is necessary because of rupture and subsequent peritonitis or multiple recurrences.

The natural history of diverticulitis follows: (1) 10% to 20% of patients with diverticulosis develop diverticulitis; (2) approximately 75% of complications of diverticular disease develop in patients with no prior colonic symptoms; and (3) approximately 25% of patients hospitalized with acute diverticulitis require surgical treatment. In the past decades the operative mortality of primary resection has dropped from 25% to less than 5%.

13. d. Treatment includes (1) nothing by mouth; (2) IV fluids with potassium; (3) NG suction if abdominal distension or vomiting is present; and (4) IV antibiotics.

14. d. See Answer 11.

15. c. The elevation of blood pressure in this patient is almost certainly directly associated with the pain that he is experiencing. Acute and chronic pain (but especially acute pain) increases the release of the "pressor hormones" such as norepinephrine. This produces vasoconstriction that ultimately results in elevated blood pressure. The patient thus experiences a vicious pain cycle that is circular in dimension: more pain, pressor hormone release, elevated blood pressure, increase in pressor hormone release, more pain, and so on.

16. a. Morphine will readily relieve the pain, decrease anxiety, and lower the elevated blood pressure.

17. d. The most common organisms involved in the development of diverticulitis are *E. coli* and *B. fragilis*.

18. a. The next step in the management of this patient is to proceed with definitive treatment.

19. e. This patient has internal hemorrhoids. The treatment of choice for the protruding internal hemorrhoids that this patient has is rubber band ligation. Rubber band ligation is especially useful in situations in which the hemorrhoids are enlarged or prolapsing.

To accomplish this procedure, the anoscope is used and the redundant mucosa above the hemorrhoid is grasped with forceps and advanced through the barrel of a special ligator. The rubber band then is placed snugly around the mucosa and the hemorrhoidal plexus. Ischemic necrosis occurs over several days, with eventual slough, fibrosis, and fixation of the tissues. One hemorrhoidal complex at a time is treated, with repeat ligations done at 2- and 4-week intervals as needed.

The major, but uncommon, complication of this procedure is pain severe enough to require removal of the band. To avoid this, the band must be placed high and well above the junction of the mucocutaneous region (dentate line). In this location the innervation is autonomic, not somatic. If pain begins and does not resolve, infection should be suspected and investigated immediately. At the time the dead tissue falls off, there may be significant bleeding; the patient should be aware of this.

20. e. Angiodysplasia is an acquired colonic condition that mainly affects elderly individuals. Pathophysiologically, angiodysplasia can be described as a focal submucosal vascular ectasis that has a high probability of producing significant bleeding. The vast majority of angiodysplastic lesions occur in the cecum and in the proximal ascending colon. In at least 25% of patients, multiple lesions are present.

The primary symptom is bright red rectal bleeding that can be extensive and that may require transfusion.

Diagnosis is made by colonoscopy. The diagnosis is made when two of the following three features are present: (1) an early-filling vein (within 4-5 seconds after injection); (2) a vascular tuft; and (3) a delayed-emptying vein.

If searched for carefully, as many as 25% of individuals older than age 60 have angiodysplasia. In many cases expectant management or colonoscopic cauterization is all that is needed. If surgery is required, the operative procedure of choice appears to be hemicolectomy.

SOLUTION TO THE CLINICAL CASE MANAGEMENT PROBLEM

Evidence-based, randomized clinical studies summarized in the two *New England Journal of Medicine* citations posted in "Suggested Reading" found no evidence that consumption of fat, fiber, or vegetables decreased the reoccurrence of colorectal cancer. However, other well-controlled studies still support fat as a risk factor (level 3aii).

Possible effects of alcohol and smoked foods are yet to be investigated.

SUMMARY OF COLORECTAL CANCER AND OTHER COLONIC DISORDERS

A. Colorectal cancer:

1. Incidence: In North America cancer of the colon and rectum ranks second after cancer of the lung in incidence and death rates. In the United States the number of new cases decreased by 1.8% per year between 1985 and 1995 but has stabilized since; the mortality, however, has continued to decrease. About 6% of Americans will develop colorectal cancer in their lifetime, and the 5-year survival rate is 62.1%.
2. Age and sex:
   a. Age: The incidence of carcinoma of the colon increases with age, starting slowly at age 40 and then doubling for each decade thereafter.
   b. Sex: Carcinoma of the colon, particularly the right colon, is more common in women, and carcinoma of the rectum is more common in men.
3. Genetic predisposition: Genetic predisposition to cancer of the large bowel is well-recognized. Relatively rare cases are inherited in a Mendelian fashion, namely: familial adenomatous polyposis and hereditary nonpolyposis colorectal cancer. However, a familial tendency also exists among the general population; by the age of 79 years a person with no affected relative has a 4% chance of developing colorectal cancer. With one first-degree relative, there is a 9% chance; with more than one first-degree relative, there is a 16% chance; and with a first-degree relative who developed cancer before the age of 45 years, there is a 15% chance.
4. Risk factors for carcinoma of the colon include the following: (a) ulcerative colitis; (b) Crohn's disease; (c) exposure to radiation; (d) colorectal polyps; (e) cigarette smoking; and high-fat diets.
5. Essentials of diagnosis: See Answer 3.
6. Distribution of cancer of the colon and rectum include the following: (a) rectum, 30% of all colorectal cancers; (b) sigmoid, 20% of all colorectal cancers; (c) descending colon, 15% of all colorectal cancers; (d) transverse colon, 10% of all colorectal cancers; and (e) ascending colon, 25% of all colorectal cancers.
7. Pathophysiology: The vast majority of colorectal cancers originate in colonic polyps. Tubular adenomas (tubulovillous adenoma) and villous adenomas are both premalignant.
8. Treatment of colorectal cancer:
   a. Basic treatment for cancer of the colon consists of wide surgical resection of the lesion and its regional lymphatic drainage after preparation of the bowel.
   b. Basic treatment for cancer of the rectum consists of abdominoperineal resection of the rectum or a low anterior resection of the rectum.
   c. Adjuvant therapy includes radiotherapy and combination chemotherapy.

B. Polyps of the colon and rectum:

1. Prevalence: Adenomatous polyps are found in approximately 25% of asymptomatic adults who undergo screening colonoscopy. The prevalence of adenomatous polyps is 30% at age 50 years, 40% at age 60 years, 50% at age 70 years, and 55% at age 80 years.
2. Malignant potential: Adenomas are a premalignant lesion, and most authorities believe that the majority of adenocarcinomas of the large bowel evolve from adenomas (adenoma-to-carcinoma sequence). The mean age of patients with polyps is 5-10 years younger than the mean age of patients with colorectal cancer.
3. Benign polyps include hematomas, inflammatory polyps, and hyperplastic polyps.
4. Essentials of diagnosis: The essentials of diagnosis of polyps of the colon and rectum include the passage of blood per rectum and sigmoidoscopic, colonoscopic, or radiologic discovery of polyps.
5. Treatment: Adenomatous polyps should be removed by methods that include electrocautery, Nd:YAG laser therapy, and laparotomy if removal through the colonoscope is unsuccessful.
6. Prevention: Eating a high-fiber diet will help prevent colonic disease.

C. Diverticulosis and diverticulitis:

1. Prevalence: Approximately 50% of individuals in the United States develop diverticula. Diverticular disease is much more common in the United States than in Japan or other Eastern countries.
2. Symptomatic versus asymptomatic: Diverticulosis probably remains asymptomatic in 80% of individuals.
3. Essentials of diagnosis of diverticulitis are as follows: (a) acute abdominal pain; (b) left lower-quadrant tenderness with or without a mass; (c) fever and leukocytosis; and (d) characteristic radiologic signs showing diverticula.

4. Treatment:
   a. Conservative: Some patients can be treated at home with oral antibiotics and analgesics.
   b. In-hospital treatment consists of NPO; insertion of an NG tube; and administration of IV fluids, antibiotics, and pentazocine for analgesia.
   c. Surgical: Surgical treatment is necessary when there is a diverticula rupture or when abscess and peritonitis ensue. Approximately 25% of hospitalized patients need surgery.
5. The "DO NOT" of diverticulitis: DO NOT do a barium enema in the acute phase (potential rupture and peritonitis).
6. Organisms associated with diverticulitis include (a) *E. coli* and (b) *B. fragilis*.
7. Prevention: Eating a high-fiber diet will help prevent colonic disease.

D. Other conditions of note:
   a. Internal hemorrhoids with prolapse: Treatment consists of rubber band ligation.
   b. Angiodysplasia: Consider angiodysplasia as another cause of rectal bleeding in elderly patients.

SUGGESTED READING

Alberts DS, et al: Lack of effect of a high fiber cereal supplement on the reoccurrence of colorectal adenomas. *N Engl J Med* 342:1156-1162, 2000.

Hobbs FD: ABC of colorectal cancer: the role of primary care. *BMJ* 321(7268):1068-1070, 2000.

McArdle C: ABC of colorectal cancer: effectiveness of follow up. *BMJ* 321(7272):1332-1335, 2000.

Pignone M, et al: Screening for colorectal cancer in adults at average risk: a summary of the evidence for the U.S. Preventive Services Task Force. *Ann Intern Med* 137(2):132-141, 2002.

Pignone M, et al: Cost-effectiveness analyses of colorectal cancer screening: a systematic review for the U.S. Preventive Services Task Force. *Ann Intern Med* 137(2):96-104, 2002 Jul 16.

Schatzkin A, et al: Lack of effect of a low-fat, high fiber diet on the reoccurrence of colorectal adenomas. *N Engl J Med* 342:1149-1155, 2000.

Walsh JM, Terdiman JP: Colorectal cancer screening: scientific review. *JAMA* 289(10):1288-1296, 2003.

Chapter 125

Breast Disease

"A lump! Does that mean mastectomy?"

CLINICAL CASE PROBLEM 1:
A 41-Year-Old Female with a Painless Breast Lump

A 41-year-old female comes to your office after finding a breast lump during a routine self-examination. She has been examining her breasts regularly for the past 5 years; this is the first lump she has found.

On examination, there is a lump located in the right breast. The lump's anatomic location is in the upper outer quadrant. It is approximately 3 cm in diameter and is not fixed to skin or muscle. It has a hard consistency. There are three axillary nodes present on the right side; each node is approximately 1 cm in diameter. No lymph nodes are present on the left.

■ SELECT THE BEST ANSWER TO THE FOLLOWING QUESTIONS:

1. At this time, what would you do?
   a. tell the patient that she has fibrocystic breast disease; ask her to return in 1 month, preferably 10 days after the next period, for a recheck
   b. tell the patient to see her lawyer and update her will; death is imminent
   c. tell the patient to go home and relax; we generally get too worked up about breast lumps
   d. order an ultrasound of the area
   e. none of the above

2. What is the first diagnostic procedure that should be performed in this patient?
   a. ultrasound of the breast
   b. mammography
   c. fine-needle biopsy
   d. all of the above
   e. none of the above

3. What is the definitive procedure that should be performed in this patient?
   a. ultrasound of the breast
   b. mammography
   c. biopsy
   d. all of the above
   e. none of the above

CLINICAL CASE PROBLEM 2:
A 49-YEAR-OLD FEMALE WITH A SUSPICIOUS LESION DISCOVERED ON MAMMOGRAPHY

A mammographic examination uncovered a very suspicious lesion in the right breast of a 49-year-old female. Clinically, the lesion is a 3-cm mass present in the left upper outer quadrant. No axillary lymph nodes are palpable. You refer her to a surgeon who books her for a surgical procedure.

4. What surgical procedure should be used for Clinical Case Problem 2?
   a. a lumpectomy
   b. a modified radical mastectomy
   c. a lumpectomy plus axillary lymph-node dissection
   d. modified radical mastectomy plus axillary lymph-node dissection
   e. none of the above

5. The risk factors for carcinoma of the breast include which of the following?
   a. a first-degree relative with breast cancer
   b. nulliparity
   c. birth of a first child after age 35
   d. early menarche
   e. all of the above

6. Current estimates suggest that one out of every how many women eventually will develop breast cancer?
   a. 1 out of 8
   b. 1 out of 15
   c. 1 out of 25
   d. 1 out of 50
   e. 1 out of 100

7. The U.S. Preventive Services Task Force on the Periodic Health Examination recommends which of the following as the preferred mammographic screening protocol for breast cancer in women?
   a. screen all women older than age 40 years every year
   b. screen all women older than age 40 years every 2 years
   c. screen all women older than age 50 years every 1-2 years
   d. screen all women older than age 40 years every 1 or 2 years
   e. screen all women between the ages of 35 and 40 years with a baseline mammogram and screen all women older than age 40 years every 1-2 years

8. Which of the following statements regarding breast-conserving surgery or lumpectomy is correct?
   a. lumpectomy and breast irradiation are just as effective as modified radical mastectomy for patients with stage I or stage II disease
   b. lumpectomy has not undergone enough testing to predict its efficacy relative to modified radical mastectomy
   c. most American surgeons are following the National Institutes of Health (NIH) recommendations concerning lumpectomy
   d. modified radical mastectomy remains the treatment of choice for most women with breast cancer
   e. nobody really knows for sure

9. What is the most common histologic type of breast cancer?
   a. infiltrating ductal carcinoma
   b. medullary carcinoma
   c. invasive lobular carcinoma
   d. noninvasive intraductal carcinoma
   e. papillary ductal carcinoma

Questions 10 to 16 consist of seven brief case histories describing seven patients with seven different combinations of breast cancer, estrogen-receptor status, and axillary lymph nodes. Match the numbered Clinical Case Problem history to the preferred treatment option. Each preferred treatment option may be used once, more than once, or not at all.

   a. tamoxifen
   b. adjuvant combination chemotherapy
   c. neither tamoxifen nor combination chemotherapy

10. A 37-year-old premenopausal woman with an estrogen receptor-positive breast cancer and positive axillary lymph nodes

11. A 34-year-old premenopausal women with an estrogen receptor-positive breast cancer with negative axillary lymph nodes

12. A 42-year-old premenopausal woman with a 1.5-cm estrogen receptor-negative breast cancer with negative axillary lymph nodes

13. A 61-year-old postmenopausal woman with a 3-cm estrogen receptor-positive breast cancer with positive axillary lymph nodes

14. A 63-year-old postmenopausal woman with a 2-cm estrogen receptor-negative breast cancer with positive axillary lymph nodes

15. A 58-year-old postmenopausal woman with a 2-cm estrogen receptor-positive breast cancer and negative axillary lymph nodes

16. A 72-year-old postmenopausal woman with a 3-cm estrogen receptor-negative breast cancer with negative axillary lymph nodes

CLINICAL CASE PROBLEM 3:

A 42-Year-Old Female with Painful Bilateral Breast Masses that Wax and Wane with Her Period

A 42-year-old female comes to your office with bilateral breast masses that are painful and seem to "come and go" depending on the stage of the menstrual cycle. There is significant pain with these masses during menstruation.

On examination, there are two areas of dense tissue, one in each breast, and each is approximately 4 cm in diameter. No axillary lymph nodes are palpable.

17. What is the most likely diagnosis in this patient?
    a. carcinoma of the breast
    b. mammary dysplasia (fibrocystic disease)
    c. fibroadenoma
    d. Paget's disease of the breast
    e. none of the above

18. If medical treatment is indicated and prescribed for the condition described in Clinical Case Problem 3, which of the following should be considered as the therapeutic agent of first choice?
    a. hormone therapy: the oral contraceptive pill
    b. hormone therapy: danazol
    c. a thiazide diuretic
    d. vitamin E
    e. none of the above

CLINICAL CASE PROBLEM 4:

A 23-Year-Old Female with a Firm but Mobile Mass

A 23-year-old female consults her physician because of a breast mass; the mass is mobile, firm, and approximately 1 cm in diameter. It is located in the upper outer quadrant of the right breast. No axillary lymph nodes are present.

19. What is the most likely diagnosis in this patient?
    a. carcinoma of the breast
    b. mammary dysplasia (fibrocystic disease)
    c. fibroadenoma
    d. Paget's disease of the breast
    e. none of the above

20. What is the treatment of choice for the condition described in Clinical Case Problem 4?
    a. modified radical mastectomy
    b. lumpectomy
    c. biopsy
    d. radical mastectomy
    e. watchful waiting

CLINICAL CASE PROBLEM 5:

A 33-Year-Old Female with a Small Lump and a Bloody Nipple Discharge

A 33-year-old female comes to your office with a 2-month history of a bloody unilateral left nipple discharge. She also has noted a small and soft lump just beneath the areola on the left side.

On examination, there is a 4-mm soft mass located just inferior to the left areola. No other abnormalities are present in either breast.

21. What is the most likely diagnosis in this patient?
    a. carcinoma of the breast
    b. fibroadenoma
    c. intraductal papilloma
    d. fibrocystic breast disease
    e. none of the above

CLINICAL CASE MANAGEMENT PROBLEM

Discuss follow-up care modalities that should be provided by the primary care physician.

ANSWERS:

1. **e.** The most likely diagnosis in this patient is carcinoma of the breast. Therefore delay is not appropriate. However, even if that were the diagnosis, it is not a death sentence. The most common presenting symptom in breast cancer is a painless lump. Although the cause of such benign lumps is generally unknown, diabetes mellitus can induce them in a condition known as diabetic mastopathy, which most commonly occurs in women who are premenopausal and have type 1 diabetes. However, diabetic mastopathy also occurs in men and type 2 diabetics.

Other symptoms that may occur in patients with breast cancer (usually at a more advanced stage) are breast pain, nipple discharge, erosions, retraction, enlargement or itching of the nipple, redness, generalized hardness of the breast, and enlargement or shrinking of the breast.

2. b. On the basis of the symptoms described, the next diagnostic procedure that should be performed in this patient is a mammogram possibly followed by an ultrasound (particularly for women younger than 35 years of age). Such imaging studies will more clearly outline the characteristics of the mass, permitting biopsy, which always must follow, using either open or fine needle. Use of the latter has improved greatly, and presently has a very low level of false-negative diagnoses.

3. c. Biopsy, by either open or needle aspiration, is the surgical procedure of choice in this patient.

4. e. The important choice of the type of surgery and the local and regional treatment needs to be made if this is a breast cancer. This is often a difficult decision and requires considerable thought on the part of both the patient and the doctor; it also requires information (education) and time.

5. e. Endogenous factors associated with an increased risk of breast cancer include (1) white race (white women have about twice the risk of Far Eastern Asian women, and the risk for Ashkenazi Jewish women is again doubled [likely because this population has a high incidence of the BRCA1 and BRCA2 cancer-causing mutations, which are inherited in a Mendelian fashion); (2) increasing age (cancer is rare among women younger than age 25 years, increases slowly thereafter, progresses more rapidly after age 40 years, and then plateaus at about 50 or 55 years of age); (3) a family history of breast cancer in a mother or sister increases risk up to four times and even more if the breast cancer was bilateral or premenopausal; (4) ataxia telangiectasia heterozygotes have a four times greater risk than average; and (5) risk also increases if there is a previous medical history of endometrial cancer, some forms of mammary dysplasia, cancer in the other breast, an early menarche (younger than age 12), a late menopause (older than age 50), a late first pregnancy (especially after 35 years of age), obesity, or nulliparity or not breastfeeding. For some reason risk is decrease in women who have had cervical cancer.

Exogenous, lifestyle–related risk factors include (a) hormonal replacement therapy (a selective estrogen receptor modulator [e.g., Raloxifene, Evista] may, in special cases, be used in place of estrogen because it has little, if any, negative effect on breast tissue and

endometrium, while retaining estrogen-agonist effects on bone and lipid metabolism], (b) estrogen-containing oral contraceptive pills, (c) use of diethylstilbestrol, (d) regular consumption of alcohol, and (e) exposure to irradiation particularly as a child.

6. a. Current estimates indicate that among North American women, approximately one woman in eight will, by the age of 80, develop breast cancer. It is 100 times less prevalent in men, but it does happen.

7. c. Yearly or biannual mammographic screening is recommended for all women starting at the age of 50 years (and by some associations at the age of 40). After the age of 65 the American Geriatrics Society recommends continuing this protocol and then cutting back to every 2-3 years after the age of 75 as long as the patient is healthy and likely to benefit from treatment of a malignancy if discovered.

8. a. The National Surgical Adjunctive Breast Project has concluded that segmental mastectomy (lumpectomy) followed by breast irradiation in all patients and adjunctive chemotherapy in women with positive nodes is appropriate therapy and is just as effective (i.e., no difference in mortality rates) as modified radical mastectomy in patients with stage I and stage II breast cancer with tumors less than 4 cm in diameter.

9. a. The most common histologic type of breast cancer is an infiltrating ductal carcinoma. This type comprises 70% to 80% of all breast cancers. The subtypes of infiltrating ductal carcinoma include medullary, colloid (mucinous), tubular, and papillary carcinoma.

Answer 10 through Answer 16: Matching Questions (Answer 10, **b**; Answer 11, **a**; Answer 12, **b**; Answer 13, **a**; Answer 14, **b**; Answer 15, **a**; and Answer 16, **b**.). The current recommendations for the use of tamoxifen and adjuvant combination chemotherapy are based on menopausal status (premenopausal or postmenopausal), estrogen receptor (ER) status, and axillary lymph-node involvement and are summarized as follows: (1) premenopausal women with positive axillary lymph nodes and either ER-positive or ER-negative tumors should be treated with adjuvant combination chemotherapy; (2) premenopausal women with negative axillary lymph nodes whose tumors are ER-positive benefit from tamoxifen; (3) premenopausal women with negative axillary lymph nodes whose tumors are ER-negative should be treated with combination chemotherapy; (4) postmenopausal women with positive axillary lymph nodes and positive hormone receptors should be treated with tamoxifen; (5) postmenopausal women with positive axillary lymph nodes whose tumors are

ER-negative should be treated with adjuvant combination chemotherapy; and (6) postmenopausal women with negative axillary lymph nodes whose tumors are ER-positive should be treated with tamoxifen; (7) however, postmenopausal women with negative axillary lymph nodes whose tumors are ER-negative should be treated with combination chemotherapy.

In addition, the NIH has issued the following statement concerning women with early-stage breast cancer: "All patients who are candidates for clinical trials should be offered the opportunity to participate in such trials [and] all node-negative patients who are not candidates for clinical trials should be made aware of the benefits and risks of adjuvant systemic therapy."

17. b. The patient in Clinical Case Problem 3 almost certainly has fibrocystic breast changes, also known as mammary dysplasia. All breast tissue contains cysts, and thus the term *fibrocystic breast disease,* as the condition previously was called, is confusing and inappropriate. The most common scenario following this label is that a woman with fibrocystic breast changes believes, in fact, that she has a serious breast disease.

Fibrocystic breast changes are most likely hormonal in origin. This may be either an estrogen or progesterone imbalance or a prolactin excess. The most common presenting symptom is pain. The pain usually begins 1 week before menstruation and is relieved following menstruation. The pain is usually bilateral and is most commonly located in the upper outer quadrants. It may be associated with breast swelling and yellow–green breast discharge.

18. a. In most women, fibrocystic breast changes do not have to be treated. If they do, the most effective treatments are a low-dose oral contraceptive pill that contains a potent progestational agent (such as Loestrin 1/20) or medroxyprogesterone acetate 5-10 mg/day from days 15 to 25 of the calendar month.

Danazol may be used to induce a pseudomenopause in patients with severe fibrocystic breast changes. It is expensive, however, and has significant side effects.

Thiazide diuretics are useful in reducing total body fluid volume and edema. In the cases of the type of "localized swelling in an enclosed cyst" that is seen in fibrocystic breast change, they are not useful.

Vitamin E has not been shown to be of value in the treatment of fibrocystic breast changes.

19. c. This patient has a fibroadenoma, or breast mouse. Fibroadenomas are the most common type of solid benign breast tumors. They are most prevalent in women younger than 25 years old. They are usually painless, well-circumscribed, completely round, and freely mobile. The classic description with respect to consistency is "rubbery."

20. c. The treatment of choice for a suspected fibroadenoma is either a fine-needle biopsy or an excisional biopsy. Although rare, malignancies occasionally have been found in fibroadenomas.

21. c. This patient has an intraductal papilloma, which is a small, soft, tumor that is found just below the areola. If a patient has a bloody nipple discharge associated with a small, soft mass, there is a 95% probability that this is an intraductal papilloma. If physical examination reveals no mass, Paget's disease of the nipple, an adenoma of the nipple, or a breast carcinoma with ductal invasion must be considered in the differential diagnosis.

The treatment of choice is surgical removal. This often is facilitated by mammography or a ductogram.

SUMMARY OF BREAST DISEASE

A. Fibrocystic breast changes:
   1. Cause: hormonal factors
   2. Symptoms: breast pain and fullness premenstrually, with or without discharge
   3. Diagnosis: breast cyst aspiration supplemented by mammography and ultrasound
   4. Treatment: supportive measures, oral contraceptives with low estrogenic activity and potent progestin, medroxyprogesterone acetate

Continued

SOLUTION TO THE CLINICAL CASE MANAGEMENT PROBLEM

The primary care physician should help manage adverse effects of therapy; monitor the response of possible metastatic disease to therapy and look for possible reoccurrence; provide psychological support; audit long- and short-term outcome of treatments; and, if necessary, provide palliative care.

SUMMARY OF BREAST DISEASE —cont'd

B. Fibroadenoma:
1. Prevalence: most frequent solid benign tumor of breast; painless, well-circumscribed, round, rubbery, freely mobile lesion; common in young women
2. Treatment: biopsy

C. Intraductal papilloma:
1. Bloody, unilateral nipple discharge with a soft mass
2. Treatment: surgical removal

D. Carcinoma of the breast:
1. Most common symptom: painless lump often diagnosed by the patient herself
2. Treatment: lumpectomy with radiation for stage I or stage II or modified radical mastectomy; adjuvant combination chemotherapy or tamoxifen for both premenopausal and postmenopausal patients (see Questions 10-16)
3. Screening: mammography every 1-2 years for women age 50-75 years old; clinical breast examination every year for all women

    All women between the ages of 50 and 75 years old should have a screening mammogram performed every 1-2 years (depending on risk factor status).

There is controversy regarding the recommendations for screening mammography beginning at age 40. Some evidence suggests that women in the 40- to 49-year-old age group may benefit from mammography as much as, or more than, women older than age 50.

SUGGESTED READING

Apantaku LM: Breast cancer diagnosis and screening. *Am Fam Physician* 62, 596-602, 605-606, 2000.

Burstein HJ, Winer EP: Primary care for survivors of breast cancer. *N Engl J Med* 343(15):1086-1094, 2000.

Hindle W: Breast cancer: introduction. *Clin Obstet Gynecol* 45(3): 738-745, 2002.

Hindle WH: Breast mass evaluation. *Clin Obstet Gynecol* 45(3):750-757, 2002.

Kerlikowske K, et al: Evaluation of abnormal mammography results and palpable breast abnormalities. *Ann Intern Med* 139(4):274-284, 2003.

Morrow M, Gradishar W: Breast cancer. *BMJ* 324(7334):410-414, 2002.

Olivotto I, Levine M: Steering Committee on Clinical Practice Guidelines for the Care and Treatment of Breast Cancer. Clinical practice guidelines for the care and treatment of breast cancer: the management of ductal carcinoma in situ (summary of the 2001 update). *CMAJ Canadian Medical Association Journal* 165(7):912-913, 2001.

Pruthi S: Detection and evaluation of a palpable breast mass. *Mayo Clin Proc* 76(6):641-647; quiz 647-648, 2001.

Zoorob R, et al: Cancer screening guidelines. *Am Fam Physician* 63:1101-1112, 2001.

Chapter 126

Ophthalmologic Problems

> "Doc, my eyes are so mucked over that I can hardly see."

CLINICAL CASE PROBLEM 1:
A 32-Year-Old Female with Bilateral Red Eyes, a Sore Throat, and a Cough

A 32-year-old female comes to your office with a 1-week history of bilateral red eyes associated with tearing and crusting, a sore throat with difficulty swallowing, and a cough that was initially nonproductive but has become productive over the last few days. The patient displays significant fatigue and lethargy and is having great difficulty performing any of her routine daily chores.

On physical examination, there is bilateral conjunctival injection. Her visual acuity is normal. There is significant pharyngeal erythema but no exudate of membrane.

Cervical lymphadenopathy is not present. Examination of the chest reveals a few expiratory crackles bilaterally.

■ **SELECT THE BEST ANSWER TO THE FOLLOWING QUESTIONS:**

1. What is the most likely cause of this patient's "red eye" condition?
   a. an autoimmune reaction secondary to the beginning of a severe systemic illness
   b. bacterial conjunctivitis related to her other symptoms
   c. bacterial conjunctivitis unrelated to her other symptoms
   d. allergic conjunctivitis secondary to a severe eosinophilic pneumonia
   e. none of the above

2. Concerning this patient's sore throat and in relation to the scenario described and the physical findings provided, what would you do?
   a. perform a throat culture and order antibiotics

b. perform a throat culture and a rapid enzyme-linked immunosorbent assay (ELISA) *Streptococcus* test and treat with an antibiotic if the ELISA test is positive
c. perform a throat culture and await the results
d. order a complete blood count and total eosinophil count
e. none of the above

3. What is the most likely organism or condition responsible for the constellation of symptoms in this patient?
a. endotoxin-producing *Staphylococcus*
b. endotoxin-producing *Streptococcus*
c. exotoxin-producing *Staphylococcus*
d. activation of the autoimmune system
e. none of the above

CLINICAL CASE PROBLEM 2:
A 17-Year-Old Female with a 1-Day History of Red Eye

A 17-year-old female comes to your office with a 1-day history of red eye. She describes a sensation of not being able to open her right eye in the morning because of the discharge. The right eye feels uncomfortable, although there is no pain.

On examination, she has a significant redness and injection of the right conjunctiva. There is a mucopurulent discharge present. No other abnormalities are present on physical examination. Her visual acuity is normal.

4. What is the most likely diagnosis in this patient?
a. bacterial conjunctivitis
b. viral conjunctivitis
c. allergic conjunctivitis
d. autoimmune conjunctivitis
e. none of the above

5. Which of the following agents is (are) a common cause(s) of bacterial conjunctivitis?
a. *Haemophilus influenzae*
b. *Staphylococcus aureus*
c. *Streptococcus pneumoniae*
d. a and b
e. a, b, and c

CLINICAL CASE PROBLEM 3:
A 29-Year-Old Male with Bilateral Red Eyes

A 29-year-old male comes to your office with bilateral red eyes. This symptom came on quite suddenly 2 hours

ago while visiting a friend's home. He describes itching and a clear discharge from both eyes. The patient mentions one previous episode that also began while visiting the same friend.

On examination, the conjunctiva are diffusely injected and edematous. On eversion of the eyelids, there are large papillae present. Visual acuity is intact.

6. What is the most likely diagnosis in this patient?
a. chemical conjunctivitis
b. toxic conjunctivitis
c. allergic conjunctivitis
d. bacterial conjunctivitis
e. none of the above

CLINICAL CASE PROBLEM 4:
A 29-Year-Old Female with a Tender, Painful, Red, and Sore Eye

A 29-year-old female comes to your office for assessment of a red eye. She describes a tender, painful, and sore right eye that began yesterday. She has had no other symptoms.

On examination, the patient has a localized area of inflammation, with dilated vessels and redness, in the lateral area of the right conjunctiva. The inflammation appears to lie beneath the conjunctival surface. Visual acuity is normal.

7. What is the most likely diagnosis in this patient?
a. localized bacterial conjunctivitis
b. acute iritis
c. acute angle closure glaucoma
d. acute episcleritis
e. none of the above

CLINICAL CASE PROBLEM 5:
A 35-Year-Old Female with an Acutely Inflamed and Painful Eye

A 35-year-old female comes to your office with an acutely inflamed and painful left eye. Her symptoms began 2 days ago. There is some visual blurring associated with the symptoms. The patient wears contact lenses.

On examination, there is a diffuse inflammation of the left conjunctiva. On fluorescein staining, there is a dendritic ulcer seen in the center of the cornea. Visual acuity is intact.

8. What is the most likely diagnosis in this patient?
a. corneal abrasion
b. herpetic corneal ulcer
c. contact lens stress ulcer
d. adenoviral ulcer
e. foreign body complicated by a viral ulcer

CLINICAL CASE PROBLEM 6:

A 36-YEAR-OLD MALE WITH ANKYLOSING SPONDYLITIS AND A PAINFUL RED EYE

A 36-year-old male with ankylosing spondylitis comes to your office for assessment of a painful, red left eye. The pain is associated with photophobia.

On examination, the redness is more pronounced around the area of the cornea. His visual acuity in the left eye has decreased to 20/60.

9. What is the most likely diagnosis in this patient?
   a. bacterial conjunctivitis
   b. viral conjunctivitis
   c. acute iridocyclitis
   d. acute episcleritis
   e. acute angle closure glaucoma

CLINICAL CASE PROBLEM 7:

A 61-YEAR-OLD MALE WITH AN EXTREMELY PAINFUL EYE

A 61-year-old male comes to your office with a 12-hour history of an extremely painful and red left eye. The patient complains that his vision is blurred and he is seeing halos around lights. He states that he has had similar but milder attacks in the past.

On examination, the eye is tender and inflamed. The cornea is hazy, and the pupil is semi-dilated and fixed. On palpation, the left eye is significantly harder than the right. Visual acuity is significantly diminished in the left eye.

10. What is the most likely diagnosis in this patient?
    a. bacterial conjunctivitis
    b. viral conjunctivitis
    c. acute iridocyclitis
    d. acute episcleritis
    e. acute angle-closure glaucoma

CLINICAL CASE PROBLEM 8:

A 23-YEAR-OLD FEMALE WITH A PAINFUL EYE AND BLURRED VISION

A 23-year-old female comes to your office with a painful left eye, conjunctival injection, and blurred vision. On examination, the visual acuity is markedly diminished in the affected eye. The conjunctival injection is primarily circumcorneal, and there is photophobia.

11. What is the most likely diagnosis in this patient?
    a. acute conjunctivitis
    b. acute iritis
    c. acute episcleritis
    d. acute angle closure glaucoma
    e. acute corneal abrasion

12. In the patient described in Clinical Case Problem 8, what will the size of the left pupil be, relative to that of the right pupil?
    a. larger than the right pupil
    b. smaller than the right pupil
    c. the same size as the right pupil
    d. indeterminate
    e. nobody really knows for sure

CLINICAL CASE MANAGEMENT PROBLEM

Compare and contrast acute conjunctivitis, acute glaucoma, acute iritis, and corneal trauma or infection with respect to the following: (1) incidence; (2) discharge; (3) vision; (4) pain; (5) conjunctival infections; (6) cornea; (7) pupil size; (8) pupillary light response; (9) intraocular pressure; and (10) smear.

ANSWERS:

1. **e.** See Answer 3.

2. **e.** See Answer 3.

3. **e.** This picture is completely consistent with adenovirus infection and a primary viral conjunctivitis. Viral agents, especially adenovirus, produce signs and symptoms of upper-respiratory tract infection, with the presence of the red eye being prominent among those symptoms.

With adenovirus there is often associated conjunctival hyperemia, eyelid edema, and a serous or seropurulent discharge. Viral conjunctivitis is self-limiting, lasting 1-3 weeks. If the conjunctivitis is definitely caused by a virus, no antibiotic treatment is necessary.

There is no indication for performing a throat culture or any other test at this time. The only theoretic concerns are the "rales" that are present in both lung bases; you could argue that if the patient is sick enough, a chest x-ray may be indicated.

4. **a.** This patient has a primary bacterial conjunctivitis. Unlike in viral conjunctivitis, bacterial conjunctivitis will produce a mucopurulent discharge from the beginning. Symptoms are more often unilateral, and associated eye discomfort is common.

In bacterial conjunctivitis, normal visual acuity always is maintained. There is usually uniform engorgement of all the conjunctival blood vessels. There is no staining of the cornea with fluorescein.

Bacterial conjunctivitis should be treated with antibiotic drops such as sodium sulfacetamide or Garamycin or the newer fluoroquinolones.

5. e. The most common organisms responsible for bacterial conjunctivitis are *Staphylococcus, Streptococcus,* and *Haemophilus. Pseudomonas* and *Moraxella* are other common bacterial isolates.

6. c. The most likely diagnosis in this patient is allergic conjunctivitis. The most common complaint with allergic conjunctivitis is itchy, red eyes. Both eyes are affected, and there is usually a clear discharge.

Examination reveals diffusely infected conjunctiva, which may be edematous (chemosis). The discharge is usually clear and stringy.

Treatment can include avoidance of allergens, immunotherapy, oral antihistamine, topical antihistamine, topical nonsteroidal antiinflammatory drugs (NSAIDs), topical mast cell stabilizer, and topical corticosteroids (use with caution).

The culprit, in this case, is most likely something in his friend's home.

7. d. This patient has episcleritis, which differs from conjunctivitis in that it usually presents as a localized area of inflammation. Although episcleritis may occur secondary to autoimmune disease such as rheumatoid arthritis, most cases of episcleritis are idiopathic. Episcleritis is almost always self-limiting; scleritis, however, may lead to serious complications such as loss of visual acuity and perforation of the globe.

Patients with episcleritis usually have a sore, red, and tender eye. Although there may be reflex lacrimation, there is usually no discharge. Scleritis is much more painful than episcleritis, and the signs of inflammation are usually more prominent.

In episcleritis there is episcleral injection, which can be nodular, sectoral, or diffuse. There is no palpebral conjunctival injection or discharge like that seen in conjunctivitis.

The symptoms of episcleritis usually resolve spontaneously in 1-2 weeks. Chilled artificial tears can be given until the redness resolves. In cases associated with systemic disease, the underlying cause is treated appropriately.

8. b. This patient has a dendritic ulcer, which almost always is caused by a herpetic infection, although other viral agents, bacterial agents, or fungal agents also may be responsible. These infections may be primary or secondary to excessive contact lens wear, a corneal abrasion, or the use of corticosteroid eye drops.

The patient with a herpetic dendritic ulcer usually has an acutely painful eye associated with conjunctival injection, discharge, and visual blurring. Visual acuity, however, depends on the location and the size of the corneal ulcer. The discharge may be watery (reflex lacrimation) or purulent (bacterial). Conjunctival injection may be generalized or localized, depending on the location of the ulcer.

Treatment consists of specific antiinfective therapy (vidarabine or trifluridine for herpes simplex ulcers and topical antibiotics for ulcers suspected of being primarily or secondarily infected by bacteria) and cycloplegic drops to relieve pain caused by ciliary muscle spasm. Topical corticosteroids are absolutely contraindicated in patients with a dendritic herpetic ulcer.

In a patient with a dendritic ulcer, referral to an ophthalmologist is recommended.

9. c. This patient has an acute iridocyclitis or anterior uveitis. Patients at risk for anterior uveitis are those patients with a history of a seronegative arthropathy, particularly if they are positive for HLA-B27. Children with seronegative arthritis are also at high risk.

Symptoms of acute iridocyclitis include a painful red eye, often associated with photophobia, and decreased visual acuity.

On examination, the affected eye is red; the inflammation is particularly prominent over the area of the inflamed ciliary body (circumcorneal). The pupil is small because of spasm of the sphincter or irregular because of adhesions of the iris to the lens (posterior synechiae). Inflammatory cells may be seen on the back of the cornea (keratitic precipitates) or may settle to form a collection of cells in the anterior chamber of the eye (hypopyon).

Treatment of anterior uveitis should include topical corticosteroids to reduce the inflammation and prevent adhesions within the eye. Mydriatics should be used to paralyze the ciliary body to relieve pain.

As with episcleritis and dendritic ulcers, a patient with iridocyclitis should be referred to an ophthalmologist.

10. e. This patient has acute angle-closure glaucoma. Acute glaucoma always should be suspected in a patient who is older than age 50 years and has a painful red eye.

Unlike the more common open-angle glaucoma, acute glaucoma usually comes on rapidly. The most common symptom is severe pain in one eye, which may or may not be accompanied by other symptoms such as nausea and vomiting. The patient complains of impaired vision and halos around lights. This is caused by edema of the cornea.

On examination, the eye is tender and inflamed. The cornea is hazy, and the pupil is partially dilated and fixed. Vision is impaired because of edema of the cornea. On palpation, the involved eye often feels significantly harder than the uninvolved eye.

Untreated, the condition can lead to blindness in 2-5 days. Initial emergent treatment to reduce intraocular pressure includes topical beta blockers, intravenous and oral carbonic anhydrase inhibitors (such as acetazolamide), and hyperosmotic agents. Once intraocular pressure is under control, a peripheral laser iridectomy is performed.

The other eye should be treated prophylactically with a laser iridotomy.

11. **b.** This patient has an acute iritis.

12. **b.** Acute iritis is characterized by incidence, common; eye discharge, none; visual acuity, slightly blurred; pain, moderate; conjunctival injection, mainly circumcorneal; cornea, usually clear; pupil size, smaller than unaffected eye; pupillary light response, poor; intraocular pressure, normal; and Gram's stain and smear, no organisms.

The treatment of acute iritis is a mydriatic to relieve ciliary spasm and a corticosteroid to decrease inflammation. Again, this patient should be referred to an ophthalmologist.

SOLUTION TO THE CLINICAL CASE MANAGEMENT PROBLEM

There are four major conditions that should be considered when a patient comes to the physician's office with a red eye: acute conjunctivitis, acute iritis, acute glaucoma, and corneal trauma or infection. Their differentiation and treatment are as follows:

1. *Incidence:* (a) acute conjunctivitis, extremely common; (b) acute iritis, common; (c) acute glaucoma, uncommon; and (d) corneal trauma or infection, common

2. *Discharge:* (a) acute conjunctivitis, moderate to copious; (b) acute iritis, none; (c) acute glaucoma, none; and (d) corneal trauma or infection, watery or purulent.

3. *Vision:* (a) acute conjunctivitis, no effect on vision; (b) acute iritis, slightly blurred; (c) acute glaucoma, markedly blurred; and (d) corneal trauma or infection, usually blurred.

4. *Pain:* (a) acute conjunctivitis, none; (b) acute iritis, moderate; (c) acute glaucoma, severe; and (d) corneal trauma or infection, moderate to severe.

5. *Conjunctival injection:* (a) acute conjunctivitis, diffuse, more toward fornices; (b) acute iritis, mainly circumcorneal; (c) acute glaucoma, diffuse; and (d) corneal trauma or infection, diffuse.

6. *Cornea:* (a) acute conjunctivitis, clear; (b) acute iritis, usually clear; (c) acute glaucoma, steamy; and (d) corneal trauma or infection, change in clarity related to cause.

7. *Pupil size:* (a) acute conjunctivitis, normal; (b) acute iritis, small; (c) acute glaucoma, moderately dilated and fixed; and (d) corneal trauma or infection, normal.

8. *Pupillary light response:* (a) acute conjunctivitis, normal; (b) acute iritis, poor; (c) acute glaucoma, none; and (d) corneal trauma or infection, normal

9. *Intraocular pressure:* (a) acute conjunctivitis, normal; (b) acute iritis, normal; (c) acute glaucoma, elevated; and (d) corneal trauma or infection, normal.

10. *Smear:* (a) acute conjunctivitis, causative organisms; (b) acute iritis, no organisms; (c) acute glaucoma, no organisms; and (d) corneal trauma or infection, organisms found only in corneal ulcers caused by infection.

SUMMARY OF OPHTHALMOLOGIC PROBLEMS

A. Infectious conjunctivitis:
1. Etiologic agents: (a) adenovirus is the most common cause of conjunctivitis; and (b) bacterial conjunctivitis, most commonly caused by *S. aureus*, *S. pneumoniae*, and *H. influenzae*
2. Symptoms: (a): watery discharge with viral infection; mucopurulent discharge with bacterial infection; (b) other symptoms as described in the Clinical Case Management Problem
3. Treatment: ciprofloxin (Ciloxan), gatifloxacin sulfacetamide, or gentamicin drops

B. Allergic conjunctivitis:
1. Symptoms: itching and clear discharge are main symptoms; conjunctiva are diffusely injected and may be associated with swelling (chemosis).
2. Treatment: avoidance of allergens, immunotherapy, topical antihistamines, topical NSAIDs, topical mast cell stabilizers, oral antihistamines, topical corticosteroids (use with caution).

C. Corneal ulcers:
1. May be bacterial, viral, or fungal in origin or also may be secondary to a corneal abrasion, contact lens wear, etc.

2. Visual acuity depends on the location and size of the ulcer. Conjunctival injection may be generalized or localized. Fluorescein must be used to stain the cornea.
3. Treatment: Cycloplegic eye drops are used to relieve ciliary muscle spasm. Trifluridine or Vidarabine are used for dendritic (herpetic) ulcer; antibiotic drops are used for suspected bacterial infection. Corticosteroid eye drops are absolutely contraindicated in herpetic ulcers.

D. Iridocyclitis (anterior uveitis):
1. Iridocyclitis often is associated with seronegative arthropathy.
2. Inflammation of the iris (iritis) and inflammation of the ciliary body (cyclitis) occur together.
3. The inflammation of anterior uveitis is circumcorneal in location, and the pupil is usually small because of associated spasm.
4. Treatment: Mydriatics are used to relieve ciliary spasm; corticosteroid drops are used to decrease inflammation.

E. Acute angle-closure glaucoma:
1. Acute, unilateral, painful red eye in a patient older than 50 years of age
2. The attack usually comes on quickly, characteristically in the evening.

3. Impaired vision caused by corneal edema and halos around lights are common.
4. Palpation reveals a hard eye.
5. Emergent treatment: Topical beta blocker, intravenous and oral carbonic anhydrase inhibitors, and hyperosmotic agents are first steps. Once intraocular pressure is under control, a peripheral laser iridectomy is performed.

SUGGESTED READING

Bielory L: Allergic and immunologic disorders of the eye. Part I: immunology of the eye. *J Allergy Clin Immunol* 106(5):805-816, 2000.
Bielory L: Allergic and immunologic disorders of the eye. Part II: ocular allergy. *J Allergy Clin Immunol* 106(6):1019-1032, 2000.
Leibowitz HM: The red eye. *N Engl J Med* 343(5):345-351, 2000.
Michael JG, et al: Management of corneal abrasion in children: a randomized clinical trial. *Ann Emerg Med* 40:67-72, 2002.
Rittichier KK, et al: Are signs and symptoms associated with persistent corneal abrasion in children? *Arch Pediatr Adolesc Med* 54:370-374, 2000.
Rodriguez JO, et al: Prevention and treatment of common eye injuries in sports. *Am Fam Physician* 67(7):1481-1488, 2003.
Shingleton BJ, O'Donoghue MW: Blurred vision. *N Engl J Med* 343(8):556-562, 2000.
Vafidis G: When is red eye not just conjunctivitis? *Practitioner* 246:469-481, 2002.

Chapter 127

Renal Stones

Stones and groans and, on occasion, bones.

CLINICAL CASE PROBLEM 1:
A 30-YEAR-OLD MALE WITH FLANK PAIN

A 30-year-old male comes to the emergency department with acute onset of severe right-side flank pain. The pain radiates down into the groin and testicle and is associated with hematuria, urinary frequency, urgency, and dysuria.

On examination, the patient is in acute distress. The patient is febrile at 101° F, pulse is 101, respirations 20, and BP 140/90. He has significant right costovertebral angle tenderness. The rest of the examination is normal. There is 2+ blood on the urine dipstick test; no casts are seen on microscopic examination.

SELECT THE BEST ANSWER TO THE FOLLOWING QUESTIONS:

1. What is the most likely diagnosis in this patient?
   a. renal colic
   b. acute pyelonephritis
   c. acute pyelitis
   d. atypical appendicitis
   e. none of the above

2. What is the most common composition of a kidney stone?
   a. calcium oxalate
   b. mixed calcium oxalate/calcium phosphate
   c. calcium phosphate
   d. struvite
   e. uric acid

3. Which of the following abnormalities is (are) usually associated with calcium oxalate stones?
   a. hypercalciuria
   b. hyperuricuria

c. hypocitraturia
d. all of the above
e. none of the above

4. What is the drug of choice for the management of idiopathic hypercalciuria?
a. cellulose sodium phosphate
b. an orthophosphate
c. potassium citrate
d. hydrochlorothiazide
e. pyridoxine

5. What is the most important component of the diagnostic workup in a patient with a kidney stone?
a. serum calcium/serum uric acid
b. serum creatinine
c. intravenous pyelography
d. 24-hour urine for volume, calcium, uric acid, citrate, oxalate, sodium, creatinine, and pH
e. serum parathyroid hormone

6. Which of the following statements regarding uric acid stones is (are) correct?
a. uric acid stones are formed in patients who are found to have an acidic urine
b. uric acid stones are formed in patients with increased uric acid secretion
c. the initial treatment for patients with uric acid stones is alkalinization of the urine
d. patients with recalcitrant uric acid stones should be treated with allopurinol
e. all of the above statements are correct

7. Which of the following statements regarding the treatment of nephrolithiasis is (are) true?
a. extracorporeal shock wave lithotripsy (ESWL) has become widely used for the treatment of renal stones
b. ureteral stones, unless large, are best managed by awaiting their spontaneous passage
c. ESWL has shown its greatest benefit in patients with stones less than 2 cm in diameter
d. all of the above statements are true
e. none of the above statements are true

8. Which of the following is (are) part of the differential diagnosis of renal colic?
a. acute pyelonephritis
b. renal adenocarcinoma
c. papillary necrosis
d. all of the above
e. none of the above

9. What is the treatment of choice for metabolic stone formation?
a. hydrochlorothiazide
b. sodium potassium citrate

c. pyridoxine
d. an organophosphate
e. none of the above

10. Magnesium-ammonium-phosphate stones are usually secondary to urinary tract infection with which of the following?
a. *Escherichia coli*
b. *Proteus* species
c. *Klebsiella*
d. Enterococcus
e. Enterobacter

CLINICAL CASE MANAGEMENT PROBLEM

A 45-year-old male comes to the emergency department with left-sided flank pain. An x-ray of the kidneys, ureter, and bladder (KUB) suggests a ureteric stone. While straining his urine, the patient discovers a stone. The pain subsides. The stone is analyzed and found to be a calcium oxalate stone. Describe the general treatment measures that you would use to prevent further stone formation in this patient.

■ **ANSWERS:**

1. **a.** This patient has renal colic. Renal colic is characterized by the sudden onset of severe flank pain radiating toward the groin. It usually is associated with hematuria, urinary frequency, urgency, and dysuria and is relieved immediately following the passage of the stone. Acute pyelonephritis, which may be associated with similar symptoms, usually is accompanied by fever and chills.

The sudden onset of severe flank pain is not typical of appendiceal disease.

2. **a.** Calcium oxalate stones are the most common type of renal stones; they constitute 60% of all stones. They are most commonly idiopathic. Other stones in order of frequency of occurrence are uric acid, mixed calcium oxalate/calcium phosphate, struvite, and cystine stones.

3. **d.** Calcium oxalate stones may be associated with hypercalciuria, hyperuricosuria, and hypocitraturia. Hypercalciuria is most common.

4. **d.** A thiazide diuretic, such as hydrochlorothiazide, is the agent of choice for the treatment of idiopathic hypercalciuria. Thiazide diuretics work by lowering urine calcium excretion. Other measures include increasing total daily fluid intake and decreasing

animal protein and salt intake. Restriction of calcium intake has not been proved to be effective.

5. d. The basic laboratory evaluation of a patient with renal colic includes urinalysis; urine culture; and blood chemistry profile including serum calcium, phosphorus, uric acid, electrolytes, and creatinine; x-ray examination of the KUB; and helical computed tomography (CT) of the abdomen. The most sensitive test for the diagnosis of metabolic abnormalities associated with nephrolithiasis, however, is the 24-hour urine collection. The 24-hour specimen should be analyzed for calcium, uric acid, citrate, oxalate, sodium, creatinine, and urine pH.

When stone composition is unknown, urine also should be obtained for qualitative cystine screening. Serum parathyroid hormone assay should be performed when hypercalcemia is present.

6. e. Uric acid stones, the second most common type of renal stone, are formed in patients with a persistent acidic urine or a high uric acid secretion (exceeding 1000 mg/day). The initial treatment of a patient with a uric acid stone involves alkalinization of the urine with either sodium bicarbonate or citrate. Patients with uric acid stones should be treated with allopurinol. A decreased purine intake (i.e., decreased consumption of red meat and, in particular, animal organs such as liver, sweetbreads, and kidney) also is recommended.

7. d. ESWL is used widely in the treatment of nephrolithiasis to break up renal stones with shock waves, permitting them to pass spontaneously.

Lithotripsy is most effective when the stone is less than 2 cm in diameter. For patients with stones larger than 2 cm, initial percutaneous nephrolithotomy followed by ESWL and a "second-look" percutaneous nephrolithotomy give the best results.

Patients with staghorn calculi, obstruction, or complex anatomy should be treated with open surgery.

Ureteral stones are best managed by awaiting spontaneous passage. If spontaneous passage is unlikely or delayed, ESWL is the first choice for stones in the upper two-thirds of the ureter; endoscopic surgery is the best alternative for lower ureteral stones.

A ureteropelvic or other obstruction, as well as stones deposited in diverticula, should be managed by endourologic techniques.

8. d. The major differential diagnosis of renal colic includes infection of the upper urinary tract (acute pyelonephritis or acute pyelitis), renal adenocarcinoma, and papillary necrosis. Papillary necrosis (ischemic necrosis of the renal papillae or of the entire renal pyramid) is usually secondary to excessive ingestion of analgesics, sickle cell trait (associated with hematuria), diabetes mellitus, obstruction with infection, or vesicoureteral reflux with infection.

9. b. Metabolic stones, including cystine stones, are best treated by giving the patient a sodium-potassium citrate solution, 4-8 ml qid. In this case the urine pH should be monitored.

10. b. Magnesium-ammonium-phosphate stones are usually secondary to urinary tract infection with bacteria that produce urease (primarily *Proteus* species). The urease hydrolyzes the urea producing ammonia and thereby raising the pH and providing the source of ammonia. Eradication of the infection prevents further stone formation. After calculi removal, prevention of stone growth is best accomplished by urinary acidification, long-term use of antibiotics, and the use of acetohydroxamic acid (a urease inhibitor that maintains an acid urinary pH).

SUMMARY OF RENAL STONES

A. Classic symptoms of renal colic: sudden, severe, flank pain with radiation to the groin; associated with hematuria, frequency, urgency, dysuria, and relief following stone passage. Diagnosis of retained stones is made by helical CT.

Continued

SOLUTION TO THE CLINICAL CASE MANAGEMENT PROBLEM

The treatment of calcium oxalate stones includes the following: (1) maintaining normal calcium intake with meals (this binds the oxalate that forms stones, increasing its loss from the gastrointestinal tract); (2) restricting dietary sodium to 2000 mg/day (6 g of salt per day); (3) limiting intake of proteins and carbohydrates; (4) using oral orthophosphates to decrease stone-forming potential; (5) using thiazide diuretics to decrease urine calcium content; and (6) using allopurinol and urinary alkalinization to reduce the formation of urate crystals.

SUMMARY OF RENAL STONES —cont'd

B. Types of stones:

1. **Calcium oxalate stones:** (a) most frequent type of stone; (b) usually idiopathic and associated with hypercalciuria, hyperuricuria, and hypocitraturia; (c) in patients with hypercalciuria, restricted intake of animal protein and salt, combined with normal calcium intake recommended to prevent recurrence

2. **Uric acid stones:** (a) second most frequent type of stone; (b) associated with urine that is persistently acidic and in conjunction with massively increased urinary uric acid secretion (greater than 1000 mg/day); (c) prevention with alkalinization of urine with bicarbonate or citrate; in addition may have to use allopurinol.

3. **Infective stones:** (a) caused by urea-splitting organisms (*Proteus* species); (b) stone should be completely removed and antibiotic therapy prescribed

4. **Cystine stones:** occur with the inherited transport disorder cystinuria

C. Stone treatment:

1. **Ureteral stones:** await spontaneous passage. If not forthcoming, then use ESWL (upper two-thirds of ureter) and endoscopic techniques (lower one-third of ureter).

2. **Renal stones:** ESWL is the treatment of choice for stones less than 2 cm and located in the upper pole of the kidney. If stones larger than 1 cm are located in the lower pole of the kidney, a combination of ESWL and percutaneous nephrolithotomy is preferred.

SUGGESTED READING

Borghi L: Comparison of two diets for the prevention of recurrent stone in idiopathic calciuria. *N Engl J Med* 346(2):77-84, 2002.

Lindbloom EJ: What is the best test to diagnose urinary tract stones? *J Fam Pract* 50(8):657-658, 2001.

Morton AR, et al: Nephrology: 1. Investigation and treatment of recurrent kidney stones. *CMAJ Canadian Medical Association Journal* 166(2):213-218, 2002.

Shokeir AA: Renal colic: new concepts related to pathophysiology, diagnosis and treatment. *Curr Opin Urol* 12(4):263-269, 2002.

Tiselius HG: Epidemiology and medical management of stone disease. *BJU Int* 91(8):758-767, 2003.

Chapter 128

Prostate Problems

| "Doc, I can hardly pee."

CLINICAL CASE PROBLEM 1:
A 75-Year-Old Male with Nocturia, Hesitancy, and a Slow Urinary Flow

A 75-year-old male comes to your office with a 6-month history of nocturia, hesitancy, a slow flow of urine, and terminal dribbling. The symptoms have been progressing. Otherwise, he is well and has had no significant medical illnesses.

On examination, his abdomen is normal. He has an enlarged prostate gland, which is smooth in contour and firm and has no nodules or irregularities.

▶ **SELECT THE BEST ANSWER TO THE FOLLOWING QUESTIONS:**

1. What is the most likely diagnosis in this patient?
   a. benign prostatic hypertrophy (BPH)
   b. carcinoma of the bladder
   c. prostatic carcinoma
   d. urethral stricture
   e. chronic prostatitis

2. Which of the following symptoms is (are) associated with the condition described in Clinical Case Problem 1?
   a. dysuria
   b. daytime frequency
   c. incomplete voiding
   d. urgency
   e. all of the above

3. Which of the following pharmacologic treatments may be indicated in the treatment of the condition described in Clinical Case Problem 1?
   a. finasteride
   b. prazosin
   c. terazosin
   d. all of the above
   e. none of the above

4. Before the medical or surgical treatment of the condition described in Clinical Case Problem 1, which of the following should be performed?
   a. digital rectal examination
   b. transrectal ultrasound

c. computed tomography (CT) scan of the pelvis
d. a and b
e. all of the above

5. Which of the following surgical procedures is the treatment of choice for severe cases of the condition described in Clinical Case Problem 1?
a. transurethral resection of the prostate (TURP)
b. open prostatectomy
c. transurethral incision of the prostate
d. hyperthermia of the prostate
e. balloon dilatation of the prostate

CLINICAL CASE PROBLEM 2:

A 58-Year-Old Male with Hesitancy of the Urinary Stream and Bone Pain

A 58-year-old male comes to your office with a 3-month history of gradually worsening hesitancy of urinary stream, urgency, nocturia, and terminal dribbling. He also complains of lumbar and pelvic bone pain present for the past 3 weeks.

On physical examination, the prostate is enlarged and very hard. There is some tenderness over the pelvic ischium on the left side and at the fourth and fifth lumbar vertebrae.

6. Which one of the following statements regarding this patient's condition is false?
a. the most likely diagnosis is prostatic carcinoma
b. radiotherapy is the most probable first line of therapy in the management of this patient
c. this patient most likely has metastatic disease
d. the evaluation of this patient should include a bone scan
e. combination chemotherapy may be indicated for the treatment of this condition

7. Which of the following statements regarding carcinoma of the prostate is (are) true?
a. prostatic cancer is a major public health problem in men
b. prostatic cancer is now the most prevalent cancer in men
c. bone is the most common site of metastatic disease
d. all of the above statements are true
e. none of the above statements are true

8. Which of the following is (are) risk factors for the disease described in the patient in Clinical Case Problem 2?
a. increased age
b. African American men
c. positive family history for the disease
d. dietary fat intake
e. all of the above

9. Which of the following statements is true regarding screening for this disorder?
a. routine digital rectal examination (DGE) in men after the age of 55 years is recommended
b. routine use of prostate specific antigen analysis (PSA) in men after the age of 55 years is recommended
c. routine combined use of PSA and DGE in men after the age of 55 years is recommended
d. routine combined use of PSA and DGE in men after the age of 65 years is recommended
e. there is insufficient evidence to recommend routine screening of men for prostate cancer at any age

10. Which of the following is the treatment of choice for stage A-1 of this disease in an 81-year-old male?
a. radiation therapy
b. radical prostatectomy
c. hormone therapy
d. combination chemotherapy
e. none of the above

11. What is the most common symptom with which a male with prostatic cancer presents?
a. a feeling of "hardness" in the rectal area
b. obstructive voiding symptoms
c. anorexia
d. weight loss
e. bone pain

CLINICAL CASE PROBLEM 3:

A 24-Year-Old Male with Fever, Suprapubic Discomfort, and Inhibited Urinary Voiding

A 24-year-old male comes to your office with a 2-day history of fever, chills, perineal and suprapubic discomfort, dysuria, and inhibited urinary voiding.

On physical examination, the lower abdomen is tender. A digital rectal examination reveals a swollen, boggy, and tender prostate. Examination of the urine reveals pus cells and bacterial rods. The man has no history of similar symptoms.

12. What is the most likely diagnosis in this patient?
a. acute prostatitis
b. acute cystitis
c. chronic prostatitis
d. acute perineal pain syndrome
e. acute nongonococcal urethritis

13. What is the most likely organism responsible for the condition described in Clinical Case Problem 3?

a. *Escherichia coli*
b. *Pseudomonas*
c. *Proteus*
d. *Serratia*
e. *Chlamydia trachomatis*

14. What is the pharmacologic agent of choice for the condition described in Clinical Case Problem 3?
    a. trimethoprim-sulfamethoxazole (TMP-SMX)
    b. erythromycin
    c. ampicillin
    d. tetracycline
    e. gentamicin

CLINICAL CASE MANAGEMENT PROBLEM

Describe the therapeutic mechanism and the therapeutic effects of the drug finasteride for the treatment of BPH.

▶ **ANSWERS:**

1. a. The most likely diagnosis in this patient is benign prostatic hypertrophy (BPH). Hyperplasia of the prostate causes increased outflow resistance.

2. e. The symptoms of BPH are described as either obstructive or irritative. Obstructive symptoms are attributed to the mechanical obstruction of the prostatic urethra by the hyperplastic tissue and include the following: (1) hesitancy; (2) weakening of the urinary stream; (3) intermittent urinary stream; (4) feeling of residual urine (incomplete bladder emptying); (5) urinary retention; and (6) postmicturition urinary dribbling.

Irritative symptoms are attributed to involuntary contractions of the vesical detrusor muscle (detrusor instability) and are associated with obstruction in approximately 50% of patients with prostatism. These symptoms include (1) nocturia; (2) daytime frequency; (3) urgency; (4) urge incontinence; and (5) dysuria.

Differential diagnosis includes carcinoma of the prostate, neuropathic bladder, chronic prostatitis, and urethral stricture.

3. d. The pharmacologic treatment of BPH is directed toward relaxation of the prostatic smooth-muscle fibers through inhibition of alpha-adrenergic receptors and toward regression of the hyperplastic tissue by hormonal suppression.

The growth of BPH depends on the presence of the androgenic hormone testosterone and its derivative dihydrotestosterone (via conversion by the enzyme 5-alpha reductase). The strategy of antiandrogenic therapy in BPH is to interfere with dihydrotestosterone production. Many antiandrogenic drugs have been tried, but at present the most promising is the 5-alpha reductase inhibitor, finasteride. Finasteride (Proscar) 5 mg/day results in a 20% reduction in prostatic size and a modest improvement of the urine's and symptom score. It also has a low incidence of adverse effects. Finasteride significantly decreases the PSA level, and detection of cancer of the prostate becomes difficult. Finasteride treatment should be considered in patients with moderate symptoms of prostatism. If the patient improves and side effects are minimal, continuation of therapy under careful urologic control is appropriate.

The tone of prostatic smooth muscle is mediated by alpha$_1$ adrenoreceptor stimulation. Selective or nonselective antagonists relax the smooth muscle, resulting in a diminution of urethral resistance, improvement of urine flow, and a significant improvement in symptoms. The results of double-blind, randomized controlled trials have demonstrated the short-term efficacy of selective alpha$_1$ blockade. Selective alpha$_1$-blocking drugs such as terazosin (Hytrin), doxazosin (Cardura), and prazosin (Minipress) represent an option for patients with moderate symptoms. The long-term efficacy remains to be established.

4. d. The following should be performed before any medical or surgical intervention for BPH: (1) a complete history; (2) a complete physical examination; (3) a DRE; (4) ultrasound (transrectal or abdominal); (5) determination of postvoiding residual urine; (6) routine urinalysis and culture; (7) electrolytes (especially urea and creatinine); (8) PSA; and (9) cystoscopy.

5. a. In general, TURP remains both safe and efficacious and is the "gold standard" against which all other treatments, both medical and surgical, must be measured. More than 80% of patients experience subjective improvement, including a significant improvement in urine flow rate. Approximately 15%, however, report no benefit 1 year after surgery. Complications of surgery can be significant, with many patients left with chronic incontinence and/or impotence.

Other surgical treatment options undergoing investigation include (1) transurethral incision of the prostate; (2) open surgery; (3) transurethral laser-induced prostatectomy; (4) transurethral balloon dilatation of the prostate; (5) laser ablation; (6) high-intensity ultrasound thermotherapy; (7) microwave thermotherapy; (8) electrovaporization; (9) radiofrequency vaporization, and (10) prostatic stents and coils.

6. b. This patient most likely has a prostatic carcinoma with osseous bone metastases. Evaluation of this patient should include a PSA level, a bone scan, plain x-rays of the pelvis and lumbar areas, and a CT scan of the pelvis. The patient should receive hormonal therapy if these investigations confirm stage D carcinoma of the prostate (pelvic lymph-node metastases or distant metastases). Although radiotherapy for stage D cancer is not entirely ruled out, it is not a first-line option.

Palliative treatment of cancer pain is discussed in Chapter 49.

7. d. Prostate cancer represents the most common tumor among men in the United States and is certainly a major public health problem; approximately 179,000 new cases were estimated to be diagnosed in 1999, and some 37,000 men were estimated to have died that year of their disease. The single most important risk factor for cancer of the prostate is age; the disease prevalence increases almost exponentially after age 50. The true prevalence is unknown, but estimates can be obtained from autopsy series or from a series of patients undergoing TURP. These series suggest that the prevalence of the disease is about 30% in men age 60-69 years and about 67% in men age 80-89 years. It approaches 100% in men older than 90 years of age. The incidence among various populations is similar in autopsy samples, but the clinical incidence various considerably. This suggests that environmental/dietary differences among various cultural groups may be important determinants of the rate of cancer growth. It has been reported that cancerous growth is promoted by high-fat diet, including the omega 3 alpha-linolenic acid and surprisingly also by high calcium intake. Conversely, growth has been reported to be inhibited by aspirin, a diet rich in fish (a rich source of longer chain omega 3 fatty acids), whole grains, lycopene and beta carotene (antioxidants), cruciferous vegetables, and vitamin D. Apparently diet plays a role, but most of these studies are preliminary in nature and need to be investigated further by well-executed, evidence-based studies.

A July 2003 study reported that finasteride reduced the risk of prostate cancer by 25%, but unfortunately patients who did develop cancer while taking finasteride had a more aggressive form of the disease; there were also sexual side effects, including reduced libido, decreased ejaculate volume, and erectile dysfunction.

The most common site of prostatic metastases is bone.

8. e. As mentioned in Answer 7, increasing age is the most important risk factor for carcinoma of the prostate. Other risk factors include African American race, dietary fat intake, positive family history for carcinoma of the prostate, and possible exposure to certain chemicals (herbicides and pesticides). Certain occupations such as farming and work in the industrial chemical industry seem to present an especially high risk.

9. e. Although the combined use of DGE and PSA has increased the accuracy of prostate cancer diagnosis, routine screening is not recommended primarily because many cancers remain asymptomatic; it also is feared that prostate screening programs may result in unnecessary biopsy and the resultant cost and risk of complications in some men, who if left alone would have suffered no symptoms for the rest of their lives. In addition, even after DGE and PSA analysis, the diagnosis is uncertain. The result of the digital examination is subjective, and BPH and other benign conditions will increase PSA values into the "gray" risk zone of 4-10 ng/ml, causing false-positive results, which again will trigger further studies. However, treatment of BPH with finasteride reduces PSA values and causes false-negative results. Rather than routine screening, it is recommended that testing be done on high-risk subjects on an individual basis at the physician's discretion.

Regular PSA analyses on high-risk subjects performed on a yearly or biyearly basis that show a gradual increase in PSA values is extremely suspicious, even if the value stays below the magic 4 ng/ml number. Also, the validity of an elevated PSA value can be further checked by a "free PSA test," a measure of unbound PSA. A free PSA value of 25% or greater means the risk of cancer is low, even if the total PSA value was higher than 4 ng/ml, whereas a free value of less than 10% means the risk is very high. However, once again there is a zone of uncertainty between 10% and 25%, making biopsy inevitable in such cases.

10. e. Multiple treatment options exist for localized prostate cancer. Studies of the natural history of untreated stages A and B disease attest to the slow progression of these lesions with disease-specific survival rates in excess of 85% at 10 years. For this reason, a watch-and-wait policy for older patients and those with significant other comorbid conditions is a reasonable option. For younger patients with a long life expectancy (greater than 10 years), treatment for cure can be accomplished with radical prostatectomy, external beam radiotherapy, or interstitial radiotherapy where the radiation source is placed close to the tumor. Radical proctectomy is the classical approach in which the prostate is removed from the urethra. Provided the tumor still is contained within the prostate, there is essentially no chance of remission or metastasis, and modern surgical technics have greatly reduced the risk of nerve damage that can result in long-term urinary incontinence and impotency. External beam radiotherapy produces equivalent results, avoids the trauma of surgery and hospitalization, but does require daily doses for 4-6 weeks and can cause fatigue and irritation; moreover, it has a non–inconsequential chance of producing impotence. Interstitial radiotherapy involves implantation of radioactive "seeds," which are permitted to slowly destroy the prostate tissue. Although it has gained in popularity during the past decade, the jury is still out concerning effectiveness and potential side effects.

11. b. The diagnosis of prostate cancer is usually a serendipitous finding. Signs and symptoms of the disease usually are encountered only at an advanced stage. These signs and symptoms include anorexia, bone pain, neurologic deficits, obstructive voiding symptoms, and weight loss. Of these, the most common initial presenting symptom is obstruction to voiding.

12. a. This patient's symptoms are classic for acute bacterial prostatitis. The symptoms include both systemic symptoms (fever and chills) and local urinary symptoms such as perineal and suprapubic discomfort, dysuria, and inhibited urinary voiding.

The DRE that reveals a swollen, tender, and boggy prostate is probably the most sensitive and specific diagnostic test for prostatitis. When performing the rectal examination in a patient with systemic symptoms, it is imperative that the prostate gland not be massaged; this may release a significant number of bacteria into the bloodstream. Only when systemic symptoms are absent can the prostate gland be safely massaged to obtain a prostatic specimen for culture.

13. a. The two bacteria responsible for most cases of bacterial prostatitis are *E. coli* and *Klebsiella*. Nonbacterial prostatitis most often is caused by *Chlamydia trachomatis* or *Ureaplasma urealyticum*.

14. a. The drugs of choice for the treatment of acute prostatitis are TMP-SMX, norfloxacin, and ciprofloxacin. Antibiotic treatment should continue for at least 4 weeks.

 ## SOLUTION TO THE CLINICAL CASE MANAGEMENT PROBLEM

The medical treatment of BPH has been revolutionized. The growth of BPH depends on the presence of the androgenic hormone testosterone and its derivative dihydrotestosterone (via conversion by the enzyme 5-alpha reductase). The strategy of antiandrogenic therapy in BPH is to interfere with dihydrotestosterone production.

As mentioned in Answer 3, finasteride results in an approximately 20% reduction in prostatic size and a modest improvement of the flow rate of urine and symptom score and has a very low rate of adverse effects.

The main adverse effects are a decrease in libido and/or erectile dysfunction. Finasteride also significantly decreases the serum PSA level and thus reduces the ability to screen for carcinoma of the prostate.

The treatment of BPH with finasteride should be considered in patients with moderate symptoms of prostatism. If the patient improves while taking the drug and does not experience significant side effects, continuation of therapy under careful physician supervision is reasonable.

 ## SUMMARY OF PROSTATE DISEASE

A. BPH:
1. Symptoms: both obstructive symptoms (hesitancy, weak stream, intermittent urinary stream, feeling of incomplete emptying, urinary retention, terminal dribbling) and irritative symptoms (nocturia, daytime frequency, urgency, urge incontinence, dysuria)

2. Investigations: complete history, physical examination, urinalysis, culture, transrectal ultrasound, residual urine, electrolytes, blood urea nitrogen, creatinine, serum PSA, cystoscopy
3. Treatment: pharmacologic treatment: 5-alpha reductase inhibitor (finasteride), alpha-receptor blocker (prazosin, terazosin); surgical treatment: TURP

B. Carcinoma of the prostate:
1. Prevalence: Carcinoma of the prostate is now

the most prevalent malignancy in men and the second leading cause of death from cancer.

2. Symptoms and signs: Symptoms and signs are the same as those of BPH, except abnormalities are found on examination of the prostate.

3. Treatment: multiple treatment trials are under way, and effective treatment strategies are a matter of great debate. Consider all options with the patient because all therapies have their pluses and minuses. One set of recommendations is as follows: (a) Stages A and B-1 (younger than age 65), prostatectomy or radiation; (b) Stages A and B-1 (older than age 65), watchful waiting; (c) Stages B and C, radiotherapy; (d) Stage D asymptomatic, await the onset of symptoms or hormone therapy; and Stage D symptomatic, hormone therapy (orchiectomy, antiandrogens, luteinizing hormone, releasing hormone analogues). Combination chemotherapy can be used in hormone-resistant cases.

C. Prostatitis:

1. **Acute bacterial prostatitis:**
   a. Symptoms: fever, chills, perineal and suprapubic discomfort, dysuria, and inhibited urinary voiding
   b. Treatment: Septra, norfloxacin, ciprofloxacin

c. Organisms: *E. coli/Klebsiella* and *Chlamydia trachomatis* are thought to be the major causes of nonbacterial prostatitis.

2. **Chronic prostatitis:**
   a. Symptoms: Either asymptomatic or symptoms are less prominent than in acute bacterial prostatitis.
   b. Investigation: Perform a three-part urine culture (third after prostatic massage).
   c. Treatment: Effective treatment is poor. Consider the same drugs as those used to treat acute bacterial prostatitis.

SUGGESTED READING

Barry MJ, Roehrborn CG: Benign prostatic hyperplasia. *BMJ* 323(7320): 1042-1046, 2001.

Batstone GR, et al: Chronic prostatitis. *Curr Opin Urol* 13(1):23-29, 2003.

Cook NR, et al: β-Carotene supplementation for patients with low baseline levels and decreased risk of total and prostate cancer. *Cancer* 86(9):1783-1792, 2001.

Harris R, Lohr KN: Screening for prostate cancer: an update of the evidence for the U.S. Preventive Services Task Force. *Ann Intern Med* 137(11):917-929, 2002.

Rosenberg J, Small EJ: Prostate cancer update. *Curr Opin Oncol* 15(3):217-221, 2003.

Thomson IM, et al: The influence of finasteride in the development of prostate cancer. *N Engl J Med* 349(3):213-222, 2003.

Chapter 129

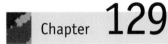

Ear, Nose, and Throat Problems

> "Doc, I can hardly hear and my head is spinning."

CLINICAL CASE PROBLEM 1:

A 38-Year-Old Female with a Feeling of Dizziness and Imbalance

A 38-year-old female comes to your office with a 1-year history of episodic dizziness, ringing in both ears, a feeling of fullness, and hearing loss. The symptoms come on every 1-2 weeks and usually last for 12 hours. Nausea and vomiting are present. When asked to describe the dizziness, the patient says that "the world is spinning around me."

On physical examination, the patient has horizontal nystagmus. The slow phase of the nystagmus is to the left, and the rapid phase is to the right. Audiograms

reveal bilateral sensorineural hearing loss in the low frequencies.

■ SELECT THE BEST ANSWER TO THE FOLLOWING QUESTIONS:

1. What is the most likely diagnosis in this patient?
   a. vestibular neuritis
   b. acute labyrinthitis
   c. benign positional vertigo
   d. orthostatic hypotension
   e. Ménière's disease

2. The treatment of this disorder includes which of the following:
   a. decrease caffeine intake
   b. decrease alcohol intake
   c. use a thiazide diuretic
   d. use an antiemetic for nausea and vomiting
   e. all of the above
   f. none of the above

CLINICAL CASE PROBLEM 2:
A 23-YEAR-OLD FEMALE WHO IS DIZZY

A 23-year-old female comes to your office with a 6-month history of dizziness. She "feels dizzy" when she stands up (as if she is going to faint). The sensation disappears within a minute.

She has a history of major depression. You started her taking doxepin 6 months ago, and she has improved much since that time.

The patient's blood pressure is 140/90 mm Hg sitting and decreases to 90/70 mm Hg when she stands. There is no ataxia, no nystagmus, and no other symptoms.

3. What is the most likely diagnosis in this patient?
   a. vestibular neuronitis
   b. acute labyrinthitis
   c. benign positional vertigo
   d. orthostatic hypotension
   e. Ménière's disease

4. What is the best treatment for the patient described in Clinical Case Problem 2?
   a. an antiemetic
   b. education and reassurance
   c. a thiazide diuretic
   d. a change in the antidepressant
   e. b and d

CLINICAL CASE PROBLEM 3:
A 30-YEAR-OLD MALE WHO BECOMES DIZZY WHEN HE ROLLS OVER

A 30-year-old male comes to your office for assessment of "dizziness." The dizziness occurs when he rolls over from the lying position to either the left side or the right side. It also occurs when he is looking up. He describes a sensation of "the world spinning around" him. The episodes usually last for 10-15 seconds. They have been occurring for the past 6 months and occur on average 1-2 times per day.

5. What is the most likely diagnosis in this patient?
   a. vestibular neuronitis
   b. acute labyrinthitis
   c. positional vertigo
   d. orthostatic hypotension
   e. Ménière's disease

6. What is the treatment of choice for the patient described in Clinical Case Problem 3?
   a. avoidance of alcohol and caffeine
   b. dimenhydrinate
   c. a thiazide diuretic
   d. reassurance and simple exercises
   e. endolymphatic surgery

CLINICAL CASE PROBLEM 4:
A 39-YEAR-OLD FEMALE WITH UNRELENTING DIZZINESS ASSOCIATED WITH NAUSEA AND VOMITING

A 39-year-old female comes to your office with a 4-day history of "unrelenting dizziness." The dizziness is associated with nausea and vomiting. There has been no hearing loss, no tinnitus, and no sensation of aural fullness. The patient has just recovered from an upper-respiratory tract infection.

On examination, nystagmus is present. The slow phase of the nystagmus is toward the left, and the rapid phase of the nystagmus is toward the right. There is a significant ataxia present.

7. What is the most likely diagnosis in this patient?
   a. vestibular neuronitis
   b. acute labyrinthitis
   c. benign positional vertigo
   d. orthostatic hypotension
   e. Ménière's disease

8. What is the treatment of choice for the patient described in Clinical Case Problem 4?
   a. avoidance of alcohol and caffeine
   b. a thiazide diuretic
   c. endolymphatic surgery
   d. reassurance and antiemetics
   e. none of the above

CLINICAL CASE PROBLEM 5:
A 26-YEAR-OLD FEMALE WITH SEVERE DIZZINESS, ATAXIA, AND HEARING LOSS

A 26-year-old female comes to your office with a 6-day history of severe dizziness associated with ataxia and right-sided hearing loss. She had an upper-respiratory tract infection 1 week ago. At that time her right ear felt plugged.

On examination, there is fluid behind the right eardrum. There is horizontal nystagmus present with the slow component to the right and the quick component to the left. Ataxia is present.

9. What is the most likely diagnosis in this patient?
   a. vestibular neuronitis
   b. acute labyrinthitis
   c. benign positional vertigo
   d. orthostatic hypotension
   e. Ménière's disease

10. What is the treatment of choice for the patient described in Clinical Case Problem 5?
    a. avoidance of caffeine and alcohol
    b. a thiazide diuretic
    c. endolymphatic surgery

d. rest and antiemetics
e. none of the above

11. What is the most common cause of sensorineural hearing loss in the adult population?
a. Ménière's disease
b. chronic otitis media
c. presbycusis
d. otosclerosis
e. mastoiditis

12. What is the most common cause of conductive hearing loss in adults who have normal-appearing tympanic membranes?
a. Ménière's disease
b. chronic otitis media
c. presbycusis
d. otosclerosis
e. mastoiditis

CLINICAL CASE PROBLEM 6:

A 37-YEAR-OLD FEMALE WITH INTERMITTENT HEARING LOSS

A 37-year-old female comes to your office for assessment of hearing loss. She has had problems intermittently for the past 12 months.

On examination, the Weber tuning fork test lateralizes to the right ear, and the Rinne tuning fork test is negative in the right ear (bone conduction is greater than air conduction [BC>AC]).

13. This suggests which one of the following hearing losses?
a. a right-sided conductive hearing loss
b. a left-sided conductive hearing loss
c. a right-sided sensorineural hearing loss
d. a left-sided sensorineural hearing loss
e. a or d

CLINICAL CASE PROBLEM 7:

A 43-YEAR-OLD MALE WITH HEARING LOSS LATERALIZED TO THE LEFT EAR

A 43-year-old male comes to your office for assessment of hearing loss. He has had hearing difficulties for the past 4 years.

On examination, the Weber tuning fork test lateralizes to the left ear. The Rinne tuning fork test is positive (AC>BC).

14. This suggests which one of the following hearing losses?
a. a right-sided conductive hearing loss
b. a left-sided conductive hearing loss

c. a right-sided sensorineural hearing loss
d. a left-sided sensorineural hearing loss
e. b or c

15. Which of the following statements is (are) true regarding the condition of acute mastoiditis?
a. it is a complication of acute otitis media
b. it most likely is caused by *Streptococcus pneumoniae*
c. otalgia, aural discharge, and fever are characteristically seen 2-3 weeks after an episode of acute suppurative otitis media
d. none of the above statements are true
e. a, b, and c are true

CLINICAL CASE PROBLEM 8:

A 42-YEAR-OLD WOMAN WITH FACIAL PAIN

A 42-year-old woman comes to your office complaining of severe facial pain in the region of her right maxilla, fever, and a purulent discharge from her right nose, all of which started after a recent upper-respiratory infection. She is taking no medications and has no known drug allergies. Her temperature is elevated to 101° F. There is tenderness over the right maxillary sinus and a greenish discharge in her right nares. The rest of her examination is normal.

16. Which of the following statements concerning sinusitis is (are) true?
a. the most common causes of sinusitis are allergic sinusitis and viral sinusitis
b. rhinovirus is the most common cause of viral sinusitis
c. viral sinusitis often is accompanied by fever, malaise, and systemic symptoms
d. a and b only
e. a, b, and c are true

17. Acute bacterial sinusitis is caused most commonly by which of the following organisms?
a. *S. pneumoniae*
b. *Haemophilus influenzae*
c. *Moraxella catarrhalis*
d. *S. pyogenes*
e. *Staphylococcus aureus*

18. Which of the following is the most predictive factor distinguishing viral sinusitis and bacterial sinusitis?
a. thick and greenish nasal discharge
b. facial pain
c. degree of fever
d. location of the pain
e. systemic symptoms

19. What is the antibacterial drug of first choice for moderate to severe acute bacterial sinusitis?
   a. amoxicillin/clavulanic acid (10-14 day course)
   b. Bactrim/Septra (10-14 day course)
   c. cefuroxime (10-day course)
   d. ciprofloxacin (10-14 day course)
   e. erythromycin (10-day course)

20. Which of the following anatomic forms of acute bacterial sinusitis is most serious?
   a. maxillary sinusitis
   b. ethmoidal sinusitis
   c. frontal sinusitis
   d. mandibular sinusitis
   e. anterior sinusitis

CLINICAL CASE MANAGEMENT PROBLEM

Describe the long-term complications of otitis media.

 ANSWERS:

1. e. This patient has Ménière's disease. The classic features of Ménière's disease are recurrent episodes of vertigo, fluctuating sensorineural hearing loss, tinnitus (ringing or buzzing in the ears), and aural fullness in the affected ear.

Ménière's disease is associated with vertigo typically lasting hours, not minutes or days. Low-tone sensorineural hearing loss also occurs. The fluctuating hearing may not be related temporally to the vertigo. In many cases, the tinnitus and fullness become severe just before the vertigo attack begins.

To make the diagnosis of Ménière's disease, the characteristic pattern of vertigo lasting a matter of hours, as well as sensorineural hearing loss, must be present. One additional factor (low-frequency hearing loss, aural fullness, or buzzing tinnitus) also should be present.

2. e. Some patients with Ménière's disease are acutely sensitive to alcohol, caffeine, or both. In these patients, alcohol and caffeine obviously should be avoided.

Ménière's disease also is known as endolymphatic hydrops. This suggests that a buildup of fluid in the endolymphatic system may be responsible for the development of the acute attack. Thus the use of a mild diuretic such as hydrochlorothiazide is a reasonable treatment (especially for patients that are having frequent attacks). A low-salt diet and alcohol restriction also is recommended.

The use of an antinauseant such as droperidol intramuscularly (IM), chlorpromazine IM, or dimen-hydrinate IM or by mouth (PO) may be extremely effective in the treatment of the acute attack. Anti-anxiety medications also have been found to be helpful in some cases. Surgery is reserved for patients who do not respond to medical management.

3. d. This patient has orthostatic hypotension. This Clinical Case Problem description illustrates the importance of obtaining an accurate history in the patient who complains of "feeling dizzy." In any patient who has this complaint, it is important to ask four specific questions: (1) Can you describe your dizziness? (2) If you had "a dollar's worth of dizziness," how much would be a sensation of the "world spinning around you," and how much would be a sensation of "things going black in front of you and a feeling that you're about to pass out?" (3) How long does the feeling of dizziness last: seconds, minutes, or hours? and (4) Are there any other symptoms present when you feel dizzy such as deafness, ear fullness, or ringing in the ears?

Orthostatic hypotension typically is initiated after standing up suddenly or, in many cases, is experienced after the patient has been up for a long time, often in closed quarters or crowded shopping malls. The feeling described is that of a subjective dizziness and is closely related to a simple faint or a syncopal episode. It often is accompanied by nausea. It is not associated with any other neurologic sensations or ear symptoms.

In this Clinical Case Problem the orthostatic hypotension is almost certainly associated with the beginning of the tricyclic antidepressant therapy 6 months ago.

4. e. The most important treatment in this patient is to reassure the patient and explain how the symptom can be minimized by slowly assuming the upright position.

Because the orthostatic hypotension developed after the initiation of the tricyclic antidepressant, doxepin, it would be reasonable to switch to an antidepressant with fewer alpha-adrenergic side effects. A good choice would be one of the new selective serotonin reuptake inhibitors such as sertraline, fluoxetine, or paroxetine.

5. c. This patient has positional vertigo, a disorder that consists of brief episodes (lasting anywhere from 2 to 10 seconds) usually caused by either rolling over toward either the right or the left when supine or looking up, such as when searching for something on a shelf.

The cause of positional vertigo is unknown but is thought to be either idiopathic or caused by trauma.

6. **d.** The treatment of choice for the patient discussed in Clinical Case Problem 3 is reassurance and the prescription of the following simple exercises:

Step 1: The patient lies on his back with his head hanging down and to the right. If this does not cause vertigo, proceed to Step 2. If it does cause vertigo, wait until it subsides. The patient then rotates his head and body slowly to the right (clockwise) until a complete 360-degree rotation is made. If further vertigo occurs, the rotation is halted until the vertigo subsides. Then the rotation is continued. If there is no vertigo after one rotation, proceed to Step 2. If vertigo reoccurs, repeat clockwise rotation until it is gone.

Step 2: The patient lies on his back with his head hanging down and to the left. If this does not cause vertigo, the exercise is finished. If vertigo occurs, wait until it subsides. Then the patient slowly rotates his head and body 360 degrees to the left (counter-clockwise). This maneuver is repeated until the vertigo is gone.

Step 3: The patient should avoid the head-dependent position for 24 hours. The exercises can be repeated at home if the positional vertigo reoccurs.

Performance of these exercises three of four times in a row (three or four times a day) often provides dramatic relief, but improvement in symptoms sometimes takes up to 10 days to occur.

Even if the exercises are not prescribed or prescribed and not performed, the condition tends to resolve with time (usually several weeks to a few months).

7. **a.** This patient has a left-vestibular neuronitis. The etiology of this disorder commonly is associated with a viral infection (such as adenovirus) following a respiratory tract infection and involves some portion of the vestibular system but with total sparing of the cochlear area. It must commonly affects young or middle-aged adults.

The disorder consists of severe vertigo with associated ataxia and nausea and vomiting. There is no hearing loss, no aural pain, and no other symptoms. Recovery usually takes 1-2 weeks.

8. **d.** The treatment of choice for a patient with vestibular neuronitis is rest, reassurance, and antiemetics. Antiemetics such as droperidol, chlorpromazine, or dimenhydrinate may be given for symptomatic relief of the vertigo; however, they should be used with caution because they may mask other less benign conditions. Rest and reassurance are sufficient in most cases.

9. **b.** This patient has acute labyrinthitis. Acute labyrinthitis usually follows an upper-respiratory tract infection accompanied by middle ear effusion. The disorder probably represents a chemical irritation of the inner ear from middle ear fluid. The features of acute labyrinthitis are similar to that of vestibular neuronitis, except it includes significant sensorineural hearing loss (with a conductive component if a middle ear effusion is present) and severe vertigo that lasts several days.

10. **d.** The treatment of choice for acute labyrinthitis includes rest, antiemetics, and, if the etiology is bacterial, antibiotics. Bacterial labyrinthitis may complicate serous labyrinthitis if antibiotics are not administered. Amoxicillin would be a good first-line agent for antibiotic prophylaxis. If symptoms do not improve, the addition of clavulanic acid to amoxicillin would be a reasonable second choice.

11. **c.** Hearing loss can be divided into sensorineural hearing loss and conductive hearing loss. The most common cause of sensorineural hearing loss in adults is presbycusis, a gradual deterioration that begins after the age of 20 years in the highest frequencies and often involves all speech frequencies by the sixth and seventh decades of life. The impaired hearing associated with presbycusis stems from degenerative changes in the hair cells, auditory neurons, and cochlear nuclei. Tinnitus is a common complaint.

Sound amplification with an electrical hearing aid does benefit some patients with relatively good speech discrimination.

12. **d.** The most common cause of conductive hearing loss in adults who have normal-appearing tympanic membranes is otosclerosis. Otosclerosis is a localized disease of the otic capsule, reducing ankylosis or fixation of the stapes footplate. The resulting conductive hearing loss starts insidiously in the third and fourth decades of life and progressively involves both ears in 80% of individuals. Otosclerosis, an inherited disease, is more common in whites and in patients with osteogenesis imperfecta.

13. **a.** Facts for Question 13: (1) BC>AC: This indicates that this is a conductive hearing loss; (2) in conductive hearing loss, the Weber test lateralizes to the affected ear and because the Weber test lateralized to the right ear in this patient, she has a unilateral right-sided conductive hearing loss.

14. **c.** The characterization of hearing loss can be localized by a combination of the Weber test and the Rinne test.

In the Weber test, placement of a 512-Hz tuning fork on the skull in the midline or on the teeth stimulates both cochleae simultaneously. If the patient has a conductive hearing loss in one ear, the sound will be perceived loudest in the affected ear (i.e., it will lateralize). When a unilateral sensorineural hearing loss is present, the tone is heard in the unaffected ear.

The Rinne test compares AC with BC. Normally AC is greater than BC. Sound stimulation by air in front of the pinna normally is perceived twice as long as sound placed on the mastoid process (AC>BC). With conductive hearing loss, the duration of AC is less than BC (i.e., negative Rinne test). In the presence of sensorineural hearing loss, the duration of both AC and BC are reduced; however, the 2:1 ratio remains the same (i.e., a positive Rinne test).

Facts for Question 14: (1) AC is greater than BC; therefore, this is a sensorineural hearing loss; (2) the Weber test lateralizes to the left ear, and in sensorineural hearing loss the Weber test lateralizes to the unaffected ear; therefore, in this case, the right ear is the affected ear. This is a unilateral right-sided sensorineural hearing loss.

15. e. Acute mastoiditis is a complication of acute otitis media that develops as a result of the retention of pus in the mastoid area. Acute mastoiditis is most commonly caused by *S. pneumoniae. S. pyogenes* and *S. aureus* are other recognized causes.

The inflammatory process in acute mastoiditis results in the destruction of bony septa (almost an osteomyelitislike process), and, as a result, there is a coalescence of mastoid air cells. This leads to subsequent erosion of the mastoid process of the petrous temporal bone.

The symptoms of acute mastoiditis include otalgia, aural discharge, and fever. These symptoms usually appear 2-3 weeks after an episode of acute suppurative otitis media. Examination reveals severe mastoid tenderness, lateral displacement of the pinna, and postauricular mastoid swelling secondary to the periosteal abscess. The treatment of choice is ceftriaxone (with or without metronidazole) and surgical drainage (for a subperiosteal abscess).

16. e. The most common causes of acute rhinosinusitis are allergic and viral. It is often extremely difficult to distinguish between the two types, although a seasonal sinusitis points to allergic sinusitis, as do symptoms such as itching and redness of the eyes.

Viral rhinitis and sinusitis may be accompanied by systemic systems including fever, chills, facial pain, malaise, and fatigue. The viruses most commonly responsible for viral sinusitis are (in order of frequency) rhinovirus, adenovirus, parainfluenzae, and influenzae.

17. a. The organisms most commonly implicated in acute bacterial sinusitis include *S. pneumoniae* (the most common), *H. influenzae, M. catarrhalis,* and *S. pyogenes.* Other organisms implicated include *S. aureus* and anaerobic organisms.

Chronic sinusitis is most often associated with *S. aureus, H. influenzae,* and anaerobic organisms.

18. a. Bacterial sinusitis can be distinguished from viral sinusitis by the thick, greenish discharge that accompanies the congestion.

19. a. The use of antibiotics in the treatment of acute sinusitis is controversial. Few well-designed, large, randomized controlled trials exist, particularly in primary care settings. Those that have been done demonstrate no better improvement in mild to moderate sinusitis with antibiotic therapy.

The antibiotic treatment of choice for moderate to severe acute bacterial sinusitis is at minimum a 10-14 day course of amoxicillin/clavulanic acid. Second-line antibiotics include trimethoprim-sulfamethoxazole (Septra/Bactrim), cefaclor (Ceclor), cefuroxime (Ceftin), and ciprofloxacin (particularly useful in repeat infections). The use of antihistamines, decongestants, and intranasal steroids are also options as adjunctive or primary therapy.

20. c. The most serious form of acute sinusitis is frontal sinusitis, which manifests as pain, tenderness, and edema of the anterior cortex of the frontal sinus. Acute frontal sinusitis usually necessitates use of high-dose intravenous antibiotics and decongestants.

Cases of chronic sinusitis not responsive to antibiotics require endoscopic sinus surgery.

SOLUTION TO THE CLINICAL CASE MANAGEMENT PROBLEM

The long-term complications of chronic otitis media include the following: (1) seventh nerve paralysis; (2) labyrinthitis; (3) petrositis; (4) intracranial suppuration; and (5) cholesteatoma.

The major complication of acute otitis media is acute mastoiditis.

SUMMARY OF EAR, NOSE, AND THROAT PROBLEMS

A. Vertigo:
1. **Ménière's disease:**
   a. Symptoms: vertigo (lasting hours), hearing loss, tinnitus, aural fullness
   b. Treatment: avoidance of caffeine, avoidance of alcohol, low-dose hydrochlorothiazide, antiemetics
2. **Acute labyrinthitis:**
   a. Symptoms: vertigo (lasting days) and associated hearing loss usually follow an upper-respiratory tract infection in which there is a middle ear effusion
   b. Treatment: rest, antiemetics, antibiotics if middle ear fluid is infected
3. **Vestibular neuronitis:**
   a. Symptoms: vertigo (lasting days), no hearing loss, no ear pain, no other symptoms; may result from upper-respiratory tract infection
   b. Treatment: rest, reassurance, antiemetics
4. **Positional vertigo:**
   a. Symptoms: vertigo (lasting for seconds), also associated with rolling over toward the left or the right when supine or when looking up
   b. Treatment: reassurance, simple exercises

B. Orthostatic hypotension:
1. Symptoms: not true vertigo (rather a sensation of lightheadedness or faintness) on assuming the upright position; often associated with antihypertensive and antidepressant medications
2. Treatment: reassurance, change in medications to one with fewer alpha-blockade properties and fewer orthostatic side effects

C. Hearing loss:
1. **Sensorineural hearing loss:**
   a. 80% of hearing loss in the United States. The pathology usually is a disorder affecting the cochlea and auditory nerves with the perception of a "distorted sound." The deficit is usually greater in the higher frequencies. There are usually degenerative changes in the hair cells, auditory neurons, and cochlear nuclei.
   b. The most common cause is presbycusis, which is a gradual deterioration that starts with high-frequency loss and often involves all speech frequencies by the sixth or seventh decade.
   c. Treatment is provision of a hearing aid, which may benefit patients with relatively good speech discrimination.
2. **Conductive hearing loss:**
   a. Pathologic condition/causation: Conductive hearing loss involves either chronic serous otitis media or otosclerosis. Otosclerosis results as a localized disease of the otic capsule where new spongy bone replaces normal bone, producing ankylosis or fixation of the stapes footplate.
   b. Treatment: The treatments for the chronic causes of conductive hearing loss are usually surgical.
   c. Interpretation of hearing loss: (i) audiogram and (ii) Weber test or Rinne test

D. Sinusitis:
1. Possible pathologic conditions include allergic, viral, bacterial; and other organisms.
   a. Rhinovirus is the most common viral cause, followed by adenovirus.
   b. *S. pneumoniae* is the most common bacterial cause, followed by *H. influenzae* and *M. catarrhalis*.
2. Symptoms: fever, chills, malaise, fatigue, facial pain
3. Bacterial sinusitis is distinguished from viral sinusitis mainly by the presence of thick, greenish nasal discharge.
4. Treatment: mild disease requires no antibiotics; only symptomatic therapy with antihistamines/decongestants, and/or intranasal steroids. Amoxicillin/clavulanic acid combination (10-14 days) or Floxin (for recurrent diseases) are reasonable drugs of choice for moderate to severe acute bacterial sinusitis.

SUGGESTED READING

Baloh RW: Vertigo. *Lancet* 352(9143):1841-1846, 1998.
Dykewicz MS: 7. Rhinitis and sinusitis. *J Allergy Clin Immunol* 111(2 Suppl):S520-529, 2003.
Elden LM, Potsic WP: Screening and prevention of hearing loss in children. *Curr Opin Pediatrics* 14(6):723-730, 2002.
El-Kashlan HK, Telia SA: Diagnosis and initiating treatment for peripheral system disorders: imbalance and dizziness with normal hearing. *Otolaryngol Clin N Am* 33:563-578, 2000.
Ioannidis JP, Lau J: Technical report: evidence for the diagnosis and treatment of acute uncomplicated sinusitis in children: a systematic overview. *Pediatrics* 108(3):E57, 2001.
Mucha SM, Baroody FM: Sinusitis update. *Curr Opin Allergy Clin Immunol* 3(1):33-38, 2003.
Osguthorpe JD: Adult rhinosinusitis: diagnosis and management. *Am Fam Physician* 63:69-71, 2001.
Parnes LS, et al: Diagnosis and management of benign paroxysmal positional vertigo (BPPV). *CMAJ Canadian Medical Association Journal* 169(7):681-693, 2003.
Strupp M, Arbusow V: Acute vestibulopathy. *Curr Opin Neurol* 14(1):11-20, 2001.
Yueh B, et al: Screening and management of adult hearing loss in primary care: scientific review. *JAMA* 289(15):1976-1985, 2003.

Chapter 130

Common Skin Cancers

> "Doc, you mean if you don't freeze that little spot I might get cancer?"

CLINICAL CASE PROBLEM 1:

A 68-Year-Old Female Who Loves Sunbathing

A 68-year-old female comes to your office and asks you to examine three shiny, pearly, semi-translucent, red nodules on her upper back. She is a light-skinned individual of Northwestern European descent. When asked if her back was ever exposed to the sun, she replied she had been sunbathing since her teens in as a skimpy bathing suit as the law permitted. When she was younger she felt a total body tan was sexy, and she still felt a tan was a sign of good health; even now at her age she thought sunbathing was a good way to get the vitamin D she needed for her old bones. In fact, she had just come from the beach.

■ SELECT THE BEST ANSWER TO THE FOLLOWING QUESTIONS:

1. Which of the following is the most likely cause of the nodules on her back?
   a. squamous cell carcinoma
   b. actinic keratosis
   c. basal cell carcinoma
   d. nodular melanoma
   e. sand flea bites

2. If left untreated the most likely outcome of the condition described in Clinical Case Problem 1 is:
   a. metastasis to bone
   b. metastasis to the liver
   c. increased size
   d. a and c
   e. b and c

CLINICAL CASE PROBLEM 2:

A 70-Year-Old Male Office Worker Who Surfed As a Youth

During a routine examination you note a circular, pinkish spot with a diameter of ¼ inch on the face of a 70-year-old patient. When you rub your finger across it you note it is dry and rough. Your patient tells you that on occasion it will become scaly and that it appeared and disappeared several times during the course of the past year before finally becoming permanent.

3. This pinkish area is most likely which of the following?
   a. squamous cell carcinoma
   b. actinic keratosis
   c. basal cell carcinoma
   d. nodular melanoma
   e. an age-related "liver spot"

4. If left untreated the most likely outcome of the condition described in Clinical Case Problem 2 is which of the following?
   a. spreading of the affected area without malignancy
   b. development of a squamous cell carcinoma
   c. development of a basal cell carcinoma
   d. development of a melanoma
   e. spontaneous remission

5. Which of the following methods is (are) used to treat the condition described in Clinical Case Problem 2?
   a. laser surgery
   b. topical medication with or without chemical peeling
   c. curettage as desiccation
   d. cryosurgery
   e. photodynamic therapy
   f. all of the above

CLINICAL CASE PROBLEM 3:

An African American Pipe Smoker

A 58-year-old dark-skinned African American male comes to your office worried about an open sore on the left side of his lower lip that occasionally bleeds. He says he has had this sore for some 3 months. However, for at least a year before developing this open sore his lip was dry, scaly, and had become paler than the surrounding area. When asked if he smoked, he said he habitually puffed on a pipe that he kept on the left side of his mouth.

6. This open sore on his lip is most likely which of the following?
   a. squamous cell carcinoma
   b. actinic keratosis
   c. basal cell carcinoma
   d. nodular melanoma
   e. a herpes infection

7. If left untreated the most likely outcome of the condition described in Clinical Case Problem 3 is which of the following?
   a. continued intermittent bleeding from the upper skin layers with no more profound consequence

b. penetration of the cancer into deeper layers of the skin
c. development of metastatic cancers
d. a and b
e. b and c

CLINICAL CASE PROBLEM 4:
A 49-YEAR-OLD FEMALE WITH A FUNNY-LOOKING MOLE

A mammography radiology technician noted a mole in the area were her patient's bra rubbed under her left breast. She became concerned because this mole was asymmetric, had an uneven border, and was colored with various shades of brown. At the technician's recommendation the patient made an appointment with her primary care physician to examine it further. The physician made a probable diagnosis.

8. The most probable diagnosis is which of the following?
   a. an unremarkable nonmalignant mole
   b. actinic keratosis
   c. a melanoma
   d. any of the above
   e. all of the above

9. Which of the following is true about the condition described in Clinical Case Problem 4?
   a. almost all of the conditions described in Clinical Case Problem 4 are caused by overexposure to sun
   b. the number of cases is increasing
   c. the number of cases is decreasing
   d. most of the conditions described in Clinical Case Problem 4 are located on the face
   e. White people are more prone to get the condition described in Clinical Case Problem 4 under the nails, the soles of their feet, or palms of their hands than African Americans or Asians.

10. Assuming the probable diagnosis in Clinical Case Problem 4 was confirmed and proper treatment was provided, which of the following is the most accurate statement concerning the likely outcome?
    a. a high probability of death
    b. a high probability of a cure
    c. it depends on the type of condition
    d. there is no way of predicting it
    e. it will depend on the patient's eating habits

ANSWERS:

1. c. Basal cell carcinoma is the most common form of skin cancer; it affects some 800,000 Americans annually. It can present in several ways: typically as a shiny, pearly, or translucent nodule; in fair-skinned individuals the nodule is red, pink, or white, whereas it might be tan, brown, or black in more deeply pigmented individuals. Fair-skinned individuals are more susceptible. The major cause is chronic exposure to sunlight, and the prevalence of the disease is increasing. Several decades ago it most commonly was found in older men who spent a lifetime working outdoors and it usually was found on the face, hands, and arms. More recently the disease has become more common in women, and as bathing suits receded in size the area of the body in which these cancers are found increased in both sexes. Because most sunbathing is done without shoes, it is not unusual to see basal cell carcinoma of the feet.

Besides presenting as a shiny, pearly, or translucent nodule, basal cell carcinomas can present in four additional ways: (1) as an open sore that bleeds, oozes, or crusts and remains open for at least 3 weeks (such open, nonhealing sores are a very common sign of early basal cell carcinoma); (2) as a reddish patch that might crust and that might itch or hurt or provide no discomfort; (3) as a slightly elevated area with a rolled border and a crusted indentation in the center in which, as the crust enlarges, tiny blood vessels develop in the center; and (4) as a white or yellow-tinted, sometimes waxy area with poorly defined borders, in which the skin appears shiny and tight. This is the least frequent sign but also may denote the presence of a particular aggressive type of basal cell carcinoma.

2. c. These cancers arise in the basal cells of the epidermis and rarely metastasize. If left untreated they will continue to grow into an increasingly unsightly mass on the skin, but only in very rare case will they metastasize into deeper tissue and cause other morbidity or death.

Treatment may be accomplished by excision, electrodesiccation and curettage, application of liquid nitrogen, Moh's surgery, radiation, or topical 5-fluorouracil cream. An advantage of excision is that this will provide a sample for biopsy. Before using a method that will destroy the sample, a specimen must be obtained for pathologic evaluation.

3. b. This is actinic keratosis (AK), which usually develops as a scaly, crusty, slightly elevated spot on the skin in an area chronically exposed to the sun, leading to the pseudonym solar keratosis. Fair-skinned individuals are more susceptible, and AK is very common in such populations, especially if they live in sunny areas. Chronic exposure to ultraviolet light is the cause, and the damage accumulates over time; thus it more commonly appears in older people.

It has been claimed that the majority of people who live into their 80s will have developed AK. Typically AK lesions appear on areas chronically exposed to the sun such as the face, ears, neck, back of the forearms, shoulders, lips, and the scalp (the latter especially on men who are bald or shave their heads). The lesions tend to start out as small circular individual spots that develop slowly, even appearing then disappearing and reappearing several times until fully established. These affected areas are often flat, but sometimes slightly elevated, always are rough, and will develop white scales that tend to come and go. They usually have a color similar to the normal skin with slightly changed pigments. Thus in fair-skinned individuals they usually have a light pinkish hue but sometimes are a deeper red or even a rusty brown or tannish color. In highly pigmented individuals they sometimes are lighter in color than the surrounding area. Several AKs may appear at the same time, and as they mature they create an area of scaly patches rather than discrete little circles.

4. a. The most likely outcome is that the affected area will increase but it will not undergo a malignant transformation. However, some 5% will undergo a malignant transformation, most commonly into a squamous cell carcinoma; so AK should be treated. AKs on the lip, known as actinic cheilitis, have a propensity for developing into a particularly aggressive type of squamous cell cancer and are therefore the most dangerous.

5. f. All the methods mentioned can be used. Cryosurgery is the most common method used when a limited number of lesions are involved. Liquid nitrogen is applied, commonly via a spraying device, although a cotton-tipped applicator also can be used. The AK becomes crusted, shrinks, and falls off within a week or 2. Sometimes some pigment is lost, particularly in highly pigmented persons.

Curettage involves taking a biopsy specimen and is particularly valuable if a malignancy is suspected.

Topical medication usually is used if a large area is involved. A cream containing 5-fluorouracil is applied by the patient on a predetermined schedule. The AK usually crusts over and falls off within a few weeks. Chemical peeling is a variation on that procedure using a more corrosive agent, usually trichloracetic acid, which is applied directly to the affected area. Within a week the skin sloughs off to be replaced by new epidermis. This method requires local anesthesia and can cause temporary discoloration and irritation.

In laser surgery a laser beam is focused on the AK, removing the epidermis and even some of the deeper areas. It is a particularly effective technique for treating small narrow arrears on the face, scalp, or ears and in particular for actinic cheilitis of the lip.

In photodynamic therapy topical 5-aminolevulinic acid (5-ALA) is applied to the affected area. On the following day the medicated area is exposed to a strong light activating the 5-ALA and selectively destroying the AK. This causes little damage to the surrounding skin.

6. a. The hallmark of a squamous cell carcinoma is an open sore that will not heal. Squamous cell carcinoma is the second most common form of skin cancer, with a yearly incidence of about 200,000 cases. As with other skin cancers, most cases occur in response to chronic exposure to the sun and are far more prevalent in the elderly, fair-skinned populations. However, they also occur in areas where skin is damaged by other agents such as burns, petroleum byproducts, radiation, and chronic irritation, such as that might be inflicted by a hot pipe; in this latter case the carcinogenic chemicals in the tobacco smoke probably play a synergistic role. Indeed squamous cell carcinoma rarely is induced by sun in dark-skinned African Americans. Such highly pigmented individuals are far less likely to develop skin cancer than less pigmented people, but when they do, about two-thirds of these cancers are squamous cell carcinoma, mostly induced by non–sun-related causes of skin damage, as in the case described. In addition a small fraction of squamous cell carcinomas may arise from an inherited condition or from white patches on the tongue or inside the mouth (leukopenia).

The dry, scaly lip described as a precursor to the open sore in Clinical Case Problem 3 was actinic cheilitis. Whether caused by chronic sun exposure or other injurious factors, some form of AK is the usually precursor; on the lip this is actinic cheilitis.

7. e. Untreated cases of SCC eventually will penetrate the underlying tissue. A small but significant fraction of these will metastasize and may become fatal. This latter outcome is much more likely to occur from SCC of the lip.

Treatment is as was described for basal cell carcinoma.

8. c. This mole bore at least three of the five typical ear marks of a melanoma (the "ABCDEs"). These are asymmetry (**A**), border irregularity (**B**), coloration that is uneven (**C**), and a diameter greater than 6 mm that is atypical of moles (**D**), and elevation or enlargement (**E**). The next step would be to arrange for a biopsy and see if the diagnosis can be confirmed.

9. b. During the past decade the number of melanoma cases diagnosed has increased more rapidly than that of any other cancer. The American Cancer Society estimates that there are at least 51,000 new cases each year. Although exposure to the sun is a risk factor, most melanomas appear to start from a chronic irritation of a preexisting mole, as in Clinical Case Problem 4. As a consequence most melanomas are found on the trunk, legs, arms, and scalp—not the face. African Americans and Asians are prone to develop a variant type of melanoma that usually appears as a black or brown discoloration under their nails, the soles of their feet, or palms of their hands.

10. c. There are four types of melanomas. Of these some tend to remain located on the uppermost part of the skin. Assuming these "in situ" cases are treated early and properly, they have almost a 100% cure rate. However, some are invasive and quickly metastasize to other tissues and as a consequence are likely to be fatal. The four basic variant types are (1) superficial spreading melanoma; (2) lentigo melanoma; (3) acral lentiginous melanoma; and (4) nodular melanoma.

Superficial spreading melanoma is the most common variant, accounting for some 70% of the total. Although these spread, it tends to be along the top layers of skin, and they only dive deeper after a considerable time. As a consequence the prognosis is favorable. This is the most prevalent form in the young adults and generally is found on trunk or legs.

Most lentigo melanomas grow in a fashion similar to the superficial spreading melanomas, but they most commonly are found on areas chronically exposed to the sun and on elderly people. Presumably, sun exposure is the precipitating factor. This form most commonly occurs in tropically/semitropical climates. A lentigo melanoma variant, called lentigo maligna melanoma, exists, which is more invasive than the more common form.

Acral lentiginous melanoma also first spreads superficially but differs from the other forms in that it appears as a black or dark brown discoloration under the nails and on the soles of the feet and palms of the hands. As mentioned earlier, it rarely is found in white people.

The fourth melanoma variant is nodular melanoma. This form is invasive from the get go, and the prognosis is not good. It is often first recognized as a bump (hence the name). As a rule, this node is black but can be almost any other color except green.

Melanoma *in situ* should be excised with margins of at least 0.5 cm. Melanoma less than 1.5 mm deep should be cut out with a margin of at least 1 cm. Lesions that are from 1.5 to 4 mm deep should be removed with margins up to 2 cm. Still deeper melanomas should have margins up to 3 cm. Sentinel node biopsy is used in patients with lesions that are more than 1 mm in depth.

SUMMARY OF COMMON SKIN CANCERS

1. Most but not all types of skin cancer are induced by exposure to ultraviolet rays from the sun. Lightly pigmented people are more susceptible to all forms of sun-induced skin lesions, and in large part these cancers appear in late maturity but got their start during an individual's first two decades.
2. The incidence of and mortality from skin cancers has increased exponentially during the past few decades. This is in part the result of high-level atmospheric protective ozone depletion, secondary to the use of aerosolized fluorocarbons. Modern dress styles also permit exposure of greater amounts of skin, particularly among younger people engaged in swimming and other sports.
3. The most common form of skin cancer is basal cell carcinoma. Theses cancers seldom metastasize.
4. The second most common form is squamous cell carcinoma. These cancers have a greater chance of penetrating the basal skin layer and metastasizing than do basal cell carcinomas, but this still is a relatively rare occurrence. The most dangerous are those on the lips or mucus membranes.
5. Actinic keratosis is a skin lesion largely derived from sun exposure. It is extremely common and has about a 5% chance of becoming malignant. As a rule the resultant malignancy is a squamous cell carcinoma.
6. Melanomas are pigmented cancers often derived from preexisting moles. Melanomas are considered likely if the lesion meets one of the five "ABCDE" criteria: Asymmetry, Border irregularity, Color variegation, Diameter > 6mm, Enlargement or Elevation. There are four types: superficial spreading melanomas, lentigo maligna, acral lentiginous melanoma, and nodular melanoma. For the most part, the first three of these are *in situ* cancers—that is, although they may spread horizontally on the skin, they only penetrate to deeper layers after being present for some time. This makes them accessible for excision and permits a respectable "cure" rate, provided they are diagnosed and treated within a reasonable time. Nodular melanomas, however, immediately go deep, making metastasis likely and the prognosis poor.
7. Most melanomas are found on the trunk and legs and are not induced by exposure to the sun. The exception is lentigo melanoma, which tends to be found on the face and other sun-exposed

Continued

SUMMARY OF COMMON
SKIN CANCERS—cont'd

areas and more often arises in the elderly in a manner analogous to basal cell and squamous cell carcinomas.

8. Acral lentiginous melanoma generally arises on soles of the feet, palms of the hands, or under the nails. It is most common in highly pigmented African Americans and Asians.

9. To reduce the risk of most skin cancers, sun burns should be avoided and exposure to ultraviolet radiation should be reduced by using a sunscreen rated 15 or higher. It is particularly important to ensure that light-skinned young children are protected from overexposure to the sun.

10. To avoid mortality from skin cancer, one should periodically perform a self-exam on all areas of the body.

SUGGESTED READING

Martinez JC, Otley CC: The management of melanoma and non-melanoma skin cancer: a review for the primary care physician. *Mayo Clin Proc* 76(12):1253-1265, 2001.

Strayer SM, Reynolds PL: Diagnosing skin malignancy: assessment of predictive clinical criteria and risk factors. *J Fam Pract* 52(3):210-218, 2003.

Wong CS, et al: Basal cell carcinoma. *BMJ* 327(7418):794-798, 2003.

GERIATRIC MEDICINE

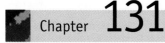 Chapter 131

Elder Abuse

"I never hit her, Doctor, but my mother keeps falling and hurting herself."

CLINICAL CASE PROBLEM 1:
A 72-YEAR-OLD FEMALE WITH A SORE RIGHT SHOULDER AND MULTIPLE BRUISES

A daughter brings her 72-year-old mother to the emergency department for assessment. The mother has Alzheimer's disease and, although able to communicate, will not answer without looking at her daughter first. The daughter tells you that her mother has had Alzheimer's disease for 5 years and has been living with her for the majority of that time. She also says that her mother is always hurting herself despite attempts to help her. Her mother lays there, tears in her eyes, and seems frightened.

The daughter tells you that her mother fell on her right shoulder approximately 3 hours ago. As you look at the patient, you notice a large bruise in the area of the head of the right humerus.

On examination, there are multiple bruises on her arms, legs, and abdomen. The head of the humerus is tender. The resident who is with you tells you that he "has things pretty well squared away." He has made the diagnosis of a rare inherited bleeding disorder on the basis of (as the nurse that is caring for the patient says) "goodness knows what."

You decide that you are not satisfied with this diagnosis and need to investigate further. Meanwhile, the patient is complaining of pain and holding her shoulder. You order an x-ray of the shoulder and diagnose a fractured head of the humerus.

SELECT THE BEST ANSWER TO THE FOLLOWING QUESTIONS:

1. At this time, what should you do?
   a. treat the patient's pain, provide a collar and cuff, and say good-bye to the patient and her daughter
   b. treat the patient's pain, provide a collar and cuff for the patient, and tell the patient that she really should be more careful
   c. treat the patient's pain and contact an orthopedic surgeon who you are sure will wish to manage this fracture with internal fixation
   d. order a complete blood count (CBC), clotting time, and all other laboratory tests vaguely associated with the hematologic and clotting system
   e. none of the above

2. What is the prevalence of elder abuse in the U.S. population?
   a. 4%
   b. 2%
   c. 10%
   d. 8%
   e. 15%

3. Regarding screening for the condition described in Clinical Case Problem 1, which of the following statements is (are) true?
   a. screening for the condition described in Clinical Case Problem 1 is recommended by the American Medical Association
   b. it is recommended that physicians incorporate routine questions related to the condition in Clinical Case Problem 1 into their daily practice
   c. direct, concrete action should be taken when a situation is identified that confirms the diagnosis described in Clinical Case Problem 1
   d. all of the above statements are true
   e. none of the above statements are true

4. Which of the following statements is (are) true when comparing the prevalence of this condition in the community setting with the prevalence of the same condition in long-term care institutions?
   a. the prevalence of this condition is much higher in institutionalized elderly patients compared to elders in the community setting
   b. the institutionalized elderly patient is at greater risk of this condition because of his or her physical or psychological status
   c. there is a high prevalence of this condition in the institutionalized elderly because of a lack of staff training and/or institutional understaffing
   d. all of the above statements are true
   e. none of the above statements are true

5. There are various forms of this condition. Which of the following would be placed in that category of forms?
   a. a physical form
   b. a psychologic form
   c. a financial form
   d. a neglect form
   e. all of the above

6. Which of the following is (are) associated with the condition described?
   a. excessive use of restraints
   b. pushing
   c. grabbing
   d. yelling
   e. all of the above

7. What is the most common manifestation of the condition described in Clinical Case Problem 1?
   a. excessive use of restraints
   b. pushing
   c. grabbing
   d. yelling
   e. slapping or hitting

8. Which of the following is not a risk factor for the condition described?
   a. unsatisfactory living arrangements
   b. low educational level of staff
   c. physical or emotional dependence on the caregiver
   d. living apart from the victim
   e. older than 75 years of age

9. Which of the following is false regarding the condition described?
   a. abusive events tend to be one-time-only events
   b. abusive events tend to escalate in the same manner in which spousal abuse escalates
   c. the situation rarely resolves spontaneously
   d. many victims refuse help
   e. serious illness, crisis, admission to an institution, or even death are all long-term sequelae of this condition

10. With respect to research priorities and the condition described, which of the following is (are) true?
    a. there should be a determination of the cause of the condition in different ethnic and cultural groups in North America
    b. there should be a comprehensive assessment of the prevalence of this condition in American long-term care institutions
    c. valid, reliable tools should be developed for use in settings such as primary care, hospital emergency departments, and long-term care institutions
    d. all of the above
    e. a and c only

11. In which of the following settings is the incidence (i.e., pick-up rate) of the condition described likely to be highest based on screening history and physical examination?
    a. in the family physician's office
    b. in the local emergency department facility
    c. in the referral-based specialist's office
    d. any of the above
    e. none of the above

12. When evaluating a patient who you feel may have been abused, what characteristics should you be looking for?
    a. a disparity in the histories between the patient and abuser
    b. a delay in treatment
    c. explanations that are vague and not realistic
    d. laboratory findings inconsistent with the history provided
    e. all of the above

CLINICAL CASE MANAGEMENT PROBLEM

Discuss a comprehensive plan to manage elder abuse in your community.

ANSWERS:

1. **e.** This patient is much more likely to have injuries inflicted as a result of abuse rather than to have a rare inherited clotting disorder or anything else.

Obviously, the patient's pain and her fractured arm have to be treated. This is not, however, the end of the treatment.

Elder abuse is extremely common and is one of those conditions that will not be diagnosed unless it is included in a differential diagnosis and thought of in all situations in which it may occur. In this case, a consult to social services is essential. With the history of physical injury, it would seem that the wisest course of action at this time is removal of the patient to a safe environment.

2. **a.** The prevalence of elder abuse in North America is estimated at 4%. This represents 700,000 to 1.2 million cases per year in those older than age 65. In many cases this abuse is long-term, repeated, or both. In one study 58% of elderly patients had suffered previous incidents of abuse.

Some studies have estimated the prevalence of elder abuse to be much higher than 4%; in reality the number might approach 10%, but there are no firm data supporting this figure.

3. d. When a situation arises that confirms elder abuse, direct action should be taken to rectify, improve, or resolve the situation.

The American Medical Association recommends that physicians screen for elder abuse in their practices and that they incorporate routine questions related to elder abuse and neglect when seeing elderly patients. For example, the physician may ask, "Is there any violence in your family that you want to tell me about?" "Has anyone tried to hurt or harm you?" "Are you afraid of anyone living in your home?" "Are you receiving enough care at home?" "Did anyone take anything from you or force you to do anything that you did not want to do?"

4. d. The prevalence of elder abuse is much higher in institutionalized elderly patients than in elderly patients who live in the community. In one study of nursing home staff, 36% had witnessed physical abuse of residents in the preceding year.

5. e. The simplest definition of elder abuse is "any act of commission or omission that results in harm to an elderly person." Elder abuse is distinguished from other crimes against elderly people by the perpetrator's occupying a position of trust. The following definition of various types elder abuse and neglect is proposed:

1. Physical abuse: assault, rough handling, sexual abuse, or the withholding of physical necessities such as food or other items of personal, hygienic, or medical care
2. Psychosocial abuse: verbal assault, social isolation, lack of affection, or denial of the person's participation in decisions affecting his or her life
3. Financial abuse: the misuse of money or property, including fraud or use of funds for purposes contrary to the needs, interests, or desires of the elderly person
4. Neglect: in active neglect, the caregiver consciously fails to meet the needs of the elderly person; in passive neglect, the caregiver does not intend to injure the dependent person. Neglect can lead to any of the other three types of abuse.

6. e. Other categories of abuse have been proposed, such as violation of rights and medical abuse (inappropriate treatment, excessive use of restraints, and withholding of treatment). Abuse may be intentional or unintentional.

7. a. As mentioned previously, a figure of 36% has been quoted as the percentage of institutionalized elderly that have been abused. In this study, the most common forms of abuse were excessive use of restraints (witnessed in the quoted study by 21% of staff); pushing, grabbing, shoving, or pinching (17%); and slapping or hitting (15%).

Psychological abuse was observed by 81% of the staff; 70% had witnessed a staff member yelling at a patient in anger; 50% had seen someone insulting or swearing at a patient; and 23% had seen a patient isolated inappropriately.

8. d. Living apart from the victim is not a risk factor for elder abuse. The risk factors for elder abuse are as follows:

A. **Situational factors:**
1. Community situational factors: (i) isolation; (ii) lack of money; (iii) lack of community resources for additional care; and (iv) unsatisfactory living arrangements
2. Institutional situational factors: (i) shortage of beds; (ii) surplus of patients; (iii) low staff-to-patient ratio; (iv) low staff compensation; and (v) staff burnout

B. **Factors relating to the victim's characteristics:** (1) physical or emotional dependence on the caregiver; (2) lack of close family ties; (3) history of family violence; (4) older than 75 years of age; and (5) recent deterioration in health

C. **Factors relating to characteristics of the perpetrator:** (1) stress caused by financial, marital, or occupational factors; (2) deterioration in health; (3) bereavement; (4) substance abuse; (5) psychopathologic illness; (6) relative of victim; (7) living with victim; and (8) long duration of care for victim (mean 9.5 years)

9. a. Elder abuse rarely resolves spontaneously; it tends to escalate in the same way as spousal abuse. Abusive events tend to be repeated and almost always will continue unless there is a major change in the environment. Such an environmental change may not occur because, in 25% to 75% of cases, victims or their families refuse help. This subsequently may result in serious illness, crisis, admission to an institution, or even death.

10. d. The research priorities for elder abuse include (1) a determination of the causes of this condition in different ethnic and cultural groups in the United States and Canada; (2) a determination of the prevalence of abuse in American and Canadian institutions; (3) the development of valid and reliable assessment tools for use in such settings as primary care, hospital emergency departments, and long-term care institutions; and (4) an evaluation of the effectiveness of interventions on the prevalence of this condition.

11. **b.** The highest incidence is likely to be observed by the local emergency department faculty. The reason is that elders are most likely to come to seek help at the time of, or shortly after, an event of abuse, and the emergency department is the most convenient place to go. This does not imply that screening should not occur at the other facilities; it should occur in all health care settings all of the time.

12. **e.** All of the above. Additional presentations may include (1) a patient who is functionally impaired coming to the emergency room or office without their primary caregiver, (2) frequent visits to the emergency room for patients with chronic diseases despite a plan for medical care and adequate resources.

SUMMARY AND SOLUTION TO THE CLINICAL CASE MANAGEMENT PROBLEM

A. A comprehensive plan to manage elder abuse should include recognition of the condition, comprehensive treatment of the condition, and a significant education component aimed at increasing public awareness of (1) the magnitude of the problem; (2) the signs and symptoms of elder abuse; and (3) the treatment options available.

B. The actual functional components of the management of elder abuse include the following:
1. Detection and risk assessment: (a) documentation of the type of abuse, the frequency and severity of abuse, the danger to the victim, and the perpetrator's intent and level of stress; (b) involvement of other health care professionals (social worker, visiting nurse, and geriatric assessment team); (c) documentation of the injuries (take photographs, if possible); and (d) assessment of the victim's overall health status, the victim's functional status, and the victim's social and financial status.
2. Assessment of decision-making capacity of the victim: Assess the cognitive state and the emotional state of the victim.
3. Measures to take if the victim is competent: (a) provide information to the victim; (b) in providing information, outline the choices or possible choices that the victim has, such as temporary relocation, home support, community agencies, and criminal charges; and (c) support the victim's decision.
4. Measures to take if the victim is not competent: (a) separate the victim and the perpetrator; (b) relocate the victim; (c) arrange advocacy services for the victim; and (d) inform a protective service agency.
5. Reduce caregiver stress.
6. Treat all medical disorders.
7. Minimize or simplify medications.
8. Seek agencies to provide respite care, support for house cleaning, personal care, and transportation.
9. Provide support groups for primary caregivers.

C. Key questions to guide intervention are as follows: (1) How safe is the patient if he or she is sent home? (2) What services of resources are available to help a stressed family? (3) Does the elderly person need to be removed to a safe environment? and (4) Does the situation need an unbiased advocate to monitor the care and finances for this patient?

Always perform an in-depth evaluation and interview when possible and carefully document physical and psychological findings. Report suspected cases to Adult Protective Services.

SUGGESTED READING

Butler RH: Warning signs of elder abuse. *Geriatrics* 54(3):3-4, 1999.

Clarke ME, Pierson W: Management of elder abuse in the emergency department. *Emerg Med Clin North Am* 17(3):631-644, 1999.

Marshall CE, et al: Elder abuse. Using clinical tools to identify clues of mistreatment. *Geriatrics* 55(2):42-44, 2000.

Paris BE, et al: Elder abuse and neglect: how to recognize warning signs and intervene. *Geriatrics* 50(4):47-51, 1995.

Reuben D, et al: *Geriatrics at your fingertips*, 5th ed. Blackwell Publishers, 2003, Oxford, England, 7, 190.

Swagerty DL Jr, et al: Elder mistreatment. *Am Fam Physician* 59(10): 2804-2808, 1999.

Chapter 132

Ethical Decision-Making Issues

> "Don't let her know, Doctor.
> It will just kill her."

CLINICAL CASE PROBLEM 1:

An 87-Year-Old Female with a Terminal Malignancy Who Has Not Been Informed of Her Condition by Her Doctors

An 87-year-old female has just been diagnosed as having inoperable cancer of the colon. The biopsied lesion that was sent to pathology following a flexible sigmoidoscopy came back as "anaplastic adenocarcinoma." A liver scan confirms metastatic disease.

A nurse on the patient's unit has told the patient's daughter and son that their mother has cancer. The daughter immediately telephones you and insists that her mother not be told. You have been the family physician to this patient for many years.

■ SELECT THE BEST ANSWER TO THE FOLLOWING QUESTIONS:

1. On the basis of the information given, what would you do?
   a. tell the daughter not to interfere; you are the boss, and you will tell the mother as soon as possible
   b. tell the daughter that this is not her decision; you will decide how the whole affair will be settled
   c. tell the daughter quite firmly that you have every intention of telling her mother when the time is right
   d. call your lawyer
   e. none of the above

CLINICAL CASE PROBLEM 2:

A 65-Year-Old Female Who Has a Terminal Illness and Has a Cardiopulmonary Arrest

You are the resident in a ward where a 65-year-old female with metastatic breast cancer has just been admitted. The patient is cachectic and exhibits Cheyne-Stokes respirations on admission. Your attending physician refuses to write a "Do Not Attempt Resuscitation" order on the chart. Three hours after admission the patient suffers a cardiopulmonary arrest and the attending physician stops the code 45 minutes after advanced cardiac life support (ACLS) has been instituted.

2. Which of the following statements concerning this case is true?
   a. this is an extremely unusual occurrence
   b. patients in the terminal phase of a malignant disease should rarely, if ever, be subjected to attempted resuscitation
   c. to not attempt resuscitation may be an ethically unacceptable decision
   d. cardiopulmonary resuscitation (CPR) has been shown to save lives in patients with terminal cancer
   e. none of the above are true

CLINICAL CASE PROBLEM 3:

A 54-Year-Old Female with Multiple Liver Metastases

You are the resident in charge of a 54-year-old female who was admitted with nausea and vomiting. The abdominal ultrasound you ordered shows multiple liver metastases from a primary pancreatic cancer. You call the attending physician, and he instructs you to "say nothing because it's better that way." The patient questions you that evening about the results of her studies.

3. At this time, what should you do?
   a. tell the patient that you know nothing
   b. tell the patient that the ultrasound machine broke
   c. tell the patient that everything will be OK
   d. tell the patient that her attending physician will break the very bad news tomorrow
   e. none of the above

CLINICAL CASE PROBLEM 4:

A 77-Year-Old Female with Malignant Melanoma

You are just completing your plastic surgery rotation. On the last day the results of a skin lesion biopsy on a 77-year-old female came back as "malignant melanoma, Clark's level IV." You also note that the patient's liver function tests are grossly elevated and conclude that she most likely already has significant metastatic disease.

You are with the attending surgeon as he sees the patient in his outpatient clinic in the afternoon. You accompany him into the room. He stands by the door flipping nervously through the chart for about 5 minutes while the patient stares at him hoping that he eventually will say something. He then looks up at the patient and says, "My dear, you have a very bad skin cancer that is probably going to kill you. It appears that it is already in your liver. If I were you I would get my affairs in order and do what you've always wanted to do as quickly as you can." You are speechless and try to console the patient after he quickly departs the room.

4. With respect to this case, which of the following statements is (are) true?
   a. this situation is not real in any way; doctors just do not do those sorts of things
   b. the remarks of the doctor described are entirely a reflection of the lack of training physicians receive in dealing with this type of scenario
   c. this situation is more common than we either admit or believe
   d. these remarks are not in any way unethical
   e. physicians are well-trained in breaking bad news; something is very wrong in this circumstance

CLINICAL CASE PROBLEM 5:

AN UNMARRIED, PREGNANT, 18-YEAR-OLD WOMAN

You have just established a family practice in the suburban area of a large city. One of your first patients is an 18-year-old girl who comes to your office for a pregnancy test. The test is positive. When you present this result to the patient she bursts into tears and requests an abortion. She is not married, does not love her boyfriend, and is sure her parents will "just die" if they find out. You have very strong feelings against abortion and are planning on becoming actively involved in your local pro-life chapter.

5. Based on this information and assuming you hold the views stated previously, what should you do?
   a. tell the patient to leave your office; you are completely opposed to her request
   b. ask the patient to find another doctor as quickly as she can; you can have nothing more to do with her care
   c. discuss the three options that the patient has: carrying through with the pregnancy and keeping the baby, carrying through with the pregnancy and giving the baby up for adoption, and therapeutic abortion; refer her for counseling and ask her to see you again following that counseling
   d. tell the patient that your religious beliefs preclude further discussion of the matter
   e. none of the above

CLINICAL CASE PROBLEM 6:

A "BRAIN DEAD" NEWBORN MALE

A male infant born at 26 weeks of gestation has been monitored in the intensive care unit for the last 8 weeks.

Unfortunately, the infant suffers a severe intraventricular hemorrhage, and the electroencephalogram demonstrates no electric activity. The infant is thought to be essentially "brain dead." When you, the attending physician, ask the parents for permission to consider discontinuing life support systems, you are accused of "just trying to get rid of our son to save money." The parents inform you that you will hear from their lawyer shortly.

6. At this time, what would you do?
   a. call your own lawyer
   b. express your displeasure at this "attitude" directly to the parents
   c. disconnect the life support system anyway
   d. arrange a family conference with significant support people for the parents present
   e. continue the life support system and promise yourself that you will not bring up the subject again

7. The right of the patient to express his or her desire for treatment following serious unforeseen complications arising out of a hospitalization is referred to as which of the following?
   a. the Patient Self-Determination Act
   b. the Desire to Live Act
   c. the Patient Emancipation Act
   d. the Patient Self-Care Act
   e. the Medical Profession Obligation Act

8. The term advance directive includes or is best described as which of the following?
   a. the legal instrument entitled "Directive to Physicians" in the Natural Death Acts enacted by various states
   b. the less formal living will
   c. the durable power of attorney
   d. all of the above
   e. none of the above

9. In the case analysis method of ethical decision making, which of the following categories must be considered?
   a. indications for medical intervention
   b. preferences of patients
   c. quality of life
   d. contextual features
   e. all of the above

10. In the case analysis method of ethical decision making, the category "Indications for Medical Intervention" includes which of the following?
    a. the concept of beneficence
    b. the concept of nonmaleficence
    c. the concept of clinical judgment

d. the concept of realistic understanding of the goals of treatment
e. all of the above

11. In the case analysis method of ethical decision making, the category "Preferences of Patients" includes which of the following?
   a. the concept of paternalism
   b. the concept of informed consent
   c. the concept of medical capacity
   d. all of the above
   e. none of the above

12. In the case analysis method of ethical decision making, the category "Quality of Life" includes which of the following?
   a. the concept of life-supporting interventions
   b. the concept of euthanasia
   c. the concept of physician-assisted suicide
   d. the concept of pain relief
   e. all of the above

13. In the case analysis method of ethical decision making, the category "Contextual Features" includes which of the following?
   a. the concept of ethical problems and public policies
   b. the concept of family, friends, and relatives
   c. the concept of the economics of care
   d. the concept of managed care plans
   e. all of the above

CLINICAL CASE MANAGEMENT PROBLEM

Using the case analysis approach to ethical decision making, consider the following case and attempt to arrive at an ethical solution.

A 71-year-old female in your care in the hospital has advanced ovarian cancer that is rapidly progressing to the point where the patient is extremely cachectic, taking almost nothing by mouth, and beginning to exhibit Cheyne-Stokes respiration. Her daughter comes to you and confronts you with the following statement: "Doctor, you are under no circumstances to offer my mother anything less than an all-out resuscitative effort in the event that she arrests while undergoing treatment in this hospital." Later on when a family meeting is held with the ethics committee of the hospital, the daughter turns to the priest of the hospital and asks, "Father don't you believe in miracles?"

ANSWERS:

1. e. The best response to this kind of request from a member of the patient's immediate family is to ask

to meet with the family as soon as possible. At that time you should gently point out the following:
1. Most patients who have a terminal disease know they have one; to refuse to discuss the patient's condition with the patient is in no one's best interest and in fact violates the Medical Code of Ethics.
2. Ask the family to be present when you discuss the results of the tests with the patient. Reassure the daughter and the rest of the family that one of the first questions you will ask of the patient is "How much do you know about your disease?" to be followed shortly by "Are you the kind of person who wants to know everything, or are you the kind of person who would rather just leave everything up to us?"

In most cases a response as described from a member of the immediate family indicates that there is some "unfinished business" that the family would rather not discuss. It is in everyone's best interest for this to be allowed to surface.

2. b. Patients in the terminal phase of a malignant disease should rarely, if ever, be subjected to a CPR attempt. It is rare that a patient with a terminal malignancy is successfully resuscitated with basic life support and ACLS protocols.

3. e. The patient has every right to ask about her results, and you have an ethical responsibility to provide her with as much information as she requests and can handle emotionally. The best plan in the case described is a call to the attending physician to let him know that the patient has "specifically asked you about the results." If the attending physician refuses to discuss the results the next day, you may have to take this to a higher level. Your best approach in this case is a telephone call to the chairman of your program and together consult your local hospital ethics committee for advice and action.

4. c. This type of situation and the remarks associated with it are a lot more common than we admit or believe. This situation can be neither accepted nor condoned.

It is at least partially attributable to the physician's lack of training in breaking bad news; however, that is not the entire picture. It is an example of a complete lack of compassion and understanding on the part of the attending physician. It is both unacceptable and unethical.

5. c. This patient has come to you as a patient, and because of the fiduciary doctor–patient relationship you have a responsibility to discuss her options with her. In this case, referral for counseling would be very appropriate and, depending on her subsequent decision, will allow you to decide how much personal involvement you wish to have. You must, however, separate your personal beliefs from your responsibilities as a physician. Even in cases in which ethical dilemmas are prominent, you usually can provide the medical care necessary for your patient's well-being and at the same time not sacrifice your personal beliefs and convictions.

6. d. The response of the parents to this request is quite typical and common. First, the parents have certainly not completed their grief work (especially if hope for a good outcome was put forward to them). Second, they may have been exposed to the criticism of their son "taking up valuable resources" potentially usable for an infant with a better prognosis by some overt or inadvertent comment. Third, parents may misinterpret something that you said or the manner in which it was said. A family conference with significant support available for the parents is the preferred method for resolving this situation. Time will be a key that will enable the parents to see the logic of your arguments and the nature and reasons for your suggestions. It is important to recognize anticipatory grieving in situations like this. Anticipatory grieving is grieving that takes place before the actual death. It is important to recognize that this may "blunt" the response of the parents at the time of the death itself.

7. a. Legislation written and passed by the U.S. Congress requires that patients be informed of their right to decide on life-supporting treatment in the event of a catastrophic complication resulting from hospitalization. This is known as the Patient Self-Determination Act.

8. d. In recent years the concept of "advance directives" has emerged and has been widely promoted as a solution to the dilemma expressed by patients concerning their potential inability to make crucial decisions about their medical care when they become mentally incapacitated. The general term advance directive covers (1) the legal instrument entitled "Directive to Physicians" enacted in the Natural Death Acts of various states in the union; (2) the less formal "living will"; and (3) the Durable Power of Attorney for Health Care (which includes medical decision-making capacity for these designated by the patient).

9. e. Clinical ethics are an intrinsic aspect of medical practice. Like diagnosis, prognosis, and treatment, ethical considerations are essential in clinical care issues. The ethics of any particular case arise out of both the facts and the values embedded in the case itself. This is most easily accomplished by dividing the considerations of the case into four categories:

(1) medical indications for interventions and treatment; (2) patient preferences (also referred to as patient autonomy); (3) quality-of-life issues; and (4) contextual features.

Details of these categories are considered later in this chapter.

10. e. Indications for medical intervention include (1) beneficence, the duty to assist patients in need; (2) nonmaleficence, the duty to "first do no harm"; (3) use of clinical judgment regarding the purely "clinical facts" of the case; (4) a realistic understanding of the goals of treatment (what exactly are you attempting to accomplish, and why are you trying to accomplish it?); (5) a realistic assessment of medical futility based on a desire to define when a proposed treatment is, in fact, useless; (6) an ability to identify the moribund patient, best defined as "eminent death"; (7) a desire to compassionately treat the patient who is terminally ill (most commonly the relevant considerations are those concerning palliative treatment in a patient with cancer or other irreversible disorder); and (8) the ability to recognize medical indications and contraindications for the performance of CPR.

Recognize that clinical judgments are made considering a matrix of facts and values that are susceptible to the influence of negative attitudes. Clinical judgments also reflect tacit inclinations about risk avoidance, skepticism about intervention, enthusiasm for innovation, peer esteem, and other personal values.

11. d. Patient preferences and patient autonomy must, by their very nature, include analysis and synthesis of the following:
1. Paternalism: overriding or ignoring a person's preferences when you believe it will benefit them or enhance their welfare
2. Informed consent: the willing acceptance of a medical intervention by a patient after adequate disclosure by the physician of the nature of the intervention. Disclosure is judged "adequate" by two standards:
   a. Information that is commonly provided by competent practitioners in the community or in the specialty
   b. Information that would allow a reasonable person to make prudent choices on their own behalf
3. Mental capacity: The ability to understand, on the basis of intelligence and comprehension, what is being said or asked of a patient on the part of that patient
4. Refusal of treatment: reasons for refusal of treatment
5. Advance directives/living wills (discussed in Answer 8)

12. **e.** Quality of life can best be defined as the subjective satisfaction expressed or experienced by an individual in his or her physical, mental, and social situation. Quality-of-life considerations include the following:

1. The distinction between quality of life (as just defined) and sanctity of life (the concept that human life is so valuable that it must be preserved at all costs, under any conditions, and for as long as possible)
2. Subjective versus objective considerations in quality of life: Who is defining quality in this case, and how does your (or someone else's) definition compare with the definition given by the patient? As well, how does a subjective determination of quality of life compare to objective criteria? These objective criteria include consideration of "restricted quality of life" and "minimal quality of life."
3. Mental retardation: Who defines quality here?
4. Issues concerning nutrition and hydration
5. Euthanasia with all its implications and definitions (active, passive, physician-assisted suicide, etc.)
6. Pain and symptom relief (especially in terminal cancer)
7. Suicide

13. **e.** Contextual features in ethical decision making are diverse, complicated, and multiple. The most important considerations include the following:

1. The possible conflict between physician responsibilities to the patient and physician responsibilities to the society. This is most clearly articulated in matters concerning cost.
2. The multiple responsibilities of physicians and methods of resolving conflict between those responsibilities: The responsibility to the patient (first and foremost); the responsibility to society; the responsibility to other health professionals; and the responsibility to self.
3. The role of the patient's next of kin in ethical decision making
4. The importance of confidentiality of patient information
5. The importance of the public welfare (i.e., is the patient a danger to others? If so, how can those "others" be identified without revealing confidential information?)
6. The concept of patient safety
7. The economics of care, including ever-decreasing health care resources, health care right versus privilege, emergency care, prospective payments and diagnostic related groups, and managed care plans

The term contextual features is also known as distributive justice.

SOLUTION TO THE CLINICAL CASE MANAGEMENT PROBLEM

A. Medical intervention:
1. Indications for medical intervention include (a) very serious and aggressive tumor; (b) advanced state of cachexia at present; (c) no likelihood that the patient will improve; and (d) symptoms objectively distressing.
2. Conclusions regarding indications for medical intervention are (a) it is very reasonable to offer interventions that will increase the comfort and reduce the pain and suffering of the patient and (b) it is illogical to offer interventions that will, in the long run, only prolong death.
B. Patient preferences:
1. Issues: (a) the patient has not been consulted as to her wishes vis-á-vis life support systems and (b) we have no indication that the wishes of the patient's daughter bear any relationship to the wishes of the patient.
2. Conclusion to patient-preference issue: The patient must, in some manner, be asked about her understanding regarding the disease process and wishes that stem from that knowledge.

C. Quality of life:
1. Issues: (a) objectively, the patient's quality of life appears to be low and decreasing daily; and (b) again, however, we have no knowledge of how the patient rates her own quality of life.
2. Conclusion to quality-of-life issue: A discussion with the patient must take place. The information that should be discussed includes the patient's knowledge of the condition and its progress, her own assessment of quality of life, and her wishes concerning treatments that are and are not acceptable.
D. Contextual features:
1. Issues: (a) in this case the main contextual feature is the insistence of the daughter to "pull out all the stops" and "spare no effort, no matter what"; and (b) no idea as to why the daughter feels this way: is there some unfinished business?
2. Conclusion regarding contextual features issue: (a) talk to the daughter; ask her why she has requested the aggressive interventions; (b) discuss with the daughter the concept of "medical futility."

Continued

SOLUTION TO THE CLINICAL CASE MANAGEMENT PROBLEM—cont'd

E. Summary of this case: This is basically an ethical situation in which the concept of indications for medical intervention indicates that aggressive resuscitative attempts are not only not indicated but also completely futile. This is counterbalanced by the concept of contextual features in which the daughter is insisting that "everything be done."

What is done will be determined by patient preferences in which the patient outlines to all not only her knowledge of the disease process and its effect on her quality of life but her desires for "heroic measures" to be or not to be undertaken on her behalf. The resolution includes a family meeting, an understanding of the patient's wishes, and comfort care.

SUMMARY OF ETHICAL DECISION-MAKING ISSUES

1. Ethical decision making can be based on a case analysis method.
2. Case analysis considers four categories: (a) indications for medical intervention; (b) patient preferences; (c) quality of life; and (d) contextual (or societal) features.
3. The most common disagreements involve indications for intervention; patient preferences; and quality-of-life disagreement between individual patient values or autonomy, indications or lack of same for treatment, and one or another of various societal pressures.
4. Golden Rule 1 of Medical Ethics: Primum non nocere—first, do no harm (nonmaleficence)
5. Golden Rule 2 of Medical Ethics: Consider first the welfare of the patient (beneficence)
6. Medical futility: A treatment that has no or an extremely remote chance of doing any good whatsoever should not be undertaken. For

purposes of security, that really should mean zero chance (as with CPR in a patient with terminal cancer with Cheyne-Stokes respiration).
7. There is absolutely no substitute for good doctor–patient communication and good interprofessional health care communication in biomedical ethics.

SUGGESTED READING

Goodman MD, et al: Effect of advanced directives on the management of elderly critically ill patients, *Crit Care Med* 26(4):701-704, 1998.

Gordon NP, Shade SB: Advanced directives are more likely among seniors asked about end-of-life preferences. *Arch Intern Med* 159(7):701-704, 1999.

Jonsen AR, et al: *Clinical ethics,* ed 3. McGraw-Hill, 1992, New York.

Kashiwagi T: Truth telling and palliative medicine. *Intern Med* 38(2):190-192, 1999.

Ott BB: Advanced directives: the emerging body of research. *Am J Crit Care* 8(1):514-519, 1999.

Post SG, et al: Physicians and patient spirituality: professional boundaries, competency, ethics, *Ann Intern Med* 132(7):578-583, 2000.

Sloan RP, et al: Religion, spirituality, and medicine. *Lancet* 53(9153): 664-667, 1999.

Chapter 133

Dementia and Delirium

> "Officer, I've lived in the same house for the past 45 years, but I can't seem to locate it today. Can you help me?"

CLINICAL CASE PROBLEM 1:

A 78-Year-Old Female with Increasing Confusion, Impairment of Memory, and Inability to Look After Herself

A 78-year-old female is brought to your office by her daughter. The patient lives alone in an apartment, and her daughter is concerned about her ability to carry on

living independently. Her daughter tells you that her mother began having difficulty with her memory 2 years ago, and since that time she has deteriorated in a slow, steady manner.

She is, however, not totally incapacitated. She is able to perform some of the activities of daily living, including dressing and bathing. When she cooks for herself, however, she often leaves burners on, and when she drives the car she often gets lost. She has had four motor vehicle accidents in the past 3 months. Her daughter became alarmed when she learned that her mother had gone to the bank and withdrawn the entire contents of her $80,000 savings account to "give to her new boyfriend." She had asked for the entire amount in $1 bills and argued with the bank teller on learning that this was impossible.

The daughter states that her mother's memory and confusion have been getting worse. Her personality has changed; her kind and caring mother now displays periods of both agitation and aggression.

On examination, the patient's "mini-mental status" examination (MMSE) is 8/30. Her blood pressure is 170/95 mm Hg, and her pulse is 84 and irregular. There is a grade II/VI systolic heart murmur heard along the left sternal edge. Examination of the respiratory system is normal. Examination of the abdomen is normal. Digital rectal examination reveals some hard stool. A detailed neurologic and musculoskeletal examination cannot be carried out.

■ SELECT THE BEST ANSWER TO THE FOLLOWING QUESTIONS:

1. Based on this history, what is the most likely diagnosis in this patient?
   a. Alzheimer's disease
   b. multiinfarct dementia
   c. major depressive disorder
   d. hypothyroidism
   e. mixed dementia

2. At this time, what would you do?
   a. order an appropriate cost-effective laboratory investigation
   b. arrange for the patient to be admitted to a chronic care facility and placate the daughter
   c. prescribe diazepam for the daughter and haloperidol for the patient
   d. refer the patient for immediate consultation with a geriatrician
   e. begin a trial of a tricyclic antidepressant

3. Which of the following diseases is the most common treatable disease confused with Alzheimer's disease in elderly patients?
   a. hypothyroidism
   b. multiinfarct dementia
   c. congestive heart failure
   d. major depressive disorder
   e. normal pressure hydrocephalus

4. Which of the following statements regarding Alzheimer's disease is true?
   a. Alzheimer's disease is present to some degree in all persons who are more than 80 years old
   b. Alzheimer's disease is a rapidly progressive dementia
   c. Alzheimer's disease is easy to differentiate from other dementias
   d. Alzheimer's disease is a pathologic diagnosis
   e. Alzheimer's disease usually has a sudden onset

5. In contrast to dementia, patients with depression often:
   a. complain about their cognitive deficits
   b. deny that their cognitive deficits exist
   c. try to conceal their cognitive deficits
   d. try to answer questions even if they do not know the answers
   e. perform consistently on tasks of equal difficulty

6. In contrast to dementia, the cognitive impairment associated with depression often:
   a. comes on more slowly
   b. comes on more rapidly
   c. is less of an impairment
   d. is not improved with the administration of an antidepressant
   e. none of the above are true

7. Diagnostic criteria for delirium include the following:
   a. disturbed consciousness
   b. cognitive change
   c. rapid onset and fluctuating course
   d. evidence of a causal physical condition
   e. all of the above

8. A cost-effective workup of a confused elderly patient does not include:
   a. a complete blood count (CBC)
   b. an electrolyte profile
   c. a plasma glucose level
   d. a computed tomography (CT) scan of the head
   e. all of the above investigations are cost-effective

9. After a complete dementia workup, you are unsure whether a patient has Alzheimer's disease or a major depressive disorder. At this time, what would you do?
   a. reexamine the patient in 3 months
   b. suggest a trial of electroconvulsive therapy
   c. arrange for the patient to be admitted to a nursing home and begin supportive psychotherapy
   d. prescribe a trial of an antidepressant
   e. none of the above

10. Which of the following is (are) an important aspect(s) of dementia management?
    a. maintaining a daily routine
    b. making the environment safe
    c. assessing family support
    d. minimizing external stimuli
    e. all of the above

11. Elderly patients frequently develop "acute confusional states." Acute confusional states also are known as which of the following?

a. dementia
b. delusional states
c. delirium
d. pseudodementia
e. pseudodelirium

12. What is the most common cause of dementia in the elderly?
    a. drug-induced dementia
    b. multiinfarct dementia
    c. pseudodementia
    d. Alzheimer's disease
    e. vascular dementia

13. What is the most common symptom and finding in patients with Alzheimer's disease?
    a. a progressive decline in intellectual function
    b. memory loss
    c. impairment in judgment
    d. impairment in problem solving
    e. impaired orientation

14. What is the most important risk factor for a patient acquiring Alzheimer's disease?
    a. history of head injury
    b. history of thyroid disease
    c. history of depression
    d. a family history of dementia
    e. history of psychiatric disease

15. Which of the following characteristics regarding the epidemiology of Alzheimer's disease is (are) true?
    a. the prevalence of Alzheimer's disease at age 65 varies from a low of 971/100,000 persons in Turku, Finland, to 10,300/100,000 persons in East Boston, Massachusetts, United States
    b. the incidence of Alzheimer's disease increases with age
    c. in the average American city or town, the prevalence of Alzheimer's disease at age 85 years is 30%
    d. there appears to be some cultural and ethnic variation in incidence and prevalence of Alzheimer's disease in the United States
    e. all of the above statements are true

16. What is (are) the histologic criteria for diagnosing Alzheimer's disease postmortem?
    a. senile plaques
    b. neuronal loss
    c. neurofibrillary tangles (NFTs)
    d. a and c
    e. all of the above

17. What pharmaceutical agents represent the best choice for treatment of Alzheimer's disease?

a. tacrine (Cognex)
b. donepezil (Aricept)
c. galanthamine (Reminyl)
d. rivastigmine (Exelon)
e. b, c, and d

18. The main predisposing factors for delirium include which of the following?
    a. age older than 65 years
    b. brain damage
    c. chronic cerebral disease
    d. b and c only
    e. a, b, and c

19. The best-documented hypothesis for delirium suggests which of the following?
    a. a serotonin deficiency
    b. a norepinephrine deficiency
    c. an acetylcholine deficiency
    d. a dopamine deficiency
    e. a catecholamine imbalance

20. What is the most important investigation for patients suspected for having delirium?
    a. a CT scan of the head
    b. a magnetic resonance imaging (MRI) scan of the head
    c. an electroencephalogram
    d. a positron emission tomography scan
    e. a CBC

21. The characteristics for mild cognitive impairment may occur in which of the following:
    a. a report by the patient (or informant) of memory loss
    b. abnormal memory performance for age (typically MMSE score of 24-28)
    c. normal general cognition
    d. normal activities of daily living
    e. all of the above

CLINICAL CASE MANAGEMENT PROBLEM

Part A: Using the mnemonic DEMENTIA and selecting at least one cause (but in some cases many causes) for each letter, construct a complete differential diagnosis of confusion in the elderly.

Part B: List and briefly describe the distinct disorders that are part of the differential diagnosis of delirium.

ANSWERS:

1. **a.** The most likely diagnosis is Alzheimer's disease. The slow, insidious course of the decline is

much more characteristic of Alzheimer's disease than of any other dementive process.

Multiinfarct dementia, in contrast, tends to produce a stepwise decline, with each step (or each decline) being temporally related to a small infarct.

Major depressive disorder tends to come on rather abruptly. This is discussed in detail in Chapter 75 and with specific relevance to the geriatric patient in Answers 5 and 6 in this chapter. Hypothyroidism always must be considered as a reversible cause of dementia, but in this case this is an unlikely cause of the symptoms.

Dementia is characterized by evidence of short-term and long-term memory impairment with impaired abstract thinking, impaired judgment, disturbances of higher cortical thinking, and personality changes. In Alzheimer's disease, short-term memory is impaired before long-term memory; consequently, patients present with repetitive thoughts or questions, forgetting daily events or people they have known for years. It is not uncommon for the "house" this patient mentioned to be the one she lived in as a child.

2. a. Alzheimer's disease is a diagnosis of exclusion. Before a patient is labeled as having Alzheimer's disease, a complete history, a complete physical examination, and a cost-effective laboratory evaluation need to be performed. It is inappropriate to arrange care in a chronic care facility and to treat patients (even with an antidepressant) until a dementia workup has been done.

An appropriate cost-effective workup of dementia includes a complete history, a complete physical examination (including a neuropsychiatric evaluation), a CBC, a blood glucose, serum electrolytes, serum calcium, serum creatinine, and serum thyroid stimulating hormone. Other tests should be done only if there is a specific indication (e.g., vitamin B_{12} and folate if macrocytosis is present). A CT or MRI scan should be performed only if there is a specific clinical indication. The likelihood of detecting a structural lesion is increased if there are focal neurologic signs or symptoms, an abrupt onset or rapid decline, onset before the age of 60 years, and concurrent medical conditions (such as cancer or use of anticoagulants).

3. d. The most common treatable disease confused with Alzheimer's disease in elderly patients is depression. It has been estimated that up to 15% of patients who are labeled with Alzheimer's disease actually have a major depressive disorder. Many more patients with Alzheimer's disease have depression as a clinical feature of the disease itself.

Depression will respond to pharmacotherapy and psychotherapy whether it is the primary diagnosis or a diagnosis secondary to Alzheimer's disease.

4. d. Alzheimer's disease is a pathologic diagnosis. The prevalence of Alzheimer's disease increases with age to a prevalence level of approximately 30% in patients older than age 80 years. It is certainly not present in all patients of any age.

The clinical progression of Alzheimer's disease is usually slow and insidious, not rapidly progressive. It is an acquired decline in memory and at least one other cognitive function (language, visual spatial, executive) sufficient to affect daily life in an alert person.

It is not easy to differentiate Alzheimer's disease from other conditions or other entities. Because of the slow and insidious onset of the disease, it often goes unnoticed by both friends and family.

5. a. In contrast to patients with dementia, patients who are depressed often complain about their cognitive deficits.

6. b. Also in contrast to dementia, the cognitive impairment associated with depression usually comes on rapidly. It is apparent that something is wrong. Other features that suggest depression include the following: (1) a personal or family history of psychiatric illness (especially major depressive disorder), bipolar affective disorder, or alcoholism; (2) depressive symptoms preceding cognitive changes (depressed mood, loss of interest or pleasure in activities, weight loss or gain, difficulty sleeping, etc.) (3) feelings of hopelessness, guilt, and/or worthlessness; and, (4) a poor affect on psychologic testing.

7. e. The *Diagnostic and Statistical Manual of Mental Disorders,* 4th edition (DSM IV) criteria for the diagnosis of delirium include the following characteristics:

In this scheme (which is expanded in the Clinical Case Management Problem), the choices offered in the question fall under the following: (1) a disturbed level of consciousness such as a decreased attention span or lack of environmental awareness; (2) cognitive change, such as a memory deficit, disorientation, or language disturbance, possibly also including visual illusions or hallucination; (3) rapid onset within hours or days with a fluctuating course; and (4) evidence of a causal physical condition.

8. e. See Answer 2.

9. d. A cautious trial of an antidepressant can be both a diagnostic test and a therapeutic trial because (1) it often can be difficult to differentiate a dementia from a depression; (2) dementia may have, as part of its symptomatology, depressive symptoms; and (3) depression is reversible, whereas dementia is not.

Selective serotonin reuptake inhibitors are the most commonly used agents for the geriatric patient. They are considered first-line choice for older patients, especially patients with heart conduction defects or ischemic disease, patients with prostatic hyperplasia, or patients with uncontrolled glaucoma. Second-line choices may include bupropion, mirtazapine, or venlafaxine. Third-line choices include nortriptyline or desipramine. These can be used for severe melancholic depression.

In an elderly patient, you want to (1) maximize the potential benefit from the antidepressant without producing an adverse drug reaction; (2) start low and go slow; and (3) select an agent that has low anticholinergic, alpha-adrenergic, and antihistaminic side effects.

10. e. The management of dementia in the elderly involves both behavioral methods and pharmacologic methods.

Regarding behavioral management, the following four principles apply to all elderly patients with a dementialike syndrome: (1) minimize external stimuli (especially external stimuli that may confuse, worry, or upset the elder); (2) establish and maintain a daily routine that does not vary by any significant degree; (3) provide support to the elder's family and offer respite care where and when needed; and (4) maximize the environmental safety of the particular residence or facility.

This latter includes attention to the maximization of lighting in the home or facility; the minimization of significant noise or distractions; the installation of handrails in hallways and rooms and at bathtub edges; and the minimization of stairs in the living accommodations of the patient.

11. c. Delirium often is referred to as an acute confusional state. (See Answer 7.)

12. d. The most common cause of dementia in the elderly is Alzheimer's disease.

The wording is important in this question. Drugs do not cause dementia; they cause delirium.

The only other cause of dementia listed in the question is multiinfarct dementia, which is equivalent to vascular dementia.

The other choice in the question, pseudodementia, is really a misnomer. Pseudodementia really represents depression that has been incorrectly diagnosed as an irreversible dementia.

13. b. Memory loss is the most common presenting feature of Alzheimer's disease, but a personality change or an impairment in the ability to perform intellectual tasks such as calculations may herald the onset.

The five major clinical manifestations of Alzheimer's disease are as follows:

1. Memory loss: Initially the memory loss is a loss for recent events only and is associated with an inability to learn new information. Recall of past events and previously acquired information becomes impaired at a somewhat later stage.
2. Language impairment: Language impairment is also common among patients with Alzheimer's disease. The term *anomia,* or "word-finding difficulty," often begins with the onset of dementia. This feature usually progresses to a transcortical, sensorylike aphasia. Severe language disturbance is a poor prognostic feature of Alzheimer's disease.
3. Visuospatial disturbance: Patients with Alzheimer's disease often are characterized by a difficulty in getting around the neighborhood or house. Practical examples of visuospatial disturbances in patients with Alzheimer's disease include difficulty following directions and getting lost in a familiar place or in familiar surroundings.
4. Loss of interest in activities: The loss of interest in activities such as personal habits or community affairs parallels the intellectual decline already discussed. This may be Alzheimer's disease first and an accompanying depression second or a primary depression manifesting itself as Alzheimer's disease.
5. Delusions and hallucinations: Delusions and hallucinations are prevalent in patients with Alzheimer's disease and tend to indicate a poor prognosis.

14. d. A family history of Alzheimer's disease is an important risk in acquiring Alzheimer's disease, especially at a younger age. Advanced age is also a risk factor, with more than 30% of those older than age 85 years developing some degree of Alzheimer's disease.

15. e. The epidemiology of Alzheimer's disease is fascinating. Because the cumulative incidence of Alzheimer's disease increases rapidly, the prevalence at age 85 in the United States averages 30% of the population (this figure includes both institutionalized and community-based elderly). There is obviously a significant difference depending on the individual's capacity to look after himself or herself, but this really becomes a circular argument.

One excellent review of the literature indicates a significant difference in prevalence depending on geographic location. For example, Turku, Finland, has a prevalence of only 971/100,000 population. East Boston has an estimated prevalence of 10,300/100,000 population. This is extremely difficult to explain, and one wonders whether there was a significant difference in diagnostic criteria or a significant difference in case-assessment criteria.

16. d. Alzheimer's disease really is a pathologic diagnosis. The National Institute on Aging's diagnostic criteria for this disease are as follows:

1. The quantity of senile plaques (age-specific): Senile plaques are microscopic lesions comprised of a significant percentage of amyloid.
2. The quantity of NFTs increases with age: NFTs, initially described in 1907, are neuronal cytoplasmic collections of tangled filaments present in abundance in the neocortex, hippocampus, amygdala, basal forebrain, substantia nigra, locus ceruleus, and other brainstem nuclei.

Although these are the two criteria on which the diagnosis of Alzheimer's disease is based, the following is a complete list of all of the microscopic lesions seen in the brain of a patient with Alzheimer's disease: (1) neuritic plaques; (2) NFTs; (3) amyloid degeneration; and (4) neuronal loss.

Most patients with Alzheimer's disease have a slight reduction in total brain weight, with the majority ranging from 900 to 1100 g. Mild to moderate cerebral atrophy often is present.

17. e. The primary treatment for patients with Alzheimer's disease includes the use of the cholinesterase inhibitors donepezil, galanthamine, and Exelon. Patients with a diagnosis of mild or moderate Alzheimer's disease should receive these medications, which increase acetylcholine levels in the brain. Only 25% of patients taking cholinesterase inhibitors show improvement, but 80% have a less rapid decline. Benefits include cognition, mood, behavioral symptoms, and daily function. Because of hepatic toxicity, tacrine would not be considered a first-line choice.

18. e. Delirium (acute confusional state) is caused by one or more organic factors that bring about widespread cerebral dysfunction.

The factors associated with delirium can be divided into the following subcategories:
1. Predisposing factors: (a) older than 65 years old; (b) brain damage; and (c) chronic cerebral disease (such as Alzheimer's disease)
2. Facilitating factors: (a) psychologic stress; (b) sleep loss or sleep deprivation; and (c) sensory deprivation or sensory overload
3. Precipitating (organic) causal factors: (a) primary cerebral diseases; and (b) systemic diseases affecting the brain secondarily, such as metabolic encephalopathies, neoplasms, infections, cardiovascular diseases, collagen vascular diseases, intoxication with exogenous substances; certain medical drugs; recreational drugs; poisons of plant, animal, or industrial origin, withdrawal from substances of abuse, alcohol, and sedative-hypnotic drugs.

One of the most common causes of delirium in the elderly is intoxication with anticholinergic drugs, such as tricyclic antidepressants given in doses that would be appropriate for a younger adult but not for a frail elderly patient.

The following are other common causes: (1) congestive cardiac failure; (2) pneumonia; (3) urinary tract infection; (4) cancer; (5) uremia; (6) hypokalemia; (7) dehydration; (8) hyponatremia; (9) epilepsy; and (10) cerebral infarction (right hemisphere).

Risk factors for delirium in hospitalized elderly patients include (1) urinary tract infections; (2) low serum albumin levels; (3) elevated white blood cell count; (4) proteinuria; (5) prior cognitive impairment; (6) limb fracture on admission; (7) symptomatic infective disease; (8) neuroleptic drugs; (9) narcotic drugs; and (10) anticholinergic drugs.

19. c. The best-documented hypothesis for delirium in the elderly suggests that the syndrome results from a widespread imbalance of neurotransmitters. It is postulated that there is a reduction in brain metabolism that results in diminished cortical function. Impairment of cerebral oxidative metabolism results in reduced synthesis of neurotransmitters, especially acetylcholine, whose relative deficiency in the brain is a common denominator in metabolic–toxic encephalopathies. Hypoxia and hypoglycemia impair acetylcholine metabolism and bring about changes in mental function. The inhibition of acetylcholine metabolism may be caused by calcium-dependent release of the neurotransmitter. Thus the cholinergic deficit is currently the most convincing pathogenic hypothesis of delirium. Numerous experimental studies have shown that the syndrome can be readily induced by anticholinergic agents.

20. e. As discussed in Answer 18, delirium is associated with many different abnormalities. One of the most important factors to rule out in the elderly is an underlying infection. Therefore a CBC would be required. It is a low-cost test that helps rule out infection, a common reversible cause of delirium in the elderly.

21. e. All of the above, although not meeting the criteria for dementia, are consistent with minimal cognitive impairment. Screening tests for patients with dementia include the MMSE and the Blessed information-memory-concentration test (IMC). Coupled with neuropsychological testing, these tests provide needed information for the diagnosis of dementia. The interpretation of scores depends on the person's age and education. A mini-mental status examination (MMSE) score of 24 or less (maximum score of 30), or an IMC test score of more than 8 (maximum score 33, minimal 0) may be an indication of an underlying dementia.

SOLUTION TO THE CLINICAL CASE MANAGEMENT PROBLEM

Part A: The following is an all-inclusive mnemonic on confusion in the elderly. This includes both reversible causes and nonreversible causes. The mnemonic is DEMENTIA.

D **D**rug intoxication (especially anticholinergic agents) but includes alcohol abuse

E **E**yes and ears (especially cataracts, diabetes mellitus, and sensorineural hearing loss)
Environment (a new environment is a sure trigger for acute confusional state.)

M **M**etabolic, including (1) hyponatremia; (2) hypokalemia; (3) hyperkalemia; (4) hypercalcemia; (5) elevated blood urea nitrogen; (6) elevated serum creatinine; and (7) elevated serum gamma glutamyl transferase (GGT) activity.

E **E**motional, including (1) major depressive disorder; (2) bipolar affective disorder; (3) schizoaffective disorder; (4) chronic schizophrenia; (5) pseudodementia (depression masking as dementia); and (6) adverse drug reaction (propranolol causes depression).
Endocrine, including (1) hypothyroidism; (2) hyperthyroidism; (3) hyperglycemia; and (4) hypoglycemia

N **N**eoplasms, including (1) benign neoplasms (rare); (2) malignancies; breast cancer, lung cancer, colon cancer, prostate cancer, lymphomas, and multiple myeloma
Neurologic: (1) normal-pressure hydrocephalus; (2) Parkinson's disease; and (3) Huntington's disease

T **T**rauma: Chronic subdural hematoma is most common. Burr holes can be lifesaving in a rural center if recognized.

I **I**nfections (in order of frequency as a cause of delirium in three groups of elderly patients):
Group 1. Infections predominating in hospitalized patients with delirium: (1) urinary tract infection; (2) bacterial pneumonia; and (3) surgical wound infections
Group 2. Infections predominating in nursing home patients who develop delirium: (1) bacterial pneumonia; (2) urinary tract infection; and (3) decubitus ulcer
Group 3. Independent, previously healthy individuals living in the community: (1) bacterial pneumonia; (2) urinary tract infection; (3) intra-abdominal infections (appendicitis, diverticulitis); and (4) infective endocarditis.

Inflammatory:
1. New onset/recurrent inflammatory bowel disease (ulcerative colitis or regional enteritis)
2. Collagen vascular disorders, including: rheumatoid arthritis and systemic lupus erythematosus
3. Musculoskeletal system
   a. Polymyalgia rheumatica (If not treated properly this can lead to serious consequences, such as blindness; for a detailed discussion see Chapter 134.)
   b. Polymyositis/dermatomyositis
4. Pericarditis
5. Pleuritis
6. Biliary colic
7. Renal colic
8. Chronic pancreatitis

A **A**nemia: (1) iron-deficiency anemia; (2) anemia of chronic disease; and (3) macrocytic anemia (vitamin B_{12} or folate deficiency)
Atherosclerotic vascular disease or cardiovascular disease: (1) myocardial infarction; (2) pulmonary embolism; (3) cerebrovascular accident (stroke); and (4) congestive cardiac failure
Alzheimer's and other dementias: (1) Alzheimer's disease; (2) multiinfarct dementia; (3) Parkinson's disease; and (4) Huntington's disease.

Part B: The distinct disorders that are part of the complex called *delirium* include the following:

1. Global disorder of cognition: this constitutes one of the essential features of delirium. In this sense, *global* refers to the main cognitive functions including (1) memory; (2) thinking; (3) perception; (4) information acquisition; (5) information processing; (6) information retention; (7) information retrieval; and (8) utilization of information.

   These cognitive deficits and abnormalities constitute an essential diagnostic feature of delirium.

2. Global disorder of attention: disturbances of the major aspects of attention are invariably present. Alertness (vigilance)—that is, readiness to respond to sensory stimuli—and the ability to mobilize, shift, sustain, and direct attention at will are always disturbed to some extent.

3. Reduced level of consciousness: This implies a diminished awareness of oneself and one's surroundings to respond to sensory inputs in a selective and sustained manner and to be able to relate the incoming information to previously acquired knowledge.

SOLUTION TO THE CLINICAL CASE MANAGEMENT PROBLEM—cont'd

4. Disordered sleep–wake cycle: Disorganization of the sleep–wake cycle is one of the essential features of delirium. Wakefulness is abnormally increased and the patient sleeps little or not at all or it is reduced during the day but excessive during the night.

5. Disorder of psychomotor behavior: A disturbance of both verbal and nonverbal psychomotor activity is the last essential feature of delirium. A patient who is delirious can be predominantly either hyperactive or hypoactive. Some patients shift unpredictably from abnormally increased psychomotor activity to lethargy and vice versa.

SUMMARY OF DEMENTIA AND DELIRIUM

The answer to Part A of the Clinical Case Management Problem (the mnemonic for confusion in the elderly) serves as the summary for this problem.

SUGGESTED READING

Chan D, Brennan NJ: Delirium making the diagnosis, improving the prognosis. *Geriatrics* 54(3):28-30, 39-42, 1999.

Cummings JL, et al: Guidelines for managing Alzheimer's disease—Part II. *Am Fam Physician* 65:2263-2276, 2002.

Doody RS, et al: Practice parameter: management of dementia (An evidence based review): Report of the quality standards subcommittee of the American Academy of Neurology: *Neurology* 56(a):1154-1166, 2001.

Inoyue S, et al: A multi component intervention to prevent delerium in hospitalized older patients. *N Engl J Med* 340(9):669-676, 1999.

Jonston CB, et al: Geriatric medicine. In: Tierny LM, et al, eds.: *Current medical diagnosis and treatment 2002*, 42nd ed. McGraw-Hill, 2003, New York, 41-58.

Kawas C: Early Alzheimer's disease. *N Engl J Med* 349:1056-1063, 2003.

Chapter 134

Polymyalgia Rheumatica and Temporal Arteritis

> "Well, Doctor, I guess arthritis has finally caught up with me."

CLINICAL CASE PROBLEM 1:

AN 82-YEAR-OLD FEMALE WITH ACHING AND STIFFNESS IN THE SHOULDER AND HIP GIRDLES

An 82-year-old female comes to your office with a 6-month history of "stiffness" and "aching" in the shoulders and hips present for the last 3 months. The onset was quite abrupt. The stiffness and aching are bilateral in both upper and lower limbs. The symptoms are especially severe in the morning. The patient says that it is difficult to get out of a chair and difficult to move her arms above her head.

The patient also mentions significant malaise and fatigue and has experienced a 20-lb weight loss. She mentions a mild fever and also a feeling of "depression."

On examination, the patient's blood pressure and pulse are normal. Although the patient describes "significant weakness," there are no objective findings.

■ SELECT THE BEST ANSWER TO THE FOLLOWING QUESTIONS:

1. What is the most likely diagnosis in this patient?
   a. osteoarthritis
   b. rheumatoid arthritis (RA)
   c. polymyalgia rheumatica (PMR)
   d. polymyositis
   e. acute degenerative arthritis

2. Which of the following disorders is most closely associated with the geriatric population?
   a. PMR
   b. osteoarthritis (OA)
   c. RA
   d. degenerative arthritis (DA)
   e. polymyositis

3. Which of the following statements regarding the condition described is (are) true?

a. the cause of the disease is unknown
b. this disease is most likely autoimmune in origin
c. the overall prevalence of this condition is approximately 17/100,000 patients
d. family aggregation of this disorder has been described
e. all of the above statements are true

4. Which of the following statements regarding this condition is (are) true?
a. there are no significant complications or related disorders of concern
b. hypothyroidism, hyperthyroidism, and hyperparathyroidism are part of the differential diagnosis
c. systemic lupus erythematosus must be considered a potential diagnostic possibility
d. b and c
e. all of the above statements are true

5. What is (are) the major difference(s) between this disorder and polymyositis?
a. marked proximal muscle weakness in polymyositis
b. marked proximal muscle tenderness in polymyositis
c. elevated muscle enzymes such as creatine kinase (CK) in polymyositis
d. a and b
e. a, b, and c

6. Which of the following is the investigation of choice in this condition?
a. muscle CK
b. erythrocyte sedimentation rate (ESR)
c. antinuclear antibody titer
d. rheumatoid factor titer
e. computed tomography scan of the shoulders and hip girdle

7. Which of the following is (are) manifestations of giant cell arteritis (GCA), also known as temporal arteritis?
a. jaw claudication
b. headaches
c. amaurosis fugax
d. scalp tenderness
e. all of the above

8. Of the symptoms listed in Question 7, which is (are) the most worrisome?
a. jaw claudication
b. headaches
c. amaurosis fugax
d. scalp tenderness
e. all of the symptoms are equally worrisome

9. The symptom(s) identified in Question 8 as most worrisome can lead to which of the following (greatly feared) complication of GCA?
a. permanent hemiplegia
b. permanent bilateral and complete sensorineural hearing loss
c. permanent monocular or binocular total blindness
d. permanent bilateral and complete sensorineural and conductive hearing losses
e. permanent quadriplegia

10. What is the treatment of choice for both PMR and GCA?
a. intravenous pulsed steroids
b. oral prednisone: 20 mg/day for PMR and 60 mg/day for GCA
c. oral methotrexate
d. cyclosporine intravenously every third day for 4 weeks
e. intravenous (IV) dihydroergotamine

11. What is the pathophysiologic cause of temporal arteritis?
a. inflammation of the middle meningeal artery
b. inflammation of the temporal artery
c. inflammation of the common carotid artery
d. inflammation of the internal carotid artery
e. inflammation of the external carotid artery

 CLINICAL CASE MANAGEMENT PROBLEM

An 82-year-old female comes to your office with a history of shoulder girdle pain and hip pain progressing to involve other joints of the upper and lower extremities. Provide a differential diagnosis for this patient's pain.

▍ **ANSWERS:**

1. **c.** The diagnosis in this patient is PMR. This is an important diagnosis to make in the elderly.

2. **a.** Of all of the musculoskeletal conditions, PMR is most closely identified with the geriatric population.

PMR is a diagnosis that is often missed, a diagnosis in which vague symptoms are present, and a diagnosis that is often characterized by the patient's seeing multiple doctors without being correctly diagnosed.

PMR is characterized by aching and stiffness in the shoulder and hip girdles. Profound morning stiffness is especially suggestive of this disorder and should be specifically sought out. The diagnosis of PMR seldom is seen before the age of 50 years; its mean age of onset is 70 years. The onset may be either abrupt or gradual. The stiffness that is present in the hips and the shoulders may become generalized, involving the neck and knees and even extending into the wrists and fingers.

There are also prominent constitutional symptoms. These include symptoms such as malaise, weight loss, low-grade fever, and depression.

3. **e.** The cause of PMR is unknown, although an autoimmune process appears to be related to the condition. The overall prevalence of PMR is 17/100,000 people. In addition, family aggregation is common.

4. **d.** The differential diagnosis of PMR in the elderly includes hypothyroidism, hyperthyroidism, hyperparathyroidism, systemic lupus erythematosus, RA, OA or DA, and polymyositis.

The single most important complication of concern in PMR is its association with giant cell arteritis (GCA). GCA will be discussed in questions 7 through 11.

5. **e.** The differences between PMR and polymyositis on clinical examination are as follows: (1) there is marked weakness associated with proximal muscle pain in polymyositis; (2) there is marked muscle tenderness associated with the proximal muscle pain in polymyositis; and (3) laboratory examination reveals elevated muscle enzymes only in polymyositis.

6. **b.** Both PMR and GCA are characterized by elevations in the ESR. Elevations to levels greater than 100 mm/hour may be seen in either disease; elevations to levels greater than 50 mm/hour are almost universal.

7. **e.** Manifestations of temporal arteritis include headache, scalp tenderness, visual symptoms, jaw claudication, constitutional symptoms (fever, weight loss, anorexia, fatigue), polymyalgia symptoms (aching and stiffness of the trunk and proximal muscle groups), cough, and amaurosis fugax.

8. **c.** Of the symptoms listed in Answer 7, the most worrisome symptom is amaurosis fugax. Amaurosis fugax, defined as brief visual loss, is related to ischemia of the posterior ciliary branch of the ophthalmic artery and can lead to blindness if not treated quickly.

9. **c.** The transient visual loss of amaurosis fugax may foretell by days, weeks, or sometimes even months the most dreaded complication, permanent monocular or binocular blindness. If any ocular involvement is present, IV methylprednisolone should be initiated immediately to try to prevent blindness.

10. **b.** Oral prednisone is the treatment of choice for both PMR and GCA. The dosage is as follows: (1) PMR: 20 mg/day by mouth (PO) for 4 weeks with gradual reduction thereafter but maintained for at least 1 year; and (2) temporal arteritis: 60 mg/day PO for 4 weeks with gradual reduction beginning at 4 weeks but with maintenance therapy for 1-2 years. Dosage should be adjusted by monitoring the ESR.

11. **b.** From a pathologic point of view, the cause of temporal arteritis is inflammation of the temporal artery. From a local anatomic standpoint, this results in temporal headache (generally unilateral and accompanied by temporal artery swelling and tenderness). Temporal artery biopsy is the definitive diagnostic procedure for GCA and should include a segment at least 2 cm long. Because of the potential for ocular involvement, treatment should be started immediately, even if biopsy cannot be done within a week. It is felt with treatment that the characteristic pathology of GCA may be present for up to 2 weeks, but do not wait for the biopsy results.

SUMMARY OF POLYMYALGIA RHEUMATICA AND TEMPORAL ARTERITIS

A. PMR:
1. **Epidemiology:** Of all the musculoskeletal conditions, none is so closely identified with the geriatric population as PMR.

Continued

SOLUTION TO THE CLINICAL CASE MANAGEMENT PROBLEM

Differential diagnosis:

A. *Nonmusculoskeletal problems:* (1) hypothyroidism; (2) hyperthyroidism; and (3) hyperparathyroidism

B. *Musculoskeletal problems:* (1) systemic lupus erythematosus; (2) RA; (3) OA or DA; (4) PMR; and (5) polymyositis

C. *Other important systemic conditions:* (1) metastatic bone cancer and (2) multiple myeloma

SUMMARY OF POLYMYALGIA RHEUMATICA AND TEMPORAL ARTERITIS—cont'd

2. **Prevalence rate:** A prevalence rate of 17/100,000 people older than age 50 years has been established (average age around 70 years old).
3. **Symptoms:** Symptoms include either sudden onset or gradual onset of pain (usually bilateral)
   a. Initial manifestations: pain, aching, and stiffness in the shoulder girdle and hip girdle; profound morning stiffness; in addition, patients may complain of fatigue, malaise, weight loss, and depression
   b. Progression: pain, aching, and stiffness progress to other joints in the upper and lower extremities
   c. Clue: patient tells you that suddenly he or she can no longer get out of bed in the morning
4. **Diagnosis:** Elevated ESR is diagnostic (almost always greater than 50 mm/hour; frequently greater than 100 mm/hour). Other findings may be a normocytic normochromic anemia, elevated platelet count, and increased C-reactive protein. Liver enzymes, especially alkaline phosphatase, are increased in one-third of the patients. Muscle enzymes are normal.
5. **Complication:** Temporal arteritis with eventual blindness is a major complication.
6. **Treatment:** Treatment involves prednisone, 20 mg/day for 1 month, and taper; maintain for 1 year. Response can be seen in 1-2 days.
7. **Differential diagnosis:** See the Clinical Case Management Problem.

B. **Temporal arteritis:**
1. **Presenting signs and symptoms:**
   a. Pain, aching, and stiffness in the shoulder and hip girdles, as described for PMR.

   b. Additional systemic signs and symptoms of inflammation include (i) fever (high spiking); (ii) weight loss; (iii) malaise; (iv) jaw claudication; (v) transient visual complaints leading to blindness if left untreated; (vi) extremity claudication; and (vii) aortic aneurysm.
   c. Significant local signs and symptoms are (i) temporal headache (unilateral); (ii) temporal artery swelling and tenderness (but not always tender); and (iii) significant neurologic symptoms (see Answers 7 to 9).
2. **Diagnosis:**
   a. ESR (as mentioned in A4 above)
   b. Temporal artery biopsy: If you suspect temporal arteritis, do not wait for a surgeon to perform a biopsy. Treat the condition with prednisone immediately. Of patients with PMR, 10% to 15% may go on and get GCA, and 40% to 60% of patients with GCA will have PMR.
3. **Complication:** Permanent monocular or binocular blindness are major complications.
4. **Treatment:** Treatment is high-dose prednisone, 60 mg/day for 4 weeks; taper slowly and maintain for 1-2 years. If symptoms are ocular, use IV methylprednisolone immediately.

SUGGESTED READING

Braunwald E, et al: *Harrison's manual of medicine,* 15th edition. McGraw-Hill, 2002, New York.

Gardner GC: Polymyalgia rheumatic and temporal arteritis. In: Rakel R, Bope E, eds.: *Conn's current therapy 2000.* WB Saunders, 2003, Philadelphia, 970-971.

Hunder GG: Giant cell arthritis and polymyalgia rheumatic. In: Ruddy S, et al, eds.: *Kelley's textbook of rheumatology,* vol 2. WB Saunders, 2001, Philadelphia, 1155-1164.

Tierney LM Jr, et al, eds.: *Current medical diagnosis and treatment, 2001.* Appleton & Lange, 2000, Stamford, CT.

Chapter 135

Hypertension in Elderly Patients

"Doc, how many pills do I have to take? That top number still is always greater than 140."

CLINICAL CASE PROBLEM 1:

AN 80-YEAR-OLD MALE WITH HYPERTENSION

An 80-year-old white male, previously healthy, comes to your office for a periodic health examination. He was last seen by a physician 20 years ago. His blood pressure is recorded as 215/95 mm Hg.

A complete history reveals no other cardiovascular risk factors. A complete physical examination reveals no evidence of end-organ damage or secondary causes of hypertension.

Basic laboratory investigations, including a complete blood count, urinalysis, electrolytes, serum calcium, fasting blood sugar, plasma cholesterol, uric acid, and an electrocardiogram are all normal.

The patient is on a fixed income and is trying to keep up with payments for his wife's nursing home care.

SELECT THE BEST ANSWER TO THE FOLLOWING QUESTIONS:

1. Based on the information given, what would you do now?
   a. begin therapy with a thiazide diuretic
   b. begin therapy with a calcium channel blocker
   c. begin therapy with an angiotensin-converting enzyme (ACE) inhibitor
   d. begin therapy with a beta blocker
   e. none of the above

Following further investigation and two more visits, his blood pressure remains elevated at 205/92 mm Hg.

You also discuss nonpharmacologic treatment with him, and it appears obvious to you that he is not really prepared to alter his"hamburgers and chips (fried in pure lard)" diet. He also states that exercise would kill him.

2. What would you do now?
   a. prescribe a thiazide diuretic
   b. prescribe a calcium channel blocker
   c. prescribe a beta blocker
   d. prescribe an ACE inhibitor
   e. prescribe a vasodilator

Appropriate therapy is prescribed for the patient, and he returns in 1 month for follow-up care. His blood pressure is now 185/90 mm Hg, and his serum potassium level has decreased from 4.0 mEq/L to 3.0 mEq/L.

3. At this time, what would you do?
   a. substitute an ACE inhibitor for the present medication
   b. substitute a calcium channel blocker for the present medication
   c. substitute a beta blocker for the present medication
   d. substitute a vasodilator for the present medication
   e. review the type and dose of the drug class being prescribed

The patient described has the necessary change to his medication treatment regimen made. When he returns next month for follow-up care, his blood pressure is 175/90 mm Hg.

4. At this time, what would you do?
   a. add an ACE inhibitor
   b. add a calcium channel blocker
   c. add a beta blocker
   d. add a vasodilator
   e. maximize the dose of a beta blocker

5. Which of the following statements regarding the treatment of hypertension in the elderly is (are) true?
   a. isolated systolic hypertension in the elderly should not be treated
   b. the benefits of treating elderly patients with hypertension have not been established
   c. no change in morbidity or mortality has been demonstrated for elderly patients treated with antihypertensives
   d. elderly patients treated for hypertension are likely to benefit only from a reduction in cerebrovascular morbidity and mortality, not cardiac morbidity or mortality
   e. none of the above are true

6. Regarding the epidemiologic importance of elevations in systolic versus diastolic blood pressure in elderly patients, which of the following statements is true?
   a. elevation of systolic blood pressure is not as important as elevation of diastolic blood pressure
   b. elevation of systolic blood pressure, although important, does not correlate well with cardiovascular morbidity and mortality
   c. elevations of systolic and diastolic blood pressure are equally important
   d. elevated systolic blood pressure is a greater risk for subsequent cardiovascular morbidity and mortality than diastolic blood pressure
   e. the relative importance of elevations in systolic blood pressure in terms of cardiovascular morbidity and mortality remains unclear

7. With respect to morbidity and mortality and treatment of systolic hypertension in the elderly, which of the following epidemiologic categories show(s) a significant decrease (compared to placebo) when systolic blood pressure is treated?
   a. total stroke morbidity
   b. total stroke mortality
   c. total coronary artery mortality
   d. a and b only
   e. a, b, and c
   f. none of the above

8. Which of the following drug combinations should be avoided in elderly patients with hypertension?
   a. hydrochlorothiazide (HCT)/amiloride and enalapril
   b. HCT/amiloride and nifedipine
   c. HCT/amiloride and atenolol
   d. HCT/amiloride and hydralazine
   e. HCT/amiloride and reserpine

CLINICAL CASE PROBLEM 2:

A 75-YEAR-OLD AFRICAN AMERICAN MALE WITH ANGINA PECTORIS

A 75-year-old African American male with angina pectoris is found, on physical examination, to have a blood pressure of 170/100 mm Hg. His angina is controlled by taking isosorbide dinitrate, 30 mg qid. His blood pressure reading is repeated on several occasions and remains unchanged.

9. At this time, what is the most reasonable treatment for this patient's blood pressure?
   a. a calcium channel blocker
   b. a beta blocker
   c. a thiazide diuretic
   d. an ACE inhibitor
   e. a and/or c

CLINICAL CASE PROBLEM 3:

A 72-YEAR-OLD WHITE FEMALE WITH HYPERTENSION AND A PREVIOUS MYOCARDIAL INFARCTION AND MILD CONGESTIVE HEART FAILURE

A 72-year-old white female with a previous myocardial infarction (MI) and mild congestive heart failure (CHF) (controlled with furosemide 40 mg qid) comes to your office for a routine assessment. She is found to have a blood pressure of 190/100 mm Hg. This reading is repeated on two occasions.

10. What would be the most appropriate treatment for her hypertension?
    a. an ACE inhibitor
    b. a calcium channel blocker
    c. a beta blocker
    d. a thiazide diuretic
    e. none of the above

CLINICAL CASE PROBLEM 4:

A 72-YEAR-OLD WHITE MALE WITH HYPERTENSION AND DIABETES

A 72-year-old white male with a 20-year history of non–insulin-dependent diabetes mellitus is found to have a blood pressure of 170/105 mm Hg. He has no history of angina pectoris or other significant vascular disease. He had never been diagnosed as hypertensive.

His blood pressure is repeated on two additional occasions, and the readings remain the same. Laboratory evaluation reveals microalbuminuria.

11. At this time, what would be the most appropriate treatment for this patient's blood pressure?
    a. a thiazide diuretic
    b. a beta blocker
    c. a calcium channel blocker
    d. an ACE inhibitor
    e. a vasodilator

12. What is the recommended dosage of HCT for the treatment of hypertension in the elderly?
    a. 12.5-25 mg
    b. 25-50 mg
    c. 50-75 mg
    d. 75-100 mg
    e. whatever you want

CLINICAL CASE MANAGEMENT PROBLEM

Part A: An 80-year-old African American male with systolic hypertension (210/85 mm Hg) is a new patient to your practice. He says he has been healthy all of his life. From three consecutive readings you determine that the patient is truly hypertensive.

Discuss your approach to this patient with respect to education and counseling regarding his hypertension. Include lifestyle advice, medication advice, and other pertinent advice that you consider important.

Part B: Discuss the medication efficacy differences that have been demonstrated with respect to race and age in the following types of patients: (1) young African American patients; (2) young white patients; (3) elderly African American patients; and (4) elderly white patients.

ANSWERS:

1. **e.** Although this patient has a systolic blood pressure of 215 mm Hg, you should consider that this is only one reading and it cannot be assumed to represent his "true blood pressure," and that even if you were able to make the diagnosis of hypertension at this time, you still would want to begin with nonpharmacologic therapy.

This patient should have his blood pressure rechecked on two other occasions before the diagnosis of hypertension is made.

2. **a.** Studies have clearly demonstrated the importance of treating systolic hypertension in the elderly, treating it, in fact, with the same rigor and aggressiveness as diastolic hypertension.

Because of the patient's fixed income and the proven efficacy of thiazide diuretics in reducing morbidity and mortality from cardiovascular disease, a low-dose (25-mg) thiazide diuretic would be the agent of choice. Thiazide diuretic has been proven to decrease morbidity and mortality.

3. e. At this time, the most reasonable alternative would be to review both the dose and the drug class.

On the positive side, this patient's systolic blood pressure has decreased significantly (from 205 to 185 mm Hg). On the negative side, his potassium also has decreased (from 4.0 to 3.0 mEq/L). This is a significant decrease and furthermore puts this patient into the danger zone for hypokalemia—the level at which dysrhythmias begin to be a serious concern.

The most reasonable strategy in this case would likely be to reduce the dose of the thiazide diuretic to an absolute minimum (12.5 mg) and add a beta blocker (such as atenolol). This combination of drugs (thiazide and beta blocker) was selected because of recommendations in the Seventh Report of the Joint National Committee on Prevention, Detection, Evaluation, and Treatment of High Blood Pressure (JNC-VII) of the National Institutes of Health. It also is discussed in Chapter 14, in which the reduction in cardiovascular morbidity and mortality induced by thiazides and beta blockers is documented. However, in the elderly a cardioselective beta blocker should be used because of side effects induced by nonspecific beta blockers in this population.

Potassium supplementation also should be considered.

4. e. Because the previous treatment reduced his systolic blood pressure to 175 mm Hg, increasing the dose of the beta blocker to its maximum should reduce his blood pressure further.

5. e. There is ample evidence to show that antihypertensive therapy prevents cerebrovascular accidents, CHF, and other blood pressure–related complications. The Systolic Hypertension in the Elderly Program (SHEP) study showed a reduction in myocardial infarcts and other coronary events in older patients with moderate to severe ischemic heart disease. Other studies confirm this.

6. c. The single most important advance in the treatment of hypertension in the elderly is the clear and unequivocal recognition that systolic hypertension is as important as diastolic hypertension as a risk factor for cardiovascular morbidity and mortality and should be treated aggressively. The goal of systolic

blood pressure reduction is a reading not exceeding 160 mm Hg. The ideal control would be a systolic blood pressure less than 140.

7. e. See Answer 5.

8. a. Of the choices provided, the drug combination that should clearly be avoided in elderly patients is HCT/amiloride and enalapril. Both amiloride and enalapril are potassium-sparing drugs. In an elderly patient with decreased renal function, this can lead to profound and rapid hyperkalemia with subsequent complications.

9. e. Calcium channel blockers and thiazide diuretics have been shown to be more effective than beta blockers in some studies in controlling hypertension in elderly African American patients; thus a calcium channel blocker (particularly diltiazem) and/or HCT would appear to be the agents of choice in this case. Be aware that verapamil may cause constipation and nifedipine may cause peripheral edema.

10. a. Considering that this elderly female has CHF as well as hypertension, the treatment of choice is an ACE inhibitor. ACE inhibitors reduce both preload and afterload in patients with hypertension and thus are the drug class of choice for the management of CHF. ACE inhibitors have minimal side effects (primarily cough with enalapril and taste disturbances with captopril). For patients with left-ventricular hypertrophy, an ACE inhibitor, a combination of hydralazine and isosorbide dinitrate, beta blockers, and spironolactone have been shown to decrease mortality. Patients started taking an ACE inhibitor should have their blood pressure checked in 1 week and serum creatine should be checked in 1 month.

11. d. Patients with diabetes mellitus and resulting renal impairment or microalbuminuria definitely should be treated with ACE inhibitors as the drug class of choice. There is some evidence that ACE inhibitors can be "renal protective agents" in patients with diabetes mellitus and even can be indicated as a prophylactic measure. Additional studies have shown that patients with microalbuminuria also may respond to angiotensin receptor blockers.

12. a. The recommended, or "correct," dose of HCT or other thiazide diuretic is the lowest dose that effectively controls the blood pressure and at the same time minimizes all of the metabolic side effects associated with thiazide diuretics.

SOLUTION TO THE CLINICAL CASE MANAGEMENT PROBLEM

Part A: Provide advice for an 80-year-old African American male with documented systolic hypertension:

1. Review the patient's diet with him. Attempt to have the patient's spouse present (if available) while discussing this.
2. Encourage the patient to adopt the general recommendations of the American Heart Association's type I diet. This includes no more than 300 mg of cholesterol per day, no more than 30% of calories from fat, and no more than 10% of calories from saturated fat.
3. Encourage the patient to begin a "gentle" aerobic exercise program. The most reasonable exercise for a man of this age would be a walking program.
4. Advise the patient to decrease his alcohol intake to no more than two drinks per day (if he drinks).
5. Encourage the patient to stop smoking (cutting down might be more reasonable) if he is a smoker.
6. Start "nonpharmacologic maneuvers" along with treatment.

Part B: Discuss age- and race-related medication efficiency:

The differentiation of efficacy of antihypertensive drugs based on age and race is extremely interesting. Interdrug differences are particularly apparent in African American patients. The following results are from a major review article on hypertension in the elderly by Massie (1994). The agents used in this study included atenolol, captopril, clonidine, diltiazem, HCT, and prazosin.

1. African American patients younger than 60 years old: diltiazem was shown in one major study to be superior to all other agents.
2. African American patients older than 60 years of age: diltiazem and HCT were the most effective agents. Captopril and atenolol were the least effective.
3. White patients younger than 60 years old: all first-line agents (thiazides, beta blockers, calcium channel blockers, and ACE inhibitors) were equally effective.
4. White patients older than 60 years of age: atenolol is the most effective agent.

SUMMARY OF HYPERTENSION IN ELDERLY PATIENTS

1. Single most important point: Systolic hypertension in the elderly (and in the young as well) is as important as diastolic hypertension.
2. Diagnosis of hypertension in the elderly: New criteria established by JNC-VII (see Answer 3).
3. Treatment of hypertension in the elderly reduces cerebrovascular morbidity, cerebrovascular mortality, cardiovascular morbidity, and cardiovascular mortality.
4. A substantial proportion of patients can have their mild and moderate hypertension controlled with a single agent, and in most this control will be maintained in the long term.
5. Assessment of cardiac risk factors: Smoking, dyslipidemia, and diabetes are important in elderly.
6. Assessment of end organ damage: Left ventricular hypertrophy, coronary artery disease, CHF, stroke or transient ischemic attacks, renal disease, peripheral arterial disease, and retinopathy may be induced by chronic hypertension and often require treatment.

7. Think renal artery stenosis if hypertension is sudden in onset, if there is a sudden increase in blood pressure, or if blood pressure is elevated with three medications. Workup would include listening for a bruit, renography, and aortogram.
8. Conditions requiring emergent reducing blood pressure include hypertensive encephalopathy, intracranial hemorrhage, unstable angina, acute MI, acute left ventricular failure with pulmonary edema, and dissecting aortic aneurysm.

SUGGESTED READING

Chobanian AV, et al: The Seventh Report of the Joint National Committee on Prevention, Detection, Evaluation, and Treatment of High Blood Pressure (JNC 7). *JAMA* 289(19):2560-2571, 2003.

Massie BM: First-line therapy for hypertension: different patients, different needs. *Geriatrics* 49(4):22-30, 1994.

Moser M: Hypertension treatment and the prevention of coronary heart disease in the elderly. *Am Fam Physician* 59(5):1248-1256, 1999.

Venkata C, et al: Hypertension. In: Rakel R, Bope E, eds.: *Conn's current therapy 2003.* WB Saunders, 2002, Philadelphia, 303-315.

World Health Organization: 1999 World Health Organization–International Society of Hypertension Guidelines for the Management of Hypertension. Guidelines subcommittee. *J Hypertension* 17(2):151-183, 1999.

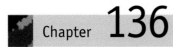

Chapter 136

Parkinson's Disease

"Doctor, my hand just sits there and quivers on its own."

CLINICAL CASE PROBLEM 1:
A 75-Year-Old Male with a Slow, Shuffling Gait, Tremors, and Depression

A 75-year-old male is brought to your office by his wife. She states that he has just been "staring into space" for the last 2 months. He has been unable to move around the house without falling over. Also, his movements appear to be very slow. According to his wife, he has been very depressed, is drooling, has difficulty swallowing, and is losing weight.

On examination, the patient has a slow, shuffling gait and walks in a "stooped-over" position. His blood pressure (lying) is 140/90 mm Hg. His standing blood pressure is 100/70 mm Hg. He has marked rigidity of his upper extremities. He also has a tremor that appears to be present only at rest.

■ SELECT THE BEST ANSWER TO THE FOLLOWING QUESTIONS:

1. What is the most likely diagnosis in this patient?
   a. Alzheimer's disease
   b. major depressive disorder with psychomotor retardation
   c. degenerative orthostatic hypotension
   d. Parkinson's disease
   e. multiple sclerosis

2. What is the most common presenting symptom in this disorder?
   a. orthostatic hypotension
   b. depression
   c. gait disturbance
   d. tremor
   e. rigidity

3. Where is the lesion associated with the described disorder located?
   a. the caudate nucleus
   b. the substantia nigra
   c. the hypothalamus
   d. the putamen
   e. the globus pallidus

4. The disorder described is associated with a central nervous system neurotransmitter deficiency. What is that neurotransmitter?
   a. acetylcholine
   b. serotonin
   c. gamma-aminobutyric acid
   d. dopamine
   e. norepinephrine

5. Many drugs are associated with side effects that mimic some of the symptoms of the described disorder. Which one of the following drugs would not produce these symptoms?
   a. diazepam
   b. haloperidol
   c. chlorpromazine
   d. perphenazine
   e. reserpine

6. Which one of the following statements regarding the condition described is false?
   a. there is marked heterogeneity in disease presentation
   b. there are at least two major subgroups of this disorder
   c. patients who have marked postural instability have a better prognosis than those who have a tremor
   d. personality changes commonly appear in the course of this disorder
   e. significant depression and dementia appear in one-third to one-half of patients with this condition.

7. What is (are) the drug(s) of choice for mild cases of the condition described (mild meaning that the main or only symptom is tremor)?
   a. amantadine
   b. trihexyphenidyl
   c. levodopa
   d. carbidopa
   e. selegiline (Deprenyl)
   f. a or b

8. If the symptoms progress to the point where another agent is needed, dose-limiting side effects develop from the drugs being used, or the drugs being used begin to lose their effectiveness, what is the next step in the treatment of the disorder described?
   a. selegiline
   b. trihexyphenidyl
   c. amantadine
   d. all of the above
   e. none of the above

9. Which of the following drugs may be indicated in the treatment of the disorder described?
   a. bromocriptine
   b. pergolide

c. amitriptyline
d. a and b
e. none of the above

10. Which of the following symptoms is not characteristic of this disorder?
a. unilateral onset of tremor
b. unilateral onset of bradykinesia
c. impaired balance
d. muscle rigidity
e. psychomotor agitation

11. Which of the following statements regarding levodopa is false?
a. levodopa in combination with carbidopa remains the primary drugs for the treatment of most patients with the condition described
b. levodopa is unlikely to lose its effectiveness over time when being used to treat the disorder described
c. levodopa is likely to produce an "on-off" phenomenon during treatment of the disorder described
d. nausea is a frequent side effect of levodopa
e. centrally mediated dyskinesia, hallucinations, dystonia, and motor fluctuations are common in patients treated with levodopa

12. Which of the following conditions is most closely associated with the condition described?
a. major depressive disorder
b. cerebrovascular disease
c. epilepsy
d. schizophrenia
e. schizoaffective disorder

13. Which of the following statements regarding benign essential tremor is (are) correct?
a. benign essential tremor is often familial
b. a nodding head and tremulousness of speech often are observed with benign essential tremor
c. benign essential tremor is a resting tremor rather than an action tremor
d. a and b only
e. all of the above statements are correct

14. Benign essential tremor frequently is treated with which of the following agents?
a. propranolol
b. alcohol
c. atenolol
d. all of the above
e. none of the above

15. What illicit drug produces symptoms closely resembling the symptoms of the condition described?
a. a meperidine analogue (MPTP)
b. crack cocaine
c. lysergic acid diethylamide
d. apomorphine
e. diamorphine (heroin)

CLINICAL CASE MANAGEMENT PROBLEM

Discuss the therapeutic choices available to treat the condition described in the patient presented in Clinical Case Problem 1. Describe a logical approach to instituting these therapeutic choices in any patient with this disorder.

■ **ANSWERS:**

1. **d.** This patient has Parkinson's disease. The most common presenting symptoms in Parkinson's disease include tremor, bradykinesia, rigidity, impaired postural reflexes, gait disturbance, autonomic dysfunction (causing orthostatic hypotension), and depression. A "masked facies" expression is typical of the disease.

Other presenting symptoms can be constipation, vague aches and pains, paresthesia, decreased smell sensation, vestibular symptoms, pedal edema, fatigue, and weight loss.

The other choices listed in this question do not explain the constellation of presenting symptoms.

2. **d.** The most common presenting symptom in Parkinson's disease is a resting tremor. This symptom is seen in 70% of patients with the disease. It initially may be confined to one hand, but it usually extends to involve all limbs.

3. **b.** The principal pathologic feature in Parkinson's disease is degeneration of the substantia nigra. Degenerative changes also are found in other brainstem nuclei.

4. **d.** Parkinson's disease is associated with a depletion of dopamine in the substantia nigrostriatal pathway system.

5. **a.** Parkinsonianlike side effects are common side effects of the neuroleptic drug class. This drug class includes chlorpromazine, haloperidol, and perphenazine. In addition, the prokinetic agent metoclopramide also can produce this side effect.

Reserpine, an older antihypertensive agent, also may produce these extrapyramidal symptoms. This is relevant because many elderly individuals who were started taking reserpine are still taking it. Diazepam does not produce any such side effects.

6. c. There is marked heterogeneity in Parkinson's disease. There are at least two major subtypes of Parkinson's disease. In one group the symptom of tremor is the most predominant clinical symptom. In the second group, postural instability and gait difficulty (PIGD) are the predominant symptoms. There is some overlap, but most patients fit into only one subgroup. Patients with tremor-predominant Parkinson's disease have slower progression of disease and have fewer problems with bradykinesia. They are also less likely to develop significant mental symptoms.

Personality changes usually occur in the early stages, and patients often become withdrawn, apathetic, and dependent on their spouses. Significant depression occurs in one-half of patients, and dementia occurs in one-third of patients. As mentioned previously, these personality and mental changes are more common in patients who present with the PIGD subtype of Parkinson's disease.

7. e. Research from three studies has supported the use of selegiline (Deprenyl) early in the course of the disease to delay the onset of the disability and the need for initiation of levodopa therapy. The combination of levodopa and carbidopa are effective and still are considered for primary treatment, but their use should be delayed as long as possible because of their side-effect profile and the eventual development of tolerance to these medications.

8. e. The next step in the pharmacologic treatment of Parkinson's disease is the combination of levodopa–carbidopa. Levodopa is a precursor of dopamine synthesis in the substantia nigra. The drug usually is administered in combination with carbidopa, which is a decarboxylase inhibitor. Obviously, treatment must be individualized: a good general rule to follow is to start low and go slow. Sinemet is most helpful for bradykinesia.

9. d. Bromocriptine and pergolide are two dopaminergic agonists. Pergolide and bromocriptine can be useful for sudden episodes of hesitancy or immobility, which patients with Parkinson's disease describe as "freezing." This can be an intermittent event or a regular event. The freezing often occurs when patients with Parkinson's disease begin to walk or they pass through a structure such as a doorway. Dyskinesias and other types of involuntary movements also are

treated by these drugs. Newer dopaminergic agents include pramipexole and ropinirole.

10. e. The unilateral onset of tremor or bradykinesia is common in patients with Parkinson's disease. Muscle rigidity and impaired balance are other important symptoms. Psychomotor agitation (although one of the characteristic symptoms of major depressive disorder) is rare. Patients with Parkinson's disease have instead psychomotor retardation.

11. b. Levodopa does lose its effectiveness over time in the treatment of Parkinson's disease. That is why, in patients who have mild symptoms, it is best to begin therapy with selegiline (Deprenyl).

Levodopa does exhibit a marked "on-off" phenomenon during treatment of Parkinson's disease. This is characterized by periods of "drug working" and "drug not working." Pramipexole may be used with Sinemet to reduce these fluctuations. Catechol-o-methyltransferases (COMTs) such as tolcapone (100 mg) or entacapone (200 mg) with each Sinemet dose may enhance the benefits of levodopa therapy.

Side effects of levodopa include nausea and vomiting, dystonias, hallucinations, dyskinesias, and motor fluctuations. Hallucinations become the most common side effect, limiting the titration of carbidopa–levodopa.

12. a. Depression is a common problem in patients with Parkinson's disease. The association between depression and Parkinson's disease generally follows this pathway: when depression occurs, the symptoms of Parkinson's disease become worse; the patient then believes that his or her disease has progressed quickly. This leads to a cycle that is difficult to break.

13. d. Benign essential tremor is the major differential diagnostic possibility when considering tremor. Benign essential tremor is familial. Typical features include generalized tremulousness, including tremulousness of speech, and a "head-nodding" motion. Benign essential tremor is, in contradistinction to the tremor of Parkinson's disease, an action tremor.

14. d. The agents of choice for treating benign essential tremor are propranolol (long acting) and primidone.

15. a. The illicitly made MPTP produces symptoms that are Parkinsonlike in presentation. This agent appears to act as a poison on the substantia nigra. Also, the symptoms appear to be irreversible, and the individual is left with a lifetime disability.

SOLUTION TO THE CLINICAL CASE MANAGEMENT PROBLEM

A reasonable therapeutic approach to the treatment of Parkinson's disease is as follows:

A. Patients with minor symptoms (not significantly impairing function): (1) no pharmacologic treatment; (2) selegiline (Deprenyl); (3) anticholinergic medications (trihexyphenidyl, benztropine; use with caution in the elderly); and (4) amantadine.

B. Patients with moderate symptoms: Levodopa–carbidopa (Sinemet); levodopa is a precursor of dopamine; carbidopa is a decarboxylase inhibitor. Although selegiline is not considered the drug of first choice, its use will increase if current research continues to support the idea that it decreases the rate of progression of Parkinson's disease or delays the use of Sinemet.

C. Patients with moderate to severe symptoms (or patients in whom the effect of levodopa has worn off): (1) in patients with a significant depressive component because of the monoamine oxidase (MAO) activity, use deprenyl (an MAO B inhibitor); (2) in patients in whom dyskinesias and other involuntary movements are prominent, use bromocriptine and pergolide (dopamine agonists)

D. Patients with Parkinson's disease with significant depression: amitriptyline or another tricyclic antidepressant with or without anticholinergic properties (balance the benefits of the anticholinergic properties of amitriptyline against the risk of increased orthostatic disturbance and imbalance)

SUMMARY OF PARKINSON'S DISEASE

1. **Epidemiology:** After stroke and Alzheimer's disease, Parkinson's disease is the most commonly encountered neurologic disorder in the elderly population.

2. **Pathologic condition:** Depigmentation of the substantia nigra results in a decrease in brain synthesis of dopamine.

3. Major symptoms include (a) resting tremor; (b) bradykinesia; (c) rigidity; (d) impaired postural reflexes; (e) gait disturbance; (f) autonomic dysfunction; and (g) depression.

4. **Major subtypes:**
   a. Parkinson's disease (group A): This group exhibits tremor (resting) as the major symptom and sign.
   b. Parkinson's disease (group B): This group exhibits PIGD as the major symptom. Progression of the disease is usually more rapid in this group; neurobehavioral changes are also more common in this group.

5. **Treatment:** See the Solution to the Clinical Case Management Problem.

6. **Other related disease entity:** Benign essential tremor is an action tremor (as opposed to the resting tremor of Parkinson's disease). It is seen most often in the extremities and sometimes is associated with head nodding and tremulousness of speech. It is familial. The drug treatment of this entity includes a beta blocker, diazepam, or alcohol (in moderation).

7. In refractory cases, unilateral pallidotomy may be effective in relieving signs of Parkinson's disease on the contralateral side; however, deep brain stimulation of the globus pallidus or subthalamic nucleus has a lower morbidity than pallidotomy and appears to improve clinical status.

SUGGESTED READING

Friedman JH: Parkinson disease. In: Rakel R, Bope E, eds.: *Conn's current therapy, 2003.* WB Saunders, 2004, Philadelphia, 918-923.

Krack P, et al: Five-year follow-up of bilateral stimulation of the subthalamic nucleus in advanced Parkinson's disease. *N Engl J Med* 349:1925-1934, 2003.

Nussbaum RL, Ellis CE: Genomic medicine: Alzheimer's disease and Parkinson's disease. *N Engl J Med* 348:1356-1364, 2003.

Young R: Update on Parkinson's disease. *Am Fam Physician* 59:2155-2160, 1999.

Chapter 137

Constipation

> "Doctor, I need a laxative. I only have three bowel movements a week."

CLINICAL CASE PROBLEM 1:
A 78-YEAR-OLD FEMALE
WITH CONSTIPATION

A 78-year-old female comes to your office with a 5-year history of "constipation." The patient, who has had significant difficulties with ischemic heart disease, is taking atenolol and verapamil.

On examination, the patient's blood pressure is 180/95 mm Hg. Her pulse is 72 and regular. On examination, the head and neck, the lungs, the cardiovascular system, and the abdomen are all normal. Digital rectal examination (DRE) reveals impacted stool.

■ SELECT THE BEST ANSWER TO THE FOLLOWING QUESTIONS:

1. Constipation is best defined as which of the following:
   a. only one bowel movement in 7 days
   b. only two bowel movements in 7 days
   c. only three bowel movements in 7 days
   d. only four bowel movements in 7 days
   e. none of the above

2. What is the most accurate patient definition of constipation?
   a. anything less than one bowel movement per day
   b. any defecation difficulty
   c. anything less than two bowel movements per day
   d. any straining at stool
   e. any of the above: constipation to patients means almost anything vaguely associated with bowel movements

3. Which of the following is (are) associated with constipation in the elderly?
   a. impaired general health status
   b. increased medication use
   c. decreased level of exercise
   d. all of the above
   e. none of the above

4. Which of the following drug classes is (are) associated with constipation?
   a. tricyclic antidepressants
   b. anticholinergic agents
   c. calcium channel blockers
   d. all of the above
   e. none of the above

5. Concerning the history and physical examination of elderly patients with constipation, which of the following should be performed?
   a. a DRE
   b. a complete medication review
   c. a functional inquiry of the gastrointestinal (GI) system
   d. all of the above
   e. a and b only

6. Which of the following is (are) a complication(s) associated with constipation in the elderly?
   a. fecal impaction
   b. diarrhea
   c. anal fissures
   d. sigmoid volvulus
   e. a and c
   f. a, b, c, and d

7. Which of the following is not a recommended treatment for constipation in the elderly?
   a. a bowel-training regimen
   b. an exercise program
   c. chronic laxative use
   d. a high-fiber diet
   e. an above-average consumption of fluids

8. Which of the following drugs is most closely associated with constipation in the elderly?
   a. hydrochlorothiazide
   b. verapamil
   c. atenolol
   d. acetaminophen
   e. fluoxetine

9. Constipation in the elderly is most closely associated with which of the following?
   a. fecal impaction
   b. diarrhea
   c. crampy back pain
   d. a and c
   e. a, b, and c

10. What is the self-reported percentage incidence of constipation in elderly Americans?
    a. 10%
    b. 20%
    c. 30%
    d. 40%
    e. 50%

11. What is the laxative group most closely associated with long-term side effects in the elderly?
a. the stimulant laxatives
b. the hyperosmolar laxatives
c. the saline laxatives
d. the emollient laxatives
e. the stool softeners

CLINICAL CASE PROBLEM 2:

AN 86-YEAR-OLD MALE WITH STAGE IV CARCINOMA OF THE PROSTATE

An 86-year-old male with stage IV carcinoma of the prostate comes to your office seeking "pain relief." He has bony metastatic disease, and his pain was well controlled taking a combination of diclofenac and morphine sulfate. With the morphine his pain decreased from 9/10 to 2/10. However, 5 days after morphine was started he began to experience more severe pain. You decide to increase the morphine dose and see him in a week. He returns after that week with worse pain than before; it is now 13/10. You increase the morphine dose even further and ask him to return in another week. He returns a week later doubled over in pain that he describes as 15/10.

12. At this time, what would you do?
a. switch the patient to hydromorphone
b. switch the patient to methadone
c. switch the patient to fentanyl (patch)
d. switch the patient to oxycodone
e. none of the above

13. At this time your physical examination maneuver of choice for the patient described in Clinical Case Problem 2 is which of the following?
a. none; you do not believe in the sensitivity, specificity, and positive predictive value of physical examination techniques any more
b. palpation of the abdomen
c. percussion of the abdomen
d. auscultation of the abdomen for bowel sounds
e. none of the above

14. At this time which of the following is the investigation of choice for the patient described in Clinical Case Problem 2?
a. a magnetic resonance imaging (MRI) scan
b. a repeat bone scan
c. a computed tomography (CT) scan of the pelvis
d. a serum calcium level to look for that ever-elusive entity, hypercalcemia
e. none of the above

15. What is the single most common cause of abdominal pain in the elderly?
a. angiodysplasia
b. diverticulitis
c. spastic colon of the elderly syndrome
d. the aging gut syndrome
e. none of the above

CLINICAL CASE MANAGEMENT PROBLEM

Name the drug in each of the drug classes listed that is most commonly responsible for constipation in the elderly: (1) antihypertensive agent; (2) antianginal agent; (3) medical diagnostic agent; (4) antacid; (5) nutritional supplement; (6) analgesic; (7) antipsychotic; (8) antidepressant; (9) anticholinergic; and (10) inexpensive osteoporotic therapy agent.

■ **ANSWERS:**

1. e. Constipation is usually medically defined as fewer than three bowel movements per week. It is a major problem for elderly patients in developed countries of the world. This is substantiated by the increase in the use of laxative therapies. Approximately 30% of patients older than age 65 years are regular laxative users. Constipation refers to infrequent, incomplete, or painful evacuation of stool.

2. e. Physicians tend to define constipation on the basis of the frequency of stooling and the consistency of stooling. To the average person, however, constipation can mean almost anything, including any difficulties in defecation such as straining at stool, anything less than one to two completely-normal-in-every-way (shape, caliber, diameter, length, color) bowel movements, and anything else vaguely related to the bowel movement. The point is, you must ask the person what he or she means by constipation.

Again, it is important to realize that there is a significant discrepancy between what physicians define as constipation in the elderly and what the elderly themselves define as constipation. For many elderly patients, a daily bowel movement is a significant mark of health.

3. d. The factors that appear to be associated with constipation in the elderly include an impaired general health status, an increased number of medications other than laxatives, diminished mobility, and diminished physical activity.

It is unclear what the true effect of diet on bowel habits is. There is epidemiologic evidence from the developed countries that greater amounts of crude dietary fiber are associated with a lesser prevalence of various GI disorders, including diverticular disease, colorectal cancer, and constipation. There may be, however, intervening variables that account for some of this difference.

4. d. There are a significant number of drug classes that are associated with constipation, especially in the elderly. These include (1) antacids (aluminum hydroxide or calcium carbonate); (2) anticholinergic agents (trihexyphenidyl); (3) antidepressants (tricyclic antidepressants, lithium carbonate, (4) antihypertensive-antiarrhythmics (calcium channel blockers [especially verapamil] and diuretics); (5) metals (bismuth, iron, and heavy metals); (6) narcotic analgesics (any narcotic analgesic, but especially codeine); (7) nonsteroidal antiinflammatory drugs (all may produce constipation in the elderly); (8) sympathomimetics (pseudoephedrine); (9) antipsychotics; and (10) anti-Parkinsonian drugs.

5. d. When an elderly patient complains of constipation, a careful history is the most important aspect of the evaluation. Sometimes all that is required is reassurance from the physician that there is a broad range of normal bowel frequency.

Symptoms of disorders that impair the motility of the large bowel should be sought. These general medical conditions include hypothyroidism, hyperparathyroidism, scleroderma, Parkinson's disease, cerebrovascular accidents, and diabetes mellitus.

Localized colorectal diseases, such as tumors or other constricting lesions that may cause constipation, often are accompanied by other symptoms. Thus the history must include questions concerning abdominal pain, weight loss, and bleeding from the rectum. In idiopathic, dietary, and drug-related constipation, there are usually no symptoms other than constipation, although a complaint of an abdominal bloating sensation is common with severe constipation.

A DRE is a sensitive screening tool in detecting anal lesions, although fissures and hemorrhoids, unless they are thrombosed or large, are found more reliably on anoscopy. Anoscopy should be performed routinely in constipated elderly patients. DRE of the anal canal and rectum is useful in assessing the tone of the internal anal sphincter and also the strength of the external sphincter and the puborectalis muscle.

The amount and the consistency of stool felt in the rectum may, in fact, indicate what type of constipation is present. Patients with a failure of the defecation mechanism tend to have much stool in the rectal vault, whereas those patients with colonic atony or irritable bowel syndrome have little or no stool in the rectum between defecations.

6. f. Although for most elderly patients constipation is just a minor annoyance, for some elders it is much more than that. The elders that are most susceptible to constipation are those who are institutionalized or bedridden.

Complications of constipation in the elderly include the following:

1. Fecal impaction is heralded by crampy, lower abdominal and lower back pain.
2. Stercoral ulcers are common in the patient who is bedridden. They are caused by pressure necrosis of the rectal or sigmoid mucosa as a result of a fecal mass. In some cases the ulcer may present as rectal bleeding.
3. Anal fissures may result from excessive straining at stool and the subsequent complications that develop, including tears and passive congestion of the tissues near the dentate line. The problem is enhanced by the irritating effect of hard stools and toilet paper. Intraabdominal pressures of up to 300 mm Hg are generated during straining. Excessive straining at stool may cause prolapse of the anal mucosa, venous distention, and internal hemorrhoids.
4. Megacolon in the elderly is almost always idiopathic. Chronic use of cathartics over a period of years may lead to an acquired degeneration of the colonic myenteric plexus and subsequent megacolon. Bacterial overgrowth may occur and further complicate matters.
5. Volvulus, especially of the sigmoid colon, occurs most commonly in elderly patients who are institutionalized and bedbound and carries a high mortality rate.
6. There is some evidence that chronic constipation is a risk factor for the development of carcinoma of the colon, particularly in women. This might be related to increased exposure time of susceptible mucosa to potentially carcinogenic substances.

7. c. The treatment of constipation is primarily nonpharmacologic. In large part, it involves inducing the patient to adopt a "healthier lifestyle." This includes a bowel-training regimen (a schedule of regular times for attempting defecation); regular exercise (bedridden patients are at great risk of constipation and often respond poorly to treatment); dietary adjustment to increase the amount of fiber in the diet; and an increased consumption of liquids, particularly water. Some foods that are exceptionally high in fiber include 100% bran cereals, beans (baked, kidney, lima, and navy), canned peas, raspberries, and broccoli.

It is not recommended that a regular or chronic laxative regimen be part of a routine prophylactic and treatment protocol for constipation.

8. b. The drug that is most closely associated with the development of constipation in the elderly is verapamil.

Verapamil is a calcium channel blocker commonly used to treat hypertension. Constipation develops in approximately 16% of patients who take verapamil for any length of time, and this percentage may be significantly higher in the elderly, especially in patients who are institutionalized or bedridden. The development of constipation-related complications already discussed may follow.

Constipation also may occur as a side effect of the use of hydrochlorothiazide, atenolol, or fluoxetine, but it does not appear to be what would be called a major side effect with those drugs. (Please refer to Answer 4.)

9. e. Constipation is often associated with fecal impaction; diarrhea; and crampy, lower abdominal and lower back pain.

Fecal impaction is the result of prolonged exposure of accumulated stool to the absorptive forces of the colon and rectum. The stool may become rocklike in consistency in the rectum (70%), in the sigmoid colon (20%), and in the distal colon (10%).

Symptoms of crampy, lower abdominal and lower back pain are common. Diarrhea may paradoxically follow the constipation, which leads to the impaction (watery material making its way around the impacted mass of stool). The impaction sometimes can be evacuated by the patient after the oral administration of polyethylene glycol (GoLYTELY), but manual disimpaction usually is required.

10. c. A survey in the United States of community-dwelling people older than age 65 years found that 30% of men and 29% of women considered themselves constipated. In the month preceding the survey, 24% of the men and 20% of the women had used laxatives.

11. a. The laxative group used to treat constipation can be divided into six major categories:

1. The bulk-forming laxatives: The bulk-forming laxatives include the various fiber-containing preparations and are thought to act in two major ways. They are hydrophilic and tend to increase the stool mass and soften the stool consistency. They are the safest laxatives and are generally well tolerated by elderly patients when introduced gradually.
2. The emollient laxatives: Emollients, or stool softeners, include mineral oil and the newer docusate salts such as dioctyl sodium sulfosuccinate (Colace). Mineral oil is generally not

recommended because safer, more effective agents are available. The newer agents reduce surface tension, allowing water to enter the stool more readily. They are generally well tolerated and may be particularly useful in elderly patients who are bedbound and at risk for fecal impaction.

3. The saline laxatives: Saline laxatives and enemas are salts of magnesium and sodium. Those in most common use are oral milk of magnesia, oral magnesium citrate, and sodium phosphate (Fleet's enema). All of these agents function as hyperosmolar agents and cause net secretion of fluid into the colon. Colonic motility is increased by these agents via release of the hormone cholecystokinin. Chronic use of magnesium-containing saline laxatives in elderly patients may contribute to hypermagnesemia (especially when there is associated impaired renal function). The phosphate-containing preparations also may induce hypocalcemia when high doses are used. The phosphate-containing enemas may cause damage to the rectum; this may occur via the nozzle part of the instrument itself or a direct toxic effect exerted by the hypertonic saline on the rectal mucosa.
4. The hyperosmotic laxatives: Hyperosmolar laxatives such as lactulose draw water into the gut lumen by an osmotic action. Lactulose is an undigestible agent that is metabolized by bacteria to hydrogen and organic acids. This causes acidification of the colon, and this, in addition to its osmotic effect, may alter electrolyte transport and colonic mobility.
5. The stimulant laxatives: The stimulant laxatives include the anthraquinone derivatives cascara, senna, and aloe; phenolphthalein; and bisacodyl (Dulcolax) tablets. Complications of the stimulant laxatives include melanosis coli from the anthraquinone group and complications such as Stevens-Johnson syndrome, dermatitis, and photosensitivity reactions from the phenolphthalein group. Although bisacodyl tablets probably are safer than the rest of the stimulant laxatives, all of the agents can cause electrolyte imbalance and precipitate hypokalemia, fluid and salt overload, and diarrhea. Thus the stimulant laxatives are the laxatives most closely associated with long-term side effects.
6. The lavage laxatives: The lavage laxatives are the newest group of laxatives. They include the agents GoLYTELY and COLyte. They work by stimulating neither secretion nor motility but by passing unimpeded through the GI tract. They are the most commonly used agents for bowel

preparation before flexible sigmoidoscopy and colonoscopy.

12. e. In this patient the increasing and different abdominal pain was caused by constipation. This patient had actually not had a bowel movement for 9 days. Thus the increasing severe abdominal pain (caused by increasing doses of morphine) completely overshadowed his previous pain (the pain caused by metastatic bone disease). Therefore switching to another painkiller is not a logical response.

13. e. The physical examination maneuver of choice in this patient is a DRE to confirm impacted stool.

14. e. The investigation of choice is an x-ray of the kidneys, ureter, and bladder (KUB) to confirm stool throughout the colon.

15. e. Remember, constipation is the single most common cause of abdominal pain in the elderly.

This patient's problem was treated by manual disimpaction, tap water enemas, and lactulose. To reduce the possibility of severe constipation, you should treat patients who you start them taking narcotic analgesics by following these two rules: (1) start a bowel regimen at the same time as you start the narcotic; and (2) maintain the bowel regimen for as long as you maintain the patient taking the narcotic.

SOLUTION TO THE CLINICAL CASE MANAGEMENT PROBLEM

The drug classes and their most common offenders are as follows:

Drug Class	Most Common Offender
Antihypertensives	Verapamil
Antianginal agents	Verapamil
Medical diagnostic agent	Barium sulfate
Antacids	Aluminum hydroxide
Nutritional supplement	Iron
Narcotic analgesics	Codeine
Antipsychotics	Thioridazine
Antidepressants	Amitriptyline
Anticholinergics	Trihexyphenidyl
Osteoporosis therapy	Calcium carbonate

SUMMARY OF CONSTIPATION

1. **Prevalence of constipation:** The reported prevalence of constipation in the elderly is 30%.
2. **Definition:** Constipation usually is defined as fewer than three bowel movements per week.
3. **Cause of constipation:** The cause of constipation includes declined or impaired general health status in the elderly, increasing number of medications (remember verapamil), and diminished mobility and physical activity.
4. **Diagnosis and investigation:** The patient's complete medical history is the most important part of the evaluation (remember to include complete functional inquiry of the GI tract). DRE is the most important part of the physical examination; anoscopy should accompany DRE. DRE and anoscopy may detect fissures, fistulas, strictures, carcinoma, or hemorrhoids.
5. **Complications:** The complications of constipation in the elderly include the following: (a) fecal impaction, crampy abdominal and back pain, and overflow diarrhea; (b) stercoral ulcers; (c) anal fissures and anal fistulas; (d) hemorrhoids (internal and external); (e) megacolon; (f) sigmoid volvulus; and (g) risk factor for carcinoma of the colon.

Continued

SUMMARY OF CONSTIPATION —cont'd

6. Treatment:
  a. Nonpharmacologic: (i) bowel training; (ii) exercise; (iii) high-fiber diet; and (iv) increased fluid intake
  b. Pharmacologic (laxatives): (i) bulk laxatives (recommended: Psyllium, methylcellulose, Polycarbophil); (ii) emollient laxatives (mineral oil is not recommended, but Colace is recommended); (iii) saline laxatives and enemas (not recommended on a long-term basis); (iv) hyperosmolar laxatives (recommended milk of magnesia [magnesium citrate], lactulose, sorbitol, glycerin, and polyethylene glycol); and (v) stimulant laxatives (not recommended [castor oil, Dulcolax, aloe, cascara, senna])

7. Rules summary:
  a. Always ask yourself the question, "Why is the patient constipated?" Constipation is not part of the normal aging process.
  b. Cancer is a common diagnosis in elderly patients. Most elderly patients with cancer eventually will require a narcotic analgesic. When that time comes, always start a constipation-correcting bowel regimen at the same time.

SUGGESTED READING

Useful information on constipation at the NIH website http://digestive. niddk.nih.gov/diseases/pubs/constipation/index.htm.
Murray FE, Bliss EM: Geriatric constipation: brief update on a common problem. *Geriatrics* 46(3):64-68, 1991.
Stark ME: Challenging problems presenting as constipation. *Am J Gastroenterol* 94(3):567-574, 1999.
Talle NJ, et al: Constipation in an elderly community: a study of prevalence and potential risk factors. *Am J Gastroenterol* 91(1):19-25, 1996.

Chapter 138

Pneumonia and Other Common Infectious Diseases of the Elderly

> "Clearly my father died because he caught pneumonia in your facility. I am going to call my attorney."

CLINICAL CASE PROBLEM 1:

AN 81-YEAR-OLD MALE WHO LIVES BY HIMSELF AND HAS INCREASING CONFUSION AND SHORTNESS OF BREATH

A previously healthy 81-year-old male is brought to the emergency department by his daughter. He lives by himself. He was well until 3 days ago. At that time, he became somewhat confused and began wandering aimlessly around the house and muttering incoherently. For the last 3 days he has had both nausea and anorexia. In addition, he became short of breath last night.

On physical examination, his blood pressure is 100/70 mm Hg. His pulse is 96 and regular. His respiratory rate is 28/minute, and his respirations appear slightly labored. On auscultation of his lung fields there are a few rales bilaterally but no other abnormalities. His white blood cell count (WBC) is 11,000/mm^3. His chest x-ray reveals right lower lobe consolidation. His PO_2 is 65 mm Hg, and his PCO_2 is 40 mm Hg.

SELECT THE BEST ANSWER TO THE FOLLOWING QUESTIONS:

1. What is the most likely diagnosis in this patient?
   a. bacterial pneumonia
   b. viral pneumonia
   c. fungal pneumonia
   d. aspiration pneumonia
   e. obstructive pneumonia

2. What is the most likely pathogen in this patient's pneumonia?
   a. *Klebsiella pneumoniae*
   b. *Haemophilus influenzae*
   c. influenza type B
   d. *Escherichia coli*
   e. *Streptococcus pneumoniae*

CLINICAL CASE PROBLEM 2:

AN 84-YEAR-OLD FEMALE WHO IS CURRENTLY RESIDING IN A LONG-TERM CARE FACILITY AND HAS INCREASING CONFUSION AND SHORTNESS OF BREATH

A presentation with almost identical symptoms and signs as the patient in Clinical Case Problem 1 occurs in an 84-year-old female who is residing in a long-term care facility and who has many chronic medical conditions. Compare her presentation to the presentation of the patient described in Clinical Case Problem 1.

3. Which of the following statements is (are) true?
   a. the prognosis is likely to be similar in both individuals
   b. the responsible organism is likely to be the same
   c. the treatment is likely to be the same
   d. all of the above statements are true
   e. none of the above statements are true

4. What is the treatment of choice for the patient described in Clinical Case Problem 1?
   a. amoxicillin
   b. erythromycin
   c. gentamicin
   d. cefixime
   e. amphotericin B

CLINICAL CASE PROBLEM 3:
AN 81-YEAR-OLD FEMALE WITH DYSURIA, FREQUENCY, URGENCY, AND INCONTINENCE

An 81-year-old female comes to your office with a 5-day history of dysuria, frequency, urgency, and incontinence. She has no other symptoms, including no costovertebral angle (CVA) tenderness or other symptoms. The patient lives at home by herself and has had no major medical problems.

On examination, her temperature is 37° C (98.6° F). Her blood pressure is 150/80 mm Hg, and her pulse is 84 and regular. No other abnormalities are found on physical examination.

5. Which of the following statements concerning this patient is (are) true?
   a. the most likely diagnosis is acute bacterial cystitis
   b. the most likely organism is *P. aeruginosa*
   c. amoxicillin is a reasonable first-choice antibiotic
   d. this patient should be treated for 14 days
   e. all of the above statements are true

6. Which of the following is (are) risk factors for the development of urinary tract infections in elderly patients?
   a. advanced age
   b. decreased bladder emptying
   c. prostatic hypertrophy
   d. decreased host defense mechanisms
   e. all of the above

7. What is the most common pathogen in urinary tract infections in noncatheterized elderly patients?
   a. *Serratia* sp.
   b. *Proteus mirabilis*
   c. *Klebsiella* sp.
   d. *E. coli*
   e. *Pseudomonas aeruginosa*

8. Concerning chronic prostatitis in elderly patients, which of the following statements is (are) true?
   a. chronic prostatitis is the most common cause of relapsing urinary tract infections in elderly males
   b. prostatic massage is not helpful in establishing a diagnosis
   c. *Klebsiella* is the most common pathogen in this condition
   d. with prolonged therapy, relapse becomes unlikely
   e. all of the above statements are true

CLINICAL CASE PROBLEM 4:
A 75-YEAR-OLD FEMALE WITH FEVER, CHILLS, CONFUSION, DYSURIA, AND DIARRHEA

A 75-year-old female comes to your office with a 2-day history of fever, chills, confusion, dysuria, and diarrhea. There are no other symptoms, including no back pain.

On examination, the patient's temperature is 38.5° C (101.3° F). Her blood pressure is 120/75 mm Hg, and her pulse is 96 and regular. There is no demonstrable CVA tenderness.

9. What is the most likely diagnosis in this patient?
   a. acute bacterial cystitis
   b. viral gastroenteritis
   c. acute pyelonephritis
   d. bacterial gastroenteritis
   e. none of the above

10. Regarding the use of antibiotics in elderly patients with indwelling catheters, which of the following statements is (are) true?
    a. indwelling urinary catheters are the leading cause of nosocomial infections
    b. indwelling urinary catheters are the most common predisposing factor in hospital-acquired, fatal, gram-negative sepsis
    c. by the time a urinary catheter has been in place for 2 weeks, 50% of catheterized patients have significant bacteriuria
    d. all of the above statements are true
    e. none of the above statements are true

11. What is the leading cause of death from infection in hospitalized elderly patients?
    a. bacterial pneumonia
    b. urinary tract infection
    c. pressure ulcers
    d. diverticulitis
    e. septic arthritis

12. What is the leading cause of death from infection in institutionalized elderly patients?

a. bacterial pneumonia
b. urinary tract infection
c. pressure ulcers
d. diverticulitis
e. septic arthritis

13. What is the leading cause of death from infection in elderly individuals living in the community?
a. bacterial pneumonia
b. urinary tract infection
c. pressure ulcers
d. diverticulitis
e. septic arthritis

14. In considering acute appendicitis in elderly patients, which of the following statements is (are) true?
a. the presenting signs and symptoms are similar to younger patients
b. gangrene of the appendix is uncommon
c. morbidity and mortality are much higher than in younger patients
d. all of the above statements are true
e. none of the above statements are true

15. Which of the following statements concerning fever in elderly patients is (are) true?
a. fever in elderly patients is more likely to be the result of a serious pathologic condition than in younger patients
b. when compared to younger patients, older adults often fail to show a temperature elevation despite having a serious infectious disease
c. in elderly patients with fever of undetermined origin (FUO), a localized infection (such as an abscess) often is found
d. all of the above statements are true
e. none of the above statements are true

CLINICAL CASE PROBLEM 5:

A 75-Year-Old Woman with an Itching and Burning Feeling on Her Face

You are called in to examine a 75-year-old female nursing home resident who has developed a rash accompanied by severe itching and a burning sensation on her face.

On examination you note that the effected area follows the course of the trigeminal nerve on the left side of her face. It leads to her left eye, which is dropping. The right side is not affected. The patient also tells you that for the past 3 or 4 days the effected areas hurt and itched but only today did a rash appear.

16. This lady most likely is suffering from:
a. Herpes zoster
b. trigeminal neuralgia

c. Bell's palsy
d. poison oak
e. none of the above

CLINICAL CASE MANAGEMENT PROBLEM

Consider the following functional states or levels of care in elderly patients and the following primary considerations in infectious or inflammatory disease. What are, in the order of frequency, the three common primary infectious diseases in each of the following groups?
1. Independent healthy elderly individuals living in the community
2. Hospitalized elderly patients
3. Nursing home or institutionalized elderly residents

■ ANSWERS:

1. **a.** The most likely diagnosis in this patient is a bacterial pneumonia. The presentation of bacterial pneumonia in elderly patients is usually much more subtle and nonspecific than in younger patients. As illustrated in this case presentation, confusion is a very common early sign. Other nonspecific early signs include disorientation and a change (decrease) in the elder's interest level. A fall is often part of the presenting symptoms and signs of elder infectious illness.

Findings on physical examination are also nonspecific. Signs of consolidation are often absent. Rales are common but not specific. An increased respiratory rate (as in this patient) may precede other signs and symptoms. Pleuritic chest pain, dyspnea, productive cough, chills, and rigors are not always present in the elderly.

The specificity of laboratory abnormalities found in elders with bacterial pneumonia is low. An increased WBC (less than 10,000 mm^3) commonly is found, but as well as being nonspecific, the WBC also has relatively low sensitivity. Hypoxemia is a common finding. In elderly patients with bacterial pneumonia the correlation between clinical findings and radiologic findings is poor. Up to 50% have a normal WBC count, but 95% have a left shift.

2. **e.** The most likely pathogen associated with community-acquired pneumonia is *S. pneumoniae*. *H. influenzae, K. pneumoniae,* and gram-negative bacilli are much less common unless there is associated chronic obstructive pulmonary disease or an immune-compromising condition. Expected organisms for community-acquired pneumonia include strep pneumonia, respiratory viruses, *H. influenzae,* gram-negative bacteria, *Moraxella catarrhalis,* legionella, tuberculosis,

and endemic fungi (listed in order of frequency of occurrence).

In summary, the difference between younger adults and older adults in community-acquired bacterial pneumonia is that *S. pneumoniae* is the responsible organism in 60% to 80% of younger patients but only 40% to 60% of elderly patients.

3. b. The most important differences between the two presentations are as follows:

1. The patient presented in Clinical Case Problem 1 resides in the community, whereas the patient presented in Clinical Case Problem 2 resides in a long-term care facility.
2. The patient presented in Clinical Case Problem 1 is otherwise healthy and has no significant medical problems, whereas the patent described in Clinical Case Problem 2 has many other chronic health problems.
3. The organism found in the patient in Clinical Case Problem 1 is likely to be *S. pneumoniae*, the most common cause of bacterial community-acquired pneumonia. The most likely organism to be found in the patient in Clinical Case Problem 2 is still *S. pneumoniae*, but other candidates should be considered, such as *H. influenzae*, *K. pneumoniae*, or other gram-negative organisms.
4. Because it is more likely to find gram-negative organisms in the patient in Clinical Case Problem 2, the treatments may be different.
5. The virulence of the organism on the host in the patient in Clinical Case Problem 2 is likely to be significantly greater than the virulence of the organism in the patient in Clinical Case Problem 1. Thus the prognosis in the patient Clinical Case Problem 2 is significantly less favorable than the prognosis in the patient in Clinical Case Problem 1.

4. b. The treatment of choice for a community-acquired bacterial pneumonia in an elderly patient is an agent that is active against *S. pneumoniae*, *H. influenzae*, *Mycoplasma pneumoniae*, *Chlamydia pneumoniae*, and *Legionella* spp. The current recommendation is a macrolide such as erythromycin, azithromycin, or clarithromycin or one of the newer quinolones such as levofloxacin. In addition, a second generation cephalosporin may be used. For outpatients at risk for drug-resistant strep pneumoniae, a beta-lactam or macrolide combination or quinolone can be used.

5. a. Regarding Clinical Case Problem 3, the following facts can be stated:

1. This appears to be an uncomplicated urinary tract infection.

2. The most likely infecting organism is *E. coli*, but *Klebsiella*, *Proteus mirabilis*, and *Pseudomonas aeruginosa* also must be considered.
3. The most likely diagnosis is acute bacterial cystitis, which is confirmed when there are no signs or symptoms of upper urinary tract infection and the bacterial count is greater than 105 organisms per milliliter of urine. The most common symptoms encountered in acute bacterial cystitis are lower abdominal or pelvic pain, dysuria, increased frequency of urination, and recent episodes of urinary incontinence.
4. The first-line drug in this case would be trimethoprim-sulfamethoxazole (TMP-SMX). A cephalosporin or quinolone (such as ciprofloxacin or levofloxacin) also would be a reasonable first-line of therapy. Amoxicillin/clavulanic acid should be reserved for those with an allergy to sulfa or where resistance is known. Although treatment with a single dose of TMP-SMX is reasonable for younger adults, it cannot be recommended for the elderly. For elders in the same situation, a 7-day course would be the best choice.

6. e. Urinary tract infections in the elderly are second only to respiratory tract infections as causes of febrile illness in patients older than age 65 years. The risk factors for urinary tract infections in the elderly include the following: (1) advanced age (the older the patient, the greater the risk, which appears to be immune-system dependent); (2) decreased functional ability resulting from cerebral vascular accidents, dementia, neurologic deficits, functional ability, and other chronic underlying illness; (3) decreased bladder emptying resulting from neurogenic bladder, bladder-outlet obstruction (such as prostatic hypertrophy), and drugs with anticholinergic side effects; (4) nosocomial spread of organisms, spread from hospitalized patients with asymptomatic bacteriuria and the use of indwelling urinary catheters; and (5) physiologic changes such as decreased vaginal glycogen and increased vaginal pH in women and decreased prostatic secretions and increased prostatic calculi in men.

7. d. The most common organism responsible for urinary tract infections in elderly patients who do not have indwelling urinary catheters is *E. coli*. Other gram-negative organisms responsible include *Klebsiella*, *Enterococcus*, *Pseudomonas*, and *Proteus mirabilis*. However, in the absence of a complication (such as an indwelling catheter), *E. coli* still predominates. In summary, the difference between younger adults and older adults with respect to the cause of uncomplicated urinary tract infections is that although *E. coli* is the most common agent in both younger adults and older patients, the percentage of infections caused by *E. coli* is lower in older patients; that is, in older patients with an acute uncomplicated urinary tract infection there is more of a chance of an infection caused by *Klebsiella, Enterococcus, Proteus mirabilis,* or *Pseudomonas.*

8. a. Chronic bacterial prostatitis is the most common cause of relapsing urinary tract infection in elderly males.

The diagnosis of chronic bacterial prostatitis is established by culturing prostatic secretions obtained by prostatic massage. The most common causative organism is *E. coli,* but *K. pneumoniae, Proteus,* and *Enterococcus* spp. are other organisms associated with the condition. The preferred antibiotic treatment is TMP-SMX or a quinolone antibiotic such as ciprofloxacin or levofloxacin. (Quinolones may be more effective and must be given for 12 weeks.) Relapses are common, even with prolonged therapy. This condition may be ameliorated by transurethral resection of the prostate.

In summary, the difference between younger adult males and older adult males with respect to prostatitis is that acute bacterial prostatitis is much more common in younger males and chronic bacterial prostatitis is much more common in older patients.

9. c. The patient described in Clinical Case Problem 4 has acute pyelonephritis. Elderly patients who develop a syndrome of fever, chills, and irritating voiding symptoms likely have acute pyelonephritis despite the absence of CVA tenderness. In fact, not more than half of elders who develop pyelonephritis have the back pain and CVA tenderness that is so classic in younger patients with the disease. Some elders do not even have fever. Geriatric patients often also have gastrointestinal symptoms such as diarrhea or pulmonary symptoms.

Bacteremia is much more common in elderly patients who develop pyelonephritis, and the urinary tract is the source of bacteremia in more than one-third of elders admitted to the hospital with generalized sepsis. Thus blood cultures are mandatory before initiating treatment. From sepsis follows septic shock in up to 20% of elders with acute pyelonephritis. As with lower urinary tract infections, the most common organisms involved are *E. coli, Klebsiella, Proteus,* and *Pseudomonas.*

For elderly patients, the best initial antibiotic choice for suspected pyelonephritis is a combination of a beta-lactamase–resistant cephalosporin and an aminoglycoside (the latter to be used with extreme caution and with careful monitoring of serum levels).

In summary, the difference between younger adults and elderly patients with respect to complicated urinary tract infections such as acute pyelonephritis is that older patients frequently do not manifest the same symptoms and signs of complicated urinary tract infections as do younger adults. Specifically, they are less likely to manifest CVA tenderness and even fever and chills. This infection must be suspected in elderly patients who are immunocompromised and incapacitated (patients who are hospitalized or in long-term care facilities).

In addition, the probability of septicemia/generalized sepsis is greatly increased in elderly patients who develop urinary tract infections.

10. d. By 2 weeks 50% of catheterized patients have significant bacteriuria, and after 1 month virtually all patients do.

Indwelling urinary catheters are the leading cause of nosocomial infection and the most common predisposing factor in hospital-acquired, gram-negative sepsis. Patients who have asymptomatic bacteriuria should not be treated with antibiotics. This applies to catheterized patients as well.

11. b. In the hospitalized elder, the most common cause of morbidity and mortality is septicemia from a urinary tract infection.

12. a. Elderly patients living in long-term care facilities are susceptible to bacterial pneumonia, which is their most common cause of death from an infective source.

13. a. The leading infective causes of morbidity and mortality in elderly patients vary depending on location of the elder's habitation.

The most common cause of death from an infective source is bacterial pneumonia in elderly patients living in the community and in long-term care facilities. This serves to illustrate the importance of preventive services designated for this age group. The United States Task Force on the Periodic Health Examination recommends that (1) all individuals older than age 65 years receive annual influenza vaccinations, and (2) all individuals older than age 65 years should receive the Pneumovax vaccination. (Consider revaccination every 6-7 years.)

Although bacterial pneumonia is discussed as the primary cause of morbidity and mortality, it must be understood that viral pneumonia frequently predates bacterial pneumonia (i.e., influenza produces a viral pneumonia that leads to a secondary bacterial pneumonia).

14. c. Acute appendicitis is primarily a disease of younger patients in their second or third decade of life. However, it also occurs with increasing frequency in males older than age 80 years. The mortality in this age group is 10%. As with other abdominal infections such as acute cholecystitis, the increased severity of disease is largely caused by the atypical presentation of the signs and symptoms of acute inflammation (or more appropriately the lack of signs and symptoms of acute inflammation). Instead of the classic time sequence of periumbilical pain; anorexia, nausea, and vomiting; and movement of the pain to the right lower quadrant seen in younger patients, the elderly male with acute appendicitis usually has a prolonged period of vague abdominal discomfort.

There may be mild nausea and anorexia, but vomiting is unusual. As localized peritonitis develops, pain may appear in the right lower quadrant. Rebound tenderness and abdominal guarding, so common in younger adults, are uncommon in the elderly.

Perforation of the appendix is much more common in the elderly because of the narrowing of the lumen and the atherosclerotic changes in the artery supplying the appendix. In elderly patients, approximately 70% of cases of acute appendicitis rupture, compared with 20% in younger patients.

In summary, critical differences between younger adults and older adults with appendicitis are that the elderly have atypical symptoms, have a high rate of perforation, and have a high mortality rate (10%).

15. **d.** In children and in young and middle-aged adults, fever is often the result of a relatively benign disease. Such is not the case with the elderly. The rapid development of an elevated body temperature in an older adult is almost invariably the result of a serious infection such as pneumonia, urinary tract infection, or an intraabdominal abscess. Although the presence of fever in an older adult usually indicates a serious infection or other serious disease process (such as neoplasia and connective tissue disorders), elderly patients are two to three times as likely to

demonstrate a lack of febrile response to the presence of serious disease.

In older adults who have FUO, the probability of a localized infection such as an abscess is high.

In summary, elders with a fever usually have a serious rather than a benign disease process going on. Always take this seriously.

16. **a.** This woman most likely is suffering from Herpes zoster (or shingles). Shingles is caused by reactivation of the varicella-zoster virus that caused chicken pox. After a primary illness with varicella-zoster, the virus can lay dormant in a dorsal root ganglion only to become reactivated at a later time. Shingles usually appears in the elderly or in immuno-compromised individuals, and it can reoccur. There usually is a prodromal period that occurs some 4-5 days before eruption of skin lesions. The route of the affected area usually follows the course of the nerve from the infected dorsal ganglion. Most commonly, areas of the trunk are involved, but the trigeminal nerve also commonly is affected. If the infection spreads into the eye, serious ophthalmitic damage can occur.

Treatment is an antiviral such as acyclovir (Zovirax), valacyclovir (Valtrex), or famciclovir (Famvir). Adjunctive treatment with oral prednisone also is used, provided there are no contraindications. It is believed that this reduces the chance of postherpetic neuralgia.

SUMMARY OF PNEUMONIA AND OTHER COMMON INFECTIOUS DISEASES OF THE ELDERLY

Because summaries are provided throughout the answers, a detailed summary will not be repeated for this chapter.

SOLUTION TO THE CLINICAL CASE MANAGEMENT PROBLEM

Primary considerations in infectious diseases in the elderly depending on the habitation status of the elder are as follows:

1. The three primary types of infection for elders living in a community setting are (a) bacterial pneumonia; (b) urinary tract infections; and (c) intraabdominal infections, including cholecystitis, diverticulitis, and appendicitis.
2. The three primary types of infection for hospitalized

elders are (a) urinary tract infections; (b) bacterial pneumonia (gram negative, anaerobes, gram positive, fungi); and (c) surgical wound infections.
3. The three primary types of infection for nursing home or other institutionalized elders are (a) bacterial pneumonia (*Streptococcal pneumoniae*, gram negative, *Staphylococcus aureus*, anaerobes, *H. influenza*, group B streptococcus, chlamydia), (b) urinary tract infection; and (c) decubitus ulcers.

SUGGESTED READING

Culligan PJ, Heit M: Urinary incontinence in women: evaluation and management. *Am Fam Physician* 62:2433-2444, 2000.

Johnston CB, et al: Geriatric medicine. In: Tierny LM, et al, eds.: *Current medical diagnosis and treatment 2003*, 42nd edition. McGraw-Hill, 2002, New York, 41-58.

Mouton CP, Bazaldua OV: Common infections in older adults. *Am Fam Physician* 63:257-268, 2001.

Whitley RJ, Gnann JW: Herpes zoster, focus on treatment in the elderly. *Anti Viral Res* 44(3):145-154, 1999.

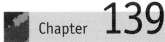

Chapter 139

Urinary Incontinence

"Doctor, I'm so embarrassed. I can't go out anywhere."

CLINICAL CASE PROBLEM 1:

AN 88-YEAR-OLD INSTITUTIONALIZED FEMALE WITH URINARY INCONTINENCE

An 88-year-old female patient who you care for and who resides in a chronic care facility is having increasing difficulties with "bedwetting." She is embarrassed to talk about this, but the nurses inform you that it is a problem and is getting progressively worse.

On your last weekly visit, the charge nurse requested permission from you to insert an indwelling urinary catheter. At that time, the patient had been incontinent continuously for 6 days. The charge nurse clearly tells you, "I haven't got enough staff to keep changing sheets 10 times a day. Please do something."

■ SELECT THE BEST ANSWER TO THE FOLLOWING QUESTIONS:

1. At this time, what should your instructions to the charge nurse be?
   a. insert the indwelling catheter; call me if there are any more problems
   b. begin intermittent 4-hour catheterization to avoid the necessity of inserting an indwelling catheter
   c. wait and see what happens over the next couple of weeks
   d. order some routine blood work to attempt to determine the cause of the problem
   e. clearly indicate that you will begin investigation of this problem now; ask the charge nurse, in return, to attempt to manage the current situation for only a short time longer

2. Regarding urinary incontinence in the elderly, which of the following statements is false?
   a. 50% of elderly patients in nursing homes have established urinary incontinence
   b. 5% to 15% of elderly patients in a community setting have developed urinary incontinence
   c. women are twice as likely as men to have urinary incontinence
   d. humiliation and embarrassment are significant life problems for the patient with urinary incontinence
   e. none of the above statements are false

3. What is the most common type of urinary incontinence in elderly patients?
   a. urge incontinence
   b. stress incontinence
   c. complex incontinence
   d. overflow incontinence
   e. functional incontinence

4. Which of the following statements regarding incontinence in the elderly is (are) true?
   a. stress incontinence usually is manifested by loss of small amounts of urine as intraabdominal pressure increases
   b. overflow incontinence occurs through bladder distention
   c. prostatic obstruction is a common cause of overflow incontinence
   d. functional incontinence is characterized by an involuntary loss of urine despite normal bladder and urethral functioning
   e. all of the above statements are true

5. Which of the following is (are) a contributing factor(s) to urinary incontinence in the elderly?
   a. a loss of the ability of the elderly to concentrate urine
   b. a decreased bladder capacity
   c. decreased urethral closing pressure
   d. decreased mobility
   e. all of the above

6. Which of the following classes of drugs have not been implicated in the pathogenesis of urinary incontinence in the elderly?
   a. thiazide diuretics
   b. neuroleptics
   c. sedatives
   d. antibiotics
   e. hypnotics

7. Which of the following nonpharmacologic treatments may be effective in the management of urinary incontinence in the elderly?
   a. Kegel exercises
   b. biofeedback
   c. behavioral toilet training
   d. clean intermittent catheterization
   e. all of the above

8. Which of the following cause(s) acute (reversible) urinary incontinence in the elderly?
   a. delirium
   b. restricted mobility
   c. infection
   d. drugs
   e. all of the above

9. Anticholinergic and narcotic drugs are most commonly associated with which of the following types of urinary incontinence?
   a. urge incontinence
   b. stress incontinence
   c. overflow incontinence
   d. complex incontinence
   e. functional incontinence

10. Which of the following components of the diagnostic evaluation of urinary incontinence is not necessary in every elderly patient with the disorder?
    a. complete history
    b. focused physical examination
    c. renal ultrasound
    d. complete urinalysis
    e. postvoiding residual (PVR) urine determination

11. PVR urine is considered definitely abnormal when it exceeds which of the following?
    a. 50 ml
    b. 100 ml
    c. 75 ml
    d. 125 ml
    e. 150 ml

12. What is (are) the drug(s) of choice for the pharmacologic management of stress incontinence?
    a. supplemental estrogen
    b. alpha-adrenergic agonists
    c. cholinergic agents
    d. a and b
    e. a, b, and c

13. Which of the following types of urinary incontinence is most amenable to surgical intervention?
    a. urge incontinence
    b. stress incontinence
    c. overflow incontinence
    d. complex incontinence
    e. functional incontinence

14. Which of the following are indications for the use of a chronic indwelling catheter in elderly patients with incontinence?
    a. urinary retention causing persistent overflow incontinence
    b. chronic skin wounds or pressure ulcers that can be contaminated by incontinent urine
    c. terminally ill or severely impaired elderly patients for whom bed and clothing changes are uncomfortable
    d. urinary retention that cannot be controlled medically or surgically
    e. none of the above statements are true
    f. a, b, c, and d

15. Alzheimer's disease, Parkinson's disease, and cerebrovascular disease usually are associated with which of the following types of urinary incontinence?
    a. urge incontinence
    b. stress incontinence
    c. overflow incontinence
    d. complex incontinence
    e. functional incontinence

CLINICAL CASE MANAGEMENT PROBLEM

List the patient-dependent (4) and caregiver-dependent (2) behaviorally oriented training procedures that may be beneficial in the management of urinary incontinence in the elderly.

ANSWERS:

1. **e.** In an elderly patient who has just become incontinent, it is inappropriate to insert a Foley catheter or do anything else until you have established the cause. The pathophysiology of urinary incontinence in the elderly population is complex, even among patients with dementia. Elderly patients deserve the same intensive investigation of the cause of incontinence as you would perform in a younger individual.

2. **e.** Of elderly patients in nursing homes, 50% have urinary incontinence. Of elderly patients in the community, 5% to 15% have urinary incontinence. Women are twice as likely as men to develop urinary incontinence. Humiliation and embarrassment are important consequences of urinary incontinence in elderly patients. This embarrassment leads to social

isolation and subsequent anxiety and depression. Incontinence is the second-leading cause of admission of elderly patients to long-term care facilities. In North America it is estimated that the total health care costs associated with urinary incontinence are more than $8 billion per year. Physical consequences, such as predisposition to skin irritations and subsequent skin ulcers and infections, are also a major problem.

3. a. The most common type of urinary incontinence in the elderly population is urge incontinence. Urge incontinence (also known as detrusor hyperreflexia) is characterized by leakage of urine caused by strong and sudden sensations of bladder urgency. Patients with urge incontinence also may experience frequency, urgency, and nocturia. Urge incontinence is also called *unstable bladder, uninhibited bladder,* and *hyperreflexic bladder.* Many conditions may predispose to urge incontinence; these include cerebrovascular accidents, Parkinson's disease, Alzheimer's disease, spinal cord injury or tumor, multiple sclerosis, prostatic hypertrophy, and interstitial cystitis.

Urge incontinence also may be present in patients in whom no neurologic or genitourinary abnormality is present.

4. e. Stress incontinence (urethral incompetence) is characterized by loss of small amounts of urine secondary to increases in intraabdominal pressure. Stress incontinence is most commonly associated with pelvic floor weakening through childbirth, obesity, injury, menopause and aging, and sphincter damage.

Overflow incontinence occurs with bladder overdistention. Overdistention results in a constant leakage of small amounts of urine or "dribbling," a physiologic situation in which the intracystic pressure exceeds the intraurethral resistance. Bladder overdistention usually is caused by an enlarged prostate, urethral stricture, or fecal impaction. A hypotonic bladder secondary to diabetes mellitus, syphilis, spinal cord compression, or anticholinergic medications also may result in overflow incontinence.

Complex incontinence refers to incontinence that has both urge and stress components.

Functional incontinence refers to involuntary loss of urine despite normal bladder and urethral functioning. This is seen most commonly with severe dementia and closed head injuries causing an inability or unwillingness to toilet because of physical, cognitive, psychologic, or environmental factors.

5. e. Many factors are associated with the development and maintenance of urinary incontinence in the elderly. These include a loss of the ability of the kidney to concentrate urine, a decreased bladder capacity, decreased urethral closing pressure following menopause, decreased mobility, decreased vision, depres-

sion, secondary inattention to bladder cues, and an inadequate environmental setting.

The importance of drugs in the causation of elderly incontinence is discussed in Answer 6.

6. d. Drug use is a common cause of incontinence in the elderly. The major drugs implicated as a cause of urinary incontinence in the elderly and the pathology involved are summarized in the table:

Drug Class	Pathology
Diuretics	Polyuria, frequency, urgency
Anticholinergics	Urinary retention, overflow incontinence, impaction
Antidepressants	Anticholinergic actions, sedation
Antipsychotics	Anticholinergic actions, sedation, rigidity, immobility
Sedative hypnotics	Sedation, delirium, immobility, muscle relaxation
Narcotic analgesics	Urinary retention, fecal impaction, sedation, delirium
Alpha-adrenergic	Urethral relaxation blockers
Alpha-adrenergic	Urinary retention agonists
Beta-adrenergic	Urinary retention blockers
Calcium channel blocker	Urinary retention
Alcohol	Polyuria, frequency, urgency, sedation, delirium, immobility

7. e. Nonpharmacologic treatments are both available and useful in the treatment of all forms of urinary incontinence in the elderly. The treatments include the following:

1. Stress incontinence: (a) pelvic muscle (Kegel) exercises, (b) biofeedback, (c) behavioral therapies (prompted voiding, habit training, and scheduled toileting), and (d) transcutaneous electrical nerve stimulation (TENS)
2. Urge incontinence: (a) biofeedback, (b) behavioral therapies (as previously listed), and (c) TENS
3. Overflow incontinence: (a) intermittent catheterization, (b) indwelling catheterization (use only for chronic urinary retention, for nonhealing pressure ulcers in patients who are incontinent, and when required by patients of families to promote comfort)
4. Functional incontinence: (a) behavioral therapies (as previously listed), (b) environmental manipulations, (c) incontinence undergarments and pads, (d) external collection devices, (e) indwelling catheters (if necessary), and (f) TENS

In the past, TENS has been used successfully to

treat chronic pain syndromes. An exciting new development provides another opportunity to avoid both surgery and pharmacologic agents in treatment of incontinence. The use of a pessary TENS unit has been shown to be effective for stress incontinence and urge incontinence. More trials need to be carried out before definitive conclusions can be made, but initial results are promising.

8. e. Causes of acute and reversible forms of urinary incontinence are provided by the DRIP mnemonic:
1. **D**elirium
2. **R**estricted mobility, retention
3. **I**nfection (urinary tract), inflammation (urethritis or atrophic vaginitis), impaction (fecal)
4. **P**olyuria (diabetes mellitus, diabetes insipidus, congestive heart failure, and venous insufficiency), pharmaceuticals

9. c. Urinary retention with overflow incontinence must be considered when any patient, who was previously completely continent, suddenly becomes incontinent. The causes include immobility, anticholinergic drugs, narcotic analgesic drugs, calcium channel blockers, beta blockers, fecal impaction, and spinal cord compression resulting from metastatic cancer.

10. c. The evaluation of urinary incontinence in the elderly should be undertaken with the same precision and care as evaluation and investigation of other urinary problems in younger patients.

All elderly patients who present with urinary incontinence should have the following procedures performed: (1) a complete history; (2) complete medication review (ideally, every elderly patient taking more than one drug should have this done every 3 months); (3) an age-specific focused physical examination (see U.S. Preventive Services Task Force recommendations); (4) complete urinalysis; (5) urine culture; and (6) a PVR urine determination.

A renal ultrasound needs to be done only if problems such as urinary obstruction (a renal tumor), uremia, or the inability of the kidneys to concentrate urine is suspected.

11. b. A PVR urine should be performed on every elderly patient with incontinence to exclude significant degrees of urinary retention. Neither the history nor the physical examination is sensitive or specific enough for this purpose in elderly patients. The PVR urine can be done either by itself as a simple one-test procedure or in conjunction with other simple urodynamic investigations.

To maximize the accuracy of PVR urine, the measurement should be performed within a few minutes of voiding. A PVR volume of 100 ml or less in the absence of straining reflects adequate bladder emptying in elderly patients. If more than 100 ml, it suggests detrusor weakness, neuropathy, outlet obstruction, or detrusor hyperactivity with impaired contractility (DHIC).

12. d. The ideal combination of pharmacologic agents for certain patients with stress incontinence involves supplemental estrogen and an alpha-adrenergic agonist.

For patients with stress incontinence, pharmacologic management is appropriate provided the following criteria are met: (1) the patient is motivated; (2) the degree of stress incontinence is "mild to moderate"; (3) there is no major associated anatomic abnormality (such as a large cystocele); and (4) the patient does not have any contraindications to the use of these drugs.

Pharmacologic treatment of stress incontinence is as efficacious as, but not more efficacious than, nonpharmacologic treatment. Approximately 75% of patients improve with each type. Combining the two modalities improves the efficacy of treatment.

Supplemental estrogen has not been found, by itself, to be as effective as when used in combination with an alpha-adrenergic agonist. If either oral or vaginal estrogen is used for a prolonged period (greater than a few months), then cyclic progesterone should be added to protect the endometrium. A combination of oral Premarin (0.3 mg/day) and oral pseudoephedrine (Sudafed), 30-60 mg bid, would be a good starting point for pharmacologic treatment of stress incontinence.

13. b. The type of incontinence that is most amenable to surgical intervention is stress incontinence. The indication for surgery in stress incontinence is continued, significant bothersome leakage that occurs after attempts at nonsurgical treatment and patients who, along with their stress incontinence, also have a significant degree of pelvic prolapse.

The second most amenable subtype of incontinence that may be significantly improved with surgery is outflow obstruction caused by prostatic hypertrophy or prostatic carcinoma in men. With benign prostatic hypertrophy it would be prudent to reduce the size of the prostate and decrease obstruction by use of a 5-alpha-reductase inhibitor or an alpha-adrenergic blocker (doxazosin, terazosin, prazosin) before contemplating surgery.

14. f. The indications for chronic indwelling catheter use include the following:
1. Urinary retention that is (a) causing persistent overflow incontinence; (b) causing symptomatic infections; (c) producing renal dysfunction;

(d) unable to be corrected surgically or medically; and (e) not practically managed with intermittent catheterization.
2. Skin wounds, pressure sores, or irritations that are being contaminated by incontinent urine
3. Care of terminally ill or severely impaired patients for whom bed and clothing changes are uncomfortable or disruptive

4. Preference of patient or caregiver when a patient has failed to respond to more specific treatments

15. **a.** Central nervous system disorders such as cerebrovascular accidents (stroke), dementia, Parkinson's disease, and suprasacral spinal cord injury are associated with detrusor motor or sensory instability resulting in urge incontinence.

 ## SOLUTION TO THE CLINICAL CASE MANAGEMENT PROBLEM

Following are examples of behaviorally oriented training procedures for urinary incontinence.
A. Patient-dependent procedures: (1) pelvic muscle (Kegel) exercises; (2) biofeedback; (3) behavioral training; and (4) bladder retraining
B. Caregiver-dependent procedures: (1) scheduled toileting or prompted voiding; and (2) habit training

---

 ## SUMMARY OF URINARY INCONTINENCE

A. **Definition:** the involuntary loss of urine in sufficient amount or frequency to be a social or health problem
B. **Subtypes of urinary incontinence:** acute (reversible) versus persistent urinary incontinence
C. **Acute (reversible) urinary incontinence: DRIP mnemonic: D**elirium; **R**estricted mobility, retention; **I**nfection, inflammation, impaction; **P**olyuria, pharmaceuticals
D. **Persistent urinary incontinence:**
   1. Stress: Involuntary loss of urine (usually small amounts) with increases in intraabdominal pressure (such as cough, laugh, or exercise). Common causes include weakness and laxity of pelvic floor musculature and bladder outlet or urethral sphincter weakness.
   2. Urge: Leakage of urine (often larger volumes, but variable) because of inability to delay voiding after sensation or bladder fullness is perceived; also known as *detrusor hyperreflexia*. Common causes include detrusor motor or sensory instability, isolated or associated with one or more of the following: cystitis, urethritis, tumors, stones, diverticula, or outflow obstruction; also central nervous system disorders such as stroke, dementia, Parkinson's disease, and suprasacral spinal cord injury.

   3. Overflow: Leakage of urine (usually small amounts) resulting from mechanical forces on an overdistended bladder or from other effects of urinary retention on either bladder or sphincter function. Common causes include anatomic obstruction by prostate, stricture, and cystocele; hypotonic bladder associated with diabetes mellitus or a spinal cord injury; neurogenic (detrusor-sphincter dyssynergy) associated with multiple sclerosis, or supraspinal cord lesions.
   4. Functional: Urinary leakage associated with the inability to toilet because of impairment of cognitive or physical functioning, psychologic unwillingness, or environmental barriers. Common causes include severe dementia and other neurologic disorders or psychologic factors such as depression, regression, anger, and hostility.
E. **Prevalence of urinary incontinence in the elderly is as follows:** (1) institutionalized elderly, 50% and (2) elderly patients living in the community, 5% to 15%.
F. **Investigations:** The basic investigations for all elderly patients with urinary incontinence are (1) complete history; (2) complete physical examination; (3) complete medication review (every 3 months); (4) complete urinalysis; (5) urine for culture and sensitivity; and (6) PVR urine determination.

G. **Primary treatments for different types of geriatric urinary incontinence:**
  1. Stress incontinence: (a) pelvic muscle (Kegel) exercises; (b) alpha-adrenergic agonists; (c) supplemental estrogen (oral or vaginal); (d) biofeedback, behavioral training; (d) surgical bladder neck suspension; and (e) periurethral injections.
  2. Urge incontinence: (a) bladder relaxants; (b) estrogen (if vaginal atrophy is present); (c) behavioral procedures (biofeedback and behavioral therapy); and (d) surgical removal of obstructing or other irritating pathologic lesions
  3. Overflow incontinence: (a) surgical removal of obstruction; (b) intermittent catheterization (if practical); and (c) indwelling catheterization.
  4. Functional incontinence: (a) behavioral therapies (prompted voiding, habit training, or scheduled toileting); (b) environmental manipulations; (c) incontinence undergarments and pads; (d) external collection devices; (e) bladder relaxants (selected patients); and (f) indwelling catheters (selected patients).

SUGGESTED READING

Culligan PJ: Urinary incontinence in women: evaluation and management. *Am Fam Physician* 62:2433-2444, 2000.

DuBeau CE: Urinary incontinence. In: Cobbs EL, et al, eds.: *Geriatric review syllabus: A core curriculum in geriatric medicine*, 5th ed. Malden MA: Blackwell Publishing for the American Geriatrics Society, 2002, Malden, MA, 139-148.

Weinstock M, Neides D: *Residents guide to ambulatory care, 2001*, 3rd ed. Anadem Publishing Inc, 2002, Columbus, OH, 335-337.

Weiss DB: Diagnostic evaluation of urinary incontinence in geriatric patients. *Am Fam Physician* 57:2675-2679, 1998.

Chapter 140

Depression in the Elderly

> "I'm dead. They just haven't buried me yet!"

CLINICAL CASE PROBLEM 1:

An 85-Year-Old Female Nursing Home Resident Who Simply "Stares into Space" and Cries Almost All of the Time

You are called to see an 85-year-old patient who moved into a nursing home 9 months ago. Previously, she was living on her own and had managed by herself since the death of her husband 6 years ago. During the past year she has become increasingly disabled with congestive heart failure and osteoarthritis. During the past 9 months the patient has lost 15 lb, has not been hungry, has lost interest in all of her social activities, and has been crying almost every day. You are aware that before moving into the nursing home she was quite active.

Her mental status examination is difficult. She does, however, describe her mood as being worse in the morning. Her short-term memory, according to the staff, also is impaired. She is taking furosemide and enalapril for her congestive heart failure and plain acetaminophen for the pain associated with osteoarthritis.

SELECT THE BEST ANSWER TO THE FOLLOWING QUESTIONS:

1. What is the most likely diagnosis in this patient?
   a. major depressive illness
   b. Alzheimer's disease
   c. multiinfarct dementia
   d. hypothyroidism
   e. none of the above

2. Regarding the diagnosis of the patient described, which of the following statements is false?
   a. this condition occurs less often in older patients than in younger patients
   b. elderly patients are less likely to recover from this illness than young adults
   c. this condition is more common among institutionalized elders than elders living at home
   d. this condition may be related to physical illness
   e. this condition may be related to the move into the nursing home itself

3. Which of the following investigations and/or assessments should be performed in the patient described?
   a. a medication review
   b. a complete blood count (CBC)
   c. a serum thyroid-stimulating hormone (TSH) level
   d. all of the above
   e. none of the above

4. Which of the following antidepressants is considered an agent of first choice for the treatment of depression in the elderly?

a. imipramine
b. nortriptyline
c. desipramine
d. amitriptyline
e. fluoxetine

5. Which of the following antidepressants specifi-cally blocks serotonin reuptake?
   a. imipramine
   b. desipramine
   c. nortriptyline
   d. amitriptyline
   e. fertraline

6. You decide to treat the patient described in Clinical Case Problem 1 with fluoxetine (Prozac). In a patient of this age, at what daily dosage would you start her?
   a. 5 mg
   b. 25 mg
   c. 50 mg
   d. 75 mg
   e. 100 mg

7. Regarding the treatment for the condition described, which of the following statements is (are) true?
   a. electroconvulsive therapy (ECT) is unlikely to be of any benefit in the treatment of this condition
   b. socialization, music therapy, and pet therapy have no role to play in the treatment of this condition
   c. cognitive and behavioral therapy may improve this condition significantly
   d. all of the above statements are true
   e. none of the above statements are true

8. Which of the following features is most com-monly associated with this diagnosis in geriatric patients?
   a. acute mania
   b. hypomania
   c. extreme anxiety
   d. psychomotor agitation or retardation
   e. hypersomnia

9. The signs and symptoms of the condition described include all except which of the following?
   a. impaired concentration
   b. guilt
   c. hopelessness
   d. suicidal ideation
   e. violent or aggressive behavior

10. The length of time recommended for the pharma-cologic treatment of this condition with the drug selected is at least
    a. 1 month
    b. 3 months
    c. 6 months
    d. 12 months
    e. 18 months

11. An elderly institutionalized patient is prescribed nortriptyline. The dose is increased up to 100 mg, but no improvement is noted. You decide to substitute fluoxetine. Which of the following side effects might you anticipate with the use of fluoxetine?
    a. constipation
    b. blurred vision
    c. urinary retention
    d. dry mouth
    e. agitation

12. If the side effect selected in Question 11 occurred, which of the following courses of action would be the most reasonable?
    a. increase the dose of the drug
    b. decrease the dose of the drug
    c. stop the drug
    d. elect ECT as your next option
    e. c and d

CLINICAL CASE MANAGEMENT PROBLEM

Part A: Discuss the differential diagnosis of depressive symptoms in the elderly.

Part B: List the three most common physical illnesses that present or manifest as depression in the elderly.

Part C: Name the most common drug associated with depression in the elderly.

Part D: Name the most common drug class associated with depression as a psychoactive substance use disorder.

▶ **ANSWERS:**

1. **a.** This patient has a major depressive illness. The criteria for major depressive illness are summarized in Chapter 75. A mnemonic that is very helpful for diagnosing depression is **A SIG: E CAPS**:

   A = **A**ffect: At least a 2-week period of a depressed mood or a depressed affect
   S = **S**leep disturbance (hyposomnia, insomnia, hypersomnia)

I = **I**nterest (lack of interest in life)
G = **G**uilt or hopelessness
E = **E**nergy level (decreased) or fatigue
C = **C**oncentration decreased
A = **A**ppetite disturbance (decreased or increased with or without weight gain or weight loss
P = **P**sychomotor retardation or agitation
S = **S**uicidal ideation

Major depressive illness is diagnosed when there is at least a 2-week period of a depressed mood or depressed affect and four of the other eight criteria are present.

Despite these criteria, depression in elderly patients is more likely to occur with weight loss and less likely to occur with feelings of worthlessness and guilt. Elderly patients are no more likely than people in midlife to report cognitive problems, although they do have more difficulties with cognition during an episode of depression.

2. b. Elderly patients are just as likely to recover from a major depressive illness as are younger adults.

Major depression is less prevalent among those aged 65 and older than in younger groups. However, suicide is not; it continues to increase in elderly patients at an alarming rate.

The prevalence of major depression in elderly patients in the community is between 1% and 2%. The majority of elderly patients who are depressed, however, do not fit the *Diagnostic and Statistical Manual of Mental Disorders,* 4th edition (DSM-IV), criteria; instead, they have depressive symptoms that are associated with an adjustment reaction (as in this patient who has just had to leave her own home) or that are associated with significant physical illness (as this patient also demonstrates).

In long-term chronic care facilities, the prevalence of major depressive illness may be as high as 10% to 20%.

3. d. The elderly patient with depressive symptoms should have the following evaluations: a complete history, a complete physical examination, and a complete medication review (both prescribed and over-the-counter medications). Some of the most common pharmacologic agents that contribute to depression include antihypertensive agents, such as propranolol and methyldopa, and cimetidine and sedative hypnotic drugs.

In addition to the complete history and physical education, the elderly patient should have the following laboratory investigations: CBC, vitamin B_{12}, serum folate level, serum TSH, chest x-ray, electrocardiogram (ECG), complete urinalysis, and serum electrolytes.

4. e. Selective serotonin reuptake inhibitors (SSRIs) should be considered medications of choice for depression in the elderly. This is especially true for patients with heart conduction defects, ischemic heart disease, prostatic hyperplasia, or uncontrolled glaucoma. Consider venlafaxine (Effexor), mirtazapine (Remeron), and bupropion (Wellbutrin, Zyban) as second-line medications and nortriptyline or desipramine as third line.

5. e. The group of antidepressant agents known as SSRIs includes fluoxetine (Prozac, Luvox), sertraline (Zoloft), and paroxetine (Paxil). These drugs are considered first choice for the treatment of depression in the elderly. They offer some significant theoretic advantages in that the common tricyclic antidepressant side effects may be averted by their use; these include dry mouth, blurred vision, tachycardia, constipation (anticholinergic), orthostatic hypotension (alpha-adrenergic blockade), and weight gain. In addition they do not increase the cardiac risk caused by blockade of impulse conduction through the atrioventricular node.

6. a. The patient described in this case, an 85-year-old female, should be started taking as low a dose of an SSRI as possible. A dose of 5 mg of Prozac would be an ideal starting dose. This dose could be increased slowly as needed to a maximum of 80 mg/day.

7. c. Elderly patients with depressive illness may be significantly improved with cognitive or behavioral psychotherapy.

Attempts at increased socialization (especially in chronic care facilities) including music therapy, pet therapy, and other therapies that serve to redirect the attention of the elderly patient appear to be effective in the treatment of depression in the elderly.

ECT may be the only effective therapy for severe depression in elderly patients, especially in patients with psychotic depression. ECT is well tolerated in geriatric patients. Indications include severe depression when a rapid response is necessary and when depression is resistant to drug therapy; it also is indicated for patients unable to tolerate antidepressants or who have psychotic depression, severe catatonia, or depression with Parkinson's disease. Contraindications to ECT include an intracranial mass, recent myocardial infarction, or a recent cardiovascular accident.

8. d. Although acute mania, hypomania, extreme anxiety, and hypersomnia may all be associated with depression in elderly patients, by far the most common symptom of those listed in elderly patients is psychomotor agitation or retardation. Psychomotor agitation is the more common presentation of the two.

9. **e.** The diagnostic symptoms of depressive illness have been covered in Answer 1. They do not include violent or aggressive behavior. If violent or aggressive behavior is found in a patient who has an underlying depression, there is likely another major diagnosis that would explain the symptom. In an elder the most common diagnosis in such a case would be Alzheimer's disease.

10. **c.** Geriatric patients with depression should be treated with antidepressants for at least 6 months.

After 6 months, if the patient is improved, the drug can be tapered and eventually discontinued.

11. **e.** The side effects of blurred vision, dry mouth, urinary retention, and constipation are all anticholinergic side effects that do not occur with the new SSRIs. Agitation, however, is a side effect that may be anticipated with these drugs, especially with fluoxetine.

12. **e.** The most reasonable course of action would be to discontinue the drug and to use ECT. Two failed drug courses (with drugs of different classes) would be a reasonable indication for the use of ECT.

SOLUTION TO THE CLINICAL CASE MANAGEMENT PROBLEM

Part A: The differential diagnosis of depressive symptoms in the elderly is lengthy. It includes four major categories: mood disorders, adjustment disorders, psychoactive substance use disorders, and somatoform disorders.
1. Mood disorders include the following: (a) major depression (single episode or recurrent); (b) dysthymia (or depressive neurosis); (c) bipolar affective disorder, depressed phase; and (d) depressive disorder not otherwise specified (NOS) (atypical depression with mild biogenic depression).
2. Adjustment disorders include the following: (a) primary degenerative dementia with associated depression; (b) organic mood disorder, depressed; (c) secondary to physical illness; and (d) secondary to pharmacologic agents.

   Pharmacologic agents that commonly induce depression in the elderly are methyldopa and propranolol.
3. Psychoactive substance use disorders, in particular

alcohol use or dependence and sedative, hypnotic, or anxiolytic abuse or dependence.
4. Somatoform disorders such as hypochondriasis and somatization disorder.

Part B: The three most common physical illnesses that present or manifest as depression in the elderly are hypothyroidism, carcinoma of the pancreas, Parkinson's disease, and cerebrovascular accident (stroke).

Part C: The most common drug associated with depression in the elderly is propranolol.

Part D: The most common drug class associated with depression is the psychoactive substance use class. This drug class includes all of the sedative–hypnotics. Sedatives and hypnotics are vastly overused in the elderly; this appears to be especially true in institutionalized elderly patients. It is much easier for nursing home staff to prescribe a sedative–hypnotic and/or a sedative than to recognize and help an elder adjust to altered sleep patterns.

SUMMARY OF DEPRESSION IN THE ELDERLY

1. Diagnosis: Follow DSM-IV criteria, except recognize that the elderly are more likely to experience weight loss and cognitive problems and less likely to experience feelings of guilt and hopelessness.
2. Recognize that depression is often an adjustment reaction to life stress, environment change (espe-

cially having to leave home), and the realization of the effects of aging itself.
3. Prevalence: Depression prevalence is 1% to 2% in a community environment and 10% to 20% in an institutional environment. Some suggest a much higher level of 50% in an institutional environment.
4. Differential diagnosis includes mood disorders, adjustment disorders, organic mental disorders,

psychoactive substance use, and somatoform disorders.

5. Investigations include mini-mental status examination; complete medication review; and laboratory evaluation including CBC, electrolytes, TSH, vitamin B_{12}, serum folate, ECG, and chest x-ray.

6. Treatment strategies include the following:
   a. Nonpharmacologic strategies: (i) relaxation techniques and mind-occupying techniques such as frequent visitors, pet therapy, and music therapy; and (ii) cognitive, supportive, and behavioral psychotherapy.
   b. Pharmacologic strategies: (i) drugs of first choice are SSRIs; (ii) drugs of second choice are venlafaxine, mirtazapine, and bupropion; (iii) drugs of third choice are tricyclic antidepressants; and (iv) if two drug classes fail, ECT should be considered. ECT has much more of a role to play in geriatric depression than it does in depression associated with younger patients.

Before committing a patient to an ECT, do a chest x-ray, ECG, serum electrolytes, and cardiac examination (may need stress test and electroencephalogram if symptoms so indicate).

Most importantly, depression in the elderly must not be treated with pharmacologic agents only; treatment should, instead, include an equal contribution from nonpharmacologic treatments and pharmacologic agents.

SUGGESTED READING

Johnston CB et al: Geriatric medicine. In Tierny et al, eds.: *Current medical diagnosis and treatment 2002,* 42nd ed. McGraw-Hill, 2003, New York, 41-59.

Mulsant BH, Pollock BG: Treatment-resistant depression in late life. *J Geriatr Psychiatr Neurol* 11(4):186-193, 1998.

Reuben D, et al: *Geriatrics at your finger tip,* 5th ed. Blackwell Publishers, 2003, United Kingdom.

 Chapter **141**

Pressure Ulcers

"Doctor, no matter what they do, the sore on my mother's back keeps on getting larger."

CLINICAL CASE PROBLEM 1:

AN 80-YEAR-OLD FEMALE NURSING HOME RESIDENT WITH A PRESSURE ULCER

You are called to a nursing home to see an 80-year-old female with a fever of 40° C (104° F). The patient is disoriented and confused. The nursing home staff has had difficulty treating her pressure ulcers, especially one on her sacrum.

On physical examination, the patient's blood pressure is 110/80 mm Hg and her pulse is 72 and regular. There is a 10 cm × 5 cm pressure ulcer on her sacrum. Also, there is a purulent, foul-smelling discharge coming from that ulcer.

■ SELECT THE BEST ANSWER TO THE FOLLOWING QUESTIONS:

1. Which of the following diseases or conditions is (are) a risk factor(s) for the development of pressure ulcers?
   a. immobility
   b. dementia
   c. Parkinson's disease
   d. congestive heart failure
   e. a, b, and c
   f. a, b, c, and d

2. Which of the following nutritional or physiologic variables increase(s) the risk of pressure ulcers?
   a. hypoalbuminemia
   b. moist skin
   c. increased pressure
   d. a and b
   e. a, b, and c

3. Regarding the pathophysiology of pressure ulcers, which of the following factors has (have) been implicated in their cause?
   a. the pressure of the body weight itself
   b. shearing forces
   c. friction
   d. moisture
   e. a, b, and d
   f. a, b, c, and d

4. Which of the following statements concerning the prevention and cause of pressure ulcers is false?

a. pressure ulcers are impossible to prevent in immobilized elderly patients
b. good nutrition in the elderly will help prevent pressure ulcers
c. anemia in the elderly patient predisposes to the formation of pressure ulcers
d. incontinence in the elderly increases the risk of pressure ulcers by a factor of five
e. patients who sit for long periods are just as likely to develop pressure ulcers as bedridden patients

5. Concerning the patient described in Clinical Case Problem 1, what amount of time would it take the large ulcer to develop from a small, untreated ulcer?
   a. 28 days
   b. 21-28 days
   c. 14-20 days
   d. 7-10 days
   e. 1-2 days

6. Which of the following anatomic sites is the least common site for the development of a pressure ulcer?
   a. the ischial tuberosity
   b. the lateral malleolus
   c. the medial malleolus
   d. the sacrum
   e. the greater trochanter

7. With respect to pathophysiology, which of the following factors contributes to the formation of pressure ulcers?
   a. blood and lymphatic vessel obstruction
   b. plasma leakage into the interstitial space
   c. hemorrhage
   d. bacterial deposition at the site of the pressure-induced injury
   e. muscle cell death
   f. all of the above

8. Which of the following statements concerning pressure ulcers and mortality in elderly patients is (are) true?
   a. there appears to be no increase in mortality among elderly individuals who develop pressure ulcers
   b. failure of a pressure ulcer to heal or improve has not been associated with a higher death rate in institutionalized elderly
   c. in-hospital death rates for patients with pressure ulcers range from 23% to 36%
   d. all of the above statements are true
   e. none of the above statements are true

9. Patients at high risk for the development of pressure ulcers should be repositioned how frequently?
   a. every 2 hours
   b. every 4 hours
   c. every 6 hours
   d. every 8 hours
   e. every 12 hours

10. Which of the following descriptions best illustrate(s) the nature of bacteria usually found in an infected pressure ulcer?
    a. gram-positive aerobic cocci alone
    b. gram-negative aerobic rods alone
    c. anaerobic bacteria alone
    d. a and c
    e. a, b, and c

11. What are the best initial antibiotic treatments for an infected pressure ulcer?
    a. tetracycline and gentamicin
    b. clindamycin and gentamicin
    c. cephalexin and doxycycline
    d. penicillin and gentamicin
    e. trimethoprim-sulfamethoxazole

12. What is the most common and serious complication of pressure ulcers in elderly patients?
    a. anemia
    b. hypoproteinemia
    c. infection
    d. contracture
    e. bone resorption

13. Bacterial sepsis leading to septic shock in pressure ulcers is associated most closely with which of the following bacteria?
    a. *Bacteroides fragilis*
    b. *Pseudomonas aeruginosa*
    c. *Proteus mirabilis*
    d. *Staphylococcus aureus*
    e. *Providencia* spp.

CLINICAL CASE PROBLEM 2:
A 78-Year-Old Immobilized Male with a Pressure Ulcer on His Heel

A 78-year-old immobilized male is seen with a 1-cm area of erythema and bruising on his left heel.

14. Which of the following is the most important aspect of the treatment of this pressure ulcer at this time?
    a. application of a full-thickness skin graft
    b. extensive débridement of the area and cleansing with an iodine-based solution

c. application of a foam pad to protect the heel from further damage

d. application of microscopic beaded dextran to the lesion

e. elevation of the left leg by 30 degrees

15. Which of the following statements concerning the use of pressure-reducing devices in the prevention and treatment of pressure ulcers is true?
a. with the proper use of pressure-reducing devices, all pressure ulcers can be prevented
b. there is consensus regarding the pressure-reducing devices of first choice
c. sheepskin can be considered a pressure-reducing device of first choice
d. there appears to be little difference between the products indicated for the prevention and treatment of pressure ulcers
e. none of the above are true

16. Which of the following factors has (have) been associated with a more favorable outcome in the prevention and treatment of pressure ulcers?
a. educational programs for health professionals
b. educational programs for families and caregivers
c. multidisciplinary health care
d. b and c
e. a, b, and c

17. Concerning local wound care in superficial pressure ulcers, which of the following is (are) acceptable for cleaning the ulcer and disinfecting the ulcer?
a. povidone–iodine
b. hydrogen peroxide
c. hypochlorite solutions
d. all of the above
e. none of the above

18. Which of the following pressure-reducing devices should not be used for the prevention and treatment of pressure ulcers?
a. an air-fluidized bed
b. a sheepskin mattress
c. a conventional foam pad
d. an air mattress
e. a water mattress

19. The débridement of moist, exudative wounds originating from the formation of pressure ulcers may be augmented by the use of which of the following?
a. hydrophilic polymers
b. enzymatic agents

c. acetic acid
d. a and b
e. a, b, and c

20. Which of the following statements concerning the use of occlusive dressings for treating pressure ulcers is (are) true?
a. hydrocolloid dressings and transparent films improve the healing rate of superficial pressure ulcers
b. hydrocolloid has proved to be effective in treating deep pressure ulcers as well as superficial pressure ulcers
c. hydrocolloid dressings and transparent films may remain in place for several days
d. a and c only
e. a, b, and c are true

◢ CLINICAL CASE MANAGEMENT PROBLEM

Pressure ulcers can be classified into four stages dependent on the degree of thickness of penetration of the epidermis and deeper tissues. Because the therapy varies depending on the stage of the ulcer, it is important to understand the difference between the four stages. Provide the definition of each of stages I, II, III, and IV pressure ulcers.

■ **ANSWERS:**

1. **f.** See discussion in Answer 2.

2. **e.** Risk factors for pressure ulcers include the following:
   1. Any disease process leading to immobility and limited activity levels, such as a spinal cord injury, dementia, Parkinson's disease, severe congestive heart failure, and chronic obstructive pulmonary disease. This can cause unrelieved pressure, which results in damage of underlying tissue.
   2. Other factors including urinary incontinence (moisture) and nutritional factors such as a decreased lymphocyte count, hypoalbuminemia, inadequate dietary intake, decreased body weight, and a depleted triceps skinfold thickness. Poor nutrition status may be secondary to immobility, poor financial status, isolation, and poor dentition.
   3. Potential risk factors identified in prospective studies include moist skin, increased body temperature, decreased blood pressure, increased age, and an altered level of consciousness. Cardiovascular disease (CVD), strokes, diabetes,

fractures, bed or wheelchair confinement, impaired level of consciousness, and hypotension are all independently associated with pressure ulcers.

3. **f.** The pathophysiology of pressure ulcers include the interaction of all of the following:
1. Pressure: Contact pressures of 60-70 mm Hg for 1-2 hours lead to degeneration of muscle fibers. Repeated exposures to pressure will cause skin necrosis because of decreased oxygen tension, vessel leakage, and lack of nutrients. Pressure is considered the most significant risk factor for developing pressure ulcers.
2. Shearing forces: Shearing forces are tangential forces that are exerted when a person is seated or when the head of the bed is elevated and the person slides toward the floor or foot of the bed. Shearing forces disrupt subcutaneous vessels and cause ischemia and subsequent necrosis.
3. Friction: Friction has been shown to cause intraepidermal blisters. When unroofed, these lesions result in superficial erosions. This kind of injury can occur when a patient is pulled across a sheet or when the patient has repetitive movements that expose a bony prominence to such frictional forces.
4. Moisture: Intermediate degrees of moisture increase the amount of friction produced by the rubbing interface, whereas extremes of moisture or dryness decrease the frictional forces between the two surfaces rubbing against each other. Moisture macerates skin tissue, predisposing the skin to breakdown.

4. **a.** Pressure ulcers are not impossible to prevent in immobilized elderly patients. It is true that it is difficult to prevent all pressure ulcers, but many of those that do develop in immobilized elderly patients are, in fact, preventable.

Good nutrition in elderly patients will help prevent pressure ulcers.

Anemia and incontinence are predisposing factors to the development of pressure ulcers.

Elderly patients who sit for long periods are just as likely to develop pressure ulcers as bedridden patients.

5. **e.** Erythema may progress to ulceration quickly. A small ulcer can progress to a large ulcer within 24-48 hours. The progression is caused by local edema or infection, the former being the most important factor. As in the patient described in Clinical Case Problem 1, severe infection can lead to septicemia, which must be

recognized and treated with appropriate systemic antibiotic therapy.

6. **c.** The most common sites for pressure ulcers to develop are as follows: (1) the sacrum; (2) the trochanters; (3) the heels; (4) the lateral malleoli; and (5) the buttocks over the ischium.

The least common site of those listed for the formation of pressure ulcers is the medial malleoli.

7. **f.** The ultimate chain of pathophysiologic events involved in the formation of pressure ulcers is as follows: (1) ischemia is associated with the occlusion of blood and lymphatic vessels; (2) as plasma leaks into the interstitium, diffusing substances increase between the cellular elements of skin and blood vessels; (3) ultimately hemorrhage occurs and leads to erythema of the skin that is unable to be blanched; (4) bacteria are deposited at sites of pressure-induced injury and set up a deep suppurative process; and (5) the accumulation of edema fluid, blood, inflammatory cells, toxic wastes, and bacteria ultimately and progressively lead to the death of muscle, subcutaneous tissue, and epidermal tissue.

The damage caused by shearing forces probably is mediated by pressure-induced ischemia in deep tissues and by direct mechanical injury to the subcutaneous tissue.

8. **c.** Increased death rates have been observed consistently in elderly patients who develop pressure ulcers. In addition, failure of an ulcer to heal or improve has been associated with a higher rate of death in nursing home residents. In-hospital death rates for patients with pressure ulcers range from 23% to 36%.

Most of these deaths are in patients who are debilitated; in many cases it is difficult to separate what contribution the actual pressure ulcer makes to the process. However, the development of a pressure sore quadruples the risk of death for institutionalized patients.

9. **a.** Data support the recommendation that high-risk patients should be repositioned every 2 hours to prevent pressure ulcers from forming and to minimize the size, thickness, and infectivity rate of pressure ulcers that have formed already.

10. **e.** Infected pressure ulcers usually are associated with *P. aeruginosa*, *Providencia* spp., *Proteus* spp., *S. aureus*, and anaerobic bacteria (particularly *B. fragilis*). The best combination of antibiotics, therefore, is one that will treat gram-positive aerobic cocci (present in

39% of isolates), gram-negative aerobic rods, and anaerobic bacteria.

11. b. One realizes the risk of using a powerful agent such as gentamicin in an elder who is debilitated; however, the elder who is debilitated most likely by that time has acquired a serious bacteremia/ septicemia. Check creatinine clearance, and adjust the gentamicin dose accordingly.

12. c. Sepsis is the most common and most serious complication of pressure ulcers in elderly patients. Contraction and bone resorption are also complications of pressure ulcers.

Anemia and hypoproteinemia are risk factors for the formation of pressure ulcers.

13. a. The following are facts concerning the infection, bacteremia, septicemia, and death associated with pressure ulcers: (1) most infected pressure ulcers are polymicrobial; (2) most infected polymicrobial pressure ulcers have *B. fragilis* as one of the major organisms involved; and (3) infected pressure ulcers also lead to other infectious complications, such as bacterial cellulitis, osteomyelitis, and septic arthritis.

14. c. The short time interval between the formation of a small area of erythema and a true pressure ulcer already has been described.

The single most important therapy at this time in this patient is to try to protect the patient's heel from progressing to any further stage of damage. This is best done by using a foam pad or other piece of protective apparatus.

15. b. Regarding the formation of pressure ulcers, the prevention of pressure ulcers, and the pressure-reducing devices available, the following facts have emerged:
1. Despite nurses' best efforts, the use of proper positioning alone is not sufficient to prevent all pressure ulcers. Even with pressure-reducing devices, this is not always possible.
2. The use of water mattresses or alternating air mattresses decreased the incidence of pressure ulcers by 50% compared with the conventional hospital mattresses.
3. Although sheepskin products are very popular, it has been demonstrated that sheepskins and 2-inch convoluted foam pad products do not have the capability of decreasing pressure enough to eliminate the risk of cutaneous injury.
4. The following have been demonstrated to have superior efficacy in preventing pressure ulcers: a

foam mattress, a static air mattress, an alternating air mattress, and a gel or water mattress. In addition, the use of air-fluidized and low-air-loss beds are recommended (especially for stage III and stage IV ulcers).

16. e. Several studies have demonstrated a significant decrease in pressure-ulcer incidence after an educational program and a multidisciplinary team approach to the problem of pressure ulcers. Such educational programs should be directed at all levels of health care professionals, patients, family, and caregivers.

17. e. Topical antiseptics such as hypochlorite solutions, povidone–iodine, acetic acid iodophor, and hydrogen peroxide should be avoided in cleaning and débriding a pressure ulcer because of the potential of these compounds for inhibiting wound healing. The preferred alternative is normal saline.

18. b. A sheepskin mattress should not be used for the prevention and treatment of pressure ulcers. See the critique in Answer 15 for further details.

19. d. The débridement of moist, exudative wounds may be augmented by using hydrophilic polymers such as dextranomer. Enzymatic agents such as collagenase, fibrinolysin, deoxyribonuclease, streptokinase, and streptodornase may be helpful in aiding débridement.

20. d. Once an ulcer is clean and granulation or epithelialization begins to occur, then a moist wound environment should be maintained without disturbing the healing tissue. Superficial lesions heal by migration of epithelial cells from the borders of an ulcer; deep lesions heal as granulation tissue fills the base of the wound. Controlled studies have shown that the use of occlusive dressing such as transparent films and hydrocolloid dressings improves healing of stage II pressure ulcers. These dressings remain in place for several days and allow a layer of serous exudate to form underneath the dressing. This facilitates the further migration of epithelial cells. Although these dressings have not been shown to improve the effective healing rate of deep ulcers, they do reduce the nursing time needed for treatment.

Clean stage III and clean stage IV ulcers should be dressed with a gauze dressing kept moistened with normal saline. Moist dressings should be kept off surrounding skin to avoid macerating normal tissues. Unless there are symptoms or signs of infection, these dressings can stay in place for several days.

SOLUTION TO THE CLINICAL CASE MANAGEMENT PROBLEM

The classification of pressure ulcers in elderly patients is as follows:

1. Stage I pressure ulcers present as erythema of intact skin that is unable to be blanched.
2. Stage II pressure ulcers involve partial-thickness skin loss involving the epidermis or the dermis.
3. Stage III pressure ulcers extend from the subcuta-

neous tissues to the deep fascia and typically show undermining.

4. Stage IV pressure ulcers involve muscle or bone. Full-thickness injury often is manifested by eschar, frequently involving muscle and bone, but cannot be staged until the eschar is removed.

SUMMARY OF PRESSURE ULCERS

A. Terminology:
1. The term *pressure ulcer* is the preferred term at this time.
2. Previous terms included the following:
   a. Decubitus ulcers
   b. Bedsores
   c. Pressure sores

B. Prevalence:
1. The prevalence of pressure ulcers among patients in acute care hospitals ranges from 1% to 10% and from 15% to 25% in long-term care facilities.
2. Among patients expected to be hospitalized and confined to bed or chair for at least 1 week, the prevalence of stage II and greater pressure ulcers is as high as 28%.
3. The prevalence of pressure ulcers in nursing homes is similar to that reported in acute care hospitals. As many as 20% to 33% of patients admitted to nursing homes have stage II or greater pressure ulcers. Less than 20% of pressure ulcers develop in the nursing home and in the home care setting; more than 60% develop in the acute care setting.
4. Pressure ulcers affect 3 million people annually, at a cost of $5 billion a year.

C. Complications:
1. Sepsis is the most serious complication of pressure ulcers.
2. Other complications include local infections, cellulitis, and osteomyelitis. As well, infected pressure ulcers may be deeply undermined and lead to osteomyelitis or penetrate into the abdominal cavity and cause peritonitis. Infected pressure ulcers lead to nosocomial reservoirs for antibiotic-resistant bacteria.

3. Pressure ulcer infections have the following characteristics:
   a. They are polymicrobial.
   b. Gram-positive anaerobic cocci, gram-negative anaerobic rods, and aerobic bacteria are the most common organisms found.
   c. Specific organisms commonly found include *P. aeruginosa, Providencia* spp., *Proteus* spp., *S. aureus,* and *B. fragilis.*

D. Mortality:
1. Failure of a pressure ulcer to heal is associated with a higher rate of death in nursing home residents.
2. In-hospital death rates for patients with pressure ulcers range from 23% to 36%. Most of these deaths are patients with severe underlying disease.

E. Risk factors:
1. Disease processes leading to immobility or reduced activity
2. Spinal cord injury
3. Dementias
4. Parkinson's disease
5. Congestive cardiac failure
6. Incontinence
7. Nutritional factors: inadequate intake of protein, vitamins, minerals, calcium, or calories leading to cachexia, hypoalbuminemia, decreased body weight, and decreased triceps skinfold thickness

F. Pathophysiology: Four factors have been implicated in the pathogenesis of pressure ulcers: (1) pressure, (2) shearing forces, (3) friction, and (4) moisture.

G. Pathophysiologic series of events in pressure ulcer formation:
1. Pressure on tissues overlying bone prominence
2. Ischemia produced by occlusion of blood vessels and lymphatic vessels

3. Endothelial cell swelling and vessel leak
4. Plasma leakage into the interstitium
5. Increased distance between cellular elements of skin and blood vessels
6. Hemorrhage
7. Erythema of the skin that is unable to be blanched
8. Continued accumulation of edema fluid, blood, inflammatory cells, toxic wastes, and bacteria
9. Death of muscle, subcutaneous tissue, and epidermal skin

H. Prevention of pressure ulcers:

1. Formal risk assessment: A formal "risk assessment" for the development of pressure ulcers should be done on all patients.
2. Frequent repositioning:
   a. Patients at highest risk should be repositioned every 2 hours.
   b. Lower risk patients should be repositioned two to four times a day.
3. Technique of repositioning: repositioning should be performed so that a person at risk is repositioned without pressure on vulnerable bony prominences. Most of these sites are avoided by positioning patients with the back at a 30-degree angle to the support surface, alternatively from the right to the left sides and to the supine position.
4. Pressure-reducing devices:
   a. Although sheepskins and 2-inch convoluted foam pads are popular, they do not have the capability to decrease pressure enough to eliminate risk of cutaneous injury.
   b. Preferred devices include static air mattresses, alternating air mattresses, gel mattresses, and water mattresses.
   c. Lifting devices or bed linen movement (not bed linen drag) will minimize friction and shear-induced injuries during transfers and position changes.

I. Education:

1. There is a significant decrease in pressure ulcer incidence after an educational program and a multidisciplinary team approach to the problem of pressure ulcers is implemented.
2. Educational interventions should be targeted to all levels of health care providers, patients, families, and caregivers.

J. Assessment of patients with pressure ulcers:

1. Appropriate assessment and treatment of underlying diseases and conditions that have put the person at risk for developing pressure ulcers
2. Nutritional assessment particularly important
3. Assessment of associated infections (as discussed)

K. Treatment of pressure ulcers:

1. Systemic treatment:
   a. Vitamin C: The patient should take 500 mg bid (84% reduction in pressure ulcer surface area in patients taking this vitamin).
   b. The drug combination of choice is clindamycin and gentamicin; monitor and watch renal function carefully while the patient is taking gentamicin.
   c. Air-fluidized bed therapy is much of an improvement over the conventional bed.
2. Local wound care:
   a. Normal saline is the agent of choice for cleaning and for gentle débridement. Avoid povidone–iodine, hypochlorite, mild acetic acid, and hydrogen peroxide.
   b. Surgical débridement is augmented with wet-to-dry dressings using normal saline.
   c. The débridement of moist, exudative lesions is facilitated by using hydrophilic polymers. Enzymatic agents should be used only until the ulcer bed becomes clean.
   d. Once clean and granulation or epithelialization begins to occur, a moist wound environment should be maintained. Occlusive dressings and hydrocolloid dressings improve healing rates for stage II ulcers. Stage III and stage IV ulcers should be dressed with a gauze soaked in normal saline.
   e. Surgical therapies should be used to remove necrotic tissue that cannot be removed any other way and that if not removed will cause septicemia and death. Surgical flaps (a more elective procedure) should be considered carefully, especially on patients who are debilitated and cachectic. Rule out osteomyelitis if clinically suspected.

SUGGESTED READING

Bates-Jensen BM, et al: The effects of exercise and incontinence intervention on skin health outcomes on nursing home residents. *J Am Geriatr Soc* 51(3):348-355, 2003.

Cullum M, et al: Beds mattresses and cushions foe pressure sore prevention and treatment (Cochrane Review). *The Cochrane Library* 2:2003, Oxford UK update software.

Ferri FF, et al, eds.: *Practical guide to the care of the geriatric patient,* ed 2. Mosby Year Book, 1997, St. Louis.

Chapter **142**

Polypharmacy and Drug Reactions

> "Gee, Mom. Do you need a trunk
> for all these medications?"

CLINICAL CASE PROBLEM 1:

*A 75-Year-Old Female with
a Bagful of Pills*

A 75-year-old female comes to your office with her daughter. Her daughter describes her mother as having undergone "a marked personality change." Apparently, her elderly mother began seeing "pink rats coming out of the wall" and she began "hearing and seeing people from outer space" floating down into her field of vision.

The patient's daughter brings in her mother's medications in a bag. She describes a visit to her mother's physician 1 week ago. At that time the doctor prescribed a number of medications including pills for her blood pressure, pills for her heart, pills for her arthritis, pills for her stomach, pills for her anxiety, pills for her depression, and pills for her insomnia.

On further questioning, the daughter states that her mother had been fairly well before the physician visit but had (unfortunately) mentioned "a few minor ailments." In response to the patient's complaints the physician prescribed hydrochlorothiazide, propranolol, nifedipine, digoxin, ibuprofen, cimetidine, Maalox, amitriptyline, and triazolam.

You are well aware of the fact that medications in the elderly often can produce significant side effects. You suspect that there is a connection between the pink rats, the space men, and the pills.

On examination, the patient is agitated and confused. Her blood pressure is 100/70 mm Hg, and her pulse is 54 and regular. She has a bruise on her head from a fall 3 days ago. Examination of the cardiovascular system reveals a normal S1 and S2 with a grade VI systolic murmur heard along the left sternal edge. There are no other abnormalities on physical examination.

▌ SELECT THE BEST ANSWER TO THE FOLLOWING QUESTIONS:

1. Which of the following statements regarding this patient's acute medical problem is true?
   a. this patient's problem is unlikely to be related to her medications
   b. this patient's presentation is unusual following the initiation of medications in the elderly
   c. this patient's problem is unlikely to lead to hospitalization
   d. this patient's problem is likely to be transient
   e. none of the above statements are true

2. Which of the following statements regarding the use of drugs in the elderly is true?
   a. elderly patients should be treated the same way as younger patients with respect to drug initiation
   b. elderly patients generally need the same dose of medications as younger patients
   c. psychotropic drugs are unlikely to produce significant side effects in elderly patients
   d. elderly patients taking multiple medications should be reassessed on a yearly basis
   e. none of the above statements are true

3. Regarding elderly patients in chronic care facilities, which of the following statements regarding medication use is (are) true?
   a. elderly patients in chronic care facilities are usually taking fewer medications than elderly patients living on their own
   b. elderly patients in chronic care facilities are usually taking between 8 and 13 different medications at any one time
   c. elderly patients in chronic care facilities are likely to experience iatrogenic side effects from medications at one time or another
   d. b and c
   e. a and c

CLINICAL CASE PROBLEM 2:

*An 85-Year-Old Female Patient with a
Dangerously High Blood Pressure*

An 85-year-old female patient of yours was placed on a combination of hydrochlorothiazide and clonidine because of a "dangerously high" blood pressure of 150/95 mm Hg. When you hear this story you are concerned about possible adverse side effects. Your worst fear comes true when you find yourself attending her in the emergency department with a serious adverse event you believe is directly related to the medications on which she was placed.

4. Which of the following specialists will you be calling to manage this adverse event?
   a. a rheumatologist
   b. a general surgeon or a general internist
   c. a gerontologist
   d. an orthopedic surgeon
   e. a psychiatrist

5. The patient becomes acutely short of breath. The adverse effect that you feared has now lead to a feared complication. What is that complication?
   a. a deep venous thrombosis (DVT) leading to a pulmonary embolus
   b. a splenic infarct

c. a cerebrovascular accident

d. aplastic anemia

e. a drug-induced psychosis

6. What is the most likely medication causing the pink rats and the people from outer space in the patient described in Clinical Case Problem 1?

a. propranolol

b. hydrochlorothiazide

c. ibuprofen

d. cimetidine

e. digoxin

7. Assume that the adverse event and its complication just described did not occur. Considering the rapid introduction of multiple medications that took place on the visit to the other physician, what would be the most appropriate course of action at this time?

a. discontinue the digoxin

b. discontinue the hydrochlorothiazide

c. discontinue the propranolol

d. discontinue the triazolam

e. discontinue all medications, observe in a geriatric day hospital environment, and reevaluate the patient continuously for the first few weeks

8. Of the drug combinations listed, which is the most likely to result in a drug–drug interaction in the elderly?

a. cimetidine and propranolol

b. digoxin and hydrochlorothiazide

c. ibuprofen and captopril

d. triazolam and amitriptyline

e. haloperidol

9. What is the most common potentially serious side effect of tricyclic antidepressants in elderly patients?

a. dry mouth

b. constipation

c. bladder spasm

d. orthostatic hypotension

e. sedation

10. Which of the following combinations of pharmacologic agents is associated most commonly with adverse drug reactions (ADRs) in the elderly?

a. cardiovascular drugs, psychotropics, and antibiotics

b. cardiovascular drugs, psychotropics, and analgesics

c. gastrointestinal drugs, psychotropics, and analgesics

d. gastrointestinal drugs, psychotropics, and antibiotics

11. Which of the following pharmacologic parameters may be associated with ADRs in the elderly?

a. altered free serum concentration of drug

b. altered volume of distribution

c. altered renal drug clearance

d. altered tissue sensitivity of the drug

e. all of the above

12. Which of the following is (are) an example(s) of ADRs in the elderly?

a. drug side effects

b. drug toxicity

c. drug–disease interaction

d. drug–drug interaction

e. all of the above

13. Some pharmacologic agents are excreted virtually unchanged by the kidneys. The dosages of these drugs must be titrated carefully in any elderly patient with renal impairment or potential renal impairment. Drugs in this category include the following:

a. cimetidine

b. gentamicin

c. lithium

d. all of the above

e. none of the above

14. Regarding antipsychotic drug therapy in the elderly, which of the following statements is (are) true?

a. antipsychotic drugs often are prescribed for behavior that chronic care staff find objectionable

b. tardive dyskinesia is a frequent side effect of antipsychotic drug use in the elderly

c. antipsychotic drugs are prescribed much more frequently in institutionalized patients than in noninstitutionalized patients

d. all of the above statements are true

e. none of the above statements are true

CLINICAL CASE MANAGEMENT PROBLEM

Provide 10 rules that will minimize ADRs in the elderly.

■ ANSWERS:

1. **e.** This patient's problem can be characterized in the following manner: (1) it is likely to be related to the bagful of medications on which she was started; (2) it is very common following the initiation of medication in the elderly, especially multiple medications; (3) it is very unlikely to be transient unless

some or all of the medications are discontinued; and (4) it will commonly lead to hospitalization.

It is believed that up to 20% of hospitalizations, and perhaps significantly more in the elderly, are a result of iatrogenic disease. Iatrogenic disease is almost always associated with multiple medication use.

2. e. The following are some helpful thoughts on the initiation of drugs in the elderly:
1. Drug initiation in the elderly should be done extremely cautiously, start very low and go very slow.
2. The elderly patient usually needs a considerably lower dose of drug than does the young adult; this is, of course, especially true of drugs that are renally excreted. The general rule on drug initiation in elderly patients is "no more than 50% of the usual adult dose; no more than one drug at a time. Increases in drugs or dosages are not any more quickly than once a week."
3. Psychotropic drugs should be used with special caution. Psychotropic medications frequently are misused in the elderly, and dosing should be monitored closely.
4. All elderly patients should have a formal drug review performed at least every 3 months. At that time, all drugs and the drug doses should be seriously considered for reduction or discontinuation, especially if the elderly patient has symptoms that suggest an ADR to one or more of the drugs that he or she is taking.

3. d. Patients in chronic care facilities have the following characteristics with respect to medication use:
1. They are usually taking multiple medications. The average number of medications used by the institutionalized elderly is 8 per day. Standard orders may increase this to 13 medications per day.
2. It has been found that the most usual scenario is that medications always are added but never subtracted. Thus the number simply continues to increase.
3. Iatrogenic side effects from medication use in chronic care facilities are extremely common. Considering the number of medications that these patients are taking, they are actually far more likely to experience at least one ADR per year than not.
4. In comparison to elderly people living on their own in the community, the number of medications used by institutional-based elderly patients is greater.

4. d. The combination of hydrochlorothiazide and clonidine is likely to produce significant orthostatic hypotension in the elderly patient. The most "adverse effect of the adverse effect" is a fall in the elder leading to a fracture of the neck of the femur. Thus the specialist that you most likely will call will be an orthopedic surgeon.

5. a. The most serious complication from a hip fracture is immobility leading to DVT. The development of a DVT is, of course, directly correlated with a subsequent pulmonary embolus.

The mortality of elders in the first year following a hip fracture approaches 25%. Prevention is the best treatment.

Prevention is best accomplished by significantly limiting the number of medications an elder is taking, especially medications that tend to produce orthostatic hypotension. It should be noted that sedative–hypnotics also increase the risk for hip fractures considerably.

6. a. The most common medication-induced cause of hallucinations in elderly patients is propranolol. Many elderly patients who are started taking propranolol develop visual or auditory hallucinations. Unfortunately, many of these patients then are prescribed antipsychotic medications to treat the hallucinations, rather than evaluating their medication list.

7. e. The most reasonable course of action at this time is to stop everything and start again. The rapid introduction of the nine medications listed was a recipe for disaster. In an attempt to counteract the imminent disaster, this logically should take place in the supervised setting of at least a geriatric day hospital. Many geriatric assessment units do exactly that when an elder is admitted for the assessment of any medical problem. With elders who have been taking multiple medications for a long time, the safest place to accomplish this is in the hospital under close observation. Of elderly hospital admissions, 10% to 17% are a result of inappropriate medication use. Use these hospitalizations to properly assess medications and to develop appropriate treatment plans.

8. b. Patients who develop ADRs are more likely to be taking six or more drugs than those who do not develop an ADR. The most commonly identified combination likely to result in a drug–drug interaction is digoxin with a diuretic. In this case the ADR most likely to be produced is hypokalemia. The hypokalemia produced often will lead to digoxin toxicity in the susceptible elder. These combinations are considered secondary drug reactions, which require at least two drugs to cause an interaction.

9. **d.** All of the side effects listed are common side effects of tricyclic antidepressant medications. The side effects that are caused by an anticholinergic mechanism include dry mouth, blurred vision, constipation, bladder spasm and urinary retention, and sedation.

The orthostatic hypotension is caused by an alpha-adrenergic blockade and is potentially the most serious because of the association described previously between the following series of events: (1) orthostatic hypotension; (2) falls in the elder; (3) fractured neck of the femur; (4) DVT; and (5) pulmonary embolism.

Excess morbidity and mortality are associated with events 3, 4, and 5 in the chain. In addition, always follow cardiac status when using digoxin, evaluating for bradycardia and dysrhythmias.

10. **b.** The three most common drug classes associated with ADRs in the elderly are cardiovascular drugs, psychotropic drugs, and analgesics (especially the nonsteroidal antiinflammatory drugs [NSAIDs]). Unfortunately, many of the drugs used in the treatment of geriatric patients are prescribed for symptoms related to the effects and the diseases of aging and not necessarily for a specific acute disease where function can be restored. This results, of course, in the elder's being on the particular agent for a longer period.

11. **e.** Many physiologic and social variables increase the incidence of ADRs in elderly patients. They include the number of drugs, compliance, absorption of drug, concentration of free drug in the serum, volume of distribution, tissue sensitivity, metabolic clearance, renal drug clearance, general homeostasis, and concentration of serum albumin.

12. **e.** An ADR is defined as any unintended or undesired effect of a drug in a patient. This may include abnormal laboratory values, patient symptoms, and signs on physical examination.

ADRs can be divided into side effects (dry mouth from tricyclic antidepressants and hypokalemia from diuretics), drug toxicity (daytime sedation from hypnotics, diarrhea from laxatives, and syncope from antihypertensive agents), drug–disease interaction (benzodiazepine and drugs with anticholinergic properties may effect the cognitive function in patients with Alzheimer's disease), drug–drug interaction (digoxin from diuretics), and secondary effects (haloperidol causing drug-induced Parkinsonism).

13. **d.** The kidney is the major source of elimination of many commonly prescribed drugs. Drugs that undergo extensive renal clearance and that are therefore likely to accumulate in the elderly include digoxin, gentamicin and other aminoglycosides, lithium, cimetidine, cotrimoxazole, disopyramide, nadolol, procainamide, and sulfonamides. Always remember that NSAIDS may increase renal toxicity, especially in high-risk patients.

14. **d.** Psychotropic drugs are commonly prescribed for geriatric patients. Indications for the use of these drugs are not well established. In nursing home situations, psychotropic drugs often are prescribed for behaviors that staff members find objectionable (i.e., for the benefit of the staff, not the patient); the patient may, in fact, continue taking this (these) drug(s) for long periods. The institutionalized elderly are 10 times as likely to receive antipsychotic agents as age-matched noninstitutionalized controls.

Double-blind, randomized, controlled trials have not established the efficacy of antipsychotic drug use in Alzheimer's disease. Tardive dyskinesia, rigidity, and excessive sedation are frequent side effects of antipsychotic drug use. In many states the use of psychotropic medication must be well documented with specific goals for behavior. The use of chemical restraints through the use of psychotropic medications is not justified.

It should be noted that the use of newer antipsychotic agents such as risperidone (Risperdal), Olanzapine (Zyprexa), and Quetiapine (Seroquel) has been shown to be effective in the treatment of psychotic behavior and neurobehavioral manifestations in patients with severe Alzheimer's disease.

SOLUTION TO THE CLINICAL CASE MANAGEMENT PROBLEM

The following is a good set of rules for prescribing medication in geriatric patients:
1. Recognize that there is no drug to treat senescence.
2. Recognize that mere prolongation of life is not a valid reason for using medications that decrease the quality of life.
3. Make sure that the effects of treatment outweigh the risks.

Continued

SOLUTION TO THE CLINICAL CASE MANAGEMENT PROBLEM—cont'd

4. Establish a priority order for treatment.

5. Keep the number of drugs administered concurrently to a minimum.

6. Know your patient well. Consider renal and hepatic impairment. Consider what else (including over-the-counter medications) is being taken and who else is prescribing drugs.

7. Always begin with nonpharmacologic therapy first if possible.

8. If you decide to prescribe a drug, know it well. Consider using a few drugs often rather than a lot of drugs infrequently.

9. Select the dose carefully: Start very low and go very slow.

10. Anticipate and minimize ADRs by considering side-effect profiles.

11. Determine whether the patient needs help using the medication.

12. Educate the patient and family.

13. Continually reevaluate whether your patient needs a specific drug.

14. Perform a drug review every 3 months on every elder taking more than one medication.

15. Use medication diaries: Have patients bring in all medications and over-the-counter and herbal medications used.

16. Check serum levels when indicated.

17. Destroy old medications.

18. Use medication cards.

SUMMARY OF POLYPHARMACY AND DRUG REACTIONS

1. Prevalence: ADRs are common, especially in institutionalized elderly who are taking an average of 8 medications. ADRs are at least twice as common in elderly patients as in younger patients.

2. Types of ADRs: (a) side effects; (b) drug toxicity; (c) drug–disease interaction; and (e) drug–drug interaction

3. Most common drugs associated with ADRs are (a) cardiovascular drugs; (b) psychotropic drugs; and (c) analgesics

4. Set of reasonable rules: Follow the set of rules listed in the Solution to the Clinical Case Management Problem.

5. Types of ADRs:
   a. Primary ADRs (one drug with one side reaction): (i) cimetidine causes psychosis and (ii) propranolol induces depression.
   b. Secondary ADR (requires at least two drugs to cause an interaction): erythromycin and theophylline used together are toxic.
   c. Drug withdrawal syndromes: (i) beta blocker withdrawal leads to angina, and (ii) addictive drugs cause withdrawal syndromes (benzodiazepines).
   d. Tertiary ADR: benzodiazepines result in a higher incidence of falls.

6. Physician factors implicated in ADRs:
   a. The physician gives a high-risk drug to a vulnerable host (NSAID for a patient with peptic ulcer disease)
   b. The physician gives a highly interactive drug to a pharmacologically vulnerable patient (i.e., captopril given to patient taking a potassium-sparing agent)
   c. The physician prescribes an inappropriate drug to treat an unrecognized drug side effect (i.e., antidepressant given to treat beta blocker depression)

7. Automatic or standard drug orders in intensive care unit, chronic care unit, or chronic care facilities should be reviewed on a regular basis.

8. Ensure appropriate follow-up.

9. Obtain a complete drug history.

10. Avoid prescribing before a diagnosis is made.

11. Review medications regularly and before adding a new medication.

12. Know the actions, adverse effects, and toxicity of the medications you prescribe.

13. Start at a low dose and titrate according to tolerability and response.

14. Attempt to maximize dose before switching to another.

15. Avoid using one drug to treat the side effects of another.

SUGGESTED READING

Weinstock M, Neides D: *Residents Guide to Ambulatory Care 2001,* 3rd ed. Medication use in the elderly. Anadem Publishing Inc, 2002, Columbus, OH, 329-332.

Williams CM: Using medications appropriately in older adults: *Am Fam Physician* 66:1917-1924, 2002.

Chapter 143

Falls

It's no longer just oopsy daisy.

CLINICAL CASE PROBLEM 1:
AN 81-YEAR-OLD FEMALE WHO IS REPEATEDLY FALLING

An 81-year-old female is brought to your office by her daughter. The elderly mother has been falling repeatedly for at least 3 months. The falling has been getting progressively worse, and the patient's daughter is very concerned about the possibility of her mother "breaking her hip."

On examination, the patient is a frail, elderly female in no acute distress. She appears somewhat depressed, but her mini-mental status examination score is 27. The patient's blood pressure is 180/75 mm Hg. Her pulse is 84 and irregular. No other abnormalities are found.

■ **SELECT THE BEST ANSWER TO THE FOLLOWING QUESTIONS:**

1. What is the prevalence of falls among community-based elderly patients between the ages of 70 and 75 years?
   a. 5% per year
   b. 10% per year
   c. 20% per year
   d. 30% per year
   e. 50% per year

2. Which of the following statements regarding falls in the elderly is (are) true?
   a. the prevalence of falling in the elderly increases with advancing age
   b. elderly patients who are physically active may be at greater risk of falling than those who are not
   c. approximately 55% of elderly patients who fall once will fall again
   d. falling in the elderly may not necessarily be a marker of functional decline
   e. all of the above statements are true

3. Which of the following is the most feared morbid outcome of falling among elderly patients?
   a. fracture of the hip
   b. fracture of the radius
   c. subdural hematoma
   d. epidural hematoma
   e. cervical fracture

4. Potential reversible causes of falling in the elderly include which of the following?
   a. medications
   b. postprandial hypotension
   c. alcohol use
   d. urinary urgency
   e. all of the above

5. Which of the following are predisposing risk factors for falls in the elderly?
   a. visual impairment
   b. cerebrovascular accidents
   c. Alzheimer's disease
   d. normal pressure hydrocephalus
   e. all of the above

6. Regarding the incidence of falling and medication use in the elderly, which of the following statements is (are) true?
   a. multiple drug use is associated with an increased incidence of falling in the elderly
   b. the higher the drug dosage, the greater the probability of falling
   c. drug interactions are a major contributing factor to an increased incidence of falling in the elderly
   d. a and b only
   e. a, b, and c are true

7. Falling in the elderly is most commonly associated with which of the following pathophysiologic factors?
   a. orthostatic hypotension
   b. decreased left-ventricular output
   c. decreased cerebral circulation
   d. increased left-ventricular output
   e. none of the above

8. Which of the following medications is most likely to lead to a serious fall in an elderly patient?
   a. amitriptyline
   b. hydrochlorothiazide
   c. enalapril
   d. nifedipine
   e. fluoxetine

9. What is the prevalence of falling among institutionalized elderly patients?
   a. 50% per year
   b. 40% per year
   c. 30% per year
   d. 20% per year
   e. 10% per year

10. Which of the following statements regarding the use of restraints in elderly patients as a means to prevent falls is (are) true?

a. restraints have been shown to reduce the incidence of falling in the elderly
b. no study has ever shown a decrease in falls with restraint use in the elderly
c. potential complications of restraint use in the elderly include strangulation, vascular damage, and neurologic damage
d. a and c
e. b and c

CLINICAL CASE MANAGEMENT PROBLEM

Describe the preventive measures that may result in a reduction in falls in the elderly.

■ **ANSWERS:**

1. d. According to several community-based surveys, about 30% of people older than age 65 experience falls each year in situations where there are no overwhelming intrinsic causes (such as syncope).

2. e. Approximately 55% of elders who fall have multiple falling episodes. The likelihood of falling increases with age. As illustrated by this very high prevalence of 30% among community-based people, falling is not just confined to the frail elderly; healthy elderly patients fall as well during ordinary daily activities. This suggests that falling is not merely a marker of functional decline in the elderly. Although the elder we all picture as falling is the frail elder with multiple medical problems, it may be the case that falling is more prevalent among the more healthy elders who are more, not less, physically active.

3. a. The most feared outcome of falls in the elderly is a fracture of the hip. This is especially common among elderly women who have significant osteoporosis.

The escalating cost of health care has resulted in increased expectations and demands concerning cost-effective health care. Hip fracture results in the death of at least 12,000 elderly Americans per year. In elderly females with hip fractures, the mortality is approximately 20% in the first year.

4. e. Potential reversible causes of falling include medication, alcohol, postprandial hypotension (30-60 minutes after a meal), urinary urgency, insomnia, peripheral edema, and environmental factors.

5. e. Vision, hearing, vestibular function, and proprioception are the major sensory modalities related to stability. Thus declines in vision, hearing, imbal-

ance leading to vertigo and dizziness, peripheral neuropathies, and cervical degenerative disease are the most common causes of falls in elderly patients.

Other associated diseases or conditions associated with falls in the elderly include cerebrovascular accidents, Parkinson's disease, normal-pressure hydrocephalus, dementia (Alzheimer's disease), severe osteoarthritis or rheumatoid arthritis, and medications causing orthostatic hypotension (discussed in Chapter 142).

6. e. Iatrogenic disease is a major cause of falls in the elderly. This iatrogenic disease, which is almost completely related to medication use, is a serious problem in elders. As discussed in Chapter 142, the average number of medications per elder (especially in the institutionalized setting) is anywhere from 8 to 13. Elderly patients taking benzodiazepines have an increased risk of falling.

Multiple drugs, increased drug dosage, and drug–drug interactions are all reasons for orthostatic hypotension (an alpha-blockade phenomenon) and sedation (the two most common predisposing pathophysiologic mechanisms associated with falling in the elderly).

7. a. Decreased left-ventricular output, most closely associated with congestive heart failure, also may play a prominent role in some cases of falling, but orthostatic hypotension is the most common.

8. a. Amitriptyline, hydrochlorothiazide, enalapril, and nifedipine all may be associated with falling in the elderly. Enalapril and hydrochlorothiazide are more likely to be associated with falling when given concomitantly. As well, the first-dose hypotensive effect of an angiotensin-converting enzyme (ACE) inhibitor should be remembered—that is, it is much safer to give the first dose of an ACE inhibitor to an elder in your office, where this possible side effect can be monitored.

Of the four medications listed, however, the most prominent predisposing to falls in the elderly is amitriptyline, a tricyclic antidepressant. Amitriptyline predisposes to falls by a combination of two mechanisms: its anticholinergic mechanism and its alpha-blockade mechanism. This drug should be used judiciously in the elderly. Starting very low and going very slowly will minimize falling as a result of drug use in elderly patients.

9. a. More than one-half of ambulatory nursing home patients fall each year. The estimated annual incidence is 1600 falls per 1000 beds. The higher frequency of falling among institutionalized elderly patients results both from the greater frailty of these patients compared to community-based elderly patients and the greater reliability of reporting in an institutional setting.

10. **e.** No study has confirmed or suggested that the risk of falling in the elderly is reduced because of the use of restraining devices. Restraining devices, however, have been shown to result in significant morbidity and mortality from strangulation, neurologic damage, and vascular damage.

In some countries in the world (such as the United Kingdom), restraints are almost forbidden. In North America the situation appears to be the opposite. In some institutions they are used routinely.

Restraints have other side effects, including anxiety, anger, agitation, and paranoia.

SOLUTION TO THE CLINICAL CASE MANAGEMENT PROBLEM

A preventive program for minimizing falls in the elderly should include the following:

1. Identification of intrinsic risk factors:
   a. A thorough clinical evaluation aimed at identifying all contributing risk factors for falling is the first, most important step. Directly observing balance and gait has been proved to be effective in identifying residents at risk for falling.
   b. A careful review of all situations may identify problem situations to be avoided in the future.
   c. A complete medication review with elimination of all unnecessary medications and a decrease in the dose of all others will minimize falls.

2. Environmental prevention:
   a. General environmental measures include ensuring adequate lighting without glare; having dry, non-slippery floors that are free of obstacles and contamination; having high, firm chairs; and having raised toilet seats.
   b. Restraints should be used only when there appears to be no other alternative. Restraints should not take the place of close supervision and attention to the risk factors discussed earlier. Alternatives to restraints, including wedges in chairs for maintenance of position and organized walking and grid barriers for prevention of wandering, may afford the necessary protection.

SUMMARY OF FALLS

1. **Prevalence:** 30% per year in community-based elders and 50% per year in institutionalized elders

2. **Major complication:** fracture of the femur and resulting morbidity and mortality from surgery, deep venous thrombosis, and pulmonary embolus

3. **Major predisposing conditions precipitating major complication:**
   a. Vision, hearing, vestibular function, and proprioception impairments
   b. Other conditions associated with increased risk include Alzheimer's disease, Parkinson's disease, and iatrogenic disease (mainly medication use, including the psychotropic agents and the cardiovascular agents, the agents with the greatest probability of producing sedation and other anticholinergic side effects

and alpha-blockade side effects [orthostatic hypotension]).
   c. 1 or 2 (above) associated with significant osteoporosis increases the risk

4. **Elder populations at greatest risk:**
   a. Active elderly patients who are at increased risk because of significant activity levels in whom even a minor impairment may be enough to cause significant problems
   b. The "frail elderly" who have concomitant chronic medical conditions
   c. The institutionalized elderly
   d. This list may, in fact, include most elders

5. **Prevention:**
   a. Prevent the development of osteoporosis in postmenopausal women whenever possible (estrogens, calcitonin, calcium, bisphosphonates).
   b. Look carefully at identifying intrinsic risk factors and environmental protection methods in helping to prevent falls.

Continued

SUMMARY OF FALLS—cont'd

c. Medications:
  i. Provide a medication review to every elder every 3 months.
  ii. Keep the number of medications to a minimum.
  iii. In starting medications, start very low and go very slow.
  iv. To minimize falls, minimize adverse drug reactions. This is covered more extensively in Chapter 142.

SUGGESTED READING

Fuller GF: Falls in the elderly. *Am Fam Physician* 61:2159-2168, 2000.
Tinetti ME: Clinical practice. Preventing falls in elderly persons. *N Engl J Med* 348(1):42-49, 2003.
Weinstock M, Neides D: *Residents guide to ambulatory care 2001,* 3rd ed. Anadem Publishing Inc, 2002, Columbus, OH, 105-106.
Woolf AD, Akesson K: Preventing fractures in elderly people. *BMJ* 327(7406):89-95, 2003.

Chapter 144

Cerebrovascular Accidents

"You say my wife has what kind of a berry in her brain?"

CLINICAL CASE PROBLEM 1:

A 67-Year-Old Male with a Sudden-Onset Left-Sided Hemiplegia, Dysphagia, and a "Visual Problem"

A 67-year-old male is brought to the emergency room (ER) by ambulance following the gradual onset of the following: inability to move his right leg, followed by his right arm; speech impairment; and a "visual problem."

On examination, the patient has a flaccid paralysis of the muscles of the right leg and the muscles (excluding the deltoid) of the right arm, a homonymous hemianopia, and dysphagia. In addition, he "does not recognize" that he is paralyzed, and he cannot he turn his eyes toward the right side. His deep tendon reflexes are hyperflexic on the right side. His right great toe is upgoing.

It is now 6 hours since the symptoms began. It appears from talking to his wife that his symptoms are "still changing."

■ SELECT THE BEST ANSWER TO THE FOLLOWING QUESTIONS:

1. What is the most likely diagnosis at this time?
   a. transient ischemic attack (TIA)
   b. completed stroke
   c. stroke-in-evolution
   d. subarachnoid hemorrhage
   e. complicated migraine

2. The location of symptoms correlates the site of the lesion to which of the following?
   a. left middle cerebral artery
   b. right middle cerebral artery
   c. left anterior cerebral artery
   d. right anterior cerebral artery
   e. left posterior cerebral artery

3. What is the most likely pathophysiologic process involved at this time?
   a. a thrombotic stroke
   b. an embolic stroke
   c. a hemorrhagic stroke
   d. a lacunar stroke
   e. a subarachnoid hemorrhage

4. What is the most common pathophysiologic process in patients who have suffered a cerebrovascular accident (CVA)?
   a. a thrombotic stroke
   b. an embolic stroke
   c. a hemorrhagic stroke
   d. a lacunar stroke
   e. a subarachnoid hemorrhage

5. In which of the following conditions would you most likely find an embolic phenomena as the pathophysiology of a CVA?
   a. hypertension
   b. atrial fibrillation
   c. ventricular fibrillation
   d. a young woman taking the oral contraceptive pill
   e. b and d

6. What is the number-one risk factor for CVAs?
   a. cigarette smoking
   b. hypertension
   c. hypercholesterolemia
   d. hypertriglyceridemia
   e. hypothyroidism

7. Lacunar strokes (lacunar infarcts) are most closely associated with which of the following?
   a. thrombosis
   b. embolization
   c. hypertension
   d. subarachnoid bleeding
   e. cerebral infarction

CLINICAL CASE PROBLEM 2:
A 67-Year-Old Patient with Mental Status Impairment, Foot Drop, and Left Sided Hemiplegia and Numbness

A 67-year-old patient develops the following symptoms and signs: impaired mental status including confusion, amnesia, perseveration, and personality changes; foot-drop; apraxia on the affected side; left-sided hemiplegia; and left-sided numbness (both muscle power and sensation retained to some degree in left upper extremity).

8. This patient most likely has had a CVA affecting which of the following arteries?
   a. right middle cerebral artery
   b. posterior cerebral artery
   c. vertebral-basilar artery
   d. right anterior cerebral artery
   e. posterior/inferior cerebellar artery

CLINICAL CASE PROBLEM 3:
A 77-Year-Old Female with Nystagmus, Homonymous Hemianopia, and Facial Numbness Weakness

A 77-year-old female presents to the ER with the following signs/symptoms: dysarthria and dysphagia, vertigo, nausea, syncope, memory loss and disorientation, and ataxic gait.

On physical examination, the patient has nystagmus, homonymous hemianopia, numbness in the area of the twelfth cranial nerve, and facial weakness. You suspect a CVA.

9. Which of the following arteries is most likely to be involved?
   a. middle cerebral artery
   b. posterior cerebral artery
   c. vertebral-basilar artery
   d. anterior cerebral artery
   e. posterior inferior cerebellar artery

10. There are many sources of potential emboli that may cause a CVA. The most common source of cerebral emboli is:
    a. from the carotid arteries
    b. from the aortic arch
    c. from the heart
    d. from vertebral basilar arteries
    e. from the middle cerebral artery

11. The role of computed tomography (CT) scanning within the first 24 hours of a stroke includes:
    a. to exclude hemorrhages
    b. to exclude tumors
    c. to exclude abscesses
    d. to diagnose stroke
    e. a, b, and c

12. The use of anticoagulation is clearly effective in preventing recurrent cardioembolic strokes from atrial fibrillation, a recent myocardial infarction, valvular disease, or a patent foramen ovale. Contraindications in the use of anticoagulation would include:
    a. hemorrhage on CT scan
    b. large cerebral infarctions
    c. evidence of bacterial endocarditis
    d. a and b above
    e. all of the above

13. A TIA is most closely associated with which of the following?
    a. amaurosis fugax
    b. subarachnoid hemorrhage
    c. lacunar hemorrhage
    d. intracranial aneurysm
    e. fusiform aneurysm

14. A ruptured berry aneurysm usually is located in which of the following?
    a. anterior cerebral artery distribution
    b. posterior cerebral artery distribution
    c. circle of Willis
    d. middle cerebral artery distribution
    e. none of the above

15. A patient is suspected of having an acute cerebral infarction. If you had the opportunity of ordering only one investigation, what investigation would that be?
    a. a regular angiogram of the cerebral circulation
    b. a CT scan of the brain without contrast
    c. magnetic resonance angiography (MRA) study of the brain
    d. a digital subtraction angiogram of the brain
    e. an immediate lumbar puncture

16. Which of the following is not a risk factor for the development of a CVA?
    a. diabetes mellitus type 1
    b. diabetes mellitus type 2
    c. African American race
    d. cigarette smoking
    e. diabetes insipidus

17. The incidence of stroke in the United States over the last 15 years has:
    a. increased significantly
    b. increased slightly
    c. decreased significantly
    d. decreased slightly
    e. nobody really knows for sure

CLINICAL CASE PROBLEM 4:

A 62-YEAR-OLD WHITE MALE WITH A CURTAIN COMING DOWN OVER HIS EYES

A 62 year-old white male presents to your office with a complaint of decreased vision, which with further questioning was described as "a curtain coming down over my eyes." The patient's past medical history included hypertension and hyperlipidemia, and he recently admitted to extensive use of cocaine. He denies intravenous drug use, vertigo, diplopia, ataxia, or an abnormal heart rate.

18. If you had the choice of one test to help determine the etiology of his symptoms, what would that be?
    a. ultrasound of the carotid arteries
    b. CT scan of the brain
    c. magnetic resonance imaging (MRI) scan of the brain
    d. fluorescein angiography of the fundi
    e. lumbar puncture

19. Which of the following statements regarding carotid endarterectomy (CEA) is (are) true?
    a. CEA is indicated in the presence of a completed stroke
    b. CEA is indicated in the presence of a complete arterial occlusion
    c. randomized, controlled trials have established the benefit of CEA over standard medical therapy for the treatment of carotid artery stenosis
    d. CEA has been established as the treatment of choice in patients with a documented TIA and a highly stenotic lesion >70%.
    e. nobody really knows for sure

20. In a patient with an asymptomatic carotid bruit, for whom evaluation reveals a high-grade stenosis, recommended treatment would include:
    a. watchful waiting
    b. anticoagulation therapy with aspirin or ticlopidine
    c. CEA
    d. CEA and aspirin
    e. none of the above

21. In the diagnostic workup of a patient with a TIA, a lumbar puncture should be used:
    a. in all diagnostic workups
    b. only when meningitis is suspected
    c. in any patient considered to have a subarachnoid hemorrhage when a CT scan is not diagnostic
    d. there are no clinical indications for a lumbar puncture in the workup of a patient with a TIA or CVA

22. Among the following, which is (are) the preferred diagnostic test(s) for evaluating patients with a cardiac embolic phenomenon?
    a. transthoracic echocardiography
    b. transesophageal echocardiography
    c. MRA
    d. all of the above
    e. none of the above

23. The main indication for the use of MRA is which of the following?
    a. to diagnose an acute stroke
    b. to evaluate for coronary artery stenosis
    c. if considering emergent thrombolytic therapy to reverse stroke progression
    d. all of the above
    e. none of the above

24. The first-line choice of antiplatelet therapy for patients with prior TIA or stroke is:
    a. acetylsalicylic acid (ASA)
    b. clopidogrel (Plavix)
    c. ticlopidine
    d. addition of dipyridamole (Persantine) and ASA
    e. warfarin

CLINICAL CASE MANAGEMENT PROBLEM

Define the following terms: (1) transient ischemic attack; (2) stroke-in-evolution; and (3) completed stroke. Describe management of acute stroke.

ANSWERS:

1. **c.** At this time, the most likely diagnosis is stroke-in-evolution. The typical development of thrombotic stroke causes a clinical syndrome known as stroke-in-evolution. An intermittent or slow progression over hours to days is characteristic of stroke-in-evolution or slow hemorrhage.

Also referred to as a progressing stroke or crescendo TIAs, some clinicians believe anticoagulation improves outcome. Aspirin would be a more conservative therapy.

2. **a.** The symptoms that this patient is experiencing suggest a lesion of the left middle cerebral artery. The signs/symptoms of middle cerebral artery occlusion are as follows: (1) dysphagia (left hemisphere involvement), dyslexia, and dysgraphia; (2) contralateral hemiparesis or hemiplegia; (3) contralateral hemisensory disturbances; (4) rapid deterioration in consciousness from confusion to coma; (5) homonymous hemianopia; (6) denial of or lack of recognition of a paralyzed extremity; and (7) eyes deviated to the side of the lesion; and (8) global aphasia if dominant hemisphere is involved.

3. **a.** Because of the slow and continuing progression of the CNS symptomatology, this is much more characteristic of a thrombotic stroke than an embolic stroke.

4. **a.** The pathophysiology of stroke in order of frequency (from most common to least common) is as follows: (1) thrombotic stroke; (2) embolic stroke; (3) hemorrhagic stroke; (4) lacunar stroke (lacunar infarct); and (5) subarachnoid hemorrhage.

5. **b.** An embolic stroke involves fragments that break from a thrombus formed outside the brain in the heart, aorta, common carotid, or thorax. Emboli infrequently arise from the ascending aorta or the common carotid artery. The embolus usually involves small vessels and obstructs at a bifurcation or other point of narrowing, thus enabling ischemia to develop and extend. An embolus may completely occlude the lumen of the vessel, or it may remain in place or break into fragments and move up the vessel. The most common source of emboli is from the heart.

Conditions associated with the onset of an embolic stroke include the following: (1) atrial fibrillation; (2) myocardial infarction; (3) endocarditis; (4) rheumatic heart disease; (5) valvular prostheses; (6) atrial septal defect; (7) disorders of the aorta; (8) disorders of the carotids; (9) disorders of the vertebral-basilar system; and (10) other embolic phenomena, such as air, fat, and tumor.

6. **b.** CVAs or strokes remain the third-leading cause of death in North America. The single most important risk factor for stroke is hypertension. The decrease in the incidence of stroke is largely the result of the successful, aggressive, and ideal treatment of hypertension in North America. The risk of stroke is three times higher in those with hypertension and is doubled in those with isolated systolic hypertension.

Other factors that are important in the etiology of stroke include the following: (1) age (the older the patient, the greater the risk); (2) other heart disease (valvular, conductive, infective, atherosclerotic); (3) cigarette smoking; (4) diabetes mellitus (type 1 and type 2); (5) the oral contraceptive pill when combined with smoking and older age; (6) race (African Americans are more prone than white Americans); (7) family history (of lipid disorders or cardiovascular diseases in general); (8) sex (strokes are more common in females than in males); and (9) dyslipidemias (puts patients at higher risk for atherogenesis).

7. **c.** Lacunar strokes (lacunar infarcts) are infarcts smaller than 1 mm in size and involve the small perforating arteries predominately in the basal ganglia pons, cerebellum, internal capsule, and (less commonly) deep cerebral white matter. Lacunar infarcts are associated primarily with hypertension. Because of the subcortical location and small area of infarction, these strokes may have pure motor and sensory deficits, ipsilateral ataxia, and dysarthria. They may appear on CT as small hypodense areas. Prognosis and recovery are usually good.

8. **d.** This patient most likely has a lesion in the territory of the right anterior cerebral artery. Signs and symptoms of a CVA in the territory of the anterior cerebral artery include the following: (1) mental status impairments including confusion, amnesia, perseveration, personality changes (flat affect, apathy), and cognitive changes (short attention span, slowness, and deterioration of intellectual function); (2) urinary continence (long duration); (3) contralateral hemiparesis or hemiplegia; (4) sensory impairments (contralateral); (5) foot and leg deficits (more frequent than arm deficits) and contralateral leg/foot paralysis; (6) apraxia on affected side; (7) expressive aphasia (for left hemisphere only); (8) deviation of the eyes and head toward the affected side; (9) abulia (lack of initiative); and (10) gait dysfunction.

9. **c.** This patient has had a CVA involving the vertebral-basilar system. The signs/symptoms of vertebral-basilar stroke are as follows: (1) dysarthria, dysphagia; (2) vertigo, nausea, and vomiting; (3) disorientation; (4) ataxic gait (ipsilateral cerebellar ataxia); (5) visual symptoms (double vision, blurred vision); (6) dysphagia; (7) ocular signs (nystagmus, conjugate gaze paralysis, ophthalmoplegia); (8) akinetic mutism (locked-in syndrome when basilar artery occlusion occurs); (9) numbness of lips and face; (10) facial weakness, alternating motor paresis; and (11) drop attacks, syncope—transcranial. (Doppler studies can detect vertebrobasilar embolic sources.)

10. **c.** The most common source of cerebral emboli is from the heart.

11. **e.** Strokes usually will not show up on a CT scan or MRI within the first 24 hours. Therefore the role of

CT scanning is to rule out structural abnormalities such as hemorrhages, tumors, or abscesses.

12. **d.** Bacterial endocarditis would not be considered a contradiction to anticoagulation therapy but would be considered a precaution with those bleeding tendencies and uncontrolled hypertension. Contraindication in this case would be a patient who has a large stroke, a hemorrhagic stroke, or severe thrombocytopenia

13. **a.** A TIA probably represents thrombotic or embolic particles causing an intermittent blockage of circulation or spasm. Amaurosis fugax, which is described by patients as "a curtain coming down in front of my eyes" or "a blackout," is really a TIA of the ophthalmic artery. This is associated primarily with the carotid circulation and also may present with contralateral weakness of the face, arm, legs, or numbness.

In the situation of a patient with a noncardio-embolic TIA, the use of ASA is indicated. Optimal dose is not known. Clopidogrel, ticlopidine, or aspirin plus dipyridamole are alternatives. In noncardioembolic TIA, full anticoagulation is generally not indicated. In possible cardioembolic TIA (e.g., atrial fibrillation, ventricular aneurysm), whether heparin should be started immediately is unknown, although most clinicians do start it. In either form of TIA, full evaluation, including carotid ultrasound Doppler imaging or MRA, is indicated. Risk factor reduction should take place. Hospitalization generally hastens the workup.

14. **c.** Intracranial aneurysms may result from arteriosclerosis, congenital abnormality, trauma, inflammation, or infection. Cocaine recently has been linked to aneurysm formation. The size may vary from 2 mm to 2 or 3 cm. Most aneurysms are located at bifurcations in or near the circle of Willis, particularly on the anterior or posterior communicating arteries. Aneurysm may be single, but in 20% of cases, more than one aneurysm is present. The peak incidence occurs between age 35 and age 60. Berry aneurysms also are known as saccular aneurysms. Berry aneurysms make up the majority of sub-arachnoid bleeds (51%).

15. **b.** The diagnostic test of choice for an acute cerebral infarction is a CT scan of the head. A CT scan of the brain without contrast will allow the exclusion of a cerebral hemorrhage. A CT scan is preferable to an MRI in the acute stages because it is quicker, and an MRI will not easily detect bleeding during the first 48 hours.

16. **e.** The risk factors for CVAs include the following: (1) hypertension (single most important risk factor), including isolated systolic hypertension; (2) hypercholesterolemia; (3) hypertriglyceridemia (because it has been found to be an independent risk factor for vascular disease); (4) African American race (probably as a result of an increased risk of hypertension); (5) obesity (also related to the increased risk of hypertension); (6) sedentary lifestyle related to obesity, which is related to hypertension; (7) cigarette smoking; (8) women in their later reproductive years (age 37-45) who are heavy cigarette smokers and taking oral contraceptives; (9) family history of CVAs; (10) family history of hyperlipidemia; (11) age older than 65 years; (12) diabetes mellitus types 1 and 2; and (13) hypothyroidism (related to hyperlipidemia).

Diabetes insipidus has nothing to do with CVA (with the possible exception of Sheenan's syndrome, postpartum pituitary necrosis).

17. **c.** Estimates vary widely; however, the incidence of stroke in the United States has declined dramatically in the last 15 years because of the relative success of the "Treatment of Hypertension" campaign. It should be noted, however, that the incidence increases almost 20-fold with age (from 100 per 100,000 people ages 45-54 to 1800 per 100,000 people at age 85).

18. **a.** This patient has had a TIA. His classic description of amaurosis fugax and his cocaine use may have contributed to this. Cocaine probably caused an intense vasospasm; it is an intensely powerful vasoconstrictor, much more powerful than either angiotensin II or thromboxane. This patient needs an ultrasound of his carotid arteries, and he needs it soon.

19. **d.** There has been a great deal of research about CEA (when to do/when not to do). Studies have demonstrated that a CEA reduces the risk of subsequent stroke in patients with high-grade stenosis who have had TIAs. Therefore, one indication for performing a CEA is a documented TIA with a highly stenotic lesion (more than 70%). If an ulcerated plaque is present even in moderate stenosis, the risk of stroke increases and patients benefit from CEA. Research is being conducted on the use of CEA for patients with asymptomatic bruits with moderate stenotic lesions. The results to date are mixed.

The current treatment recommendations for carotid stenosis include the following: (1) prior TIA or stroke with a stenosis of more than 70% (carotid endarterectomy is superior to medical management); (2) prior TIA or stroke with a stenosis or 50% to 60%, carotid endarterectomy preferred at high volume, good outcome centers or medical management with serial carotid Dopplers to identify developing plaques; (3) prior TIA or stroke with stenosis of less than 50%, medical management (CEA of no proven benefit); (4) asymptomatic patient with stenosis of 80% or more, CEA should be considered, particularly at high-volume centers; and (5) asymptomatic with less than 80% stenosis should consider medical management.

Carotid angioplasty with stenting (CAS) is an emerging treatment at many centers. CAS has had favorable results in several studies, particularly when combined with antiplatelet medications. Whether this therapy will supplant CEA remains to be seen.

20. d. Studies report that in asymptomatic patients with a high-grade carotid artery stenosis, a CEA at a high volume center in combination with aspirin therapy and risk-factor reduction may be the treatment of choice. This combination may reduce the relative risk of stroke when compared to medical therapy alone.

21. c. A lumbar puncture should be done in any patient considered to have a subarachnoid hemorrhage when a CT scan is not diagnostic. It should be performed in patients suspected of having infective endocarditis, meningitis, or inflammatory vasculitis, looking for the presence of cerebrospinal fluid leukocytosis.

22. a. Transesophageal echocardiography is preferred for the evaluation of cardiogenic emboli.

23. c. MRA is indicated if one is considering emergent thrombolytic therapy to reverse stroke progression. It should be noted that thrombolytic therapy is still unproven in the elderly population.

24. a. Aspirin is considered first-line antiplatelet therapy for patients with a prior stoke. Plavix is used if patients are intolerant to ASA or if ASA fails. Ticlid requires regular blood monitoring, and Aggrenox, a combination of ASA and dipyridamole, is also available. The efficacy of warfarin therapy in the absence of atrial fibrillation is unproven.

SUMMARY OF CEREBROVASCULAR ACCIDENTS

1. **Incidence:** very significant decrease over last 15 years. The reason: hypertension control
2. **Pathologic classification (in order of frequency):** (a) thrombotic stroke; (b) embolic stroke; (c) hemorrhagic stroke; (d) lacunar stroke; and (e) subarachnoid hemorrhage
3. **Risk factors for CVA:** (a) hypertension is the single most important risk factor; (b) there is no longer any such entity as mild hypertension; and (c) see also Answer 17

Continued

SOLUTION TO THE CLINICAL CASE MANAGEMENT PROBLEM

Definitions:

1. *Transient ischemic attack:* a disturbance of cerebrovascular system in which neurologic symptoms both appear and then disappear within 24 hours
2. *Stroke-in-evolution:* the typical course of a thrombotic stroke. This is also known as a progressive stroke. It is best defined as an intermittent progression of a neurologic deficit over hours to days.
3. *Completed stroke:* a CVA that has reached its maximum destructiveness in producing neurologic deficits, although cerebral edema may not have reached its maximum

Management of Acute Stroke:

1. *Thrombolysis:* For patients with ischemic deficits of no more than 3 hours duration, with hemorrhage ruled out by CT scanning, thrombolysis with intravenous recombinant tissue plasminogen activator is

recanalization therapy of choice. Unfortunately, many people are not seen early enough to effectively use this treatment option.

2. *Blood pressure:* Blood pressure never should be lowered precipitously. In extreme cases (systolic more than 220 mm hg), gradual reduction to 180 mm hg should be undertaken. Intravascular volume should be maintained, and, in some cases, cerebral edema should be controlled with mannitol. For patients with cerebellar infarction, neurosurgical consult should be sought because of the risk of brainstem compression.

3. *Antiplatelet agents:* Aspirin has a small but definite benefit in acute stroke and can reduce the risk of further TIAs and stroke in symptomatic patients. As discussed previously, clopidogrel and dipyridamole also can be used. Antiplatelet agents may reduce the risk of new strokes by 25% to 30%.

SUMMARY OF CEREBROVASCULAR ACCIDENTS—cont'd

4. **Classification of CVAs:** see the Solution to the Clinical Case Management Problem.

   It is important to evaluate and workup TIAs. Recent research concerning the benefits of CEA and aspirin therapy may prevent future TIAs or strokes.

5. **Signs/symptoms:** see details on arteries in Answers 2, 8, and 9.

6. **Investigations/treatment:** (a) history; (b) physical examination; (c) immediate MRI angio or CT; (d) if not hemorrhagic and if not a completed stroke, and if within a 3-hour window, consider a recanalization strategy (see treatment later in this chapter); if it is already complete, do not follow this approach; (e) cerebral edema may become a major problem and corticosteroid therapy may be required; (f) unless contraindicated, all patients with TIAs, history of stroke, and risk factors for stroke (major) should be undergoing aspirin prophylaxis; and (g) rehabilitation (aggressive, early, and forceful)

7. **Concomitant conditions:** depression is the single most important coexisting or concomitant condition. Remember also that this applies to both the patient and the patient's caregiver.

8. **The biopsychosocial model of illness:** Few diseases are as devastating to a patient and a patient's family as stroke. Often the person that really gets lost in this whole ordeal is the spouse. Please remember the spouse.

9. **Prevention:** (a) treat hypertension aggressively; (b) treat obesity and sedentary lifestyle aggressively; (c) stop smoking; and (d) remember, an aspirin a day keeps the neurologist away.

10. **Acute ischemic stroke management:** see acute management in the Solution to the Clinical Case Management Problem.

11. **Prevention of embolic stroke:** In patients with atrial fibrillation, the choice between warfarin and ASA prophylaxis is determined by age and risk factors such as increased chance of falling and compliance. Warfarin is most effective and should be used unless contraindications exist.

SUGGESTED READING

Akopov S, Cohen SN: Preventing stroke: a review of current guidelines. *J Am Med Dir Assoc* 4(5 Suppl):S127-132, 2003.

Broderick JP, Hacke W: Treatment of acute ischemic stroke: Part I: Treatment of Acute Ischemic Stroke: Part I: Recanalization Strategies. *Circulation* 106(12):1563-1569, 2002.

Broderick JP, Hacke W: Treatment of acute ischemic stroke: Part II: neuroprotection and medical management. *Circulation* 106(13):1736-1740, 2002.

Connolly SJ: Preventing stroke in patients with atrial fibrillation: current treatments and new concepts. *Am Heart J* 145(3):418-423, 2003.

Corvol JC, et al: Differential effects of lipid-lowering therapies on stroke prevention: a meta-analysis of randomized trials. *Arch Intern Med* 163(6):669-676, 2003.

De Schryver EL, et al: Cochrane review: dipyridamole for preventing major vascular events in patients with vascular disease. *Stroke* 34(8):2072-2080, 2003.

Johnston SC: Clinical practice. Transient ischemic attack. *N Engl J Med* 347(21):1687-1692, 2002.

Kastrup A, et al: Early outcome of carotid angioplasty and stenting with and without cerebral protection devices: a systematic review of the literature. *Stroke* 34(3):813-819, 2003.

Teasell R: Stroke recovery and rehabilitation. *Stroke* 34(2):365-366, 2003.

Chapter 145

Erectile Dysfunction in the Elderly

| "Doctor, could I speak to you privately?"

CLINICAL CASE PROBLEM 1:

A RELUCTANT 72-YEAR-OLD MALE

Mr. R is a 72-year-old male with past medical history of type 2 diabetes mellitus for 15 years. During a routine office visit he seemed distracted, and although he said everything was fine, his wife seemed concerned when he replied that he did not have any problems with erectile dysfunction (ED).

When the doctor left the room, Mr. R turned to his wife and said, "I did not want to say anything in front of the medical student!" She understood, and they both agreed they should talk to the doctor privately.

■ SELECT THE BEST ANSWER TO THE FOLLOWING QUESTIONS:

1. The percentage of men with ED between the ages of 40 and 70 years in the United States is approximately?
   a. 15%
   b. 32%
   c. 42%
   d. 52%
   e. 60%

2. Risk factors for ED include all of the following except for:
   a. alcohol abuse
   b. hypoglycemia
   c. depression
   d. trauma to the perineum
   e. Peyronie's disease

3. Which of the following is (are) a component(s) in the erectile cycle?
   a. cyclic guanosine monophosphate (cGMP)
   b. cyclic adenosine monophosphate (cAMP)
   c. nitrous oxide
   d. endothelin
   e. a and c

4. True or false: A low testosterone level represents a major cause of ED.

5. The prevalence of ED at age 70 is estimated to be:
   a. 55%
   b. 65%
   c. 70%
   d. 75%
   e. 80%

6. The percentage of men seeking an evaluation or examination for ED is:
   a. 10%
   b. 20%
   c. 30%
   d. 40%
   e. 60%

7. Physical finding(s) that may be associated with ED include which of the following?
   a. penile plaques
   b. decreased male pattern hair
   c. absent cremasteric reflex
   d. gynecomastia
   e. none of the above
   f. a, b, c, and d

8. Medications associated with ED include which of the following?
   a. antihypertensives
   b. antidepressants
   c. cytotoxic drugs
   d. H_2 receptor blockers
   e. all of the above

9. To check for a libido problem associated with ED, which hormone(s) should you check?
   a. testosterone
   b. thyroid stimulating hormone (TSH)
   c. luteinizing hormone (LH)
   d. none of the above
   e. a, b, and c

10. A reduced penile brachial index is indicative of which of the following causes for ED?
    a. neurologic
    b. hormonal
    c. vascular
    d. all of the above
    e. none of the above

11. First-line treatment options for ED include:
    a. oral medications
    b. vacuum devices
    c. psychosexual counseling if indicated
    d. intracavernosal injections
    e. a, b, and c
    f. a, b, c, and d

12. The mechanism of action of sildenafil includes the following:
    a. release of nitric oxide
    b. enhanced smooth-muscle relaxation
    c. increase in cGMP levels
    d. all of the above
    e. b and c

13. Side effects of sildenafil include:
    a. headache
    b. flushing
    c. dyspepsia
    d. color tinge in vision
    e. all of the above

14. Second-line therapy for ED includes all of the following except:
    a. intracavernosal injections
    b. intraurethral instillation
    c. penile prosthesis
    d. vascular reconstructive surgery
    e. a and b

■ ANSWERS:

1. **d.** The approximate percentage of men with ED between the ages of 40 and 70 years in the United States is 52%.

2. **b.** ED more commonly occurs with diabetes and not hypoglycemia. Risk factors for ED include disease status that can affect the vascular system, neurologic system, and smooth muscles. These typically include alcohol abuse, anemia, coronary artery or peripheral

vascular disease, depression, hyperlipidemia, hypertension, hypogonadism, Peyronie's disease, hyperprolactinemia, smoking, trauma or surgery to the pelvis or spine, and vascular surgery. In addition, medications always should be reviewed and considered.

3. a. The initial substance released in the erectile sequence is nitric oxide (NO), not to be confused with nitrous acid (N$_2$O, laughing gas). This short-lived hormone then interacts with a cytoplasmic receptor and stimulates guanylate cyclase activity increasing the concentration of cGMP. The cGMP then activates a specific phosphokinase (protein kinase G), which phosphorylates vascular smooth-muscle components, causing vasodilation and thereby inducing an erection.

4. False. A low serum testosterone level rarely is a sole cause for ED. It, however, may lead to a decrease in libido. Research may reveal that a circulating testosterone threshold maybe important because nitric oxide synthase, which leads to the formation of nitric oxide, is an androgen-dependent enzyme.

5. c. The estimated prevalence of ED by age 70 years is 70%.

6. a. Although the prevalence of men with ED between the ages of 40 and 70 years is 52%, and 70% for those older than age 70, only 10% seek attention for this disorder.

7. e. Neuropathies that may be associated with ED may include orthostatic hypotension, impaired response to Valsalva maneuver, absent bulbocavernosus, or cremasteric reflex. Peyronie's disease may present with penile bands or plaques. Hypogonadism may present with diminished male pattern hair, gynecomastia, and small testes (less than 20-25 mm long).

8. e. There are many medications that may cause ED. Antihypertensive medications and antidepressants may cause ED by interfering with blood flow or in response to neurotransmitter. Other medications or drugs that may cause ED include estrogens, antiandrogens, H$_2$ receptor blockers, ketoconazole, beta blockers, psychotropics, spironolactone, lipid-lowering agents, nonsteroidal antiinflammatory agents, cytotoxic drugs, and diuretics. In addition, alcohol, cocaine, cigarettes, and marijuana may cause ED.

9. a. If a decline in libido also is associated with ED, the testosterone level should be checked.

10. c. A reduced penile brachial pressure index suggests vascular disease as an underlying cause of ED.

11. e. Oral medications, vacuum devices, and psychosexual counseling when indicated are considered first-line treatment based on the diagnosis. Second-line treatment options include intracavernosal injection and intraurethral instillation. Third-line treatment options include penile prosthesis and vascular reconstructive surgery.

12. e. (Also see Answer 3.) The normal sequence in getting an erection is sexual stimulation, which causes synthesis of NO from arginine and its release. NO then stimulates guanylate cyclase activity increasing the concentration of cGMP. The cGMP stimulates phosphorylation of vascular muscles, causing vasodilation and permitting blood to rush into the corpus spongiosa. Some 40% to 50% of the tissue in the corpus spongiosa is vascular, and the expansion of this vascular component compresses the base of the blood-filled corpus spongiosa inhibiting outflow and increasing the internal pressure. A full erection occurs when the intracorpus spongiosa pressure reaches 200 mm Hg or more. Normally the cGMP is rapidly destroyed by the action of phosphodiesterase 5 (PDE-5). Sildenafil acts by inhibiting PDE-5 and in that way maintains high cGMP levels, which in turn maintains vascular dilation, high intracorpus spongiosa blood pressure, and a hard erection. However, it does not stimulate the release of NO, and because guanylate cyclase activity is dependent on the synthesis and release of NO after sexual stimulation, sildenafil cannot act in the absence of sexual arousal.

13. e. Side effects of sildenafil include headache, flushing, dyspepsia, and a color tinge in vision. Less common side effects may include nasal congestion, diarrhea, dizziness, and rash. Many of these side effects stem from the fact that although sildenafil's phosphodiesterase activity is relatively specific for the penile phosphodiesterase isozyme, it does have some cross reactivity with other PDE isozymes. A potentially important side effect is that it is a weak systemic vasodilator and can react synergistically with nitrates, causing hypotension. Therefore its use by men undergoing nitrate therapy is contraindicated. The blue haze often observed at the periphery of the visual field is because it also is a weak inhibitor of the retinal phosphodiesterase, PDE-6. However, this transitory effect has stopped few from taking the drug.

Presently there are three PDE-5 inhibitors approved by the FDA. They are sildenafil (Viagra), vardenafil (Levitra), and tadalafil (Cialis). All three have the same mode of action, although vardenafil and tadalafil have longer durations of action, thus perhaps permitting greater spontaneity in initiating sexual activity. Contraindications for use of all three include nitrate and alpha blocker use.

14. Answers a and b are the correct choices, with c and d being considered third-line therapy. Alprostadil (Caverject) is a vasoactive intracavernosal-type pharmacotherapy. This vasodilating drug is injected into the shaft of the penis to activate smooth-muscle relaxation. Potential side effects include corporal fibrosis, penile deformity, and priapism. Muse (medicated urethral system for erection) is the intraurethral instillation of alprostadil. It has a low efficacy rate (30% to 50%) and a high level of pain. A penile prosthesis should be considered an option of last resort but may be effective with neurovascular disorders or corporal fibrosis. Patient and partner satisfaction with a prosthesis remain the highest of all therapies at 90% at 98%.

SUMMARY OF ERECTILE DYSFUNCTION IN THE ELDERLY

ED is a common problem, and prevalence increases with age. Although the prevalence of ED between the ages of 40 and 70 years is 52%, and it is 70% for those older than age 70 years, only 10% of patients seek attention for this disorder. Therefore, clinicians should ask about erectile functioning as part of the sexual history.

Risk factors for ED include disease states that can affect the vascular system, neurologic system, and smooth muscles and medication use, particularly antihypertensives. Disease states or behaviors that increase risk typically include alcohol use, smoking, anemia, coronary artery or peripheral vascular disease, depression, hyperlipidemia, hypertension, hypogonadism, Peyronie's disease, hyperprolactinemia, trauma or surgery to the pelvis or spine, and vascular surgery.

If a decline in libido also is associated with ED, the testosterone level should be checked.

The type 5 phosphodiesterase inhibitors, such as sildenafil, are effective treatment in all age groups and particularly in elderly men with common comorbidities such as diabetes. Common side effects include headache flushing and dyspepsia. They are contraindicated in patients taking nitrates because of the possibility of inducing hypotension and subsequently compromising cardiac perfusion.

SUGGESTED READING

Montorsi F, et al: The ageing male and erectile dysfunction. *BJU Int* 92(5):516-520, 2003.

Mulhall JP: Deciphering erectile dysfunction drug trials. *J Urol* 170(2 Pt 1): 353-358, 2003.

Seftel AD: Erectile dysfunction in the elderly: epidemiology, etiology and approaches to treatment. *J Urol* 169(6):1999-2007, 2003.

EMERGENCY AND SPORTS MEDICINE

 Chapter **146**

Treatment of the Patient in Cardiac Arrest

> "I know it's hard to believe, but this is the second time I've died and here I am back again."

CLINICAL CASE PROBLEM 1:

A 55-Year-Old Male Found Collapsed in the Street

A 55-year-old male is found collapsed in the street by a passerby. The passerby begins cardiopulmonary resuscitation (CPR) and is joined shortly by another citizen. Someone calls 911, and CPR is continued until the paramedics arrive and initiate ACLS.

Despite complete advanced cardiac life support (ACLS) maneuvers, the patient remains pulseless and breathless as the paramedics hand over care to the emergency room (ER) doctor on duty at the closest hospital.

■ SELECT THE BEST ANSWER TO THE FOLLOWING QUESTIONS:

1. What is the most common rhythm initially responsible for cardiac arrest?
   a. ventricular tachycardia (VT)
   b. ventricular fibrillation (VF)
   c. ventricular standstill
   d. asystole
   e. complete heart block

2. What is the most common rhythm leading directly to death in cardiac arrest?
   a. VT
   b. VF
   c. second-degree heart block-Mobitz type II
   d. ventricular asystole
   e. complete heart block

3. A "quick-look paddles" is performed on the patient in Clinical Case Problem 1. You diagnose VF. What should be your first step?
   a. defibrillate with 200 joules
   b. defibrillate with 360 joules
   c. administer epinephrine 1.0 mg intravenous (IV) push

   d. administer vasopressin 40 units IV bolus
   e. intubate the trachea

4. What is the antiarrhythmic of choice in the management of VF?
   a. bretylium
   b. lidocaine
   c. procainamide
   d. magnesium
   e. amiodarone

5. The patient is successfully converted to sinus rhythm. Unfortunately, on the way to the coronary care unit he arrests again. The rhythm strip reveals asystole. CPR is restarted. Which of the following is the next logical step in treatment?
   a. administer epinephrine 1.0 mg IV push
   b. administer calcium chloride 10 cc of a 10% solution IV push
   c. administer sodium bicarbonate 1 mEq/kg IV push
   d. administer isoproterenol 2-20 μg/kg/min
   e. administer lidocaine 75 mg IV push

6. With appropriate treatment the patient again converts to sinus rhythm. He is stabilized in the coronary care unit. Unfortunately, 2 hours later he develops VT. His blood pressure is 100/60 mm Hg, and he has a palpable pulse. Your next step should be to administer which of the following?
   a. lidocaine 1-1.5 mg/kg IV
   b. procainamide 20-30 mg/min up to a maximum of 50 mg/min
   c. bretylium 5 mg IV bolus
   d. verapamil 5 mg IV bolus
   e. none of the above

7. Sinus rhythm is restored again, and his condition returns to satisfactory. Unfortunately, he develops a second-degree atrioventricular (AV) block (Mobitz type II). His pulse is 40 beats/minute and his blood pressure drops to 70/40 mm Hg. Given this change, what would you do now?
   a. observe the patient only
   b. administer isoproterenol 2-10 mg/min
   c. administer atropine 0.5-1.0 mg
   d. administer epinephrine 0.5-1.0 mg
   e. none of the above

8. What is the definitive therapy for the dysrrhyth-mia described in the previous question?
   a. a constant infusion of isoproterenol 2-20 mg/min
   b. a constant infusion of lidocaine 2-4 mg/min
   c. a constant infusion of procainamide 2-4 mg/min
   d. a transvenous pacemaker
   e. none of the above

9. CPR is in progress on a 70-kg man who collapsed in the street (witnessed arrest). Basic life support (BLS) was begun, as was ACLS, when the para-medics arrived. He was brought immediately to the ER, and a blood gas sample was drawn. The results were as follows: pH=7.10, P_{CO_2}= 60 mm Hg, P_{O_2}=75 mm Hg, HCO_3^-=15 mEq/L. This represents which of the following:
   a. metabolic acidosis with respiratory alkalosis
   b. respiratory acidosis with metabolic alkalosis
   c. pure metabolic acidosis
   d. pure respiratory acidosis
   e. mixed respiratory and metabolic acidosis

10. What is the most appropriate treatment of the patient described in Question 9?
    a. sodium bicarbonate 1.0 mEq/kg
    b. sodium bicarbonate 0.5 mEq/kg
    c. increased ventilation
    d. both a and c
    e. both b and c

11. Which of the following should be treated first in this patient?
    a. respiratory acidosis
    b. metabolic acidosis
    c. respiratory alkalosis
    d. metabolic alkalosis
    e. all of the above

12. A 53-year-old male presents to your ER with a 2-hour history of a "rapid heartbeat," nausea, and dizziness. A 12-lead electrocardiogram (ECG) shows atrial flutter with variable AV conduction. As you are taking his history he becomes dis-oriented. You are only able to obtain his systolic blood pressure (40 mm Hg). At this time, what should you do?
    a. administer epinephrine 1.0 mg IV
    b. administer isoproterenol 2-20 mg/min IV
    c. defibrillate with 300 joules
    d. cardiovert with 300 joules
    e. cardiovert with 100 joules

13. What is the first step in initiation of resuscitation following a witnessed or unwitnessed cardiac arrest in the community?
    a. begin rescue breathing
    b. begin rescue compression
    c. initiate a call to 911
    d. check pulse
    e. go for help

14. Which of the following statements concerning BLS is false?
    a. the prompt administration of BLS is the key to success
    b. mouth-to-mouth resuscitation is the recom-mended method of respiratory exchange in performing BLS
    c. BLS is used most commonly in family situations—one family member resuscitating another
    d. BLS succeeds no more frequently than in 15% of out-of-hospital attempts
    e. infectious diseases such as acquired immuno-deficiency syndrome (AIDS) and serum hepatitis pose little, if any, risk to rescuers

15. What is the recommended BLS compression/ven-tilation rescue sequence in one- or two-person CPR?
    a. 15/2
    b. 15/1
    c. 20/4
    d. 10/1
    e. 10/3

■ ANSWERS:

1. **b.** See Answer 2.

2. **d.** The most common initial rhythm diagnosed in patients who suffer a cardiac arrest is VF. The usual course of events is as follows: coarse VF to fine VF to ventricular asystole. If cardiopulmonary resusci-tation is started within 4 minutes after collapse, the likelihood of survival to hospital discharge doubles. Early defibrillation is essential. An out-of-hospital goal of defibrillation within 5 minutes of a telephone call is recommended. An in-hospital goal of defibril-lation within 3 minutes of collapse is recommended. Communities report survival rates for out-of-hospital cardiac arrest ranging from 4% to 34%. Once ven-tricular asystole develops, the probability of successful resuscitation is virtually zero. Thus, although VF is the most common initial rhythm, ventricular asystole is the most common arrhythmia leading directly to death.

3. **a.** The first step in the treatment of VF is defib-rillation with an energy level of 200 joules. If the first attempt is unsuccessful, two further defibrillations (200-300, 360 joules) should follow immediately. If defibrillation is not successful, the trachea is intubated,

an IV is established, and epinephrine or vasopressin is given. Defibrillations also may be given via biphasic nonescalating shocks at 150-200 joules.

4. **e.** The antiarrhythmic agent of choice is amiodarone. Amiodarone is a class IIb intervention (supported by "fair to good" scientific evidence) for VF/pulseless (VT) after defibrillation, and epinephrine or vasopressin have failed to restore a perfusing rhythm. Amiodarone is administered in a dosage of 300 mg IV push and repeated doses of 150 mg may be given if required.

Bretylium is not recommended as an antidysrhythmic agent in CPR because of a lack of demonstrated efficacy and its high side-effect profile.

Lidocaine is classified as an indeterminate intervention because of little evidence supporting its use.

Procainamide is given for recurrent or intermittent VF or pulseless VT. Patients who convert from VF to a perfusing rhythm and then revert back to VF may benefit.

Procainamide is administered in a dose of 20-30 mg/min until one of the following is observed: (1) the arrhythmia is suppressed; (2) hypotension ensues; (3) the QRS complex is widened by 50% of its original width; or (4) a total of 17 mg/kg of drug has been administered.

Magnesium is given for VF or VT only if an underlying rhythm is caused by hypomagnesemia.

5. **a.** The next step in the management of the original patient is the administration of epinephrine 1.0 mg IV push. This should be repeated every 3-5 minutes. If intubation has not been performed, it should be done. Atropine in a dose of 1.0 mg IV push should be given as well and repeated every 3-5 minutes to a total of 3 mg. Transcutaneous cardiac pacing if available should be performed early. Termination of resuscitation efforts should be considered if asystole lasts more than 10 minutes and no treatable condition exists. The rate of survival in patients with asystole is close to zero.

6. **a.** The treatment of choice for patients with VT who are hemodynamically stable is lidocaine 1-1.5 mg/kg. This can be repeated until a total of 3 mg/kg has been given.

The second-line drug in this case is procainamide in a dose of 20-30 mg/min until the VT resolves or a total of 17 mg/kg has been given.

Bretylium is no longer recommended for use in CPR.

Verapamil, a calcium channel blocker, may be used in the treatment of stable narrow complex tachycardia.

7. **c.** See Answer 8.

8. **d.** Second-degree heart block (Mobitz type II) occurs below the level of the AV node either at the bundle of His (uncommon) or bundle branch level (more common). It usually is associated with an organic lesion in the conduction pathway. Its usual progression is to a third-degree (complete) heart block.

Initial treatment is aimed at increasing the heart rate in an attempt to increase cardiac output. Thus atropine in a dose of 0.5-1.0 mg is the drug of choice. The maximum dose of atropine is 0.04 mg/kg. Transcutaneous pacing should be used early on if available. Dopamine and epinephrine can be given if signs or symptoms persist. The definitive treatment in this patient is a transvenous pacemaker.

9. **e.** See Answer 11.

10. **c.** See Answer 11.

11. **a.** Most patients who have arrested and who are undergoing CPR have a mixed respiratory and metabolic acidosis. The normal P_{CO_2} is 40 mm Hg. The patient in this case has a markedly elevated P_{CO_2} of 60 mm Hg and thus is being hypoventilated. The patient's bicarbonate level of 15 mEq/L is below the normal range of 21-28 mEq/L; thus he has a metabolic acidosis as well.

Recommendations are that bicarbonate should be used with caution. Although cardiac function is depressed by acidosis, the determining factor is intracellular pH, not extracellular pH, as is measured by arterial pH. Hypoxia, not acidosis, accounts for most of the cardiac depression. Respiratory acidosis, however, produces immediate and profound depression. Thus increasing ventilation should be used as the primary means of correcting acidosis, and respiratory acidosis should be treated first.

By contrast, the use of bicarbonate has long been known to present risks that are not limited to alkalosis but include hypernatremia and hyperosmolarity. The accumulation of metabolic byproducts, not bicarbonate deficits, produces the acidosis. Giving bicarbonate to buffer the arterial pH will not benefit the patient.

12. **e.** The treatment of choice for acute unstable atrial flutter is synchronized cardioversion. The initial energy chosen should be 100 joules. If unsuccessful, this should be followed by cardioversion at 200, 300, and 360 joules. If the patient is stable, vagal maneuvers can be attempted, followed by medications (calcium channel blockers, beta blockers)

13. **c.** When witnessing a collapse or seeing an unresponsive victim, the first step in cardiac resuscitation is to access the Emergency Medical Service

(EMS) system by dialing 911 or the emergency number in your area. In children younger than age 8 years, however, before calling EMS, 1 minute of CPR should follow the initial assessment.

14. b. Until recently, the recommended method of BLS ventilation was mouth-to-mouth. However, as a result of increased fear of contact of infectious diseases (especially AIDS), the recommendation has been changed to a primary recommendation of mouth-to-mask ventilation. (However, if masks are not available, mouth-to-mouth resuscitation must be started immediately). The risk of contacting an infectious disease through mouth-to-mouth resuscitation is extremely remote.

15. a. For one or two rescuers providing CPR, the compression/ventilation ratio recommended is 15/2. The compression rate should be approximately 100/minute.

SUMMARY OF THE TREATMENT OF THE PATIENT IN CARDIAC ARREST

A. VF/pulseless VT:
1. Defibrillation: 200, 200-300, 360 joules
2. Epinephrine 1.0 mg IV push (repeat q 3-5 min) or vasopressin 40 units IV (single dose)
3. Defibrillate again (360 joules)
4. Amiodarone (IIb—good to very good scientific evidence)
5. Lidocaine (indeterminate—lack of scientific evidence)
6. Procainamide (indeterminate—lack of scientific evidence)

B. Asystole:
1. Consider immediate transcutaneous pacing
2. Epinephrine 1.0 mg IV push (repeat q 3-5 min)
3. Atropine 1.0 mg IV push (repeat q 3-5 min up to total 3 mg)
4. Identify and treat potential causes
5. Consider termination of resuscitation if confirmed asystole lasts longer than 10 minutes

C. VT: stable
1. Depends if monomorphic or polymorphic VT
   a. Monomorphic VT with normal left-ventricular function: (i) procainamide; (ii) amiodarone; (iii) lidocaine
   b. Monomorphic VT with impaired left-ventricular function: (i) amiodarone; (ii) lidocaine; or (iii) cardioversion
2. a. Polymorphic VT (normal QT): (i) treat underlying cause (e.g., metabolic disorders, ischemia, drug toxicities); (ii) beta blockers; (iii) lidocaine; (iv) amiodarone; and (v) procainamide
   b. Polymorphic VT (prolonged QT—torsades de pointes): (i) treat cause; (ii) magnesium; (iii) overdrive pacing; (iv) isoproterenol; (v) phenytoin; and (vi) lidocaine
   c. Polymorphic VT (impaired left-ventricular function): (i) amiodarone; (ii) lidocaine; and (iii) cardioversion

D. Heart block (second-degree Mobitz II and third degree):
1. Atropine 0.5-1.0 mg IV q 3-5 min up to 0.04 mg/kg
2. Transcutaneous pacing
3. Dopamine 5-20 μg/kg per minute
4. Epinephrine 2-10 μg per minute

E. Supraventricular tachycardia
1. Vagal maneuvers such as carotid sinus pressure
2. Adenosine 6 mg rapid IV push and repeated in 1-2 minutes at 12 mg if no therapeutic response
3. Treatment guidelines next depend if junctional tachycardia, AV nodal reentrant tachycardia, ectopic atrial tachycardia, or multifocal atrial tachycardia

F. Pulseless electrical activity
1. Rhythm exists but no blood pressure or pulse
2. Identify a cause: hypovolemia, hypoxia, acidosis, electrolyte abnormalities, hypothermia, drug overdose, cardiac tamponade, tension pneumothorax, coronary thrombosis
3. Intervention sequence: CPR, airway management, epinephrine, atropine, and in some cases sodium bicarbonate

---

SUGGESTED READING

American Heart Association: Guidelines 2000 for cardiopulmonary resuscitation and emergency cardiovascular care. *Circulation* 102 (suppl): I1-I384, 2000.

Eisenberg MS, Mengert TJ: Primary care: Cardiac resuscitation. *N Engl J Med* 344(17):1304-1313, 2001.

Kern KB, et al: New guidelines for cardiopulmonary resuscitation and emergency cardiac care: changes in the management of cardiac arrest. *JAMA* 285(10):1267-1269, 2001.

Xavier LC, Kern KB: Cardiopulmonary Resuscitation Guidelines 2000 Update: What's happened since? *Curr Opin Crit Care* 9(3):218-221, 2003.

Chapter 147

Advanced Trauma Life Support

"Too bad she didn't fasten her safety belt. She had such a bright future."

CLINICAL CASE PROBLEM 1:
A 27-Year-Old Female Injured in a Motor Vehicle Accident

A 27-year-old female is injured in a head-on two-car collision. She is transported to your emergency room (ER) in critical condition. You are the duty doctor in a small, rural hospital. The nearest trauma center is 180 miles away.

As she is wheeled through the ER doors, you note that her C-spine appears to be adequately immobilized. On examination, the patient is in acute respiratory distress. Her respiratory rate is 32/minute. Breath sounds are absent in the right lung field. She is pale, and her blood pressure is 90/60 mm Hg. Her pulse is 106/minute. Her heart sounds are distant and muffled. Her jugular venous pressure (JVP) is elevated. There is blood and pink-tinged fluid leaking from her nose, and a large scalp laceration is present.

Her neurologic examination reveals a dilated right pupil. She is responsive to deep sternal pressure and palpation of the abdomen. When you touch her abdomen, she pulls back in pain. This appears to be maximal over the left upper quadrant. Her right hip is in a posture of external rotation. There also is blood present at the urethral meatus, and her pelvis appears to be in an "odd position."

SELECT THE BEST ANSWER TO THE FOLLOWING QUESTIONS:

1. At this time, what should be your first priority?
   a. carry on with the rest of the complete assessment
   b. establish an intravenous (IV) infusion
   c. send the patient to x-ray for a stat chest x-ray
   d. send the patient to x-ray for a lateral x-ray of the cervical spine
   e. none of the above

2. What is the most likely cause of this patient's respiratory distress?
   a. flail chest
   b. tension pneumothorax
   c. acute pulmonary embolus
   d. pericardial tamponade
   e. none of the above

3. After establishing an airway and dealing with the patient's respiratory status, what should you do?
   a. complete the neurologic examination
   b. perform a Glasgow coma scale
   c. establish a central venous pressure (CVP) line or two large peripheral IVs
   d. perform a diagnostic paracentesis
   e. perform a stat electrocardiogram (ECG)

4. What is the most likely cause of this patient's dilated (R) pupil?
   a. a middle meningeal artery tear
   b. a chronic subdural hematoma
   c. an acute subdural hematoma
   d. a or c
   e. none of the above

5. The patient's neurologic status changes are as follows: (1) eyes: closed, no response to verbal commands but eyes open in response to pain; (2) best verbal response: none; and (3) best motor response: flexion withdrawal to pressure on the brachial plexus. What is the patient's Glasgow coma scale?
   a. 12
   b. 8
   c. 7
   d. 4
   e. 2

6. A diagnostic peritoneal lavage is performed and draws bloody fluid. On examination, pain is maximal in the left upper quadrant. What is the most likely cause of this patient's abdominal pain?
   a. liver laceration
   b. duodenal rupture
   c. renal hematoma
   d. splenic rupture
   e. pancreatic tear

CLINICAL CASE PROBLEM 2:
A 31-Year-Old Male Involved in a Car–Motorcycle Accident

A 31-year-old male is brought to the ER after having been involved in a car–motorcycle accident.

On examination, he is drowsy but conscious. His respiratory rate is 40/minute. His blood pressure is 70/50 mm Hg. His heart sounds are muffled. He has significant elevation of the JVP and a large contusion over the sternal area. There is a laceration seen over the precordial region. No other significant abnormalities are noted on primary survey.

7. What is the most likely diagnosis in this patient?
   a. myocardial contusion
   b. pericardial tamponade

c. aortic rupture
d. pulmonary contusion
e. pneumothorax

8. What is the treatment of choice for the patient's diagnosis from Question 7?
   a. pericardiocentesis
   b. increased rate of crystalloid infusion
   c. crystalloid infusion plus blood
   d. urgent thoracotomy
   e. chest tube insertion

9. What is the minimal gauge of a peripheral IV catheter that should be inserted in a patient in shock?
   a. #25 gauge
   b. #22 gauge
   c. #18 gauge
   d. #16 gauge
   e. #12 gauge

CLINICAL CASE MANAGEMENT PROBLEM

What is a reasonable probable problem list for the patient in Clinical Case Problem 1?

▶ **ANSWERS:**

1. e. Your first priority is to attend to the ABCs (airway, breathing, circulation) of resuscitation. Thus the establishment of an airway is first. Following that, breathing should be assessed (this includes assessment of breath sounds in both lung fields and respiratory rate). Finally, the patient's circulatory status must be attended to with the establishment of either a CVP line or two large bore IV lines.

2. b. The most likely cause of this patient's respiratory distress is a tension pneumothorax. Tension pneumothorax occurs from air in the pleural space under pressure. It is a common life-threatening injury that needs to be assessed and treated immediately. Clues to the high probability of a tension pneumothorax include complete absence of breath sounds in a lung field and hypotension in the presence of distended neck veins.

The most common error in this situation would be to transport the patient to x-ray without a physician. In fact, with the history and physical findings it would be entirely appropriate to treat the patient on the basis of your presumed diagnosis without an x-ray. A needle can be inserted into the chest wall cavity to decompress the potentially life-threatening tension pneumothorax. A "rush of air" will confirm the diag-

nosis. Subsequent management requires a chest tube thoracostomy.

3. c. As mentioned earlier, the priority following A and B is C, which is circulation. A CVP line or two large bore (#16 gauge IV catheters) should be inserted to maximize the ability to replace intravascular volume.

4. d. The dilated (R) pupil is most likely caused by an initial skull fracture producing tearing of either veins (subdural hematoma) or the middle meningeal artery (epidural hematoma). If CT scanning is unavailable and the patient is comatose with decerebrate or decorticate posturing that is unresponsive to mannitol or hyperventilation, a burr hole should be placed. The burr hole is placed in the temporal region on the ipsilateral side of the dilated pupil.

5. c. This patient's Glasgow coma scale is 7.
The Glasgow coma scale rating is as follows:
1. Eyes opening: spontaneously, 4; in response to verbal command, 3; in response to pain, 2; no response (stay closed), 1.
2. Best verbal response: orientated and converses, 5; disoriented and converses, 4; inappropriate words, 3; incomprehensible sounds, 2; no response, 1.
3. Best motor response: obeys verbal command, 6; localizes pain in response to painful stimulus, 5; flexion withdrawal, 4; abnormal flexion, 3; (decorticate rigidity) extension, 2; (decerebrate rigidity) no response, 1.
Total 2+1+4=7

6. d. A diagnostic peritoneal lavage that draws bloody fluid suggests an intraabdominal bleed most likely resulting from organ laceration or organ rupture. Pain maximal in the left upper quadrant suggests that this is most likely the result of splenic rupture. Splenic rupture is one of the most common abdominal injuries seen in multiple trauma victims.

In many trauma centers ultrasound has replaced diagnostic peritoneal lavage for the emergency evaluation of trauma patients. The technique known as the FAST (Focused Assessment with Sonography for Trauma) examination is rapid and accurate for detection of intraabdominal fluid or blood. In addition to the peritoneal cavity, the FAST examination also can scan the pericardium and pleural space.

7. b. See Answer 8.

8. d. This patient has a pericardial tamponade. Pericardial tamponade is an injury that is often missed. It also is a frequent injury in motor vehicle accidents in which multiple injuries are sustained. It is particularly common in car–motorcycle accidents where the motorcyclist is often thrown a significant distance.

In stable patients, diagnosis can be confirmed by echocardiography. Pericardiocentesis (the removal of fluid from around the heart) is the treatment. Unstable patients require urgent thoracotomy.

9. **d.** The minimum gauge of an IV catheter that should be inserted in a patient in shock is #16 gauge. It is recommended two #16 gauge catheters be inserted, one in each arm.

SOLUTION TO THE CLINICAL CASE MANAGEMENT PROBLEM

A probable problem list for patient in Clinical Case Problem 1 is as follows: (1) motor vehicle accident—patient in critical condition; (2) cervical spine injury until proved otherwise; (3) hypovolemic shock; (4) tension pneumothorax; (5) pericardial tamponade; (6) skull fracture, with acute epidural or subdural hematoma; (7) cerebrospinal fluid leak secondary to item 6; (8) probable splenic rupture or tear; (9) probable pelvic fracture; (10) probable femoral fracture; (11) probable urethral tear secondary to item 9; and (12) scalp laceration

SUMMARY OF ADVANCED TRAUMA LIFE SUPPORT

The major interventions that should be undertaken when a patient presents with traumatic shock are as follows:

1. Remember the ABCs (airway, breathing, circulation) and assess and treat those priorities first.
   A = Airway: airway management with protection of the cervical spine. Techniques to maintain an airway include chin lift, jaw thrust, artificial airway placement, and suctioning. Supplemental oxygen should be provided to patients with multiple trauma. Intubation is often necessary.
   B = Breathing: ensure breath sounds heard on both sides of the chest. Evaluate for degree of chest expansion, tachypnea, crepitus from rib fractures, subcutaneous emphysema, and the presence of penetrating or open wounds. Acute life-threatening pulmonary conditions are tension pneumothorax, open pneumothorax, flail chest, and in some cases massive hemothorax.
   C = Circulation: establish CVP line or two large bore IV lines. Intraarterial catheter is preferable for monitoring vital signs, but if not, attempt continuous monitoring by other means as necessary. Begin fluid resuscitation with Ringer's lactate or normal saline. Crossmatch for immediate blood.
   D = Deficits of neurologic function. Perform a brief neurologic examination. Assess level of consciousness, pupil size and reactivity, and motor and sensory function.
   E = Exposure = Completely undress all trauma patients.
2. Monitor input and output: urinary catheter, nasogastric tube
3. Perform primary survey of all systems, and pay particular attention to the following:
   a. Neurologic status: the Glasgow coma scale: is there any sign of increased intracranial pressure (ICP)? Consider IV mannitol and hyperventilation, and also maintain PO_2 >80 mmHg, and control blood pressure. Burr holes should be used in dire circumstances when indicated.
   b. Cardiovascular system: low blood pressure, elevated JVP, and muffled heart sounds suggest pericardial tamponade; consider other myocardial injuries, such as contusion.
   c. Respiratory system: is there any evidence of pneumothorax? Is a flail chest present? Are there any other injuries?
   d. Abdomen: is there any abdominal tenderness or bruising? Is there any tenderness in the right upper quadrant (RUQ) (possible liver laceration) or left upper quadrant (LUQ) (splenic laceration or rupture)? Is there any other injury? Is computed tomography scan or ultrasound available in the ER?

Continued

SUMMARY OF ADVANCED TRAUMA LIFE SUPPORT—cont'd

e. Reassess ABCs at regular intervals.
f. Musculoskeletal: are there any obvious fractures, especially open? Is there any evidence of pelvic fracture? Is there blood at the urethral meatus?
g. Maxillary-facial trauma: do not let injuries that look worse than they are detract your attention from more serious injuries.
h. Perform secondary survey.
i. Contact tertiary care facility and arrange transfer if this has not already been done.
j. Order investigations: complete blood count, electrolytes, chest x-ray, C-spine x-ray, skull x-ray, ECG, amylase, urinalysis, x-rays of abdomen, abdominal ultrasound, and any other appropriate investigations deemed necessary for the individual patient (x-rays of long bones, and so on). If computed tomography or magnetic resonance imaging facilities are available, other investigations may be ordered.
k. Treat non–life-threatening injuries when the patient has been stabilized.

The major mistakes (in order of frequency) in treating patients with trauma are as follows:
1. Inadequate airway management
2. Inadequate shock therapy
3. Inadequate C-spine immobilization
4. Failure to recognize and decompress pneumothorax
5. Distracting visually impressive but not life-threatening injuries (maxillofacial trauma, open fractures)
6. Delay in transfer to tertiary care facility
7. Failure to transfer patients to tertiary care center at all

SUGGESTED READING

Macho JR, et al: Management of the injured patient. In: Way LW, Doherty GM, eds.: *Current surgical diagnosis and treatment,* 11th ed. Lange Medical Books, 2003, New York, 230-267.
Scalea T: What's new in trauma in the past 10 years. *Int Anesthesiol Clin* 40(3):1-17, 2002.

Chapter **148**

Diabetic Ketoacidosis

> "I just hate sticking my fingers! Don't try to make me do it."

CLINICAL CASE PROBLEM 148:

A 17-Year-Old Male with Abdominal Pain

A 17-year-old male presents to the emergency room (ER) with acute abdominal pain. He describes the pain as follows: quality, dull; pain level, baseline 8/10 and ranging from 6 to 10/10; location, central abdominal with some radiation through to the back; chronology, began approximately 4 days ago and has been getting progressively worse, especially over the last 18 hours; it is constant rather than intermittent; it is aggravated by movement and relieved by rest. Associated manifestations include nausea, vomiting, and significantly increased thirst. His previous pain history includes no similar episodes. Execution of a provocative maneuver, superficial palpation to the abdomen, reproduces the pain.

On examination, he appears dehydrated. His skin and tongue are dry. His blood pressure is 140/70 mm Hg, and his pulse is 84 and regular. He is hyperventilating, and his respiratory rate is 32/minute. His abdomen is tender to touch. The tenderness is generalized. There is no rebound tenderness.

■ SELECT THE BEST ANSWER TO THE FOLLOWING QUESTIONS:

1. The laboratory tests that you should perform at this time include which of the following?
   a. complete blood count (CBC)/differential (diff)
   b. electrolytes
   c. urinalysis
   d. serum lipase
   e. serum glucose
   f. all of the above

2. Of the laboratory tests just listed, which one is likely to be abnormal to the greatest degree?
   a. CBC/diff
   b. serum potassium
   c. serum sodium
   d. serum lipase
   e. serum glucose

3. The laboratory investigations ordered produce the following results:

1) Blood pH, 7.1; lipase pending; blood sugar 450 mg/dL; CBC 17,500 with 20% bands; potassium 5.9 mEq/L; chloride 76 mEq/L; sodium 132 mEq/L; and bicarbonate 9 mEq/L.

2) Urinalysis, pH = 4.5; leukocytes (+); sugar (+); and ketones (+).

What is the most likely diagnosis at this time in this patient?

a. diabetic hyperosmolar state
b. diabetic ketoacidosis
c. acute pancreatitis
d. acute peritonitis
e. none of the above

4. At this time, what should you do?
a. rehydrate the patient in the ER with oral fluids and discharge him
b. rehydrate the patient in the ER with intravenous (IV) fluids and discharge him
c. observe the patient for 2 hours before discharge
d. admit the patient for active treatment
e. it depends on the patient's condition

5. In the condition described, which one of the following situations regarding the serum/body potassium is usually true?
a. the serum potassium is low; total body potassium is low
b. the serum potassium is elevated; total body potassium is low
c. the serum potassium is low; total body potassium is high
d. the serum potassium is low; total body potassium is high
e. neither the serum potassium nor the total body potassium usually are altered

6. Electrolyte and fluid replacement in the condition described should initially be which of the following?
a. dextrose 5% normal saline
b. hypertonic saline
c. Ringer's lactate
d. one-half normal saline
e. normal saline

7. In this condition, which of the following pathophysiologic abnormalities usually does not occur?
a. elevated serum potassium
b. depressed pH
c. elevated serum insulin level
d. elevated blood sugar
e. depressed serum bicarbonate level

8. Insulin usually is administered in this condition in a recommended dosage of approximately:

a. 0.1 units/kg IV/hour
b. 1.0 units/kg IV/hour
c. 1.5 units/kg IV/hour
d. 2.5 units/kg IV/hour
e. 0.5 units/kg IV/hour

9. In this condition, glucose usually is added to the IV solution when the serum glucose is lowered to which of the following?
a. 600 mg/dL
b. 500 mg/dL
c. 400 mg/dL
d. 250 mg/dL
e. 125 mg/dL

10. Which of the following is not characteristic of the condition described?
a. Kussmaul's respirations
b. significant dehydration
c. decreased respiratory rate
d. acetone breath
e. increased sweating

CLINICAL CASE MANAGEMENT PROBLEM

Describe the basic therapeutic methods used to treat the condition described in Clinical Case Problem 1.

■ ANSWERS:

1. **f.** This patient presented to the ER with acute abdominal pain. In addition to either an x-ray of the kidney, ureter, and bladder (KUB) or three x-ray views of the abdomen, this patient should have a complete blood chemistry workup, including at least a CBC with diff, electrolytes, serum glucose, serum amylase or serum lipase, blood urea nitrogen (BUN) and creatinine, serum calcium, serum uric acid, and arterial blood gases.

2. **e.** This patient has the signs and symptoms compatible with diabetic ketoacidosis (DKA). Although the CBC and diff, the serum electrolytes (sodium, potassium, HCO_3^-, and BUN), and the pH and the Pco_2 may be abnormal, the serum glucose value is likely to be the test that is abnormal to the greatest degree.

3. **b.** This patient most likely has DKA. DKA, in its initial presentation to the ER, often presents with abdominal pain being the major symptom. Diabetes may often be overlooked in this situation, and the patient may not be adequately evaluated. This may result in the patient being discharged without the correct diagnosis being made. Ultimately, this could be catastrophic.

4. d. This patient needs to be hospitalized now. He needs acute, active treatment in a highly monitored area, if not an intensive care unit. At the present time he has severe disturbances of his intravascular volume (he is significantly dehydrated), electrolyte balance, arterial blood gases, blood sugar, and serum insulin level.

5. b. The serum potassium in a patient with DKA is often significantly elevated. This, however, is deceptive. Although the serum potassium is usually elevated, the total body potassium is usually low and the patient needs potassium added to the IV fluids.

This is true for two basic reasons. First, there exists a general total body potassium deficit because of urinary losses; however, since the vast majority of the body's potassium is intracellular, this loss is not reflected in the extracellular compartment. Second, acidosis causes a spurious elevation in serum potassium because much of the excess extracellular hydrogen ion is exchanged by the cells for potassium—that is hydrogen ion flows into cells and potassium flows out.

6. e. The requirements of fluid resuscitation usually can be met if therapy begins with normal saline at a rate of 10-20 mL/kg/hour for the first 2 hours. Amounts at the higher end of this range are used in cases with hypotension or severe acidosis. The subsequent rate is calculated from the estimated deficit; a rate of 3-6 mL/kg/hr usually will suffice. After the first 2-4 hours, saline can be replaced by ½ normal saline (0.5 NS).

When the serum glucose approaches 250 mg/dL, 5% glucose solutions should be used to maintain glucose between 200-300 mg/dL.

7. c. The serum insulin level in DKA is depressed. The basic principles of therapy are to replace deficits of fluid, replace deficits of electrolytes, replace CHO deficits, and reverse the catabolic state with insulin.

8. a. There are many alternative methods for delivering insulin during the treatment of DKA; probably any method that delivers a dose of at least 0.1 units/kg/hour is acceptable. A constant intravenous insulin infusion offers many advantages, including simplicity of dosing, predictable insulin effect, and ease of dose adjustment. A convenient way to achieve a dose of 0.1 units/kg/hour in a constant infusion is to add 100 units of regular insulin to 100 mL of saline (1 unit per mL). This solution should be piggybacked onto replacement fluids so that each can be adjusted independently. Before the insulin infusion begins, 10-20 mL of insulin-saline mixture should be run through the tubing to saturate insulin binding on the plastic; the infusion then is begun at 0.1 mL/kg/hour.

9. d. As mentioned earlier, when the serum glucose level approaches 250 mg/dL, the fluid replacement can be changed from isotonic saline to 5% glucose solutions.

10. c. In an attempt to compensate for the metabolic acidosis, the respiratory rate in DKA is increased, not decreased. Kussmaul breathing is a rapid, deep, breathing pattern that usually is associated with metabolic acidosis.

Increased sweating and dehydration are common. Acetone breath, as a result of the production of acetone as a byproduct of the pathophysiologic process that produces DKA, is also common.

SOLUTION TO THE CLINICAL CASE MANAGEMENT PROBLEM

The basic therapeutic principles of treating the condition described are as follows:

1. Replace lost intravascular fluid volume (often several liters because of dehydration).
2. Replace lost electrolytes (potassium, magnesium, phosphate, calcium), although electrolyte panel suggests elevated potassium and sodium levels.
3. Provide insulin (beginning at 0.1 unit/kg/IV/hour).
4. Correct the metabolic acidotic state (by actions 1-3 listed here, the metabolic acidotic state usually will

be corrected). Bicarbonate administration should be considered only in patients with a blood pH less than 7.0. Studies have not shown any decrease in morbidity/mortality when bicarbonate is given to patients with different degrees of acidosis.

5. Begin IV solution with normal saline; after the first 2-4 hours, this can be changed to ½ normal saline. When the blood sugar reaches 250 mg/dl, ½ normal saline can be switched to dextrose 5% water or dextrose 5%, ½ normal saline.

SUMMARY OF DIABETIC KETOACIDOSIS

1. **Diagnosis:** DKA most frequently occurs in the patient with type 1 diabetes. Infection is a major precipitating factor. DKA can also occur in patients with type 2 diabetes and may be associated with any type of stress, such as sepsis or gastrointestinal bleeding. About 25% of all episodes of DKA occur in patients whose diabetes was previously undiagnosed. Often a young person presents to the ER with the most common complaints being polyuria, polydipsia, abdominal tenderness and rigidity, increased sweating, and in severe cases altered levels of consciousness.

   A common error in DKA is not thinking of the diagnosis because of "concentration on the abdominal pain" and a failure to associate abdominal pain with diabetes.

2. **Pathophysiology:** DKA is caused by insulin deficiency. Its development is promoted by an excess of counter-regulatory hormones, including glucagon, catecholamines, cortisol, and growth hormone; these hormones act synergistically with insulin deficiency to reduce glucose utilization, increase hepatic glucose production, and increase lipolysis and hepatic ketogenesis.

3. **Laboratory evaluation:** investigations should include the following: CBC with differential, electrolytes (potassium, magnesium, phosphate, and calcium), BUN/creatinine, bicarbonate, serum amylase or lipase, serum/plasma glucose, urinalysis, and arterial blood gases.
4. **Management:** see the Clinical Case Management Problem.
5. **Complications:**
   a. Cerebral edema: an uncommon complication but there is an increased risk in children and adolescents. It may be caused by too aggressive fluid replacement therapy. This is best prevented by maintaining blood glucose levels between 200-300 mg/dL for the initial 24 hours of therapy.
   b. Hypoxemia
   c. Hypoglycemia
   d. Hypokalemia
   e. Noncardiogenic pulmonary edema

SUGGESTED READING

Cydnlka RK, Siff J: Diabetes mellitus and disorders of glucose homeostasis. In: Marx JA, ed: *Rosen's emergency medicine: concepts and clinical practice,* 5th ed. Mosby, Inc., 2002, Philadelphia.
Umpierrez GE, Fisher JN: Diabetic ketoacidosis and the hyperosmolar, hyperglycemic state. In: Rakel RE, ed. *Conn's current therapy,* 55th ed. Elsevier, 2003, Philadelphia.

Chapter 149

Emergency Treatment of Abdominal Pain in the Elderly

"In my 80 plus years I've had many hurts, but this belly ache beats all."

CLINICAL CASE PROBLEM 1:

AN 84-YEAR-OLD MALE WITH ABDOMINAL PAIN

An 84-year-old male presents with a 6-hour history of severe abdominal pain. The pain is described as follows: quality, dull, aching; quantity severe, baseline 9/10, range 8 to 10/10; location, epigastric, radiating through to the back and flank; chronology, began suddenly after supper 6 hours ago. Aggravating factor is movement; relieving factor is rest; provocative maneuver is deep palpation to abdomen. He had no previous episodes like this; no

history of similar pain; and no previous significant history of angina pectoris. Associated manifestations are "faintness and dizziness" along with nausea.

On examination, the patient's blood pressure is 90/70 mm Hg, and his pulse is 96 and regular. His respiratory rate is 16. He is breathing normally. Examination of the abdomen reveals no distention and normal bowel sounds. There is, however, marked central abdominal tenderness to palpation.

SELECT THE BEST ANSWER TO THE FOLLOWING QUESTIONS:

1. What is the major differential diagnosis in this patient's case?
   a. ruptured aortic aneurysm
   b. intestinal ischemia or infarction
   c. perforated viscus
   d. splenic infarction
   e. all of the above

2. Given the history and physical examination findings, which of the following diagnostic possibilities is most likely?
   a. ruptured aortic aneurysm
   b. intestinal ischemia or infarction
   c. perforated viscus
   d. splenic infarction
   e. myocardial infarction

3. The diagnosis of the condition described can best be confirmed by which of the following?
   a. ultrasonography
   b. computed tomography (CT) scan of the abdomen
   c. magnetic resonance imaging (MRI) scan of the abdomen
   d. 12-lead electrocardiogram (ECG)
   e. laparotomy

4. What is the most important diagnostic clue that leads you to arrive at the diagnosis?
   a. the patient's hypotension
   b. the location of the abdominal pain
   c. hypotension with back and flank pain
   d. the periumbilical tenderness
   e. none of the above

5. What is the most critical early intervention that must take place in this patient?
   a. the placement of an endotracheal tube
   b. the establishment of intravenous (IV) access for fluid and blood replacement
   c. an abdominal paracentesis
   d. the administration of a thrombolytic agent
   e. the establishment of an arterial line

6. In which of the following conditions do pharmacotherapy and the adverse effects of same (i.e., iatrogenic disease) play the greatest role?
   a. ruptured aortic aneurysm
   b. intestinal ischemia or infarction
   c. peptic ulcer perforation
   d. splenic infarction
   e. diverticulitis

7. Which drug is most often closely associated with peptic ulcer perforation?
   a. ibuprofen
   b. piroxicam
   c. naproxen
   d. aspirin
   e. sulindac

8. What is the treatment of choice for the patient described in the problem?

   a. monitoring in the intensive care unit, thrombolytic therapy, aspirin, beta blockers, and antiarrhythmic therapy
   b. laparotomy—oversew perforation
   c. laparotomy—removal of ischemic bowel
   d. laparotomy—surgical repair of aortic aneurysm
   e. laparotomy and splenectomy

9. Which of the following statements is (are) true regarding ruptured aortic aneurysm?
   a. more than 80% of abdominal aortic aneurysms are asymptomatic when first diagnosed
   b. the diagnosis is often missed because physicians do not consider it
   c. most abdominal aortic aneurysms are atherosclerotic in nature
   d. all of the above are true
   e. none of the above are true

10. What is the key to reducing morbidity and mortality in the condition described?
    a. enhanced tertiary prevention
    b. enhanced secondary prevention
    c. regular yearly checkups
    d. early diagnosis and intervention
    e. early administration of thrombolytic agents

CLINICAL CASE MANAGEMENT PROBLEM

Provide the differential for acute abdominal pain in the elderly as an ER presentation.

ANSWERS:

1. **e.** The differential diagnosis of abdominal pain in the elderly is extensive. In this case the sudden onset of the pain and the severity of the pain strongly suggest an acute abdomen. At the top of the list would be ruptured aortic aneurysm, perforated viscus, intestinal ischemia or infarction, a perforated diverticulum, and pancreatitis.

2. **a.** Given the history and physical findings, the most likely diagnosis is ruptured aortic aneurysm. The clue to ruptured aortic aneurysm in this case is the hypotension and location of pain. The signs and symptoms suggest at least a leaking aneurysm.

3. **b.** The working diagnosis can best be confirmed by the performance of a CT scan of the abdomen. Ultrasound and CT are both close to 100% accurate in diagnosing an abdominal aortic aneurysm. The CT scan is subject to less technical and interpretation errors than an ultrasound. The CT scan also better detects retroperitoneal hemorrhage associated with an aneurysm rupture.

4. c. See Answer 2.

5. b. Remember the ABCs. Because this patient is breathing normally, the next most important step is circulation. You should immediately place either a central venous pressure line or two large bore IV lines (two lines of at least #16 gauge).

6. c. See Answer 7.

7. d. Iatrogenic disease (in the form of a nonsteroidal antiinflammatory drug [NSAID] prescription) is closely associated with perforated peptic ulcer. Many thousands of Americans die each year from perforated and bleeding peptic ulcers caused by the prescription of NSAIDs.

The NSAID that causes more peptic ulcers and is associated with more perforated peptic ulcers than any other agent (on a prevalence/administration rate basis) is acetylsalicylic acid (aspirin). The risk appears to be dose related.

8. d. The treatment of choice in this patient is removal of the segment of the aorta affected by the aneurysm and replacement with a graft.

9. d. More than 80% of aortic aneurysms are asymptomatic when first diagnosed. The diagnosis often is missed because the possibility is not considered.

Most aortic aneurysms are atherosclerotic in nature and result from a generalized atherosclerotic process.

10. d. The key to reducing morbidity and mortality from aortic aneurysm is early diagnosis and intervention. Although routine screening for aortic aneurysms in the elderly is not recommended by the United States Preventive Services Task Force on the Periodic Health Examination, it is wise to consider this on a risk-factor basis in the patients you see. High-risk patients and patients with symptoms that even vaguely suggest aortic aneurysm probably should be evaluated by both physical examination and ultrasound.

SOLUTION TO THE CLINICAL CASE MANAGEMENT PROBLEM

The following is a differential diagnosis of abdominal pain in the elderly as an ER presentation.
1. Nonabdominal-related causes: (a) myocardial infarction; (b) pneumonia; and (c) pericarditis.
2. Abdominal-related causes: (a) constipation (major cause); (b) diverticulitis; (c) cholecystitis/cholelithiasis; (d) peptic ulcer disease/gastritis; (e) pancreatitis; (f) appendicitis; (g) bowel obstruction (large bowel, small bowel); (h) inflammatory bowel disease; (i) carcinoma (stomach, pancreas, colon); (j) ruptured aortic aneurysm; (k) intestinal ischemia or infarction; and (l) urinary tract sepsis.

SUMMARY OF EMERGENCY TREATMENT OF ABDOMINAL PAIN IN THE ELDERLY

1. **Diagnosis:**
   a. Life-threatening causes of abdominal pain may present with few findings in the elderly.
   b. The elderly are less likely to have rebound or guarding because of decreased abdominal musculature.
   c. In general, compared to younger patients, abdominal pain in the elderly often has a vague presentation and higher rates of serious disease.
   d. Constipation is the single most common cause of abdominal pain in the elderly.
   e. When elderly patients present to the ER with sudden onset of abdominal pain, think of the following: (i) nonabdominal causes: myocardial infarction; (ii) abdominal causes: see Solution to Clinical Case Management Problem.

2. **Investigations:** basic investigations in an elderly patient with abdominal pain: CBC; electrolytes; amylase; lipase; liver function tests; ECG; kidney, ureter, and bladder x-ray (KUB); urinalysis; ultrasonography; and CT scan
3. **Treatment:**
   a. Treat the cause.
   b. Remember ABCs in acutely ill elderly patients.
   c. Remember that elderly patients present quite differently from younger patients—they often lack the classic signs and symptoms of any acute abdominal condition.
   d. A major error in acutely ill elderly patients seen in community or rural hospitals is the failure to transfer to a tertiary care center soon enough.

SUGGESTED READING

Birnbaumer DM: The elder patient. In: Marx JA, et al, eds.: *Rosen's emergency medicine,* 5th ed. Mosby, 2002, St. Louis.
McQuaid KR: Alimentary tract. In: Tierney LM, et al, eds.: *Current medical diagnosis and treatment.* Lange Medical Books, 2003, New York.

Chapter 150

Acute and Chronic Poisoning

> "It was an accident. I didn't go to sleep after taking one pill, so I took 10."

CLINICAL CASE PROBLEM 1:
A 24-Year-Old Female Brought In with a Suspected Drug Overdose

A 24-year-old female is brought into the emergency room (ER) of your local hospital with a suspected drug overdose. She was found by a friend, unconscious beside her bed, with a number of unmarked pill containers beside her. Her friend does not know any other details. Her friend is hysterical and has to be restrained. You are called by the intern, who is on his first day of service. He asks you, "What should I do now?"

You come down immediately and examine the patient. The patient has a Glasgow coma scale score of 7.

The vital signs are as follows: blood pressure, 90/70 mm Hg; pulse, 84 and regular; and respirations, 16 and regular. No other abnormalities are evident. Her pupils are equal and reactive to light and accommodation.

▶ SELECT THE BEST ANSWER TO THE FOLLOWING QUESTIONS:

1. What is the first step in the management of the victim of a potential drug overdose?
   a. administration of syrup of ipecac
   b. administration of naloxone
   c. administration of dextrose 5% water
   d. administration of activated charcoal
   e. none of the above

2. Accidental poisonings make up what percentage of total poisoning episodes in children and adults?
   a. 20%
   b. 40%
   c. 60%
   d. 70%
   e. 85%

3. The majority of drug-related suicide attempts involve which of the following?
   a. central nervous system stimulants
   b. central nervous system depressants
   c. amphetamines
   d. over-the-counter analgesics
   e. none of the above

4. What is the most common cause of death in patients with a drug overdose outside the hospital?
   a. lower airway obstruction
   b. upper airway obstruction
   c. cardiac arrest
   d. ventricular fibrillation
   e. complete heart block

5. Which of the following conditions resulting in coma or altered level of consciousness can be treated quickly if recognized immediately?
   a. hypoxia
   b. hypoglycemia
   c. opioid overdose
   d. b and c
   e. a, b, and c

6. After the ABC's of life support, which of the following is indicated in the initial assessment of the patient with possible overdose?
   a. a history from anyone who has knowledge of the patient
   b. physical examination with particular attention to vital signs and neurologic status
   c. serum electrolytes
   d. acetaminophen plasma concentration
   e. all of the above

7. The anion gap is defined as which of the following?
   a. anion gap=$[K^+ + Cl^-] - [Na^+ + HCO_3^-]$
   b. anion gap=$[Na^+] - [Cl^- + HCO_3]$
   c. anion gap=$[Cl^-] + [Na^+ + K^+] - [HCO_3^-]$
   d. anion gap=$[pH] + [Na^+ + Cl^-]$
   e. anion gap=$[HCO_3^-] - [Cl^- + Na^+]$

8. Which of the following is (are) associated with an increased anion gap?
   a. salicylates
   b. methanol
   c. ethylene glycol
   d. organic solvents
   e. all of the above

9. Following the assessment and maintenance of vital functions, which of the following is (are) the next step(s)?
   a. antidote administration (if poison known)
   b. prevention of absorption
   c. reduction of local damage
   d. b and c
   e. a, b, and c

10. Which of the following gastrointestinal decontamination procedures should be performed routinely in all poisonings?
    a. syrup of ipecac
    b. gastric lavage
    c. activated charcoal
    d. dilution of poison with intravenous fluids
    e. none of the above

11. What is the specific antidote for the treatment of acetaminophen poisoning?
    a. N-acetyl coenzyme A
    b. N-acetyl ATPase
    c. N-acetylcysteine
    d. calcium disodium etidronate
    e. atropine

12. What is the specific antidote for the treatment of benzodiazepine poisoning?
    a. Antabuse
    b. naloxone
    c. carbamazepine
    d. flumazenil
    e. naltrexone

13. What is the specific antidote for the treatment of methanol or ethylene glycol poisoning?
    a. Antabuse
    b. naloxone
    c. fomepizole
    d. flumazenil
    e. naltrexone

14. What is the specific antidote for the treatment of opioid intoxication (poisoning)?
    a. Antabuse
    b. naloxone
    c. carbamazepine
    d. flumazenil
    e. naltrexone

15. What is the specific antidote for the treatment of organophosphate poisoning?
    a. ethanol
    b. naloxone
    c. naltrexone
    d. atropine
    e. arginine

ANSWERS:

1. **e.** The first step in the management of the potential overdose victim is the assessment and support of the ABCs (airway, breathing, circulation) of life support. Before any medications are administered, a secure airway must be established, respiratory and circulatory system function should be assessed and supported, and intravenous and/or central venous lines should be inserted.

2. **e.** The severity of the manifestations of acute poisoning exposures varies greatly with the age and intent of the victims. Accidental poisoning exposures make up 80% to 85% of all poisoning episodes and are most frequent in children younger than age 5 years. Intentional poisonings constitute 15% to 20% of all poisonings, and often these patients require more intensive therapy. Suicide attempts represent a significant number of these poisonings, and the use of toxic substances often is involved.

3. **b.** The majority of drug-related suicide attempts involve a central nervous system depressant.

4. **b.** The most common cause of death in patients with drug overdose outside the hospital is upper airway obstruction. Any patient who is comatose and has absent protective airway reflexes is able to tolerate an endotracheal tube and should have one inserted immediately.

5. **e.** The second step in the management of the victim of a potential overdose is the treatment of specific conditions with specific antidotes. Because it is almost impossible to differentiate one overdose from another at this time, give the following: (1) naloxone (antidote for opioid intoxication); (2) thiamine (antidote for Wernicke's encephalopathy); (3) glucose (antidote for hypoglycemia, secondary to insulin overdose); (4) oxygen; and (5) antidotes if toxins identified.

6. **e.** All of the above. Remember that the initial assessment of all patients follows the principles of basic and advanced cardiac life support.

A physical examination with emphasis on vital signs (and particular attention to pupil size and reaction to light and accommodation), temperature, and a complete neurologic examination should be done.

Although the patient often will not be able to supply accurate (if any) information, as much information as possible should be obtained from the family, friends, the patient's physician, or anyone else that knows the patient.

Laboratory testing should include the following: serum electrolytes (and measurement of anion gap), arterial blood gases, blood glucose, renal and liver tests, acetaminophen plasma concentration, and a 12-lead electrocardiogram (ECG). Radiography of the chest and abdomen also may be useful.

7. **b.** See Answer 8.

8. e. The term anion gap was developed to indicate the difference between the measured sodium level and the measured chloride and bicarbonate level (really the CO_2 content). This is very important, especially in diabetic ketoacidosis and toxic acidic chemicals. The definition is: anion gap = $[Na^+] - [Cl^- + HCO_3^-]$.

The causes of an increased anion gap are as follows: (1) an accumulation of organic acids, such as that seen in lactic acidosis; (2) an accumulation of organic acids, such as that seen in diabetic ketoacidosis; (3) an accumulation of organic acids, such as that seen in acute renal failure and toxic ingestions; (4) exogenous anions; (5) reduced inorganic acid excretion, such as seen in chronic renal failure; (6) an increase in the anionic contribution of unmeasured weak acids; and (8) a decrease in unmeasured cations. Hyponatremia will cause a decreased anion gap.

The etiology of metabolic acidosis is dependent on the determination of the presence or absence of a normal anion gap. The normal anion gap is 8 to 12. An increased anion gap usually can be traced to one of the following: (1) toxic amounts of salicylates; (2) any amount of methanol; (3) any amount of ethylene glycol; (4) an overdose of iron (as in ferrous sulfate); (5) any amount of paraldehyde; (6) an overdose of phenformin; (7) an overdose of isoniazid; and (8) certain organic solvents such as toluene.

9. e. See Answer 10.

10. e. The prevention of absorption and the reduction of local damage are important in the treatment of poison ingestions.

Reduction of local damage applies primarily to the eye (with a caustic acid or a caustic base) and the skin (with a significant burn).

The prevention of absorption is best accomplished by gastrointestinal decontamination. No procedure for gastrointestinal decontamination is routine. Decisions need to be individualized for each case. Syrup of ipecac has a very limited role in the management of poison ingestions. The risk of use outweighs the benefits. Gastric lavage is considered only when it can be performed within 1 hour of ingestion and only if there are no known contraindications to its use. Gastric lavage is contraindicated, for example, in the ingestion of caustic substances or if there are uncontrolled convulsions or significant cardiac dysrhythmias. Recent guidelines from the American Academy of Clinical Toxicology suggest that activated charcoal should not be given routinely in all cases of toxic ingestion. However, in general, activated charcoal is the gastrointestinal decontamination procedure of choice.

11. c. N-acetylcysteine is the specific antidote that should be administered in cases of acetaminophen poisoning. It is given orally. The intravenous route is still investigational.

12. d. Flumazenil binds competitively and reversibly to the gamma-aminobutyric acid (GABA)-benzodiazepine receptor complex and inhibits the effects of benzodiazepine. The drug is approved for the treatment of benzodiazepine overdose and/or for the reversal of benzodiazepine oversedation.

13. c. Ethanol and fomepizole are antidotes for methanol or ethylene glycol poisoning. Both of these poisons are oxidized by alcohol dehydrogenase (ADH) before becoming converted to toxic products. Ethanol act as a competitive inhibitor because it has a greater affinity for ADH than either poison; fomepizole acts by directly inhibiting ADH.

14. b. The antidote for opioid overdose is naloxone.

15. d. The specific antidote for organophosphate and carbamate (pesticides) poisoning is atropine.

SUMMARY OF ACUTE AND CHRONIC POISONING

A. Assessment and maintenance of vital functions:
  1. The ABCs of resuscitation:
     A = Airway management (endotracheal tube in unconscious patient)
     B = Breathing (assisted ventilation if the respiratory rate and depth are inadequate)
     C = Circulation (assessed by blood pressure, heart rate, and heart rhythm); volume expansion may be indicated if there is hypotension or other measurements of decreased cardiac function; Ringer's lactate or normal saline is preferred for hypovolemia; plasma expanders and vasopressors are indicated if intravenous fluids are not sufficient.
  2. History/physical examination/laboratory investigations:
     a. History: attempt to elicit history from any family member or friend who happens to be there. Attempt to search for empty pill containers.
     b. Physical examination: pay particular attention to vital signs and neurologic examination with emphasis on the Glasgow coma scale.

c. Laboratory investigations:
  i. 12-lead ECG
  ii. electrolytes, blood urea nitrogen, creatinine, glucose, left-ventricular tachycardias, arterial blood gases, acetaminophen plasma concentration
  iii. radiographs of chest and abdomen may be useful
3. Calculate the anion gap = $(Na^+) - (Cl^- + HCO_3^-)$. Remember that the normal anion gap is 8 to 12.

B. Treatment:
1. Immediate treatment to all victims: (a) ABCs (may include endotracheal tube, intravenous fluids); (b) naloxone; (c) thiamine; (d) glucose; (e) supplemental oxygen; and (f) antidotes
2. Decontamination: Decision making for procedure of choice is different in each case. Gastric emptying procedures using syrup of ipecac or gastric lavage are used infrequently. Gastric lavage may have some benefit if performed within 1 hour of ingestion and there are no contraindications. Activated charcoal is the gastrointestinal gastrodecontaminating agent of choice. However, it should not be given routinely in all cases.
3. Enhancement of elimination (used sometimes in life-threatening circumstances): (a) dialysis, hemodialysis; (b) hemoperfusion; (c) exchange transfusion; and (d) plasmapheresis

4. Specific antidotes:
  a. Substance : acetaminophen
     Antidote : N-acetylcysteine
  b. Substance : opioid analgesics
     Antidote : naloxone
  c. Substance : methanol or ethylene glycol
     Antidote : ethanol
  d. Substance : benzodiazepines
     Antidote : flumazenil
  e. Substance : organophosphates
     Antidote : atropine

C. Common drug overdoses:
1. Over-the-counter analgesics (acetaminophen is number one)
2. Prescribed hypnotics–sedatives
3. Prescribed benzodiazepines

D. Prevention of complications: anticipate and treat complications such as seizures, coma, hypotension, and hyperthermia.

SUGGESTED READING

Kulig K: General approach to the poisoned patient. In: Marx JA, et al, eds.: *Rosen's emergency medicine,* 5th ed. Mosby, 2002, St. Louis.

Mofenson HC, et al: Medical toxicology: ingestions, inhalations, and dermal and ocular absorptions. In: Rakel R, Bope ET, eds.: *Conn's current therapy.* WB Saunders, 2003, Philadelphia.

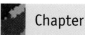

Chapter **151**

Urticaria and Angioneurotic Edema

"You mean my nephew may die because I fed him a peanut butter sandwich?"

CLINICAL CASE PROBLEM 1:

A 24-Year-Old Male Who Developed a "Skin Rash" While Playing Football

A 24-year-old male was playing football with his friends on a hot summer afternoon. Approximately 10 minutes into the game, he began to "feel funny," and he began to itch all over. He sat down, but the itch did not go away; it only got worse. Within 10 minutes he was covered with a "raised" rash all over his body, with individual lesions varying from 2 cm to 5 cm in diameter. His lips also became very swollen, and he began to have trouble breathing.

His friend called 911, and he was brought to the local hospital, located only 3 minutes from the football field. The friend who works with the patient tells you that "he is certain that the problem has arisen because of stress"; the patient apparently had a very bad day at work today.

On examination, his respiratory rate is 42/minute and he is gasping. His lips are swollen, and he has a very prominent, raised skin rash with lesions of various sizes covering his entire body. His blood pressure is 75/50 mm Hg.

SELECT THE BEST ANSWER TO THE FOLLOWING QUESTIONS:

1. At this time, what is your first priority?
   a. give the patient PO (oral) steroids
   b. give the patient IV (intravenous) steroids
   c. give the patient IV diphenhydramine
   d. give the patient PO diphenhydramine
   e. none of the above

2. What is the most likely diagnosis in this patient?
   a. chronic urticaria with angioedema
   b. exercise-induced bronchospasm
   c. exercise-induced anaphylaxis and urticaria
   d. urticarial vasculitis
   e. stress-induced urticaria with esterase inhibitor deficiency

3. What is the first priority in this patient?
   a. establish a large-gauge IV line
   b. establish a central venous pressure (CVP) line if possible; if not possible, establish two large IV lines
   c. intubate the patient
   d. administer 100% oxygen to the patient by nasal specs
   e. draw blood gases

4. What is the second priority in the management of this patient?
   a. auscultate both lung fields
   b. forget this "tube and airway" business—get with the IV lines and get with them now!
   c. draw blood gases
   d. perform a chest x-ray to check the position of the endotracheal tube
   e. administer 100% oxygen

5. What is the third priority in the management of this patient?
   a. draw blood gases
   b. draw serum electrolytes
   c. put in two large peripheral IV lines
   d. put medical anti-shock trousers (MAST) on the patient
   e. administer "pretty much every pressor agent you can think of"

6. Which of the following also is indicated in the management of this patient?
   a. administer isotonic fluids
   b. administer epinephrine intravenously, subcutaneously (SQ), or intramuscularly (IM)
   c. administer Solumedrol intravenously
   d. administer vasopressor agents if blood pressure does not rise with the measures outlined in a, b, and c
   e. a, b, c, and d

7. With respect to exercise in the future, what should your advice be to this patient?
   a. take an antihistamine before exercise
   b. carry an epinephrine kit during exercise at all times
   c. do not exercise within 4 hours after eating
   d. do not exercise alone
   e. all of the above

CLINICAL CASE PROBLEM 2:
A 38-YEAR-OLD FEMALE WITH A RAISED, ITCHY RASH

A 38-year-old women comes to your office with a raised, itchy rash over her entire body that has been present for 9 weeks. She cannot remember any unusual exposures and has not traveled outside the country. She has had a few episodes of lip and tongue swelling. On examination there are diffuse, erythematous wheals that measure up to 3 inches in diameter.

8. What is the most likely diagnosis in this patient?
   a. chronic urticaria and angioedema
   b. dermatographism
   c. cholinergic urticaria
   d. cold urticaria
   e. solar urticaria

9. Angioedema is most likely to occur in which of the following situations?
   a. allergy to peanuts
   b. allergy to chocolate
   c. allergy to milk
   d. allergy to red wine
   e. allergy to monosodium glutamate

10. What is the most common drug to cause urticaria and angioedema?
    a. acetaminophen
    b. sulfonamide antibiotic
    c. ampicillin antibiotic
    d. aspirin
    e. Naprosyn

11. Which of the following form part of an allergic triad?
    a. nasal polyps
    b. asthma
    c. aspirin sensitivity
    d. all of the above
    e. none of the above

■ **ANSWERS:**

1. **e.** The first priority is to go through the ABCs of cardiopulmonary resuscitation as follows. Priority 1: establish an airway. This patient, from the history given, is very close to having his airway completely obstructed. The placement of a properly sized endotracheal tube is the first priority. Priority 2: establish proper ventilation. Make sure that the endotracheal tube is in the trachea and not in the esophagus, and

establish that there is bilateral airflow through auscultation of both lung fields. Priority 3: establish circulation. Establish access with two large-bore IVs. Start isotonic fluids (Ringer's lactate or normal saline).

2. **c.** The diagnosis in this case is exercise-induced anaphylaxis and urticaria. Certain foods and medication can coprecipitate an episode of exercise-induced anaphylaxis.

3. **c.** As described in Answer 1, the first priority is to insert a properly sized endotracheal tube.

4. **a.** Again to emphasize the ABCs as described in Answer 1, the second priority is to auscultate both lung fields to make sure they are clear.

5. **c.** The C in the ABCs is circulation, so put in two large peripheral IV lines.

6. **e.** Treatment also should include the following: subcutaneous epinephrine 0.2-1.0 mg (for patients with severe respiratory symptoms and/or low blood pressure [<70 mm Hg], epinephrine should be given intravenously), intravenous corticosteroids. Pressor agents (such as dopamine or dobutamine) may be administered as necessary if the blood pressure does not rise after giving fluids, epinephrin, and corticosteroids.

7. **e.** This patient should be careful in participating in any sports that will bring on physical urticaria; whether he decides to abstain is a personal risk/benefit decision. However, if he is going to begin exercise again he should (1) begin with a short period of exercise only (the more intense the exercise, the more likely symptoms will occur); (2) take an antihistamine before exercise; (3) carry an epinephrine kit during exercise at all times; (4) not exercise alone; and, (5) not eat anything for at least 4 hours before exercise.

8. **a.** The condition of chronic urticaria is characterized by hives that occur on a regular basis for more than 6 weeks. In about 40% of patients with chronic urticaria, angioedema will also be present. Hives associated with chronic urticaria last for 4-36 hours. Hives associated with dermatographism and physical urticaria last 30 minutes to 2 hours. In some cases, chronic urticaria and angioedema can be associated with Hashimoto's disease. An association with Graves' disease is less common.

9. **a.** Angioedema is life threatening. It occurs most commonly in association with food allergy. The two most common foods implicated in angioneurotic edema are nuts (of all kinds) and fish and shellfish.

In the case of the latter, even the odor of the cooking of the fish or shellfish may be enough to set off a life-threatening reaction.

10. **d.** The most common drug causing angioedema is aspirin.

11. **d.** Many of the patients who develop aspirin anaphylaxis have the following allergic triad: (1) aspirin sensitivity; (2) asthma; and (3) nasal polyps. Any individual who has developed a significant allergic reaction or angioedema to aspirin should never take another nonsteroidal antiinflammatory drug (NSAID). There is a very high cross-reactivity.

SUMMARY OF URTICARIA AND ANGIONEUROTIC EDEMA

A. Classification of urticaria
1. Ordinary urticaria: (a) acute (up to 6 weeks of continuous activity); (b) chronic (6 weeks or more of continuous activity); and (c) episodic (intermittent)
2. Physical urticaria (induced by a physical stimulus): (a) cholinergic urticaria; (b) cold urticaria; (c) dermatographism; (d) localized heat urticaria; and (e) solar urticaria
3. Contact urticaria (caused by biologic or chemical skin contact)
4. Urticarial vasculitis (skin biopsy reveals vasculitis)

B. Difference between urticaria and angioedema:
1. Urticaria ("hives"): result of capillary vasodilation followed by plasma leakage into the superficial dermis
2. Angioedema: plasma leakage in the deeper layers of the skin and subcutaneous tissues; Results in formation of thick, firm plaques

C. Pathophysiology of exercise-induced anaphylaxis and cholinergic urticaria: likely a result of vasoactive mediators released by mast cells. Plasma histamine, tryptase, and leukotriene levels are increased.

D. Skin lesion characteristics are as follows: (1) usually total body; (2) lesions begin as "small wheals" and eventually coalesce; and (3) lesions are very pruritic and erythematous

E. Treatment of angioedema: (1) airway management (intubate if necessary); (2) 100% oxygen; (3) epinephrine; (4) antihistamine; (5) corticosteroid; (6) isotonic fluids (Ringer's lactate, normal saline); and (7) vasopressor agents if hypotension is not corrected.

Continued

SUMMARY OF URTICARIA AND ANGIONEUROTIC EDEMA—cont'd

F. Treatment of exercise-induced anaphylaxis and urticaria: (1) modification of activities; (2) exercise with a partner; (3) do not exercise within 4 hours of eating; (4) do not take aspirin or NSAIDs before exercising; (5) administer subcutaneous epinephrine at first sign of symptoms; and (6) take an antihistamine prior to exercise (cromolyn or leukotriene modifying agents may be effective).

G. Treatment of chronic urticaria and angio-edema: medications used are (a) antihistamines; (b) H$_2$ blockers (i.e., cimetidine); (c) leukotriene modifying agents; and (d) corticosteroids (avoid prolonged use)

SUGGESTED READING

Grattan C, et al: Management and diagnostic guidelines for urticaria and angioedema. *Br J Dermatol* 144(4):708-714, 2001.

Hosey RG, et al: Exercise-induced anaphylaxis and urticaria. *Am Fam Physician* 64:1367-1374, 2001.

Kaplan AP: Chronic urticaria and angioedema. *N Engl J Med* 346(3): 175-179, 2002.

Chapter 152

Fracture Management

> "You mean I am supposed to wear that heavy, ugly cast for 6 weeks?"

CLINICAL CASE PROBLEM 1:

A 75-Year-Old Female Who Slipped and Fell on Her Outstretched Hand

A 75-year-old female is brought to the emergency room (ER) after having fallen on her outstretched hand. She complains of pain in the area of the right wrist.

On examination, there is a deformity in the area of the right wrist. The wrist has the appearance of a dinner fork. There is significant tenderness over the distal radius. Both pulses and sensation distally to the injury are completely normal.

■ SELECT THE BEST ANSWER TO THE FOLLOWING QUESTIONS:

1. What is the most likely diagnosis in this patient?
   a. fracture of the distal ulna with dislocation of the radial head
   b. fracture of the carpal scaphoid
   c. fracture of the carpal lumate
   d. Colles' fracture
   e. fracture of the shaft of the radius with dislocation of the ulnar head

2. What is the treatment of choice for the patient described?
   a. internal reduction and immobilization
   b. internal reduction and fixation
   c. external reduction and immobilization
   d. external reduction and fixation
   e. none of the above

CLINICAL CASE PROBLEM 2:

The Team's Top Scorer Fell and Hurt His Hand

An 18-year-old basketball player is brought to the ER after having fallen on his outstretched hand. He is the league's leading scorer, and his coach directs you to "fix it and fix it fast."

On examination, there is slight tenderness and swelling just distal to the radius, in the "snuffbox." No other abnormalities are found. X-ray examination of the wrist and hand are normal.

3. What is the most likely diagnosis in this patient?
   a. second-degree wrist sprain
   b. avulsion fracture of the distal radius
   c. fractured scaphoid
   d. fractured triquetrum
   e. none of the above

4. What is the treatment of choice for the patient described in Clinical Case Problem 2?
   a. active physiotherapy
   b. passive physiotherapy
   c. nonsteroidal antiinflammatory drugs
   d. surgical exploration of the wrist
   e. none of the above

5. What is the major complication of the injury described in Clinical Case Problem 2?
   a. peripheral nerve injury
   b. local muscle damage
   c. peripheral arterial injury
   d. avascular necrosis of the bone
   e. septic arthritis of the joint

CLINICAL CASE PROBLEM 3:

A 25-Year-Old Male with Pain in His Ankle

A 25-year-old male is brought to the ER after having been thrown from his motorcycle. He complains of severe pain in the area of the right ankle and is unable to bear weight on the foot.

On examination, there is swelling of the entire right ankle, with more prominent swelling on the lateral side. There is point tenderness over the lateral malleolus. There does not appear to be any other deformity or abnormality.

6. What is the most likely diagnosis in this patient?
   a. second-degree ankle sprain
   b. third-degree ankle sprain
   c. fractured distal tibia
   d. fractured distal fibula
   e. fractured talus

7. What is the treatment of choice for the patient described in Clinical Case Problem 3?
   a. internal reduction and fixation
   b. external reduction and fixation
   c. active physiotherapy
   d. ice, compression, and elevation
   e. immobilization of the ankle

8. Which of the following statements regarding acute compartment syndrome is (are) true?
   a. acute compartment syndrome is caused by increasing pressure within a closed fascial space as a result of effects of the injury
   b. acute compartment syndrome is found primarily in the lower leg and the forearm
   c. acute compartment syndrome may lead to muscle and nerve ischemia
   d. acute compartment syndrome may lead to muscle and nerve death
   e. all of the above

9. The emergency treatment of orthopedic injuries includes which of the following?
   a. assessment of all injuries, many of which are multiple
   b. assessment of vascular and neurologic injury in the involved region
   c. correction of deformities
   d. splinting or immobilization of all injured areas
   e. all of the above

10. Which of the following is/are part of the Ottawa Ankle Rules for determining the need for x-rays when evaluating ankle injuries?
    a. bone tenderness at the distal lateral malleolus
    b. bone tenderness at the distal medial malleolus

c. inability to bear weight both immediately at time of injury and at time of assessment
d. patient is age 18 years or older
e. all of the above

► ANSWERS:

1. d. This patient has a Colles' fracture, a fracture of the distal radius. It occurs most commonly in elderly patients, especially women, after falling onto an outstretched hand. It is most often associated with osteoporosis. The typical displacement is reflected in a characteristic appearance that has been termed the dinner-fork deformity. The clinical history and deformity are not compatible with any of the other choices listed.

2. c. The treatment of choice for the patient described in the question is external reduction under a regional block or a local hematoma block, followed by immobilization in a splint or bivalve cast. Because of the age of the patient, the cast probably will have to remain for 6 weeks to ensure complete healing.

3. c. This young man most likely has a fractured scaphoid bone. This is an injury that is significantly more common in younger adults. The most common cause of a scaphoid fracture is a fall on an outstretched hand.

Fracture of the scaphoid bone should be suspected if there is tenderness in the "anatomical snuff box" and at the scaphoid tubercle. Radiographs may be negative initially. If a fracture is suspected, despite negative x-rays, the region should be immobilized in a thumb spica cast. After 2 weeks reevaluate the injured area and repeat x-rays. If there is a fracture of the scaphoid, x-rays will be positive at 2 weeks (a bone scan will be positive within 72 hours of a scaphoid fracture). A nondisplaced fracture of the scaphoid requires 8-12 weeks of cast immobilization.

4. e. See Answer 5.

5. d. Failure to properly treat a scaphoid fracture likely will lead to complications. The major complication is avascular necrosis.

6. d. The history of trauma, the symptoms elicited, and the signs present suggest a fracture of the lateral malleolus. Although the physical findings of a major (second- or third-degree) ankle sprain may be somewhat similar, the injury (being thrown from a motorcycle) and his inability to bear weight is definitely more suggestive of a fracture injury than a sprain injury.

7. **e.** The treatment of choice for the patient described in Clinical Case Problem 3 is immobilization. Initially it should be in a posterior splint, and then, after swelling adequately diminished, a walking cast or boot is to be applied for 4-6 weeks. Weightbearing is allowed as tolerated by patient. In the absence of significant deformity and confirmation on x-ray of a nondisplaced fracture to the lateral malleolus, no other treatment is indicated. An x-ray should be repeated in 1-2 weeks after the injury to check for any displacement of the fracture.

8. **e.** Acute compartment syndromes are caused by increasing tissue pressure in a closed fascial space. The fascial compartments of the leg and forearm are most frequently involved. Acute compartment syndromes are usually the result of a fracture with subsequent hemorrhage, limb compression, or a crushing injury. In an acute compartment syndrome, fluid pressure is increased. This leads to muscle and tissue ischemia. Severe ischemia for a period of 6-8 hours results in subsequent muscle and nerve death.

Physical examination reveals swelling and definitive palpable tenseness over the muscle compartment. The signs on physical examination include paresis in the involved area and a sensory deficit over the involved area. Acute compartment syndrome should be treated with immediate fasciotomy.

9. **e.** In treating orthopedic injuries in a patient who has been involved in a traumatic event, it is very important to remember that these injuries must be seen and treated within the overall context of the patient's condition. Thus the ABCs of resuscitation, which are discussed in other chapters in this book, must take first priority. Associated cardiac dysrhythmias must be treated according to basic cardiac life support (BLS) and advanced cardiac life support (ACLS) protocols. Traumatic injuries must be treated according to basic trauma life support (BTLS) and advanced trauma life support (ATLS) protocols.

First, the trauma patient must be suspected of having multiple injuries rather than a single injury. Cervical spine injuries should be assumed to be present until they have been excluded. Primary and secondary surveys must be performed as per ATLS protocol.

Second, with any injured extremity, arterial injury must be suspected and pulses must be assessed quickly. Acute compartment syndromes must be ruled out.

Third, deformities should be corrected as soon as possible under local (hematoma block), regional, or general anesthesia. Ideally, the injured limb(s) should be splinted before the patient arrives in the ER. Open fractures and surrounding tissue must be thoroughly debrided and cleaned as quickly as possible.

Fourth, after stabilization is complete, tetanus prophylaxis should be given and antibiotics active against coagulase positive staphylococcus must be started.

10. **e.** The Ottawa Ankle Rules are guidelines to determine the need for ankle radiographs in patients who have sustained an ankle injury. If there is boney tenderness on the tip or posterior aspect of the lateral or medial malleolus, or an inability to bear weight both immediately at time of injury and at time of assessment, x-rays should be obtained. The Ottawa Ankle Rules do not apply to patients younger than age 18 years. It is important to also use clinical judgment when deciding when to obtain x-rays.

SUMMARY OF FRACTURE MANAGEMENT

A. Fall on an outstretched hand:
   1. Elderly: possible Colles' fracture
   2. Young adult: possible scaphoid fracture

B. Colles' fracture
   1. Fracture of distal metaphysis of radius, which is dorsally displaced and angulated
   2. "Dinner fork" deformity: requires immediate reduction (closed reduction usually adequate) and immobilization

C. Scaphoid fracture: tenderness in "snuff box":
   1. Radiographs may take more than 2 weeks to reveal fracture
   2. If scaphoid fracture is suspected, must immobilize even if initial x-rays are negative
   3. Bone scan or magnetic resonance imaging studies will show scaphoid fractures earlier than x-rays
   4. Must immobilize for period of 8-12 weeks; some scaphoid fractures require internal fixation
   5. Possible complications: avascular necrosis and nonunion of fracture

D. Nondisplaced lateral ankle fracture
   1. Immobilize in posterior splint until swelling adequately diminished, then place in short leg cast or walking cast boot for 4 to 6 weeks
   2. Advance weightbearing as tolerated

E. The basics of fracture management and other orthopedic and trauma injuries are as follows:
   1. Remember the ABCs of resuscitation.
   2. Suspect and search for multiple injuries.
   3. Suspect and prevent potential spine injuries. Immobilize cervical spine in trauma patients.

4. Rule out arterial injury in the affected limb.
5. Rule out a compartment syndrome.
6. Recognize and treat open fractures with copious irrigation, débridement, and initiation of IV antibiotics.
7. Correct deformities whenever possible.
8. Splint each injured area.
9. If there is significant swelling in a limb, consider either a bivalve cast or splint until swelling has decreased significantly. A full cast can lead to complications such as compartment

syndrome if applied too soon after injury when there is significant swelling.
10. If one fracture is found, always check the joint above and the joint below for additional fractures, dislocations, or other injuries.

SUGGESTED READING

DeLee JC, et al, eds.: *DeLee and Drez's orthopaedic sports medicine: principles and practice.* WB Saunders, 2003, Philadelphia.

Mellion MB, et al, eds.: *Team physician's handbook,* 3rd ed. Hanley & Belfus, 2002, Philadelphia.

 Chapter **153**

Heat and Cold Illness

"Thank God the cold saved my little boy's brain function."

CLINICAL CASE PROBLEM 1:

A 51-Year-Old Alcoholic Male Brought into the Emergency Room

A 51-year-old alcoholic male is brought into the emergency room (ER) after having been found in a snow bank. He is unconscious, and no history can be obtained. No family is known.

On physical examination, his blood pressure is 90/60 mm Hg. His pulse is 36 and regular. His core body temperature is 28° C (82.4° F). His electrocardiogram (ECG) reveals sinus bradycardia and a J wave after the QRS complex.

■ **SELECT THE BEST ANSWER TO THE FOLLOWING QUESTIONS:**

1. Which of the following statements regarding the hypothermia in this patient is false?
   a. most patients with hypothermia are intoxicated with ethanol or other drugs
   b. body temperatures from 32° C to 35° C constitute mild hypothermia
   c. the Osborne J wave on the ECG is characteristic of hypothermia
   d. arrhythmias and dysrhythmias are common when the core body temperature drops below 30° C (86° F)
   e. intravascular volume usually is not maintained in patients with hypothermia
   f. all of the above

2. What is the treatment of choice for the patient described?
   a. passive rewarming
   b. active external rewarming
   c. active core rewarming
   d. a and b
   e. none of the above

CLINICAL CASE PROBLEM 2:

A 46-Year-Old Male with Blanched Feet

A 46-year-old male is brought into the ER from his worksite with numbness of both feet after working in 0° C (32° F) weather for 6 hours.

On examination, both feet are blanched. Sensation is decreased in both feet to the level of the ankles. Both feet are cold to touch and are bloodless. You suspect frostbite.

3. What is the most appropriate treatment of this patient at this time?
   a. passive rewarming
   b. vigorous rubbing
   c. immersion in water at 42° C (107.6° F)
   d. placement close to a radiant heater
   e. immersion in water at 30° C (86° F)

CLINICAL CASE PROBLEM 3:

A 4-Year-Old Male with a Core Temperature of 28° C

A 4-year-old male is brought into the ER after having fallen through the ice into a lake. He was rescued approximately 15 minutes later. Cardiopulmonary resuscitation (CPR) was begun at the scene and is in progress as the patient is wheeled through the ER doors.

On examination, there is no spontaneous breathing or cardiac activity. The child's core temperature is 28° C (82.4° F).

4. At this time, what would be the most appropriate action?
   a. stop CPR
   b. continue CPR while rewarming the patient with active external rewarming
   c. continue CPR while rewarming the patient with inhalation warming therapy
   d. continue CPR while rewarming the patient with peritoneal dialysis
   e. activate the advanced cardiac life support (ACLS) protocol

5. Following the initial treatment just selected, what would be your next step?
   a. stop CPR
   b. continue CPR while rewarming the patient with active external rewarming
   c. continue CPR while rewarming the patient with inhalation warming therapy
   d. continue CPR while rewarming the patient with active core rewarming
   e. none of the above

CLINICAL CASE PROBLEM 4:

AN OVERHEATED 34-YEAR-OLD MALE

A 34-year-old male soldier is brought into the ER by a friend after having been outdoors on patrol all day in temperatures exceeding 42° C (107.6° F). He complains of painful spasms of the skeletal muscles, most prominent in the lower extremities and the abdomen. No other symptoms are associated with these spasms.

On physical examination, the patient is alert and cooperative. His blood pressure is 120/80 mm Hg, and his pulse is 108/minute. His temperature is 38° C (100.4° F). The remainder of the physical examination is normal.

6. Which of the following conditions does this patient have?
   a. heat cramps
   b. heatstroke
   c. heat exhaustion
   d. b or c
   e. none of the above

7. What is the treatment of choice for this patient at this time?
   a. oral electrolyte replacement therapy
   b. core body cooling
   c. warm intravenous (IV) fluids
   d. intensive care unit monitoring and Swan-Ganz catheterization
   e. none of the above

CLINICAL CASE PROBLEM 5:

AN EXHAUSTED 23-YEAR-OLD FEMALE MARATHON RUNNER

A 23-year-old female marathon runner presents to the ER after completing a marathon. During the last mile, she began to develop lightheadedness, nausea, vomiting, severe headache, rapid heart rate, and rapid respiratory rate.

On examination, the patient's blood pressure is 90/70 mm Hg. Her pulse is 120/min and regular. She is orthostatic. Her temperature is 37.5° C (99.5° F). The rest of the physical examination is normal.

8. Which of the following conditions does the patient described in Clinical Case Problem 5 have?
   a. heat cramps
   b. heatstroke
   c. heat exhaustion
   d. b or c
   e. none of the above

9. Which of the following statements regarding this patient's condition is (are) true?
   a. rapid IV volume and electrolyte replacement are indicated in this patient
   b. this patient can be safely discharged without any active treatment; oral fluids will suffice
   c. this patient's temperature will likely go up significantly in the next few hours
   d. serum potassium and serum sodium levels are likely to be normal in this patient
   e. none of the above are true

CLINICAL CASE PROBLEM 6:

AN 34-YEAR-OLD MALE MARATHON RUNNER WHO COLLAPSED

A 34-year-old male is brought to the ER by paramedics after having collapsed in a marathon. Apparently, at approximately the eighteenth mile he fell to the ground in an unconscious state.

On physical examination, his blood pressure is 90/60 mm Hg. His pulse is 128 beats/minute, and his respiratory rate is 45/minute. The patient's temperature is 41° C (105.8° F).

10. Which of the following statements about this patient is (are) true?
    a. this patient has heat stroke
    b. hepatic and renal abnormalities are common in this condition
    c. treatment should be directed at lowering the core temperature as quickly as possible
    d. all of the above
    e. none of the above

ANSWERS:

1. f. The majority of patients with hypothermia are intoxicated with ethanol or other drugs. Ethanol is a vasodilator, and because of its anesthetic and central nervous system (CNS)–depressant effects, intoxicated subjects do not feel the cold. Other factors that increase susceptibility to cold are certain drugs (including sedatives, meperidine, clonidine, and neuroleptics), hypothyroidism, diabetes, infancy, advanced age, malnutrition, exhaustion, spinal cord damage, and sepsis.

Hypothermia is defined as mild if the body temperature is between 32° C and 35° C (89.6° F to 95.0° F), moderate if the body temperature is between 28° C and 32° C (82.4° F and 89.6° F), and severe if below 28° C (82.4° F). Shivering stops at 31° C (87.8° F).

Hypothermia causes characteristic ECG changes and may induce certain life-threatening dysrhythmias, including ventricular fibrillation and asystole. The Osborne (J) wave, a slow, positive deflection at the end of the QRS complex, is characteristic, although not pathognomonic, of hypothermia. The probability of dysrhythmias increases with decreasing body temperature. Oxygen delivery to the tissues is impaired, and intravascular volume is lost because of a plasma shift to the extravascular space.

Hypothermia produces a depression of CNS function resulting in confusion, lethargy, and (in severe cases) coma.

2. c. Because of the severity of the hypothermia (core temperature of 28° C), active core rewarming is the method of choice for the correction of this patient's hypothermia. Core rewarming will warm all of this patient's internal organs preferentially and at the expense of other areas of the body. Core rewarming also will decrease myocardial irritability and the risk of dysrhythmias and improve cardiac function.

The methods of active core rewarming include inhalation rewarming; heated IV fluids; heated irrigation of the peritoneum, thorax, and gastrointestinal tract; and extracorporeal warming.

Passive rewarming includes removing wet clothing and insulating patients with blankets. Core temperature increases slowly with this method, and therefore rewarming cannot be recommended in a patient, as presented, with cardiovascular compromise.

Active external rewarming (warm-water immersion, heating blankets, radiant heat) may be successful in rapidly raising body temperature. The application of external heat, however, may cause peripheral vasodilatation and return cold blood to the core. It is thus not appropriate for this patient.

The method of choice for rewarming a patient depends on the duration, degree, and cause of the hypothermia. Simple cold-water immersion, for example, produces little disturbance of intravascular volume, electrolyte balance, and acid–base status. In these patients, rapid external rewarming, therefore, is usually both safe and successful.

In patients who are in the early phase of hypothermia, improvement usually occurs irrespective of the method chosen. At temperatures higher than 30° C (86° F) there is a very low incidence of arrhythmias, and rapid rewarming is unnecessary.

The most important consideration in the choice of rewarming method is the patient's cardiovascular status. Patients who have stable cardiac function do not need rapid rewarming. Passive rewarming and noninvasive internal modalities (moist warm oxygen and warm IV fluids) will suffice.

Patients with cardiovascular compromise, including persistent hypotension and life-threatening dysrhythmias, need to be rewarmed rapidly. The initial management of patients with hypothermia always begins with the ABCs.

3. c. The initial clinical response to cold is known as frostnip. Frostnip, a superficial and reversible injury, begins as a blanching and numbness of the involved area, followed by a sudden cessation of cold and discomfort. The sudden loss of cold sensation at the injury site is a very reliable sign of impending frostbite. If treatment is initiated at this point, frostnip will not progress to frostbite.

The best initial treatment for frostnip and frostbite is rapid rewarming of the involved extremity in a circulating warm-water bath (42° C, 107.6° F). Slow rewarming is less effective and actually may increase tissue damage.

4. e. The first step in the resuscitation of this patient should be the activation of the ACLS protocol. Again, remember the ABCs (in that order). The cardiac status of a drowning victim is the first priority. With the activation of the ACLS protocol, CPR should not be stopped until the core temperature is higher than 32° C (89.6° F).

5. d. Death in hypothermia is confirmed only when the patient has failed to respond to basic cardiac life support and ACLS and the core temperature is higher than 32° C. In this case, the rewarming recommended is active core rewarming.

6. a. This patient has heat cramps.

7. a. This patient has heat cramps. Heat cramps usually are associated with strenuous physical activity. The painful spasm of skeletal muscles, including muscles of the extremities and abdomen, occurs.

Other symptoms include weakness, fatigue, nausea, vomiting, and tachycardia. On physical examination, the body temperature is normal. The pathophysiology is a total body salt deficiency (Na^+ deficiency).

Heat cramps are benign and respond well to oral electrolyte replacement and mild cooling.

8. c. See Answer 9.

9. a. This patient has heat exhaustion. Heat exhaustion is characterized by volume depletion, fluid and electrolyte losses from sweating, and tissue hypoperfusion secondary to the hypovolemia. Heat exhaustion usually presents with fatigue, lightheadedness, nausea, and/or vomiting, and headache. Significant hypovolemia with associated tachycardia, hyperventilation, and hypotension also occurs. The patient's body temperature is usually normal or only slightly elevated. Sweating may be profuse.

The treatment of choice in this patient is IV fluid replacement (normal saline or lactated Ringer's). Treatment also includes removal to a cool environment, removal of excess clothing, spraying with tepid water (40° C, 104° F), and cooling with fans.

10. d. This patient has heat stroke. Heat stroke is defined as the combination of hyperpyrexia (>40° C) with associated neurologic symptoms. Classic heat stroke, seen primarily in the elderly, is characterized by altered mental status and absence of sweating. In exertional heat stroke, seen in younger patients undergoing rigorous exercise, there is commonly profuse sweating. All patients have tachycardia and hyperventilation. Heat stroke is a medical emergency.

Risk factors for heat stroke include the following: (1) the extremes of age; (2) preexisting cardiovascular disease; (3) high environmental temperature and humidity; (4) occupations such as professional athletes, laborers, and military recruits; and (5) use of pharmacologic agents, including anticholinergic drugs, phenothiazines, tricyclic antidepressants, monoamine oxidase inhibitors, and antihistamines.

Heat stroke usually presents abruptly, with the rapid onset of neurologic dysfunction.

Hepatic, renal, and hematologic abnormalities are common in heatstroke. Hepatic failure, renal failure, and disseminated intravascular coagulation may occur. Fluid and electrolyte abnormalities vary with the onset and duration of heatstroke, underlying disease, and the prior use of medications (especially diuretics). Unlike in heat exhaustion, dehydration and volume depletion may not occur in heatstroke. Vigorous fluid replacement may result in pulmonary edema.

Heat stroke is treated by removing all clothing; applying cool water to the entire skin prior to reaching the ER; followed by treatment in the ER consisting of spraying with a mist of tepid water while using a high-volume fan, ice packs applied to the groin and axillae, ice water gastric lavage, and iced peritoneal lavage. Ice-water immersion makes it difficult to monitor the patient and initiate CPR or defibrillation if necessary. As with all emergencies the initial treatment begins with the ABCs.

SUMMARY OF HEAT AND COLD ILLNESS

1. **Cold injuries and syndromes:**
   a. Frostnip and frostbite: frostnip is superficial, really an "early frostbite" and completely reversible; frostbite is superficial or deep but usually associated with some tissue damage. Treatment of both syndromes involves immersion of the extremity in a circulating warm-water bath (42° C, 107.6° F).
   b. Hypothermia: Mild hypothermia is defined by a core temperature between 32° C and 35° C; moderate hypothermia is defined by a core temperature between 28° C and 32° C; severe hypothermia is defined by a core temperature lower than 28° C. Mild hypothermia should be treated by passive external rewarming. In some cases, active external rewarming may be necessary. Moderate hypothermia is treated by active external rewarming applied to the trunk rather than the extremities; active core rewarming (warmed IV fluids) may be necessary. Treatment of severe hypothermia requires active core rewarming. Cardiac resuscitation should be continued until core temperature is higher than 32° C.

2. **Heat syndromes:**
   a. Heat cramps: no disturbance of core body temperature. There is a salt (Na^+) deficiency. Treatment is by oral electrolyte replacement.
   b. Heat exhaustion: volume and electrolyte depletion. The core temperature is normal or slightly elevated. Treatment is giving IV fluids (normal saline/Ringer's lactate), removing excess clothing, moving to a cool environment, spraying tepid water, and cooling with fans.
   c. Heat stroke: hyperpyrexia and neurologic symptoms; absence of sweating is characteristic. In exertional heat stroke there may be profuse sweating. Treatment of choice is a rapid, aggressive lowering of body temperature.

This includes iced gastric lavage, iced peritoneal lavage, and in some cases ice-water immersion (however, it is difficult with ice-water immersion to monitor the patient and initiate CPR).

SUGGESTED READING

Biem J, et al: Out of the cold: management of hypothermia and frostbite. *Can Med Assoc J* 168(3):305-311, 2003.
Bouchama A, Knochel JP: Medical progress: heat stroke. *N Engl J Med* 346(25):1978-1988, 2002.
Mellion MB, et al, eds.: *Team physician's handbook,* 3rd ed. Hanley & Belfus, 2002, Philadelphia.

 Chapter **154**

Upper Extremity Injuries

"I always thought tennis elbow was a joke."

CLINICAL CASE PROBLEM 1:

A 42-Year-Old Male with Right Shoulder Pain

A 42-year-old male comes to your office with complaints of right shoulder pain. He does not remember any specific injury but has been playing a lot of tennis over the past 4 months. He tells you that "opposing players no longer fear my serve." It has become difficult and painful for him to reach overhead and behind him. Even rolling onto his shoulder in bed is painful.

On examination of the right shoulder there is full range of motion in all planes with obvious discomfort at end ranges of flexion, abduction, and internal rotation. There is significant pain when you place the shoulder in a position of 90 degrees flexion and then internally rotate. There is also moderate weakness with abduction and external rotation of the shoulder. The rest of the musculoskeletal examination is normal.

■ SELECT THE BEST ANSWER TO THE FOLLOWING QUESTIONS:

1. The most likely diagnosis is:
   a. acromioclavicular sprain
   b. rotator cuff tear
   c. adhesive capsulitis
   d. rotator cuff impingement
   e. cervical radiculopathy

2. The best initial treatment is:
   a. corticosteroid injection
   b. arthroscopic subacromial decompression
   c. strengthening and range-of-motion exercises
   d. elbow sling
   e. cervical collar

3. Predisposing factors for this problem include which of the following:
   a. repetitive motion of the shoulder above the horizontal plane
   b. hooked acromion
   c. acromioclavicular spurring
   d. shoulder instability
   e. all of the above

CLINICAL CASE PROBLEM 2:

A 37-Year-Old Man with Right Elbow Pain

A 37-year-old man comes into the office complaining of right elbow pain. He has been painting the walls of his kitchen for the past 5 days. He tells you that the colors came out beautiful, his wife is very happy, but he is "really paying the price." It hurts him when lifting things, when shaking hands, and even when trying to fully straighten his elbow.

On examination there is full range of motion of the elbow but there is pain when the elbow is fully extended. There is also pain and weakness when you stress test the wrist extensor and supinator muscles. Palpation reveals tenderness over the dorsum of the forearm extending proximally to the elbow. The rest of the musculoskeletal examination is normal.

4. The most likely diagnosis is:
   a. lateral epicondylitis
   b. olecranon bursitis
   c. wrist strain
   d. cubital tunnel syndrome
   e. olecranon stress fracture

5. The primary muscle involved in this condition is the:
   a. triceps
   b. extensor carpi radialis brevis
   c. extensor carpi ulnaris
   d. flexor digitorum profundus
   e. pronator teres

6. Which of the following is the best initial treatment?
   a. corticosteroid injection
   b. surgical débridement

c. short arm cast
d. rest and a progressive stretching and strengthening program
e. elbow sling

CLINICAL CASE PROBLEM 3:

A 29-Year-Old Woman with Severe Wrist Pain

A 29-year-old woman comes into the office with severe wrist pain. She has had the pain for a few months, but over the past month it has worsened significantly. She denies any trauma, and other than having a cesarean section 4 months ago, her past medical and surgical histories are negative.

On examination there is tenderness just distal to the radial styloid. Finkelstein's test is positive. Phalen's test is negative. There is full range of motion of the wrist.

7. The most likely diagnosis is:
   a. carpal tunnel syndrome
   b. scaphoid fracture
   c. ulnar nerve entrapment
   d. Kienböck's disease
   e. De Quervain's tenosynovitis

8. The best initial treatment is:
   a. thumb spica splint
   b. surgical release
   c. long arm cast
   d. volar wrist splint
   e. low-dose amitriptyline

CLINICAL CASE PROBLEM 4:

A 23-Year-Old Female with a Painful Thumb

A 23-year-old female injured her hand while skiing 1 day ago. She "caught an edge" and fell onto her right hand. She notices swelling at the base of her thumb and has pain when she moves or bangs the thumb.

On examination there is tenderness over the ulnar aspect of the first carpometacarpal joint. When you stress test the ulnar collateral ligament you note laxity compared to the opposite hand, but there is a firm endpoint. There is no tenderness in the snuff box.

9. The most likely diagnosis is:
   a. grade I sprain of the ulnar collateral ligament
   b. grade II sprain of the ulnar collateral ligament
   c. grade III sprain of the ulnar collateral ligament
   d. fracture of the head of the first metacarpal
   e. fracture of the scaphoid

10. The best initial treatment is:
    a. surgical repair
    b. physical therapy

c. corticosteroid injection
d. nonsteroidal antiinflammatory drugs (NSAIDs)
e. cast immobilization

► ANSWERS:

1. d. Rotator cuff impingement, also known as "painful arc syndrome," is a common shoulder disorder. It is often the result of the supraspinatus tendon impinging on the undersurface of the cora-coacromial arch. This may be the result of a curved or hooked acromion, acromioclavicular spurring, repetitive motion of the shoulder above the horizontal plane, or instability of the glenohumeral joint leading to a functional loss of the subacromial space. Physical examination often reveals a limitation in shoulder range-of-motion and positive provocative maneuvers including the Neer's and Hawkin's impingement signs. In the Neer's impingement sign the shoulder is passively moved into a position of flexion and internal rotation. In the Hawkin's impingement sign the shoulder is passively moved into a position of forward flexion to 90 degrees and internal rotation.

2. c. Strengthening and range-of-motion exercises are essential in the treatment of rotator cuff impingement syndrome and are prescribed early in the course of treatment. Corticosteroid injection to the subacromial space typically is given later in the course of treatment, if more conservative therapeutic modalities have failed. Arthroscopic subacromial decompression is considered if conservative treatment fails after 3-6 months. An elbow sling is not indicated. If the shoulder is immobilized for an extended period, the patient is at risk for developing adhesive capsulitis.

3. e. All are predisposing factors for rotator cuff impingement syndrome.

4. a. Lateral epicondylitis, an injury to the wrist extensor and supinator muscles, results from either repetitive strain or a single traumatic event. Patients typically complain of pain in the elbow or dorsum of the forearm that is aggravated with activity. Physical examination reveals tenderness on the lateral epicondyle, pain with passive wrist flexion, and pain with resisted wrist extension and supination.

5. b. The primary muscle involved in this condition is the extensor carpi radialis brevis.

6. d. The best initial treatment is rest and a progressive stretching and strengthening program. Other treatments include NSAIDs, a compression strap or counter-force bracing, and modifying aggravating activities. Corticosteroid injection may be given later in the course of treatment. Surgical débridement is reserved for patients who have failed all conservative therapy. Immobilization of the elbow and a short arm cast are not part of the treatment for lateral epicondylitis.

7. e. De Quervain's disease is a stenosing tenosynovitis of the first dorsal compartment of the wrist. The involved tendons are the abductor pollicis longus and the extensor pollicis brevis. The condition is caused by repetitive grasping or repetitive use of the thumb. Mothers with newborns, for example, are at increased risk of developing De Quervain's disease from the repetitive lifting of their child. On physical examination there is tenderness to palpation in the region of the radial styloid and there is a positive Finkelstein's test. This test is performed by having the patient make a fist with the thumb tucked inside and then passively moving the wrist into a position of ulnar deviation.

8. a. The best initial treatment is a thumb spica splint. The patient's wrist should be immobilized for a period of approximately 3 weeks. Additional treatment includes NSAIDs, modifying aggravating activities, and possibly physical therapy. For resistant cases a corticosteroid injection may be beneficial. Surgery is indicated when all conservative management fails.

9. b. The most likely diagnosis is a grade II sprain of the ulnar collateral ligament. This injury is commonly referred to as "skier's thumb" or "gamekeeper's thumb." The mechanism of injury is usually a fall on an outstretched hand with the thumb in an abducted position. Tenderness is elicited when palpating at the insertion of the ulnar collateral ligament on the proximal phalanx. It is important to stress test the ulnar collateral ligament to grade the degree of injury. Compared to a grade II sprain, a grade I sprain has no laxity when stress testing and a grade III sprain does not have a firm endpoint when stress testing.

10. e. The best initial treatment is cast immobilization for a period of 5-6 weeks. A grade III sprain of the ulnar collateral ligament may require surgical treatment.

SUMMARY OF UPPER EXTREMITY INJURIES

1. Rotator cuff impingement is a common shoulder disorder caused by the supraspinatus tendon impinging on the undersurface of the coraco-acromial arch.

   a. **Predisposing factors:** curved or hooked acromion; acromioclavicular spurring; repetitive motion of the shoulder above the horizontal plane; and instability of the glenohumeral joint
   b. **Clues on examination:** painful arc; decreased range of motion; and Neer's and Hawkin's signs are positive.
   c. **Treatment:** strengthening and range-of-motion exercises; avoidance of aggravating activities; NSAIDs; corticosteroid injection; and arthroscopic subacromial decompression if conservative treatment fails.
2. Lateral epicondylitis is caused by injury to wrist extensor and supinator muscles as the result of repetitive strain or single traumatic event. The extensor carpi radialis brevis is most commonly involved.
   a. **Clues on examination:** tenderness over lateral epicondyle; pain with passive wrist flexion; and pain with resisted wrist extension and supination
   b. **Treatment:** rest; progressive stretching and strengthening program; counter-force bracing; modifying aggravating activities; and corticosteroid injection if necessary
3. De Quervain's tenosynovitis is stenosing tenosynovitis of the first dorsal compartment of the wrist and is caused by repetitive grasping or repetitive use of the thumb.
   a. **Clues on examination:** tenderness in region of radial styloid and a positive Finkelstein's test
   b. **Treatment:** thumb spica brace; NSAIDs; modifying aggravating activities; physical therapy; corticosteroid injection if necessary; and surgery if conservative treatment fails
4. Ulnar collateral ligament sprain of thumb (aka skier's thumb or gamekeeper's thumb) is caused by a traumatic injury, usually a fall on an outstretched hand.
   a. **Clues on examination:** tenderness at insertion of ulnar collateral ligament; and stress testing on the ulnar collateral ligament to check for laxity and severity of injury.
   b. **Treatment:** thumb spica cast immobilization; surgery is sometimes necessary in grade III injuries

SUGGESTED READING
Mellion MB, et al, eds.: *Team physician's handbook*, 3rd ed. Hanley & Belfus, 2002, Philadelphia.
Sallis RE, Massimino F, eds.: *ACSM's essentials of sports medicine*. Mosby, 1997, St. Louis.

Chapter **155**

Lower Extremity: Strains and Sprains

> "It's that darned ankle again."

CLINICAL CASE PROBLEM 1:
A 21-Year-Old Female with a Swollen Ankle

A 21-year-old female comes to the emergency room (ER) after "twisting" her ankle while playing lacrosse. She tells you her ankle "rolled in" at the time of injury, and she says she has pain at her right ankle. She is able to walk without any assistance.

On examination, there is mild ecchymosis and swelling on the lateral side of her right ankle. There is pain with inversion of the right ankle. Ankle tenderness is maximal just anterior to the tip of the lateral malleolus. There is no actual bone tenderness. There is no ligamentous laxity.

■ **SELECT THE BEST ANSWER TO THE FOLLOWING QUESTIONS:**

1. The injury in this patient is most likely which of the following?
   a. a grade I sprain of the ligament complex on the medial side of the right ankle
   b. a grade III sprain of the ligament complex on the lateral side of the right ankle
   c. a grade I sprain of the ligament complex on the lateral side of the right ankle
   d. a strain of the peroneus brevis tendon
   e. a fracture of the distal fibula

2. What is the most likely ligament involved in this injury?
   a. anterior inferior tibiofibular ligament
   b. calcaneofibular ligament
   c. anterior talofibular ligament
   d. dorsal calcaneocuboid ligament
   e. interosseous talocalcaneal ligament

3. What is the treatment of choice in this patient?
   a. a fiberglass cast
   b. weightbearing as tolerated with active range-of-motion exercises
   c. nonweightbearing and a posterior splint
   d. a corticosteroid injection
   e. surgical repair of the ligament

CLINICAL CASE PROBLEM 2:
A 26-Year-Old Football Player Hit on the Lateral Side of the Knee

A 26-year-old professional football player is brought to the ER after being hit on the lateral side of the left knee. His knee buckled, and he is now in severe pain.

On examination, there is swelling over the medial aspect of the left knee. There is laxity when a valgus stress test is performed on the knee. There is a negative Lachman's test and McMurray's test.

4. What is the most likely injury in this patient?
   a. lateral meniscus tear
   b. medial meniscus tear
   c. lateral collateral ligament sprain
   d. medial collateral ligament sprain
   e. tibial plateau fracture

5. Based on your diagnosis in Question 4, what is the initial treatment of choice?
   a. corticosteroid injection
   b. knee brace
   c. fiberglass cast
   d. complete bed rest
   e. surgical repair

CLINICAL CASE PROBLEM 3:
A 22-Year-Old Male Who Twisted His Right Knee

A 22-year-old is brought to the ER 8 hours after twisting his right knee while playing in a soccer match. At the time of injury he felt a sharp pain on the "inner" part of his right knee. He has been unable to straighten his knee fully and had to be carried off the field by his teammates.

On examination, there is a moderate joint effusion, tenderness at the medial joint line, and limitation of the last 20 degrees of extension by a springy resistance. There is sharp anteromedial knee pain when passive extension is forced.

6. What is the most likely diagnosis in this patient?
   a. medial meniscus tear
   b. lateral meniscus tear
   c. medial collateral ligament sprain
   d. anterior cruciate ligament sprain
   e. fractured patella

7. The radiologic procedure of choice to confirm the diagnosis in the patient described in Clinical Case Problem 3 is which of the following?

a. a plain anterior posterior (AP) and lateral x-ray of the right knee
b. a cone-view c-ray of the right knee
c. an arthrogram
d. a computed tomography (CT) scan
e. a magnetic resonance imaging (MRI) scan

8. What is the treatment of choice for the injury to the patient described in Clinical Case Problem 3?
a. nonweightbearing and a knee immobilizer
b. nonweightbearing and a full cast
c. ice, elevation, and an elastic bandage
d. arthroscopic surgery
e. physical therapy

CLINICAL CASE PROBLEM 4:

A 23-YEAR-OLD FEMALE WITH RIGHT POSTERIOR THIGH PAIN

A 23-year-old female comes to your office with right posterior thigh pain. She was running in a 100-meter race when she felt a "pop" in her thigh.

On examination, there is tenderness over the mid-portion of the right hamstring muscles and pain with resisted stress testing. There is mild swelling and discoloration. There is no bony tenderness and no palpable defect.

9. What is the most likely diagnosis in this patient?
a. right hamstring strain
b. right hamstring sprain
c. popliteus artery hemorrhage
d. right hamstring avulsion
e. none of the above

10. What is the initial treatment of choice for the patient described in Clinical Case Problem 4?
a. surgical repair
b. splint
c. a full cast
d. ice, rest, elevation, and compression
e. none of the above

CLINICAL CASE PROBLEM 5:

A 16-YEAR-OLD FEMALE WHO INJURED HER KNEE WHILE PIVOTING

A 16-year-old female, the star on her high school basketball team, sustains a knee injury after pivoting on her right knee during a game. She collapses to the floor in pain and is immediately taken to the ER.

She arrives at the ER approximately 45 minutes after the injury, and her right knee is already very swollen. There is significant laxity when a Lachman test is performed.

11. What is the most likely diagnosis in this patient?
a. anterior cruciate ligament sprain
b. posterior cruciate ligament sprain
c. quadriceps tendon tear
d. lateral collateral ligament sprain
e. medial collateral ligament sprain

12. The diagnosis of this injury is best confirmed in the ER by which of the following?
a. history of the injury
b. anterior drawer test
c. the Lachman test
d. aspiration of the knee joint
e. MRI of the knee

13. What is the definitive treatment of choice in this patient for her injury?
a. ice, elevation, compression
b. a long leg cast
c. corticosteroid injection
d. reconstruction surgery
e. none of the above

◢ CLINICAL CASE MANAGEMENT PROBLEM

Differentiate a collateral ligament tear from a meniscus tear.

▪ ANSWERS:

1. **c.** This patient most likely has a grade I sprain of the ligament complex on the lateral side of the ankle.

A sprain is defined as a complete or partial tear of a ligament (intrasubstance or at origin/insertion). Swelling and tenderness over a ligament and pain when it is stretched suggest a sprain. Note that when a ligament is completely torn, as in a grade III injury, there may be no pain when the involved ligament is passively stretched. Excessive motion of the joint when the ligament is stretched confirms the diagnosis of a grade III sprain. Sprains are graded according to the following criteria:

Grade I: a tear of a few ligament fibers. The joint is tender and painful, but there is no laxity. Swelling and ecchymosis are usually minimal.

Grade II: a tear of a moderate number of ligament fibers. On physical examination, there is a moderate amount of swelling and pain. There is little to no instability of joint.

Grade III: total disruption or tear of the ligament involved. No endpoint is felt when the joint is stressed. Swelling and ecchymosis are prominent.

The most common ankle injury is an inversion-type injury with partial or complete disruption of the lateral ligament complex.

2. c. Most ankle sprains are caused by inversion-type injuries. The lateral ligaments are most commonly involved. Specifically, the anterior talofibular ligament is the most commonly injured ligament. Tenderness is maximal anterior to the tip of the lateral malleolus.

3. b. The treatment of choice in this patient is ice, elevation, weightbearing as tolerated, active range-of-motion exercises, and an ankle support brace. Early weightbearing hastens healing and return to activity.

A cast is inappropriate and can lead to complications if the swelling worsens. Surgical intervention is not indicated in most ankle sprains. Corticosteroid injection also is not indicated in the acute management of ankle sprains.

4. d. The most likely injury in this patient is a sprain of the medial collateral ligament. The mechanism of injury (a blow to the lateral side of the knee), the swelling demonstrated on the medial side of the knee, and the laxity with valgus stress testing suggest a sprain of the medial collateral ligament complex. The Lachman's test is used to diagnose injuries to the anterior cruciate ligament. The McMurray's test is used to diagnose tears of the menisci.

5. b. Initial treatment consists of a knee brace, ice, elevation, and straight leg raise exercises in the brace. The patient may ambulate as tolerated in the brace. It is not necessary to apply a cast. Surgery and corticosteroid injection are not indicated. The patient does not need to be on bed rest.

6. a. This patient has a torn right medial meniscus. The history of the injury is quite characteristic. Often a torn meniscus is the result of a twisting or squatting type injury. The patient then has pain along the affected joint line. The knee usually swells over the first 12 hours, and there is sometimes a sensation of "locking." This locking can be from a displaced meniscal fragment or from hamstring spasm ("pseudolocking").

On physical examination, there is joint line tenderness and an effusion may be present. There is a positive McMurray's test and Apley's test. For McMurray's test, with the patient in a supine position, the clinician holds the lower leg, flexing and extending the knee while simultaneously internally and externally rotating the tibia on the femur. A positive test is a "clicking" sensation felt with the other hand along the joint line or the patient experiencing pain. For Apley's test, the patient lies prone with the knee flexed 90 degrees. The leg is internally and externally rotated with pressure applied to the heel. Pain with downward pressure is a positive test for meniscal

disease. In addition to meniscal tears, twisting injuries also may give rise to anterior cruciate ligament tears.

7. e. The diagnostic test of choice for a suspected medial meniscal tear and locking is an MRI scan.

8. d. The treatment of choice for the patient described in Question 6 is arthroscopic surgery. With the use of an arthroscope, the torn fragment either can be removed or repaired.

9. a. This patient most likely has a right hamstring muscle strain. A strain is defined as an "overstretching" of some portion of muscle or tendon. As with sprains, every degree of strain, ranging from the overstretching of just a few muscle fibers to the complete rupture of a muscle or tendon, may occur.

10. d. The initial treatment of choice for the patient discussed in Clinical Case Problem 4 is ice, rest, elevation, and compression bandage. This is followed with a gradually progressive stretching and strengthening program.

11. a. This is an injury to the anterior cruciate ligament.

12. c. The mechanism of injury to the anterior cruciate ligament is usually noncontact: a deceleration, hyperextension, or marked internal rotation of the involved knee. It also may be associated with a medial meniscus tear. Because the anterior cruciate ligament is a very vascular structure, a tear will cause an immediate knee effusion.

Injury to the anterior cruciate ligament is diagnosed by performing the Lachman test, the anterior drawer test, and the pivot shift test. Although the anterior drawer test is a time-honored test, it turns out not to be very sensitive. The Lachman test is much more sensitive. In this test, the examiner places the knee in 20-30 degrees of flexion by resting it on a pillow and stabilizes the femur, just above the knee, with his or her nondominant hand. The dominant hand of the examiner is placed behind the leg at the level of the tibial tubercle, and the examiner introduces an anterior force, attempting to displace the tibia forward. If there is excessive anterior translation of the tibia and lack of a firm endpoint, a tear in the anterior cruciate ligament has occurred.

13. d. The initial treatment includes a knee brace, ice packs, and elevation, followed by isometric and range-of-motion exercises. The definitive treatment in young active patients is most often reconstruction. Surgery usually is delayed 3 weeks postinjury to allow for increased range-of-motion and strength and decreased swelling.

SOLUTION TO THE CLINICAL CASE MANAGEMENT PROBLEM

To help differentiate a collateral ligament tear from a meniscus tear make note of the following: a positive varus or valgus stress test present on clinical exami-nation is consistent with a collateral ligament injury, whereas joint line tenderness is consistent with a meniscus tear.

SUMMARY OF LOWER EXTREMITY: STRAINS AND SPRAINS

1. **Definitions:**
   a. Sprain: a ligament injury. Sprains are classified as follows: first-degree: tear of only a few liga-ment fibers with no joint instability; second-degree: tear of a moderate number of ligament fibers with little or no joint instability; third-degree: complete rupture of ligament with joint instability.
   b. Strain: a muscle-tendon injury. Strain injuries are classified as follows, ranging from tearing only a few fibers to a complete rupture of the muscle-tendon unit: first-degree, second-degree, third-degree.
2. **Common sites:**
   a. Ankle sprain: lateral ligament complex injured more frequently than medial ligament complex (tenderness is usually maximal anterior to tip of lateral malleolus over the anterior talofibular ligament)
   b. Knee sprain: (1) medial and lateral collateral ligaments: varus and valgus stress testing; (2) anterior cruciate ligament: Lachman's test.

3. **Other significant injury:** medial and lateral meniscal injuries of the knee:
   a. Clinical clue: joint line tenderness, positive McMurray's test, Apley's test (see A6).
   b. Diagnosis: if further diagnostic procedure is needed, MRI is the radiologic test of choice.
4. **Treatments:** sprain (ankle)—conservative; RICE: **R**est: stop physical activity; protected weight-bearing as tolerated; **I**ce: apply ice to the injury for 15-20 minutes each hour while awake for the first 24 hours. Wrap the ice in a wet towel or other buffer to prevent skin damage. Ice reduces swelling and pain. To prevent nerve injuries do not leave ice on longer than 20 minutes; **C**ompression: use an elastic bandage or air-filled splint to apply pressure to an injury. Wear it all day long. Compression helps control swelling; **E**levation: keep the injured area elevated. This allows fluid to drain from the injury site, reducing swelling.

SUGGESTED READING

Mellion MB, et al: *Team physician's handbook,* 3rd ed. Hanley & Belfus, 2002, Philadelphia.

Chapter 156

Low Back Pain

> "I don't care if you can't find anything wrong. There is no way I can go back to work with that bum back."

CLINICAL CASE PROBLEM 1:

A 28-YEAR-OLD MALE WITH CHRONIC LOW BACK PAIN

A 28-year-old male with chronic low back pain (LBP) comes to your office for renewal of his medication. He was injured at work 5 years ago while attempting to lift a box of very heavy tools. Since that time, he has been off work, living on compensation insurance payments, and has not been able to find a job that does not aggravate his back.

On physical examination, the patient demonstrates some vague tenderness in the paravertebral area around L3 to L5. He has some limitations on both flexion and extension.

▶ SELECT THE BEST ANSWER TO THE FOLLOWING QUESTIONS:

1. Which of the following statements regarding the epidemiology of LBP is (are) true?
   a. the annual incidence of acute LBP is 5%
   b. approximately 2% of all workers injure their backs each year

c. the lifetime prevalence of LBP is 90%

d. all of the above are true

e. none of the above are true

2. Which of the following statements regarding chronic LBP is (are) true?

a. chronic LBP is the most common cause of disability among people younger than 45 years of age

b. back injuries account for the majority of claims to compensation boards

c. in terms of expense to society, LBP peaks at approximately 40 years of age

d. all of the above

e. none of the above

3. Regarding the pathogenesis of chronic LBP, which of the following statements is (are) true?

a. in up to 85% of cases of chronic LBP, a definite anatomic or pathophysiologic diagnosis cannot be made

b. approximately 10% of patients with acute LBP eventually will require surgery

c. patients with acute LBP and no previous surgical procedures have a 20% to 25% chance of recovering after 6 weeks, regardless of the treatment used

d. the anatomic structures causing LBP are identified clearly

e. none of the above statements are true

4. Regarding the pathogenesis of chronic LBP, which of the following statements is (are) true?

a. researchers continue to debate the exact origin of the pain

b. no diagnostic test can definitively distinguish among neural, discogenic, bony, muscular, and ligamentous pain

c. ordinary radiographs, computed tomography (CT) scans, and magnetic resonance imaging (MRI) scans of the lumbar spine have low specificity

d. all of the above

e. none of the above

5. Which of the following is the most common cause of LBP?

a. metastatic bone disease

b. inflammatory back pain

c. lumbosacral sprain or strain

d. posterior facet strain

e. none of the above

CLINICAL CASE PROBLEM 2:

A 64-Year-Old Male with Back and Leg Pain Aggravated by Walking

A 64-year-old male comes into the office complaining of back and leg pain that is aggravated by walking. He tells you that the pain starts after walking two blocks. He gets relief when sitting or when walking and leaning forward. Physical examination reveals pain and decreased motion with backward bending of the lumbosacral spine. There is a negative straight leg raise test, and there are no neurologic deficits.

6. What is the most likely diagnosis?

a. vascular claudication

b. Reiter syndrome

c. spinal stenosis

d. herniated disc L5

e. mechanical LBP

7. Which of the following is not indicative of inflammatory back pain such as ankylosing spondylitis?

a. insidious onset

b. onset before age 40 years

c. pain for more than 3 months

d. morning stiffness

e. aggravation of pain with activity

8. Which of the following statements regarding the history and physical examination of a patient with LBP is (are) true?

a. the positive predictive value of the history in LBP is high

b. the positive predictive value of the physical examination in LBP is high

c. the positive predictive value of the radiographic investigations for patients with LBP is high

d. the positive predictive value of serum blood and chemistry for LBP is high

e. none of the above are true

9. Which of the following is (are) characteristic of a history of mechanical LBP?

a. relatively acute onset

b. a history of overuse or a precipitating injury

c. pain worse during the day

d. a and b only

e. a, b, and c

10. Which of the following is (are) a "red flag(s)" or danger signal(s) relative to the diagnosis of LBP?

a. bowel or bladder dysfunction

b. impotence

c. weight loss
d. significant night pain
e. all of the above

11. Which of the following statements regarding plain spinal x-rays of patients with LBP is false?
   a. osteophyte formation in the intervertebral space is predictive of discogenic disease
   b. there is little justification for the extensive use of radiography in LBP
   c. there is a poor relationship between most radiographic abnormalities and symptoms of LBP
   d. x-rays of the lumbar spine are associated with gonadal radiation exposure
   e. there is a low yield of findings on plain x-rays that alter management of LBP

12. Which of the following statements regarding the use of CT or MRI scanning in the diagnosis of disc herniation and spinal stenosis is false?
   a. CT and MRI scanning have largely replaced myelography in the diagnosis of disc herniation
   b. as many as 25% of asymptomatic people will have findings of a herniated disc on MRI
   c. CT scanning is better at imaging soft tissues compared to MRI
   d. if CT or MRI scanning is to be used in the diagnosis of a disc herniation and/or spinal stenosis, then surgery should be a serious pretest consideration
   e. none of the above statements are false

13. What is the most cost-effective and crucial aspect of the treatment of chronic LBP?
   a. patient education
   b. physiotherapy
   c. bed rest
   d. muscle relaxants
   e. nonsteroidal antiinflammatory drugs (NSAIDs)

14. Regarding the use of exercises in the treatment of chronic LBP, which of the following statements is true?
   a. exercises allow patients to participate in their treatment program
   b. exercises should follow a graduated progression
   c. following the beginning of an exercise program for LBP, a temporary increase in pain may occur
   d. stretching exercises are recommended in the initial exercise program; isometric strengthening exercises follow
   e. all of the above

15. Which of the following statements regarding the treatment of LBP is true?
   a. bed rest for seven days is recommended
   b. transcutaneous electrical nerve stimulation (TENS) is an effective treatment for chronic LBP
   c. specific exercises are effective for the treatment of acute LBP
   d. NSAIDs are effective for short term symptomatic relief in acute LBP
   e. muscle relaxants are more effective than NSAIDs in the treatment of LBP

■ **ANSWERS:**

1. **d.** The annual incidence of acute LBP is 5%. Approximately 2% of all workers injure their backs each year. The lifetime prevalence of LBP is approximately 90%. Back pain is considered to be one of the most expensive ailments seen in advanced industrial societies. Costs are estimated to be more than $20 billion each year in the United States alone. About 80% of these costs are incurred by those 7% to 10% of patients who go on to develop chronic LBP.

2. **d.** There is increasing concern (and frustration) expressed about the epidemic of LBP disability in Western industrialized countries, where approximately 1% of the population is considered totally disabled as a result of back problems. Back injuries account for the vast majority of Worker's Compensation Board claims and the highest dollar amount paid out to injured workers. Chronic LBP is the most common cause of disability among people younger than the age of 45 years and the third most common cause of disability among people aged 45-64 years.

3. **a.** For up to 85% of cases of LBP a definite anatomic or pathophysiologic diagnosis cannot be made. Only 1% of patients with acute LBP eventually require surgery. Patients with acute LBP and no previous surgical procedure have an 80% to 90% chance of recovering after 6 weeks, no matter what treatment is prescribed.

4. **d.** The anatomic structures causing LBP are not clearly identified. Researchers continue to debate whether the pain originates from the spine (facet joints and disks) or soft tissues (supporting muscles and ligaments). The well-entrenched axiom that pain on flexion originates in the disk and pain on extension originates in the facet joints is difficult to prove and does not necessarily hold true. In many of these cases, several spinal conditions may coexist.

No diagnostic test can definitively distinguish among discogenic, facetogenic, and musculoligamentous pain. Physicians should focus on injured musculoligamentous structures as common causes of chronic LBP. Despite improved radiographic diagnostic techniques, there are still significant limitations correlating clinical symptoms with radiologic interpretations. Radiographs, CT scans, and MRIs suffer from poor specificity (many false-positive results).

Often the debate over musculoligamentous or spinal LBP is resolved with the diagnosis of "mechanical LBP." This does not suggest a pathologic source but does indicate that back pain is aggravated by the effects of activity or sustained postures on already injured but unidentified structures.

5. c. The most common diagnosis in LBP is lumbosacral sprain or strain, or mechanical LBP. Injury is thought to result from abnormal stress on normal tissues or normal stress on damaged or degenerated tissues.

6. c. The most likely diagnosis is spinal stenosis. Back pain that is associated with exertional leg pain (claudication) often represents spinal stenosis. On examination there is usually pain with backward bending or extension of the lumbosacral spine. To differentiate from vascular claudication: symptoms often occur when standing up, and to relieve symptoms patients need to sit down (just stopping walking usually will not relieve symptoms).

7. e. Inflammatory back pain (ankylosing spondylitis) is an important subset of chronic LBP, although it accounts for very few cases of acute or chronic LBP. Diagnostic clues to inflammatory LBP include the following: (1) insidious onset of back pain; (2) onset before the age of 40 years; (3) pain 3 months in duration; (4) morning stiffness (longer than 30 minutes); (5) pain relief with activity; (6) pain forcing patient from bed; (7) a history of psoriasis, Reiter's disease, colitis, or ankylosing spondylitis; (8) limitation of lumbar spine in sagittal and frontal planes; (9) chest inspiratory expansion less than 2 cm; (10) evidence of sacroiliitis during physical examination; and (11) evidence of peripheral inflammatory joint disease. However, activity does not increase the pain.

8. e. One of the problems with the diagnosis, physical examination, laboratory investigation, and radiographic investigation of chronic LBP is that the sensitivity, specificity, and positive predictive value of the assessments, procedures, and other diagnostic modalities produce false-positive results and many false-negative results. From that follows that the patient ends up with misinformation that actually may "create" disease (anxiety, worry, and increased pain) where none existed before.

9. e. The history of mechanical back pain is typically one of relatively acute onset of pain, often with known precipitating injury or history of overuse. The pain is worse during the day, is relieved by rest (although the pain might worsen with prolonged rest), and is worse with activity.

In contrast, the history of inflammatory back pain classically presents with an insidious onset of pain and stiffness, worse at rest and improved with activity and often worse at night and in the morning. Many patients need to get up at night to find a comfortable position to partially relieve the pain and stiffness.

10. e. Danger signals in patients with acute or chronic LBP include the following: (1) bowel or bladder dysfunction; (2) impotence; (3) ankle clonus; (4) color change in extremities; (5) considerable night pain; (6) constant and progressive symptoms; (7) fever and chills; (8) weight loss; (9) lymphadenopathy; (10) distended abdominal veins; (11) buttock claudication; and (12) new-onset LBP in children/adolescents and individuals older than age 50.

11. a. Plain x-rays of the lumbar spine frequently are ordered for LBP. There is, however, little justification for such extensive use of radiography. A much more cost-effective and selective approach should be undertaken.

Apart from the cost factor, routine radiographs of the lumbar spine have three important drawbacks: a very low yield of findings that do not alter management in any way, a poor relationship between most radiographic abnormalities and signs and symptoms of LBP, and the potential of gonadal irradiation. Abnormalities seen on x-ray, particularly changes such as degenerative osteoarthritis, spondylosis, and congenital abnormalities, are often as common in asymptomatic individuals as they are in symptomatic individuals. Also, many patients who present with chronic LBP have normal x-ray examination results. There is no direct correlation between intervertebral osteophyte formation and discogenic disease. Most importantly, radiographs rarely alter treatment plans.

Specific indications for radiographic studies include the following: (1) ruling out an infectious or malignant process; (2) assessing a patient with objective evidence of neurologic abnormalities in the lower extremities, with loss of bowel or bladder control, or with loss of sexual function unexplained by another cause; (3) identifying a compression fracture; and (4) chronic sacroiliitis.

12. **c.** CT scanning and MRI have largely replaced myelography and are valuable for diagnosing disc disease and spinal stenosis. If the test is to influence management, then surgery must be considered a serious option before the test is performed. Consider obtaining an MRI or CT scan in patients with intractable pain or progressive neurologic deficits or if a systemic cause of back pain such as infection or neoplasm is suspected. MRI scans will reveal herniated discs in up to 25% of asymptomatic people. The presence of abnormal findings on MRI scan does not correlate well with clinical symptoms.

13. **a.** Patient education is the most crucial and cost-effective aspect of the treatment protocol for LBP. Many patients are very worried that they have a "serious illness" that is causing their pain and are dissatisfied by what they perceive as an inadequate explanation of their symptoms.

Most patients with mild to moderate LBP do not even consult physicians, and many symptomatic patients are more interested in seeking information and reassurance (the diagnosis and prognosis) than they are in "finding a cure." It is extremely important to reassure patients that "hurt is not equal to harm" in almost all cases. Older treatment regimens recommended bed rest, but studies have shown that early activity as tolerated leads to a better outcome.

14. **e.** A cornerstone of treating LBP is physical exercise. The Cochrane Review of exercise for LBP concluded that there was no evidence to indicate that specific exercises are effective for the treatment of acute LBP, but exercises may be helpful for chronic LBP. Scientific information about the method of action exerted by physical exercise is limited, which reflects the uncertainty regarding the pathophysiology of LBP. Exercises allow patients to participate in the treatment program and serve to prevent contractures, deconditioning, and weakness. Contrary to popular belief, exercise programs can safely begin within hours of developing LBP or an exacerbation of chronic LBP, even with the persisting muscle spasm.

The exercise programs that have been developed tend to emphasize repeated flexion and extension exercises and abdominal and lumbar strengthening exercises.

Any exercise program that is developed and begun should follow a graduated course. Patients need to be warned about a temporary increase in pain; otherwise they will tend to stop the program when it occurs. Stretching exercises are recommended first, followed by isometric strengthening exercises. One of the most important aspects of any exercise program is regularity.

15. **d.** In the treatment of acute LBP and sciatica there is no good evidence to support the recommendation of bed rest or exercise therapy. TENS has not been shown to be effective in the treatment of chronic LBP. Although muscle relaxants are effective in managing LBP, they have not been shown to be more effective than NSAIDs. NSAIDs are effective for short-term relief of symptoms from acute LBP.

Physical therapy and spinal manipulation are other modalities used in the treatment of LBP. At 6 months the functional status of patients with LBP demonstrates no difference regardless of the type of therapy that had been used. Patient satisfaction, however, is higher with hands-on types of therapy.

SUMMARY OF LOW BACK PAIN

1. **Incidence:** 5% per year. Lifetime prevalence is approximately 90%. LBP is considered one of the most expensive ailments in advanced industrial societies. LBP in industrialized countries can be labeled an epidemic.
2. **History/physical examination:** both the history and the physical examination lack both sensitivity and specificity.
3. **Pathophysiology:** LBP has been described as "an illness in search of a disease." Specific medical diagnosis and specific medical therapy are seldom possible. It is very difficult to specifically identify if chronic LBP is muscular, ligamentous/tendinous, facet joint, or discogenic in origin.
4. **Common diagnoses:**
   a. Mechanical LBP or back strain: pain in low back, buttock, or posterior thigh increased with activity or bending. Examination: localized tenderness, limited spinal motion.
   b. Acute disc herniation: usually acute onset of sharp, burning, radiating pain. Pain aggravated with coughing, sneezing, straining, sitting, and forward bending. Examination: positive straight leg raise test in seated and supine positions, possible weakness or asymmetric reflexes.
   c. Spinal stenosis: pain aggravated with standing and walking and relieved with sitting, spinal flexion, or walking uphill. Examination: limited and/or painful spinal extension.
   d. Spondylolysis: stress fracture of the pars interarticularis, seen mostly in athletes who perform repetitive spinal extension movements (e.g., gymnasts, football offensive linemen). Examination: pain with extension (single leg hyperextension test).

Continued

SUMMARY OF LOW BACK PAIN —cont'd

5. **Investigations:** radiographs, CT scans, and MRIs are the most commonly used tests but are over-used and suffer from a lack of specificity. Plain spine x-rays in most cases are virtually useless.
6. **Nomenclature:** the debate over musculoligamentous or spinal LBP is resolved with the diagnosis of "mechanical" LBP.
7. **Treatment:**
   a. Education of patients: education is the most crucial and cost-effective treatment. This often alleviates the patient's worry that the pain is caused by a "serious illness."
   b. The Cochrane Collaboration systematic reviews for "best evidence" for treatment of acute and chronic LBP recommends that for acute LBP stay active and use NSAIDs, muscle relaxants, or analgesics. For chronic LBP "back schools" are recommended to learn behavioral treatments and exercise therapy.
   c. Medications: NSAIDs are effective for short-term symptomatic relief of symptoms caused by acute LBP. Acetaminophen may relieve pain symptoms, but more studies comparing them with NSAIDs are needed. Muscle relaxants are effective in management of nonspecific LBP.

Narcotic analgesics may be necessary for management of acute LBP but should be avoided in patients with chronic LBP.
   d. Physical treatments: physical therapy and manipulation do not change outcome but improve patient satisfaction.
   e. Supports (including lumbar braces and corsets): there is no evidence to support their use for LBP.
   f. Epidural corticosteroids: there is no evidence of any long-term benefit.
   g. Surgery: This is the final resort. It is indicated for intractable discogenic pain, progressive neurologic deficits, and advanced symptoms and signs of spinal stenosis unresponsive to other modalities. For herniated disc disease, the long-term outcomes are not any better for surgical versus conservative therapy.

SUGGESTED READING

Patel AT, Ogle AA: Diagnosis and management of acute low back pain. *Am Fam Physician* 61:1779-1786, 1789-1790, 2000.
Sierpina VS, et al: An integrative approach to low back pain. *Clin Inv Fam Pract* 4(4), 2002.
Swink HG, et al: Low Back Pain Symposium. *Am J Med Sci* 324(4):207-211, 2002.
The Cochrane Database of Systematic Reviews. *The Cochrane Collaboration* Vol 3, 2003.

Chapter 157

Acceleration and Deceleration Neck Injuries

"I always wanted a fur neck piece, but I had a different style in mind."

CLINICAL CASE PROBLEM 1:

A 32-Year-Old Female with Very Severe Neck Pain

A 32-year-old female comes into your office complaining of "very severe" neck pain that radiates to the region of the left shoulder. She was involved in a motor vehicle accident 1 day ago. Her car was struck from behind while stopped at a traffic light. The pain did not start until this morning and has gotten progressively worse. Over-the-counter analgesics have given no relief. Past medical history is negative, including no previous history of neck pain.

On examination there is significantly decreased range of motion of the neck in all planes. There is tenderness to palpation in the cervical paraspinal muscles bilaterally. There is no bony tenderness. You try to perform a Sperling's test, but the patient has too much pain when you attempt to put the neck into the provocative position. There are no neurologic deficits.

■ SELECT THE BEST ANSWER TO THE FOLLOWING QUESTIONS:

1. Which of the following statements regarding whiplash injury is correct?
   a. symptoms are often out of proportion to physical findings
   b. only about 1% of patients will have an abnormality on magnetic resonance imaging (MRI) scan related to the trauma
   c. x-rays often show a slight flattening of the normal lordotic curvature of the cervical spine

d. the annual economic cost in the United States related to whiplash injury is in the billions of dollars

e. all of the above

2. Which of the following statements regarding the mechanism of whiplash injury is correct?
   a. most commonly results from motor vehicle accident
   b. after a rear impact, the lower cervical vertebrae appear to move into extension and the upper cervical vertebrae appear to move into relative flexion
   c. the cervical paraspinal muscles are not involved
   d. a and b
   e. all of the above

3. Which of the following is the best treatment option for the patient in Clinical Case Problem 1?
   a. soft cervical collar
   b. hard cervical collar
   c. early exercise therapy
   d. bed rest
   e. none of the above

4. Which of the following is a predictor of delayed recovery from a whiplash injury?
   a. older age
   b. severe pain
   c. radicular symptoms
   d. a and c
   e. a, b, and c

5. Which of the following is a correct statement regarding whiplash injury?
   a. insurance and compensation systems have no impact on prognosis
   b. without any treatment, a large number of patients will get better within 6 months
   c. patients rarely have loss of neck motion
   d. all of the above
   e. none of the above

ANSWERS:

1. **e.** All of the above. The symptoms of whiplash injury are often out of proportion to the findings on examination. Only about 1% of patients with a whiplash injury will have an abnormality related to trauma, such as prevertebral edema, on MRI. After an acceleration–deceleration injury, radiographs often show a slight flattening of the normal lordotic curve of the cervical spine. Whiplash injuries pose a tremendous economic cost, in the billions of the dollars, in the United States.

2. **d.** Whiplash injuries most commonly result when a person in a stopped car is struck from behind. Recent studies have demonstrated that with a rear impact the cervical spine moves into an abnormal S-shaped pattern, with the lower cervical vertebrae moving into an extended position and the upper cervical vertebrae moving into a flexed position. The cervical paraspinal muscles respond by contracting.

3. **c.** The best treatment is early exercise therapy. This has been shown to reduce pain and increase motion of the cervical spine. Bed rest and cervical collars have been shown to slow healing.

4. **e.** Predictors of delayed recovery from a whiplash injury include older age, radicular symptoms, and severe neck or head pain.

5. **b.** Insurance and compensation systems significantly influence the prognosis of whiplash injuries. Even without any treatment, a large number of patients will get better within 6 months after sustaining a whiplash injury. Patients commonly have restricted motion of the cervical spine after sustaining an acceleration–deceleration type neck injury.

SUMMARY OF ACCELERATION AND DECELERATION NECK INJURIES

1. The neck injury most commonly results when the patient is in a stopped car that is struck from behind by another vehicle.
2. Such injuries have a major economic cost (billions of dollars).
3. Radiographs frequently show a slight flattening of the normal lordotic curve of the cervical spine.
4. MRI usually shows no abnormality related to the trauma sustained in an acceleration–deceleration injury.
5. The cervical spine assumes an S-shaped pattern immediately on impact, with the lower cervical vertebrae moving into an extended position and the upper cervical vertebrae moving into a flexed position.
6. Predictors of delayed recovery include older age, radicular symptoms, and severe neck or head pain.
7. Insurance and compensation systems influence the prognosis of these injuries.
8. Exercise therapy is recommended early on in the treatment.
9. Even without treatment, most people will get better within 6 months.

SUGGESTED READING

Cote P, et al: A systematic review of the prognosis of acute whiplash and a new conceptual framework to synthesize the literature. *Spine* 26(19):E445-E458, 2001.

Eck JC, et al: Whiplash: a review of a commonly misunderstood injury. *Am J Med* 110(8):651-656, 2001.

Rao R: Neck pain, cervical radiculopathy, and cervical myelopathy: pathophysiology, natural history, and clinical evaluation. *J Bone Joint Sci* 84-A(10):1872-1881, 2002.

 Chapter 158

Concussions

"I don't want to wear a helmet. None of the big boys do."

CLINICAL CASE PROBLEM 1:
AN UNCONSCIOUS FOOTBALL PLAYER

As team physician for a high school football team, you are standing on the sideline during a game when you note that one player does not rise after a play. When you reach him, he is lying on his back with his eyes closed. He is not moving.

■ SELECT THE BEST ANSWER TO THE FOLLOWING QUESTIONS:

1. The first thing to do for this patient is:
   a. establish that the patient has a patent airway and is breathing.
   b. place a roll under the patient's neck for support
   c. check the pupils
   d. take off the patient's helmet and pads
   e. place an intravenous line

2. After approximately 10 seconds, the patient awakens. He is disoriented and confused but can tell you his name and what he had for breakfast. He does not, however, remember anything about the game. He denies any neck pain and is allowed to sit up. With help, he walks to the sideline and sits down again for your evaluation. He says that he feels perfectly fine and wants to go back into the game. Your evaluation should include:
   a. a complete neurologic evaluation
   b. immediate and long-term memory recall
   c. balance testing
   d. serial subtraction testing
   e. all of the above

3. After a few moments of evaluation, the athlete begins to complain of a severe right-sided headache. He becomes lethargic and lapses again into unconsciousness. He is immediately taken to the emergency room by the ambulance on the sideline. What injury is he most likely to account for his second collapse?

   a. subdural hematoma
   b. epidural hematoma
   c. diffuse axonal injury
   d. second-impact syndrome
   e. subarachnoid hemorrhage

CLINICAL CASE PROBLEM 2:
A CONFUSED FOOTBALL PLAYER

You are covering a college football game as a team physician. A player sustains a hard hit to the head while being tackled by two other players. He stands up directly after the play, shakes his head for a moment, and then joins the huddle for the next play. He appears confused and runs to the wrong spot. After a few more plays, one of his teammates tells the trainer that he is not remembering the plays.

4. When the trainer tells you this information, you:
   a. allow him to continue play because he had no loss of consciousness and the game is almost over
   b. have the trainer check to make sure that there is enough air in his helmet
   c. watch him more carefully on the next play
   d. remove him immediately from play for evaluation
   e. remind the trainer that this particular player failed most of his classes the previous semester

5. When you speak to the athlete, he states that he feels fine and wants to go back to play. He denies headache or dizziness and has a normal neurologic examination. He cannot recall three objects 2 minutes after being told them. He also cannot subtract serial 7s accurately. You now should:
   a. allow him to return to play because he has a normal neurologic examination
   b. send him directly to the hospital for a computed tomography (CT) scan of the head
   c. have the athlete sit down quietly and retest him in 15 minutes
   d. send him to the showers
   e. send him home with his parents

6. The most important reason for not allowing an athlete with symptoms of a concussion to play is:

a. he has not been checked for a neck injury
b. the athlete may experience headache and dizziness with exertion
c. if the athlete is injured, the physician is likely to be sued
d. if the patient cannot remember the plays, the team is likely to lose the game
e. the athlete is at risk for much more severe injury if he sustains another hit

7. Choose the following statement that is false:
   a. approximately 10% of college football players will sustain a concussion each season
   b. multiple concussions can result in cumulative brain damage
   c. there does not have to be a loss of consciousness for there to be a diagnosis of concussion
   d. athletes readily admit to symptoms of a concussion
   e. close observation of the athlete is of critical importance after a head injury

8. Warning signs for which an athlete who has sustained a concussion should seek immediate medical evaluation include:
   a. difficulty in staying awake
   b. seizures
   c. urinary or bowel incontinence
   d. weakness or numbness of any part of the body
   e. all of the above

CLINICAL CASE PROBLEM 3:
A Gymnast Who Fell and Hit Her Head

A gymnast fell off of the uneven bars during a competition and hit her head on the ground. She had a 2-minute loss of consciousness and had posttraumatic amnesia for 2 hours, which completely resolved. She was sent to the emergency room and had a CT scan of the head, which was negative for any intracranial bleeding. She was discharged to home. She now comes 2 days later to your office complaining of headache and the inability to concentrate in class.

9. This patient has signs and symptoms of:
   a. postconcussive syndrome
   b. continuing symptoms of a concussion
   c. second-impact syndrome
   d. epidural hematoma
   e. malingering

10. The athlete in Clinical Case Problem 3 has an important competition coming up in 2 days. She should be:

a. allowed to participate because her CT scan was negative for any bleeding
b. allowed to do any event except for the uneven bars
c. restricted from any activity until she has been asymptomatic for 1 week and has no symptoms on exertion
d. restricted until her headache goes away at rest
e. readmitted to the hospital for another CT scan of the head

11. The athlete in Clinical Case Problem 3 recovers and returns to competition after 1 week. Two weeks later, she receives a glancing blow to the head and sustains another loss of consciousness, this time of less than 30 seconds. She has no amnesia and recovers quickly with no symptoms of headache or difficulty concentrating. She should:
    a. return to competition as soon as she is asymptomatic
    b. return to competition when she has been asymptomatic for 1 week
    c. be restricted for activity for at least 1 month, then only may return if she is asymptomatic for more than 1 week
    d. return to competition but wear a helmet
    e. exercise on a stationary bicycle for 2 weeks

12. Which one of the following statements is not true?
    a. the Glasgow coma scale is a useful adjunct for evaluating an athlete after a head injury
    b. despite the guidelines for return to play as compiled by Cantu and others, the final decision should be based on the individual situation and the best clinical judgment
    c. types of intracranial injuries that can be encountered in the athlete include epidural hematomas, subdural hematomas, subarachnoid hemorrhages, diffuse axonal injury, and intracerebral hematomas
    d. concussions can have longlasting effects on cognitive abilities and concentration
    e. concussions can be prevented by proper helmet use

■ ANSWERS:

1. **a.** No matter what the situation, the ABCs of airway, breathing, and circulation should be the clinician's first concern. Once these are established, other concerns can be addressed. An unconscious football player cannot tell the physician if his neck is hurting; therefore, any unconscious player is assumed

to have a cervical spine injury until proved otherwise. The spine should be immobilized, and if the patient is prone, experienced team members can help to log-roll the patient. Football pads and helmet are specially designed to keep the head and neck in a proper position, so they should not be removed until the patient is under controlled circumstances where the entire head and spine can be stabilized. The face mask of the helmet can be removed if the athlete's airway is an issue. A roll should not be placed under the patient's neck. Checking the pupils will be a part of the later assessment.

2. **e.** Evaluation after a head injury should include a complete neurologic examination. Concussion is described by the Congress of Neurological Surgeons as "a clinical syndrome characterized by immediate and transient post-traumatic impairment of neural functions, such as alteration of consciousness, disturbance of vision, equilibrium, etc. due to brainstem involvement." Any loss or alteration of consciousness requires a complete examination. Neuropsychological testing is critical to determine the athlete's cognitive function and coordination. Athletes can be apparently asymptomatic after a concussion and still have severe problems with memory, concentration, and coordination. Asking patients to recall what they had for breakfast tests long-term memory. Giving the athlete several items to remember and then asking for them a few moments later tests immediate recall. Asking the athlete to subtract serial 7s from 100 assesses figuring and concentration. Balancing on one foot with the eyes closed tests coordination.

3. **b.** This case shows a common presentation of an epidural hematoma. The typical scenario is that of an athlete sustaining a head injury, commonly on the temple. The athlete has a brief period of confusion or unconsciousness and then has a "lucid period," during which the athlete feels fine. Rapid deterioration, lethargy, and unconsciousness occurs in the next stage. This is caused by a high-pressure arterial bleed into the epidural space, often from rupture of the middle meningeal artery as it passes behind the temporal bone. Prompt neurosurgical evacuation of the hematoma is critical and must be done emergently. If the hematoma can be recognized and evacuated in a timely manner, the prognosis is good for these patients because there is usually little underlying brain damage. Failure to recognize and evacuate this hematoma can lead to coma and death.

4. **d.** The player should be immediately removed from play for evaluation. Despite having no loss of consciousness, he is symptomatic with amnesia and

has sustained at least a Grade I concussion. He must be evaluated and protected from subsequent hits, which could worsen his condition. Hits such as the one that this athlete sustained often are referred to as "dings" or having one's "bell rung." Safety equipment such as helmets should regularly be checked, but in this situation the athlete has already sustained the hit. The athlete's academic performance has no bearing on whether he can remember his regular plays.

There are several different systems of scoring concussions. One of the most widely known was developed by Dr. Robert C. Cantu. By his scoring system, a Grade I concussion consists of no loss of consciousness and posttraumatic amnesia lasting less than 30 minutes. Grade II concussion consists of a loss of consciousness of less than 5 minutes and/or posttraumatic amnesia lasting more than 30 minutes but less than 24 hours. Grade III concussion consists of a loss of consciousness of 5 minutes or greater and/or posttraumatic amnesia lasting 24 hours or more.

5. **c.** The athlete is still experiencing posttraumatic amnesia and must continue to be evaluated. There are no focal deficits on neurologic examination to cause concern. The athlete should sit quietly on the bench (and not exert himself on the sideline) under close observation. In about 15-20 minutes, he can be reevaluated for amnesia. In most cases without a loss of consciousness, the posttraumatic amnesia will resolve in less than 30 minutes and therefore be scored as a Grade I concussion. He should not go home with his parents until his symptoms have resolved, and he should definitely not go to the showers, where he will be unobserved. At this time, there is no indication for a CT scan of the head.

6. **e.** Athletes still suffering symptoms from a concussion should not be allowed to play. The effects of multiple head injuries have been found to be cumulative. Also, after an athlete sustains one concussion, he or she is more likely to sustain another concussion, sometimes with a mild hit. The most significant cause for concern would be the so-called "second-impact syndrome." This entity has been observed in athletes sustaining a second hit while still recovering from the first. When this occurs, the autoregulation of the brain is lost, and there is an intense reaction of brain swelling and edema. There is a greater than 50% mortality rate with this condition. This catastrophic possibility is the reasoning behind limiting the activity of all athletes continuing to be symptomatic after a head injury.

7. **d.** Often, athletes are so enthusiastic about their sport that they wish to participate even after a significant

head injury. Athletes may not understand the dangers of participation and may lie about their symptoms so as to return to play. This is where accurate neuropsychological testing is critical; if an athlete has amnesia, they cannot "fake" memory. If hand–eye coordination or balance have not yet recovered, this also will be obvious on testing.

Prevalence studies have shown about a 10% rate of concussion per season for college football players. Other risky sports include ice hockey, soccer, boxing, gymnastics, and wrestling.

As discussed previously, according to the Cantu scoring system, there does not need to be a loss of consciousness for a diagnosis of concussion. Multiple head injuries can cause cumulative brain damage. Close observation is of critical importance for any athlete with any type of head injury.

8. e. Any athlete who develops the following symptoms should seek immediate medical attention, even if he or she has been asymptomatic after a head injury: lethargy or difficulty in staying awake, loss of bowel or bladder function, vomiting, severe or worsening headache, neck pain, seizures, weakness or numbness, or difficulties with vision. Any of these symptoms could indicate a more serious injury.

9. a. This patient has signs and symptoms of postconcussive syndrome. These symptoms include headache, dizziness, inability to concentrate, irritability, tinnitus, problems with balance, fatigue, or difficulty sleeping. These symptoms can last for days to weeks after a concussion.

Because this patient recovered her memory within 2 hours of the injury, she is no longer experiencing the actual concussion. This injury would be classified as a Grade II concussion by the Cantu criteria because her loss of consciousness was less than 5 minutes and her posttraumatic amnesia was less than 24 hours.

The patient, by history, has not sustained another head injury, so second-impact syndrome would be highly unlikely.

10. c. The athlete should be restricted from activity until she has been asymptomatic for 1 week. When she has been asymptomatic, she may begin light exercise. If the headache or other symptoms recur, she should cease the activity and rest. Symptoms may recur with exertion, even when the athlete feels normal at rest. Allowing her to participate puts her at risk for another head injury, especially in a sport such as gymnastics, in which precision and balance are critical for safety.

Even without bleeding on CT scan, the athlete may have sustained significant shearing injury or diffuse axonal injury. These injuries can cause disability and place the athlete at risk for further head injuries.

It is relatively common for an athlete to experience symptoms like this after a significant concussion as described. If the symptoms do not improve over the following days, however, a repeat CT or magnetic resonance imaging (MRI) or the head may be warranted to rule out any further injury such as cerebral contusion or slow bleeding subdural hematoma.

11. c. Separate guidelines exist for return to play guidelines after multiple concussions. The athlete in this case has sustained two Grade II concussions and therefore must be restricted for at least 1 month to prevent her from sustaining further injury. All exertional physical activity, including stationary bicycling, should be restricted. The Cantu guidelines for return to play are as follows: For the first Grade I concussion, the athlete may return to play if asymptomatic for one week. For the second concussion, the athlete may return to play in 2 weeks if asymptomatic for 1 week. After the third concussion in one season, the athlete's season should be terminated, with return the next season if asymptomatic.

For the first Grade II concussion, the athlete may return to play if asymptomatic for 1 week. After the second concussion, the athlete must wait a minimum of 1 month and may return at that point if asymptomatic for 1 week. After the third concussion, the season should be terminated.

For the first Grade III concussion, the athlete should wait a minimum of 1 month and then may return if asymptomatic for 1 week. After the second concussion, the season should be terminated.

12. e. Proper helmet and other safety equipment use can decrease the likelihood of concussion, but no helmets or safety measures have been found to eliminate risk altogether. Certain sports carry a small but definite risk of serious, even fatal, injury. Athletes and parents should be aware of this. The Glasgow coma scale should be used as a helpful tool in evaluating an athlete with a head injury. Types of intracranial injuries that can be encountered in the athlete include epidural hematomas, subdural hematomas, subarachnoid hemorrhages, diffuse axonal injury, and intracerebral hematomas. Cognitive deficits and impaired concentration can linger for weeks after a concussion, as described as a part of the postconcussion syndrome. It must be remembered that the guidelines for return to play, as published by Cantu and others, are comprehensive and of great use but are only guidelines. Each athlete is an individual, and clinical judgment must be the deciding factor in decisions to return to play safely.

SUMMARY OF CONCUSSIONS

Concussion is described by the Congress of Neurological Surgeons as "a clinical syndrome characterized by immediate and transient posttraumatic impairment of neural functions, such as alteration of consciousness, disturbance of vision, equilibrium, etc. due to brainstem involvement." Participation in certain sports, especially contact sports, places the athlete at risk for concussion. Several grading systems have been developed for evaluating the severity of a concussion. One of the most widely used was developed with Dr. Robert C. Cantu.

Grade I: no loss of consciousness and posttraumatic amnesia for less than 30 minutes.

Grade II: loss of consciousness of less than 5 minutes and/or posttraumatic amnesia for more than 30 minutes but less than 24 hours

Grade III: loss of consciousness of greater than 5 minutes and/or posttraumatic amnesia for greater than 24 hours

Concussion can represent different types of brain injury, and the clinician must be considering epidural hematomas, subdural hematomas, subarachnoid hemorrhages, diffuse axonal injury, and intracerebral hematomas in the differential examination. Suspicion of intracranial bleeding, lethargy, emesis, worsening headaches, neck injury, bowel or bladder incontinence, and focal neurologic signs should elicit prompt referral to a hospital with a neurosurgical service.

Postconcussion syndrome is characterized by continuing headache, dizziness, inability to concentrate, impaired balance or cognitive ability, irritability, fatigue, and difficulties sleeping. Patients should be followed closely and kept at rest because exercise may exacerbate the symptoms.

Return-to-play guidelines were listed earlier in the chapter and are very useful to the clinician, but individual clinical judgment should be the deciding factor. Athletes who have sustained one concussion are more likely than others to sustain another concussion. In addition, the "second-impact syndrome" is a catastrophic syndrome of sudden brain edema after a second head injury, in which the athlete had not yet recovered from the first head injury. This carries a high mortality rate and is the basis for keeping an athlete out of activity until completely recovered.

SUGGESTED READING

Cantu RC: Return to play guidelines after a head injury. *Clin Sports Med* 17(1):Jan 1998, 45-60.

Kelly JP, Rosenberg JH: The development of guidelines for the management of concussion in sports. *J Head Trauma Rehabil* 13:53-65, 1998.

Kuschner DS: Concussion in sports: minimizing the risk for complications. *Am Fam Physician* 64(6):1007-1018, 2001.

Solomos NJ: Management guidelines for sport related concussions. *Am Fam Physician* 65(12):2435-2436, 2002.

Chapter 159

Exercise Prescription

"I don't want to do all that jumping up and down. Isn't there a pill that will work just as well?"

CLINICAL CASE PROBLEM 1:

A 48-Year-Woman Wanting to Start an Exercise Program

A 48-year-old woman comes into the office with questions and concerns about starting an exercise program. Although she has been sedentary most of her life she is very determined to change. She has heard about all the benefits of exercise. Her past medical history is positive for hypertension that is well controlled by taking a low dose of hydrochlorothiazide, and she has a history of irregular heavy menses now controlled by low-dose oral contraceptives.

On physical examination her blood pressure is 125/85 and her pulse is 82 beats/minute. Her cardiovascular examination reveals regular rhythm and rate (RRR) with a mid-systolic click. Her lungs are clear and her abdomen is benign. The rest of the examination is normal.

■ SELECT THE BEST ANSWER TO THE FOLLOWING QUESTIONS:

1. Which of the following would be an appropriate intervention prior to this patient's commencement of an exercise program?
   a. echocardiography
   b. complete blood count (CBC)
   c. ferritin level
   d. exercise stress test
   e. no testing is indicated

2. Exercise improves outcomes for which of the following conditions:

a. type 2 diabetes mellitus
b. depression
c. obesity
d. hypertension
e. all of the above

3. Which one of the following statements regarding exercise is true?
   a. about 40% of adults in the United Stated exercise enough to derive health benefits from physical activity
   b. previous athletic performance or exercise provides lasting protection
   c. increased levels of physical activity are inversely proportional to long-term cardiovascular mortality
   d. about 70% of physicians counsel their patients about exercise
   e. there is no evidence to support exercise as a primary intervention to promote health

4. The cardiovascular benefits of exercise include which of the following:
   a. reduced systolic and diastolic blood pressure
   b. reduced serum triglyceride level
   c. increased serum high-density lipoprotein (HDL) level
   d. reduced arterial stiffness
   e. all of the above

5. Which one of the following statements about exercise, heart rate, and autonomic function is true?
   a. regular exercise does not lower resting heart rates
   b. exercise increases heart rate variability
   c. endurance training results in decreased parasympathetic (vagal) tone
   d. endurance training results in a less rapid decrease in heart rate after exercise
   e. all of the above

6. The exercise prescription should include which of the following:
   a. flexibility training
   b. resistance or weight training
   c. duration of exercise
   d. intensity of exercise
   e. all of the above

7. Which one of the following statements about the exercise prescription is true?
   a. exercise should be performed 2 days every week
   b. exercise should be performed continuously for 90 minutes to gain any health benefits
   c. resistance training is not recommended for people older than 60 age years

d. increasing the intensity of exercise does not reduce the risk of coronary heart disease
e. there is a lack of evidence regarding the benefit of flexibility exercises in the prevention and treatment of musculoskeletal injuries

8. Which one of the following statements about exercise intensity is true?
   a. high-intensity exercise is defined as 65% of an individual's maximum heart rate
   b. exercise intensity can be measured in METs (metabolic equivalents); a MET is the amount of oxygen consumed during low-intensity exercise
   c. low-intensity exercise has no health benefits
   d. the formula, 220 minus the age of the patient, underestimates the maximum heart rate, especially in people older than age 55 years
   e. if a person can hold a conversation while exercising, they are exercising at an intensity too low to derive any health benefits

9. About 50% of people stop an exercise program within 6-12 months. Which of the following has been shown to increase adherence to an exercise program?
   a. a high-intensity exercise program
   b. exercising alone
   c. increasing the intensity and duration of an exercise program by 40% each week
   d. alternating activities
   e. exercising just before bedtime

10. Which of the following are normal responses during exercise?
    a. the diastolic blood pressure remains the same or decreases
    b. the systolic blood pressure increases
    c. heart rate decreases by 12 beats or more during the first minute after peak exercise
    d. heart rate increases with exercise secondary to a withdrawal of vagal tone and increasing sympathetic tone
    e. all of the above

■ ANSWERS:

1. **e.** No testing is indicated. According to the American College of Sports Medicine guidelines, a woman younger than age 55 years who is asymptomatic and has only one risk factor for coronary artery disease does not need an exercise stress test prior to the start of an exercise program. Unless an individual is at high risk for coronary artery disease, an exercise stress test is not necessary before beginning a

moderate exercise program. Moderate exercise is defined as an intensity well within the individual's capacity and one that can be sustained for a prolonged period (45 minutes). There is no evidence that an exercise stress test or echocardiogram at this age will predict increased mortality or morbidity. An exercise stress test can have false-positive results. Despite the history of heavy menses, there is no need to check for anemia because she is taking an oral contraceptive.

2. e. All of the above. Exercise improves outcomes for many conditions including the following: atherosclerosis; ischemic heart disease; hypertension; type 2 diabetes mellitus; osteoarthritis; obesity; asthma; chronic obstructive pulmonary disease; osteoporosis; depression; anxiety; and cancer of the colon, breast, prostate, and rectum.

3. c. Increased levels of physical activity are inversely proportional to long-term cardiovascular mortality. Only 20% to 25% of adults exercise enough to derive health benefits from physical activity. Vigorous exercise early in life does not provide lasting protection. A physically active lifestyle throughout life confers significant health benefits. Less than 35% of physicians counsel their patients about exercise. Evidence supports exercise as a primary intervention to promote health.

4. e. All of the above. The cardiovascular benefits of exercise include the following: reduced systolic and diastolic blood pressure, decreased low-density lipoprotein levels, increased HDL levels, reduced triglyceride levels, reduced obesity, increased maximal volume of oxygen utilization (VO_2 max), increased insulin sensitivity, improved fibrinolysis and lowered levels of fibrinogen, reduced arterial stiffness and improved arterial compliance, and increased heart rate variability. It also improves myocardial function, including increased contractility, faster relaxation rates, enzymatic alterations, increased calcium availability, and improved autonomic and hormonal function.

5. b. Exercise increases heart rate variability. A delayed recovery of heart rate after exercise significantly increases mortality. Regular exercise lowers resting and submaximal heart rates. Endurance training results in an increased parasympathetic tone (vagal) tone and a more rapid decrease in heart rate after exercise.

6. e. All of the above. An exercise prescription should include mention of the following:

1. The type of activity. This should take into account a patient's medical status, level of fitness, interests, available exercise facilities, climate, and geographic location.
2. The frequency of exercise. The current recommendation is for people to exercise on most, preferably all, days of the week.
3. The duration of exercise. People should engage in 20-60 minutes of continuous or intermittent aerobic activity throughout the day.
4. The intensity of exercise. Moderate-intensity exercise, exercising at a level equal to 65% to 75% of a person's maximum heart rate, is recommended. Several methods are used to calculate the proper intensity. These include the following:
   a. The commonly used formula "220 minus age" to measure the maximal heart rate. This formula, however, underestimates the maximum heart rate especially in people older than age 55 years.
   b. The Karvonen method to calculate exercise intensity is as follows: Training heart rate = (HRmax − RHR) × 0.7 + RHR. (HRmax, maximum heart rate; RHR, resting heart rate.)
   c. The "talk test" can be used to avoid exercising at too high an intensity. People should exercise at an intensity not to exceed that of being able to carry on a conversation.
   d. Exercise intensity also can be measured in METs. A MET is the resting metabolic rate or the amount of oxygen consumed at rest, which is approximately 3.5 ml O_2/kg/min. Metabolic equivalents are determined by treadmill testing.
5. Resistance training or weight lifting. Resistance training results in lower heart rate and blood pressure response to any given load and can improve aerobic endurance. Weight training reduces risk of coronary heart disease. Recommendation is a minimum of 8-10 exercises involving major muscle groups performed 2-3 days per week using a minimum of one set of 8-12 repetitions. For older people 10-15 repetitions at lower resistance is more desirable because muscle strength declines by 15% per decade after age 50 and 30% per decade after age 70. The goal is to lift weight that is 70% to 80% of one maximum lift.

Contraindications to resistance training are unstable angina, uncontrolled hypertension, uncontrolled dysrhythmias, uncontrolled chronic heart failure, severe stenotic or regurgitant valvular disease, and hypertrophic cardiomyopathy.

6. Flexibility training: Although there is a lack of evidence regarding benefit of flexibility exercises in prevention and treatment of musculoskeletal injuries, it still is recommended to stretch major muscle/tendon groups, four repetitions per muscle group, a minimum of 2-3 days per week. Static stretches should be held for 10-30 seconds.

7. Warm-up and cool-down periods. Before and after exercise there should be a 5-10 minute period of stretching and low-level aerobic exercise.

7. e. As stated earlier, there is a lack of evidence regarding the benefit of flexibility exercises in the prevention and treatment of musculoskeletal injuries. Exercise should be performed on all or most days of the week. Exercise does not have to be continuous to gain health benefits. Short bouts of exercise throughout the day are just as beneficial as continuous exercise. Resistance training is recommended for all adult age groups. Increasing the intensity of exercise does reduce the risk of coronary artery disease.

8. d. As stated earlier, the formula "220 minus age" underestimates the maximum heart rate, especially in people older than age 55 years. High-intensity exercise is defined as 75% to 90% of a person's maximum heart rate. A MET is the amount of oxygen consumed at rest. Low-intensity exercise has health benefits. Exercising at an intensity still permitting one to hold a conversation has health benefits and prevents exercising at too high an intensity.

9. d. Alternating activities has been shown to increase adherence to an exercise program. Other interventions to increase adherence to an exercise program include the following: setting specific goals; physician's active interest; repeated counseling and educating patients about health benefits of exercise; encouragement of family and friends; limiting increases in duration and intensity to 5% to 10% per week to reduce risk of injury; and exercising with others. Patients are also more likely to adhere to moderate-intensity program than a high-intensity one.

10. e. All of the above.

SUMMARY OF EXERCISE PRESCRIPTION

1. Exercise is a primary intervention to promote health and is as powerful as smoking cessation, blood pressure control, and lipid management in lowering mortality from coronary artery disease.
2. Exercise has a favorable influence on multiple body systems and improves outcomes for many chronic diseases, including diabetes, hypertension, obesity, and depression.
3. Exercise training results in increased parasympathetic (vagal) tone and a subsequent more rapid decrease in heart rate after exercise, lower resting and submaximal heart rates, and increased heart rate variability.
4. Components of exercise prescription include the following: (a) type of activity; (b) frequency; (c) duration; (e) intensity; (f) resistance training; (g) flexibility training; (h) and warmup and cooldown.
5. Encourage adherence to an exercise program.
6. Increasing physical activity is a major goal in the health initiative *Healthy People 2010* by the U.S. Department of Health and Human Services.

SUGGESTED READING

American College of Sports Medicine: ACSM Position Stand: The recommended quantity and quality of exercise for developing and maintaining cardiorespiratory and muscular fitness, and flexibility in healthy adults. *Med Sci Sport Exer* 30(6):975-991, 1998.

Andersen RE, et al: Encouraging patients to become more physically active: the physician's role. *Ann Intern Med* 127(5):395-400, 1997.

Blair SN, et al: Changes in physical fitness and all-cause mortality. *JAMA* 273:1093-1098, 1995.

Cole CR, et al: Heart rate recovery immediately after exercise as a predictor of mortality. *N Engl J Med* 341:1351-1357, 1999.

Dustan D, et al: High intensity resistance training improves glycemic control in older patients with type 2 diabetes. *Diabetes Care* 25(10):1729-1736, 2002.

Manson JE, et al: Walking compared with vigorous exercise for the prevention of cardiovascular events in women. *N Engl J Med* 347(10):716-725, 2002.

Rosenwinkel ET, et al: Exercise and autonomic function in health and cardiovascular disease. *Cardiol Clin* 19(3):369-387, 2001.

Stein PK, et al: Effect of exercise training on heart rate variability in healthy older adults. *Am Heart J* 138(3):567-576, 1999.

Tanasescu M, et al: Exercise type and intensity in relation to coronary heart disease in men. *JAMA* 288(16):1994-2000, 2002.

U.S. Department of Health and Human Services: *Healthy People 2010: Understanding and Improving Health,* 2nd ed. U.S. Government Printing Office, November 2000, Washington, DC.

U.S. Preventive Services Task Force: Behavioral counseling in primary care to promote physical activity: recommendations and rationale. *Am Fam Physician* 66(10):1931-1936, 2002.

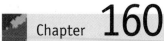

Chapter **160**

Female Athlete Triad

"You mean I exercise too much?"

CLINICAL CASE PROBLEM 1:
A 20-YEAR-OLD FEMALE RUNNER WITH "SHIN SPLINTS"

A 20-year-old cross-country runner presents for evaluation of "shin splints." She is a very competitive runner, averaging about 50-60 miles per week. On examination, the patient is a small, thin female with very well-defined musculature. She has some tenderness over both medial tibias but has one discrete area of increased point tenderness 3 cm proximal to the medial malleolus. Her coach is waiting outside to see when she will be able to return to running because they have an important meet next weekend.

■ **SELECT THE BEST ANSWER TO THE FOLLOWING QUESTIONS:**

1. What is the most important piece of history to obtain from this patient when suspecting a stress fracture?
   a. whether she has been icing the painful areas
   b. complete menstrual history
   c. how much she stretches before exercise
   d. medications that she is taking
   e. types of surfaces on which she runs

2. The female athlete triad consists of:
   a. anorexia, oligomenorrhea, calcium deficiency
   b. osteoporosis, stress fractures, calcium deficiency
   c. disordered eating, amenorrhea, osteoporosis
   d. disordered eating, use of laxatives, osteoporosis
   e. metamenorrhagia, hypothalamic dysfunction, osteoporosis

3. The best time to screen female athletes for risk factors for the female athlete triad is:
   a. at the preparticipation physical examination
   b. when the patient presents with an injury
   c. when the clinician notices that the patient is underweight or losing weight
   d. when the patient presents for a routine Pap test and pelvic examination
   e. after competition is complete for the season

4. When obtaining a history from a female athlete, critical questions to ask include:
   a. age of menarche, regularity, and date of last menstrual period
   b. whether the patient is happy with her weight and the patient's idea of her ideal body weight
   c. maximum and minimum weights that the patient has achieved
   d. history of any stress injuries or stress fractures
   e. all of the above

CLINICAL CASE PROBLEM 2:
AN 18-YEAR-OLD FEMALE WITH AMENORRHEA

An 18-year-old girl comes to the office with a complaint of amenorrhea. She experienced menarche at age 14, and since that time has been having about 4-6 menses per year. However, her last menstrual period was 9 months ago. She is a competitive gymnast and travels a great deal with her team and coaches. She says that she knows that it is "normal" for athletes to miss their periods but that her mother had wanted her to come in. She wants to know if there is any medication that you can give her that "won't make me fat."

5. Amenorrhea in the athlete is most specifically associated with:
   a. decreased levels of estrogen
   b. increased levels of progesterone
   c. calcium deficiency
   d. use of laxatives to lose weight
   e. exercise

6. Workup for amenorrhea for greater than 6 months duration in a female athlete could include the following except which one of the following?
   a. dual-energy x-ray absorptiometry (DEXA) bone mineral density scan
   b. serum electrolytes, complete blood count, thyroid panel and hormonal evaluation
   c. pelvic examination
   d. ultrasound of the abdomen and pelvis
   e. psychological evaluation

7. The following are characteristics of anorexia nervosa except which one of the following?
   a. distorted body image and excessive fear of gaining weight
   b. amenorrhea
   c. complete recovery in 50% of patients with counseling
   d. weight of less than the 85th percentile for age and height
   e. severe restriction of calories

8. Choose the true statement from the following:
   a. there are optimal body fat percentages specific for each sport

b. athletes with disordered eating habits often disclose this information on the first visit

c. teammates are almost always aware of another athlete's disordered eating behaviors

d. coaches and parents may promote and perpetuate disordered eating by emphasizing the importance of winning and slim physiques

e. caloric needs are the same for each athlete

9. Choose the true statement from the following:

a. the primary care provider usually is able to care for a patient with the female athlete triad without the involvement of others

b. treatment should include a multidisciplinary team including the primary care physician, a nutritionist, a psychologist or psychiatrist, coaches, trainers, and parents.

c. for a diagnosis of the female athlete triad, the patient must meet the *Diagnostic and Statistical Manual of Mental Disorders*, 4th edition (DSM-IV) criteria for either anorexia or bulimia

d. societal pressures concerning the importance of thinness have no effect on athletes

e. continuing to vigorously exercise through illness and injury demonstrates toughness and a healthy attitude

10. The most important intervention for an athlete diagnosed with female athlete triad is which one of the following?

a. hormone replacement therapy

b. psychologic counseling

c. calcium and vitamin D replacement

d. monthly x-rays

e. changes in eating behaviors and training regimens

■ ANSWERS:

1. **b.** The most important piece of history from the choices listed would be a complete menstrual history. The patient's thin physique, high running mileage, and obvious competitive nature place her at risk for the female athlete triad of disordered eating, amenorrhea, and osteoporosis. The coach's active involvement in the waiting room suggests pressure for success. The menstrual history should include age at menarche, frequency and duration of periods, dysmenorrhea or associated symptoms with menses, last menstrual period, longest gap between menses, and any birth control pills or other hormonal therapy taken previously.

Shoe type, running surfaces, preseason conditioning, icing, and stretching are all important questions to ask when evaluating a patient for stress injury. In the

female patient with so many red flags, however, the menstrual history is the most critical.

2. **c.** The female athlete triad consists of disordered eating, amenorrhea, and osteoporosis.

3. **a.** The optimal time to screen female patients for the female athlete triad is during the preparticipation physical examination, before the season has begun. At this time, athletes at risk can be identified for further evaluation and treatment. The sports that place athletes at most risk are those that place pressure on athletes to maintain a slim physique, especially gymnastics, dance, figure-skating, track, and cross-country. However, studies have shown that all female athletes may be at risk, and the prevalence of disordered eating behaviors has been reported to be between 15% and 62% of female college athletes.

After a stress injury, it is obviously too late to screen a patient for the female athlete triad, but if a patient was missed, a stress injury gives a very opportune time for an evaluation. A stress fracture can be a very serious injury, and this may convince the patient that disordered eating and excessive exercise place their bodies at risk.

4. **e.** All of the choices provided are crucial to ask during a complete evaluation of a female athlete. A complete menstrual history, as described earlier, cannot be emphasized enough. A weight history is also critical. Obtaining the athlete's perception of her own weight is critical for diagnosis. Minimum and maximum weights achieved and perceived ideal body weight also are important. An attempt to elicit weight loss techniques should be made, although many patients are initially reluctant to answer honestly. An exercise history should include training schedule, extracurricular activity, and time commitment. A history of previous stress injury, including "shin splints," stress fractures, compartment syndromes, and other overuse injuries should be elicited.

5. **a.** Amenorrhea in the athlete is associated most specifically with decreased levels of estrogen. Changes in the hypothalamus cause decreased secretion of estrogen. Researchers are still trying to delineate the causative factors of decreased estrogen production. Caloric restriction and excessive exercise training regimens have been associated with low estrogen levels, but the exact mechanism of this disruption has yet to be elucidated.

6. **d.** Workup for a patient with suspected female athlete triad could include a DEXA bone scan. This will delineate areas of osteopenia and can be compared to age-related norms. X-rays will show old

fractures and may show acute stress fractures. A three-phase bone scan also can find areas of stress injury where the athlete is at risk for frank stress fractures. Serum electrolytes and complete blood count are critical, especially in a patient suspected of restricting calories and/or fluids. A thyroid panel and hormonal panel (follicle-stimulating hormone, luteinizing hormone, prolactin) will help with the diagnosis of amenorrhea. A complete pelvic examination is also part of the workup. A complete psychological evaluation is also indicated at this time to delineate harmful eating and exercise behaviors and to explore the reasoning behind this behavior. An ultrasound of the abdomen and pelvis is not indicated at this time unless the clinician has other diagnostic suspicions.

7. **c.** Anorexia is characterized by the DSM-IV as a refusal to maintain body weight more than 85% of expected weight for age and height. It also is characterized by an intense fear of gaining weight, a distorted body image, and amenorrhea (in post-menarcheal females). The prognosis for anorexia nervosa is, unfortunately, generally poor. Approximately 25% of patients may recover fully, with about 50% having some improvement over time but still suffering symptoms, and about 25% with chronic symptoms. Researchers have estimated between 2% and 10% mortality for the disease. This is a long-term disease, and recovery can take upwards of 5-10 years. These numbers are elusive, and further studies may show more specific outcomes.

8. **d.** There is no such thing as an ideal body weight percentage specific for each sport. Individual athletes can excel in the same sport with widely different body types. Caloric needs are different for each individual and depend on activity level, percentage lean body mass, and individual metabolism. Teammates are often not aware of an athlete's eating disorder. Behaviors associated with eating disorders are often secretive, and athletes may eat normally in public and then perform purging behaviors later in private. Coaches and parents are sometimes not aware of the pressures that they are placing on athletes. Constant reminders on the need to succeed and win at all costs may make eating disorder behaviors seem necessary and almost normal to an athlete. The concentration in many sports and in society in general on thinness puts further pressure on athletes to achieve success by any method necessary.

9. **b.** Treatment for a patient diagnosed with the female athlete triad should include a multidisciplinary team. The primary care or team physician must act as a coordinator for all services. The nutritionist is critical to advise the patient on meal plans and eating techniques that will work with the athlete's desires and also maintain a healthy diet. A psychiatrist/psychologist is also critical to explore eating behavior issues and other stressors that may contribute to pathology. Coaches, trainers, and parents should be involved as much as the patient wishes for them to be involved. Usually, however, open communication and education produce the best results.

Disordered eating behaviors for the female athlete triad do not have to specifically meet the DSM-IV criteria for anorexia nervosa or bulimia nervosa. Any type of disordered eating behavior will qualify and usually can be referred to as an eating disorder not otherwise specified.

Another critical myth to debunk is the myth of "no pain, no gain." Continuing to exercise vigorously through serious illness or injury demonstrates pathology, not "mental toughness." Athletes need to understand that discomfort is common in exercise and can be overcome. Actual pain, however, is a sign that there is something wrong, something that requires stopping the activity and seeking medical attention.

10. **e.** The most important intervention to make for an athlete with female athlete triad is to convince the athlete to make significant changes in their eating behaviors and exercise regimens. This is often the hardest intervention to achieve but clearly the most critical and longlasting. Hormone replacement therapy is an important adjunct and is commonly used to allow patients to resume normal menses. A balanced diet with calcium supplementation and vitamin D is also important for general bone health. Psychological counseling can be an important "lifeline" for these patients. X-rays should be performed according to specific complaints and diagnostic suspicions, not as a screening tool.

SUMMARY OF FEMALE ATHLETE TRIAD

1. The female athlete triad consists of disordered eating, amenorrhea, and osteoporosis. Disordered eating can refer to a wide range of eating behaviors and can include restricting, binging, purging, and the use of laxatives and diuretics. The key factors for these athletes are lower energy intake and higher energy expenditures through exercise.

2. Amenorrhea can be common among female athletes, but this does not make it "normal." Amenorrhea can be primary (patient has never had menarche) or secondary (patient has had menarche but now has stopped having menses for >6 months). In the general female population,

studies estimate a prevalence of 2% to 5% for amenorrhea. Among athletes, this number increases to 34% to 66%. Accurate prevalence data are very difficult to obtain because of the secretive nature of eating disorders. Studies have tried to determine the exact cause for the amenorrhea. Athletes whose energy expenditure is significantly greater than their energy intake have lower estrogen levels and also fail to have appropriate release of follicle-stimulating hormone and luteinizing hormone. Lower body fat percentages also contribute to lower levels of estrogen. Some studies have estimated the lowest body fat percentage, which would allow an athlete to have menses to be around 18%. Although other studies have shown that the percentage of body fat necessary for menses is different in different patients, it is an important indicator of normal menstrual and reproductive function.

3. Osteoporosis is the third component of the female athlete triad. Amenorrhea and low levels of gonadal hormones have been shown to be associated with low bone mass. Decreased bone mass results in cortical thinning, increased fragility, and increased risk of fractures. One area of current study is trying to determine if these bone losses are reversible. Some studies have shown that resumption of menses does cause an increase in bone mineral density but that values may still remain below age-matched norms.

4. Prevalence is difficult to determine because of the secretive nature of disordered behavior and athletes' intense desire to continue to compete.

5. For screening, clinicians must remember to question the athlete, especially during the pre-participation examination. A compete menstrual history, a history of previous stress injuries, and presence or history of eating behaviors should be asked.

6. For diagnosis, patients with amenorrhea should have complete histories taken, as mentioned earlier. Athletes with suspected female athlete triad should have x-rays and/or bone scans to delineate current symptomatic fractures. A DEXA scan also can be used to determine overall bone mineral density. A complete blood count, metabolic panel, thyroid panel, and hormone levels should be checked. A complete pelvic examination should be performed. A history of eating behaviors and sample daily intake should be elicited.

7. Treatment should involve a multidisciplinary team of a primary care doctor, a nutritionist, a psychologist or psychiatrist, coaches, trainers and parents. The single most important intervention is to convince the athlete to modify her eating and exercise behavior. Other interventions can include hormonal therapy to induce menses, calcium supplements and vitamin D for better bone health, close work with a nutritionist, and work with a psychologist/psychiatrist. Agreeing on a goal weight or body fat percentage with the athlete can be one method, but this can be controversial because it encourages the athlete to concentrate excessively on the "numbers" instead of general good nutrition and reasonable exercise goals. Dispelling myths about the importance of thinness and excessive exercise are critical. Eating disorders in general represent long-term pathology, and constant and close supervision will be necessary to ensure the best outcomes.

SUGGESTED READING

Hobart JA, Smucker DR: The female athlete triad. *Am Fam Physician* 61(11):3357-3364, 2000.

Otis CL, et al: American College of Sports Medicine position stand. The female athlete triad. *Med Sci Sports Exer* 29:i-ix, 1997.

Sanborn CF, et al: Disordered eating and the female athlete triad. *Clin Sports Med* 19(2):199-213, 2000.

Chapter 161

Infectious Disease and Sports

> "No way! You just have to let me play. This game is for the league championship."

CLINICAL CASE PROBLEM 1:

A 17-Year-Old Soccer Player with Aches, Pains, and Fever

A 17-year-old high school student comes into the office complaining of having generalized body aches, feeling "feverish," and having a dry cough for the past 2 days. She has been taking acetaminophen to help relieve symptoms. She tells you that she is the leading scorer on the school's soccer team and that there is a big game against a rival school in 3 days.

On examination her blood pressure is 100/70, pulse 94, respiration 20, and temperature 101.0° F. Examination of her head, ears, eyes, nose, and throat show a mild pharyngeal erythema. Her neck is supple, with no adenopathy; cardiovascular regular rhythm and rate is S1, S2, with no murmurs. Her lungs are clear; her abdomen is soft and not tender; there is no organomegaly; and bowel sounds are active.

SELECT THE BEST ANSWER TO THE FOLLOWING QUESTIONS:

1. Which of the following statements regarding exercise and viral upper-respiratory tract infections is true?
   a. exercising during a viral illness can decrease the duration and severity of illness
   b. all over-the-counter cold medications are approved by sports governing bodies for use during competition
   c. a fever decreases strength and endurance
   d. athletes with a fever less than 103° F can safely participate in sports
   e. none of the above

2. After you complete your examination she asks if she can practice with the soccer team later that day. Which of the following is the best response?
   a. she should not exercise until the fever has resolved
   b. she may exercise but only at a moderate intensity
   c. to decrease the duration of illness she should exercise at a high intensity
   d. she may play only noncontact sports until her symptoms resolve
   e. none of the above

3. Which of the following statements regarding exercising during a febrile viral illness is true?
   a. the athlete is at an increased risk for myocarditis
   b. the athlete is at an increased risk for heat illness
   c. recovery from the illness is quickest for the athlete who allows for adequate rest
   d. all of the above
   e. none of the above

4. Which of the following statements regarding exercise and the immune system is true?
   a. white blood cells decrease during exercise
   b. salivary and nasal immunoglobulin A (IgA) is increased for 24 hours after strenuous exercise
   c. exercising at moderate intensity appears to enhance immune function
   d. lymphocytes decrease during exercise
   e. none of the above

CLINICAL CASE PROBLEM 2:

A 20-YEAR-OLD FOOTBALL PLAYER WITH MONONUCLEOSIS

A 20-year-old male with mononucleosis follows up in your office 3 weeks after the start of symptoms. He tells you that he "feels fine." The examination is normal. The spleen does not feel enlarged, and all lab tests are normal. He plays on his college football team and wants to immediately start practicing with the team.

5. Regarding return to play, which of the following is recommended in athletes with mononucleosis (assuming the spleen is not enlarged, the athlete is afebrile, and liver function tests [LFTs] are normal)?
   a. the athlete may return to contact and strenuous activity at 8 weeks after the onset of illness
   b. the athlete may return to contact and strenuous activity at 12 weeks after the onset of illness
   c. the athlete may return to noncontact practice and nonstrenuous activity at 3 weeks after the onset of illness
   d. the athlete may return to noncontact practice and nonstrenuous activity at 6 weeks after the onset of illness
   e. none of the above

CLINICAL CASE PROBLEM 3:

THREE WRESTLERS WITH HERPES GLADIATORUM

Three members of the college wrestling team have herpes gladiatorum. The coach is concerned that the breakout is going to "ruin the season" and his chance to get into the Coaches Hall of Fame.

6. Which of the following statements regarding herpes gladiatorum is true?
   a. athletes with a history of recurrent herpes gladiatorum may benefit from prophylactic acyclovir
   b. wrestlers may continue to compete as long as the lesions are covered with a gauze dressing
   c. a Tzanck smear of scrapings from the wound will always be negative
   d. herpes gladiatorum is caused only by herpes simplex virus 1
   e. none of the above

7. Which of the following is true regarding exercise and human immunodeficiency virus (HIV) infection?
   a. exercise is a safe and beneficial activity for people with HIV
   b. there have been no documented cases of HIV transmission in sports
   c. exercise can increase the number of CD4 cells in people with HIV
   d. mild to moderate exercise has been shown to limit or decelerate the body wasting seen in people with acquired immune deficiency syndrome (AIDS)
   e. all of the above

8. Which of the following statements regarding hepatitis B infection (HBV) and sports is true?
   a. there have been no documented cases of HBV transmission in sports
   b. the risk of HBV transmission in sports is greater than that for HIV
   c. an athlete who is asymptomatic and is a chronic HBV carrier with the e-antigen present should be restricted from strenuous activity
   d. the hepatitis B vaccine should not be given to elite athletes
   e. all of the above

9. Which of the following statements regarding the athlete and myocarditis is true?
   a. the most common cause of myocarditis is a virus
   b. myocarditis can cause sudden death in athletes
   c. according to the 26th Bethesda Conference, athletes suspected of having myocarditis should be kept out of sports for 6 months
   d. the coxsackie virus appears to have a predilection for the heart in exercising individuals
   e. all of the above

10. A 15-year-old comes to your office complaining of vomiting and diarrhea for the past 2 days. You diagnose viral gastroenteritis. Which of the following statements regarding viral gastroenteritis and sports is true?
    a. athletes with viral gastroenteritis are at an increased risk for heat injuries
    b. athletes should not be allowed to return to play until they are well-hydrated and afebrile
    c. the most common agents are the rotavirus and Norwalk virus
    d. antimotility drugs may prolong the gastrointestinal infection
    e. all of the above

ANSWERS:

1. **c.** During the course of an viral upper-respiratory infection, an athlete's performance is adversely affected. Muscle strength, aerobic power, and endurance are decreased. Exercising during a viral illness can prolong and increase the severity of the illness. Certain over-the-counter medications are banned by sports governing bodies, and if taken during competition can lead to disqualification of an athlete. Certain medications also can impair athletic performance and increase the risk of injury. Athletes with a temperature of 100.8° F or higher should not participate in sports.

2. **a.** As discussed, she should not exercise until the fever has resolved.

3. **d.** Exercising during a febrile viral illness increases an athlete's risk of developing heat illness, injury, and myocarditis. Performance also will be impaired.

4. **c.** Exercising at moderate intensity appears to enhance immune function. When exercising at moderate levels, athletes tend to experience fewer viral infections. Elite or high-level athletes, however, complain of frequent viral infections when training hard or after competitions. There is a transient increase in white blood cells and lymphocytes during exercise. Salivary and nasal IgA levels decrease after strenuous exercise and return to normal within 24 hours of rest. This may explain the increased susceptibility to viral illness after strenuous exercise.

5. **c.** The current return-to-play recommendations for athletes with mononucleosis are that if an athlete is afebrile, the spleen is not enlarged, lab tests including LFTs are normal, and there are no other complications the athlete may return to noncontact and nonstrenuous sports at 3 weeks after the onset of symptoms. The athlete may return to full-contact sports and strenuous activity at 4 weeks after the onset of symptoms.

6. **a.** Herpes gladiatorum is a herpes infection of the skin caused by herpes simplex virus 1 and 2. The skin lesions usually are found on the face and body and are transmitted via direct skin-to-skin contact as seen in such sports as wrestling and rugby. Wrestlers and other athletes with herpes gladiatorum are prohibited from competition until skin lesions have resolved. Treatment includes antiviral agents, such as acyclovir, famciclovir, and valacyclovir. Prophylactic therapy should be considered if recurrences are frequent and before any important competition.

7. **e.** Exercise is safe and beneficial for people with HIV. In addition to psychological benefits, exercise can increase the number of CD4 cells and can limit or slow down the body wasting seen in AIDS. There have been no documented cases of HIV transmission in sports.

8. **b.** Like HIV, the HBV is transmitted via direct contact with infected blood and body fluids. The risk of transmission is much greater for HBV than HIV. HBV transmission in sports has been reported in the literature. People who are chronic HBV carriers with e-antigen present may fully participate in all levels of activity. Hepatitis B vaccine should be considered in all athletes who participate in contact sports.

9. **e.** Myocarditis is most commonly the result of a virus and can cause sudden death in athletes. The

coxsackie virus has been shown to have a predilection for the heart in exercising individuals. The 26th Bethesda Conference recommends that athletes with myocarditis not be allowed to return to sports for 6 months. Before returning to sports the athlete needs to have normal ventricular function, normal cardiac size, and no arrhythmias.

10. **e.** Viral gastroenteritis most commonly is caused by the rotavirus and Norwalk virus. There is an increased risk of heat injuries in athletes with viral gastroenteritis because of dehydration from fever, diarrhea, or vomiting and an impaired thirst drive because of nausea. Antimotility drugs have the potential to prolong the infection because of resulting decreased bowel motility and transit time. Athletes with viral gastroenteritis should be afebrile and well-hydrated before returning to sports.

SUMMARY OF INFECTIOUS DISEASE AND SPORTS

1. Effects of exercise on the immune system:
   a. Transient increase in white blood cells and lymphocytes during exercise (lymphocytes may decrease for a short time after exercise to below preexercise levels).
   b. Salivary and nasal IgA are decreased for 24 hours after strenuous activity.
   c. Exercising at moderate levels enhances immune function.
   d. Strenuous exercise can increase susceptibility to upper-respiratory infections.
2. Exercise and viral respiratory infections:
   a. Exercise during a viral illness can increase the duration and severity of illness.
   b. Fever decreases the strength and performance of athletes.
   c. Athletes with a fever of 100.8° F or higher or myalgias should not participate in sports. There is an increased risk for heat illness, injury, and myocarditis.
3. Mononucleosis and return-to-play decisions (assuming there is no spleen enlargement, no fever, normal LFTs, and no complications)
   a. Athletes may return to noncontact and non-strenuous activity at 3 weeks after the onset of symptoms.
   b. Athletes may return to contact and strenuous activities at 4 weeks after the onset of symptoms.
4. Herpes gladiatorum
   a. Caused by herpes simplex virus 1 and 2.
   b. Transmission is a result of direct skin-to-skin contact.
   c. Virus is seen in sports such as wrestling and rugby.
   d. Skin lesions are seen on the face and body.
   e. Tzanck smear can confirm diagnosis.
   f. Treat with an antiviral medication such as acyclovir.
   g. Consider prophylactic treatment if recurrences are frequent or before important matches.
5. HIV infection and sports
   a. Exercise is safe and has many health benefits.
   b. Exercise can increase number of CD4 cells and limit or slow down body wasting seen in AIDS.
   c. There are no documented cases of HIV transmission in sports.
6. HBV infection and sports
   a. The risk of transmission in sports is greater than for HIV.
   b. Consider giving vaccine to all athletes participating in contact sports.
7. Viral gastroenteritis and sports
   a. Most common agents are rotavirus and Norwalk virus.
   b. Athletes with viral gastroenteritis are at increased risk of heat illness.
   c. Athletes should not be allowed to return to sports until they are afebrile and well hydrated.
   d. Antimotility drugs may prolong the illness.

SUGGESTED READING

Martin TJ: Infections in athletes. In: Mellion MB, et al, eds.: *Team physician's handbook.* Hanley & Belfus, 2002, Philadelphia.

Wilckens JH, Glorioso JE: Viral disease. In: DeLee JC, et al, eds.: *DeLee and Drez's orthopaedic sports medicine: principles and practice.* Elsevier, 2003, Philadelphia.

Chapter 162

Preparticipation Evaluation

> "Just because I am a girl you can't keep me
> from trying out for the varsity football team."

CLINICAL CASE PROBLEM 1:
THE FIRST YEAR TEAM'S PHYSICIAN'S DILEMMA

This is your first year as team physician for the local high school. All the talk in the community is about the school's football team, which is expected to win the state championship this season. The coach of the football team "doesn't like to lose" and was known to put pressure on the previous team physician to give medical clearance to players before games.

■ **SELECT THE BEST ANSWER TO THE FOLLOWING QUESTIONS:**

1. Which of the following is a contraindication to participation in contact sports?
   a. sickle cell trait
   b. human immunodeficiency virus (HIV) infection
   c. solitary testicle
   d. fever of 102° F
   e. convulsive disorder, well-controlled

2. The most common cause of sudden death in an athlete younger than age 35 years is:
   a. coronary artery anomaly
   b. premature coronary artery disease
   c. myocarditis
   d. hypertrophic cardiomyopathy
   e. rupture of the aorta

3. Which of the following tests is recommended for routine screening of athletes during the preparticipation evaluation (PPE)?
   a. electrocardiography
   b. echocardiography
   c. exercise stress testing
   d. vision screen
   e. urinalysis

4. During the PPE, you note that the 17-year-old star quarterback of the high school football team has a blood pressure of 148/95 mm Hg. His past medical history is negative, and he has never been told that he has high blood pressure. He is 6 foot 2 inches and weighs 175 lb. As the team physician you tell him that:

   a. he cannot play any contact sports
   b. he cannot play football until his blood pressure is under control
   c. he is cleared to play but must have his blood pressure measured twice during the next month
   d. if he begins taking antihypertensive medication immediately, then he is cleared to play
   e. he must lose 10 lb before he will be cleared to play football

5. The school's wrestling team has had an unusually high amount of injuries this season. Which of the following conditions is reason to disqualify a wrestler from competition?
   a. herpes simplex
   b. HIV
   c. hepatitis C
   d. inguinal hernia
   e. diabetes mellitus

6. When performing a PPE on a female athlete, certain considerations should be taken for gender-specific predispositions. Which of the following conditions are more common in female athletes compared to male athletes?
   a. eating disorders
   b. stress fractures in runners
   c. anterior cruciate ligament injuries in basketball players
   d. osteoporosis
   e. all of the above

7. Which one of the following statements concerning the PPE is true?
   a. about 10% of athletes are denied clearance during the PPE
   b. the PPE ideally should be performed 6 months prior to preseason practice
   c. a primary objective of the PPE is to detect conditions that may predispose an athlete to injury
   d. a primary objective of the PPE is to counsel athletes on health-related issues such as tobacco and drug use
   e. a complete history will identify approximately 95% of problems affecting athletes

8. Which one of the following sports is considered limited contact?
   a. downhill skiing
   b. basketball
   c. soccer
   d. diving
   e. lacrosse

9. You are the physician for the town's football league and are performing PPEs for the senior division (13- to 15-year-old boys). You note that one of the players is much smaller than the rest. He is 4 foot 10 inches, weighs 100 lb, and is Tanner stage 1. Regarding clearance to play, which of the following is recommended?
   a. clearance only after evaluation by an endocrinologist
   b. may play but limited to only certain positions on the field
   c. no clearance until has grown in size and weight and is at Tanner stage 2
   d. recommend he plays this season with the younger division
   e. full clearance to play

10. When performing a PPE on an athlete with a spinal cord injury, which of the following is important to ask about in the history:
    a. use of adaptive equipment
    b. heat illness
    c. autonomic dysreflexia
    d. medication use
    e. all of the above

■ ANSWERS:

   1. **d.** Fever of 102° F. A fever in an athlete or exercising individual can have negative effects including increased cardiopulmonary effort, reduced maximum exercise capacity, orthostatic hypotension, and increased risk for heat illness and myocarditis (especially if the fever is caused by the coxsackie virus).

   Athletes with sickle cell trait can participate in all sports. These athletes have an increased risk of developing exertional rhabdomyolysis and should be counseled regarding proper conditioning, hydration, and acclimatization.

   There have been no known cases of transmission of HIV infection during sports. The risk of transmission of HIV in football has been estimated to be less than one transmission per 1 million games.

   An athlete with a solitary testicle may be cleared for contact sports. The athlete should be informed of the risk of injury and should wear a protective cup.

   Athletes with well-controlled convulsive disorders may be cleared for most school-sponsored sports. Neurologic consultation is recommended for high-risk sports such as skiing, gymnastics, and high diving.

   2. **d.** The most common cause of sudden death in an athlete younger than age 35 years is hypertrophic cardiomyopathy. Coronary artery disease is the most common cause of sudden death in athletes 35 years of age and older. Coronary artery anomalies, premature coronary artery disease, myocarditis, and rupture of the aorta all can cause sudden death in an athlete.

   3. **d.** A vision screen should be performed in all athletes and should be 20/40 or better in each eye with or without corrective lenses. Athletes with only one eye or corrected vision worse than 20/40 in either eye should wear protective eye gear when playing in sports with high risk of eye injury.

   Routine electrocardiography is not recommended as a screening tool for the PPE.

   Echocardiography and exercise stress testing are not cost effective in large screening programs of athletes.

   Urinalysis is not recommended. This test has a low yield in an asymptomatic, healthy population.

   4. **c.** He is cleared to play but must have his blood pressure measured twice during the next month. Athlete's with severe hypertension (i.e., adolescents 16-18 years old with systolic blood pressure ≥150 and diastolic blood pressure ≥98) need to have their blood pressure controlled before being allowed to participate in sports. When measuring an athlete's blood pressure, be certain that the cuff fits properly.

   5. **a.** A wrestler could be disqualified for having herpes simplex. While an athlete is contagious with such conditions as herpes simplex, scabies, impetigo, or molluscum contagiosum, he or she is disqualified from certain contact/collision sports. HIV, hepatitis C, inguinal hernia, and diabetes mellitus are not reasons to disqualify an athlete from sports.

   6. **e.** All of the above. Anorexia nervosa, bulimia nervosa, and other eating disorders are more common in female athletes. Disordered eating is reported in 15% to 62% of college female athletes. All athletes should be questioned about a desire to lose weight or displeasure with body habitus.

   Stress fractures are more common in female runners. The reason is probably multifactorial and includes such factors as muscle strength and balance, limb alignment, and medical factors such as nutrition, eating habits, menstrual dysfunction, and osteopenia or osteoporosis.

   Noncontact anterior cruciate ligament injury rates are higher in female athletes. Risk factors probably include such things as anatomic, biomechanical, and neuromuscular differences. These injuries occur commonly during deceleration, landing, or pivoting.

Osteoporosis is more common in female athletes, and along with osteopenia can exist in the young female athlete. Disordered eating and menstrual dysfunction are risk factors that should be screened for during the PPE.

7. c. A primary objective of the PPE is to detect conditions that may predispose an athlete for injury. Other primary objectives are to detect conditions that may be life threatening or disabling and to meet legal and insurance requirements.

About 0.3% to 1.3% of athletes are denied clearance during the PPE.

The best time to perform the PPE is 6 weeks prior to the start of preseason practice. This gives enough time to rehabilitate any injuries or workup and treat other conditions.

Counseling athletes on health-related issues, such as tobacco and drug use, is not a primary objective of the PPE. This is because of time constraints. When time permits, physicians should counsel athletes on such health-related topics.

A complete history identifies approximately 75% of problems affecting athletes. It is a very important part of the PPE. To obtain a more accurate history, the athlete and parents should complete a history form prior to the examination.

8. a. Downhill skiing is considered limited contact. Sports are classified as noncontact, limited contact, and full contact/collision. The categories are based on the potential for injury from collision. In some cases, athletes may not be able to safely participate in some sports but may be able to do so in others. The classifications can help the physician make return-to-play decisions.

Noncontact sports include golf, running, swimming, and tennis.

Limited contact sports include baseball, bicycling, volleyball, in-line skating, and downhill skiing.

Contact/collision sports include basketball, soccer, diving, lacrosse, football, wrestling, and ice hockey.

9. e. The patient should be given full clearance to play. There is no evidence that assessing physical maturity and separating athletes according to stage of development decreases the rate of injuries. Therefore, Tanner staging is not a recommended part of the PPE.

10. e. All of the above. Athletes with spinal cord injuries are at risk of injury from adaptive equipment such as wheelchairs and prostheses.

Heat illness is a concern in athletes with a spinal cord injury, especially when lesions are above T8.

These athletes are more susceptible to heat illness because of abnormal sweating below the lesion level; venous pooling and decreased venous return in the lower limbs; and certain medications, such as sympathomimetics and anticholinergics, that they may be taking. Athletes with spinal cord injuries are also more susceptible to hypothermia.

Autonomic dysreflexia is a serious condition that can occur in athletes with spinal cord injuries. It occurs more commonly in athletes with lesions above T6. An uncontrolled sympathetic response leads to cardiac dysrrhythmias, sweating above the lesion, chest tightness, headache, an acute increase in blood pressure, hyperthermia, and gastrointestinal disturbances. Autonomic dysreflexia can be triggered from such things as urinary tract infection, bladder or bowel distension, pressure sores, and exercising in hot or cold weather. At the first sign of symptoms athletes should be removed from the sports activity, potential triggers should be treated, and athletes should be transported to the nearest hospital.

It is important to know all the medications, prescription and over-the-counter, and nutritional supplements that an athlete is taking. Athletes with a spinal cord injury may be taking medications that make them more susceptible to heat and cold injuries, dehydration, sedation, and cardiovascular events. Also, be aware of potential drug side effects and drug interactions.

SUMMARY OF PREPARTICIPATION EVALUATION

1. Primary objectives are as follows:
   a. Detect conditions that may predispose to injury
   b. Detect conditions that may be life threatening or disabling
   c. Meet legal and insurance requirements
2. Only about 0.3% to 1.3% of athletes are denied clearance during the PPE.
3. The best time to perform the PPE is 6 weeks before the start of preseason practice.
4. Most common causes of sudden death in athletes are as follows:
   a. Hypertrophic cardiomyopathy (younger than 35 years old)
   b. Coronary artery disease (35 years and older)
5. Contraindications to participation in sports include the following (partial list):
   a. Fever
   b. Acute myocarditis or pericarditis

Continued

SUMMARY OF PREPARTICIPATION EVALUATION—cont'd

c. Hypertrophic cardiomyopathy

d. Long QT interval syndrome

e. History of recent concussion and symptoms of postconcussion syndrome

f. Acute enlargement of spleen or liver (such as splenomegaly seen in infectious mononucleosis)

g. Contagious skin infections such as herpes simplex, impetigo, and molluscum contagiosum

6. PPE should include vision screen, height, weight, blood pressure, and pulse.

7. Tanner staging is not a recommended part of the PPE.

8. Physicians should be aware of certain conditions that are more common in female athletes:

a. Eating disorders

b. Noncontact anterior cruciate ligament injuries

c. Stress fractures in runners

d. Osteopenia and osteoporosis

9. When performing a PPE on an athlete with a spinal cord injury it is important to ask about the following:

a. Use of adaptive equipment

b. History of heat or cold illness

c. History of autonomic hyperreflexia

d. Medications (prescription and over-the-counter) and nutritional supplements

SUGGESTED READING

Kurowski K, Chandran S: The preparticipation athletic evaluation. *Am Fam Physician* 61:2683-2690, 2696-2698, 2000.

Patel DR, Greydanus DE: The pediatric athlete with disabilities. *Ped Clin N Am* 49(4), 2002.

Smith DM, et al: *Preparticipation physical examination,* 2nd ed. Physician and Sports Medicine, 1997, Minneapolis.

Chapter 163

High Altitude and Barotrauma

"I was too tired to ski the moguls."

CLINICAL CASE PROBLEM 1:

A 37-Year-Old Male Requesting Travel Advice

A 37-year-old male comes into the office seeking travel advice. He is planning a ski trip to Colorado in 2 weeks. He tells you that 5 years ago he went on a similar vacation and had a headache, had difficulty sleeping, and felt nauseous and tired during the entire trip. This time he wants to get in as much skiing as possible and does not want to be "sick." His past medical history is significant for mild intermittent asthma and well-controlled type 1 diabetes mellitus.

▌ SELECT THE BEST ANSWER TO THE FOLLOWING QUESTIONS:

1. This patient was likely suffering from which of the following conditions during his ski trip 5 years ago:

a. acute mountain sickness (AMS)

b. high-altitude pulmonary edema (HAPE)

c. high-altitude cerebral edema (HACE)

d. hypoglycemia

e. acute exacerbation of asthma

2. You recommend he take which of the following medications to prevent a similar illness during his upcoming trip?

a. ergotamine

b. albuterol inhaler

c. glyburide

d. acetazolamide

e. nifedipine

3. Which of the following is true regarding this condition?

a. children and adolescents are more susceptible than adults

b. elderly people are more susceptible

c. people with asthma are more susceptible

d. people with diabetes mellitus are more susceptible

e. people living at low altitudes (below 900 meters) are more susceptible

CLINICAL CASE PROBLEM 2:

A 34-Year-Old Male Would-Be Mountain Climber

A 34-year-old male has been camping and climbing at an altitude of 9500 feet for the past 3 days. He notices that it has become more and more difficult to "catch his breath," even at rest, and in addition he feels very weak and has developed a dry cough.

4. The most likely diagnosis in Clinical Case Problem 2 is:
   a. AME
   b. HACE
   c. HAPE
   d. pneumonia
   e. altitude-induced congestive heart failure

5. The treatment for the condition diagnosed in response to Question 4 is:
   a. supplemental oxygen
   b. descent
   c. hyperbaric chamber
   d. nifedipine
   e. all of the above

6. A common early sign of HACE is:
   a. seizures
   b. ataxia
   c. raccoon eyes
   d. focal neurologic deficits
   e. coma

CLINICAL CASE PROBLEM 3:
A 56-YEAR-OLD FEMALE SCUBA DIVER WITH PAINS

A 56-year-old female with no significant past medical history is brought into the emergency room complaining of extreme fatigue, headache, arm and leg pain, and itching. She tells you her symptoms started this morning just 30 minutes after scuba diving to depths of more than 50 feet. This was her first dive without an instructor present.

7. The most likely diagnosis is:
   a. decompression sickness
   b. arterial gas embolism
   c. oxygen toxicity
   d. inert gas narcosis
   e. hyponatremia

8. In scuba diving the most common cause of pulmonary barotrauma in recreational divers is related to which of the following?
   a. rapid descent
   b. breath holding
   c. a prolonged dive
   d. low oxygen concentrations
   e. poor fitting mask

9. Which of the following is (are) proper treatment(s) for a scuba diver with arterial gas embolism?
   a. cardiac life support
   b. 100% oxygen

c. hydration
d. recompression therapy
e. all of the above

ANSWERS:

1. **a.** AMS is a type of altitude illness that is self-limited and affects about 25% of unacclimatized people traveling to altitudes of 9000 feet. Symptoms are varied and develop within the first 36 hours of arrival at a moderate altitude (7000-9000 feet). Common symptoms include headache, anorexia, nausea or vomiting, insomnia, dizziness, and fatigue.

2. **d.** Acetazolamide, a carbonic anhydrase inhibitor, can prevent or reduce the severity of AMS if taken at least 1 day prior to ascent and continued until adequate acclimatization has occurred. In people allergic to sulfa drugs, dexamethasone is an alternative. The best way to prevent altitude illness is by ascending at a slower rate and allowing the body to acclimatize to the lower barometric pressure present at high altitude.

Nifedipine has been shown to be effective in the prevention and treatment of HAPE.

3. **e.** People living at low altitudes (below 900 meters) are more susceptible to altitude illness. Children, adolescents, the elderly, and people with asthma or diabetes are not at increased risk for developing altitude illness.

4. **c.** HAPE is a severe form of altitude illness associated with pulmonary hypertension and elevated capillary pressure. Risk factors for developing HAPE are similar to AMS and include rate of ascent, altitude, individual susceptibility, exertion, and cold temperatures. HAPE usually occurs at higher altitudes than AMS. Symptoms commonly start the second night at a new altitude and include dry cough, shortness of breath, and decreased exercise tolerance. Without treatment, HAPE can progress to severe dyspnea, pink or bloody sputum, coma, and death.

5. **e.** All of the above. Immediate descent is the highest priority. Supplemental oxygen reduces pulmonary artery pressure and increases arterial oxygen pressure. Nifedipine also helps reduce pulmonary pressure. If available, a portable hyperbaric chamber is effective in the treatment of HAPE.

6. **b.** HACE is the most severe form of altitude illness and is recognized by the onset of ataxia or altered consciousness in a person with AMS or HAPE. Coma is a later finding. Seizures and focal neurologic signs

are less common. Raccoon eyes are a physical finding seen in trauma patients with basilar skull fractures.

7. a. Decompression sickness develops after ascent from depth, when a diver does not follow established guidelines to prevent the release of inert gas bubbles, usually nitrogen, into the bloodstream and tissues. Symptoms of mild decompression sickness can include itching, rash, headache, joint and muscle pain, and extreme fatigue.

Arterial gas embolism is a serious form of pulmonary barotrauma seen in divers. The most common signs and symptoms are confusion, coma, seizures, focal weakness, and visual loss.

Oxygen toxicity can occur in divers. Symptoms usually develop underwater without warning and include focal seizures, vertigo, nausea and vomiting, paresthesias, and visual and respiratory changes.

Inert gas narcosis, also known as nitrogen narcosis, occurs at depths greater than 100 feet. Symptoms may include loss of motor and cognitive skills, bizarre behavior, hostility, and unconsciousness.

8. b. Breath holding is one of the most common causes of pulmonary barotrauma among recreational divers. During ascent, if expanding gas is not allowed to escape via exhalation, pulmonary barotrauma will result. Other causes of pulmonary barotrauma are rapid ascent, heavy physical exertion while diving, and pulmonary obstructive diseases.

9. e. All of the above. The treatment of arterial gas embolism consists of cardiac life support, 100% oxygen, hydration, and recompression therapy. Recompression therapy reduces the size of air bubbles by increasing ambient pressure.

SUMMARY OF HIGH ALTITUDE AND BAROTRAUMA

A. AMS a self-limited altitude illness.
1. **Symptoms:** headache, anorexia, nausea or vomiting, fatigue or weakness, and insomnia
2. **Treatment:** stopping any further ascent, rest at same or lower altitude for 1-2 days, analgesics, antiemetics, and in some cases acetazolamide or dexamethasone
3. **Prevention:** acclimatization, slow ascent, and drug treatment with acetazolamide or dexamethasone as necessary

B. HAPE is a severe form of altitude illness
1. **Pathophysiology:** noncardiogenic pulmonary edema associated with pulmonary hypertension and elevated capillary pressure
2. **Risk factors:** rate of ascent, high altitudes, individual susceptibility, exertion, and cold temperatures; usually occurs at higher altitudes than AMS
3. **Symptoms:** dry cough, shortness of breath, and decreased exercise tolerance; can progress to severe dyspnea, pink or bloody sputum, coma, and death; symptoms usually start the second night at a new and higher altitude
4. **Treatment:** immediate descent, supplemental oxygen, nifedipine, and hyperbaric chamber
5. **Prevention:** slow and gradual ascent, avoid overexertion, consider taking acetazolamide beginning 1 day prior to ascent and continuing for 2 days at the new altitudes; treat symptoms of AMS early on.

C. HACE is the most severe form of altitude illness:
1. **Signs at onset:** ataxia or altered consciousness in a person with AMS or HAPE
2. **Treatment:** immediate descent, oxygen supplementation, hyperbaric chamber, and dexamethasone; acetazolamide if descent is delayed
3. **Prevention:** same as for HAPE

D. Decompression sickness can develop in scuba divers after ascent from depth.
1. **Factors that can increase risk of developing decompression sickness:** rate of ascent, hypothermia, fatigue, increased age, dehydration, alcohol use, female sex, obesity, and patent foramen ovale
2. **Cause:** inert gas bubbles, usually nitrogen, released into the bloodstream and tissues
3. **Signs/symptoms:** itching, rash, headache, joint and muscle pain, and extreme fatigue; in severe cases there can be sensory loss and paresthesias in the trunk and extremities, ascending leg weakness, and loss of bowel and/or bladder control
4. **Treatment:** hyperbaric chamber, oxygen supplementation, and intravenous hydration

E. Pulmonary barotrauma can occur in scuba divers during ascent.
1. **Cause:** most common cause in recreational divers is breath holding; other causes are rapid ascent, strenuous exertion while diving, and pulmonary obstructive diseases

2. **Arterial gas embolism:** most serious form of pulmonary barotrauma; signs and symptoms can include focal weakness, visual loss, confusion, seizures, and coma
3. **Treatment:** cardiac life support, oxygen supplementation, hydration, and transport to a facility with a hyperbaric chamber

SUGGESTED READING

Barry PW, Pollard AJ: Altitude illness. *BMJ* 326(7395):915-919, 2003.

Bove AA, Neuman TS: Diving-related illnesses. In: Safran MR, et al, eds.: *Manual of sports medicine*. Lippincott-Raven, 1998, Philadelphia.

Hackett PH, Roach RC: Current concepts: high-altitude illness. *N Engl J Med* 345(2):107-114, 2001.

Krieger BP: Diving: what to tell the patient with asthma and why. *Curr Opin Pulm Med* 7(1):32-38, 2001.

Newton HB: Neurologic complications of scuba diving. *Am Fam Physician* 63:2211-2218, 2225-2226, 2001.

Woodward GA: Altitude illness. *Clin Ped Emerg Med* 2:168-178, 2001.

ILLUSTRATED REVIEW

Chapter 164

Illustrated Review

Each picture in this section is accompanied by a brief clinical vignette. For each picture, determine the diagnosis. Wherever a figure relates directly to a previously discussed topic in an earlier chapter, that chapter and page is cross-referenced for you. Answers are at the end of this section.

Primary Dermatological Conditions

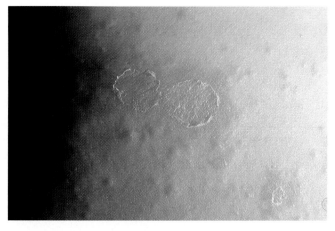

1. A 26-year-old man presents with this rash, which subsequently spreads in a Christmas-tree fashion over his entire back, and resolves with conservative treatment in some 6 to 8 weeks.

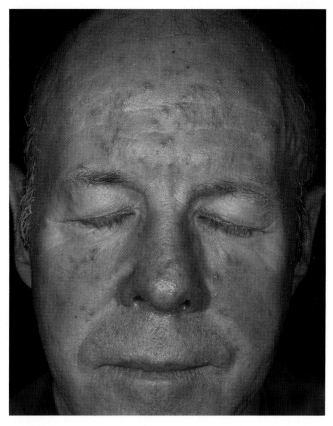

2. This 57-year-old man presents to your office with a many year history of this facial eruption that has never been treated.

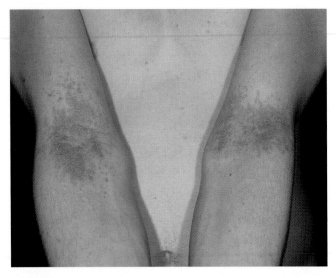

3. This 15-year-old teenager has a history of mild persistent asthma.

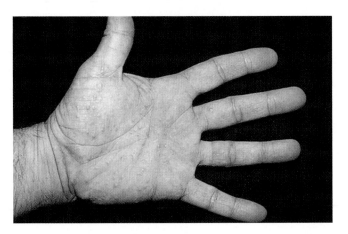

4. This 29-year-old auto mechanic has had this outbreak for several years. He finds mild over-the-counter topical steroid creams somewhat effective.

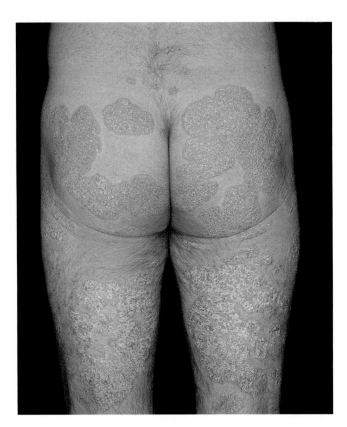

5. This individual finds these eruptions improve somewhat in the summertime.

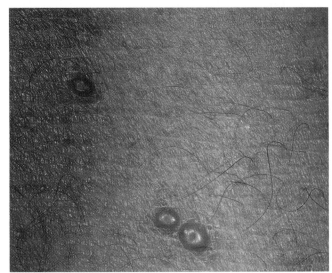

6. This painless rash presents in a 16-year-old high school wrestler.

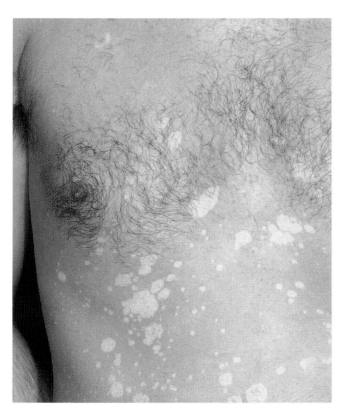

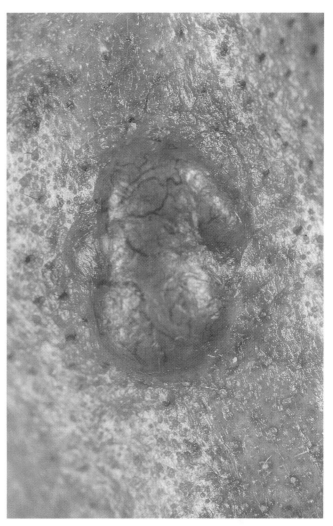

7. This gentleman's rash has been present for several months, is slowly spreading, and has worsened with over-the-counter steroids.

8. This lesion on a chronically sun-exposed area has been slowly enlarging for 9 months.

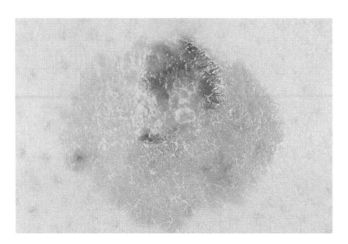

9. This lesion recently changed color in this 48-year-old lifeguard.

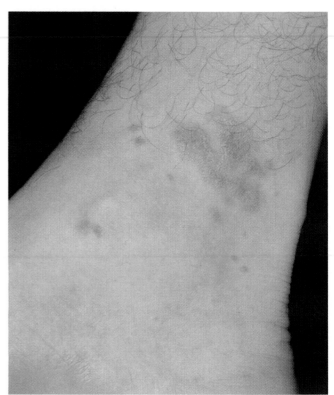

10. This 40-year-old man developed this lesion once before, but it went away. This lesion is characterized by five P's: pruritic, planar (flat-topped), polyangular, purple papules.

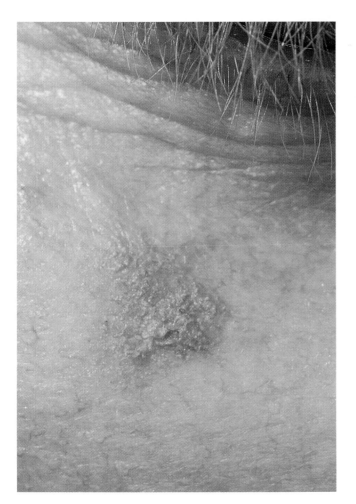

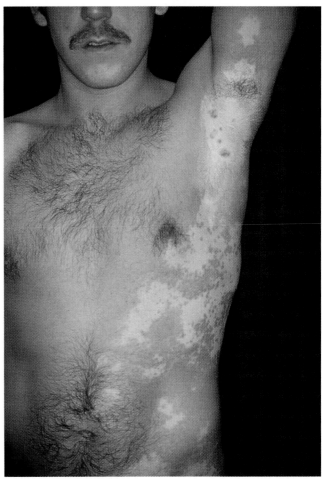

11. This lesion, on a yachting captain's neck, is one of many in sun-exposed areas of his head and neck.

12. This condition has been slowly worsening and affects all areas of his skin.

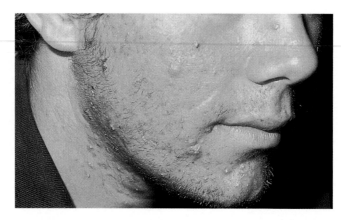

13. This teenager was told by his grandmother to avoid chocolate and wash his face more often to alleviate this condition.

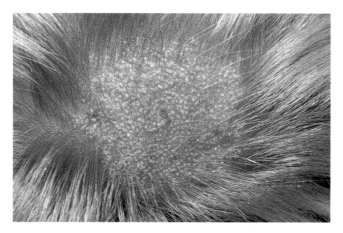

14. This third-grade student was sent home by the school nurse and told to seek treatment for the condition, which is pruritic.

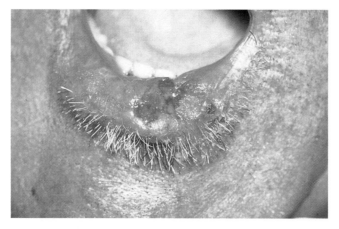

15. This smoker noticed this growing lesion about five months ago.

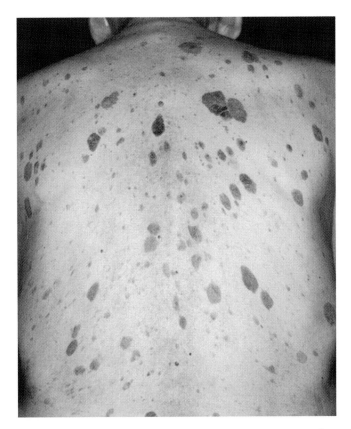

16. These growths have become more common as this patient ages.

Dermatologic Manifestations of Underlying Disease

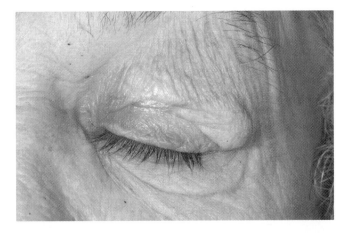

17. This patient had a total cholesterol level of 450 mg/dl and a family history of premature cardiovascular mortality.

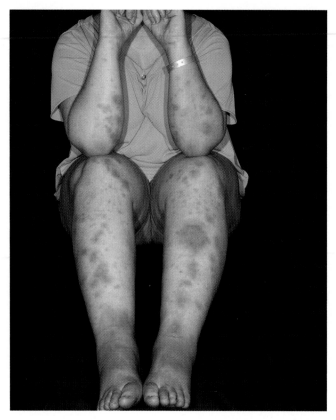

18. These nodular eruptions, thought to be an inflammatory hypersensitivity reaction in subcutaneous fat, began after a course of sulfonamide antibiotics.

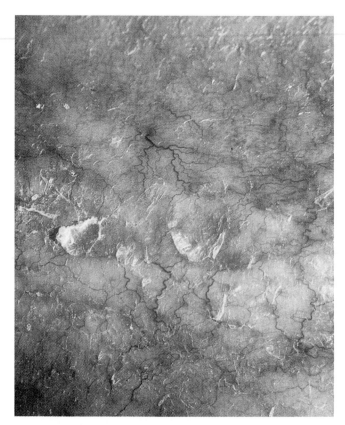

19. This chronic eruption is on the shin of this 24-year-old woman with type 1 diabetes.

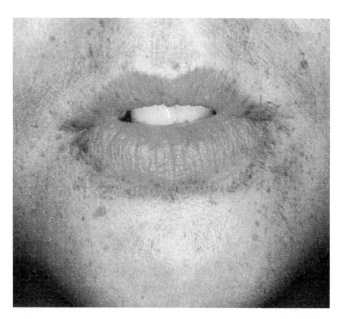

20. This patient has multiple hamartomatous polyps throughout the gastrointestinal tract, from the stomach to the rectum, and an iron deficiency anemia.

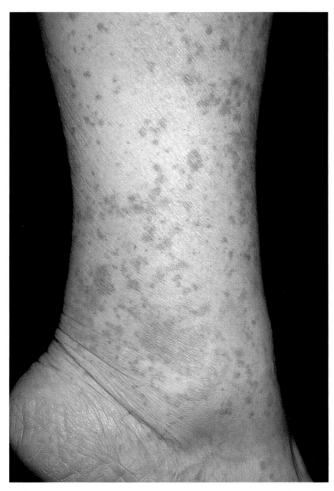

21. This eruption is palpable in a 35-year-old with leukemia.

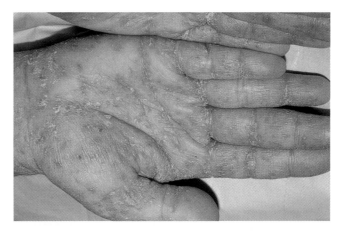

22. This intensely pruritic eruption is also present in a close contact of this patient.

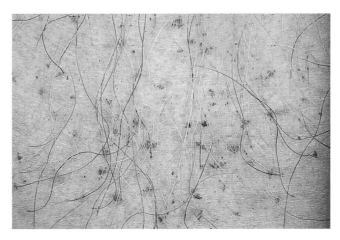

23. This patient's pubic area shown here has been the source of constant irritation and itching for several weeks.

Viral Exanthems

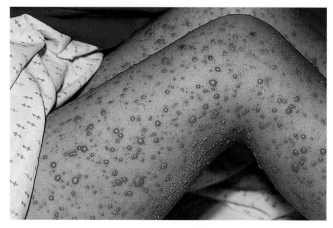

24. The pruritic lesions of this disease erupted initially on the face and trunk, and then spread to the extremities.

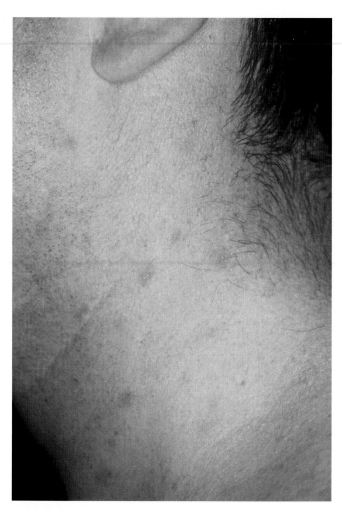

25. This infection is spread by aerosolized particles from respiratory secretions of infected individuals. Patients with this disease are most infectious from the prodrome (days 7–10 postexposure) through the fourth day after rash onset.

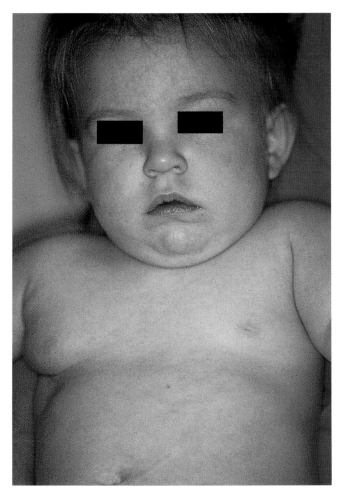

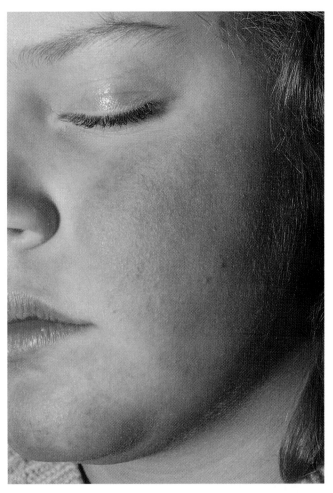

26. This disease, caused by human herpesvirus 6 and 7, is characterized by high fever (37.9 to 40° C, 101 to 106° F) that ends abruptly and is followed by onset of the rash depicted.

27. The infection that causes this rash, characterized by a slapped face appearance, is parvovirus B19. The prodrome to the rash is usually mild with low-grade fever, headache, and mild upper respiratory tract infection symptoms.

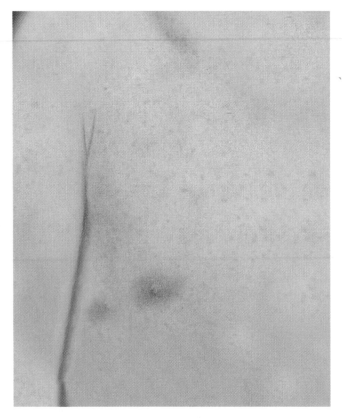

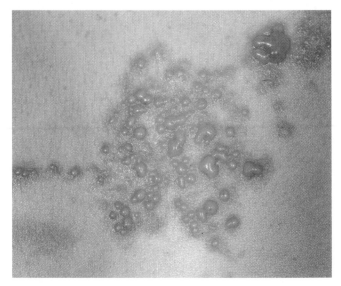

28. The variable rash of this mild to moderate disease, which usually begins on the face and spreads cephalocaudal over 24 hours, belies the serious complications the underlying virus can cause to the fetus of a pregnant woman. Characteristic findings include lymphadenopathy, particularly posterior auricular and suboccipital.

29. This rash, which occurs in a dermatomal distribution, is usually preceded by paresthesias of the affected area. Pain can be quite intense and last long after the rash has resolved.

Ophthalmoscopy

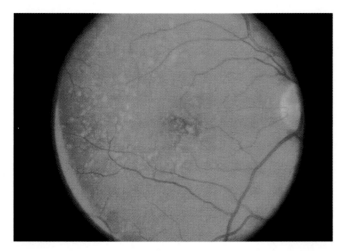

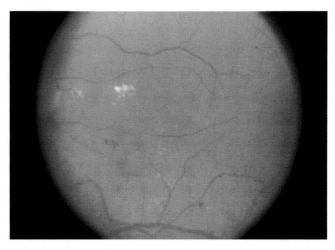

30. The condition seen here is now the main cause of blindness in the U.S. Decreased central vision is the hallmark of this condition whose prevalence increases with age. Yellowish deposits on the retina shown here are characteristic.

31. These eye grounds are of a 54-year-old woman with a long-standing chronic disease that has compromised her vision.

Microscopy

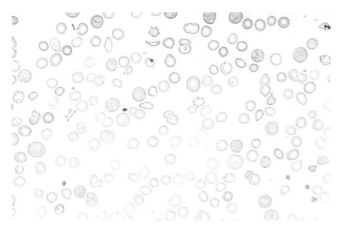

32. This smear was obtained on a 36-year-old woman who has been having heavy menstrual bleeding for years.

ANSWERS:

1. Herald patch, pityriasis rosea (see Chapter 103, Answer 25).

   From Miller RG, Sisson SD, Ashar B: The Johns Hopkins Internal Medicine Board Review. Philadelphia, Mosby, 2004, Fig. 63-9.

2. Rosacea (see Chapter 31, Answers 16, 17, 18, and 19).

   From Miller RG, Sisson SD, Ashar B: The Johns Hopkins Internal Medicine Board Review. Philadelphia, Mosby, 2004, Fig. 63-1.

3. Atopic dermatitis (see Chapter 113, Answers 1 through 5). Note that although 90% of children resolve their symptoms by adolescence, people with asthma often have a persistent history of atopy.

   From Miller RG, Sisson SD, Ashar B: The Johns Hopkins Internal Medicine Board Review. Philadelphia, Mosby, 2004, Fig. 63-2.

4. Dyshidrotic eczema, pictured here, is a vesicular pattern of eczema generally affecting the hands and occasionally the feet. Affected individuals may have a history of contact dermatitis, often induced by nickel. However, in many cases no specific allergen can be identified and a history of atopic dermatitis is rare. The condition tends to be aggravated by sweating and may arise secondary to a fungal infection.

   From Miller RG, Sisson SD, Ashar B: The Johns Hopkins Internal Medicine Board Review. Philadelphia, Mosby, 2004, Fig. 63-4.

5. Chronic plaque psoriasis. This is a chronic auto-immune condition with a strong genetic component. The skin lesions are caused by dermal hyperproliferation causing the skin to literally "pile up." It affects more than 4 million Americans and has a wide range of symptoms. Most individuals have the relatively mild plaque type similar to that pictured, which tends to localize to the elbows and knees. However, some individuals have severe cases covering most of the body and gross open lesions may occur. Psoriatic arthritis, a condition similar to rheumatic arthritis, develops in about 23% of the cases.

   From Miller RG, Sisson SD, Ashar B: The Johns Hopkins Internal Medicine Board Review. Philadelphia, Mosby, 2004, Fig. 63-6.

6. Molluscum (see Chapter 103, Answer 26).

   From Miller RG, Sisson SD, Ashar B: The Johns Hopkins Internal Medicine Board Review. Philadelphia, Mosby, 2004, Fig. 63-12.

7. Tinea versicolor (see Chapter 103, Answer 23).

   From Miller RG, Sisson SD, Ashar B: The Johns Hopkins Internal Medicine Board Review. Philadelphia, Mosby, 2004, Fig. 62-13.

8. Basal cell carcinoma (see Chapter 130, Answers 1 and 2).

   From Miller RG, Sisson SD, Ashar B: The Johns Hopkins Internal Medicine Board Review. Philadelphia, Mosby, 2004, Fig. 63-15.

9. Melanoma (see Chapter 130, Answers 8–10).

   From Miller RG, Sisson SD, Ashar B: The Johns Hopkins Internal Medicine Board Review. Philadelphia, Mosby, 2004, Fig. 63-14B.

10. Lichen planus. A pruritic, papular skin eruption usually found on the genitalia, mucous membranes, or flexor surfaces of the extremities, lichen planus occurs most commonly between the ages of 30 and 60. Diagnosis may be confirmed by biopsy. The cause is unknown, although some eruptions have been associated with antibiotic use, and spontaneous remissions occur in up to 65% of cases within one year. Topical steroids are often used for cutaneous lesions, although no randomized controlled trials have been performed to demonstrate efficacy.

    From Miller RG, Sisson SD, Ashar B: The Johns Hopkins Internal Medicine Board Review. Philadelphia, Mosby, 2004, Fig. 63-18.

11. Actinic keratosis (see Chapter 130, Answers 3–5).

    From Miller RG, Sisson SD, Ashar B: The Johns Hopkins Internal Medicine Board Review. Philadelphia, Mosby, 2004, Fig. 63-16.

12. Vitiligo. A probable autoimmune disease related to destruction of melanocytes, vitiligo is a disease of hypopigmentation. Approximately 1% of the population is affected, with half of cases beginning before adulthood. Thyroid disease is seen in some 30% of patients with vitiligo. Oral photo-chemotherapy and topical steroids have been used for treatment with some success.

    From Miller RG, Sisson SD, Ashar B: The Johns Hopkins Internal Medicine Board Review. Philadelphia, Mosby, 2004, Fig. 63-24.

13. Acne vulgaris (Chapter 31, Clinical Case Problem and Answers 1–14).

    From Hooper BJ, Goldman MP: Primary Dermatologic Care. St. Louis, Mosby, 1999, p 12.

14. Tinea capitis. Scalp ringworm is a common occurrence in grade school children. It may resemble seborrheic dermatitis, but more often presents with broken off hair shafts and smooth plaques. They may be surrounded with inflammation, and secondary lymphadenitis is common. Oral antifungals are generally required for successful treatment.

From White G, Cox N: Diseases of the Skin: Color Atlas and Text. St. Louis, Mosby, p 371, Fig. 23-12.b.

15. Squamous cell carcinoma (see Chapter 130, Answers 6 and 7).

From Lawrence CM, Cox NH. Physical Signs in Dermatology. St. Louis, Mosby, 2002, p 184, Fig. 9-96.

16. Seborrheic keratosis. These, the most common of benign skin neoplasms, have a characteristic stuck-on appearance with a well-circumscribed border. They are typically tan-brown to dark brown in color, and increasing numbers often appear with aging. Sudden appearance of large numbers has been associated with the presence of internal malignancy (mostly adenocarcinoma of the stomach) in some case reports, although this observation has not been substantiated in other epidemiologic studies.

From Miller RG, Sisson SD, Ashar B: The Johns Hopkins Internal Medicine Board Review. Philadelphia, Mosby, 2004, Fig. 63-8.

17. Xanthoma. These yellowish nodular skin lesions are typically seen in patients with type I or type V hyperlipoproteinemia.

From Miller RG, Sisson SD, Ashar B: The Johns Hopkins Internal Medicine Board Review. Philadelphia, Mosby, 2004, Fig. 2-1.

18. Erythema nodosum. An acute, nodular, and tender skin eruption that results from inflammation of subcutaneous fat, erythema nodosum is the result of a cell-mediated immune reaction to a variety of stimuli including various infectious agents (bacteria, fungi, viruses), drugs (antibiotics, aspirin, oral contraceptives, antihypertensives), and diseases (sarcoidosis, lymphomas, reactive arthropathies). Nodules usually resolve within 8 weeks.

From Miller RG, Sisson SD, Ashar B: The Johns Hopkins Internal Medicine Board Review. Philadelphia, Mosby, 2004, Fig. 63-10.

19. Necrobiosis lipoidica. These plaque-like reddened areas that fade over time and take on a mottled yellowish appearance are found on the anterior surfaces of the legs of diabetics, and may ulcerate with very little trauma to the area.

From Miller RG, Sisson SD, Ashar B: The Johns Hopkins Internal Medicine Board Review. Philadelphia, Mosby, 2004, Fig. 63-23.

20. Peutz-Jeghers syndrome. An autosomal dominant genetically transmitted disease with incomplete penetrance. In addition to the polyposis, these patients have pigmented lesions of the lips, buccal mucosa, nose, hands, feet, and genital area. They are at high risk for gastrointestinal, breast, pancreatic, ovarian and Sertoli cell malignancies.

From Gawkrodger DJ: An Illustrated Colour Text: Dermatology. Edinburgh, Churchill-Livingstone, 1992, p 67, Fig. 4.

21. Palpable purpura. A circumscribed collection of blood greater than 0.5 cm. Diagnostic considerations for palpable purpura are numerous, and include malignancies, infection, drug reactions, disseminated intravascular coagulation, collagen-vascular diseases, trauma, cryoglobulinemias, and embolization.

From Miller RG, Sisson SD, Ashar B: The Johns Hopkins Internal Medicine Board Review. Philadelphia, Mosby, 2004, Fig. 63-29.

22. Scabies. This eruption is caused by a mite that burrows under the skin surface and travels through the stratum corneum depositing eggs and feces. Contagious, it is commonly spread among close contacts, especially through infested bedding. Primary lesions are intensely pruritic, and common in the web spaces of the hands and feet, genitals, wrists, and buttocks. Treated with topical insecticide applied as a cream (lindane in adults or permethrin in children and pregnant women). Itching may last for weeks after mites are successfully treated and may also require treatment.

From White G, Cox N: Diseases of the Skin: Color Atlas and Text. St. Louis, Mosby, p 371, Fig. 23-12.b.

23. Pediculosis pubis. Pubic lice are a common infestation frequently spread between sexual partners. Patients complain about itching, and the infection is apparent upon inspection. Live nits fluoresce white or gray with a Wood's lamp. Permethrin or lindane are effective as treatments.

From Callen JP, Greer KE, Paller AS, Swinyer LJ: Color Atlas of Dermatology, 2nd ed. Philadelphia, W.B. Saunders, 2000, p 309, Fig. 20-28.

24. Chickenpox (varicella) (Chapter 103, Answers 1–3).

From Callen JP, Greer KE, Paller AS, Swinyer LJ: Color Atlas of Dermatology, 2nd ed. Philadelphia, W.B. Saunders, 2000, p 143, Fig. 5-43.

25. Measles (rubeola) (Chapter 103, Answers 6–10).

From Hooper BJ, Goldman MP: Primary Dermatologic Care. St. Louis, Mosby, 1999, p 166, Fig. 4-26.

26. Roseola (exanthema subitum; sixth disease), exanthem subitum (roseola infantum) (Chapter 103). Note: antibiotics have essentially eliminated scarlet fever, one of the earlier major exanthemas, leaving roseola (the sixth disease) as one of the big five exanthems.

From Hooper BJ, Goldman MP: Primary Dermatologic Care. St. Louis, Mosby, 1999, p 173, Fig. 4-34.

27. Erythema infectiosum (fifth disease) (Chapter 103, Answers 11–15).

From Hooper BJ, Goldman MP: Primary Dermatologic Care. St. Louis, Mosby, 1999, p 157, Fig. 4-13.

28. Rubella (Chapter 103, Summary; and Chapter 64, Answer 1). Fetuses exposed during gestation may develop congenital rubella syndrome. Common abnormalities include deafness, eye defects, CNS anomalies, cardiac malformations (patent ductus arteriosis, pulmonic stenosis), and mental retardation.

From Hooper BJ, Goldman MP. Primary Dermatologic Care. St. Louis, Mosby, 1999, p 57, Fig. 2-7.

29. Herpes zoster (Chapter 103, Answers 4 and 5).

From Miller RG, Sisson SD, Ashar B: The Johns Hopkins Internal Medicine Board Review. Philadelphia, Mosby, 2004, Fig. 63-11.

30. Macular degeneration. Two forms exist: wet and dry. Degenerative changes occur with aging in the vascular neural and pigmented layers of the macula. Wet form is more common and is associated with fluid leakage from the blood vessels. Dry form is thought to be ischemic in origin. Laser treatment slows the course of the disease somewhat, but in most cases progression occurs.

From Miller RG, Sisson SD, Ashar B: The Johns Hopkins Internal Medicine Board Review. Philadelphia, Mosby, 2004, Fig. 65-2.

31. Nonproliferative diabetic retinopathy. Diabetic retinopathy is an eye disorder manifested by microaneurysms, hemorrhages, exudates, and neovascularity. Found in 80% of those who have had diabetes for 15 or more years, it is a leading cause of blindness. Treatment is by laser photocoagulation.

From Miller RG, Sisson SD, Ashar B: The Johns Hopkins Internal Medicine Board Review. Philadelphia, Mosby, 2004, Fig. 65-3.

32. Hypochromic, microcytic red cells characteristic of iron deficiency anemia (Chapter 34, Answers 1–11).

From Miller RG, Sisson SD, Ashar B: The Johns Hopkins Internal Medicine Board Review. Philadelphia, Mosby, 2004, Plate 2.

INDEX

Page numbers followed by f, t, and b indicate figures, tables, and boxed material, respectively.

H